Diseases of the Nails and their Management

Diseases of the Nails and their Management

EDITED BY

R. BARAN MD
Head of the Dermatological Unit
General Hospital, Cannes

AND

R. P. R. DAWBER
MA, MB, ChB, FRCP
Consultant Dermatologist, Oxford Hospitals
and Clinical Lecturer in Dermatology
University of Oxford

SECOND EDITION

OXFORD
BLACKWELL SCIENTIFIC PUBLICATIONS
LONDON EDINBURGH BOSTON
MELBOURNE PARIS BERLIN VIENNA

Editorial Offices:
Osney Mead, Oxford OX2 0EL
25 John Street, London WC1N 2BL
23 Ainslie Place, Edinburgh EH3 6AJ
238 Main Street, Cambridge, Massachusetts 02142, USA
54 University Street, Carlton, Victoria 3053, Australia

Other Editorial Offices

Librairie Arnette SA
1, rue de Lille, 75007 Paris, France

Blackwell Wissenschafts-Verlag GmbH
Düsseldorfer Str. 38, D-10707 Berlin, Germany

Blackwell MZV
Feldgasse 13, A-1238 Wien, Austria

First published 1984
Second edition 1994

Set by Excel Typesetters Company, Hong Kong
Printed and bound in Spain

DISTRIBUTORS

Marston Book Services Ltd
PO Box 87
Oxford OX2 0DT
(*Orders*: Tel: 0865 791155
Fax: 0865 791927
Telex: 837515)

USA
Blackwell Scientific Publications, Inc.
238 Main Street
Cambridge, MA 02142
(*Orders*: Tel: 800 759-6102
617 876-7000)

Canada
Times Mirror Professional Publishing, Ltd
130 Flaska Drive
Markham, Ontario L6G 1B8
(*Orders*: Tel: 800 268-4178)
416 470-6739)

Australia
Blackwell Scientific Publications Pty Ltd
54 University Street
Carlton, Victoria 3053
(*Orders*: Tel: 03 347-5552)

A catalogue record for this title
is available from the British Library

ISBN 0-632-03754-7

Library of Congress
Cataloging in Publication Data

Diseases of the nails and their management/
edited by R. Baran and
R.P.R. Dawber. – 2nd ed.
p. cm.
Includes bibliographical references
and index.
ISBN 0-632-03754-7
1. Nails (Anatomy) – Diseases.
2. Nail manifestations of general diseases.
I. Baran, R. (Robert)
II. Dawber, R. P. R. (Rodney P. R.)
[DNLM: 1. Nail Diseases – therapy.
2. Nails – abnormalities. WR 475 D611 1994]
RL 165.D57 1994
617.6′92 – dc20
DNLM/DLC
for Library of Congress

Contents

Contributors, vii

Preface to the Second Edition, ix

Preface to the First Edition, xi

1 Science of the Nail Apparatus, 1
R. P. R. DAWBER, D. A. R. DE BERKER & R. BARAN

2 Physical Signs, 35
R. BARAN & R. P. R. DAWBER

3 The Nail in Childhood and Old Age, 81
R. BARAN & R. P. R. DAWBER

4 Fungal (Onychomycosis) and Other Infections Involving the Nail Apparatus, 97
R. J. HAY, R. BARAN & E. HANEKE

5 The Nail in Dermatological Diseases, 135
R. BARAN & R. P. R. DAWBER

6 The Nail in Systemic Diseases and Drug-induced Changes, 175
A. TOSTI, R. BARAN & R. P. R. DAWBER

7 Occupational Abnormalities and Contact Dermatitis, 263
R. J. G. RYCROFT & R. BARAN

8 Cosmetics: The Care and Adornment of the Nail, 285
E. BRAUER & R. BARAN

9 Hereditary and Congenital Nail Disorders, 297
L. JUHLIN & R. BARAN

10 Nail Surgery and Traumatic Abnormalities, 345
E. HANEKE & R. BARAN (with the participation of G. J. BRAUNER)

11 Tumours of the Nail Apparatus and Adjacent Tissues, 417
R. BARAN & E. HANEKE

Index, 499

Contributors

R. BARAN MD *Head of the Dermatology Unit, General Hospital Cannes, France*

E. BRAUER MD (*Deceased*) *Formerly Associate Professor of Clinical Dermatology, New York University School of Medicine, New York, USA*

G.J. BRAUNER MD *Associate Clinical Professor of Dermatology, New York Medical College, Valhalla, New York, USA*

R.P.R. DAWBER MA, MB, ChB, FRCP *Consultant Dermatologist, Oxford Hospitals and Clinical Lecturer in Dermatology, University of Oxford, Oxford, UK*

D.A.R. de BERKER MB, BS, MRCP *Department of Dermatology, Royal Victoria Infirmary, Newcastle upon Tyne, UK*

E. HANEKE Prof Dr Med *Department of Dermatology, Ferdinand Sauerbruch Klinikum, Wuppertal, Germany*

R.J. HAY MA, DM, FRCP, MRCPath *Mary Dunhill Professor of Cutaneous Medicine, Department of Dermatology, Guy's Hospital, London, UK*

L. JUHLIN MD *Professor and Head, Department of Dermatology, Uppsala University, Uppsala, Sweden*

R.J.G. RYCROFT MD, FFCP, FFOM, DH *Consultant Dermatologist, Institute of Dermatology and St John's Dermatology Centre, St Thomas's Hospital, London, UK*

A. TOSTI MD *Professor of Dermatology, Istituto di Clinica Dermatologica dell' Universita di Bologna, Bologna, Italy*

Preface to the Second Edition

The first edition was aimed mainly at those involved in nail care, diagnosis and treatment – dermatologists, surgeons, podiatrists, industrial and cosmetic experts, geneticists and related scientists in all these disciplines. Our hope was to give enough detail and referenced information to enable onychologists to deal with all aspects of the nail in disease. We were grateful to find that it has gone some way towards satisfying these needs.

Much has changed in recent years that has enabled us to expand many sections, particularly the area of nail surgery. The use of full colour illustrations has been an exciting new development in this edition. Many more rare and often unique clinical pictures have been included. We hope that these additions will help those requiring diagnostic and therapeutic help with difficult cases.

It is our very sad duty to record the death of our dear colleague Earl Brauer who contributed eruditely to the first edition. The best epitaph that we can provide for Earl is that his chapter has required very little change despite the passing years.

We welcome three new contributors, Gary Brauner who has written the section on lasers, David de Berker who has added his great skill and knowledge to the scientific sections and Antonella Tosti for her expertise on the nail in systemic disease.

The book remains a group activity and *not* simply a collection of chapters written entirely by individuals – we hope this will be evident from the structure of the many sections. Many of our dermatological colleagues around the world have loaned us material for this edition – if we have failed to acknowledge this in the text we sincerely apologize for this inadvertent omission.

Robert Baran
Rodney Dawber

Preface to the First Edition

Since the earliest publication by Heller there have been several books written on diseases of the nail: in particular the works of Alkiewicz and Pfister; Pardo-Castello and Pardo; Samman, Sertoli and Zaïas must be mentioned as they are of high quality and extremely useful, mainly to dermatologists.

For many years we have felt that there is a need for a comprehensive reference book on all aspects of the nail in health and disease. It is evident that in different cultures nail abnormalities are often seen by a variety of specialists, e.g. traumatic and genetic dystrophies are rarely seen initially by dermatologists whilst cosmetic and industrial problems may be handled by dermatologists, industrial health experts, cosmetologists or chiropodists. These are a few examples of the need for a reference book to 'cross' speciality, and even more important, parochial, national medical barriers. We believe that a satisfactory book on the nail must do this. The world is small! We have both travelled widely in recent years and do hope that the content and style of the book succeeds in this aim.

Some people may be surprised to find a Frenchman and Englishman apparently having agreed with each other for long enough to produce a book of this nature – not all French and English are enemies! We have worked diligently to benefit from our language differences and to combine the differences in training and interests and hope that this first truly international book, including authors from France, Germany, Sweden, UK and USA, will be of use world wide.

Though the chapters have been contributed by specific authors, we must point out that the book is very much a group activity; in particular, the editors have contributed much from their own files to every section. This applies to the script, references and figures, and therefore any errors of fact, emphasis or quality of picture may be the fault of the editors rather than the named chapter writers!

The inclusion of colour pictures has obviously made the book more expensive than with black and white pictures alone. We gave considerable thought to this and decided to include them as important diagnostic aids because of the photogenic nature of the nail; and the fact that between the ten authors we had a unique opportunity to pool material collected over many years.

Acknowledgements

An undertaking of this kind is quite impossible without the help of a vast number of colleagues the world over who have encouraged, cajoled and constructively disagreed with us over the many years that we have been interested in nails; and more specifically we must thank those who have provided details and pictures of their patients – these are acknowledged in the script.

We are deeply indebted to Georges Achten, Peter Samman and Nardo Zaïas who at various times have stimulated our interest in this field; without their help in our careers this book would not have materialized in any shape or form.

We are very grateful to Dr Gerald Godfrey and Chris Gummer who gave great assistance in formulating the final text.

Robert Baran
Rodney Dawber

Chapter 1
Science of the Nail Apparatus

R.P.R. DAWBER, D. DE BERKER & R. BARAN

Gross anatomy
Embryology
Regional anatomy
Matrix
Nail bed
Hyponychium
Nail plate
Nail fold
Vasculature
Nerve supply
Comparative anatomy
Physiology
Nail growth
Systemic influences
Biochemistry
Elemental analysis
Physical properties
Mechanics
Permeability
Radiation and light
Imaging

Gross anatomy

The nail is an opalescent organic window through to the vascular nail bed. It is held in place at the lateral margins by the soft tissue of the lateral nail folds and emerges from the matrix via the proximal nail fold. It ends at a free edge distally, overlying the hyponychium. These structures are illustrated in Figs 1.1(a), 1.1(b) and 1.2. The definition of the components of the nail unit are as follows:

Nail plate (nail): durable keratinized structure which continues growing throughout life.

Lateral nail folds (nail walls): the cutaneous folded structures providing the lateral borders to the nail.

Proximal nail fold (posterior or dorsal nail fold): this is the cutaneous folded structure providing the visible proximal border of the nail, continuous with the cuticle. On the undersurface the proximal one-quarter of this becomes the proximal or dorsal matrix; the distal ventral part of the proximal nail fold is often termed the eponychium.

Cuticle: the horny layer extending from the dorsal and ventral aspects of the proximal nail fold and adhering to the dorsal aspect of the nail plate.

Nail matrix (nail root): traditionally, this can be split into three parts (Lewis, 1954). The dorsal matrix overlies the proximal part of the nail plate and is continuous with the ventral aspect of the proximal nail fold; the intermediate (synonyms: distal or germinative) matrix is the epithelial structure starting at the point that the dorsal matrix folds back on itself to underlie the proximal nail. The so-called ventral matrix is synonymous with the nail bed and starts at the distal border of the lunula, where the intermediate (distal) matrix stops. It is limited distally by the onychodermal band proximal to the hyponychium.

Lunula (half moon): the convex margin of the intermediate (distal) matrix seen through the nail. It is more pale than adjacent nail bed. It is most commonly visible on the thumbs and great toes. It may be concealed by the proximal nail fold.

Nail bed (ventral matrix): the vascular bed upon which the nail rests extending from the lunula to the hyponychium. This is the major territory seen through the nail plate. The nail plate is firmly bonded to the nail bed, less so proximal to the lunula margin.

Onychodermal band: the distal margin of the nail bed has a contrasting hue in comparison with the rest of the nail bed (Terry, 1955). Normally, this is a transverse band of 1–1.5 mm of a deeper pink (Caucasian) or brown (Afro-Caribbean). Its colour, or presence, may vary with disease or compression which influences the vascular supply (Fig. 1.3(a)&(b)).

Sonnex *et al.* (1991), having described the confusing terminology of the various distal colour bands on normal nails, undertook to re-emphasize the nature of these (Fig. 1.3(b)) – the distal yellow line traversing the nail is ascribed to Pinkus, but is often left out of standard texts. Clinical and histological studies presented by Sonnex *et al.* (1991) showed that the band is present in more than 90% of normal adult fingernails and represents the most proximal point of the attachment of the fingertip stratum corneum to the nail plate – they suggested that this should therefore be termed the onychocorneal band or junction. This region has distinctive histological features and is the first major barrier to material or organisms passing proxi-

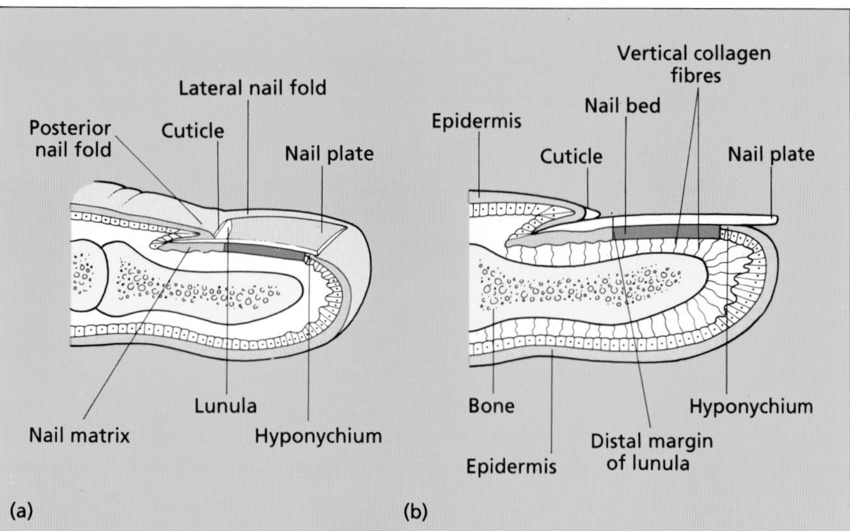

Fig. 1.1. (a & b) Longitudinal section of a digit showing the dorsal nail apparatus.

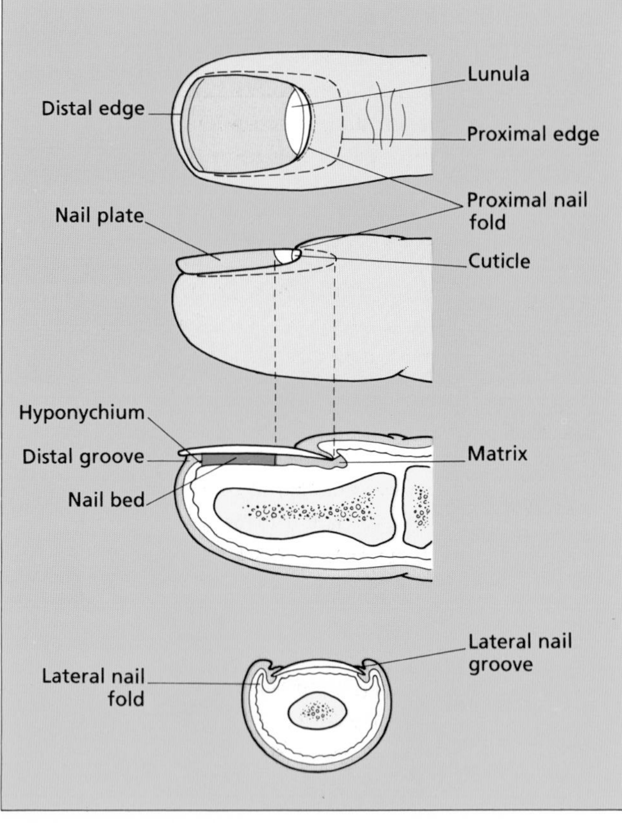

Fig. 1.2. The tip of a digit showing the component parts of the nail apparatus.

mally beneath the nail plate. They suggested that abnormalities of this structure may result in onycholysis, pachyonychia congenita and pterygium inversum unguis.

Hyponychium: the cutaneous margin underlying free nail, bordered distally by the distal groove. In this region the separation of the nail plate and nail bed begins.

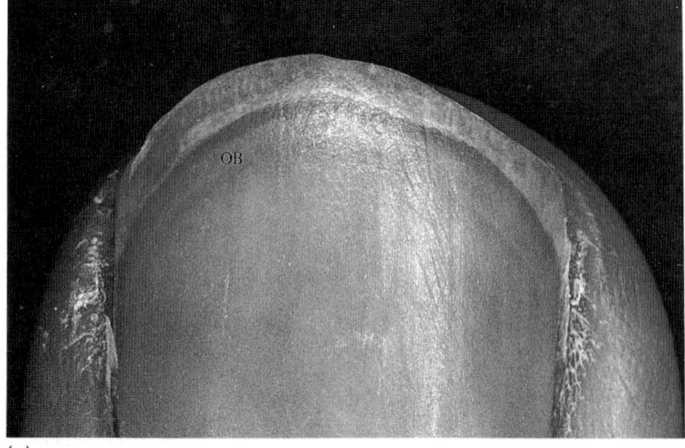

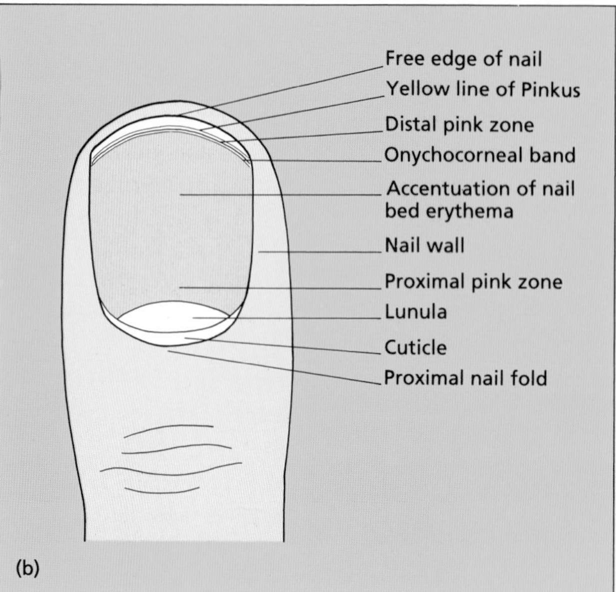

Fig. 1.3. (a) Onychocorneal band (OB). (b) Diagrammatic representation of the morphological features of the normal nail; detail of the distal physiological colour bands are shown (courtesy of Dr T.S. Sonnex & Dr W.A.D. Griffiths, St John's Institute of Dermatology).

Distal groove (limiting furrow): this is a cutaneous ridge demarcating the border between subungual structures and the finger pulp. It is convex-shaped distally.

References

Lewis B.L. (1954) Microscopic studies of fetal and mature nail and surrounding soft tissue. *Arch. Dermatol. Syphilol.* **70**, 732–744.

Terry R.B. (1955) The onychodermal band in health and disease. *Lancet* **i**, 179–181.

Sonnex T.S., Griffiths W.A.D. & Nicol W.J. (1991) The nature and significance of the transverse white band of human nails. *Semin. Dermatol.* **10**, 12–16.

Embryology

Morphogenesis

8–12 weeks

Individual digits are discernible from the eighth week of gestation (Lewis, 1954). The first embryonic element of the nail unit is the nail anlage present from 9 weeks as the epidermis overlying the dorsal tip of the digit. At 10 weeks a distinct region can be seen and is described as the primary nail field. This almost overlies the tip of the terminal phalanx, with clear proximal and lateral grooves in addition to a well-defined distal groove. The prominence of this groove is partly due to the distal ridge, thrown up proximally, accentuating the contour. The primary nail field grows proximally by a wedge of germinative matrix cells extending back from the tip of the digit. These cells are proximal to both the distal groove and ridge. The spatial relationship of these two latter structures remains relatively constant as the former becomes the vestigial distal groove and the latter, the hyponychium (Fig. 1.4).

13–14 weeks

Differential growth of the slowly developing primary nail field and surrounding tissue results in the emergence of overhanging proximal and lateral nail folds. Depending on the point of reference, the nail folds may be interpreted as overhanging (Warwick & Williams, 1973) or the matrix as invaginating. By 13 weeks the nail field is well defined in the finger, with the matrix primordium underlying a proximal nail fold. By 14 weeks the nail plate is seen emerging from beneath the proximal nail fold, with elements arising from the lunula as well as more proximal matrix.

17 weeks–birth

At 17 weeks, the nail plate covers most of the nail bed and the distal ridge has flattened. From 20 weeks, the nail unit and finger grow in tandem, with the nail plate abutting the distal ridge. This now becomes termed the hyponychium. The nail bed epithelium no longer produces keratohyalin, with a more parakeratotic appearance. By birth the nail plate extends to the distal groove, which becomes progressively less prominent. The nail may curve over the volar surface of the finger. It may also demonstrate koilonychia. This deformity is normal in the very young and a function of the thinness of the nail plate. It reverses with age.

Tissue differentiation

Keratin synthesis can be identified in the nail unit from the earliest stages of its differentiation (Moll *et al.*, 1988). In 12 and 13 week embryos, the nail matrix anlage is a thin epithelial wedge penetrating from the dorsal epidermis into the dermis. This wedge was thought to represent the 'ventral matrix primordium'. Trichocyte ('hard'), or T-keratins, are found co-expressed with the epithelial ('soft') or E-keratins at this site. At other sites, such as the lunula and parts of the nail bed, there is exclusive expression of T-keratin epibasally with E-keratins 10/11 found at a suprabasal location appropriate for normal skin.

By week 15, T-keratins are found throughout the nail bed and matrix. This could have significance concerning theories of nail embryogenesis and growth, where debate exists as to the contribution made by the nail bed to nail

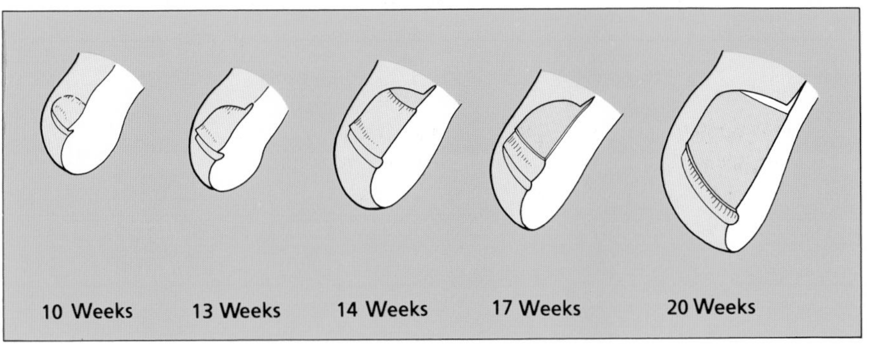

Fig. 1.4. Embryogenesis of the nail apparatus. 10 weeks: The primary nail field can be seen with proximal, lateral and distal grooves. The latter is accentuated by a distal ridge. 13 weeks: A wedge of matrix primordium moves proximally, with the invagination of the proximal nail fold above. 14 weeks: The nail plate emerges. 17 weeks: The nail plate covers most of the nail bed and the distal ridge starts to flatten. 20 weeks: The nail plate extends to the distal ridge, now termed hyponychium. Finger and nail grow roughly in tandem from now on.

growth (Lewis, 1954; Hashimoto *et al.*, 1966; Zaias, 1963; Zaias & Alvarez, 1968; Johnson *et al.*, 1991). However, at 22 weeks, the layer of T-keratin-positive cells remains very thin in the nail bed, whereas it is considerably thickened in the intermediate matrix. In the adult nail, there have been reports of both the presence (Baden & Kubilus, 1984) and absence (Heid *et al.*, 1988; Moll *et al.*, 1988) of T-keratins in the nail bed.

Histological observation at 13 and 14 weeks reveals parakeratotic cells just distal to this nail plate primordium staining for disulphydryl groups. This contrasts to adjacent epithelium, suggesting the start of nail plate differentiation. Such differentiation is consistent with the coincident changes in the T-keratins. The embryonic nail bed epithelium produces keratohyalin at this stage.

By 25 weeks, most features of nail unit differentiation are complete. Changes may still occur in the chemical constitution of the nail plate after this date. A decrease in sulphur and aluminium and a rise in chlorine has been noted as a feature of fullterm newborns in comparison with the nail plate of premature babies (Sirota *et al.*, 1988). An elevated aluminium may correspond to bone abnormalities which lead to osteopenia.

Moll and Moll (1993) found increasing numbers of Merkel cells in the nail anlagen from 9–15 weeks; by 22 weeks these had decreased and were rare in adult nail biopsies.

Factors in embryogenesis

The nail plate grows from the fifteenth week of gestation until death. Many factors act upon it in this time and influence its appearance. Because it is a rugged structure, growing over a cycle of 6–18 months, it provides a record of the effects of these influences. To consider the different formative mechanisms, it is important to distinguish:

1 embryogenesis;
2 regrowth;
3 growth.

There is overlap in all these processes, with the main clues concerning embryogenesis deriving from fetal studies and analysis of congenital abnormalities. Regrowth is the growth of the nail plate following its removal. This may be for therapeutic reasons or following accidental trauma with associated damage. Observations of this process add to our understanding of both growth and embryogenesis. Growth is the continuous process of nail plate generation over a fully differentiated nail bed and hyponychium. Embryogenesis is the subject of this section.

In the chick limb bud formation there is a complex interaction between mesoderm and ectoderm. Initially, the mesoderm induces the development of the apical ectodermal ridge (AER). The mesoderm then becomes dependent upon the AER for the creation of the limb. Removal of the AER results in a halt of mesodermal differentiation. Replacing the underlying mesoderm with mesoderm from another part of the limb primordium still results in normal differentiation (Zwilling, 1968). However, the AER continues to be dependent upon the mesoderm, which must be of limb type. Replacement of limb mesoderm with somite mesoderm causes flattening of the AER. These morphogenetic interactions occur prior to cytodifferentiation (Grant, 1978). In the human, cases of anonychia secondary to phenytoin (Johnson, 1981) might implicate the drug at this stage, prior to 8 weeks. Drugs have been argued as being contributory to congenital nail dystrophies, mainly affecting the index finger (Higashi *et al.*, 1975).

Other congenital abnormalities highlight the debate that spans embryogenesis, growth and regrowth (Telfer *et al.*, 1988; Telfer, 1991). Congenital onychodysplasia of the index fingers (COIF) is frequently associated with abnormalities of the terminal phalanges (Baran, 1980). The nail may be absent, small or composed of several small nails on the dorsal tip of the affected finger. The bony abnormality varies, with the most marked change being bifurcation of the terminal phalanx on lateral X-ray (Millman & Strier, 1982). However, a bony abnormality is not mandatory in this condition or other conditions with ectopic nail (Aoki & Sozuki, 1984). A normal nail may overly an abnormal bone on other than the index finger (Kinoshita & Nagano, 1976); but more often abnormal bone is associated with altered overlying nail. COIF appears to demonstrate an association between abnormalities of bone and nail, rather than the presence of a strict contingent relationship. It may represent a fault of mesoderm/ectoderm interaction at the stage when these layers are mutually dependent. It has been suggested that a vascular abnormality may provide the common factor between pathology in the two embryonic layers (Kitayama & Tsukada, 1983).

An interpretation based upon a mutual mesodermal and ectodermal fault would fit with the observation of two cases of congenital anonychia and hypoplastic nails combined with hypoplastic phalanges (Baran & Juhlin, 1986). These cases were used as a foil for the suggestion of a mechanism of 'bone-dependent nail formation'. It might also be argued in reverse, that the bone was dependent upon the nail. One must state however that the bone develops before the nail and bone and nail become intimately and directly bonded by vertical connective tissue. The shape of the nail is certainly closely dependent on the terminal phalanx shape both in health and disease.

References

Aoki K. & Suzuki H. (1984) The morphology and hardness of the nail in two cases of congenital onychoheterotopia. *Br. J. Dermatol.* **110**, 717–723.

Baden H.P. & Kubilus J. (1984) A comparative study of the immunologic properties of hoof and nail fibrous proteins. *J. Invest. Dermatol.* **83**, 327–331.

Baran R. & Juhlin L. (1986) Bone dependent nail formation. *Br. J. Dermatol.* **114**, 371–375.

Baran R. (1980) Syndrome d'Iso et Kikuchi (COIF syndrome). 2 cas avec revue de la littérature (44 cas). *Ann. Dermatol. Venereol.* **107**, 431–435.

Grant P. (1978) Limb morphogenesis: a dialog between an ectodermal sheet and mesoderm. In: *Biology of Developing Systems*, pp. 414–421. Holt Rinehart and Winston, New York.

Hashimoto K., Gross B.G., Nelson R. & Lever W.F. (1966) The ultrastructure of the skin of human embryos. III. The formation of the nail in 16–18 week old embryos. *J. Invest. Dermatol.* **47**, 205–207.

Heid H.W., Moll I. & Franke W.W. (1988) Patterns of trichocytic and epithelial cytokeratins in mammalian tissues. II. Concomitant and mutually exclusive synthesis of trichocytic and epthelial cytokeratins in diverse human and bovine tissues. *Differentiation* **37**, 215–230.

Higashi N., Ikegami T. & Asada Y. (1975) Congenital nail defects of the index finger. *Jpn. J. Clin. Dermatol.* **29**, 699–701.

Johnson M., Comaish J.S. & Shuster S. (1991) Nail is produced by the normal nail bed: a controversy resolved. *Br. J. Dermatol.* **125**, 27–29.

Johnson R.B. & Goldsmith I.A. (1981) Dilantin digital defects. *J. Am. Dermatol.* **5**, 191.

Kinoshita Y. & Nagano T. (1976) Congenital defects of the index finger. *Jpn. J. Plast. Reconstr. Surg.* **19**, 23.

Kitayama Y. & Tsukada S. (1983) Congenital onychodysplasia. Report of 11 cases. *Arch. Dermatol.* **119**, 8–12.

Lewis B.L. (1954) Microscopic studies of fetal and mature nail and surrounding soft tissue. *Arch. Dermatol. Syphilol.* **70**, 732–744.

Millman A.J. & Strier R.P. (1982) Congenital onychodysplasia of the index fingers. *J. Am. Acad. Dermatol.* **7**, 57–65.

Moll I., Heid H.W., Franke W.W. & Moll R. (1988) Patterns of expression of trichocytic and epithelial cytokeratins in mammalian tissues. *Differentiation* **39**, 167–184.

Moll I. & Moll R. (1993) Merkel cells in ontogenesis of human nails. *Arch. Dermatol. Research* **285**, 366–377.

Sirota L., Straussberg R., Fishman P. *et al.* (1988) X-ray microanalysis of the fingernails in term and preterm infants. *Pediatric Dermatol.* **5**, 184–186.

Telfer N.R., Barth J.H. & Dawber R.P.R. (1988) Congenital and hereditary nail dystrophies: an embryological approach to classification. *Clin. Exp. Dermatol.* **13**, 160–163.

Telfer N.R. (1991) Congenital and hereditary nail disorders. In: *Seminars in Dermatology*, ed. Baran R., Vol. 10(1), pp. 2–7. W.B. Saunders, Philadelphia.

Warwick R. & Williams P.L., eds (1973) *Gray's Anatomy*, 35th edn. Longman, London.

Zaias N. & Alvarez J. (1968) The formation of the primate nail plate. An autoradiographic study in the squirrel monkey. *J. Invest. Dermatol.* **51**, 120–136.

Zaias N. (1963) Embryology of the human nail. *Arch. Dermatol.* **87**, 37–53.

Zwilling E. (1968) Morphogenetic phases in development. *The Emergence of Order in Developing Systems*, ed. Locke M., pp. 184–207. Academic Press, New York.

Regional anatomy

Histological preparation

High quality sections of the nail unit are difficult to obtain. Nail keratin is very hard and tends to split or tear. In biopsies containing nail plate and soft subungual and periungual tissue, the nail plate is often torn from the matrix and other adjacent structures by the microtome. This effect can be diminished by softening the nail.

Nail softening techniques

Nail alone

There are several different techniques to soften the nail plate. Lewis (1954) recommended routine fixation in 10% formalin and processing as usual. Early techniques used fixation with potassium bichromate, sodium sulphate and water. The section is then decalcified with nitric acid and embedded in colloidin. Alkiewicz and Pfister (1976) recommended softening the nail with thioglycollate or hydrogen peroxide. Nail fragments are kept in 10% potassium thioglycollate at 37°C for 5 days or in 20–30% hydrogen peroxide for 5–6 days. The nail is then fixed by boiling in formalin for 1 min. Ten to 15 μm sections are cut with the cryomicrotome.

Although softening of nail clippings for histology is not mandatory, it is possible and may be helpful. Suarez *et al.* (1991) suggest soaking the clipping for 2 days in a mix of mercuric chloride, chromic acid, nitric acid and 95% alcohol. The specimen is then transferred to absolute alcohol, xylene, successive paraffin mixtures, sectioned at 4 μm and placed on gelatinized slides.

Nail and soft tissue

In nail biopsies containing soft tissue, more gentle methods of preparation are necessary. Adequate softening may be achieved by using a special fixative of 5% trichloroacetic acid and 10% formalin (Alvarez & Zaias, 1967). Alternatively, the specimen can be soaked in distilled water for a few hours before placing in formalin (Bennett, 1976). Good results are obtained with routine fixation and embedding if permanent wave solution, thioglycollate or 10% potassium hydroxide solution is applied with a cotton swab to the surface of the paraffin block every two or three sections. Lewin *et al.* (1973) suggest applying 1% aqueous polysorbate 40 to the cut surface of the block for 1 h at 4°C.

Routine staining with haematoxylin and eosin is sufficient for many cases. Periodic acid Schiff (PAS) and Grocott's silver stain can be used to demonstrate fungi; a blancophore fluorochromation selectively delineates fungal

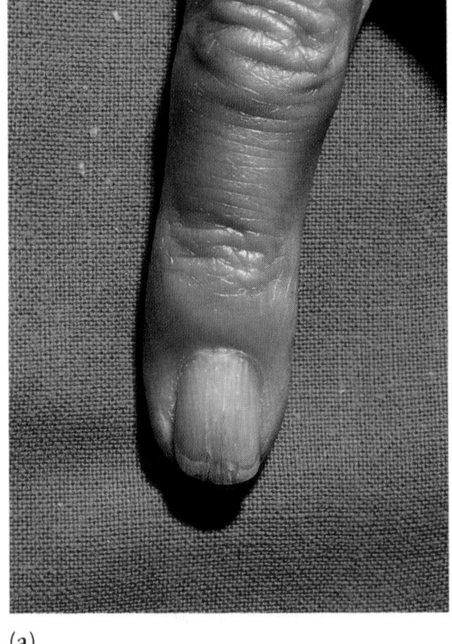

(a)

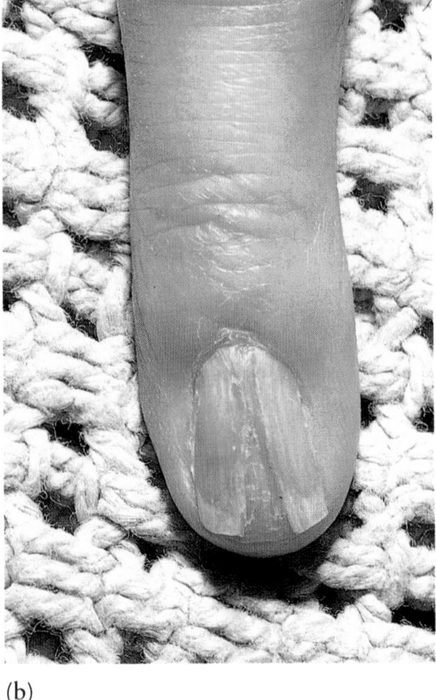

(b)

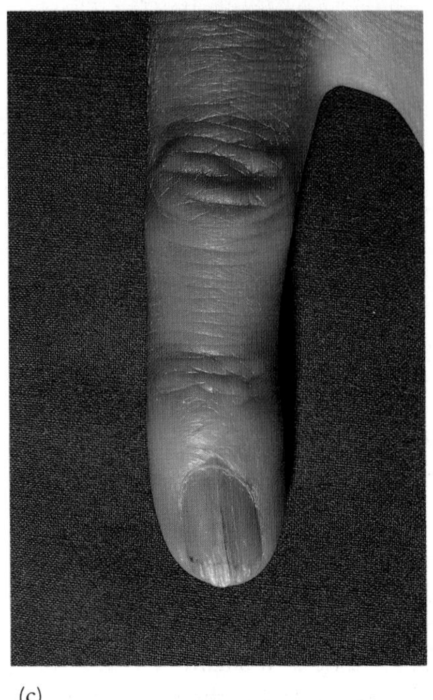

(c)

Fig. 1.5. (a)–(c) Longitudinal nail biopsy of Zaias. (a) Before biopsy; (b) 5 weeks after; (c) 3 months later.

walls (Haneke, 1991). Toluidine blue at pH 5 allows better visualization of the details of the nail plate (Achten, 1963, 1991). Fontana's argentaffin reaction demonstrates melanin. Haemoglobin is identified using a peroxidase reaction. Prussian blue and Perl stains are not helpful in the identification of blood in the nail. They are specific to the haemosiderin product of haemoglobin breakdown caused by macrophages. This does not occur in the nail (Achten & Wanet, 1973; Alkiewicz & Pfister, 1976; Baran & Haneke, 1984). Masson–Goldner's trichrome stain is very useful to study the keratinization process and Giemsa stain reveals slight changes in the nail keratin.

Polarization microscopy shows the regular arrangement of keratin filaments and birefringence is said to be absent in disorders of nail formation such as leuconychia.

Nail matrix

The sites of nail production (nail matrix) are described on p. 21. The intermediate matrix underlying the nail plate is generally considered to be the source of the bulk of the nail plate thickness (approx. two-thirds), although further contributions may come from other parts of the nail unit (see nail growth, p. 25). Contrast with these other regions helps characterize the intermediate matrix.

The matrix is vulnerable to surgical and accidental trauma; a longitudinal biopsy of greater than 3 mm width is likely to leave a permanent dystrophy (Zaias, 1967) (Fig. 1.5(a)–(c)). Once matrix damage has occurred, it is difficult to provide an aesthetic repair (Nakayama *et al.*, 1990; Pessa *et al.*, 1990). This accounts for the relatively small amount of histological information on normal nail matrix.

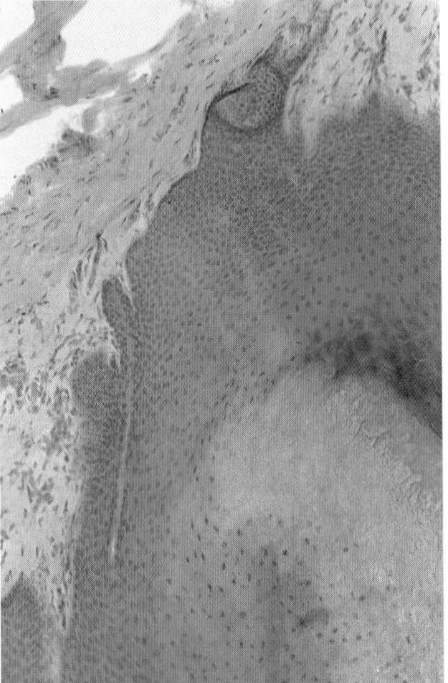

Fig. 1.6. Junction between the intermediate matrix and the proximal nail fold. The latter has a granular layer.

Routine histology

The cells of the intermediate matrix are distinct from the adjacent nail bed (ventral matrix) distally and the ventral surface of the nail fold (dorsal matrix), lying at an angle

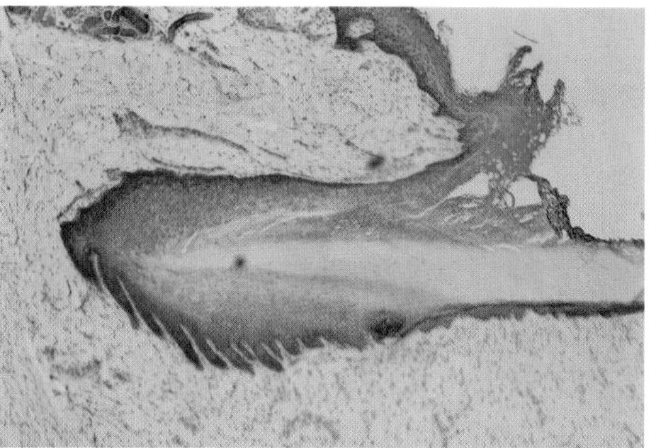

Fig. 1.7. Keratin stain of the nail apparatus delineating the epithelial structures of the matrix and proximal nail fold.

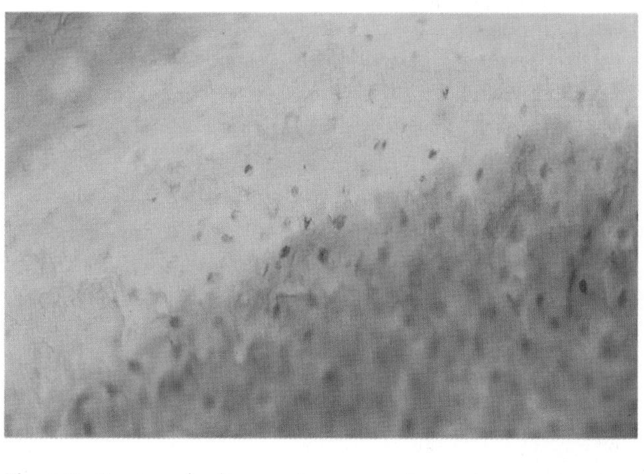

Fig. 1.8. Pertinax bodies can be seen as the nuclear remnants within the nail plate (see also Fig. 3.14).

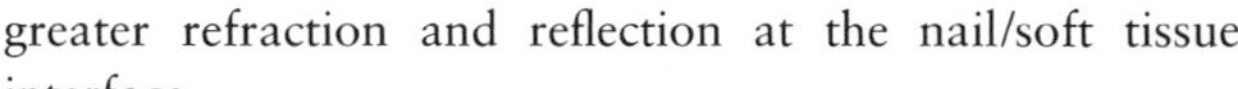

above. It is the thickest area of stratified squamous epithelium in the mid-line of the nail unit, comparable with the hyponychium. There are long rete ridges characteristically descending at a slightly oblique angle, their tips pointing distally. Laterally, the intermediate matrix rete ridges are less marked, whereas those of the nail bed and nail folds become prominent.

Unlike the dorsal matrix, but like the nail bed, the intermediate (distal) matrix has no granular layer (Fig. 1.6). The demarcation between dorsal and intermediate matrix is enhanced by the altered morphology of the rete ridges. At their junction in the mid-zone of the nail, the first intermediate matrix epithelial ridge may have a bobbed appearance, like a lopped sheep's tail. PAS staining is marked at both the distal and proximal margins of the intermediate matrix (Fig. 1.7).

Distally, there is often a step reduction in the epithelial thickness at the transition of the intermediate matrix with the nail bed. This represents the edge of the lunula, which may be visible clinically, particularly in the thumb. The thinner epidermis of the nail bed may account for the contrast between white and pink appearance of the lunula and bed, respectively (Burrows, 1917). Diminished vascularity and increased dermal collagen beneath the intermediate matrix may also be contributory (Lewin, 1965). These factors seem likely to be the most relevant in this observation, but many other suggestions have been made (Burrows, 1917, 1919; Ham & Leeson, 1961; Achten, 1963; Lewin, 1965; Baran & Gioanni, 1969).

1 The matrix epithelium in the lunula has more nuclei than the nail bed, making it appear parakeratotic with an altered colour.

2 The surface of the nail is smoother and more shiny proximally.

3 The thicker epidermis of the lunula obscures the underlying vasculature.

4 The nail attachment at the lunula is less firm, allowing greater refraction and reflection at the nail/soft tissue interface.

5 The underlying dermis has less capillaries in it.

6 The underlying dermis is of looser texture.

The presence of a lunula is not universal, even if the nail fold is retracted. In addition, the edge of the lunula may be blurred and not coincide with the distal margin of the intermediate matrix. All these factors oblige us to keep an open mind concerning its aetiology and significance.

Nail is formed from the intermediate (germinal or distal) matrix as the cells initially become larger and more pale and the nucleus disintegrates. There is progression with flattening, elongation and further pallor (Picardo *et al.*, 1992). Occasionally retained shrunken or fragmented nuclei persist to be included into the nail plate. Lewis (1954) called these 'pertinax bodies'. They can give an impression of the longitudinal progression of growth in the nail plate (Fig. 1.8).

Melanocytes are present in the intermediate matrix where they reach a density of 300 mm^2 (Higashi, 1968; Higashi & Saito, 1969); they are less numerous in the more proximal matrix. They are dendritic cells found in the epibasal layers. This differs from normal epidermis, where melanocytes are found only in the basal layer. Melanin in the nail plate is composed of granules derived from matrix melanocytes (Zaias, 1963). Longitudinal melanonychia may be a benign phenomenon, particularly in Afro-Caribbeans. Seventy-seven per cent of black people will have melanonychia by the age of 20 and almost 100% by the age of 50 (Monash, 1932; Leyden *et al.*, 1972; Baran & Kechijian, 1989). The Japanese also have a high prevalence of longitudinal melanonychia, it being present in 10–20% of adults (Kopf & Waldo, 1980). In a study of 15 benign melanonychia lesions in Japanese patients, the lesions were found to arise from an increase in activity and number of DOPA-positive melanocytes in the intermediate matrix, not a melanocytic naevus

(Higashi, 1968). Longitudinal melanonychia in Caucasians is more sinister. Oropeza (1986) stated that a subungual pigmented lesion in this group has a higher chance of being malignant than of being benign.

Langerhans cells are demonstrable in the nail apparatus, mainly in the epithelial components, including the dorsal and intermediate matrix.

There is only a thin layer of dermis dividing the intermediate matrix from the terminal phalanx. This has a rich vascular supply and an elastin and collagen infrastructure giving direct, vertically orientated attachment to periosteum.

Electron microscopy

Transmission electron microscopy confirms that in many respects, intermediate matrix epithelium is similar to normal cutaneous epithelium (Hashimoto, 1971a–d). The basal cells contain desmosomes and hemidesmosomes and interdigitate freely. Differentiating cells are rich in ribosomes and polysomes and contain more RNA than equivalent cutaneous epidermal cells. As cell differentiation proceeds towards the nail plate, there is an accumulation of cytoplasmic microfibrils (7.5–10 nm). These fibrils are haphazardly arranged within the cells up to the transitional zone. Beyond this, they become aligned with the axis of nail plate growth.

Membrane coating granules (Odland bodies) are formed within the differentiating cells. They are discharged onto the cell surface in the transitional zone and have been thought to contribute to the thickness of the plasma membrane. They may also have a role in the firm adherence of the squamous cells within the nail plate, which is a notable characteristic (Parent *et al.*, 1985). The glycoprotein characteristics of cell membrane complexes isolated from nail plate may reflect the constituents of these granules (Allen *et al.*, 1991).

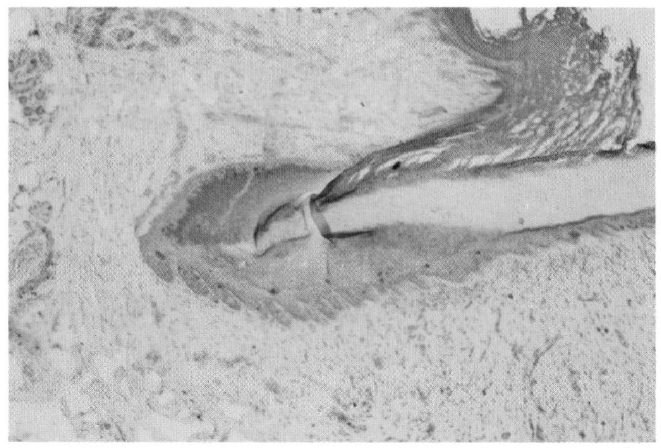

Fig. 1.9. Peroxidase immunostaining of keratin 10 in the nail apparatus. The nail bed is left unlabelled, whilst other structures express this suprabasal keratin.

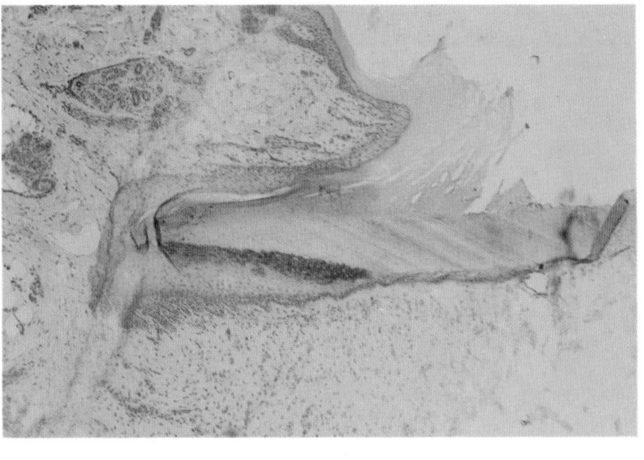

Fig. 1.10. Peroxidase immunostaining of the nail apparatus labelled with a trichocyte keratin antibody. It is found only in the intermediate matrix.

Mitochondria are degraded during the transitional phase whilst RNA-containing ribosomes are evident up to the stage of plasma membrane thickening. Vacuoles containing lipid and other products of cytolysis are seen at the transitional stage. Dorsal matrix cells start to show nuclear shrinkage at this point, whereas the nuclei in the intermediate matrix remain intact to a higher level.

Immunohistochemistry

The most extensive immunohistological investigations of the nail unit have utilized keratin antibodies. The nail plate (Lynch *et al.*, 1986; Heid *et al.*, 1988), human embryonic nail unit (Heid *et al.*, 1988; Moll, 1988), accessory digit nail unit (de Berker *et al.*, 1993) and adult nail unit (Haneke, 1990) have all been examined.

Using the antibody 34βE12, Haneke (1990) demonstrated positivity of the basal two-thirds of the intermediate matrix. This antibody detects keratins 5, 10 and 11, indicating the presence of one or more of these at this location. Using monospecific antibodies, de Berker *et al.* (1993) detected keratins 1 and 10 in a suprabasal location in the intermediate matrix and noted their absence from the nail bed (Fig. 1.9) (ventral matrix). Keratins 1 and 10 are 'soft' epithelial keratins found suprabasally in normal skin (Purkis *et al.*, 1990). Keratin 7 and Ha-1 were found in the intermediate matrix. Ha-1 is a trichocyte, or 'hard' keratin. Keratin 7 was found at other sites in the nail unit and hair follicle, whereas Ha-1 was limited to the intermediate matrix of the nail (Fig. 1.10) and the germinal matrix of the hair follicle. de Berker *et al.* (1993) also detected keratin 19 basally and suprabasally in the intermediate matrix, not a consistent finding in the work of Haneke (1990) or Moll (1988) where different antibodies were used. However, Moll (1988) did detect keratin 19 at this site in 15 week embryo nail units. Keratin 19 is also

Table 1.1. Analysis of nail unit basement membrane zone using monoclonal and polyclonal antibodies

	Digit 1					Digit 2				Digit 3	
	Nail apparatus					Nail apparatus					
	Fold	Matrix	Bed	HN	Proximal phalangeal skin	Fold	Matrix	Bed	HN	Split skin	Intact skin
Mono. Ab											
LH7:2	+	+	+	+	+	+	+	+	+	epi	+
L3d	+	+	+	+	+	+	+	+	+	epi	+
Col IV	+	+	+	+	+	+	+	+	+	epi	+
GB3	+	+	+	+	+	+	+	+	+	epi	+
LH24	+	+	+	+	+	+	+	+	+	epi	+
LH39	+	+	+	+	+	+	+	+	+	epi	+
GDA	+	+	+	+	+	+	+	+	+	epi	+
Tenascin	+	+	+	+	+	+	+	+	+	epi	+
a6	+	+	+	+	+	+	+	+	+	epi	+
G71	+	+	+	+	+	+	+	+	+	epi	+
Poly. Ab											
Fibronectin	–	–	–	–	–	–	–	–	–	–	–
Laminin	+	+	+	+	+	+	+	+	+	derm	+
BP 220 kDa	+	+	+	+	+	+	+	+	+	epi	+
EBA 250 kDa	+	+	+	+	+	+	+	+	+	derm	+
LAD 285 kDa	+	+	+	+	+	+	+	+	+	epi	+
LAD ? kDa	+	+	+	+	+	+	+	+	+	derm	+

HN: Hyponychium

found in the outer root sheath of the hair follicle and lingual papilla (Heid *et al.*, 1988).

Haneke (1990) has provided a review of other important immunohistochemically detectable antigens. Involucrin is a protein necessary for the formation of the cellular envelope in keratinizing epithelia. It is strongly positive in the upper two-thirds of the matrix and weakly detected in the suprabasal layers. The antibody HHF35 is considered specific to actin. It shows a strong membranous staining and weak cytoplasmic staining of intermediate matrix cells.

In the dermis, vimentin is strongly positive in fibroblasts and vascular endothelial cells. Vimentin and desmin are expressed in the smooth muscle wall of some vessels. S100 stain, for cells of neural crest origin, reveals perivascular nerves, glomus bodies and Meissner's corpuscles distally. Filaggrin cannot be demonstrated in the matrix.

The basement membrane zone of the entire nail unit has been examined, employing a wide range of monoclonal and polyclonal antibodies (Sinclair *et al.*, 1993). Collagen VII, fibronectin, chondroitin sulphate and tenascin were among the antigens detected. All were present in a quantity and pattern indistinguishable from normal skin (Table 1.1).

References

Achten G. (1963) L'ongle normal et pathologique. *Dermatologica* **126**, 229–245.

Achten G. & Wanet J. (1973) Pathologie der Nagel. In: *Spezielle Pathologische Anatomie*, eds Doerr W., Seifert G. & Uehlinger E. Vol. 7, pp. 487–528. Springer-Verlag, New York.

Achten G., André J. & Laporte M. (1991) Nails in light and electron microscopy. *Sem. Dermatol.* **10**, 54–64.

Alkiewicz J. & Pfister R. (1976) *Atlas der Nagelkrankheiten.* Schattauer-Verlag, Stuttgart.

Allen K.A., Ellis J. & Rivett D.E. (1991) The presence of glycoproteins in the cell membrane complex of variety of keratin fibres. *Biochim. Biophys. Acta.* **1074**, 331–333.

Alvarez R. & Zaias N. (1967) A modified polyethylene glycol-pyroxylin embedding method specially suited for nails. *J. Invest. Dermatol.* **49**, 409–410.

Baran R. & Gioanni T. (1969) Les dyschromies ungueales. *Hôpital (Paris)* **57**, 101–107.

Baran R. & Haneke E. (1984) Diagnostik und Therapie der streifenförmigen Nagelpigmentierung. *Hautarzt* **35**, 359–365.

Baran R. & Kechijian P. (1989) Longitudinal melanonychia: diagnosis and management. *J. Am. Acad. Dermatol.* **21**, 1165–1175.

Bennett J. (1976) Technique of biopsy of nails. *J. Derm. Surg. Oncol.* **2**, 325–326.

Burrows M.T. (1917) The significance of the lunula of the nail. *Anat. Rec.* **12**, 161–166.

Burrows M.T. (1919) The significance of the lunula of the nail. *Johns Hopkins Med. J.* **18**, 357–361.

de Berker D., Leigh I., Wojnarowska F. *et al.* (1993) Pattern of keratin expression in the nail unit – an indicator of regional matrix differentiation (in press).

Ham A.W. & Leeson T.S. (1961) *Histology*, 4th edn. Pitman Medical, London.

Haneke E. (1990) The human nail matrix – flow cytometric and immunohistochemical studies. *Clinical Dermatology in the Year 2000*, London, May 1990. Book of Abstracts.

Haneke E. (1991) Fungal infections of the nail. In: *Seminars in Dermatology*, ed. Baran R., Vol. 10, pp. 41–53. W.B. Saunders, Philadelphia.

Hashimoto K. (1971a) Ultrastructure of the human toenail: cell migration, keratinization and formation of the intercellular cement. *Arch. Dermatol. Forsch.* **240**, 1–22.

Hashimoto K. (1971b) The marginal band: A demonstration of the thickened cellular envelope of the human nail. *Arch. Dermatol.* **103**, 387–393.

Hashimoto K. (1971c) Ultrastructure of the human toenail: I. Proximal nail matrix. *J. Invest. Dermatol.* **56**, 235–246.

Hashimoto K. (1971d) Ultrastructure of the human toenail: II. *J. Ultrastruct. Res.* **36**, 391–410.

Heid W.H., Moll I. & Franke W.W. (1988) Patterns of expression of trichocytic and epithelial cytokeratins in mammalian tissues. II. Concomitant and mutually exclusive synthesis of trichocytic and epithelial cytokeratins in diverse human and bovine tissues. *Differentiation* **37**, 215–230.

Higashi N. (1968) Melanocytes of nail matrix and nail pigmentation. *Arch. Dermatol.* **97**, 570–574.

Higashi N. & Saito T. (1969) Horizontal distribution of the DOPA positive melanocytes in the nail matrix. *J. Invest. Dermatol.* **53**, 163–165.

Kopf A.W. & Waldo F. (1980) Melanonychia striata. *Austr. J. Dermatol.* **21**, 59–70.

Lewin K. (1965) The normal finger nail. *Br. J. Dermatol.* **77**, 421–430.

Lewin K., Dewitt S. & Lawson R. (1973) Softening techniques for nail biopsy. *Arch. Dermatol.* **107**, 223–224.

Lewis B.L. (1954) Microscopic studies of fetal and mature nail and the surrounding soft tissue. *Arch. Dermatol. Syphilol.* **70**, 732–744.

Leyden J.J., Spot D.A. & Goldsmith H. (1972) Diffuse banded melanin pigmentation in nails. *Arch. Dermatol.* **105**, 548–550.

Lynch M.H., O'Guin W.M., Hardy C. *et al.* (1986) Acid and basic hair/nail ('hard') keratins: Their co-localisation in upper corticle and cuticle cells of the human hair follicle and their relationship to 'soft' keratins. *J. Cell Biol.* **103**, 2593–2606.

Moll I., Heid H.W., Franke W.W. & Moll R. (1988) Patterns of expression of trichocytic and epithelial cytokeratins in mammalian tissue. *Differentiation* **39**, 167–184.

Monash S. (1932) Normal pigmentation in the nails of negroes. *Arch. Dermatol.* **25**, 876–881.

Nakayama Y., Iino T., Uchida A. *et al.* (1990) Vascularised free nail grafts nourished by arterial inflow from the venous system. *Plast. Reconstr. Surg.* **85**, 239–245.

Oropeza R. (1986) Melanomas of special sites. In: *Cancer of the Skin: Biology, Diagnosis, Management*, Vol. 2, pp. 974–987. Blackwell Scientific Publications, Oxford.

Parent D., Achten G. & Stouffs-Vanhoof F. (1985) Ultrastructure of the normal human nail. *Am. J. Dermatopathol.* **7**, 529–535.

Pessa J.E., Tsai T.M., Li Y. & Kleinert H.E. (1990) The repair of nail deformities with the non-vascularised nail bed graft: Indications and results. *J. Hand Surg.* **15A**, 466–470.

Picardo M., Marchese C., Zompetta C., Camelli N., Fanti P. & Tosti A. (1992) Characterisation of human matrix cells in vitro. *J. Invest. Dermatol.* **98**, 523–528.

Purkis P.E., Steel J.B., Mackenzie I.C. *et al.* (1990) Antibody markers of basal cells in complex epithelia. *J. Cell Sci.* **97**, 39–50.

Sinclair R.D., Wojnarowska F. & Dawber R.P.R. (1993) The basement membrane zone of the nail, in press.

Suarez S.M., Silvers D.N. & Scher R.K. (1991) Histologic evaluation of nail clippings for diagnosing onychomycosis. *Arch. Dermatol.* **127**, 1517–1519.

Zaias N. (1963) Embryology of the human nail. *Arch. Dermatol.* **87**, 37–53.

Zaias N. (1967) The longitudinal nail biopsy. *J. Invest. Dermatol.* **49**, 406–408.

Nail bed and hyponychium

The nail bed extends from the distal margin of the lunula to the hyponychium. It is also called the ventral or sterile matrix depending on whether or not you believe that it contributes to the substance of the nail plate (see nail growth, p. 21). Avulsion of the nail plate reveals a pattern of longitudinal epidermal ridges stretching to the lunula.

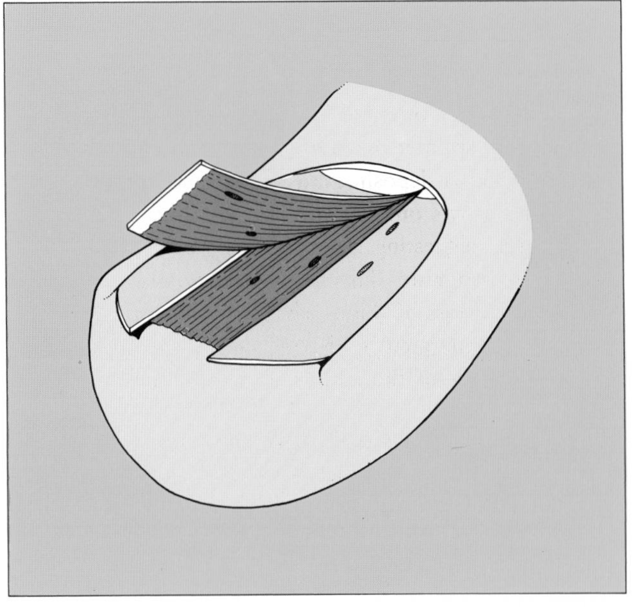

Fig. 1.11. The appearance of splinter haemorrhages. Haem from longitudinal nail bed vessels is deposited on the underside of the nail plate. This grows out in the shape of a splinter.

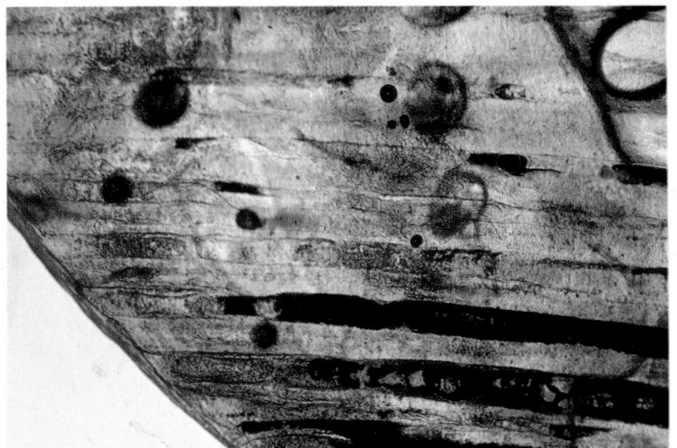

Fig. 1.12. The nail plate has longitudinal ridges on its lower aspect.

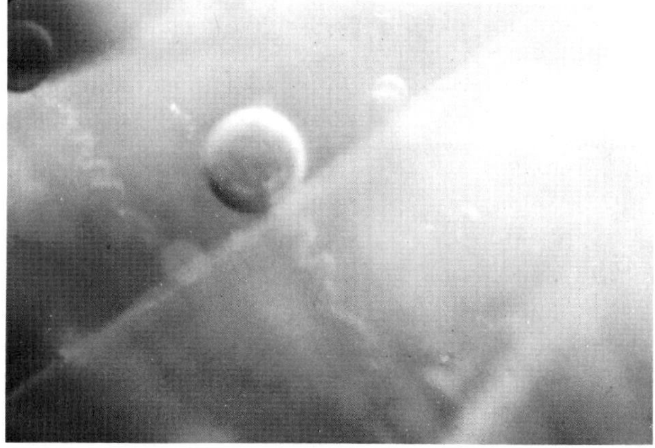

Fig. 1.13. Sweat pores in the distal nail bed (Maricq, 1967).

On the underside of the nail plate is a complementary set of ridges, which has led to the description of the nail being led up the nail bed as if on rails. The small vessels of the nail bed are oriented in the same axis. This is demonstrated by splinter haemorrhages (Figs 1.11 & 1.12), where blood is deposited on the undersurface of the nail plate and grows out with it. The free edge of a nail loses the ridges, suggesting that they are softer than the main nail plate structure. The nail bed also loses these ridges shortly after loss of the overlying nail. It is likely that the ridges are generated at the margin of the lunula on the ventral surface of the nail to be imprinted upon the nail bed.

The epidermis of the nail bed is thin over its main territory. It becomes thicker at the nail folds where it develops rete ridges. It has no granular layer. The dermis is sparse, with little fat, firm collagenous adherence to the underlying periosteum and no sebaceous or follicular appendages (Lewin, 1965). Sweat ducts can be seen at the distal margin of the nail bed using *in vivo* magnification (Fig. 1.13) (Maricq, 1967).

The hyponychium is the residuum of the distal ridge (embryogenesis) seen from the tenth week of gestation onwards. It may be the seat of subungual hyperkeratosis in some diseases such as pityriasis rubra pilaris or pachyonychia congenita. In these instances, and in some elderly people, it can be thought of as the solenhorn described by Pinkus (1927).

Pterygium inversum unguis is a further condition characterized by changes in the distal nail bed and hyponychium (Caputo & Prandi, 1973). There is tough, fibrotic tissue tethering the free edge of the nail plate to the underlying soft structures. It is found in both congenital (Odom *et al.*, 1974) and acquired forms (Patterson, 1977). The aetiology is not clear. Patterson proposed that it was a combination of a genetic predisposition and microvascular ischaemia.

The hyponychium and overhanging free nail provide a crevice. This is a reservoir for microbes, relevant in surgery and the dissemination of infection. After 10 min of scrubbing the fingers with povidone iodine, nail clippings cultured for bacteria, yeasts and moulds revealed *Staphylococcus epidermidis* in 19 out of 20 patients (Rayan & Flournoy, 1987). Seven out of 20 patients had an additional bacteria, eight had moulds and three had yeasts. These findings could have significance to both surgeons and patients.

Nail plate

The nail plate is composed of compacted keratinized epithelial cells (Kitahara & Ogawa, 1992). It covers the

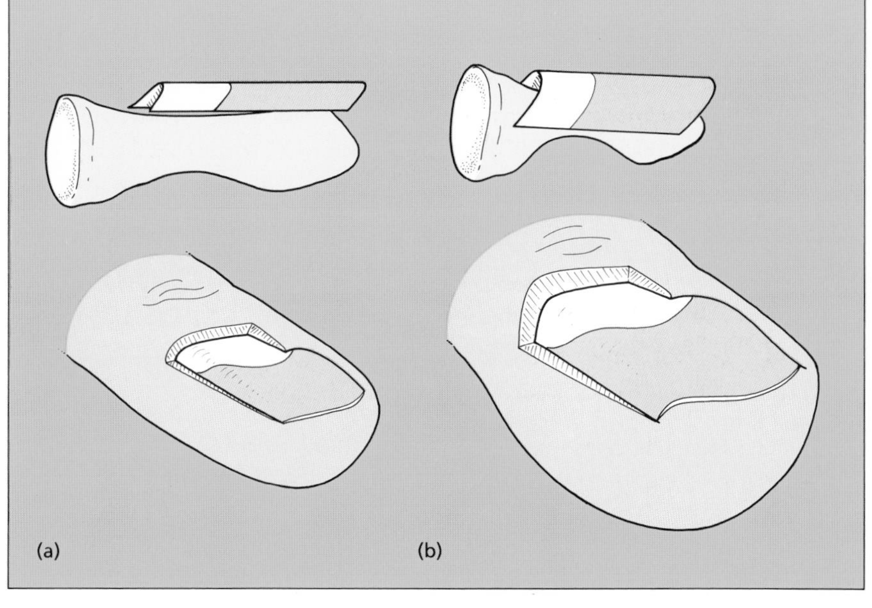

Fig. 1.14. Nail plate association with soft tissue and bone in the finger and toe. (a) In the finger the nail plate has modest transverse curvature and shallow association with soft tissues. (b) In the great toe the nail plate has more marked transverse curvature and deep soft tissue association. This makes it strong – appropriate to the foot – but also accounts for the tendency to ingrow and the need for deep lateral extirpation at lateral matricectomy.

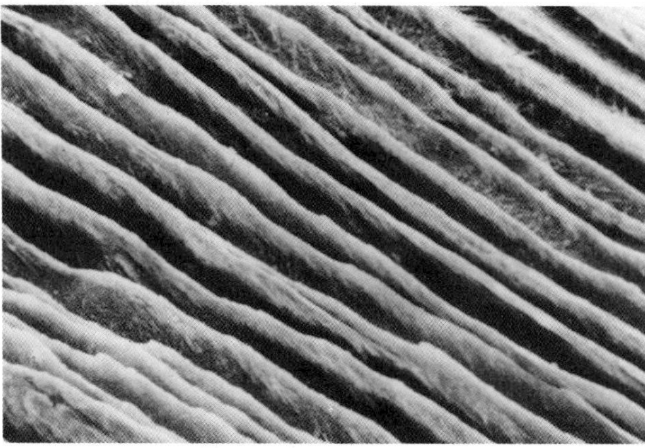

Fig. 1.15. Scaning electron micrograph of the nail bed demonstrating longitudinal ridges.

nail bed and intermediate (distal) matrix. It is curved in both the longitudinal and transverse axes. This allows it to be embedded in nail folds at its proximal and lateral margins, which provide strong attachment and make the free edge a useful tool. This feature is more marked in the toes than the fingers. In the great toe, the lateral margins of the matrix and nail extend almost half way around the terminal phalanx. This provides strength appropriate to the foot (Fig. 1.14).

The upper surface of the nail plate is smooth and may have a variable number of longitudinal ridges that change with age. These ridges are sufficiently specific to allow forensic identification and the distinction between identical twins (Diaz *et al.*, 1990). The ventral surface also has longitudinal ridges that correspond to complementary ridges on the upper aspect of the nail bed (see nail bed, p. 10) to which it is bonded (Fig. 1.15). These nail ridges may be best examined using polarized light. They can also be used for forensic identification (Apolinar & Rowe, 1980) as can blood groups from fragments of nail plate (Garg, 1983). These interdigitating ridges are a likely explanation for the marked adherence of the nail plate to the nail bed in comparison with the intermediate matrix. Independent of the embedding function of the nail folds described earlier, the nail bed demonstrates a strong bonding to the undersurface of the nail plate. This is evident at avulsion. Proximal hemiavulsion to visualize the matrix alone meets with little resistance.

The onychocorneal band is the firmest point of nail bed adherence which is of great functional significance (Sonnex *et al.*, 1991). Once this band has been disrupted, the nail unit is vulnerable, with sequestration of debris and microbes resulting in progressive onycholysis. The physical nature of this seal is seen in cosmetic onycholysis, where the increasing overhanging length of the nail plate means that greater leverage is exerted upon the onychocorneal

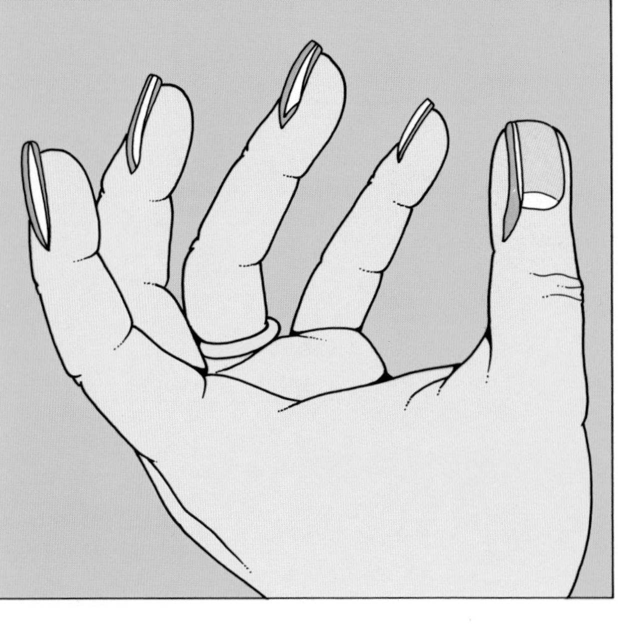

Fig. 1.16. The histochemistry of the human nail plate (Jarrett & Spearman, 1966). Nail plates were sectioned and stained, purple represents positive staining. Index, calcium; middle: phospholipid; ring: sulphydryl; little: disulphide; thumb: acid phosphatase.

band until it is eventually disrupted. Probing with manicure instruments often supplements this damaging process.

The nail plate gains thickness and density as it grows distally (Johnson *et al.*, 1991) according to analysis of surgical specimens. *In vivo* ultrasound suggests that there may be an 8.8% reduction in thickness distally (Finlay *et al.*, 1987). A thick nail plate may imply a long intermediate matrix. This stems from the process whereby the longitudinal axis of the intermediate matrix becomes the vertical axis of the nail plate. Other factors, like linear rate of nail growth (Samman & White, 1964), vascular supply, subungual hyperkeratosis and drugs also influence thickness.

The tendency to describe a dorsal, intermediate and ventral matrix, has generated descriptions of corresponding layers of the nail plate deriving from the different matrix zones. Whether or not the three demarcations of the nail matrix exist, it is important to recognize the basic principle that proximal regions of matrix produce dorsal nail plate and distal matrix, ventral nail plate.

Light microscopy

Lewis (1954) described a silver stain that delineates the nail plate zones. Three regions of nail plate have been histochemically defined (Jarrett & Spearman, 1966) (Fig. 1.16). The dorsal plate has a relatively high calcium, phospholipid and sulphhydryl group content. It has little acid phosphatase activity and is physically hard. The

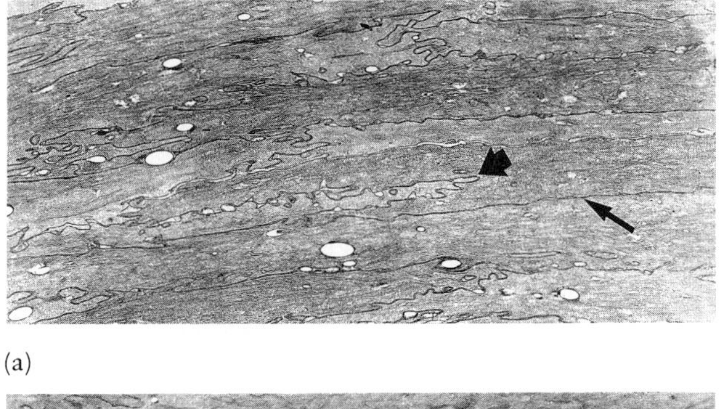

(a)

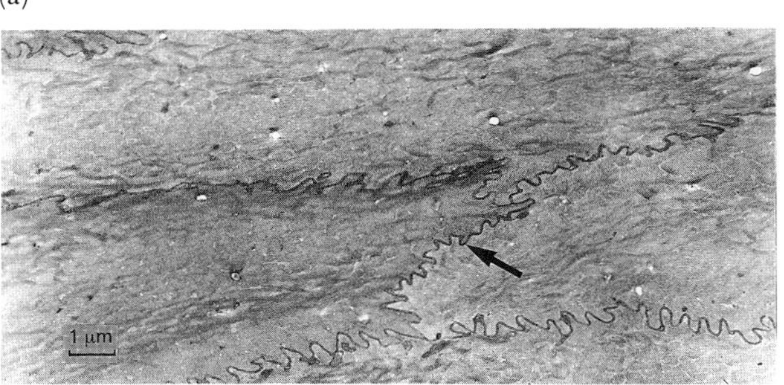

(b)

Fig. 1.17. (a) Transmission electron micrograph of the upper part of the nail plate. The corneocytes are flattened and joined laterally by infrequent deep interdigitations (broad arrow). (b) The cell membranes between adjacent cell layers are discretely indented and in parts without invaginations – Thierry's technique (Prof. Achten, Brussels, Belgium).

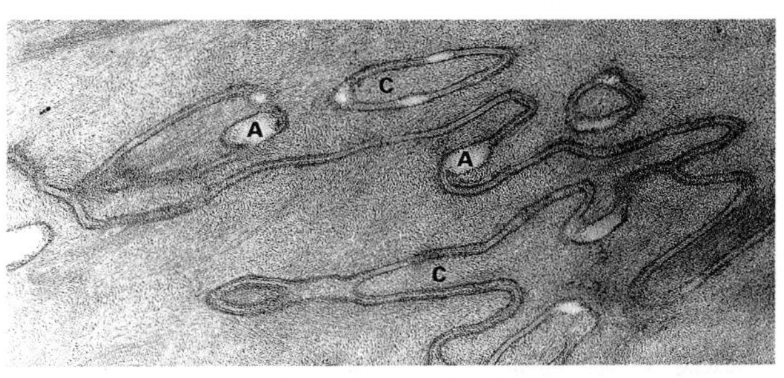

(a)

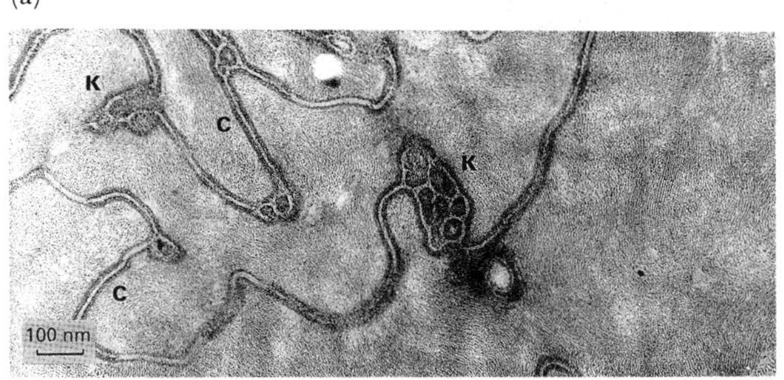

(b)

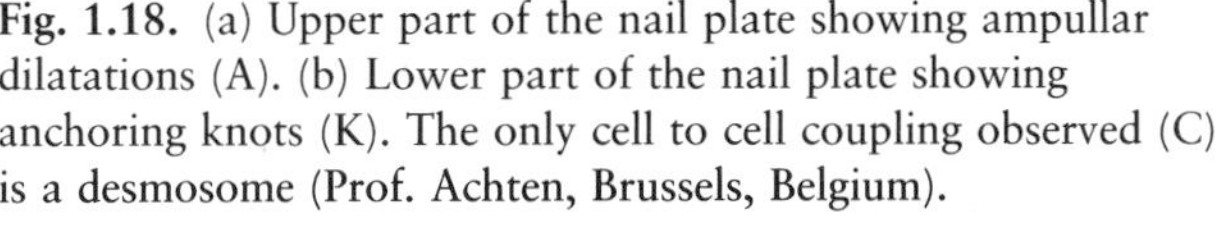

Fig. 1.18. (a) Upper part of the nail plate showing ampullar dilatations (A). (b) Lower part of the nail plate showing anchoring knots (K). The only cell to cell coupling observed (C) is a desmosome (Prof. Achten, Brussels, Belgium).

phospholipid content may provide some water resistance. The intermediate nail plate has a high acid phosphatase activity, probably corresponding to the number of retained nuclear remnants. There is a high number of disulphide bonds, and low content of bound sulphhydryl groups, phospholipid and calcium. Controversy allows that the ventral nail plate may be a variable entity (Samman, 1961). Jarrett and Spearman (1966) described it as a layer only one or two cells thick. These cells are eosinophilic and move both upwards and forward with nail growth. With respect to calcium, phospholipid and sulphhydryl groups it is the same as the dorsal nail plate. It shares a high acid phosphatase and frequency of disulphide bonds with the intermediate nail plate.

Ultrasound examination of *in vivo* and avulsed nail plates suggests that it has the physical characteristics of a bi-lamellar structure (Jemec & Serup, 1989). There is a superficial dry compartment and a deep humid one. This has been given as evidence against the existence of a ventral matrix contribution to the nail plate.

In clinical practice, histology of the nail plate may be useful in the identification of fungal infections in culture negative specimens (Haneke, 1991; Suarez *et al.*, 1991) (see section on onychomychosis). It may also be used to identify the dorso-ventral location of melanin in the nail clipping of a longitudinal melanonychia and hence allow

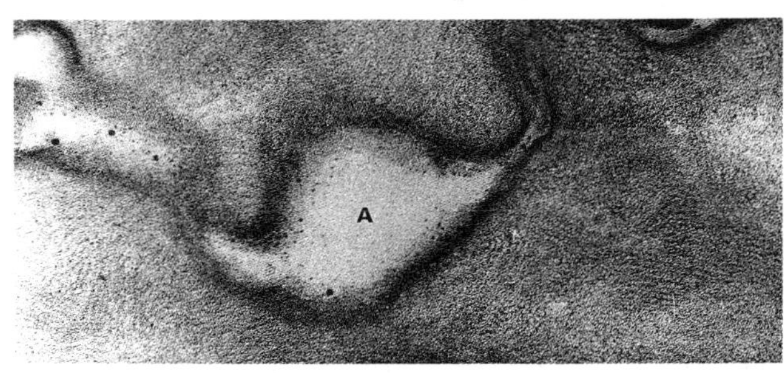

(a)

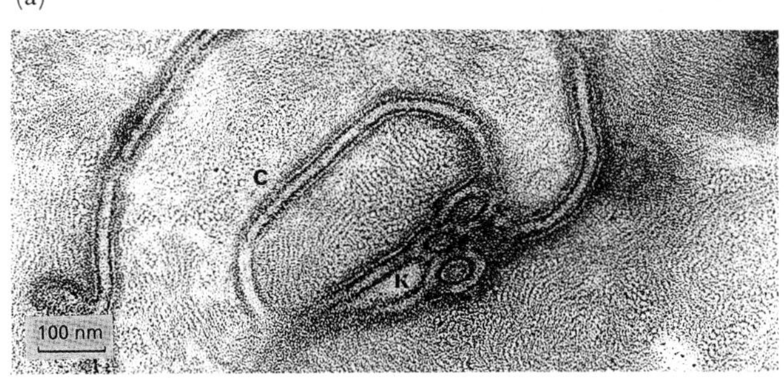

(b)

Fig. 1.19. (I) Upper part of the nail plate as in Fig. 1.18, in greater detail (Prof. Achten, Brussels, Belgium).

prediction of the site of melanocyte activity in the intermediate matrix (Baran & Kechijian, 1989; Dawber & Colver, 1991).

Germann *et al.* (1980) utilized a form of tape-stripping

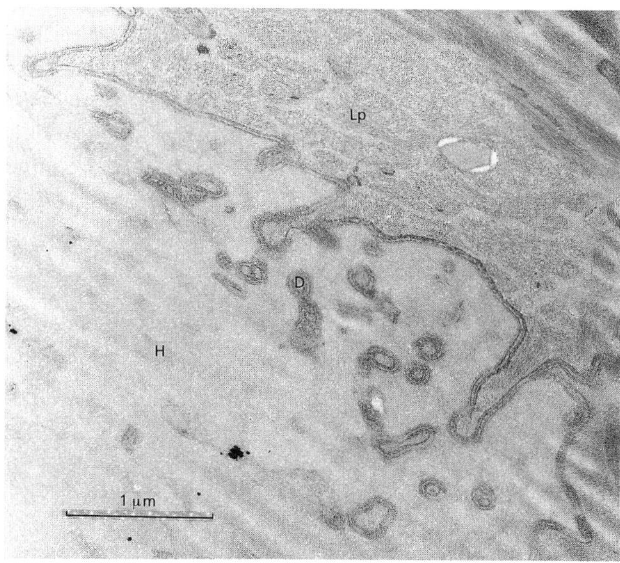

Fig. 1.20. Corneocytes of the lowest part of the nail plate (Lp) sending out numerous digitations (D) penetrating the hyponychial nail bed cells (Prof. Achten, Brussels, Belgium).

in conjunction with light microscopy to examine dorsal nail plate corneocyte morphology in disease and health. They found that conditions of rapid nail growth (psoriasis and infancy) resulted in smaller cell size.

Electron microscopy

Scanning electron microscopy has added to our understanding of onychoschizia (Shelley & Shelley, 1984; Wallis *et al.*, 1991) as well as basic nail plate structure (Forslind & Thyresson, 1975; Dawber, 1980). In the normal nail corneocytes can be seen adherent to the dorsal aspect of the nail plate. In cross section, the compaction of the lamellar structure is visible. Both these features can be seen to be disrupted in onychoschizia following repeated immersion and drying of the nail plates.

Transmission electron microscopy has been used to identify the relationship between the corneocytes of the nail plate (Parent *et al.*, 1985). Using Thierry's tissue processing techniques, material with the following description has been provided. Cell membranes and intercellular junctions are easily discernible (Fig. 1.17). Even though at low magnification one can differentiate the dorsal and intermediate layers of the nail plate, the exact boundary is unclear using transmission electron microscopy. Cells on the dorsal (34 × 60 × 2.2 μm) aspect are half as thick as ventral cells (40 × 50 × 5.5 μm), with a gradation of sizes in between. In the dorsal nail plate, large intercellular spaces are present corresponding to ampullar dilatations (Figs 1.18 & 1.19). These gradually diminish in the deeper layers and are absent in the ventral region. At this site,

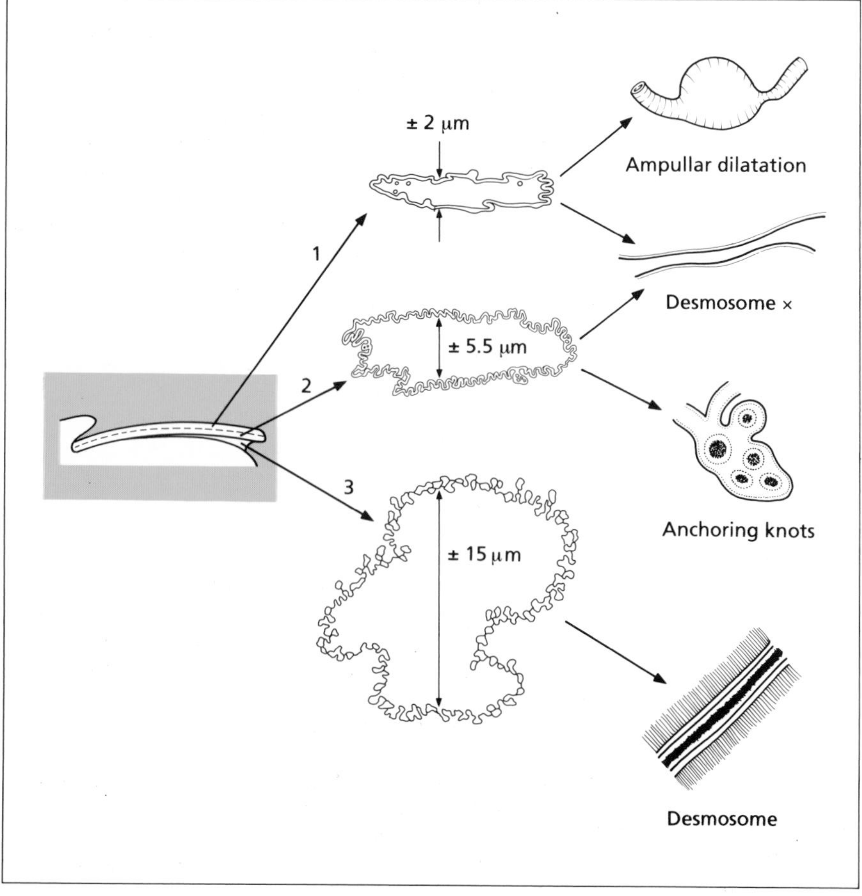

Fig. 1.21. Intercellular junctions of the three parts of the nail: (1) upper plate; (2) lower plate; (3) hyponychial ventral nail with desmosome as seen by Thiery's technique (Prof. Achten, Brussels, Belgium).

cells are joined by complete folds, membranes of adjacent cells appearing to penetrate each other to form 'anchoring knots'.

Corneocytes of the dorsal nail plate are joined laterally by infrequent deep interdigitations. The plasma membranes between adjacent cell layers are more discretely indented, often with no invaginations (Fig. 1.17). In the deeper parts of the nail plate the interdigitations are more numerous, but more shallow (Fig. 1.17). No tight gap junctions are seen in either of the major nail layers in this series (Parent *et al.*, 1985), although they were identified previously by Forslind and Thyresson (1975). The intercellular material is homogeneous and separated from the cell membrane by two thin electron-dense lines. The space between the cell membranes varies from 25 to 35 nm (Figs 1.18 & 1.19). No complete desmosomal structures are seen.

Nail bed cells show considerable infolding and interdigitation at their junction with the nail plate cells (Fig. 1.20). They are polygonal and show no specific alignment. They are between 6 and 20 μm across and show neither tight nor gap junctions. They do, however, have desmosomal connections of the type seen in normal epidermis (Fig. 1.21).

Cells of the hyponychium are distinguished from the nail plate on the basis of morphology, staining affinities and size.

Using different preparation techniques, other workers have demonstrated other anatomical details. On the cytoplasmic side of the cell membranes of nail plate cells lies a layer of protein particles (Hashimoto, 1971a,b). Other staining techniques suggest that the single type of intercellular bond described by Parent *et al.* (1985) may be a spot desmosome (Arnn & Stoehelin, 1981).

Nail folds

The proximal and lateral nail folds give purchase to the nail plate by enclosing more than 75% of its periphery. They also provide a physical seal against the penetration of materials to vulnerable subungual and proximal regions.

The epidermal structure of the lateral nail folds is unremarkable, and comparable with normal skin. There is a tendency to hyperkeratosis, sometimes associated with trauma. When the trauma arises from the ingrowth of the nail, considerable hypertrophy can result, with repeated infection.

The proximal nail fold has three parts. Its upper aspect is glabrous skin, providing no direct influence upon the nail plate. At the point where its distal margin meets the nail plate it forms the cuticle. In health, the cuticle adheres firmly to the dorsal aspect of the nail plate, achieving a seal. Its disruption may be associated with systemic disorders (collagen vascular) or local dermatoses. In the latter it may be the avenue of contact allergens or microbes. The ventral aspect of the proximal nail fold (eponychium) is apposed to the dorsal aspect of the nail. It contrasts with the adjacent intermediate matrix by being thinner, with shorter rete ridges, and having a granular layer. Keratins expressed in the proximal nail fold may differ on its dorsal and ventral aspects and can contrast with expression elsewhere in the nail unit (de Berker *et al.*, 1993).

The proximal nail fold has significance in three main areas.

1 It contributes to the generation of nail plate through dorsal matrix on the lower segment of its ventral aspect.

2 It may influence the direction of growth of the nail plate by directing it obliquely over the nail bed (Kligman, 1961).

3 Nail fold microvasculature can provide useful information in some pathological conditions.

The first two issues are dealt with in the section on nail growth (see nail growth), the latter under vasculature (see vasculature).

References

Apolinar E. & Rowe W.F. (1980) Examination of human fingernail ridges by means of polarized light. *J. Forensic Sci. CA* **25**, 154–161.

Arnn Y. & Stoehelin L.A. (1981) The structure and function of spot desmosomes. *Int. J. Dermatol.* **20**, 331–339.

Caputo R. & Prandi G. (1973) Pterygium inversum unguis. *Arch. Dermatol.* **108**, 817–818.

Dawber R.P.R. (1980) The ultrastructure and growth of human nails. *Arch. Dermatol. Res.* **269**, 197–204.

Dawber R.P.R. & Colver G.B. (1991) The spectrum of malignant melanoma of the nail apparatus. *Sem. Dermatol.* **10**, 82–87.

de Berker D., Leigh I. & Wojnarowska F. (1993) Patterns of keratin expression in the nail unit – an indicator of regional matrix differentiation. *Br. J. Dermatol.*, in press.

Baran R. & Kechijian P. (1989) Longitudinal melanonychia diagnosis and management. *J. Am. Acad. Dermatol.* **21**, 1165–1175.

Diaz A.A., Boehm A.F. & Rowe W.F. (1990) Comparison of fingernail ridge patterns of monozygotic twins. *J. Forensic Sci. CA* **35**, 97–102.

Finlay A.Y., Moseley H. & Duggan T.C. (1987) Ultrasound transmission time: an in vivo guide to nail thickness. *Br. J. Dermatol.* **117**, 765–770.

Forslind B. & Thyresson N. (1975) On the structures of the normal nail. *Arch. Dermatol. Forsch.* **251**, 199–204.

Garg R.K. (1983) Determination of ABO(H) blood group substances from finger and toenails. *Z. Rechtsmed.* **91**, 17–19.

Germann H., Barran W. & Plewig G. (1980) Morphology of corneocytes from human nail plates. *J. Invest. Dermatol.* **74**, 115–118.

Haneke E. (1991) Fungal infections of the nail. *Semin. Dermatol.* **10**, 41–51.

Hashimoto K. (1971a) The marginal band: A demonstration of the thickened cellular envelope of the human nail. *Arch. Dermatol.* **103**, 387–393.

Hashimoto K. (1971b) Ultrastructure of the human toenail: II. *J. Ultrastruct. Res.* **36**, 391–410.

Jarrett A. & Spearman R.I.C. (1966) The histochemistry of the human nail. *Arch. Dermatol.* **94**, 652–657.
Jemec G.B.E. & Serup J. (1989) Ultrasound structure of the human nail plate. *Arch. Dermatol.* **125**, 643–646.
Johnson M., Comaish J.S. & Shuster S. (1991) Nail is produced by the normal nail bed: a controversy resolved. *Br. J. Dermatol.* **125**, 27–29.
Kitahara T. & Ogawa H. (1992) Cultured nail keratinocytes express hard keratins characteristic of nail and hair in vivo. *Arch. Dermatol. Res.* **1**, 253–256.
Kligman A. (1961) Why do nails grow out instead of up? *Arch. Dermatol.* **84**, 181–183.
Lewin K. (1965) The normal finger nail. *Br. J. Dermatol.* **77**, 421–30.
Lewis B.L. (1954) Microscopic studies of fetal and mature nail and surrounding soft tissue. *Arch. Dermatol. Syphilol.* **70**, 732–44.
Maricq H.R. (1967) Observation and photography of sweat ducts of the fingers in vivo. *J. Invest. Dermatol.* **48**, 399–401.
Odom R.B., Stein K.M. & Maibach H.I. (1974) Congenital, painful aberrant hyponychium. *Arch. Dermatol.* **110**, 89–90.
Parent D., Achten G. & Stouffs-Vamhoof F. (1985) Ultrastructure of the normal human nail. *Am. J. Dermatopathol.* **7**, 529–535.
Patterson J.W. (1977) Pterygium inversum unguis-like changes in scleroderma. *Arch. Dermatol.* **113**, 1429–1430.
Pinkus F. (1927) In: *Handbuch der Haut und Geschlechtskrankheiten*, ed. Jadassohn J., pp. 267–289. Springer, Berlin.
Rayan G.M. & Flournoy D.J. (1987) Microbiologic flora of human fingernails. *J. Hand Surg.* **12A**, 605–607.
Samman P.D. (1961) The ventral nail. *Arch. Dermatol.* **84**, 1030–1033.
Samman P.D. & White W.F. (1964) The 'yellow nail' syndrome. *Br. J. Dermatol.* **76**, 153–157.
Shelley W.B. & Shelley D. (1984) Onychoschizia: Scanning electron microscopy. *J. Am. Acad. Dermatol.* **10**, 623–627.
Sonnex T.S., Griffiths W.A.D. & Nicol W.J. (1991) The nature and significance of the transverse white band of human nails. In: *Seminars in Dermatology*, ed. Baran R., **10** (1), pp. 12–16. WB Saunders, Philadelphia.
Suarez S.M., Silvers D.N., Scher R.K. *et al.* (1991) Histologic evaluation of nail clippings for diagnosing onychomycosis. *Arch. Dermatol.* **127**, 1517–1519.
Wallis M.S., Bowen W.R. & Guin J.D. (1991) Pathogenesis of onychoschizia (lamellar dystrophy). *J. Am. Acad. Dermatol.* **24**, 44–48.

Vascular supply

Arterial supply

The vascular supply of the finger is considered in detail here. Many of the anatomical principles may be extended to the anatomy of the foot and toe, whilst details can be sought elsewhere (Warwick & Williams, 1973).

The radial and ulnar arteries supply deep and superficial palmar arcades that act as large anastamoses between the two vessels. From these arcades extend branches aligned with the phalanges. Four arteries supply each digit, two on either side. The dorsal digital arteries are small and arise as branches of the radial artery. They undertake anastomoses with the superficial and deep palmar arches and the palmar digital vessels before passing distally into the finger. The palmar digital arteries provide the main blood supply to the fingers. They receive contributions from the deep and superficial palmar arcades. Although paired, one is normally dominant (Smith *et al.*, 1991a). They anastomose via dorsal and palmar arches around the distal phalanx. The palmar arch is located in a protected position, beneath the maximal padding of the finger pulp and tucked into a recess behind the protuberant phalangeal boss (Fig. 1.22).

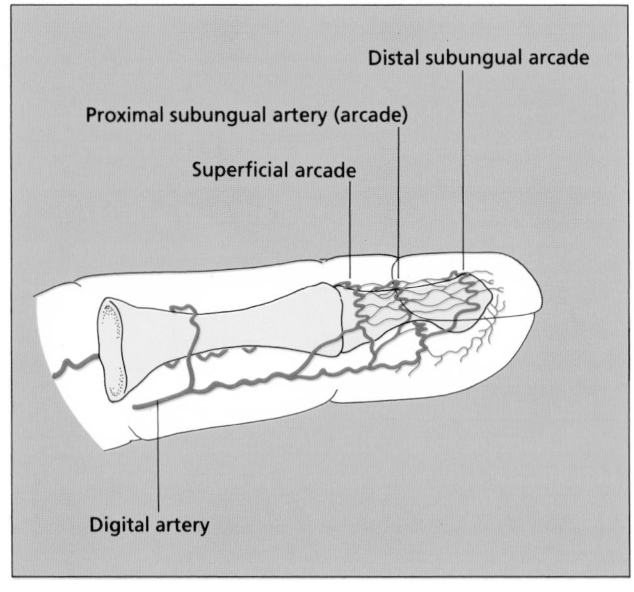

Fig. 1.22. Arterial supply of the distal finger.

The dorsal nail fold arch (superficial arcade) lies just distal to the distal interphalangeal joint. It supplies the nail fold and extensor tendon insertion. It is tortuous, with numerous branches to the intermediate nail matrix. Its transverse passage across the finger can be roughly located by pushing proximally on the free edge of the nail plate. This produces a faint crease about 5 mm proximal to the cuticle and is both the cul de sac of the proximal nail fold and the line of the dorsal nail fold arch.

The subungual region is supplied by distal and proximal subungual arcades, arising in turn from an anastomosis of the palmar arch and the dorsal nail fold arch. A helpful study on adults and fetuses was performed by Flint (1955).

The tortuosity of the main vessels in the finger is a notable feature. Vessels may turn through 270° and resemble a coiled spring (Smith *et al.*, 1991a). Functionally, this can be interpreted as protection against occlusion by kinking in an articulated longitudinal structure.

Venous drainage

Venous drainage of the finger is by deep and superficial systems. The deep system corresponds to the arterial supply. Superficially, there exist the dorsal and palmar digital veins. These are in a prominent branching network, particularly on the dorsal aspect. However, in the microsurgical techniques needed to restore amputations, it appears that distally, the palmar superficial veins are largest (Smith *et al.*, 1991b).

Although the arterial supply to the nail unit is substantial, the intermediate matrix will tolerate only limited trauma before scarring (Zaias, 1967). A longitudinal biopsy of greater than 3 mm is likely to leave a permanent dystrophy. Equally, it appears to need a precise, not just abundant, blood supply. Non-vascularized split thickness nail bed grafting is moderately successful for the nail bed, but not for intermediate matrix (Pessa *et al.*, 1990). This is in the presence of otherwise adequate local blood supply at sites of previous trauma. Toenail intermediate matrix grafts can be made successfully if they are transplanted with associated soft tissue and a venous pedicle (Nakayama *et al.*, 1990). The local arterial supply is then anastomosed through this pedicle.

Lymphatics

The lymphatic vessels of the nail bed are very numerous, particularly near the free edge of the nail – the superficial network joins the deep trunks by anastomotic rami (Pardo-Castello, 1960).

Effects of altered vascular supply

Impaired arterial supply can have a considerable effect upon the finger pulp and nail unit. Lynn *et al.* (1955) claimed that there was almost complete correlation between occluded arteriographic findings and the presence of paronychial infection or ulceration, ridged brittle fingernails or phlyctenular gangrene. Samman *et al.* (1962) reviewed the nail dystrophies of 41 patients with features of peripheral vascular disease. In this uncontrolled study, they observed that onycholysis, Beau's lines, thin brittle nails and yellow discoloration were all attributable to ischaemia in the absence of other causes. It has also been suggested that congenital onychodysplasias may result from digital ischaemia *in utero* (Kitayama & Tsukada, 1983). Immobilization might be associated with diminished local blood supply and has been noted to reduce nail growth (Dawber, 1981). Conversely, the increased growth associated with arteriovenous shunts may reflect the role of greater blood flow (Orentreich *et al.*, 1979). Clubbing constitutes a change in both the nail and nail bed. It is believed that it arises secondary to neurovascular pathology. Post mortem studies suggest that it is due to increased blood flow with vasodilatation rather than vessel hyperplasia (Currie & Gallagher, 1988).

Nail fold vessels

The nail fold capillary network (Gilje *et al.*, 1974) is seen easily with a ×4 magnifying lens or an ophthalmoscope. With the latter it should be set at +40 and the lens held very close to a drop of oil on the nail fold. It is similar to the normal cutaneous plexus in health, except that the capillary loops are more horizontal and visible throughout their length. The loops are in tiers of uniform size, with peaks equidistant from the base of the cuticle (Fig. 1.23) (Ryan, 1973). The venous arm is more dilated and tortuous than the arterial arm. There is a wide range of morphologies within the normal population (Davies & Landau, 1966). Features in some disorders may be sufficiently gross to be useful without magnification; erythema and haemorrhages being the most obvious.

Microscopy of small vessels can be of diagnostic value in some connective tissue diseases (Buchanan & Humpston, 1968; Grainier *et al.*, 1986). Pathological features include venous plexus visibility, density of capillary population, avascular fields, haemorrhages, giant capillaries and cessation of blood flow following cooling. When determined quantitatively, using television microscopy, Studer *et al.* (1991) found it possible to distinguish between systemic and disseminated cutaneous lupus erythematosus, and between localized and systemic sclerosis. The mechanism of their evolution may in part arise from impaired fibrino-

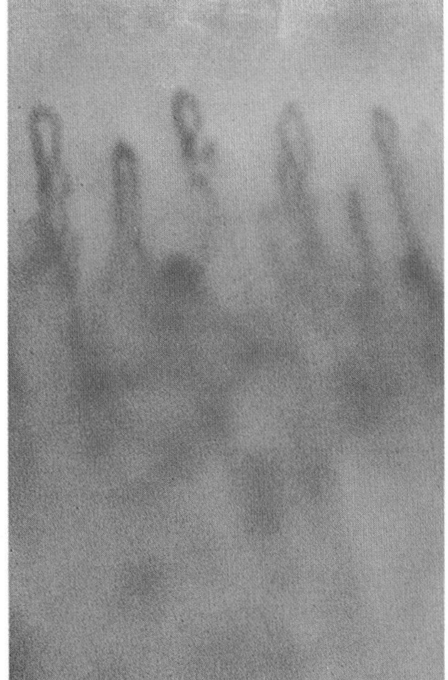

Fig. 1.23. Capillary loops visible in the proximal nail fold.

lysis, macroglobulinaemia and cryoglobulinaemia (Ryan, 1973).

The capillary networks in the normal nail fold of toes and fingers have been compared using video-microscopy. This has revealed a greater density of capillaries in the toe nail fold, but with a reduced rate of flow (Richardson & Schwartz, 1984).

Intravenous bolus doses of Na-fluorescein dye have been followed through nail fold microscopy (Bollinger *et al.*, 1979). There is rapid and uniform leakage from the capillaries in normal subjects to within 10 μm of the capillaries. It is suggested that a sheath of collagen may prevent diffusion beyond this point. The same procedure has been followed in patients with rheumatoid arthritis demonstrating decreased flow rates and abnormal flow patterns, but no change in vessel leakage (Grassi *et al.*, 1989).

Nail fold microscopy has been used for the investigation of Raynaud's phenomenon (Mahler *et al.*, 1987). Recently, it has been possible to assess vascular toxicity affecting nail fold vessels following chemotherapy, using the same method (Hansen *et al.*, 1990). Gasser (1991) used nail fold video-microscopy to study the effects of drugs on microcirculation in normal and ischaemic skin areas, showing that nifedipine and ketanserin are able to inhibit cold-induced 'flow stops'.

Ultimately, histological information on the vessels and tissue of the nail folds may be helpful. The technique and benefits of nail fold biopsy have been described (Schnitzler *et al.*, 1976, 1980a,b). Amyloid deposits, sub-intimal hyalinosis and severe dermal fibrosis are cited as useful information yielded by biopsy (see Chapter 6).

Glomus bodies

The word glomus is defined as a ball, tuft or cluster, a small conglomeration or plexus of cavernous blood vessels. In the skin it is an end organ apparatus in which there is an arteriovenous anastamosis bypassing the intermediary capillary bed. This anastamosis includes that afferent artery, the Sucquet–Hoyer canal, the latter is surrounded by structures including cuboidal epithelioid cells, and cells possibly of smooth muscle or pericyte (Zimmerman type) origin. These are surrounded by a rich nerve supply and then the efferent vein which connects with the venous system outside the glomus capsule.

The nail bed is richly supplied with glomus bodies. These are neurovascular bodies which act as arteriovenous anastomoses (AVA). AVAs are connections between the arterial and venous side of the circulation with no intervening capillaries. Each glomus body is an encapsulated oval organ 300 μm long comprised of a tortuous vessel uniting an artery and venule, a nerve supply and a capsule. It contains many modified large muscle cells, resembling epithelioid cells, and cholinergic nerves. Digital nail beds contain 93–501 glomus bodies/cm^3. They lie parallel to the capillary reservoirs which they bypass. They are able to contract asynchronously with their associated arterioles such that in the cold, arterioles constrict and glomus bodies dilate. They can thus serve as regulators of capillary circulation, acquiring the name 'the peripheral heart of Masson' (Masson, 1937). They are particularly important in the preservation of blood supply to the peripheries in cold conditions.

Nerve supply

The perionychial area is innervated by dorsal branches of the paired digital nerves. Wilgis and Maxwell (1979) stated that the digital nerve consists of three major fascicles and divides into three branches just distal to the distal interphalangeal joint – one of these going to the nail fold. The commonest nail apparatus supply is from a branch that passes under the nail edge and into the deeper layer of the nail bed at lunular level (Zook, 1988). Winkelmann (1960) showed many nerve endings adjacent to the epithelial surface, mainly in the nail folds.

References

Bollinger A., Jager K., Roten A., Timeus C. & Mahler F. (1979) Diffusion, pericapillary distribution and clearance of Na-fluorescein in the human nailfold. *Pflügers Arch.* **382**, 137–143.

Buchanan I. & Humpston D.J. (1968) Nail fold capillaries in connective tissue disorders. *Lancet* **41**, 845–847.

Currie A.E. & Gallagher P.J. (1988) The pathology of clubbing: vascular changes in the nail bed. *Br. J. Chest.* **82**, 382–385.

Davies E. & Landau J. (1966) *Clinical Capillary Microscopy.* C.C. Thomas, Springfield, IL.

Dawber R.P.R. (1981) The effect of immobilization upon finger nail growth. *Clin. Exp. Dermatol.* **6**, 533–535.

Flint M.H. (1955–56) Some observations on the vascular supply of the nail bed and terminal segments of the finger. *Br. J. Plast. Surg.* **8**, 186–195.

Gasser P. (1991) Reaction of capillary blood cell velocity in nailfold capillaries to nifedipine and ketanserin in patients with vasospastic disease. *J. Int. Med. Res.* **19**, 24–31.

Gilje O., Kierland R. & Baldes E.J. (1974) Capillary microscopy in the diagnosis of dermatologic diseases. *J. Invest. Dermatol.* **22**, 199–206.

Granier F., Vayssairat M., Priollet P. *et al.* (1986) Nailfold capillary microsopy in mixed connective tissue disease. *Arthritis Rheum.* **29**, 189–195.

Grassi W., Felder M., Thuring-Vollenweider U. & Bollinger A. (1989) Microvascular dynamics at the nailfold in rheumatoid arthritis. *Clin. Exp. Rheum.* **7**, 47–53.

Hansen S.W., Olsen N., Rossing N. & Rorth M. (1990) Vascular toxicity and the mechanism underlying Raynaud's phenomenon in patients treated with cisplatin, vinblastine and bleomycin. *Ann. Oncol.* **1**, 289–292.

Kitayama Y. & Tsukada S. (1983) Congenital onychodysplasia. Report of 11 cases. *Arch. Dermatol.* **119**, 8–12.

Lynn R.B., Steiner R.E. & Van Wyck F.A.F. (1955) Arteriographic appearances of the digital arteries of the hands in Raynaud's disease. *Lancet* **i**, 471–474.

Mahler F., Saner H., Boss C. *et al.* (1987) Local cold exposure test for capillaroscopic examination of patients with Raynaud's syndrome. *Microvasc. Res.* **33**, 422–427.

Masson P. (1937) *Les Glomus neurovasculaires*. Hermann et Cie, Paris.

Nakayama Y., Iino T., Uchida A., Kiyosawa T. & Soeda S. (1990) Vascularised free nail grafts nourished by arterial inflow from the venous system. *Plast. Reconstr. Surg.* **85**, 239–245.

Orentreich N., Markofsky J. & Vogelman J.H. (1979) The effect of ageing on linear nail growth. *J. Invest. Dermatol.* **73**, 126–130.

Pardo-Castello V. (1960) *Diseases of the Nail*, 3rd edn. Charles C. Thomas, Springfield, IL.

Pessa J.E., Tsai T.M., Li Y. & Kleinert H.E. (1990) The repair of nail deformities with the non-vascularised nail bed graft: indications and results. *J. Hand Surg.* **15A**, 466–470.

Richardson D. & Schwartz R. (1984) Comparison of resting capillary flow dynamics in the finger and toe nailfolds. *Microcirc. Endothel. Lymphatics* **1**, 645–656.

Ryan T.J. (1973) Direct observations of blood vessels in the superficial vasculature system of the skin. In: *The Physiology and Pathophysiology of the Skin*, ed. Jarrett A., Vol. 2, pp. 658–659. Academic Press, London.

Samman P. & Strickland B. (1962) Abnormalities of the finger nails associated with impaired peripheral blood supply. *Br. J. Dermatol.* **74**, 165–173.

Schnitzler L., Baran R., Civatte J., Schubert B., Verret J.L. & Hurez D. (1976) Biopsy of the proximal nail fold in collagen diseases. *J. Dermatol. Surg.* **2**, 313–315.

Schnitzler L., Civatte J., Baran R. *et al.* (1980a) Le repli sus-unquéal normal. *Ann. Dermatol. Venereol.* **107**, 771–776.

Schnitzler L., Baran R. & Vernet J.L. (1980b) Le repli sus-unquéal dans les maladies dites du collagène. Etude histologique, ultrastructurale et en immunofluorescence. *Ann. Dermatol. Venereol.* **107**, 777–785.

Smith D.O., Oura C., Kimura C. & Toshimori K. (1991a) Artery anatomy and tortuosity in the distal finger. *J. Hand Surg.* **16A**, 297–302.

Smith D.O., Oura C., Kimura C. & Toshimori K. (1991b) The distal venous anatomy of the finger. *J. Hand Surg.* **16A**, 303–307.

Studer A., Hunziker T., Lutolf O. *et al.* (1991) Quantitative nailfold capillary microscopy in cutaneous and systemic lupus erythematosus and localised and systemic scleroderma. *J. Am. Acad. Dermatol.* **24**, 941–945.

Warwick R. & Williams P.L. (1973) *Gray's Anatomy*, 35th edn. Longman, London.

Wilgis E.F.S. & Maxwell G.P. (1979) Distal digital nerve graft. *J. Hand Surg.* **4**, 439–443.

Winkelmann R.K. (1960) *Nerve Endings in Normal and Pathological Skin*, p. 100. C.C. Thomas, Springfield, IL.

Zaias N. (1967) The longitudinal nail biopsy. *J. Invest. Dermatol.* **49**, 406–408.

Zook E.G. (1988) Injuries of the fingernail. In: *Operative Hand Surgery*, 2nd edn. Churchill-Livingstone, New York.

Comparative anatomy and function

The comparative anatomy of the nail unit can be considered from two aspects. There is the comparison of the nail with other ectodermal structures and most particularly hair and its follicle. The nail can also be viewed in an evolutionary setting alongside such structures as the hoof and claw. In this respect the functional qualities of the nail or its equivalent are exemplified by the morphological differences in different species. The human nail can be considered to have many mechanical and social functions, the most prominent of which are:

- fine manipulation
- scratching
- physical protection of the extremity
- a vehicle for cosmetics and aesthetic manipulation.

In comparison with other species, the first three functions have evolved with detailed physical modifications in the form of the hoof, claw and nail.

Hair and nail

It was noted by Achten (1968) that the nail unit was comparable in some respects to a hair follicle, sectioned longitudinally and laid on its side (Fig. 1.24). The hair bulb was considered analagous to the intermediate nail matrix and the cortex to the nail plate. As a model to stimulate thought, this idea is helpful. It also encourages the consideration of other manipulations of the hair follicle that might fit the analogy more tightly. The nail unit could be seen as an unfolded form of the hair follicle, producing a hair with no cortex, just hard cuticle. Scanning electron microscopy of the nail confirms that its structure is more similar to compacted cuticular cells than cortical fibres. A third model could represent the nail unit as a form of follicle abbreviated on one side, providing a modified form of outer root sheath to mould and direct nail growth in the manner of the proximal nail fold (Fig. 1.24).

A considerable amount of biochemical work on hair and nail confirms their common ground (Lynch *et al.*, 1986; Shono *et al.*, 1987; Kitaharo & Ogawa, 1992). In one study (Dekio & Jidoi, 1989) two-dimensional electrophoresis was used to determine the presence of nine keratins in human hair and nail. Those of molecular weights 76 000, 73 000, 64 000, 61 000 and 55 000 were common to hair and nail. One component of 61 000 was specific to hair, and two components, both with a molecular weight of 50 000, were specific to nail. Further definition of these proteins was given by Heid *et al.* (1988) who employed gel electrophoresis, immunoblotting, peptide mapping and complementary keratin binding analysis. They found that whilst nail plate contained both 'soft' epithelial and 'hard' trichocyte keratins, plucked hairs contained only the latter. By contrast, 'soft' epithelial keratins could be detected in the hair follicle and co-expressed with 'hard' keratins in a pattern also seen in the intermediate nail matrix. Although these 'hard' keratins

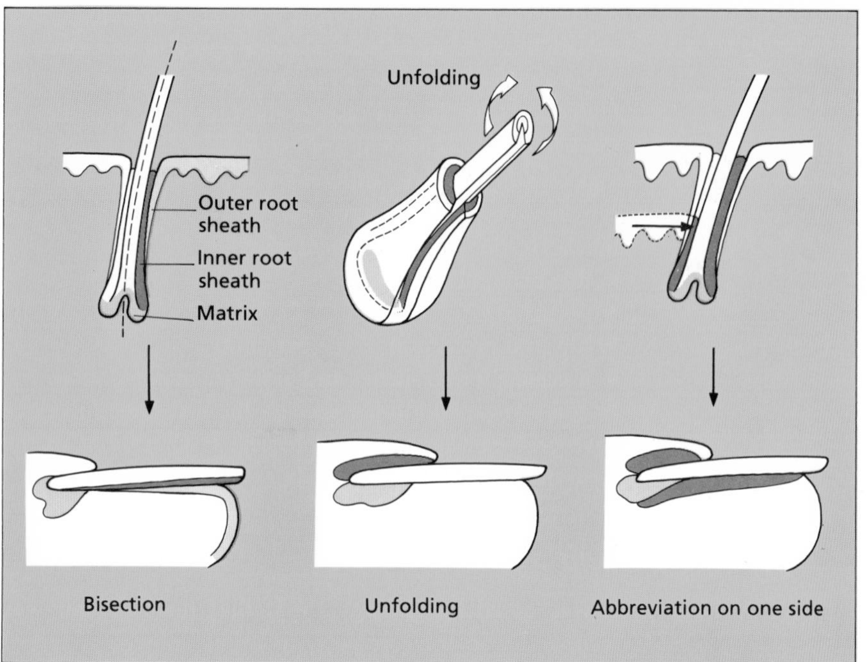

Fig. 1.24. Models of hair follicle/nail unit homology (de Berker after Prof. Achten, Belgium, Brussels).

are found in small amounts in the embryonic thymus and lingual papilla, they can generally be thought to be a feature of the hair/nail differentiation. This thesis was pursued further by Lynch *et al.* (1986) who suggested that the precursor cells of hair cortex and nail plate share a major pathway of epithelial differentiation. They felt that the acidic 44 Kd/46 Kd and basic 56–60 Kd 'hard' keratins represent a co-expressed keratin pair that defines hair/nail tissue.

The character of the nail plate and hair has led to their use in assays of circulating metabolites. They both lend themselves to this because they are long-lasting structures that may afford historical information. Additionally, their protein constituents bind metabolites and they provide accessible specimens. This allows both hair and nail to be used in the detection of systemic metabolites which may have disappeared from the blood many weeks previously (see nail analysis, p. 30).

Phylogenetic comparisons

The structure of claws and hooves and their evolutionary relationship to the human nail have been well reviewed (Spearman, 1978). In higher primates, nails have developed with the acquisition of manual dexterity. Other mammals do not possess such flattened claws from which nails have evolved (Fig. 1.25).

The lowest evolutionary level at which claws are seen is in the amphibia (Lucas & Strettenheim, 1972). The intermediate matrix contributes the greatest mass to the nail plate in man and other primates with a lesser contribution from the dorsal and nail bed matrices. Claws

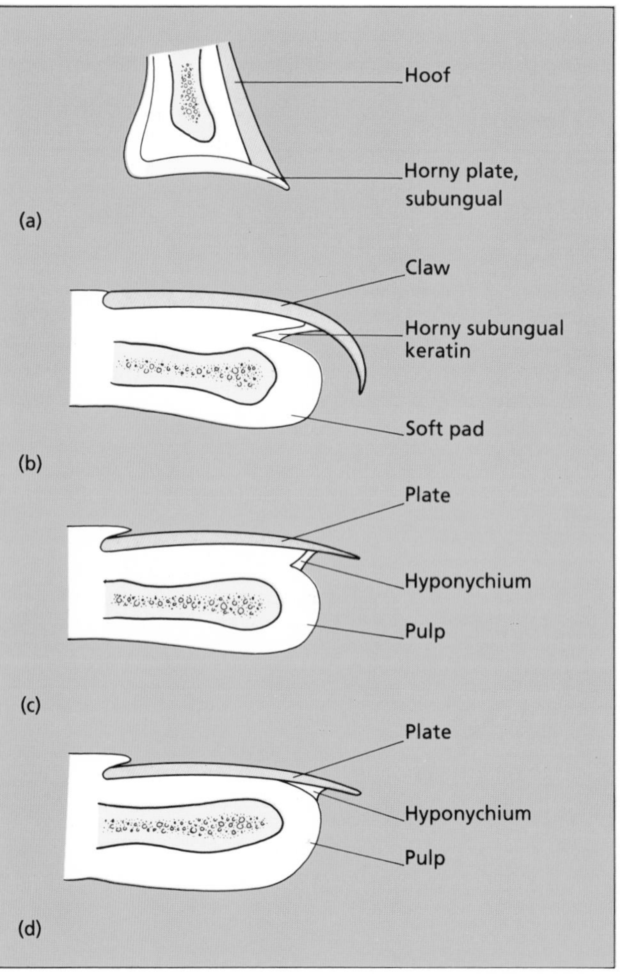

Fig. 1.25. Structure of a typical hoof, claw and nail (after Prof. Achten, Belgium, Brussels). (a) Hoof. (b) Claw. (c) Monkey. (d) Human.

(Kato, 1977) are formed from an extensive germinal matrix, which occupies the territory of the nail bed in primates. The shape of the cat claw may partly be determined by the sickle shape of the underlying phalanx (Kato, 1977) and achieved by differential growth made possible by a dorsal matrix contribution. It is postulated that their sharp tip is produced by a dominant midline matrix.

Claws and talons are harder than nails, probably because the content of calcium as crystalline hydroxyapatite within keratinocytes (Pautard, 1964). Altered orientation of keratin microfibrils may contribute to their strength. Bird and reptile claws are made up of β-keratin.

Claws and nails have many similarities but both have little in common with hooves. Hooves have evolved to provide a 'bulky claw' for weight bearing and locomotion over hard ground (Sisson & Grossman, 1953). It is interesting that among the prosimians, tarsiers have nails on all digits apart from the second and third digits of the hindlimb which bear claws (Spearman, 1978). In hooves the nail fold and root have been displaced backwards with a forwards extension of the nail bed. The hard 'soft plate' under hooves is produced from an area equivalent to the subungual part of the claw. In some animals, cloven hooves have only developed on the digits that touch the ground. In horses, the single large hoof is produced from the third digit. The typical hoof shape is due to a deep, backwardly placed root matrix with the ventral plate formed from the subungual epidermis. The microfibrils in hooves are from 25 to 100 μm in diameter. The orientation of the fibrils is along the main axis of the hoof similar to the hair cortex. Gorillas have oblique lines which are permanent; they converge toward the centre distally—human nails only show this characteristic in childhood.

References

Achten G. (1968) Normale Histologie und Histochemie des Nagels. In: *Handbuch der Haut- und Geschlechtskrankheiten*, ed. Jadassohn J., Vol. 1, p. 339–376, Springer-Verlag, Berlin.

Dekio S. & Jidoi J. (1989) Comparison of human hair and nail Low-sulfur protein compositions on two-dimensional electrophoresis. *J. Dermatol.* **16**, 284–288.

Heid H.W., Moll I. & Franke W.W. (1988) Patterns of expression of trichocytic and epithelial cytokeratins in mammalian tissues. *Differentiation* **37**, 215–230.

Kato T. (1977) A study on the development of the cat claw. *Hiroshima J. Med. Sci.* **26**, 103–126.

Kitahara T. & Ogawa H. (1992) Cultured nail keratinocytes express hard keratins characteristic of nail and hair. *Arch. Dermatol. Res.* **1**, 253–256.

Lucas A.M. & Strettenheim P.R. (1972) Avian anatomy integument. Pt. 2. *Agricultural Handbook*, 362. US Govt. Printing, Office, Washington, DC.

Lynch M.H., O'Guin W.M., Hardy C. *et al.* (1986) Acidic and basic hair/nail ('hard') keratins: Their co-localization in upper cortical and cuticle cells and the human hair follicle and their relationship to 'soft' keratins. *J. Cell Biol.* **103**, 2593–2606.

Pautard F.G.E. (1964) Calcification of keratin. In: *Progress in Biological Sciences in Relation to Dermatology*, eds Rook A.J. & Champion R.E., Vol. 2, p. 227. Cambridge University Press, Cambridge.

Shono S., Mataga N. & Toda K. (1987) The two dimensional peptide mappings of the nail low-sulfur S-carboxy-methyl keratins. *J. Dermatol.* **14**, 419–426.

Sisson S. & Grossman J.D. (1953) *The Anatomy of the Domestic Animals*. W.B. Saunders, Philadelphia.

Spearman R.I.C. (1978) The physiology of the nail. In: *The Physiology and Pathophysiogy of the Skin*, ed. Jarrett A., Vol. 5, p. 1827. Academic Press, New York.

Physiology

Nail growth

Matrix kinetics

Study of intermediate matrix cells is made difficult by the natural reluctance to biopsy normal living nail matrix. In some studies this has been overcome by the use of squirrel monkeys (Zaias & Alvarez, 1968), the careful use of human volunteers (Norton, 1971) and use of matrix excisions acquired at matricectomy for ingrowing toenails (Picardo *et al.*, 1992). Analysis of nail plate mass and growth has allowed inductive proposals concerning matrix function (Johnson, 1991; Johnson *et al.*, 1991).

In cultured explants of intermediate nail matrix cells, they have been characterized morphologically, in terms of keratin differentiation and with respect to colony growth behaviour (Nagae *et al.*, 1991; Picardo *et al.*, 1992; Kitahara & Ogawa, 1992). In comparison with normal skin epidermis, the cells divide more rapidly and are larger. They show the presence of both 'hard' and 'soft' keratins.

E. Haneke and F. Kiesewetter (personal communication) performed flow cytometry on matrix cells obtained in the same way. This demonstrated 94% of the matrix cells were in G0/1 phase, 3.4% in S phase and 2% in G2+M phase. The corresponding values for matrix connective tissue cells were 96.6% for G0/1, 2.3% for S and 1.1% for G2+M phases. The differences between matrix cells and associated connective tissue were statistically significant. This suggests that the percentage of cells in the phase of DNA synthesis and mitosis (S plus G2+M phases) in the nail matrix is much lower than that of hair matrix cells and equals that of the cells in the hair root sheath.

Definition of the nail matrix

Controversy remains as to the relative contributions of the three putative nail matrices to the nail plate. The three contenders are the dorsal, intermediate and ventral matrix (Fig. 1.26). The first is part of the proximal nail fold, the latter is the nail bed. Lewis (1954) claimed that the

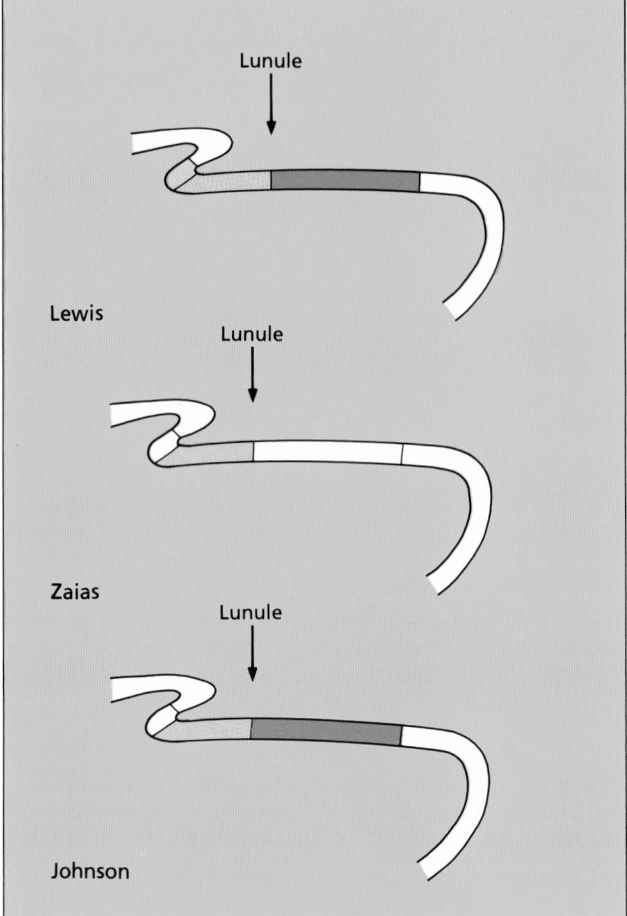

Fig. 1.26. Theories of nail plate origin.

nail plate demonstrated a three layer structure on silver staining and that each layer derived from one of the possible matrices. Zaias and Alvarez (1968) dismissed this on the basis of *in vivo* autoradiographic work on squirrel monkeys. They were only able to find circulating radiolabelled glycine deriving from the intermediate matrix contributing to the nail plate. Johnson (1991) and Johnson *et al.* (1991) in turn dismissed the evidence of Zaias and Alvarez, claiming that the methodology was flawed. It is also reasonable to comment that the nail bed of squirrel monkeys is less developed than that of humans and may not provide a direct model. Norton (1971) used human subjects and although there was some incorporation of radiolabelled glycine in the area of the nail bed, it was in a poorly defined location, making clear statements impossible. A modest contribution from the nail bed, with the major element from the intermediate matrix, would be consistent with measurements of mitotic rate using tritiated thymidine (Zaias, 1990). These show mitosis as being frequent in the latter and seldom in the former.

Those used to observing regrowth after nail plate removal will be very well aware that the nail bed alone is incapable of producing a good, flat, functionally useful nail plate.

Ultrasound

Ultrasound studies of the nail plate have done little to support the notion that the nail bed contributes significantly to its substance (Finlay, 1987; Jemec & Serup, 1989). Jemec claimed that the nail plate had a clear two part structure, neither of which appeared to come from the nail bed. Finlay observed that the nail plate had a more rapid ultrasound transmission distally; paradoxical if one imagines a nail bed contribution. This last comment is almost diametrically opposite to that of Johnson *et al.* (1991). They examined the thickness and mass of 21 nail plates lost through trauma. The thickness almost doubled from the mid-lunula to the distal edge and the mass increased by 20%. These changes are taken as evidence of a contribution derived from the nail plate. A weakness in the argument arises from the character of traumatic avulsion. In this situation part of the nail plate might remain adherent to the nail matrix, giving the avulsed specimen a spuriously thin proximal region. Indeed, the increase in nail plate thickness from the nail plate overlying the proximal nail bed to free edge was 15% and could be attributable to compaction through terminal microtrauma.

Keratin studies

Keratin studies on the whole of the nail unit have demonstrated a paucity of suprabasal markers in the nail bed (de Berker *et al.*, 1993). Trichocyte 'hard' nail keratins have been found thinly in the ventral matrix at embryonic stages, but not later (Heid *et al.*, 1988; de Berker *et al.*, 1993). These two features might fit with a ventral matrix contribution early in life, but less so later on. Alternatively, it might be the 'soft' epidermal keratins that are contributed to the nail plate by the nail bed in adulthood, as these are known to constitute 20% of the nail plate keratins (Lynch *et al.*, 1986). A distinction between the nail bed in the child and adult can also be made in the context of regrowth. Children are able to regenerate the amputated tips of fingers with nail, so long as the intermediate (germinal or distal) matrix remains intact. Adults are much less able to do this (Libbin & Neufeld, 1988).

In some circumstances, most commonly old age, there is a pattern of subungual hyperkeratosis associated with nail thickening which gives the impression of a nail bed contribution to the nail plate. Historically, this has been referred to as the solehorn (Fig. 1.27) (Solenhorn) and considered a germinal element of the hyponychium. Samman (1961) considered this issue in the context of a patient with pustular psoriasis: he concluded that the

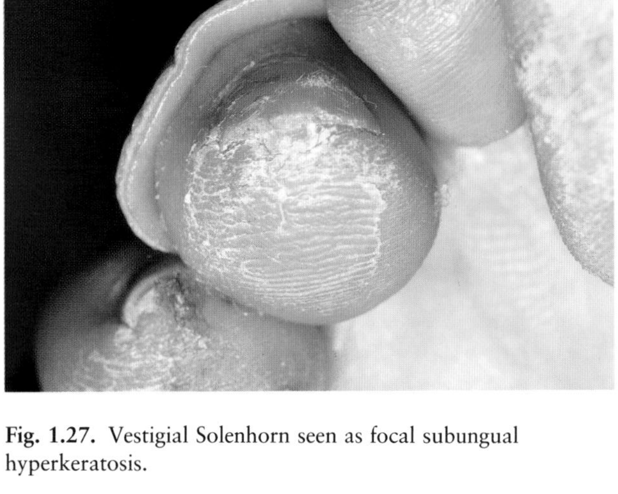

Fig. 1.27. Vestigial Solenhorn seen as focal subungual hyperkeratosis.

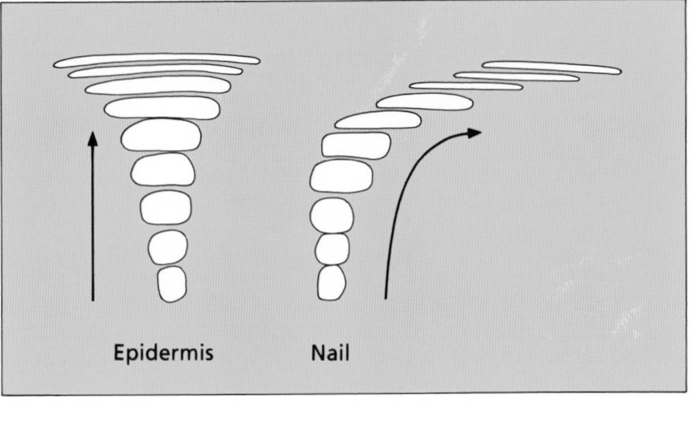

Fig. 1.28. Change in shape and direction of the cells within the epidermis and the nail matrix (after Kligman).

ventral nail is a movable feast, manifesting itself in certain pathological circumstances.

The dorsal matrix, at the base of the proximal nail fold, is less favoured in the debates concerning nail genesis. The epithelium may have a granular layer, distinguishing it from the intermediate and ventral matrix. However, in common with the intermediate (germinal) matrix, it expresses keratin 7, which is not seen in the ventral matrix (de Berker *et al.*, 1993). Lewis (1954) also noted that one of the three silver-staining layers of the nail plate appeared to derive from the dorsal matrix. Neither Zaias and Alvarez (1968) nor Norton (1971) noted incorporation of labelled glycine into the nail plate via the dorsal matrix.

Normal nail morphology

The main issues in normal nail morphology are, why is the nail flat, and why is the free edge rounded and not pointed? Factors influencing nail plate thickness are dealt with earlier.

The first question was addressed by Kligman (1961) and Hashimoto (1971). Kligman's hypothesis was that the proximal nail fold acts to mould the nail as it moves distally. From observing other keratinizing epithelia, he noted that growth is normally parallel to the axis of keratinization. From this, he considered it anomalous that nails grow out along the nail bed and not upwards (Fig. 1.28). A patient with the nervous habit of chewing off the proximal nail fold did not provide an adequate experiment to demonstrate its function. However, when given the opportunity to autograft 4 mm matrix punch biopsies from digit to forearm, nail tissue was seen to grow upwards like a cutaneous horn. This was presented as proof of the hypothesis.

Baran (1981) was in disagreement, and presented evidence from surgical experience in the removal of the proximal nail fold and the lack of subsequent change in the nail. He also challenged the validity of Kligman's experiment on the basis that the underlying terminal phalanx has a great influence upon nail growth (Baran & Juhlin, 1986) and this was lost in transplanting the graft to the arm. Further examples of ectopic nail growth do not resolve the issue (Kikuchi *et al.*, 1984).

All the models demonstrating the influence of the different elements of the nail unit upon the nail are flawed. Those above do not acknowledge the adherent quality of the nail bed as an influential factor, or the guiding influence of the lateral nail being embedded in the lateral nail folds. It is reasonable with our present knowledge to consider horizontal nail growth as being attributable to more than one part of the nail unit (Fig. 1.29).

The second issue is why are nails rounded and not pointed? This has generally been accepted as being a function of the shape of the lunula, as illustrated in Fig. 1.30. Given that nails are growing continuously throughout life, it is possible to argue that we rarely see the true free edge, but observe the eroded or manicured outline. However, there are two instances when we see the genuine free edge; at birth and with regrowth following avulsion (Fig. 1.31(a)–(d)). These appear to follow the margin of the lunula. Finally, the nail bed may have some role in determining the shape of the free edge. Trauma to the nail bed can result in nail plate dystrophies giving the free edge a scalloped contour. This can be corrected with nail bed grafts (Pessa *et al.*, 1990). In the Iso–Kikuchi syndrome the abnormal lunula may give rise to hemionychogryphosis. Hemionychogryphosis observed in Iso–Kikuchi syndrome results from abnormally shaped lunula (Baran & Stroud, 1984).

References

Baran R. (1981) Nail growth direction revisited. *J. Am. Acad. Dermatol.* **4**, 78–83.

Baran R. & Juhlin L. (1986) Bone dependent nail formation. *Br. J. Dermatol.* **114**, 371–375.

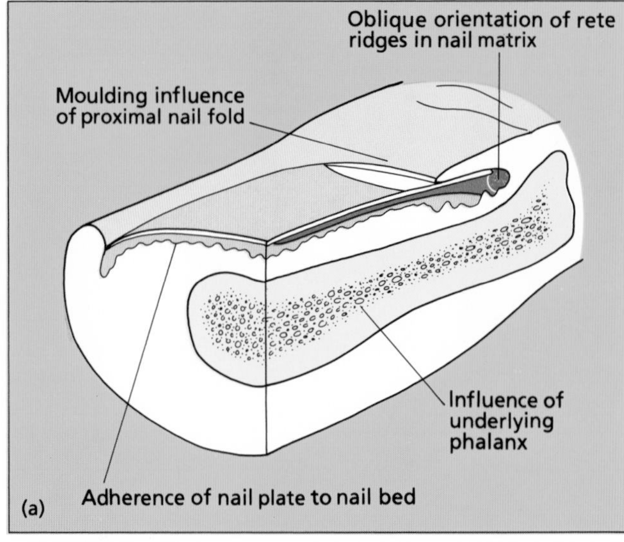

Fig. 1.29. (a) Why do nails grow out instead of up? (i) Guiding restraint of proximal nail fold; (ii) inductive influence of underlying phalanx; (iii) containment by lateral nail folds; (iv) adherence to nail bed.

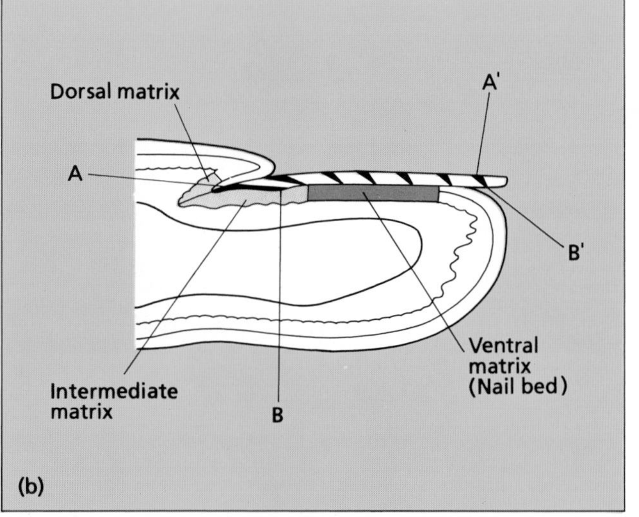

Fig. 1.29. (b) Generation of nail plate marked at monthly intervals. The horizontal axis of the intermediate axis is transformed into an oblique axis. Proximal matrix, A, generates dorsal nail A^1. Distal intermediate matrix, B, generates ventral nail B^1.

Baran R. & Stroud J.D. (1984) Congenital onychodysplasia of the index fingers. *Arch. Dermatol.* **128**, 243–244.

de Berker D., Leigh I., Wojnarowska F. *et al.* (1993) Patterns of keratin expression in the nail unit – an indicator of regional matrix differentiation *Br. J. Dermatol.*, in press.

Finlay A.Y., Moseley H. & Duggan T.C. (1987) Ultrasound transmission time: an in vivo guide to nail thickness. *Br. J. Dermatol.* **117**, 765–770.

Hashimoto K. (1971) Ultrastructure of the human toenail: proximal nail matrix. *J. Invest. Dermatol.* **56**, 235–246.

Heid H.W., Moll I. & Franke W.W. (1988) Patterns of expression of trichocytic and epithelial cytokeratins in mammalian tissues. *Differentiation* **37**, 215–230.

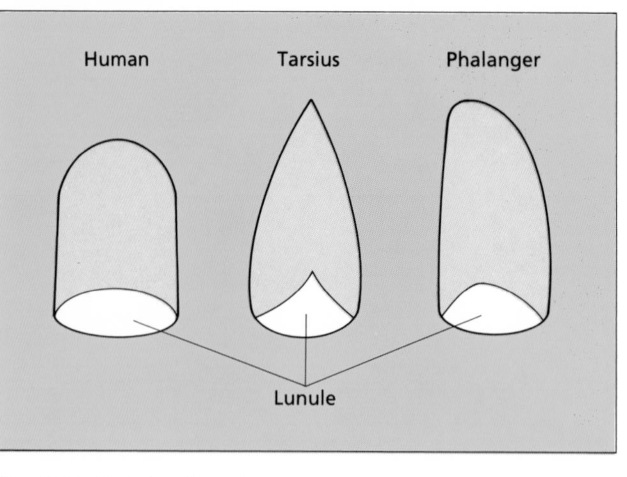

Fig. 1.30. Relationship of lunula to nail tip shape.

Jemec G.B.E. & Serup J. (1989) Ultrasound structure of the human nail plate. *Arch. Dermatol.* **125**, 643–646.

Johnson M. (1991) The formation and permeability of the human nail plate. D.Phil. Thesis, Univ. of Newcastle, UK, pp. 3–29.

Johnson M., Comaish J.S. & Shuster S. (1991) Nail is produced by the normal nail bed: a controversy resolved. *Br. J. Dermatol.* **125**, 27–28.

Kikuchi I., Ogata K. & Idemori M. (1984) Vertically growing ectopic nail. *J. Am. Acad. Dermatol.* **10**, 114–116.

Kitahara T. & Ogawa H. (1992) Cultured nail keratinocytes express hard keratins characteristic of hair and nail in vivo. *Arch. Dermatol. Res.* **1**, 253–256.

Kligman A. (1961) Why do nails grow out instead of up? *Arch. Dermatol.* **84**, 181–183.

Le Gros Clark W.E. (1936) The problem of the claw in primates. *Proc. Zool. Soc. Lond.* **1**, 1–24.

Lewis B.L. (1954) Microscopic studies of fetal and mature nail and the surrounding soft tissue. *Arch. Dermatol. Syphilol.* **70**, 732–744.

Libbin R.M. & Neufeld D.A. (1988) Regeneration of the nail bed. *Plastic Reconstr. Surg.* **81**, 1001–1002.

Lynch M., O'Guin W.M., Hardy C. *et al.* (1986) Acidic and basic hair/nail keratins: Their co-localisation in upper cortical cells and cuticle cells of the human hair follicle and their relationship to 'soft' keratins. *J. Cell Biol.* **103**, 2593–2606.

Nagae H., Arase S., Nakanishi H. & Takeda K. (1991) Culture of human nail matrix cells on collagen type IV and in a collagen matrix. *Jpn. J. Dermatol.* **101**, 1377–1388.

Norton L.A. (1971) Incorporation of thymidine-methyl-H^3 and glycine-2-H^3 in the nail matrix and bed of humans. *J. Invest. Dermatol.* **56**, 61–68.

Pessa J.E., Tsai T.M., Li Y. & Kleinert H.E. (1990) The repair of nail bed deformities with the nonvascularised nail bed graft: Indications and results. *J. Hand Surg.* **15A**, 466–470.

Picardo M., Marchese C., Zompetta C. *et al.* (1992) Characterisation of human nail matrix cells in vitro. *J. Invest. Dermatol.* **98**, 523–528.

Samman P. (1961) The ventral nail. *Arch. Dermatol.* **84**, 192–195.

Zaias N. & Alvarez J. (1968) The formation of the primate nail plate. An autoradiographic study in the squirrel monkey. *J. Invest. Dermatol.* **51**, 120–136.

Zaias N. (1990) *The Nail in Health and Disease.* 2 edn, Appleton & Lange, CN.

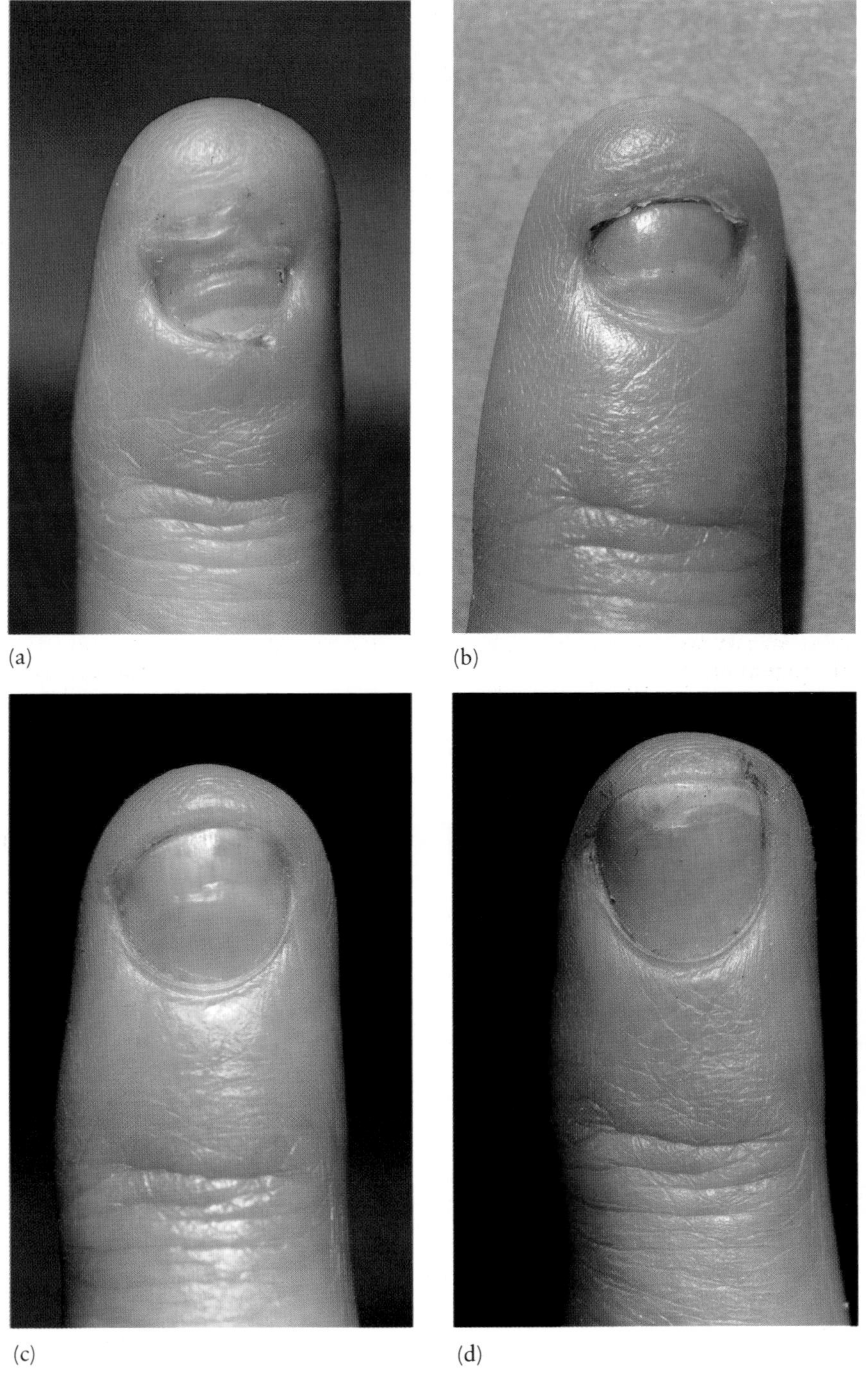

Fig. 1.31. (a)–(d) Regrowth of the fingernail following traumatic avulsion. The free edge is parallel to the lunula.

Nail growth measurement

A range of quantitative methods have been employed to measure nail growth, mostly requiring the imprint of a fixed reference mark on the nail and measuring its change in location relative to a fixed structure separate from the nail after a study period. Gilchrist *et al.* (1938–39) made a transverse scratch about 2 mm from the most distal margin of the lunula. This distance was then measured using a rule and magnifier. Changes in the distance with time provided a record of growth rate. There have been variants of this, with the scratch being made at the convex apogee of the lunula and subsequent measurements made with reference to the lunula (Hillman, 1955), or alternaltively making a scratch a fixed 3 mm from the cuticle and noting the change with time (Dawber, 1970a) (Fig. 1.32). The precision of these methods was increased by the introduction of magnified photographs before and after, and comparison of the photographs (Babcock, 1955). This was modified further by Sibinga (1959) who increased the

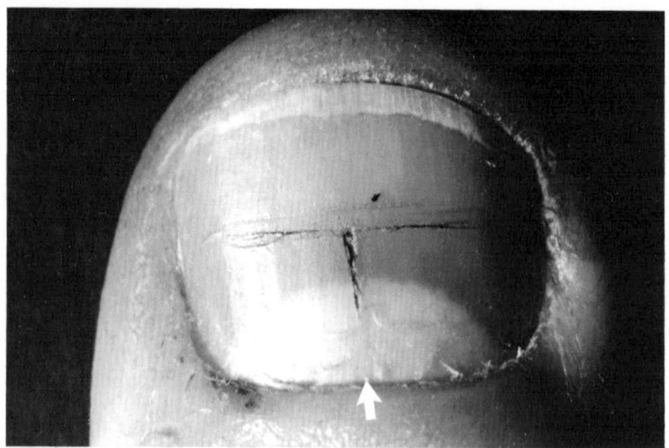

Fig. 1.32. T-shaped mark etched on nail for nail growth measurement (Dawber, 1970a). Arrow points to posterior nail fold reference point. Note the absence of a cuticle.

photographic magnification from a factor of 6 to 35. This made it possible to conduct studies of nail growth over a period as short as 1 month.

Babcock (1955) understood the problems in the methods involving the lunula and cuticle as reference points, as they both might conceivably change during the study. The method suggested for overcoming this was inventive, but unacceptable these days for ethical reasons. The nail was marked with a deep scratch which was then filled with bismuth amalgam. This made it radio-opaque and allowed comparison with the underlying bony reference points on X-ray. A follow-up X-ray, after re-filling the scratch with amalgam, allowed growth estimation. The concern over variation in the non-nail plate reference point can be partly surmounted by using two reference points and possibly halving the error. This can be done by making a scratch at the tip of the lunula and measuring the distance to the distal limit of the nail plate attachment, visible through the nail plate. Subsequent measurements are made from both the lunula and the edge of nail plate attachment. Their sum should always be equal as a way of verifying the method (Fig. 1.33). All these methods involve estimation of linear growth. As a measure of total matrix activity this could be misleading. Hamilton *et al.* (1955) sought to measure volume by the following equation:

thickness (mm) × breadth (mm) × length grown/day
= volume

Johnson *et al.* (1991) also tried to measure volumetric growth with respect to linear growth, ignoring time. This entailed the measurement of thickness and mass at different points in the avulsed nail plate. The method presumed that linear measurements in the longitudinal axis of the nail plate were proportional to time and that no element of compaction complicated the issue.

Attempts to measure volume take on particular significance in disease states provoking Beau's lines. In a condition where the bulk of the nail is manifestly affected, measurement of linear growth alone is of little help (Fig. 1.34). Van Noord (1993) measured the length and weight of clippings.

Physiological factors and nail growth

Most studies concern fingernails. Their rate of growth can vary between 1.9 and 4.4 mm/month (Sibinga, 1959). A reasonable guide is 3 mm/month or 0.1 mm/day. Toenails are estimated to grow around 1 mm/month. Population studies on nail growth have given the general findings

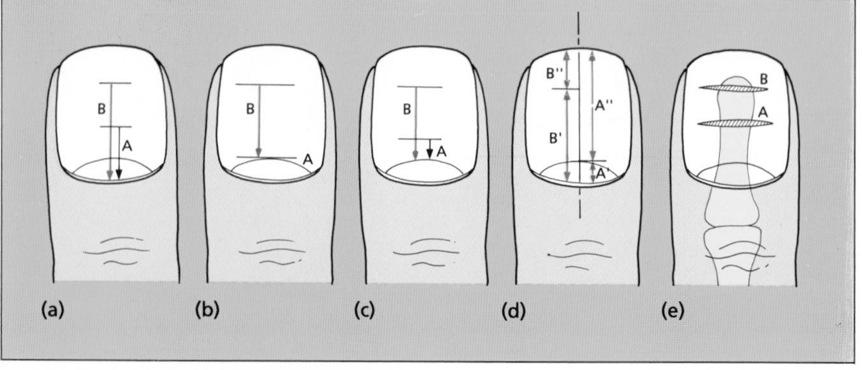

Fig. 1.33. Methods of nail growth measurement. (a) Reference, cuticle; growth, B – A; c̄ magnifier, Dawber (1970). (b) Reference, lunula; growth, B; Hillman (1955); c̄ × 6 reference photo, Babcock (1955), c̄ × 35 reference photo, Sibinga (1959). (c) Reference, lunula; growth, B – A; c̄ magnifier, Gilchrist (1938). (d) Reference; cuticle and nail attachment margin; growth,

$$\frac{(B' - A') + (A'' - B'')}{2};$$

verification by A′ + A″ = B′ + B″, de Berker (1990). (e) Reference; bone feature on X-ray, bismuth amalgam in nail scratch; growth, depends on landmark.

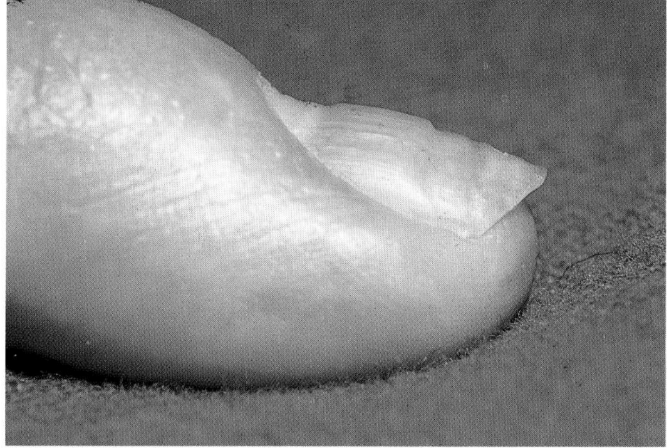

Fig. 1.34. Side view of a nail with Beau's line, indicating the change in nail bulk.

that there is little marked seasonal change and nails are unaffected by mild intercurrent illnesses (Hillman, 1955; Sibinga, 1959). The height or weight of the individual made no significant difference (Hillman, 1955; Hewitt & Hillman, 1966). Sex makes a small difference in early adulthood, with men having significantly ($p < 0.001$) faster linear nail growth up to the age of 19 (Hamilton *et al.*, 1955). They continue to do so with gradually diminishing significance levels, up to the age of 69, when there is a crossover and women's nails grow faster than men's. There is rough agreement from Hillman (1955) in an earlier study, although he found that the crossover age was around 40. However, males continued to have a greater rate of nail growth throughout life if volume was measured, and not length (Hamilton *et al.*, 1955). Children under 14 have faster growth than adults. Pregnancy may increase the rate of nail growth (Hewitt & Hillman, 1966) and poor nutrition may retard it (Gilchrist *et al.*, 1938–39).

Temperature is an influence with unclear effects. Bean (1980) kept a slightly idiosyncratic record of his own fingernail growth by making a scratch at the free edge of his cuticle on the first day of each month for 35 years. His record showed a gradual slowing with age. It initially showed a seasonal variation with heightened growth in the warm months. This variation became less marked with age, combining with a move from Iowa to Texas where seasonal contrasts are reduced. Other studies to determine the influence of temperature have compared nail growth rates for people in temperate and polar conditions. An original study in 1958 (Geoghegan *et al.*, 1958) found that nail growth was significantly retarded by living in the Arctic. Subsequent studies from the Antarctic found that there was no change in nail growth (Donovan, 1977; Gormly & Ledingham, 1983). These studies are not scientific, and it is unclear whether they are commenting on the improvement in thermal insulation since 1958 or nail physiology.

Nail growth in disease

Systemic disease

Insufficient numbers of seriously ill people have been followed as part of a larger study to give good statistical evidence concerning the influence of disease on nail growth. There is plenty of evidence from small numbers that some severe systemic upsets disturb nail formation. The observations of Justin Honoré Simon Beau in 1836 (Weismann, 1977) detailed the development of transverse depressions upon the nails of people surviving typhoid. The form of nail growth interference represented by Beau's lines is seen in many conditions. Severe illness in the form of mumps has been noted to bring linear growth to a standstill (Sibinga, 1959). Other acute infections are quite variable, with 10 cases of acute febrile tuberculosis failing to have significant effect (Sibinga, 1959). In the same study, chronic nephrosis produced exceptionally slow nail growth. Paradoxically, Sibinga also found that cadavers appeared to continue the growth of their nails in the 10

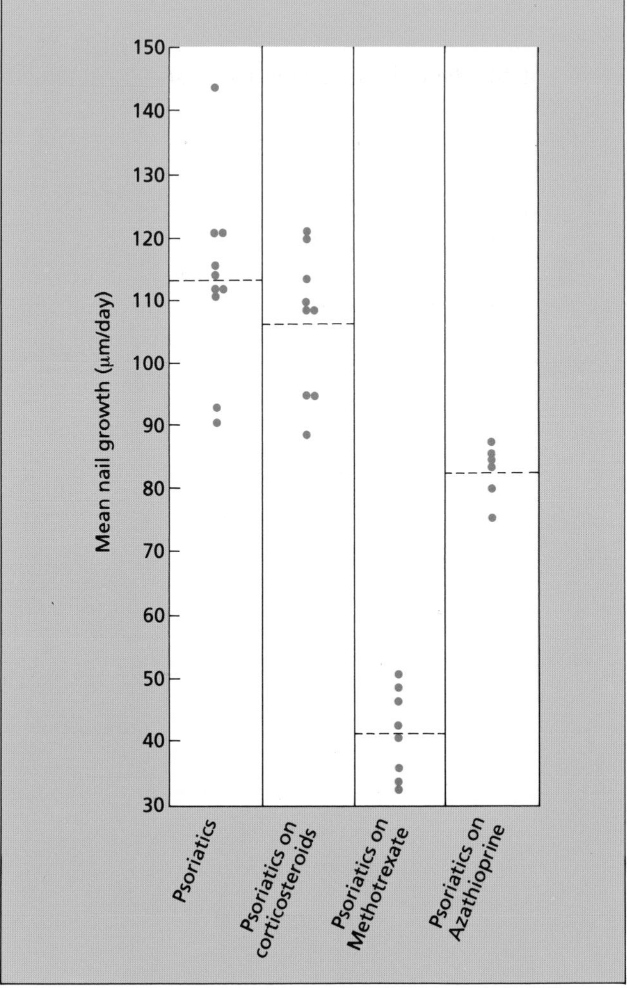

Fig. 1.35. Effect of therapy on nail growth in psoriasis (Dawber, 1970b).

days post mortem during which they were assessed. The effect of death was less marked than mumps, something adults with mumps might agree with!

Local disease

Local diseases can influence nail growth. Dawber *et al.* (1971) noted that onycholysis increased nail growth. This was true whether it was related to psoriasis or idiopathic. It is interesting that psoriasis may also produce Beau's lines and so reduce the bulk of the nail. It is not even clear whether Beau's lines represent a reduction in linear growth. They have been noted after retinoid therapy, and yet this group of drugs has been noted to increase nail growth in psoriasis (Galosi *et al.*, 1985). Perhaps a nail that is growing faster is unable to accumulate bulk. Other systemic psoriasis treatments may reduce the rate of nail growth (Dawber, 1970b) (Fig. 1.35).

Table 1.2 includes influences upon nail growth that are reported, but not always of statistical significance.

References

Babcock M.J. (1955) Methods for measuring fingernail growth rates in nutritional studies. *J. Nutrition* **55**, 323–336.

Baran R. (1982) Action thérapeutique et complications dues au rétinoide aromatique sur l'appareil unguéal. *Ann. Derm. Venereol.* **109**, 367–371.

Bean, W.B. (1974) Nail growth: 30 years of observations. *Arch. Int. Medicine* **134**, 497–502.

Bean W.B. (1980) Nail growth. Thirty-five years of observation. *Arch. Intern. Med.* **140**, 73–76.

Dawber R. (1970a) Fingernail growth in normal and psoriatic subjects. *Br. J. Dermatol.* **82**, 454–457.

Dawber R.P.R. (1970b) The effect of methotrexate, corticosteroids and azathioprine on fingernail growth in psoriasis. *Br. J. Dermatol.* **83**, 680–683.

Dawber R.P.R. (1980) Ultrastructure and growth of human nails. *Arch. Derm. Research* **269**, 197–204.

Table 1.2. Influences on nail growth

Faster	Slower
Daytime	Night
Pregnancy (Hewitt & Hillman, 1966)	1st day of life (Schnick, 1908)
Minor trauma/nail biting (Gilchrist *et al.*, 1938–39; Hamilton *et al.*, 1955)	
Right hand/dominant	Left hand/non-dominant
Youth	Old age (Hamilton *et al.*, 1955)
Fingers	Toes (Pfister, 1969)
Summer (Bean, 1980)	Winter/cold (Geoghegan, 1958)
Middle finger	Thumb and little finger (LeGros Clark & Boxton, 1938; Orentreich *et al.*, 1979)
Men	Women (LeGros Clark & Boxton, 1938; Hamilton *et al.*, 1955)
Psoriasis (Landherr *et al.*, 1982) Pitting (Dawber, 1970a) Normal nails (Dawber, 1970a) Onycholysis (Dawber *et al.*, 1971)	Finger immobilization (Dawber, 1981) Fever (Sibinga, 1959) Beau's lines (Weismann, 1977)
Pityriasis rubra pilaris (Dawber, 1980)	Methotrexate, azathioprine (Dawber, 1970b)
Total leuconychia	
Etretinate (Baran, 1982)	Etretinate (Baran, 1982)
Idiopathic onycholysis of women (Dawber *et al.*, 1971)	Denervation (Head & Sherrin, 1905)
Bullous ichthyosiform erythroderma (Samman, 1978)	Poor nutrition (Gilchrist *et al.*, 1938–39)
Hyperthyroidism (Orentreich *et al.*, 1979)	
L-Dopa (Miller, 1973)	
AV shunts (Orentreich *et al.*, 1979)	Yellow nail syndrome (Samman, 1978)
Itraconazole; fluconazole (Shelley & Shelley, 1992)	
Calcium/vit. D (Hogan *et al.*, 1984)	Relapsing polychondritis (Estes, 1983)
Cyclosporin A (Baran, unpublished data)	
Benoxaprofen (Fenton & Wilkinson, 1983)	

Dawber, R.P.R. (1981) Effects of immobilization on nail growth. *Clin. Exp. Derm.* **6**, 1–4.

Dawber R.P.R., Samman P. & Bottoms E. (1971) Fingernail growth in idiopathic and psoriatic onycholysis. *Br. J. Dermatol.* **85**, 558–560.

Dawber, R.P.R. & Baran, R. (1987) Nail growth. *Cutis* **39**, 99–104.

Donovan K.M. (1977) Antarctic environment and nail growth. *Br. J. Dermatol.* **96**, 507–510.

Estes S.A. (1983) Relapsing polychondritis. *Cutis* **32**, 471–476.

Fenton D.A. & Wilkinson J.D. (1983) Milia, increased nail growth and hypertrichosis following treatment with Benoxaprofen. *J.R. Soc. Med.* **76**, 525–527.

Galosi A., Plewig G. & Braun-Falco O. (1985) The effect of aromatic retinoid RO 10-9359 on fingernail growth. *Arch. Dermatol. Res.* **277**, 138–140.

Geoghegan B., Roberts D.F. & Sampford M.R. (1958) A possible climatic effect on nail growth. *J. Appl. Physiol.* **13**, 135–138.

Gilchrist M. & Dudley Buxton L.H. (1938–39) The relation of fingernail growth to nutritional status. *J. Anat.* **73**, 575–582.

Gormly P.J. & Ledingham J.E. (1983) Nail growth in antarctic conditions. *Aust. J. Dermatol.* **24**, 86–89.

Hamilton J.B., Terada H. & Mestler G.E. (1955) Studies of growth throughout the lifespan in Japanese: Growth and size of nails and their relationship to age, sex heredity and other factors. *J. Gerontol.* **10**, 401–415.

Head H. & Sherrin J. (1905) The consequence of injury to peripheral nerves in man. *Brain* **28**, 116.

Hewitt D. & Hillman R.W. (1966) Relation between rate of nail growth in pregnant women and estimated previous general growth rate. *Am. J. Clin. Nutrition* **19**, 436–439.

Hillman R. (1955) Fingernail growth in the human subject. *Human Biol.* **27**, 274–283.

Hogan D.B., McNair S., Young J. & Crilly R. (1984) Nail growth, calcium and vitamin D. *Ann. Int. Med.* **101**, 283.

Johnson M., Comaish J.S. & Shuster S. (1991) Nail is produced by the normal nail bed: a controversy resolved. *Br. J. Dermatol.* **125**, 27–28.

Landherr G., Braun-Falco O., Hofmann C. *et al.* (1982) Fingernagelwachstum bei Psoriatikern unter Puva-Therapie. *Hautarzt.* **33**, 210–213.

LeGros Clarke W.E. & Buxton L.H.D. (1938) Studies in nail growth. *Br. J. Dermatol.* **50**, 221–229.

Miller E. (1973) Levodopa and nail growth. *New Engl. J. Med.* **288**, 916.

Orentreich N., Markofsky J. & Vogelman J.H. (1979) The effect of ageing on the rate of linear nail growth. *J. Invest. Dermatol.* **73**, 126–130.

Pfister R. & Heneka J. (1969) Wachstum und Gestaltung der Zehennägel bei Gesunden. *Arch. Klin. Exp. Derm.* **223**, 263–274.

Samman P.D. (1978) *The Nails in Disease*, 3rd edn. p. 14. Heinemann, London.

Schnick B. (1908) Die physiologische Nagelline des Säuglings. *Säuglings Jahr Kinderh.* **67**, 146.

Shelley W.B. & Shelley E.D. (1992) Portrait of a practice. *Cutis* **49**, 386.

Sibinga M.S. (1959) Observations on growth of fingernails in health and disease. *Pediatrics* **24**, 225–233.

Van Noord P.A.H. (1993) The growth of nails from hands and feet by length and weight in one individual over 9 years of aging. Personal Communication.

Weismann K. (1977) J.H.S. Beau and his descriptions of transverse depressions on nails. *Br. J. Dermatol.* **97**, 571–572.

Nail plate inorganic and biochemical analysis

Methods of analysis

A great range of methods have been used to analyse the organic and inorganic content of nails. Table 1.3 gives a guide, indicating how particular methods are appropriate for different constituents.

Nail proteins

From Table 1.3 on analytical methods it is clear that a considerable number of endogenous and exogenous materials can be sought in the nail plate. The protein mesh into which the elements fit is made primarily of keratin and associated proteins. These fall into three categories:

1 low sulphur keratins (40–60 K);
2 high sulphur proteins (10–25 K);
3 high glycine/tyrosine proteins (6–9 K).

It is believed that the low sulphur keratins form 10 nm filaments and the latter two groups of proteins form an interfilamentous matrix. The diversity of keratins within humans and between different species, lies in the permutations of these three proteins (Gillespie & Frenkel, 1974) and the diversity of the keratins themselves. Over 30 high sulphur proteins have been identified in human nail by polyacrylamide gel electrophoresis (Marshall, 1980).

Nail plate keratin fibrils appear oriented in a plane parallel to the surface and in the transverse axis (Forslind, 1970). They fall roughly into an 80:20 split between 'hard' hair type (trichocyte) keratin and 'soft', epithelial keratin (Lynch *et al.*, 1986). These two variants are similar in many respects and share an X-ray diffraction pattern of α-helices in a coiled conformation. Hard keratins also split into the classical association of acidic and basic pairs, with extensive amino acid homologies with the epithelial forms (Hanukoglu & Fuchs, 1983). In spite of regions of homology, the 'hard' and 'soft' keratins are distinguishable by immunohistochemistry (Lynch *et al.*, 1986; Heid *et al.*, 1988). The relative resilience of the two groups of keratins is also reflected in their solubility in 2-mercaptoethanol. At 50 mmol concentrations, only epthelial 'soft' keratins are extracted from nail clippings. The concentration needs to be raised to 200 mmol before significant quantities of 'hard' keratin dissolve (Kitahara & Ogawa, 1991).

The main lipid of nail is cholesterol. The total fat content is 0.1–1%, contrasting with the 10% found in the stratum corneum. The water content is less than that of skin, being 7–12% compared with 15–25%.

Mineral constituents of nail

X-ray diffraction is one of the most frequently used methods of elemental nail analysis. Much of the initial

Table 1.3. Different methods of nail constituent analysis

Method	Element	Reference
Immunohistochemistry	Keratin	Heid *et al.*, 1988
Enzymic assay	Steroid sulphatase	Matsumoto *et al.*, 1990
Electron microscopy	Lipid, cystine	Salamon *et al.*, 1988
Neutron activation analysis	Zinc, selenium	Van Noord *et al.*, 1987; Rogers *et al.*, 1991
Mass fragmentography	Metamphetamine	Suzuki *et al.*, 1989
X-ray diffraction	Mg, Cl, Na, Ca, S, Cu	Forslind, 1970; Sirota *et al.*, 1988
High performance liquid chromatography	Furosine (glycosylated keratin), terbinafine	Sueki *et al.*, 1989; Dykes *et al.*, 1990; Melnik *et al.*, 1990
Atomic absorption spectometry	Cd, Pb, Zn, Ca, Mg	Forslind, 1970; Helsby, 1976; Wilhelm *et al.*, 1991
Colorimetry	Fe	Jacobs & Jenkins, 1960
Adsorption differential pulse voltametry	Ni	Gammelgaard & Veien, 1990
Gas chromatography	Amphetamine	Suzuki *et al.*, 1984

work was done by Forslind (1970). He observed that the hardness of the nail plate is unlikely to be due to calcium, which the analogy with bone has suggested. Detailed resumés of normal nail mineral content have been made (Zaias, 1990).

Much interest has been demonstrated in the analysis of nails as a source of information concerning health. A significant increase in the nail content of Na, Mg and P was noted in a survey of 50 patients with cirrhosis (Djaldetti *et al.*, 1987). In a comparison of term and preterm infants, a decrease of aluminium and sulphur was found in term deliveries. The high aluminium content in preterm infants was considered of possible relevance to the osteopenia observed in this group (Sirota *et al.*, 1988). Copper and iron have been observed at higher levels in the nails of male 6–11 year olds in comparison with females (Alexiou *et al.*, 1980). Iron levels in the general population were found to be equal in men and women, but higher in children and highest in the neonate (Jacobs & Jenkins, 1960).

Disease prognostication and nail analysis

In some respect, nail analysis can be compared with a blood test, but involving the examination of a less labile source of information. An analysis of chloride in nail clippings of a juvenile control population and those suffering from cystic fibrosis, revealed a significant increase of chloride, by a factor of 5, in the latter. This has led to the suggestion of 'screening nail by mail' for inaccessible regions, where sending nails would be relatively easy.

The glycosylated globin molecule, used for estimation of long-term diabetic control, has been used as a model in studies measuring nail furosine in diabetes mellitus. The nail fructose-lysine content is raised in this disease and has shown a correlation with the severity of diabetic retinopathy and neuropathy (Oimomi *et al.*, 1985). Nail furosine levels have also shown a good correlation with fasting glucose and may even compete with glycosylated haemoglobin as an indicator of long-term diabetic control (Sueki *et al.*, 1989).

Steroid sulphatase and its substrate, cholesterol sulphate, have been assayed in the nails of children being screened for X-linked ichthyosis and found to have adequate sensitivity and accuracy to be useful (Matsumoto *et al.*, 1990; Serizawa *et al.*, 1990). Sudan IV-positive material in nails has been measured as a guide to serum triglycerides (Salamon *et al.*, 1988) and selenium in those being screened for oral cancer (Rogers *et al.*, 1991) and carcinoma of the breast (Van Noord *et al.*, 1987). The last two studies were inconclusive.

Exogenous materials in nail analysis

Exogenous materials can be considered in two groups; environmental and ingested substances. In the first category, cadmium, copper, lead and zinc were examined in the hair and nails of young children (Wihelm *et al.*, 1991). This was done to gauge the exposure to these substances sustained in rural and industrialized areas of Germany. Both hair and nail reflected the different environments, although the multiple correlation coefficient was higher for hair than nails. Nickel analysis has been performed to establish occupational exposure (Gammelgaard & Veien, 1990).

The use of forensic nail drug analysis has been reported

by the Japanese where over 20 000 people were arrested for the abuse of methamphetamine in 1987 (Suzuki *et al.*, 1984, 1989). It was found that the drug was included to the nail via both the intermediate matrix and nail bed. Chronic drug abusers could be distinguished from those with a single recent ingestion by scraping the under surface of the nail before analysis. This would remove the nail bed contribution and the drug it contained in the 'one off' abuser. Following single large doses of methamphetamine, it could be detected by mass fragmentography in saliva up to 2 days later, in hair up to 18 days and in nails for the next 45 days (Suzuki *et al.*, 1989) Chloroquine has also been measured in nail clippings for research purposes up to a year after ingestion (Ofori-Adjei *et al.*, 1985). Inclusion of the antifungal, terbinafine, via the nail bed has also been observed (Dykes *et al.*, 1990). This is one of the reasons that the duration of courses of antifungal therapy has fallen.

References

Alexiou D., Koutsclinis A., Manolidis C. *et al.* (1980) The content of trace elements in fingernails of children. *Dermatologica* **160**, 380–382.

Djaldetti M., Fishman P., Harpaz D. & Lurie B. (1987) X-ray microanalysis of the fingernails in cirrhotic patients. *Dermatologica* **174**, 114–116.

Dykes P.J., Thomas R. & Finlay A.Y. (1990) Determination of terbinafine in nail samples during treatment for onychmycoses. *Br. J. Dermatol.* **123**, 481–486.

Forslind B. (1970) Biophysical studies of the normal nail. *Acta Dermatov. (Stockh.)* **50**, 161–168.

Gammelgaard B. & Veien N.K. (1990) Nickel in nails, hair and plasma from nickel-hypersensitive women. *Acta. Dermatol. Venereol. (Stockh.)* **70**, 417–420.

Gillespie J.M. & Frenkel M.J. (1974) The diversity of keratins. *Comp. Biochem. Physiol.* **47B**, 339–346.

Hanukoglu I. & Fuchs E. (1983) The cDNA sequence of a human epidermal keratin: divergence of sequence but conservation of structure among intermediate filaments. *Cell* **31**, 243–251.

Heid H.W., Moll I. & Franke W.W. (1988) Patterns of expression of trichocytic and epithelial cytokeratins in mammalian tissues. *Differentiation* **37**, 215–230.

Helsby C.A. (1976) Determination of mercury in fingernails and body hair. *Analyt. Chim. Acta.* **82**, 427–430.

Jacobs A. & Jenkins D.J. (1960) The iron content of finger nails. *Br. J. Dermatol.* **72**, 145–148.

Kitahara T. & Ogawa H. (1991) The extraction and characterisation of human nail keratin. *J. Dermatol. Sci.* **2**, 402–406.

Lynch M.H., O'Guin W.M., Hardy C. *et al.* (1986) Acidic and basic hair/nail 'hard' keratins: Their co-localisation in upper cortical and cuticle cells of the human hair follicle and their relationship to 'soft' keratins. *J. Cell Biol.* **103**, 2593–2606.

Marshall R.C. (1980) Genetic variation in the proteins of the human nail. *J. Invest. Dermatol.* **75**, 264–269.

Matsumoto T., Sakura N. & Ueda K. (1990) Steroid sulphatase activity in nails: screening for X-linked ichthyosis. *Pediatr. Dermatol.* **7**, 266–269.

Melnik B., Hollmann J., Hofmann U. *et al.* (1990) Lipid composition of outer stratum corneum and nails in atopic and control subjects. *Arch. Dermatol. Res.* **282**, 549–551.

Ofori-Adjei D. & Ericsson O. (1985) Chloroquine in nail clip pings. *Lancet* **ii**, 331.

Oimomi M., Maeda Y, Hata F. *et al.* (1985) Glycosylation levels of nail proteins in diabetic patients with retinopathy and neuropathy. *Kobe J. Med. Sci.* **31**, 183–188.

Rogers M., Thomas D.B., Davis S. *et al.* (1991) A case control study of oral cancer and pre-diagnostic concentrations of selenium and zinc in nail tissue. *Int. J. Cancer.* **48**, 182–188.

Salamon T., Lazovic-Tepavac O., Nikulin A. *et al.* (1988) Sudan IV positive material of the nail plate related to plasma triglycerides. *Dermatologica* **176**, 52–54.

Serizawa S., Nagai T., Ito M. & Sato Y. (1990) Cholesterol sulphate levels in the hair and nails of patients with recessive X-linked ichthyosis. *Clin. Exp. Dermatol.* **15**, 13–15.

Sirota L., Straussberg R., Fishman P., Dulitzky F. & Djaldetti M. (1988) X-ray microanalysis of the fingernails in term and preterm infants. *Pediatr. Dermatol.* **5**, 184–186.

Sueki H., Nozaki S., Fujisawa R. *et al.* (1989) Glycosylated proteins of skin, nail and hair: Application as an index for long-term control of diabetes mellitus. *J. Dermatol.* **16**, 103–110.

Suzuki O., Hattori H. & Asano M. (1984) Nails as useful materials for detection of metamphetamine or amphetamine abuse. *Forensic Sci. Int.* **24**, 9–16.

Suzuki S., Inoue T., Hori H. & Inayama S. (1989) Analysis of methamphetamine in hair, nail, sweat and saliva by mass fragmentography. *J. Anal. Toxicol.* **13**, 176–178.

Van Noord P.A.H., Collette H.J.A., Maas M.J. & de Waard F. (1987) Selenium levels in nails of premenopausal breast cancer patients assessed prediagnostically in a cohort-nested case-referent study among women screened in the DOM project. *Int. J. Epidemiol.* **16** (suppl), 318–322.

Wilhelm M., Hafner D., Lombeck I. & Ohnesorge F.K. (1991) Monitoring of cadmium, copper, lead and zinc status in young children using toenails: comparison with scalp hair. *Sci. Total Environ.* **103**, 199–207.

Zaias N. (1990) *The Nail in Health and Disease*, 2nd edn. Appleton & Lange, Norwalk, CN.

Physical properties of nails

Strength

The strength and physical character of the nail plate are attributable to both its constituents and design. The features of design worthy of note are the double curvature, in transverse and longitudinal axes and the flexibility of the ventral plate compared with the dorsal aspect. The first provides rigidity, whereas the latter allows moderate flexion deformity and slightly less extension. The dorsal matrix produces corneocytes that contribute to the shininess of the nail plate – when it is absent due to trauma or disease, the nail has a rough surface.

Measuring nail strength

Several techniques have been developed to study the physical properties of nails (Baden, 1970; Maloney & Paquette,

1977; Finlay *et al.*, 1980). Maloney and Paquette's studies showed changes of tensile, flexural and tearing strength with age, sex and the digit from which the nail derived. Finlay *et al.* devised a 'nail flexometer' able to repeatedly flex longitudinal nail sections through 90°, recording the number it took to fracture the nail. In this way, the strength could be quantified. They noted that the immersion of nails in water for an hour increased their weight by 21%. It also made them significantly more flexible. After 2 h, the flexibility was still increasing, whilst the water content reached a plateau. Mineral oil had no effect on flexibility, although it could act to maintain some of the flexibility imbued by water. This principle is applied in the treatment of onychoschizia, where repeated hydration and drying of the nail plate results in splitting at the free edge (Wallis *et al.*, 1991). Splitting can be partially overcome by applications of emollient after soaking the nails in water. The use of nail varnish can also decrease water loss (Spruit, 1971).

Permeability

The degree of nail plate swelling in alkali has been suggested as an index of disease (Zaun & Becker, 1976). Normal, onychomycotic and psoriatic nails differ in the time it takes them to stop swelling, and what percentage volume increase they sustain.

Nail permeability is relevant to topical drugs. Transonychial water loss can be measured *in vivo* (Spruit, 1971; Jemec *et al.*, 1989; Johnson, 1991) but drug penetration assay is more complicated. The simplest method is to use cadaver nails. Using this method, the permeability coefficient for water has been estimated at 16.5×10^{-3} cm/h and that for ethanol, 5.8×10^{-3} cm/h (Walters *et al.*, 1983, 1985a,b). This demonstrates that the hydrated nail is more permeable to water than to alcohol and behaves like a hydrogel of high ionic strength to polar and semipolar alcohols. Combining alcohols with water may increase the permeation by the alcohol.

In spite of the high water permeability of the nail (10 times that of the skin), there is possibly a parallel lipid pathway that allows permeation of hydrophobic molecules (Walters, 1985b). The dense matrix of keratin and as sociated proteins is considered an obstacle to DMSO penetration in the nail plate, contrasting with its easier access through skin (Walters, 1985b). However, it appears to facilitate the penetration of some topical antimycotics (Stüttgen & Baver, 1982). Some medicated lacquers are also able to penetrate sufficiently to be of clinical use, even though their access is not increased by abrading the dorsal surface of the nail plate (Ceschin-Roques *et al.*, 1991; Mensing & Splanemann, 1991).

In a study of topical application of sodium pyrithione, Mayer *et al.* (1992) found only insignificant amounts in the systemic circulation. Munro and Shuster (1992) have shown that drugs can penetrate rapidly into the distal nail plate via the nail bed.

Radiation penetration

The permeability of the nail plate to radiation has both advantages and drawbacks. It is the basis for treating 20 nail dystrophy with topical PUVA (Halkier–Sørensen, 1990) and also the cause of photo-onycholysis. This may be in association with photosensitizing drugs (Baran & Juhlin, 1987). Benign longitudinal melanonychia can complicate photo-therapy for psoriasis; less commonly nail bed pigmentation develops (Beltrani & Scher, 1991).

Chronic X-irradiation is associated with carcinoma *in situ* and invasive squamous cell carcinoma (Onukak, 1980). The polydactylous form of Bowen's disease is commonly related to some source of radiation (Baran & Gormley, 1987). Parker and Diffey (1983) have investigated the transmission of light through the toenails of cadavers. Examining wavelengths between 300 and 600 nm, it appears that transmission at the shorter wavelength is minimal; this corresponds to UVB. If the nail plate is acting as a sunscreen it is fortuitous, but the character of the toenails studied may not be the same as fingernails, which are more commonly exposed.

References

Baden H.P. (1970) The physical properties of nail. *J. Invest. Dermatol.* **55**, 115.

Baran R. & Gormley D.E. (1987) Polydactylous Bowen's disease of the nail. *J. Am. Acad. Dermatol.* **17**, 201–204.

Baran R. & Juhlin L. (1987) Drug induced photo-onycholysis. *J. Am. Acad. Dermatol.* **17**, 1012–1016.

Beltrani V. & Scher R. (1991) Evaluation and management of melanonychia striata in a patient receiving phototherapy. *Arch. Dermatol.* **127**, 319–320.

Ceschin-Roques C.G., Hanel H., Pruja-Bougaret S.M., Luc J., Vandermander J. & Michel G. (1991) Ciclopirox nail lacquer 8%: in vivo penetration into and through nails. *Skin Pharmacol.* **4**, 89–94.

Finlay A.F., Frost P., Keith A.C. & Snipes W. (1980) An as sessment of factors influencing flexibility of human fingernails. *Br. J. Dermatol.* **103**, 357–365.

Halkier–Sørensen L., Cramers M. & Kragballe K. (1990) Twenty-nail dystrophy treated with topical PUVA. *Acta Derm. Venereol (Stockh)* **70**, 510–511.

Jemec G.B.E., Agner T. & Serup J. (1989) Transonychial water loss: relation to sex, age and nail plate thickness. *Br. J. Dermatol.* **121**, 441–446.

Johnson M. (1991) The formation and permeability of the human nail plate. D.Phil. Thesis, Univ. of Newcastle, UK.

Maloney M.J. & Paquette E.G. (1977) The physical properties of fingernails. I. Apparatus for physical measurements. *J. Soc. Com. Chem.* **28**, 415.

Mayer P.R., Couch R.C., Erickson M.K., Wooldridge C.B. & Brazzell R.K. (1992) Topical and systemic absorption of sodium pyrithione following topical application to the nails of the rhesus monkey. *Skin Pharmacol.* **5**, 154–159.

Mensing H. & Splanemann V. (1991) Evaluation of the antimycotic activity of the pathological substance under the nail after treatment with RO 14-4767 Nail Lacquer. *Proc. 1st Congress EADV Congress*, pp. 921–922. Blackwell Scientific Publications, Oxford.

Munro C.S. & Shuster S. (1992) The route of rapid access of drugs to the distal nail plate. *Acta Dermatol. Venereol.* **72**, 387–388.

Onukak E.E. (1980) Squamous cell carcinoma of the nail bed. Diagnosis and therapeutic problems. *Br. J. Surg.* **67**, 893–895.

Parker S.G. & Diffey B.L. (1983) The transmission of optical radiation through human nails. *Br. J. Dermatol.* **108**, 11–16.

Spruit D. (1971) Measurement of water vapour loss through the human nail in vivo. *J. Invest. Dermatol.* **56**, 359–361.

Spruit D. (1972) The effect of nail polish on hydration of the fingernail. *Am. Cosmet. Perfumery* **87**, 57–58.

Stüttgen G. & Bauer E. (1982) Bioavailability, skin and nail penetration of topically applied antimycotics. *Mykosen.* **25**, 74–80.

Wallis M.S., Bowen W.R. & Guin J.D. (1991) Pathogenesis of onychoschizia (lamellar dystrophy) *J. Am. Acad. Dermatol.* **24**, 44–48.

Walters K.A., Flynn G.L. & Marvel J.R. (1983) Physicochemical characterisation of the human nail: permeation pattern for water and the homologous alcohols and differences with respect to the stratum corneum. *J. Pharm. Pharmacol.* **35**, 28–33.

Walters K.A., Flynn G.L. & Marvel J.R. (1985a) Physicochemical characterisation of the human nail: solvent effects on the permeation of homologous alcohols. *J. Pharm. Pharmacol.* 37, 771–775.

Walters R.A., Flynn G.L. & Marvel J.R. (1985b) Penetration of the human nail plate: effects of vehicle pH on permeation of miconazole. *J. Pharm. Pharmacol.* 37, 498–499.

Zaun H. & Becker H. (1976) Die Quelleigenschaften von Nagelmaterial in Natronlauge bei Bestimmug mit einer standardisierten Methode. *Ärztl. Kosmetologie.* **6**, 115–119.

Imaging of the nail apparatus

Radiology

X-ray reveals little of the soft structures of the nail unit under normal circumstances. Most isolated nail dystrophies should be X-rayed prior to surgical exploration. Clues to an exostosis, bone cyst, acro-osteolysis or psoriatic arthropathy might be found. In invasive subungual squamous cell carcinoma up to 55% of patients will have radiological evidence of changes in the underlying phalanx (Lumpkin *et al.*, 1984).

Glomus tumours may provide particular radiological features. Mathis and Schulz (1948) reviewed 15 such tumours on the digit and found that nine had characteristic changes of bony erosion. This was smooth and concave in most cases, but occasionally with a punched out appearance on the phalangeal tuft. Supplementation of routine X-rays with arteriography may reveal a star-shaped telangiectatic zone (Camirand & Giroux, 1970). More recently magnetic resonance imaging (MRI) has proven a very satisfying method of locating the tumour, particularly where there is diagnostic difficulty (Jablon *et al.*, 1990; Holzberg, 1992; Goettman *et al.*, 1994); Zemtsov and Lorig (1991) also showed MRI to be useful in a variety of cutaneous neoplasms.

Xeroradiography is another imaging method for soft tissue lesions although there is no constructive literature applied particularly to the nail apparatus.

Ultrasound

Ultrasound has been used in the nail unit both as a research tool and to aid clinical diagnosis. Finlay *et al.* (1987, 1990) used a 20 MHz pulse echo ultrasound to measure nail thickness *in vivo*, proximally and distally. The latter measurement correlated well with a micrometer gauge measurement of the free edge. Pulse transmission time was reduced by 8.8% distally, in comparison to the proximal measurement. This implies that the nail becomes thinner as it emerges, which is contrary to findings on avulsed nails (see nail growth). They also found that the nails ranked in thickness sequentially around the hand, with the thumb being top and the little finger bottom.

Jemec and Serup's (1989) study of cadaver nails, *in situ* and avulsed, showed that nail desiccation destroyed the correlation between ultrasound thickness measurements and screwgauge micrometer. This could have significance in quantification when the water content of nails can vary by 10%.

Clinically, high frequency ultrasound has been used in the diagnosis of glomus tumours. Fornage examined 12 patients and could depict the tumour in nine. The resolution of his transducer meant that lesions smaller than 3 mm could not be seen (Fornage, 1988).

Photography

Many sophisticated systems are available for taking good photographs of the nail unit. Whilst their function might be sophisticated, their operation should be simple. It is not possible to deal with complicated equipment and tend to patients at the same time. The essentials involve a 1:1 macrolens, with a further magnifying filter if great detail within the nail unit is desired. This can be part of a zoom or supplemented by a further 50 mm lens. If one has a mobile system, a hand-held flash is necessary, which is usually superior to a ring flash. It gives greater flexibility than the ring flash and allows oblique lighting if needed. However, in general, the light should be directed from the tip of the finger up the arm to avoid shadows.

As with all medical photography, it is necessary to run off several films with practise shots at different settings and on different coloured skins. A dark, matt background cloth is preferable.

Light

A good pocket torch is useful in the diagnostic transillumination of a myxoid cyst. Transillumination (Goldman, 1962) should also be used to distinguish between intrinsic nail plate chromonychia and surface changes. Wood's light may enhance the colour changes, induced by tetracycline and give a yellow fluorescence. Demethylchlortetracycline appears reddish, and *Pseudomonas*, yellowish-green: atebrine gives a yellow colour.

Polarized light can be helpful in the examination of the underside of nails. This is done with the aid of a light microscope to identify the longitudinal ridge pattern (Apolinar & Rowe, 1980).

Laser doppler can be used to assess the blood flow in the nail unit.

References

Apolinar E. & Rowe W.F. (1980) Examination of human finger nail ridges by means of polarized light. *J. Forensic Sci. CA* **25**, 156–161.

Camirand P. & Giroux J.M. (1970) Subungual glomus tumour. Radiological manifestations. *Arch. Dermatol.* **102**, 677–679.

Finlay A.Y., Moseley H. & Duggan T.C. (1987) Ultrasound transmission time: an in vivo guide to nail thickness. *Br. J. Dermatol.* **117**, 765–770.

Finlay A.Y., Western B. & Edwards C. (1990) Ultrasound velocity in human fingernail and effects of hydration: validation of in vivo nail thickness measurement techniques. *Br. J. Dermatol.* **123**, 365–373.

Fornage B.D. (1988) Glomus tumours in the fingers: Diagnosis with ultrasound. *Radiology* **167**, 183–185.

Holzberg M. (1992) Glomus tumor of the nail. *Arch. Dermatol.* **128**, 160–162.

Goettman S., Drapé J.L., Idy–Peretti I. *et al.* (1994) Magnetic resonance imaging: a new tool in the diagnosis of nail tumours. *Br. J. Dermatol.*, in press.

Goldman L. (1962) Transillumination of the fingertip as aid in examination of nail changes. *Archiv. Derm. Chicago* **85**, 644.

Jablon M., Horowitz A. & Bernstein D.A. (1990) Magnetic resonance imaging of a glomus tumor of the finger tip. *J. Hand Surg.* **15A**, 507–509.

Jemec G.B.E. & Serup J. (1989) Ultrasound of the human nail plate. *Arch. Dermatol.* **125**, 643–646.

Lumpkin L.R., Rosen T. & Tschen J.A. (1984) Subungual squamous cell carcinoma. *J. Am. Acad. Dermatol.* **11**, 735–738.

Mathis W.H. & Schulz M.D. (1948) Roentgen diagnosis of glomus tumours. *Radiology* **51**, 71–76.

Zemtsov A. & Lorig R. (1991) Magnetic resonance imaging of cutaneous neoplasms. *J. Dermatol. Surg. Oncol.* **17**, 416–422.

Chapter 2
Physical Signs

R. BARAN & R. P. R. DAWBER

Modifications of nail configuration
- Clubbing
- Koilonychia
- Transverse overcurvature
- Dolichonychia
- Brachyonychia (short nails)
- Parrot beak nails
- Claw-like nails
- Circumferential nail
- Macro- and micronychia
- Worn-down nails
- Onychatrophy
- Anonychia
- Hypertrophy
  - Pachyonychia, onychauxis
  - Onychogryphosis

Modifications of nail surface
- Longitudinal lines
- Transverse groove (Beau's lines) and onychomadesis
- Pitting
- Trachyonychia
- Lamellar splitting (onychoschizia lamellina)
- Elkonyxis

Modifications of nail plate and soft tissue attachments
- Pterygium
- Nail shedding
- Onycholysis
- Subungual hyperkeratosis

Modifications of perionychial tissue

Modifications of nail consistency
- Hard
- Soft
- Brittle
- Friable

Colour changes (chromonychia or dyschromia)

Modifications in the configuration of the nail

Clubbing or hippocratic digits

Clubbed fingers have been known since the first century BC, when Hippocrates first described the sign in patients suffering from empyema. The morphological changes combine (1) increased longitudinal and transverse curvature of the nails, and (2) enlargement of the soft tissue structures, strictly confined to the fingertips (Coury, 1960). The increased nail curvature which characterizes this disorder affects all the nails, but has a predilection for the radial three digits.

The appearance of the curvature is variable; the deformity may be fusiform, shaped like a bird's beak, or clubbed. These types can be found in all forms of clubbing. There are four main categories of finger clubbing.

The simple type

This is the most common category. It has several elements.

1 Increased nail curvature with a transverse furrow which separates it from the rest of the nail both in the early stage and on resolution. The onset is usually gradual and painless, except in some cases of carcinoma of the lung where clubbing may develop abruptly and may be associated with severe pain.

2 Hypertrophy of the soft parts of the terminal segment due to a firm, elastic, oedematous infitration of the pulp, which may spread on to the dorsal surface forming a periungual swelling.

3 Hyperplasia of the dermal fibrovascular tissue which readily extends to involve the adjacent matrix. This accounts for one of the earliest signs of clubbing, i.e. an abnormal mobility of the nail base which can be rocked back and forth giving the impression that it is floating on a soft oedematous pad (Lovibond, 1938). The increased vascularity is responsible for the slow return of colour when the nail is pressed.

4 Local cyanosis, present in 60% of the cases described by Coury (1960).

In the early stages clubbing may involve one hand only, though eventually both hands become affected symmetrically. Several stages of clubbing or acropachy may be distinguished: suspected, slight, average and severe. In practice the degree of the deformity may be determined by Lovibond's 'profile sign' which measures the angle between the curved nail plate and the proximal nail fold when the finger is viewed from the radial aspect. This is normally 160° but exceeds 180° in clubbing (Fig. 2.1). With a modified profile sign one measures the angle between the middle and the terminal phalanx at the interphalangeal joint (Curth *et al.*, 1961). In normal fingers the distal phalanx forms an almost straight (180°) extension of the middle phalanx, whereas in severe clubbing this angle may be reduced to 160° or even 140° (Fig. 2.2). However

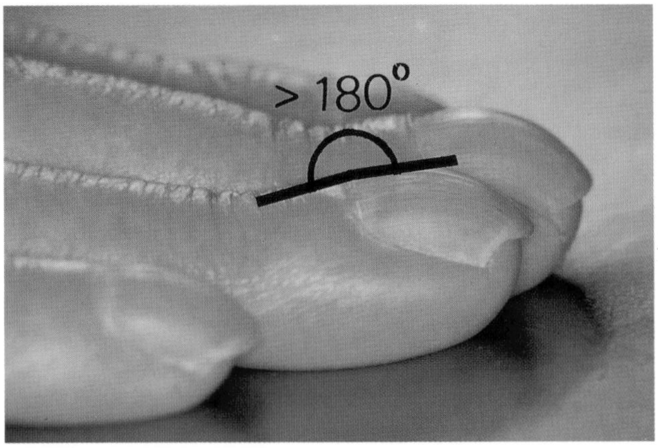

Fig. 2.1. Clubbing – Lovibond's 'profile' sign: the angle is normally less than 160° but exceeds 180° in clubbing.

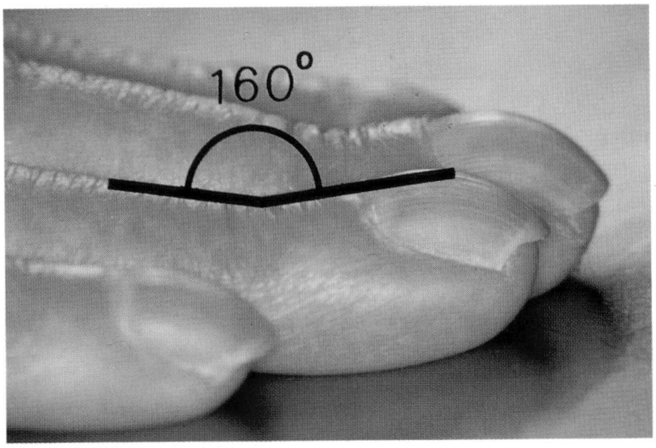

Fig. 2.2. Clubbing – Curth's modified profile sign.

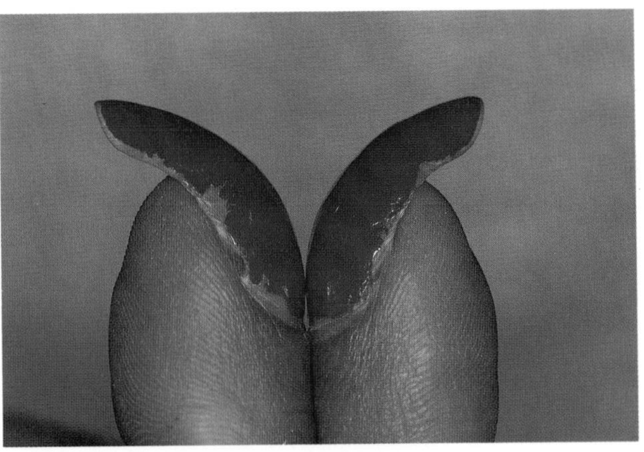

(a)

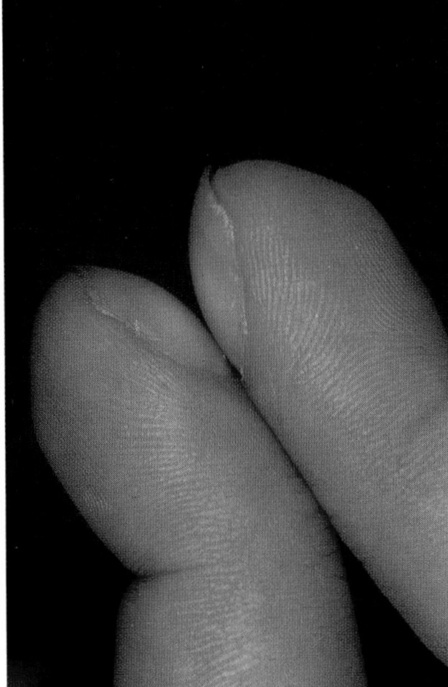

(b)

Fig. 2.3. (a & b) Clubbing – Schamroth's sign. 'Window' lost in clubbing, with prominant distal angle between the ends of the nail.

the best indicator may well be the measurement of the hyponychial angle (Regan *et al.*, 1967). This may be assessed either clinically or with the aid of a clubbing shadowgraph (Bentley *et al.*, 1976) which may allow serial measurements of the angles to record any progression of finger clubbing. Other methods are described by Blumsohn (1981). In fact fixing the limits of true clubbing in minimal cases is ultimately a matter of clinical sense and habit (Coury, 1960); therefore a simple clinical method was adopted by Schamroth (1976). In the normal individual a distinct aperture or 'window', usually diamond shaped, is formed at the base of the nail beds; early clubbing obliterates this window and demonstrates a prominent distal angle between the ends of the nails (Lampe & Kagan, 1983) (Fig. 2.3).

Radiological changes occur in less than one-fifth of cases. They include phalangeal demineralization and irregular thickening of the cortical diaphysis. Ungual tufts generally show considerable variations and may be prominent in advanced stages of the disease. Atrophy may be present.

Congenital clubbed fingers may be accompanied by abnormalities and deformities such as hyperkeratosis of the palms and soles, and cortical hypertrophy of the long bones. Familial clubbing may occur in conjunction with familial, hypertrophic osteoarthropathy; for some authors, simple clubbing is regarded as a mild form of the latter (Curth *et al.*, 1961). Isolated watch-glass nails without their accompanying deformities are also constitutionally determined.

Very rare cases of unilateral hippocratic nails have been reported due to obstructed circulation, causalgia (Saunders & Hanna, 1988), oedema of the soft tissues and dystrophies of the affected parts. Asymmetric clubbing may be a manifestation of sarcoid bone disease (Hashmi & Kaplan, 1992).

The pathological process which appears to be responsible for clubbing and its associated changes, is increasing blood flow as a result of vasodilatation rather than hyperplasia of vessels in the nail bed (Currie & Gallagher, 1988). In Bigler's series (1958), a thickness of the nail bed of the thumb greater than 2.0 mm was found only in clubbed digits.

Hypertrophic osteoarthropathy

This disorder may be divided into two categories:
1 hypertrophic pulmonary osteoarthropathy;
2 hypertrophic osteoarthropathy confined to the lower extremities.

Hypertrophic pulmonary osteoarthropathy (Bamberger–Pierre–Marie syndrome)

This disorder is characterized by the six following signs (Coury, 1960).
1 Clubbing of the nails on hands and feet.
2 Hypertrophy of the upper and lower extremities, which is similar to the deformity found in acromegaly (spade-like enlargement of the hands).
3 Joint manifestations with pseudo-inflammatory, symmetrical, painful arthropathy of the large limb joints, especially those of the lower limbs. This syndrome is almost pathognomonic of malignant chest tumours, especially lung carcinoma, mesotheliomata of the pleura and less commonly bronchiectasis. Associated gynaecomastia is a further indication of malignancy.
4 There may be bone changes which consist of bilateral, proliferative periostitis with a translucent thin line between the periosteal reaction and the thickened cortex especially over the distal ends of the long bones (Fisher *et al.*, 1964). Moderate, diffuse decalcification may also be present.
5 Peripheral neurovascular disorders are common, such as local cyanosis and paraesthesia.
6 The pain and swelling often disappear with successful therapy of the underlying disease process.

Hypertrophic osteoarthropathy confined to the lower extremities

Recurrent infections of the lower extremities after an aortofemoral bypass graft is associated with pain in the legs and X-ray findings of severe hypertrophic osteoarthropathy (Gibson *et al.*, 1974; Sorin *et al.*, 1980; Stock, 1986). This condition is restricted to the legs when the flow of blood is reversed through a patent ductus arteriosus or when sepsis occurs in the presence of an abdominal aortic prosthesis with an intestinal fistula (Stein & Little, 1978).

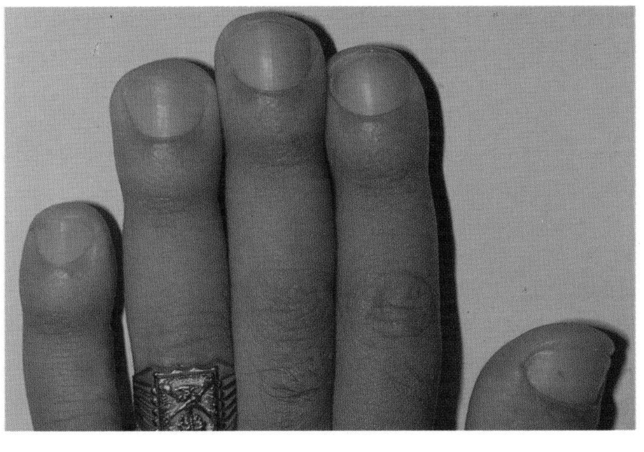

Fig. 2.4. (a) Clubbing in pachydermoperiostosis (courtesy of P.Y. Venencie, Paris).

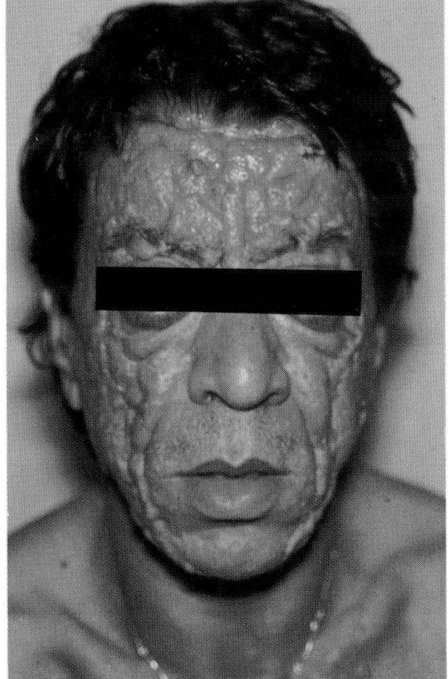

Fig. 2.4. (b) Pachydermoperiostosis, severe skin changes.

Pachydermoperiostosis (Touraine–Solente–Golé syndrome) (Touraine *et al.*, 1935)

Pachydermoperiostosis or idiopathic hypertrophic osteoarthropathy is very rare. In most of the reported cases the digital changes begin at or about time of puberty. The ends of fingers and toes are bulbous and often grotesque, with hyperhidrosis of the hands and the feet. This clubbing stops abruptly at the distal interphalangeal joint (Rimoin, 1965) (Fig. 2.4(a) & (b)). In this type the lesions of the fingertips are clinically identical to those of hypertrophic pulmonary osteoarthropathy. However, in pachydermoperiostosis, the thickened cortex appears homogeneous radiologically and does not encroach on the medullary space (Fisher *et al.*, 1964). Acro-osteolysis of the distal phalanges has been reported with increased blood flow through clubbed fingers (Fam *et al.*, 1983). The pachydermal change of the extremities and face, with furrowing and oiliness of the skin, is the most characteristic feature of this disorder (Fig. 2.4(b)). Nevertheless in hypertrophic pulmonary osteoarthropathy there may be facial skin and scalp changes which are indistinguishable from those seen in primary pachydermoperiostosis; this could be explained by a common genetic factor (Vogl & Goldfischer, 1962; Lindmaier *et al.*, 1989). The differential diagnosis includes acromegaly, which enhances tufting of the terminal phalanges, but does not cause acro-osteolysis in contrast to pachydermoperiostosis (Guyer *et al.*, 1978). Thyroid acropachy is usually associated with exophthalmus, pretibial myxoedema and disturbed thyroid function.

The shell nail syndrome

First reported by Cornelius and Shelley (1967), this syndrome occurs in some cases of bronchiectasis and is similar to clubbing, but there is associated atrophy of the nail bed and the underlying bone.

Table 2.1. Classification of clubbing

Idiopathic forms

Hereditary and congenital forms, sometimes associated with other anomalies (see Table 9.5) Familial and racial forms (black people, North Africans)

Acquired forms

1 Thoracic organ disorders (involved in about 80% of cases of clubbing, often with the common denominator of hypoxia)
- (a) Bronchopulmonary diseases, especially chronic and infective bronchiectasis, abscess and cyst of the lung, pulmonary tuberculosis
  - Sarcoidosis, pulmonary fibrosis, emphysema, Ayerza's syndrome, chronic pulmonary venous congestion, asthma in infancy
  - Blastomycosis, pneumonia, pneumocystis carinii
- (b) Thoracic tumours:
  - Primary or metastatic bronchopulmonary cancers, pleural tumours, mediastinal tumours (an infrequent cause), Hodgkin's disease, lymphoma, pseudo-tumour due to oesophageal dilatation
- (c) Cardiovascular diseases:
  - Congenital heart disease associated with cyanosis (rarely non-cyanotic)
  - Thoracic vascular malformations: stenoses and arteriovenous aneurysms
  - Osler's disease (subacute bacterial endocarditis)
  - Congestive cardiac failure
  - Myxoma
  - Raynaud's syndrome, erythromelalgia, Maffucci's syndrome

continued

Table 2.1. *Continued*

2 Disorders of the alimentary tract (5% of cases):
- (a) Oesophageal, gastric and colonic cancer
- (b) Diseases of the small intestine
- (c) Colonic diseases with:
  - Amoebiasis and inflammatory states of the colon
  - Ulcerative colitis
  - Familial polyposis, Gardner's syndrome
  - Ascardiasis
- (d) Chronic active hepatitis
  - Primary or secondary cirrhoses

3 Endocrine origin:
- POEMS syndrome (Myers, 1991)
- Graves' disease (pretibial myxoedema, exophthalmus and finger clubbing)

4 Haematological causes:
- Primary polycythaemia or secondary polycythaemia associated with hypoxia
- Poisoning by phosphorus, arsenic, alcohol, mercury or beryllium

5 Hypervitaminosis A

6 Malnutrition, kwashiorkor

7 Syringomyelia

8 Lupus erythematosus

9 Unilateral or limited to a few digits:
- Subluxation of the shoulder (with paralysis of the brachial phexus), median nerve neuritis
- Causalgia (Saunders & Hanna, 1988)
- Pancoast–Tobias syndrome
- Aneurysm of the aorta or the subclavian artery
- Sarcoidosis (Hashmi & Kaplan, 1992)
- Tophaceous gout

10 Confined to the lower extremities: abdominal aortic graft with sepsis

11 Isolated forms:
- Local injury, whitlow, lymphangitis
- Subungual epidermoid inclusions, osteoid osteoma, enchondroma

12 Transitory form:
- Physiological in the newborn child (due to reversal of the circulation at birth)

13 Occupational acro-osteolysis (exposure to vinyl choride)

References

Bentley D., Moore A. & Schwachman H. (1976) Finger clubbing: a quantitative survey by analysis of the shadowgraph. *Lancet* **ii**, 164.

Bigler F.C. (1958) The morphology of clubbing. *Am. J. Pathol.* **34**, 237.

Blumsohn D. (1981) Clubbing of the fingers with special reference to Schamroth's diagnostic method. *Heart and Lung* **10**, 1069–1072.

Cornelius C.E. & Shelley W.B. (1967) Shell nail syndrome associated with bronchiectasis. *Arch. Dermatol.* **96**, 694.

Coury C. (1960) Hippocratic fingers and hypertrophic osteoarthropathy. *Br. J. Dis. Chest* **54**, 202.

Currie A.E. & Gallagher P.J. (1988) The pathology of clubbing: vascular changes in the nail bed. *Br. J. Dis. Chest* **82**, 382–385.

Curth H.O., Firschein I.L. & Alphert M. (1961) Familial clubbed fingers. *Arch. Dermatol.* **83**, 829.

Fam A.G., Chin-Sang H. & Ramsay C.A. (1983) Pachydermoperiostosis: scintigraphic, thermographic, plethysmographic, and capillaroscopic observations. *Ann. Rheum. Dis.* **42**, 98–102.

Fisher D.S., Singer D.H. & Feldman S.M. (1964) Clubbing: A review with emphasis on hereditary acropachy. *Medicine* **43**, 459.

Gibson T., Joye J. & Schumauer H.R. (1974) Localized hypertrophic osteoarthropathy with abdominal aortic prosthesis and infection. *Ann. Intern. Med.* **81**, 556–557.

Guyer P.B., Brunton F.J. & Wren M.W.G. (1978) Pachydermoperiostosis with acro-osteolysis. A report of five cases. *J. Bone Joint Surg.* **60B**, 219.

Hashmi S. & Kaplan D. (1992) Asymmetric clubbing as a manifestation of sarcoid bone disease. *Am. J. Med.* **93**, 471.

Lampe R.M. & Kagan A. (1983) Detection of clubbing—Schamroth's sign. *Clin. Pediatr.* **22**, 125.

Lindmaier A., Raff M., Seidl G. *et al.* (1989) Pachydermoperiostose (Klinik, Klassifikation und Pathogenese) *Hautarzt* **40**, 752–757.

Lovibond J.L. (1938) Diagnosis of clubbed fingers. *Lancet* **i**, 363.

Myers B.M. (1991) POEMS syndrome with idiopathic flushing mimicking carcinoid syndrome. *Am. J. Med.* **90**, 646–648.

Regan G.M., Tagg B. & Thomson M.L. (1967) Subjective assessment and objective measurement of finger clubbing. *Lancet* **i**, 530.

Rimoin D.L. (1965) Pachydermoperiostosis (idiopathic clubbing and periostosis). *New Engl. J. Med.* **272**, 923.

Saunders P.R. & Hanna M. (1988) Unilateral clubbing of fingers associated with causalgia. *Br. Med. J.* **297**, 1635.

Schamroth L. (1976) Personal experience. *S. Afr. Med. J.* **50**, 297–300.

Sorin S.B., Askari A. & Rhodes R.S. (1980) Hypertrophic osteoarthropathy of the lower extremities as a manifestation of arterial graft septis. *Arthr. Rheum.* **23**, 768–770.

Stein H.B. & Little H.A. (1978) Localized hypertrophic osteoarthropathy in the presence of an abdominal aortic prosthesis. *CMA J.* **118**, 947–948.

Stock C.M. (1986) Trommel schlegelfinger. Ein Symptom. *Z. Hautkr.* **61**, 1745–1748.

Touraine A., Solente G. & Gole A. (1935) Un syndrome ostéodermopathique, la pachydermie plicaturée avec pachypériostose des extrémités. *Presse Medicale* **43**, 1830.

Vogl A. & Goldfischer S. (1962) Primary or idiopathic osteoarthropathy. *Am. J. Med.* **33**, 166.

Koilonychia (Table 2.2)

Koilonychia is the converse of clubbing, the nail being concave with the edges everted, the so-called 'spoon nail' (Fig. 2.5). This dystrophy, which becomes more apparent when the nail is viewed laterally, normally affects several fingers, especially the thumb. All the fingers may be involved and, less frequently, the toes. The underlying tissues may be healthy or affected by subungual hyperkeratosis, which is clearly visible at the margin. This would suggest psoriasis, or an occupational origin of the deformity; the first three digits are frequently involved in the latter case. The nail, which may be normal, thinned or thickened and sometimes soft, has a smooth surface when the koilonychia is idiopathic. Longitudinal splitting with koilonychia in each of the separated parts of the nail plate appears in some cases of lichen striatus, and in certain inherited conditions (Fig. 2.6). Some or all of the fingernails may, in contrast, present with a central, longitudinal ridge in place of the fissure. In the trichoonychotic hidrotic ectodermal dysplasias, for example, there is a peculiar longitudinal fold increasing distally. This divides the nail plate with separated koilonychia on each side and without abnormalities elsewhere (Fig. 2.6).

The 'serrated koilonychia' syndrome (Runne, 1978) combines spoon nail and transverse grooves involving all the digits; steroid injections in the proximal nail fold lead to temporary improvement.

The petaloid nail is a variant of an early stage of koilonychia, in which flattening of the nail is the

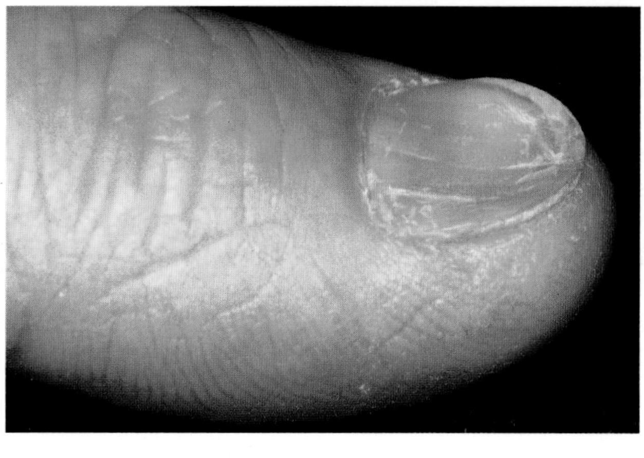

Fig. 2.5. Koilonychia.

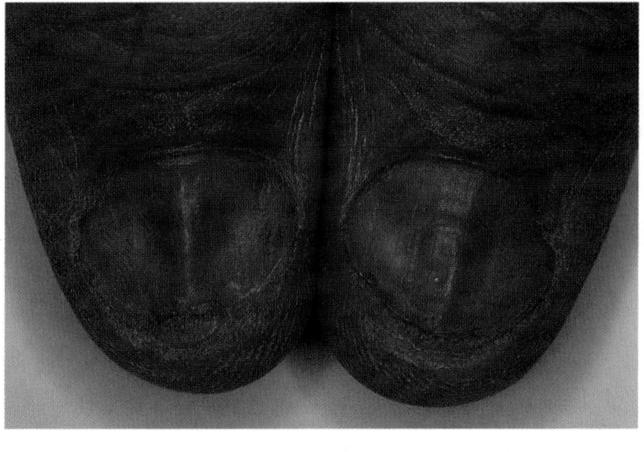

Fig. 2.6. Koilonychia in trichonychotic hidrotic ectodermal dysplasia.

characteristic sign. A variety of koilonychia is the type known as 'ongle en fermoir d'epingle de nourrice', in which the deformity is shaped like the catch on a safety pin. Koilonychia is commonly found in the toenails of normal children but this defect usually disappears spontaneously. In infants there is a significant correlation between koilonychia and iron deficiency; it may be noted before clinical and laboratory signs of anaemia develop (Hogan & Jones, 1970). Spoon nails can be seen also in haemochromatosis, therefore iron deficiency *per se* is not the cause of the deformity. Cystine content of the nail substance is said to be lower than normal (Jalili & Al-kassab, 1959). Familial cases have been reported (Bergeron & Stone, 1967; Almagor & Haim, 1981) sometimes with associated abnormalities; these include leukonychia (Baran & Achten, 1969; Crosby & Petersen, 1989), onychogryphosis and monilethrix. Koilonychia may be a racial characteristic, seen mainly in Tibetan populations (Anan & Harris, 1988). In Ladakh, koilonychia has been attributed to exposure to cold mud while repairing walls and irrigation canals. It appears that a tendency to koilonychia may be a racial characteristic of the Sherpa population, especially women, and the manual activities play a role in the development of this deformity (Murdoch, 1993). According to Stone (1975), nail changes in clubbing and spooning are the result of an angulation of the matrix secondary to connective tissue changes. Clubbing occurs if the distal portion of the matrix is relatively high compared with the proximal end; in spooning, the distal portion is relatively low compared with the proximal end. The lifting up of the former results from connective tissue proliferation and at times from the increase in vascular flow. The depressed distal portion of the latter may be due to distal, connective tissue anoxia and atrophy. In psoriasis or onychomycosis, the hyperkeratotic reaction in the nail bed exerts an upward pressure which is transmitted to the area of keratinization and results in a spoon nail-type deformity. Minimal expansion of the dorsal aspect of the distal portion of the bony phalanx is capable of producing this effect.

Since koilonychia is frequently found in the thumb, index and middle fingernails, Higashi (1985) believes that it is related to the pressure-bearing function of the fingers. As the distal phalanx is only the heart of the distal portion of the finger, upward pressure causes upward deformation of distal and lateral portion of the nail plate.

Table 2.2. Classification of koilonychia

Idiopathic forms
Hereditary and congenital forms, sometimes occurring with other anomalies
 Fissured nails, in adenoma sebaceum
 Monilethrix; hyperkeratosis of the palm (Meleda type); leukonychia
 Hereditary osteoonychodysplasia (nail–patella syndrome)
 Nezelof's syndrome (immunological defect)
 Oliver–McFerlane syndrome (Zaun *et al.*, 1984)

Acquired forms
Cardiovascular and haematological
 Iron deficiency anaemia (following gastrectomy; Plummer–Vinson syndrome)
 Iron malabsorption by the intestinal mucosa
 Haemaglobinopathy SC
 Polycythaemia
 Haemochromatosis
 Banti's syndrome (the nails heal after splenectomy)
 Coronary disease.
Infections
 Syphilis, fungal diseases
Endocrine forms
 Acromegaly
 Diabetes (Beaven & Brooks, 1984)
 Hypothyroidism
 Thyrotoxicosis
Traumatic and occupational forms
 Petrol, various solvents, engine oils
 Acids and alkalis, thioglycolate (hairdressers)
 Housewives, chimney sweeps, rickshaw boys (toes)
 Nail biting
Avitaminoses (B_2 and especially C)
Dermatoses, Raynaud's disease, connective tissue diseases, lichen planus, acanthosis nigricans, psoriasis alopecia areata
 Porphyria cutanea tarda, Darier's disease, incontinentia pigmenti
Toenails
 Physiological in toes of otherwise normal young children (temporary)
Kidney transplantation
Carpal tunnel syndrome

References

Almagor G. & Haim S. (1981) Familial koilonychia. *Dermatologica* **162**, 400.

Anan I.S. & Harris P. (1988) Koilonychia in Ladakhis. *Br. J. Dermatol.* **119**, 267–268.

Baran R. & Achten G. (1969) Les associations congénitales de koilonychie et de leuconychie totale. *Arch. Belges Dermatol. Syphil.* **XXV**, 13.

Beaven D.W. & Brooks S.E. (1984) *A Colour Atlas of the Nail in Clinical Diagnosis.* Wolfe Medical Books, London.

Bergeron J.R. & Stone O.J. (1967) Koilonychia. A report of familial spoon nails. *Arch. Dermatol.* **95**, 351.

Crosby D.L. & Petersen M.J. (1989) Familial koilonychia. *Cutis* **44**, 209–210.

Higashi N. (1985) Pathogenesis of the spooning. *Hifu* **27**, 29–34.

Hogan G.R. & Jones B. (1970) The relationship of koilonychia and iron deficiency in infants. *J. Pediatr.* 77, 1054.

Jalili M.A. & Al-kassab S. (1959) Koilonychia and cystine content of nail. *Lancet* **ii**, 108–110.

Murdoch D. (1993) Koilonychia in Sherpas. *Br. J. Dermatol.* **128**, 592–593.

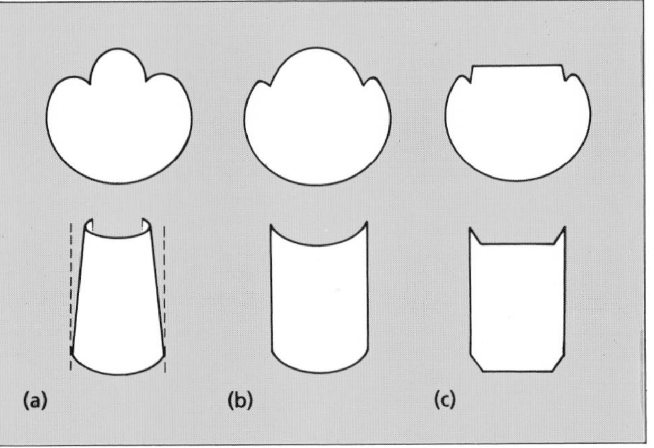

Fig. 2.7. Transverse overcurvature showing the three subtypes: (a) pincer or trumpet nail; (b) tileshaped nail; and (c) plicated nail with sharply angled lateral margins.

Runne U. (1978) Koilonychia serrata Syndrom. *Z. Hautkr.* 53, 623.

Stone O.J. (1975) Spoon nails and clubbing, significance and mechanisms. *Cutis* **16**, 235–241.

Zaun H., Strenger D., Zabransky S. *et al.* (1984) Das Syndrom der langen Wimpern (Trichomegalie Syndrom Oliver-McFerlane). *Hautarzt* 35, 162–165.

Transverse overcurvature of the nail

There are three main types of this condition (Fig. 2.7): the arched, pincer, trumpet or omega nail (Fig. 2.8); the tile-shaped nail; and a third less common variety, the 'plicated' nail (Fig. 2.9).

1 Pincer nail is a dystrophy characterized by transverse overcurvature that increases along the longitudinal axis of the nail and reaches its greatest proportion at the distal part. At this point, the lateral borders tighten around the soft tissues which are pinched without necessarily breaking through the epidermis (Fig. 2.8). In extreme cases, they may join together, forming a tunnel; or they may roll about themselves taking the form of a cone. In certain varieties, the nails are shaped like claws, sometimes resembling pachyonychia congenita. After a while, the soft tissue may actually disappear and this may be accompanied by a resorption of the underlying bone (Cornelius & Shelley, 1968). Pincer nail is probably due to selective widening of the proximal region of the lateral matrix horns by juxta-articular osteophytes. As the shape of the distal matrix does not change, the nail plate assumes a conical shape which rises above the nail bed. As the nail is tightly bound to the periosteum it lifts a traction osteophyte from the dorsum of the underlying phalanx (Haneke, 1992). This morphological abnormality would be no more than a curiosity if the constriction were not occasionally accompanied by pain which is sometimes provoked by the lightest of touch, e.g. the weight of a bedsheet (Baran, 1974). The origin of this dystrophy probably resides in a

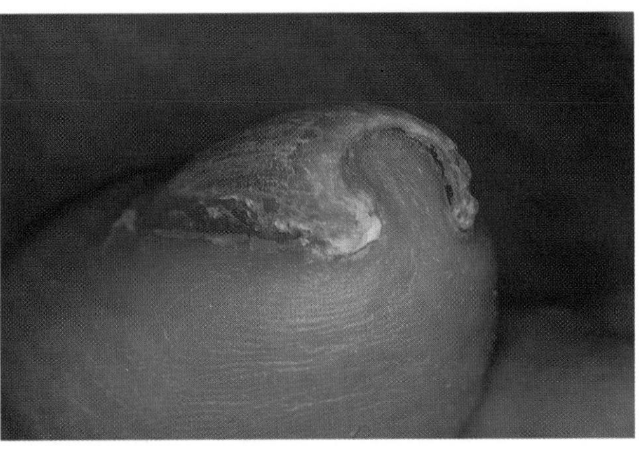

Fig. 2.8. Pincer nail deformity.

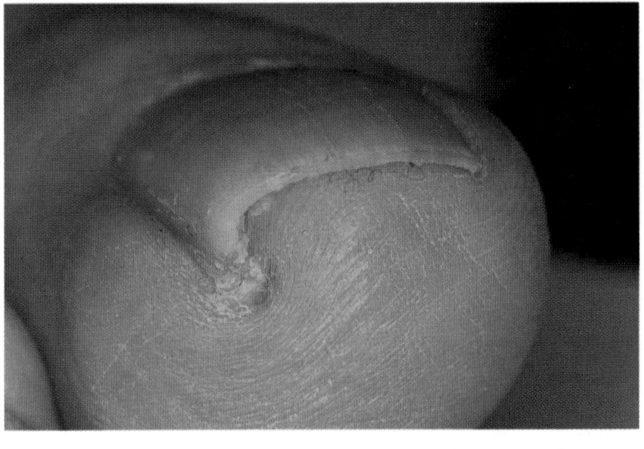

Fig. 2.9. Unilateral variety – may have lateral pincer or plicated lateral change.

developmental anomaly and may be an inherited disorder (Chapman, 1973). Some cases have been attributed to the wearing of ill-fitting shoes. Underlying pathology, such as subungual exostosis in the toes and inflammatory osteoarthritis should always be looked for, especially where the fingers are involved. Higashi (1990) reported on six patients with pincer nail due to tinea unguium. The deformity was cured with oral griseofulvin.

2 The tile-shaped nail presents with an increase in the tranverse curvature; the lateral edges of the nail remain parallel.

3 In the plicated variety the surface of the nail plate is almost flat, while one or both lateral margins are sharply angled forming vertical sides which are parallel (Fig. 2.9).

Although these deformities may be associated with ingrowing nails, inflammatory oedema due to the constriction of the soft tissue is unusual. For treatment, see Chapter 9.

In terms of aetiology and pathogenesis, three different types have to be differentiated.

1 A symmetrical form, often hereditary and seen in several generations of a family and in several family members of the same generation; it is usually seen in toenails with both the great and the lesser nails being affected. It is usually associated with a malalignment of the nail's long axis; the great toenail is deviated laterally, the other nails medially. X-ray films show that the distal phalanx of the big toe also shows a slight lateral deviation, the base of the last phalanx is very wide and exhibits bony outgrowths pointing distally, and there is a small traction osteophyte on the dorsal tuft of the tip of the distal phalanx. Its histological examination reveals amorphous dense osseous material. From proximal to distal, the nail bed epithelium becomes progressively more acanthotic, papillomatous and hyperkeratotic with a marked hypergranulosis and round to oval globules of inspissated serous exudate in the subungual horn. There is also a marked dilatation of capillaries in the tip of the nail bed's papillary dermis (Haneke, 1992).

2 An asymmetrical form, that is acquired and associated with degenerative osteoarthritis of the distal interphalangeal joints of the fingers or foot deformation; this type is more frequently seen in elderly women. Radiography of the big toe also reveals a wide base of the distal phalanx with lateral and medial exostoses and sometimes also irregular subperiostal bone appositions on the processus unguicularis and a small osteophyte on the dorsal aspect of the tip of the distal phalanx.

3 Repeated nail avulsions, injury to the distal phalanx and the nail organ as well as some dermatoses, particularly psoriasis and total dystrophic onychomycosis with secondary shrinking of the nail field may cause transverse overcurvature of the involved nail (Higashi, 1990).

References

Baran R. (1974) Pincer and trumpet nails. *Arch. Dermatol.* **110**, 639.

Chapman R.S. (1973) Overcurvature of the nails. An inherited disorder. *Br. J. Dermatol.* **89**, 211–213.

Cornelius C.E. & Shelley W.B. (1968) Pincer nails syndrome. *Arch. Surg.* **96**, 321.

Haneke E. (1992) Etiopathogenie et traitement de l'hypercourbure transversale de l'ongle du gros orteil. *J. Med. Esthet.* **29**, 123–127.

Higashi N. (1990) Pincer nail due to tinea unguium. *Hifu* **32**, 40–44.

Dolichonychia

Normally the ratio between the length and the width of the nail is 1 ± 0.1. In dolichonychia this is greater: 1.9 (Alkiewicz & Pfister, 1976). It may be seen in Ehlers–Danlos syndrome, in Marfan's syndrome, in association with eunuchoidism or with hypopituitarism.

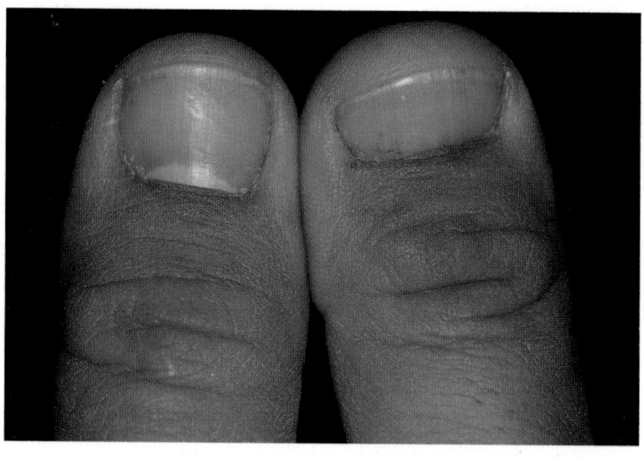

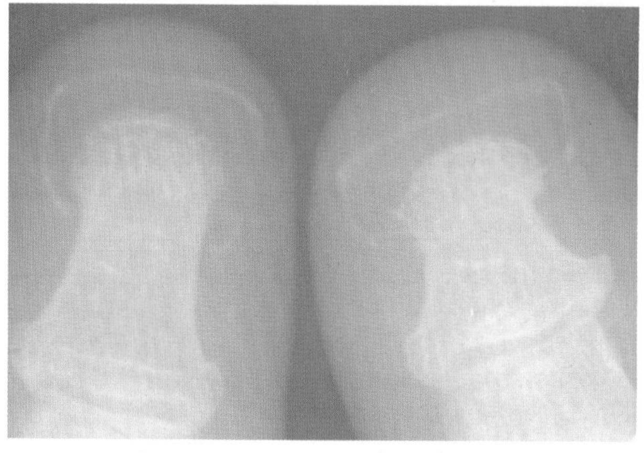

Fig. 2.10. (a) Brachyonychia – unilateral (right). (b) X-ray of (a) showing the shortened terminal phalanx (right).

Reference

Alkiewicz J. & Pfister R. (1976) *Atlas des Nagelkrankheiten*, pp. 52–53. Schattauer Verlag, Stuttgart, New York.

Short nails (brachyonychia) (see acroosteolysis and Table 9.6)

Short nails should be divided into true brachyonychia and raquet nails. The width of the nail plate (and the nail bed) is greater than the length (Fig. 2.10(a)). It may occur in isolation or associated with a shortening of the terminal phalanx (Basset, 1962) (Fig. 2.10(b)). This condition may be acquired in nail biters, or associated with bone resorption in hyperparathyroidism and psoriatic arthropathy. Thickened and large cuticle extending on the nail may mimic brachyonychia.

The 'racquet thumb' is usually inherited as an autosomal dominant trait. All the fingers may be involved. The epiphyses of the terminal phalanx of the thumb are normally closing at the age of 13–14 in girls and slightly later in boys. In individuals with this hereditary defect the epiphyseal line is prematurely obliterated on the affected side at the age of 7–10 years, while it is still present according to age in the normal thumb. Johnson (1966) recorded the syndrome of broad thumbs, broad great toes, facial abnormalities and mental retardation.

Racquet nails have been reported in association with brachydactylia and multiple malignant Spiegler tumours (Tsambaos *et al.*, 1979).

References

Basset H. (1962) Trois formes génotypiques d'ongles courts, le pouce en raquette, les doigts en raquette, les ongles courts simples. *Bull. Soc. Fr. Dermatol. Syphil.* **69**, 15.

Johnson C.F. (1966) Broad thumbs and broad great toes with facial abnormalities and mental retardation. *Pediatrics* **68**, 942.

Tsambaos D., Greither A. & Orfanos C.E. (1979) Multiple malignant Spiegler tumors with brachydactyly and racket-nails. *J. Cut. Pathol.* **6**, 31.

Parrot beak nails

This peculiar, symmetrical overcurvature of the free margin of some fingernails simulates the beak of a parrot (Kandil, 1971; Fig. 2.11(a) & (b)). If the patient trims the affected nails close to the line of separation from the nail bed, no abnormality would be noted clinically.

Soaking the nails in tepid warm water for about 30 min causes this overcurvature to disappear temporarily. Distal hemitorsion of the nail plate observed in porphyria cutanea tarda (Baran, 1981) could be clinically related to the parrot beak nail.

References

Baran R. (1981) Porphyria. In: *The Nail*, ed. Pierre M., p. 51. Churchill Livingstone, Edinburgh.

Kandil E. (1971) Parrot beak nails. *Leb. Med. J.* **24**, 433–436.

Claw-like nail

One or both little toenails are often rounded like a claw. This condition predominates in women wearing high heels and narrow shoes and is often associated with the development of hyperkeratosis such as calluses on the feet. Congenital claw-like finger- and toenails have been reported (Egawa, 1977). Claw nails may be curved dorsally showing a concave upper surface. This condition resembles onychogryphosis or post-traumatic hook nail (Chapters 9 and 10).

Reference

Egawa T. (1977) Congenital claw-like fingers and toes. *Plast. Reconstr. Surg.* **59**, 569.

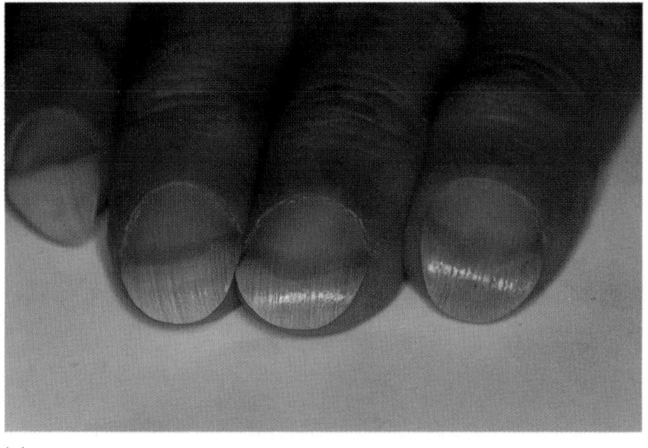

(a)

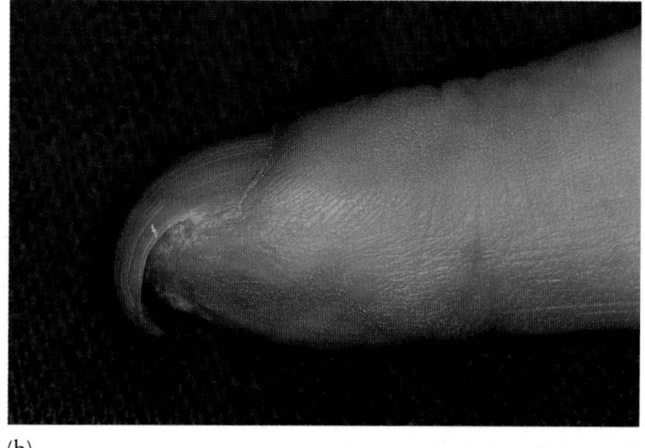

(b)

Fig. 2.11. Parrot beak nails – different degrees between (a) and (b).

Circumferential nail (see Chapter 9)

This exceptional malformation is congenital and may be seen in siblings (Chauda & Crosby, 1993).

Reference

Chavda D.V. & Crosby L.A. (1993) Circumferential toenail. *Foot Ankle* **14**, 111–112.

Macronychia and micronychia

The nails are larger or smaller than normal and affect one or more digits with wide or narrow nail bed areas and matrices. They may occur as an isolated defect or in association with megadactyly (Fig. 2.12) as in Recklinghausen's disease or in epiloia. In fact macrodactyly may be the form fruste of a wide variety of connective tissue abnormalities. It has been associated with the Proteus syndrome (partial gigantism, hemihypertrophy, etc.), Maffucci's syndrome and Klippel–Trenaunay–Weber syndrome. Greenberg *et al.* (1987) reported on a patient with

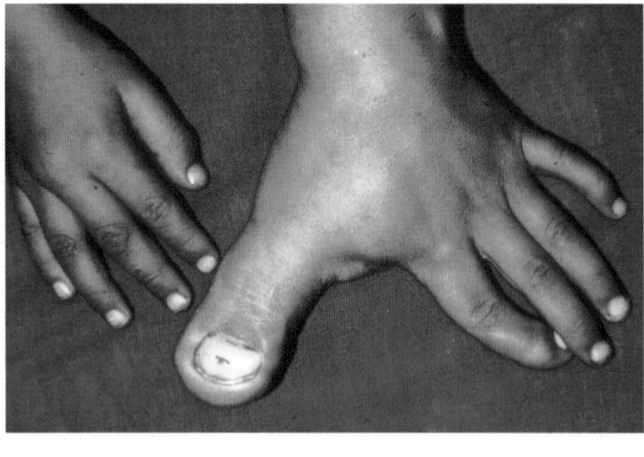

Fig. 2.12. Macronychia associated with megadactyly (courtesy, Prof. A. Tosti, Bologna).

epidermal naevus syndrome who also exhibited bilateral, four finger megadactyly. Involvement of both hands and both feet of the same patient is unique (Keret *et al.*, 1987).

Macrodactyly of the middle and index fingers continue to maintain their overwhelming majority (Barsky, 1967); in most cases, the area of involvement corresponds to the territory supplied by the sensory branches of the median nerve which was designated as nerve territory-oriented macrodactyly (NTOM) (Kelikian, 1974). Macrodactyly associated with plexiform neurofibroma of the medial plantar nerve of the right foot is an unusual localization (Turra *et al.*, 1986). About one-third of neural fibrolipomas are associated with overgrowth of bone and macrodactyly (Silverman & Enzinger, 1985; Wu, 1991). Distant benign lipoblastomatosis in the axilla has been reported (Colot *et al.*, 1984). As a rule, the involvement by macrodactylia fibrolipomatosis is almost always unilateral.

Pseudomegadactyly is an anecdotal presentation of chronic granulomatous paronychia resulting in hypertrophy of nail plate and bed (Mittal & Mittal, 1984). Pseudomacronychia has been reported in congenital aphalangia as a large dorsal distal mass of hyperkeratotic tissue (Zimmerman *et al.*, 1992).

Duplication of the distal phalanx is usually accompanied by a wide digit with a bifid nail, fissured or confluent (Robertson, 1987; Tosti *et al.*, 1992) (Fig. 2.13(a) & (b)).

In Iso–Kikuchi's syndrome the micronychia is usually medially sited instead of a centrally placed small nail, except for a less common type termed 'rolled micronychia' (Millman & Strier, 1982) where the nail is centrally sited.

Apparent micronychia may be due to overlapping of the nail surface by the lateral nail folds. This is sometimes seen in Turner's syndrome in which the whole paronychium may be affected as in recalcitrant chronic paronychia (Zaias, 1990). Micronychia is often observed in Zimmerman–Laband syndrome (Laband *et al.*, 1964).

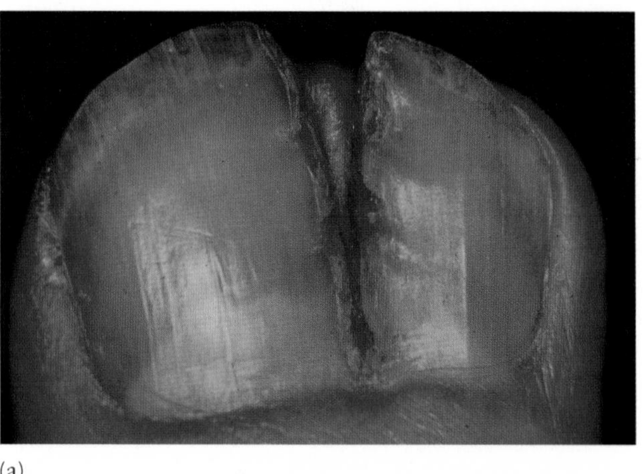

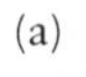

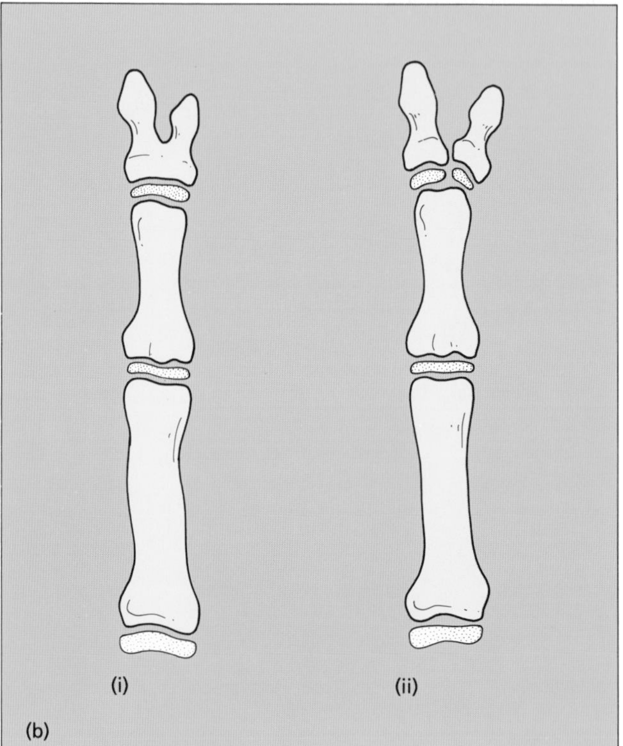

Fig. 2.13. (a) Duplication of the nail (Prof. A. Tosti, Bologna). (b) Duplication of the nail – diagram of associated bony changes. (i) Bifid distal phalanx; (ii) duplicated distal phalanx.

References

Barsky A.J. (1967) Macrodactyly. *J. Bone Joint Surg.* **49A**, 1255–1256.

Colot G., Castmans-Elias S. & Philippet G. (1984) Macrodactylie associée a une lipoblastomatose bénigne. *Ann. Chir. Main* **3**, 262–265.

Greenberg B.M., Pess G.M. & May J.W. (1987) Macrodactyly and the epidermal naevus syndrome. *J. Hand Surg.* **12A**, 730–733.

Kelikian H. (1974) *Congenital Deformities of the Hand and Forearm*, pp. 610–660. W.B. Saunders, Philadelphia.

Laband P.F., Habib G. & Humprey G.S. (1964) Hereditary gingival fibromatosis. Report of an affected family with

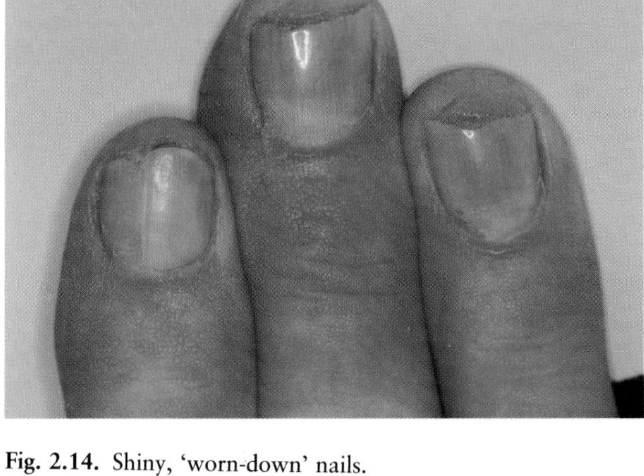

Fig. 2.14. Shiny, 'worn-down' nails.

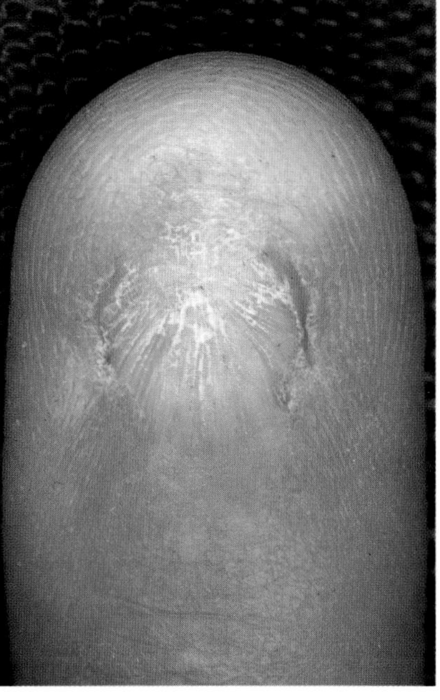

Fig. 2.15. Scleroatrophy, here associated with lichen planus.

associated splenomegaly and skeletal and soft tissue abnormalities. *Oral Surg.* **17**, 339–351.
Millman A.J. & Strier R.P. (1982) Congenital onychodysplasia of the index fingers. *J. Am. Acad. Dermatol.* 7, 57–65.
Mittal R.L. & Mittal R. (1984) Pseudomegadactyly. *Dermatologica* **169**, 86–87.
Robertson W.W. (1987) The bifid great toe, a surgical approach. *J. Pediatr. Orthop.* 7, 25–28.
Silverman T.A. & Enziger F.M. (1985) Fibrolipomatous hamartoma of nerve. A clinicopathologic analysis of 26 cases. *Am. J. Surg. Pathol.* 9, 7.
Tosti A. Paoluzzi P. & Baran R. (1992) Doubled nail of the thumb. A rare form of polydactyly. *Dermatology* **184**, 216–218.
Turra S., Frizziero P., Cagnoni G. *et al.* (1986) Macrodactyly of the foot associated with plexiform neurofibroma of the medial plantar nerve. *J. Pediatr. Orthop.* **6**, 489–492.
Wu K.K. (1991) Macrodactylia fibrolipomatosis of the foot. *J. Foot Surg.* **30**, 402–405.
Zaias N. (1990) *The Nail in Health and Disease.* Lange & Appleton, Norwalk, CN.
Zimmerman P., Prior J., McGuire J. *et al.* (1992) Onychia of a

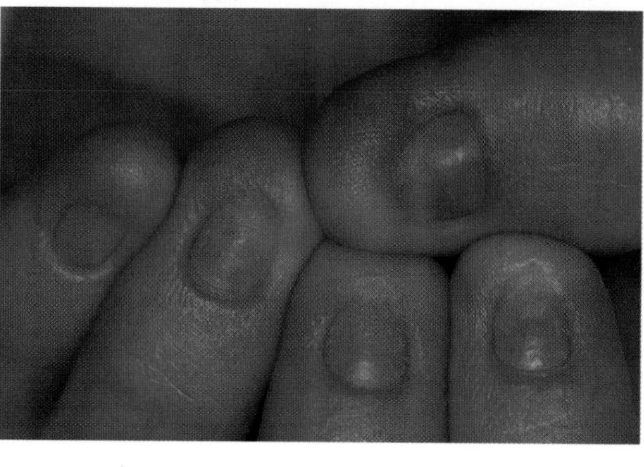

Fig. 2.16. Anonychia.

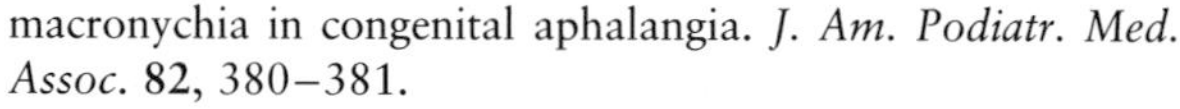

macronychia in congenital aphalangia. *J. Am. Podiatr. Med. Assoc.* **82**, 380–381.

Worn-down nails

Patients with atopic dermatitis or chronic erythroderma may be 'chronic scratchers and rubbers'. The surface of the nail plate becomes glossy and shiny and the free edge is worn away (Fig. 2.14). 'Usure des ongles' may also occur in many different, manual occupations (Ronchese, 1962). This condition has been described as an occupational hazard of mushroom pickers handling heavy, plastic bags (Schulbert *et al.*, 1977), and in an amateur trout fisher who tied his own flies.

References

Ronchese F. (1962) Nails – injuries and disease. In: *Traumatic Medicine and Surgery for the Attorney*, Vol. 6, p. 626. Butterworth, Washington.
Schubert B., Minard J.J., Baran R. *et al.* (1977) Onychopathie des champignonnistes. *Ann. Dermatol. Vener.* **104**, 627.

Onychatrophy

Acquired (e.g. lichen planus) and congenital onychatrophy present as a reduction in size and thickness of the nail plate, often accompanied by fragmentation and splitting. This condition may progressively worsen, scar tissue eventually replacing the atrophic nail plate (Fig. 2.15).

Anonychia

This implies absence of all or part of one or several nails (Fig. 2.16). In aplastic anonychia, a rare congenital disorder occasionally associated with other defects such as ectrodactyly, the nail never forms (Solammadevi, 1981). Loose horny masses are produced by the metaplastic, squamous epithelium of the matrix and the nail bed in anonychia keratodes. Hypoplasia of the nail plates is a hallmark of the nail–patella syndrome. In the least af-

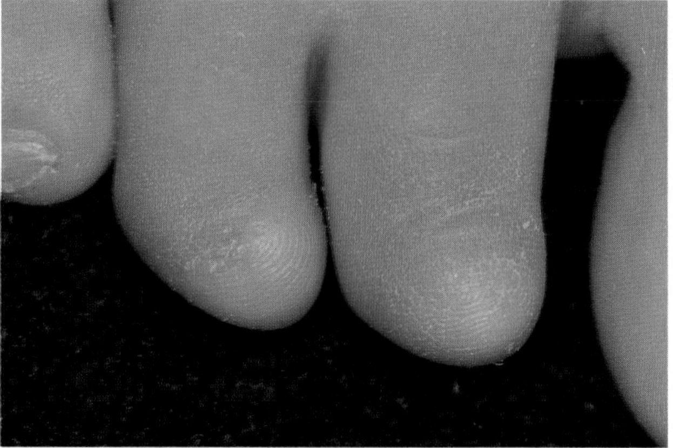
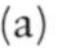

(a)

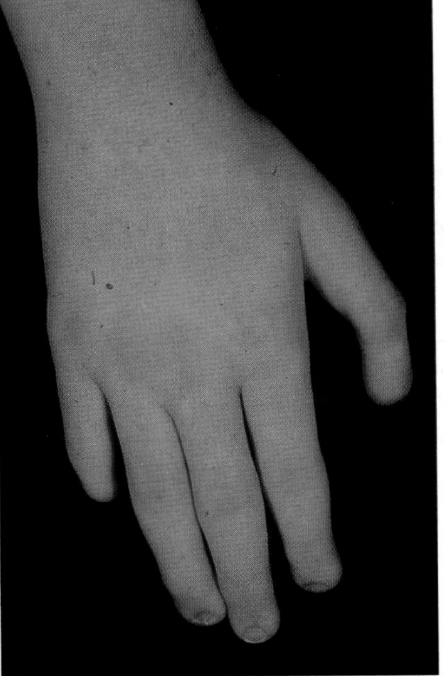

(b)

Fig. 2.17. Severe anonychia: (a) associated with absent distal phalanges; (b) in the DOOR syndrome (Prof. Nevin, Belfast).

fected cases only the ulnar half of each thumb nail is missing.

Kelikian (1974) states that 'one cannot conceive of a normal nail above an anomalous ungual phalanx'. It would appear that congenital anonychia and hyponychia may represent 'bone territory'-dependent disorders (Baran & Juhlin, 1986). The development of a normal nail is not only dependent on the underlying bone but this dependence may also extend to the middle phalanx. Anonychia or hyponychia may result when the underlying phalanx is either hypoplastic or completely absent (Fig. 2.17).

In acquired nail atrophy (anonychia atrophica), the damage to the matrix can result in a rudimentary nail reduced to a corneal layer or to progressive scar formation; it is impossible to draw a strict line between anonychia and onychatrophy. In contrast to these permanent types, a transient anonychia can be due to a local or systemic condition, for example, after etretinate therapy.

References

Baran R. & Juhlin L. (1986) Bone dependent nail formation. *Br. J. Dermatol.* **114**, 371–375.

Kelikian H. (1974) *Congenital Deformities of the Hand and Forearm.* W.B. Saunders, Philadelphia.

Solammadevi S.V. (1981) Simple anonychia. *South. Med. J.* **74**, 1555.

Hypertrophy of the nail

Hypertrophy of the nail may be acquired, the result of dermatological or systemic conditions, including trauma, or occur as a developmental abnormality.

Onychauxis or pachyonychia represent a thickening of the nail plate, often brownish, with an irregular surface. This has been reported in association with the eunuchoid state (Hollander, 1920; Lisser, 1924).

Sometimes the aspect of the nail is that of a horn and the condition is called onychogryphosis.

Hyperplastic subungual tissues, especially of the hyponychium, can arise, the nail plate and the nail consistency may be hard, as in pachyonychia congenita, or soft, as in psoriasis, pityriasis rubra pilaris, chronic eczema and onychomycosis.

In pachyonychia congenita (Jadassohn–Lewandowsky syndrome) the nails are yellow-brown in colour and extremely hard (Fig. 2.18). They present an overcurvature with a free edge shaped like a horseshoe or a barrel. All the nails are affected but the toenails are less severely involved. Recurrent paronychia results in repeated shedding of the nails.

Histology shows normal proximal nail fold and matrix. The nail plate is normal or moderately thickened, but its structure is normal. The nail bed shows marked acanthosis, papillomatosis and huge hyperkeratosis. Groups of amorphous periodic acid Schiff (PAS)-positive globules are arranged in vertical columns between the keratin masses of the subungual hyperkeratosis (Alkiewicz & Lebioda, 1961); they are very similar to those seen in pincer nails and probably represent serum inclusions. Electron microscopy confirms the acanthosis and also shows hypergranulosis. There is no difference between classical and late-onset pachyonychia congenita (Forslind *et al.*, 1973; Paller *et al.*, 1991).

Onychogryphosis (see Table 2.3) may rarely occur as a developmental abnormality but is usually acquired. It is most common in the toenail and presents as an uneven, thickened, opaque nail plate without attachment to the nail bed. The hallux is particularly vulnerable and the nail is often shaped like a ram's horn and is brownish in colour. Its irregular surface is marked by striations which are most frequently transverse. Sometimes this onychodystrophy is oyster-like. The matrix produces the nail plate at uneven rates; the faster growing side determines

(a)

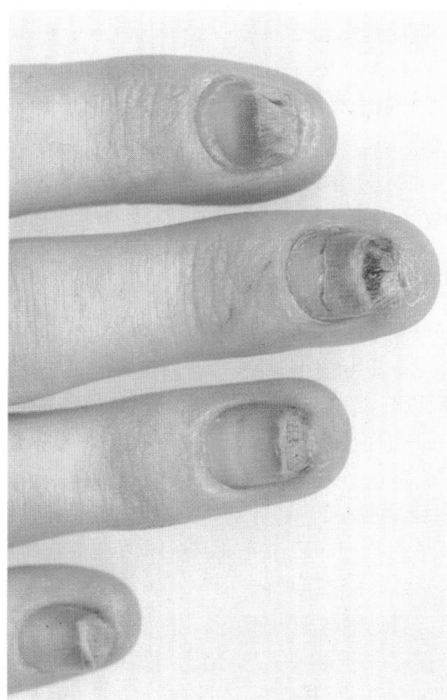

(b)

Fig. 2.18. Pachyonychia congenita (Jadassohn–Lewandowsky syndrome). (a) Side view; (b) showing uniformity of thickening on several digits.

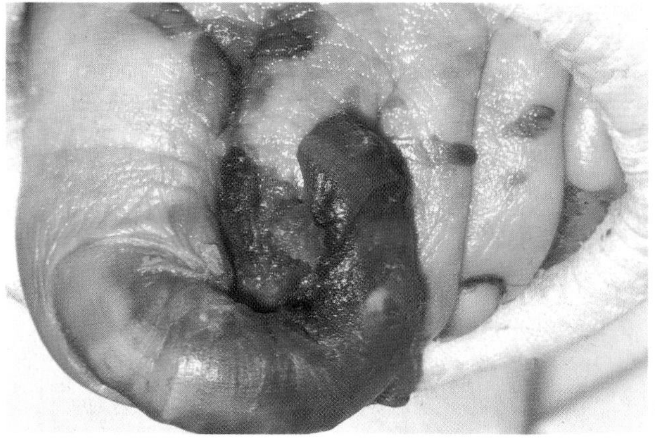

Fig. 2.19. Onychogryphosis.

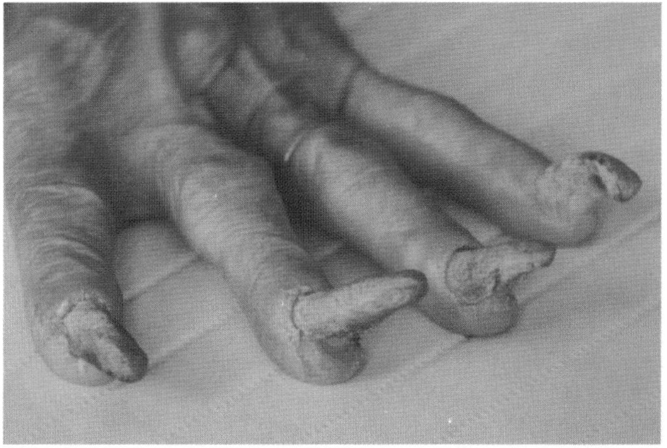

Fig. 2.20. Onychogryphosis, in this case due to psoriasis.

the direction of the deformity (Zaias, 1990). The condition is obvious when the changes are marked (Fig. 2.19). In the early stages, however, when there is just a mild hypertrophy of the nail plate, diagnosis may present some difficulty.

In the elderly the dystrophy is usually caused by pressure from footwear. The bend of the nail is laterally directed, accentuated by hypertrophy of the nail bed (Zaias, 1990), and favoured by secondary foot anomalies such as hallux valgus. Onychogryphosis may be related to weight-bearing function of the great toe, especially at the step-off phase. In cases where the free edge of the great toenail is considerably shorter than the tip of the great toe, the distal tissue bulge causes the onychogryphosis, which is due to improper nail cutting (Higashi & Matsumura, 1988).

Onychogryphosis appears in cases of self-neglect and is often seen in tramps and in senile dementia. Although this dystrophy may be a source of discomfort, or even pain when shoes are worn, it is usually accepted without complaint. In old age, fungal infection associated with onychogryphosis is not unusual (Tanaka *et al.*, 1986). It may be restricted to a single fingernail. Symptomatic onychogryphosis may be due to diseases such as ichthyosis and psoriasis (Fig. 2.20). Pemphigus, syphilis and variola (Heller, 1927) are exceptional causes.

Impairment of the peripheral circulation may produce onychogryphosis. Occasionally in the elderly, the pressure on the thickened onychogryphotic nail will initiate subungual gangrene (Douglas & Krull, 1981).

Onychogryphosis may result from an injury to the matrix, scarring of the nail bed, and pathology in the central, or peripheral nervous system. The traumatic type is common in young people.

In hereditary onychogryphosis (Videbaek, 1948; Schmidt, 1965; Lubach, 1982) all the nails of both hands and feet may be involved. The deformity is congenital and particularly marked during the first years of life. The disease is inherited as an autosomal dominant trait. Hemionychogryphosis may result from congenital mala-

Table 2.3. Causes of onychogryphosis (see references p. 47)

Dermatological diseases
Ichthyosis
Psoriasis
Infectious conditions
Onychomycosis
Syphilis, pemphigus, variola (Heller, 1927)
Local causes
Injury to the nail apparatus
Repeated minor trauma caused by footwear
Foot anomalies such as hallux valgus
Regional causes
Associated varicose veins
Thrombophlebitis, even in the upper limb
Aneurysms
Elephantiasis
Pathology in the peripheral nervous system
General causes
Old age
Uricaemia
Tramps and senile dementia
Diseases involving the central nervous system
Idiopathic forms
Acquired
Hereditary

lignment of the big toenail and can be prevented by surgical correction of the deformity. One of the signs of the Iso–Kikuchi syndrome is hemionychogryphosis of the index finger.

Onychogryphosis may be considered as one of the manifestations of hyperuricaemia (Horvath & Vlcek, 1986).

References

Alkiewicz J. & Lebioda J. (1961) Zur Klinik und Histologie der Pachyonychia congenita. *Arch. Klin. Exp. Dermatol.* **112**, 140–147.

Douglas M.C. & Krull E.A. (1981) Diseases of the nails. *Current Therapy*, p. 712. W.B. Saunders, Philadelphia.

Forslind B., Nylen B., Swanbeck G., Thyresson M. & Thyresson N. (1973) Pachyonychia congenita. A histologic and microradiographic study. *Acta Dermatol. Venereol.* **53**, 211–216.

Higashi N. & Matsumura T. (1988) The aetiology of onychogryphosis of the great toe nail and of ingrowing nail. *Hifu* **30**, 620–623.

Hollander L. (1920) Onychauxis due to hypopituitarism. *Arch. Dermatol. Syph.* **2**, 35–43.

Horvath G. & Vlcek F. (1986) Uricaemia and onychogryphosis. *Cesk. Dermatol.* **81**, 388–390.

Heller J. (1927) Die Krankheiten der Nägel. In: *Handbuch der Haut-und Geschlechtskrankheiten*, ed. Jadassohn, Vol. XIII/2. Springer, Berlin.

Lisser H. (1924) Onychauxis in a eunuchoid. *Arch. Dermatol. Syph.* **10**, 180–182.

Lubach D. (1982) Erbliche Onychogryphosis. *Hautarzt* **33**, 331.

Paller A.S., Moore J.A. & Scher R. (1991) Pachyonychia congenita tarda. A late-onset form of pachyonychia congenita. *Arch. Dermatol.* **127**, 701–703.

Schmidt H. (1965) Total onychogryphosis traced during 6 generations. *Proc. Fenno-Scand. Assoc. Dermatol.* 36–37.

Tanaka T., Sohba S. & Tanida Y. (1986) Onychogryphosis considered to be due to tinea unguium. *Hifuka no Rinsho* **28**, 1333–1337.

Videbaek A. (1948) Hereditary onychogryphosis. *Ann. Eugen.* **14**, 139.

Zaias N. (1990) *The Nail in Health and Disease*, 2nd edn, p. 164. Lange & Appleton, Norwalk, CN.

Modifications of the nail surface

Longitudinal lines

Longitudinal lines, or striations, may appear as indented grooves or projecting ridges.

Longitudinal grooves

Longitudinal grooves represent long-lasting abnormalities and can occur under the following conditions.

1 Physiological, as shallow and delicate furrows, usually parallel, and separated by low, projecting ridges. They become more prominent with age and in certain pathological states, such as lichen planus, rheumatoid arthritis, peripheral circulatory disorders, Darier's disease and other genetic anomalies.

2 Onychorrhexis is a series of narrow, longitudinal parallel furrows which have the appearance of having been scratched by an awl or by sandpaper. Sometimes dust becomes ingrained on the nail surface. Splitting of the free edge is common.

3 Tumours, such as myxoid cysts and warts, located in the proximal nail fold area, may exert pressure on the nail matrix and produce a wide, deep, longitudinal groove or canal, which will disappear if the cause is removed.

4 Median nail dystrophy. This uncommon condition consists of a longitudinal defect of the thumbnails in the mid-line or just off centre, starting at the cuticle and growing out of the free edge. It may be associated with an enlarged lunula (Zelger *et al.*, 1974). In the cases described by Heller (1928), the base of the 2–5 mm wide groove with steep edges showed numerous transverse defects (Fig. 2.21(a)–(c)). Ronchese (1951) reported cases showing longitudinal fissures as 'dystrophia longitudinalis fissuriformis'. In some cases median longitudinal ridges have been observed, occasionally combined with fissures and/or a groove, developed from the distal edge of the nail plate to the matrix. Often a few, short feathery cracks, chevron-shaped, extend laterally from the split. The so-called

(a)

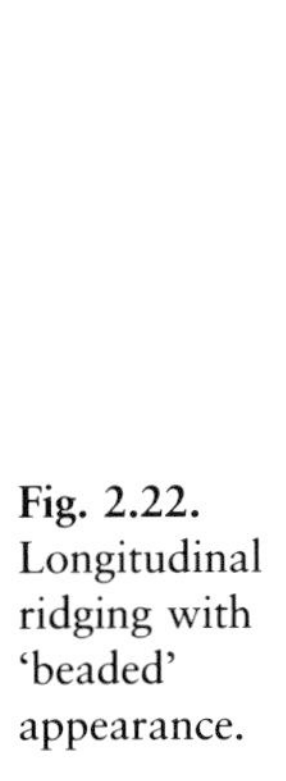

(b)

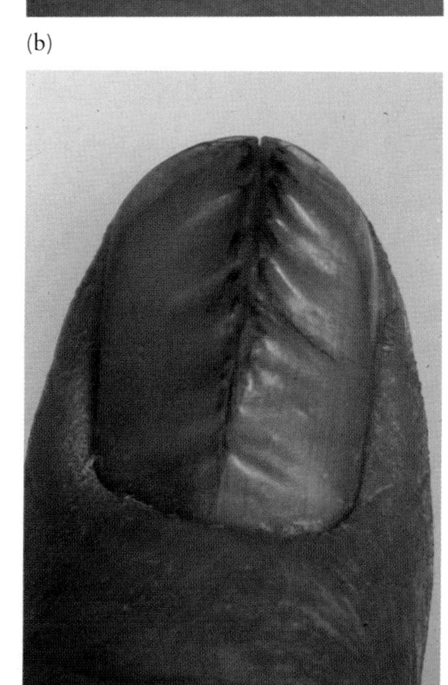

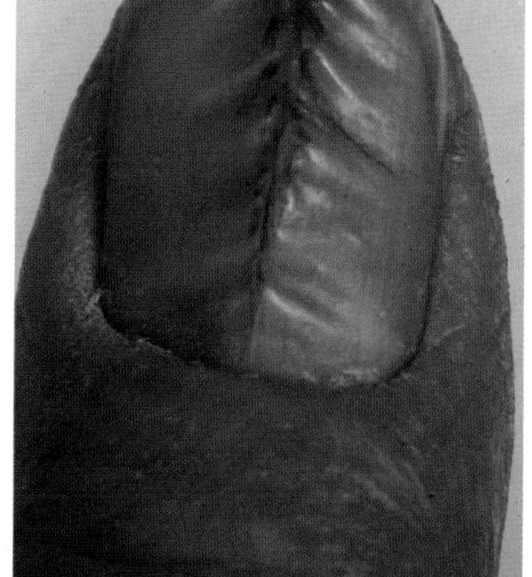

(c)

Fig. 2.21. Median canaliform (Heller's) dystrophy: (a) early; (b) later; (c) inverted 'fir tree' appearance.

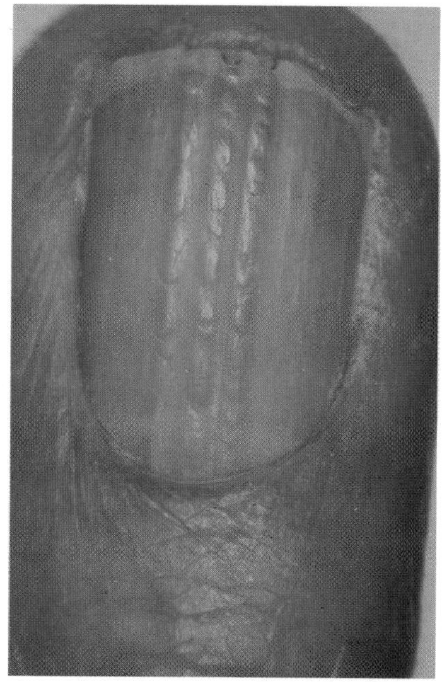

Fig. 2.22. Longitudinal ridging with 'beaded' appearance.

'naevus striatus symmetricus of the thumbs' (Oppenheim & Cohen, 1942) corresponds to this form (Leclercq, 1964). Median nail dystrophy is usually symmetrical and most often affects the thumbs. Sometimes other fingers are involved, seldom the toes (usually the big toe). After several months or years, the nail returns to normal but recurrences are not exceptional. Sutton and Waisman (1975) reported a case that they termed 'solenonychia' with a flabby filament of fleshy tissue present in the toenail canal. Familial cases have been recorded (Rehtijarvi, 1971; Seller, 1974). In all cases the aetiology is unknown, but Zaias (1990) suggests that the deformity is usually due to self-inflicted trauma resulting from a tic or habit. Pressure repeatedly exerted on the base of the nail probably explains the appearance of this condition as well as its enlarged reddish lunula.

It has been suggested that treatment of recalcitrant cases be identical to that of post-traumatic nail splitting. We do not advocate this view.

Differential diagnosis

A central longitudinal depression is found in 'washboard nail plates' (MacAulay, 1966) caused by chronic, mechanical injury. Unlike Heller's dystrophy, the cuticle is pushed back and there is accompanying inflammation of the proximal nail fold (see p. 51). Splits due to trauma, or those occurring in the nail–patella syndrome and in pterygium, are generally obvious. Longitudinal splits may also result from Raynaud's disease, lichen striatus and trachyonychia.

Nail wrapping (Chapter 8) may reduce the disability produced by the fissure. The proximal nail fold must be protected from repeated minor trauma.

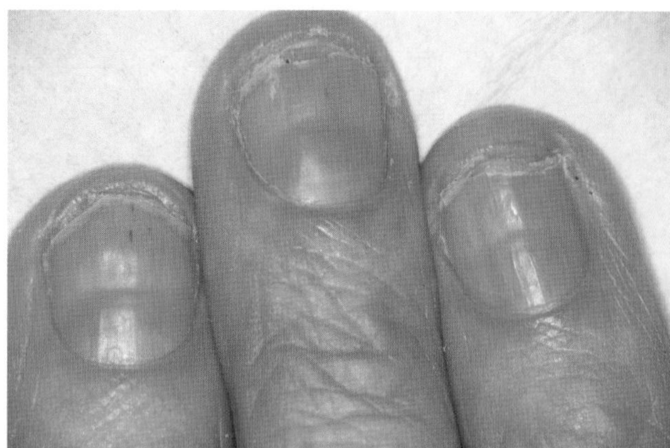

Fig. 2.23. Beau's lines.

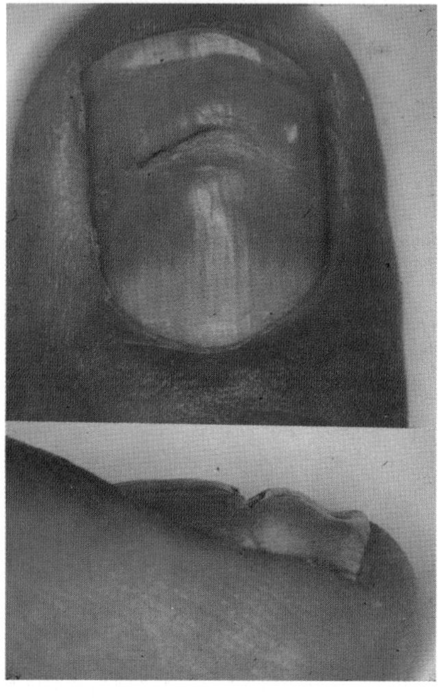

Fig. 2.24. Beau's lines – wider depression than in Fig. 2.23.

Longitudinal ridges

Small rectilinear projections extend from the proximal nail fold as far as the free edge of the nail, or they may stop short. They may be interrupted at regular intervals giving rise to a beaded appearance (Fig. 2.22). Sometimes a wide, longitudinal median ridge has the appearance, in cross section, of a circumflex accent. This condition is usually post-traumatic, but may be inherited and affect mainly the thumb and fingers of both hands.

References

Heller J. (1928) Dystrophia unguium mediana canaliformis. *Dermatol. Z.* **51**, 416–419.

Leclercq R. (1964) Naevus striatus symmetricus unguis, dystrophie ungueale mediane canaliforme de Heller ou dystropie ungueale mediane en chevrons. A propos de 2 cas. *Bull. Soc. Fr. Dermatol. Syphil.* **71**, 655.

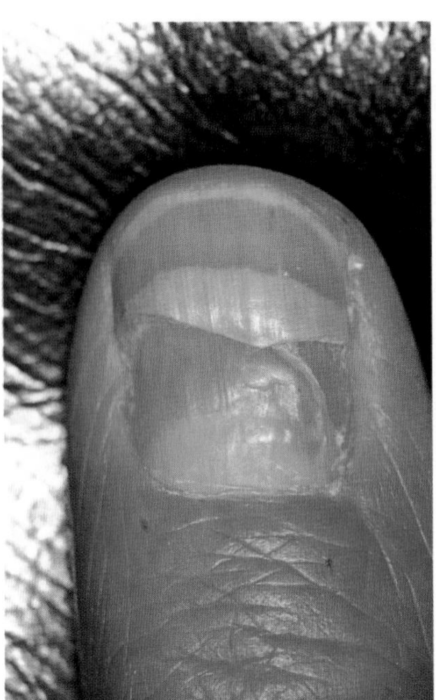

Fig. 2.25. Latent onychomadesis.

MacAulay W.L. (1966) Transverse ridging of the thumbnails. *Arch. Dermatol.* **93**, 421.

Oppenheim M. & Cohen D. (1942) Naevus striatus symmetricus unguis. *Arch. Dermatol. Syphil.* **45**, 253.

Rehtijarvi K. (1971) Dystrophia unguis mediana canaliformis (Heller). *Acta Dermatol. Venereol.* **51**, 315.

Ronchese F. (1951) Peculiar nail anomalies. *Arch. Dermatol.* **63**, 565.

Seller H. (1974) Dystrophia unguis mediana canaliformis. Familiäres Vorkommen. *Hautarzt* **25**, 456.

Sutton R.L. Jr & Waisman M. (1975) *The Practitioner's Dermatology.* Yorke Medical Books, New York.

Zaias N. (1990) *The Nail in Health and Disease*, 2nd edn. Appleton & Lange, CN.

Zelger J., Wohlfarth P. & Putz R. (1974) Dystrophia unguium mediana canaliformis Heller. *Hautarzt* **25**, 629.

Beau's lines and transverse grooves (Fig. 2.23)

Transverse lines in the form of sulci, limited proximally by a slightly elevated ridge and affecting the surface of all nails at corresponding levels (Fig. 2.23) were described by Beau (1846) as 'retrospective indicators' of a number of pathological states. The condition is sometimes restricted to the thumbs and big toes. The grooves are superficial, but more marked in the middle aspect of the nail.

The transverse depression, sometimes involving the whole depth of the nail plate, appears some weeks after illness (e.g. fever). As the approximate growth rate is known (Chapter 1), it is possible to assess the approximate time of the prior causative disease which has marked the nails; the thumbnail supplies information for the previous 5–6 months, and the big toenail evidence of disease for up to 2 years. As the thumb- and toenails are most frequently affected they are the most reliable indicators of

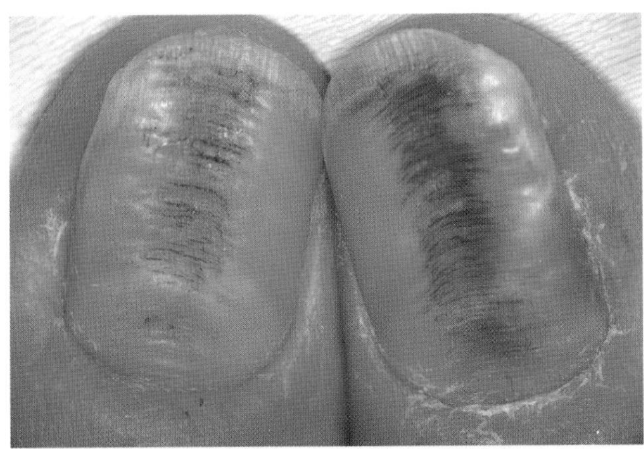

Fig. 2.26. Multiple transverse grooves of thumbs – 'habit-tic' deformity.

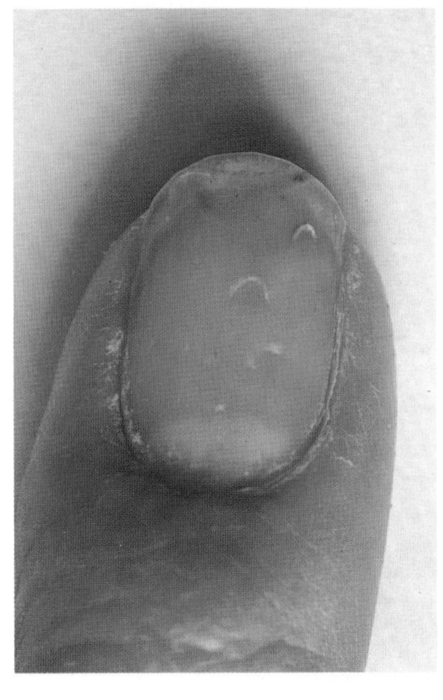

Fig. 2.27. Pitting of the nails, due to eczema in this case – irregular sized pits seen.

previous disease. Markings occur inconsistently on the other digits.

The width of the furrow is an indicator of the duration of the disease which has affected the matrix. If abrupt, the distal limit of the depression represents a more acute onset (Fig. 2.24). If the activity of the entire matrix is inhibited for a period of 1–2 weeks, for example, Beau's line will reach its maximum depth causing a total division of the nail plate. This is seen in *latent* onychomadesis (Fig. 2.25) and leads to a temporay shedding of the nail (Runne & Orfanos, 1981). Beau's lines are analogous to the Pohl–Pincus line found in the hair which shows decreased diameter of the shaft and loss of medulla.

Physiological Beau's lines may occur in 4–5-week-old babies, marking the transition from intrauterine to extra-uterine life, and monthly with each menstrual cycle. Cyclical transverse nail grooves occurring simultaneously with groups of knots in the hair have been reported (Fabry, 1965). Colver and Dawber (1984) reported multiple transverse ridges at monthly intervals in association with severe dysmenorrhoea. Beau's lines may be due to any severe disability and, particularly, to measles in childhood; zinc deficiency, whatever the cause, may produce multiple transverse grooves. Transverse depressions restricted to one or two digits may indicate one of the following causes: injury, carpal tunnel syndrome, or extremes of cold in Raynaud's disease. Beau's line may develop after hand trauma involving damage to nerves and flexor tendons (Ward *et al.*, 1988). A transverse groove is the most common ischaemic deformity of the nail seen by the hand surgeon following the use of the upper extremity tourniquet (Zook & Russell, 1990). Fine transverse grooves, a few millimetres wide, and starting at one lateral edge of the nail plate may appear on the whole length from its proximal part to the free margin in chronic paronychia; they may be dark or have a greenish tinge. When the transverse depressions are the consequence of a chronic condition, such as eczema they may lead to latent onychomadesis. When a series of transverse grooves parallels the proximal fold rather than the distal convex curve of the lunula the cause is likely to be repeated injury to the matrix from overzealous manicuring (Sutton & Waisman, 1975). The grooves are separated by ridges of healthy nail.

A nervous habit of repeatedly pushing back the cuticle on one or several fingers can create 'washboard nails' (MacAulay, 1966). Usually the proximal nail fold of the thumb on the same hand is damaged by the index finger and shows redness, swelling and scaling. This chronic, mechanical injury results in a series of transverse grooves and a large central depression running down the nail (Fig. 2.26). When the central depression does not exist, psoriasis should be suspected.

The 'serrated koilonychia' syndrome (Runne & Orfanos, 1981) consists of a combination of saw-like transverse grooving of all nails with koilonychia.

References

Beau J.H.S. (1846) Note sur certains caractères de séméiologie rétrospective présentés par les ongles. *Arch. Gen. Med.* **11**, 447.

Colver G.B. Dawber R.P.R. (1984) Multiple Beau's lines due to dysmenorrhoea. *Br. J. Dermatol.* **111**, 111–113.

Fabry H. (1965) Gleichzeitiges rhythmisches Auftreten von Querfurchen der Nägel und gruppierten Knotenbildungen der Haare. *Z Haut-Geschl. Krankh.* **39**, 336–338.

MacAulay W.L. (1966) Transverse ridging of the thumbnails – 'washboard thumbnails'. *Arch. Dermatol.* **93**, 421–432.

Runne V. & Orfanos C.E. (1981) The human nail. *Curr. Prob. Dermatol.* **9**, 102–149.

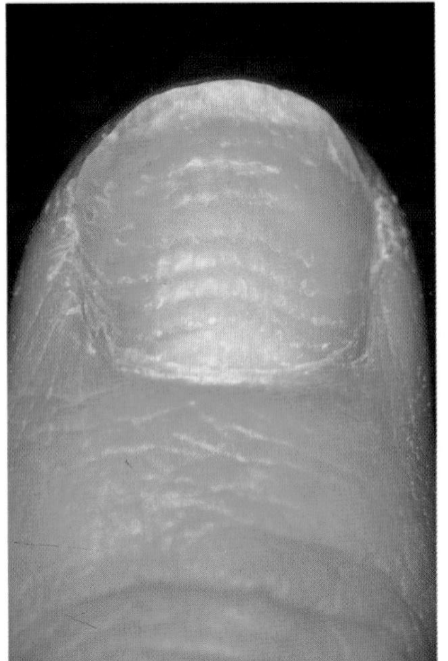

(a)

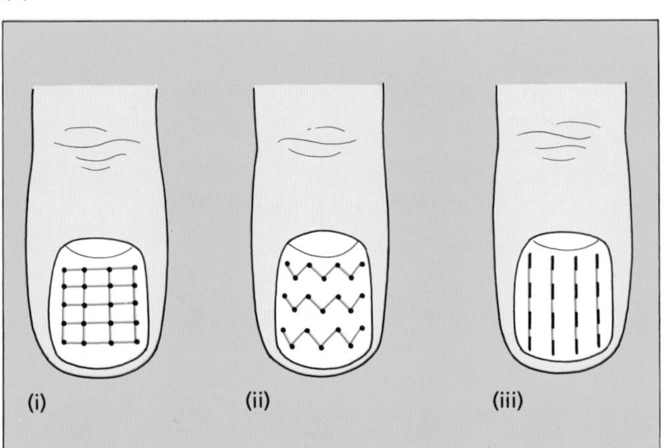

(b)

Fig. 2.28. (a) Rippled lines of pits. (b) Pitting; (i) regular; (ii) rippled. (iii) Ridged varieties.

Sutton R.L. & Waisman M. (1975) *The Practitioner's Dermatology*. Yorke Medical Books, New York.

Ward D.J., Hudson I. & Jeffs J.V. (1988) Beau's lines following hand trauma. *J. Hand Surg.* **13B**, 411–414.

Zook E.G. & Russell R.C. (1990) Reconstitution of a functional and esthetic nail. *Hand Clin.* **6**, 59–68.

Pitting (pits, onychia punctata, erosions, Rosenau's depressions)

Pits develop as a result of defective nail formation in punctate areas located in the proximal portion of the matrix. The surface of the nail plate is covered by small punctate depressions which vary in number, size, depth and shape (Fig. 2.27). The depth and width of the pits relates to the extent of the matrix involved; their length is determined by the duration of the matrix damage.

They are randomly distributed or uniformly arranged in series along one or several longitudinal lines, or sometimes arranged in a criss-cross pattern. They may resemble the external surface of a thimble.

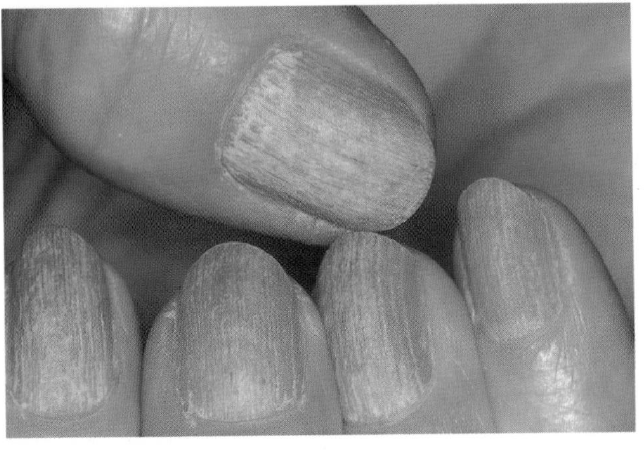

Fig. 2.29. Trachyonychia – sandpapered appearance.

Samman (1978) has shown that regular pitting could be converted to rippling or ridging (Fig. 2.28(a) & (b)) and these two conditions appear, at times, to be variants of uniform pitting. Nails showing pitting grow faster than the apparently normal nails. Shelley and Shelley (1985) have described 'shoreline nails' as a sign of drug-induced erythroderma.

Occasional pits occur on normal nails. Deep pits can be attributed to psoriasis. Shallow pits are usually seen in alopecia areata, dermatitis or occupational trauma. In some cases a genetic basis is possible. In secondary syphilis and pityriasis rosea pitting occurs rarely. We have seen one case of the latter, with the pits distributed on all the fingernails at corresponding levels, in a manner analogous to Beau's lines.

References

Samman P.D. (1978) *The Nails in Disease*, 3rd edn, p. 180. Heinemann, London.

Shelley W.B. & Shelley D.E. (1985) Shoreline nails, sign of drug-induced erythroderma. *Cutis* **35**, 220–224.

Trachyonychia (rough nails)

This dystrophy was described by Alkiewicz (1950) and then Achten and Wanet-Rouard (1974) especially in relation to congenital nail atrophies, and more recently by Samman (1979). It is characterized by a roughness of the nail surface and a grey opacity of the nail, which becomes brittle and splits at the free edge. One form may result from external chemical action (Alkiewicz, 1950); other types are idiopathic, familial (Arias *et al.*, 1982), congenital or acquired. The latter type involving all the digits, the so-called 'twenty-nail dystrophy', affects both children and

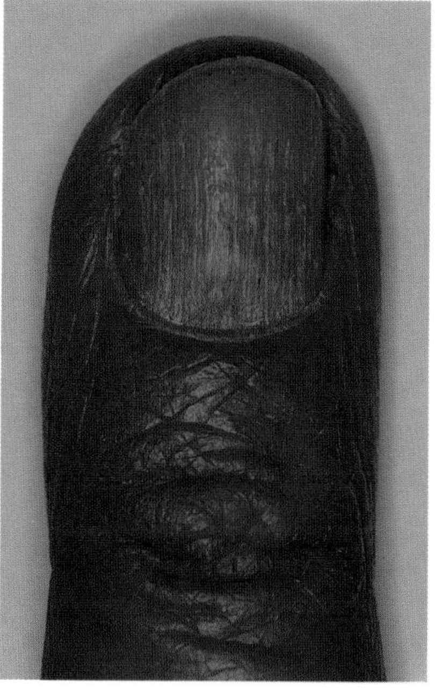

Fig. 2.30. Trachyonychia – nail shiny but fine, stippled opalescent, longitudinal ridging.

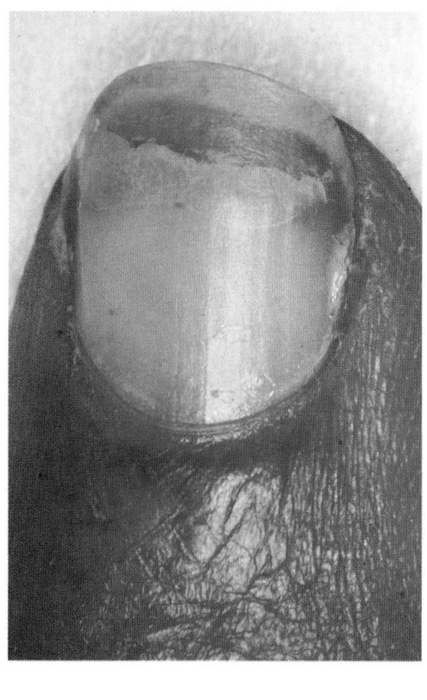

Fig. 2.31. Onychoschizia lamellina (lamellar splitting).

adults. It may be related to a known dermatological disorder, such as lichen planus, psoriasis or alopecia areata, although these conditions may not yet be manifest. Identical nail changes have been described in ichthyosis vulgaris (James *et al.*, 1981): dark red lunulae and knuckle pads (Runne, 1980), selective IgA deficiency (Leong *et al.*, 1982) and ectodermal dysplasia.

Some clarification of the confusion in the literature regarding this condition is indicated. It can be divided into two main types (Baran, 1981).

1 The whole nail gives the appearance of having been sandpapered in a longitudinal direction (Fig. 2.29). There is excessive ridging and a roughness which deprives the nail of its natural lustre. We have designated this 'vertical striated sandpaper twenty-nail dystrophy' (Baran & Dupre, 1977). It is most frequently associated with alopecia areata, when a specific aetiology exists. It is difficult to demonstrate the condition adequately by photography.

2 In the second type, the nail plate is shiny, with opalescent longitudinal ridging (Fig. 2.30). The fine stippled aspect of the nail reflects the camera flash and is clearly evident on photography. Alopecia areata may occur in association with both types.

Tosti *et al.* (1991) have detected spongiotic inflammation of the nail apparatus in the nail biopsy specimens from each of 13 patients affected by severe trachyonychia involving all 20 nails. Spongiotic trachyonychia is due to a T-cell-mediated immune response. The possibility that idiopathic spongiotic trachyonychia is actually a variety of alopecia areata limited to the nails is suggested by clinical and immunohistochemical data.

References

Achten G. & Wanet-Rouard J.J. (1974) Atrophie ungueale et trachyonychie. *Arch. Belges Dermatol.* **30**, 201.

Alkiewicz J. (1950) Trachyonychie. *Ann. Dermatol. Syphil.* **10**, 136.

Arias A.M., Yung C.W., Rendler S. *et al.* (1982) Familial severe twenty-nail dystrophy. *J. Am. Acad. Dermatol.* **7**, 349.

Baran R. (1981) Twenty-nail dystrophy of alopecia areata. *Arch. Dermatol.* **117**, 1.

Baran R. & Dupré A. (1977) Vertical striated sandpaper nails. *Arch. Dermatol.* **113**, 1613.

James W.D., Odom R.B. & Horm R.T. (1981) Twenty-nail dystrophy and ichthyosis vulgaris. *Arch. Dermatol.* **117**, 316.

Leong A.B., Gange R.W. & O'Connor R.D. (1982) Twenty-nail dystrophy (trachyonychia) associated with selective IgA deficiency. *Pediatrics* **100**, 418.

Runne V. (1980) Twenty-nail dystrophy mit knuckle pads. *Z. Hautkr.* **55**, 901.

Samman P.D. (1979) Trachyonychia (rough nails) *Br. J. Dermatol.* **101**, 701.

Tosti A., Fanti P.A., Morelli R. *et al.* (1991) Spongiotic trachyonychia. *Arch. Dermatol.* **127**, 584–585.

Onychoschizia lamellina (lamellar nail splitting)

In this condition, found in 27–35% of normal adult women, the distal portion of the nail splits horizontally (Fig. 2.31). The nail is formed in layers analogous to the formation of scales in the skin; the thin lamellae then break off. Exogenous factors contribute to the cause of the defect. It is common in those whose nails are repeatedly soaked in water and then dried. Splitting into layers has

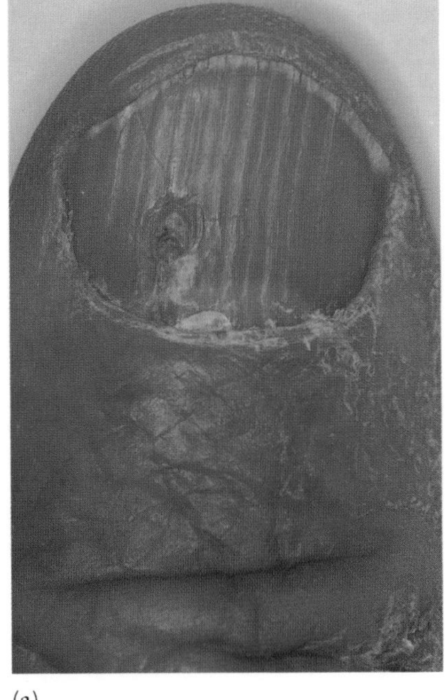
(a)

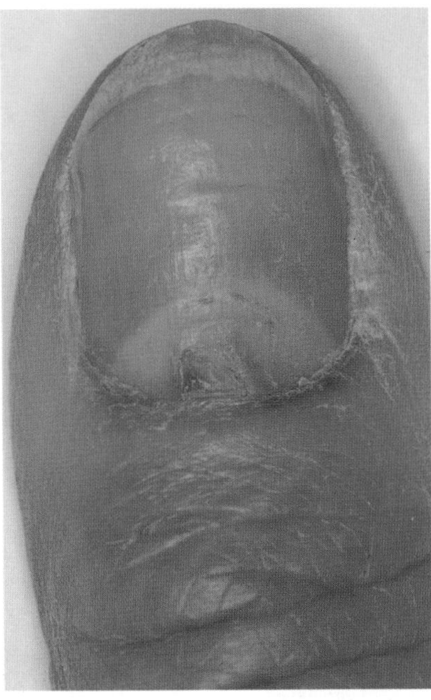
(b)

Fig. 2.32. (a & b) Elkonyxis.

been reported in X-linked dominant chondrodysplasia punctata (Happle, 1979) and in polycythaemia vera (Graham-Brown & Homes, 1980). In lichen planus, in psoriasis, and due to aromatic retinoid therapy, onychoschizia may be seen in the proximal portion of the nail (Baran, 1990).

Shelley and Shelley (1984) studied the distal ends of the nails of four women, demonstrating onychoschizia, with scanning electron microscopy. The dorsal surface and tip of each nail showed horizontal lamellar separations representing single cell layers. Some cleavage lines extended proximally into the nail plate, revealing remarkable sculptured cell surfaces deep within the plate. These observations indicate that the lamellar splitting of onychoschizia occurs between cell layers. This presumably results from repeated trauma to a nail with diminished adherence between cell layers, secondary to the dissolution of intercellular cement by detergents and nail polish solvent.

Wallis *et al.* (1991) studied the *in vitro* nail changes produced by several organic solvents, detergents, other polar materials, and both acidic and basic solutions. Although other factors may influence onychoschizia, the typical changes can be produced in normal nails after a 21 day challenge of repeated exposure to water followed by dehydratation. Scanning electron microscopy demonstrated unattached individual cells in empty spaces in which separation was more prominent. The prominent *in vitro* changes from wetting and drying suggest that lamellar dystrophy could be managed by hydration followed by an occlusive topical agent that promotes water retention. Wallis *et al.* (1991) have successfully combined protection from exposure with hydrophilic petrolatum (Aquaphor) as a nail cream applied to the wet nails to maintain a relatively constant level of hydration.

References

Baran R. (1990) Retinoids and the nails. *J. Dermatol. Treat.* **1**, 151–154.

Happle R. (1979) X-linked dominant chondrodysplasia punctata. *Humangenetik* **53**, 65.

Graham-Brown R.A.C. & Homes R. (1980) Polycythaemia rubra vera with lamellar dystrophy of the nails, a report of two cases. *Clin. Exp. Dermatol.* **5**, 209.

Shelley W.B. & Shelley E.D. (1984) Onychoschizia, scanning electron microscopy. *J. Am. Acad. Dermatol.* **10**, 623–627.

Wallis M.S., Bowen W.R. & Guin J.R. (1991) Pathogenesis of onychoschizia (lamellar dystrophy) *J. Am. Acad. Dermatol.* **24**, 44–48.

Elkonyxis (Fig. 2.32(a) & (b))

In this condition the nail appears initially pinched out at the lunula and subsequently the disorder moves distally with the growth of the nail. It has been described in secondary syphilis, psoriasis, Reiter's syndrome, and after trauma. It may be produced by etretinate (Cannata & Gambetti, 1990).

Reference

Cannata G. & Gambetti M. (1990) Elconyxis, une complication inconnue de l'étrétinate. *Nouv. Dermatol.* **9**, 251.

Modifications of the nail plate and soft tissue attachments

The proximal nail fold is closely applied to the dorsal surface of the newly formed nail plate. At the free border of the proximal nail fold, the cuticle should adhere to the dorsal surface of the nail and seal the cul-de-sac. Inflam-

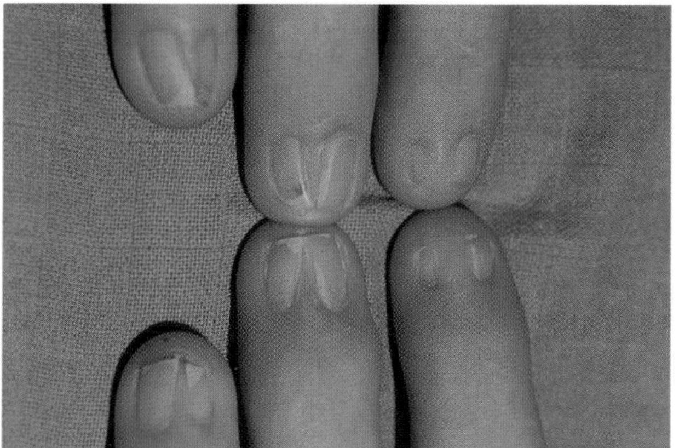

(a)

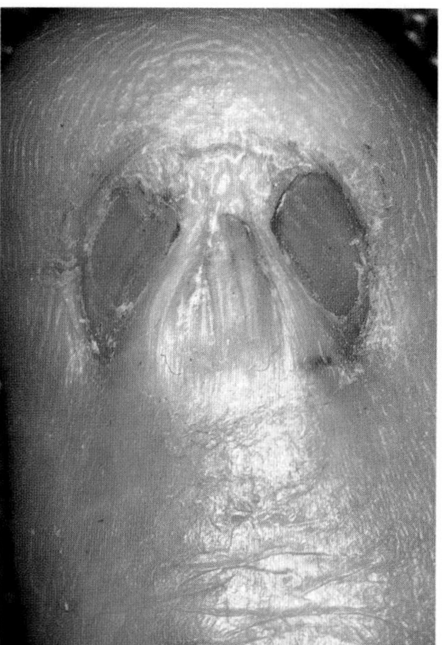

(b)

Fig. 2.33. (a) Congenital dorsal pterygium (courtesy G. Moulin, Lyon, France) (b) dorsal pterygium in lichen planus.

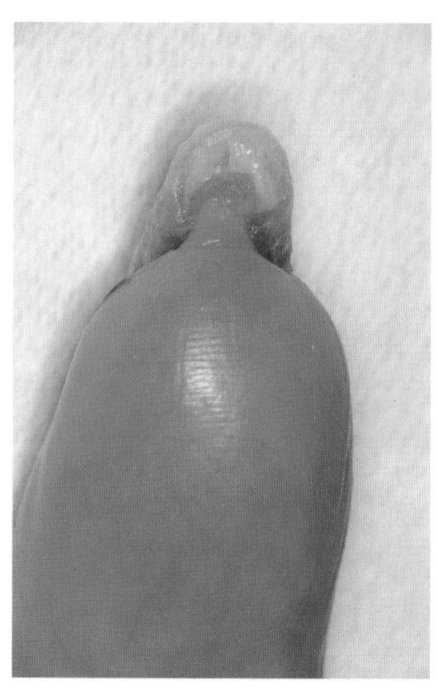

Fig. 2.34. Ventral pterygium (pterygium inversum unguis).

mation of the proximal nail fold is called paronychia and is described elsewhere; when this condition becomes chronic, the cuticle disappears and a 'pocket' is created between the ventral surface of the posterior nail fold and the nail.

Pterygium

Dorsal pterygium (Fig. 2.33(a) & (b)) consists of a gradual shortening of the cul-de-sac under the proximal nail fold with associated thinning of the nail plate until the latter becomes fissured because of the fusion of the proximal nail fold to the matrix and subsequently to the nail bed; the divided nail plate portions progressively decrease in size as the pterygium widens. This results in two small nail remnants. Complete involvement of the matrix and nail bed in the pathological process leads to total loss of the nail plate, with permanent atrophy and sometimes scarring in the nail area. Pterygium is characteristic of lichen planus and, less often, of peripheral vascular ischaemia. It also occurs after severe bullous dermatoses, radiotherapy and on the hands of radiologists; it may follow injury, and rarely is congenital (Fig. 2.33(a)).

Ventral pterygium, or pterygium inversum unguis (Fig. 2.34), is a distal extension of the hyponychial tissue which anchors to the under surface of the nail, thereby eliminating the distal groove (Caputo & Prandi, 1973; Caputo *et al.*, 1978; Amblard & Reymond, 1980). Scarring in the vicinity of the distal groove, causing it to be obliterated, may produce secondary pterygium inversum unguis (Catterall & White, 1978). This type may be seen in scleroderma associated with Raynaud's phenomenon (Patterson, 1977), disseminated lupus erythematosus, and causalgia of the median nerve. Unilateral pterygium inversum unguis affected the right fingers and toes in a 50-year-old man after a stroke resulting in paresis of the same side (Morimoto & Gurevitch, 1988). The possibility of a traumatic origin should also be considered (Runne & Orfanos, 1981). Pterygium inversum has been reported as a reaction to a formaldehyde-containing nail fortifier (Daly & Johnson, 1986). The condition may also be idiopathic, congenital, and sometimes familial. A congenital, aberrant, painful hyponychium has been described associated with oblique, deep fractures of the nails (Odom *et al.*, 1974). There are some reports of familial forms of the disease (Christophers, 1975; Dugois *et al.*, 1975; Chams-Davatchi, 1980). Toenails are only rarely involved (Amblard & Reymond, 1980; Nogita *et al.*, 1991). Dupré *et al.* (1981) described an unusual acquired association of pterygium inversum unguis and lenticular atrophy of the palmar creases (Fig. 2.35(a) & (b)). Pain in the fingertip from minor trauma and haemorrhages may appear when the distal, subungual

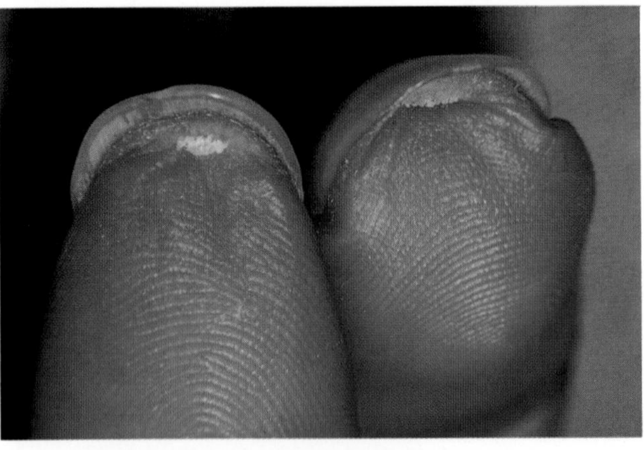

(a)

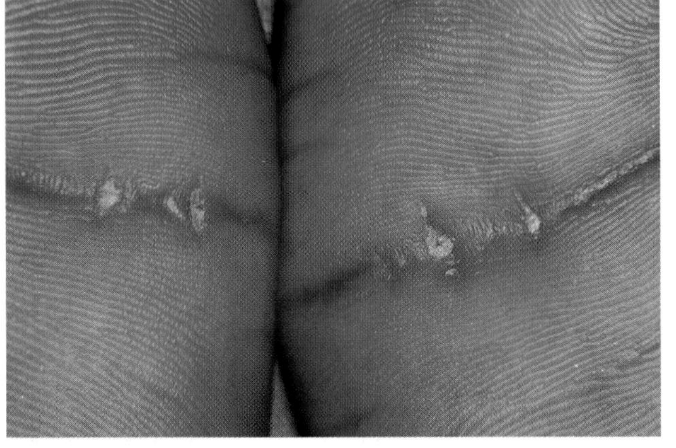

(b)

Fig. 2.35. (a) Ventral pterygium, here associated with (b) lenticular atrophy of the palmar creases (courtesy of A. Dupré, Toulouse, France).

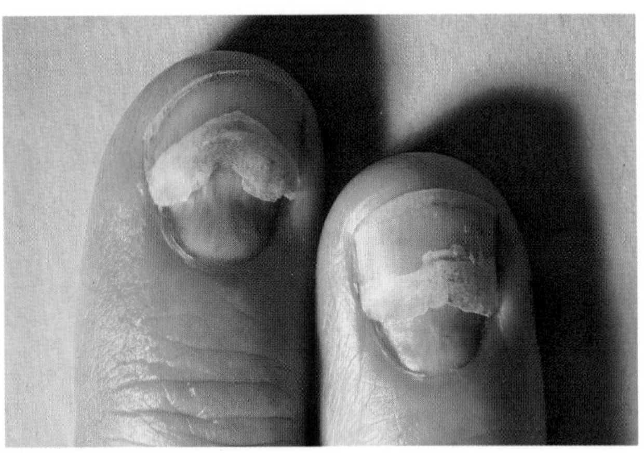

Fig. 2.36. Nail shedding – onychomadesis type (courtesy A. Krebs, Basel, Switzerland).

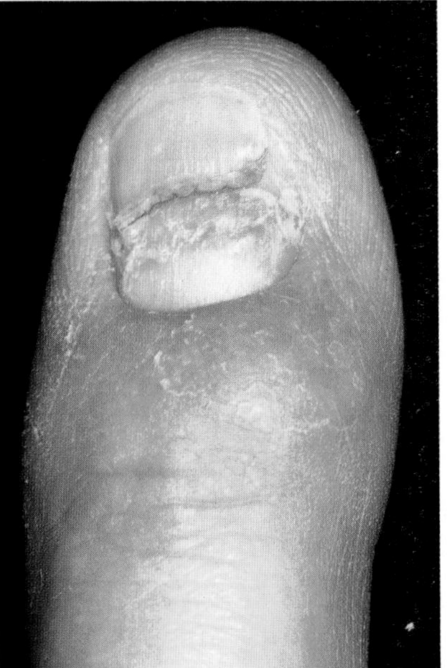

Fig. 2.37. Nail shedding – latent onychomadesis type (Dr Van Neste, Belgium).

area is repeatedly pushed back or the nail cut short. Subungual pterygium is analogous to the claw of lower primates.

In patients suffering from dorsal pterygium (except of the traumatic or congenital type) the main characteristic is a dilatation in the nail fold capillary loops and the formation of a slender microvascular shunt system in the more dilated loops (Trevisan & Talocchi, 1980). These changes are visible using capillaroscopy.

References

Amblard P. & Reymond J.L. (1980) Letter. *Ann. Dermatol. Venereol.* **107**, 949.

Caputo R. & Prandi G. (1973) Pterygium inversum unguis. *Arch. Dermatol.* **108**, 817.

Caputo R., Crosti C. & Menni S. (1978) Pterygio inverso delle unguie. *G. Ital. Dermatol. Minerva Dermatol.* **113**, 559–562.

Catterall M.D. & White J.E. (1978) Pterygium inversum unguis. *Clin. Exp. Dermatol.* **3**, 437.

Chams-Davatchi C. (1980) Pterygium inversum unguéal. A propos de 3 cas. *Ann. Dermatol. Venereol.* **107**, 83.

Christophers E. (1975) Familiäre subunguale Pterygien. *Hautarzt* **26**, 543.

Daly B.M. & Johnson M. (1986) Pterygium inversum due to nail fortifier. *Contact Dermatitis* **15**, 256–257.

Dugois P., Amblard P., Martel C. *et al.* (1975) Pterygium inversum unguis familial. *Bull. Soc. Fr. Dermatol. Venereol.* **82**, 283.

Dupré A., Christol B., Bonafe J.L. *et al.* (1981) Pterygium inversum unguis et atrophie ponctuée des plis palmaires. *Dermatologica* **162**, 209.

Morimoto S.S. & Gurevitch A.W. (1988) Unilateral pterygium inversum unguis. *Int. J. Dermatol.* **27**, 491–494.

Nogita T., Yamashita H., Kawashima M. *et al.* (1991) Pterygium inversum unguis. *J. Am. Acad. Dermatol.* **24**, 787–788.

Odom R.B., Kenneth M.S. & Maibach H.I. (1974) Congenital painful, aberrant hyponychium. *Arch. Dermatol.* **110**, 89.

Patterson J.W. (1977) Pterygium inversum unguis-like changes in scleroderma. *Arch. Dermatol.* **113**, 1429–1430.

Runne U. & Orfanos C.E. (1981) The human nail. *Curr. Prob. Dermatol.* **9**, 102.

Trevisan G. & Talocchi G. (1980) Pterygium unguis senza alterazioni acroasfittiche clinicamente rilevabili: 20 casi studiati con capillaroscopia. *Ann. Ital. Dermatol. Clin. Speriment* **34**, 361.

Nail shedding

Spontaneous separation of the nail from the matrix area is called onychomadesis (Fig. 2.36). At first, a cleavage appears under the proximal portion of the nail, followed by the disappearance of the juxtamatricial portion of the surface of the nail. A sort of surface ulcer is thus formed, which does not usually involve the deeper layers. It is due to a limited lesion of the proximal part of the matrix. The terms onychoptosis defluvium or alopecia unguium are sometimes used to describe atraumatic nail loss. In latent onychomadesis (Runne & Orfanos, 1981) the nail plate shows a transverse split (Fig. 2.37) because of transient, complete inhibition of nail growth for at least 1–2 weeks. It may be characterized by a Beau's line which has reached its maximum dimension; nevertheless the nail continues growing for some time because there is no disruption in its attachment to the nail bed. Growth ceases when it is cast off after losing this connection. In some, very severe, general acute diseases, such as Lyell's syndrome, the proximal edge of all the nail plates may be elevated.

Onychomadesis usually results from serious generalized disease, bullous dermatoses, drug reactions, intensive X-ray therapy, acute paronychia, severe psychological stress or it may be idiopathic. When the disease is inherited (as a dominant characteristic) the shedding may be periodic, and rarely associated with the dental condition amelogenesis imperfecta. Longitudinal fissures, recurrent onychomadesis and onychogryphosis may be associated with mild degrees of keratosis punctata. In toenails, onychomadesis may be produced by minor traumatic episodes, as in sportsman's toe.

Total nail loss with scarring may be due to permanent damage of the matrix following trauma, or late stages of acquired onychatrophia following lichen planus, bullous diseases, or where there is defective peripheral circulation.

In texts on congenital anomalies, this defect is sometimes referred to as aplastic anonychia, which does not always produce scarring.

Temporary, total nail loss may also result from severe progressive onycholysis.

Reference

Runne U. & Orfanos C.E. (1981) The human nail. *Curr. Prob. Dermatol.* **9**, 102.

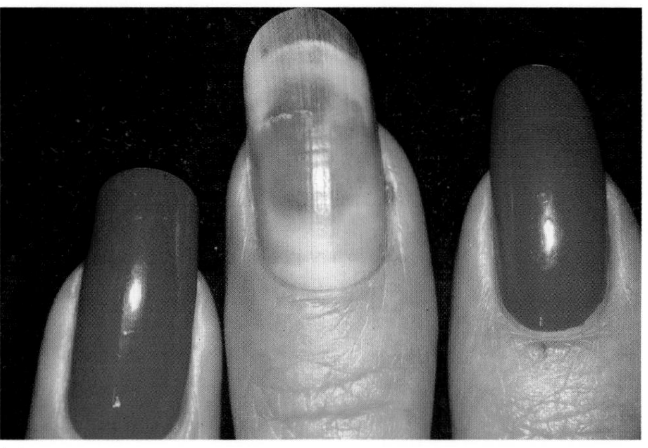

(a)

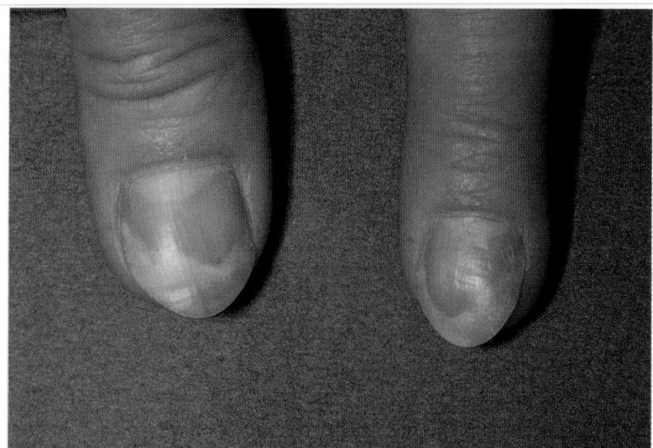

(b)

Fig. 2.38. (a & b) Onycholysis.

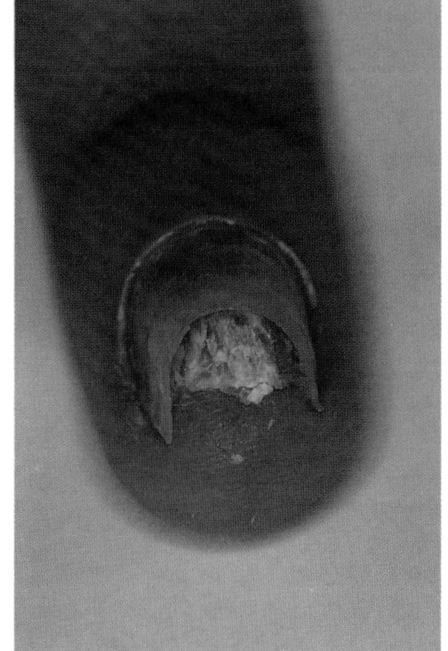

Fig. 2.39. Onycholysis, with rolling or coiling of the nail plate.

Onycholysis

Onycholysis refers to the detachment of the nail from its bed at its distal end and/or its lateral attachments (Fig. 2.38). The pattern of separation of the plate from the nail bed takes many forms. Sometimes it closely resembles the damage from a splinter under the nail, or the detachment extending proximally along a convex line, giving the appearance of a half-moon. When the process reaches the matrix, onycholysis becomes complete. Involvement of the lateral edge of the nail plate alone is less common. In certain cases, the free edge rises up like a hood, or coils up on itself like a roll of paper (Fig. 2.39). Onycholysis creates a subungual space that gathers dirt and keratin debris; the greyish-white colour is due to the presence of air under the nail but the colour may vary from yellow to brown, depending on the aetiology. This area is sometimes malodorous.

In psoriasis there is usually a yellow margin visible between the pink, normal nail and the white separated area. In the 'oily spot' or 'salmon-patch' variety, the nail plate–nail bed separation may start in the middle of the nail; this is sometimes surrounded by a yellow margin. The accumulation of large amounts of serum-like exudate containing glycoprotein, in and under the affected nails (Zaias, 1990), explains the colour change in this kind of onycholysis. Glycoprotein deposition is commonly found in inflammatory and eczematous diseases affecting the nail bed. Oil patches have been reported in systemic lupus erythematosus; they may be extensive in lectitis purulenta et granulomatosa (Runne *et al.*, 1978). Onycholysis is usually symptomless and it is mainly the appearance of the nail which brings the patient to the doctor; occasionally there is slight pain associated with inflammation in the early stages. The extent of onycholysis increases progressively and can be estimated by measuring the distance separating the distal edge of the lunula from the limit of proximal detachment (Taft, 1968). Transillumination of the terminal phalanx gives a good view of the area.

The onset of this condition may be sudden, as in photo-onycholysis (Baran & Juhlin, 1987) where there may be a triad of 'photosensitization, onycholysis and dyschromia' (Segal, 1963), or when the cause is contact with chemical irritants such as hydrofluoric acid (Shewmake & Anderson, 1979) or thioglycolate (Baran, 1980). Sculptured onycholysis (Zaias, 1990) is a self-induced nail abnormality produced by cleaning the underside of the nail plate with a sharp instrument. This results in an opaque, dead portion of the nail with a gently curved proximal, 'lytic' border.

Onycholysis of the toes demonstrates some differences from the condition on the fingers: the major distinctions are governed by:

1 the lack of occupational hazards;
2 the reduced use of cosmetics on the feet;
3 the protection afforded by footwear which reduces the risk of photoonycholysis;
4 mechanical factors.

The two main causes of onycholysis of the toenail, especially the great toenail are: (i) onychomycosis, since mycotic infection has always been considered to be the main causative condition involving the toenails; and (ii) repeated minor traumas.

'Primary' candida onycholysis is almost exclusively confined the fingernails.

Traumatic onycholysis of the toenails may present differently to onycholysis in the fingernails.

1 The diagnosis is conspicuous when the nail is lifted up by a bulla after strenous exercise in new footwear, not necessarily platform shoes. The bulla may have disappeared leaving an oozing nail bed. Sometimes there is only a blackish hue or thorough examination finds a distal worn-down great toenail.
2 Sometimes the diagnosis is not self-evident. A careful search must look for a discrete brownish tinge, the signature of the trauma.
3 In distal and subungual onychomycosis of the toenails, the horny thickening raises the free edge with disruption of the normal nail plate–nail bed attachment; this gives rise to secondary onycholysis in this common presentation.

Baran and Badillet (1982) have questioned whether big toenail onycholysis is ever truly primary. Its presence should always lead to a search for abnormalities of the foot such as hyperkeratosis of the metatarsal heads, large thickening of the ball of the foot or pressure on the big toe by an overriding second toe, this being fully developed when shoes are worn. All these disorders are frequently combined with high heels, narrow and slanting shoes.

Treatment consists of a silicone rubber-moulded toe cap, silicone rubber orthodigital splint, or direct moulding splint, the device being produced *in situ*.

In summary, dermatophyte infection and plantar anomalies are the main cause of onycholysis. In instances where it is idiopathic or traumatic, dermatophytes may act as commensal agents. We suggest that therapy should above all remove the pressure and help to restore proper balance to the foot with fitted shoes and padding or accommodative shields.

The various conditions which can produce onycholysis are listed in Table 2.4.

References

Baran R. (1980) Acute onycholysis from rust-removing agents. *Arch. Dermatol.* **116**, 382–383.

Baran R. & Badillet G. (1982) Primary onycholysis of the big toenails. A review of 113 cases. *Br. J. Dermatol.* **106**, 526.

Baran R. & Juhlin L. (1987) Drug-induced photo-onycholysis. Three subtypes identified in a study of 15 cases. *J. Am. Acad.*

Table 2.4. Classification of onycholysis (modified from Ray, 1963). See appropriate text for references

1 *Idiopathic*
- 1.1 Leukoonycholysis paradentotica (Schuppli, 1963)

2 *Systemic* (Chapter 6)
- 2.1 Circulatory (lupus erythematosus, Raynaud's syndrome, etc.)
- 2.2 Yellow nail syndrome
- 2.3 Endocrine (hypothyroidism, thyrotoxicosis, etc.)
- 2.4 Pregnancy
- 2.5 Syphilis (Chapter 4)
- 2.6 Iron deficiency anaemia, pellagra
- 2.7 Carcinoma of the lung (Hickman, 1977)
- 2.8 Shell nail syndrome (Cornelius, 1967)

3 *Congenital and/or hereditary* (Chapter 9)
- 3.1 Partial hereditary onycholysis (Schulze, 1966; Bazex 1990)
- 3.2 Hereditary nail dysplasia of the fifth toe (Hundeiker, 1969)
- 3.3 Malalignment of the big toenail (Baran, 1983)
- 3.4 Speckled hyperpigmentation, palmoplantar punctate keratoses and childhood blistering (Boss, 1981).
- 3.5 Hereditary ectodermal dystrophy (Clouston, 1929)
- 3.6 Pachyonychia congenita
- 3.7 Hyperpigmentation and hypohidrosis (Sparrow, 1976)
- 3.8 Hypoplastic enamel, onycholysis and hypohidrosis inherited as an autosomal dominant trait (Witkop, 1975)
- 3.9 Periodic shedding, leprechaunism, Darier's disease

4 *Cutaneous diseases*
- 4.1 Psoriasis, Reiter's syndrome, vesiculous or bullous disease, lichen planus, alopecia areata, multicentric reticulohistiocysis
- 4.2 Atopic dermatitis, contact dermatitis (accidental or occupational)
- 4.3 Hyperhidrosis
- 4.4 Tumours of the nail bed, histiocytosis-X (Chapter 10)
  Pyogenic granuloma
  Bowen's disease, mycosis fungoides (Kechijian, 1985, Mikhail, 1984)
- 4.5 Drugs: bleomycin, doxorubicin, 5-fluorouracil, retinoids, oral contraceptives (Byrne, 1976; Zaun, 1985)
  Indomethacin, captopril (Brueggemeyer & Ramirez, 1984) (Chapter 6)
- 4.6 Drug-induced photoonycholysis: trypaflavine, chlorpromazine, chloramphenicol, cephaloridine, cloxacillin (exceptional), clorazepate dipotassium (Torras *et al.*, 1989), allopurinol (Shelley, 1985)
  Tetracylines: especially demethylchlortetracycline and doxycycline but also minocyline (Angeloni *et al.*, 1987)
  Fluoroquinolones (Baran, 1986)
  Photochemotherapy with psoralens (sunlight or PUVA)
  Benoxaprofen, thiazide diuretics, flumequine (Revuz & Pouget, 1983)

5 *Local causes* (Chapters 7, 8, 10)
- 5.1 Traumatic (accidental, occupational, self-inflicted or mixed) – Chapter 7

continued

Table 2.4. *Continued*

- 5.1.1 As when clawing, pinching or stabbing causes trauma to the nails
- 5.1.2 Foreign bodies
- 5.2 Infections – see Chapter 4
  - 5.2.1 Fungal
  - 5.2.2 Bacterial (granulomatous purulent nail bed inflammation, Chapter 10)
  - 5.2.3 Viral (e.g. warts; herpes simplex)
- 5.3 Chemical (accidental or occupational – Chapter 9)
  - 5.3.1 Prolonged immersion in (hot) water with alkalis and detergents, sodium hypochlorite, etc.
  - 5.3.2 Paint removers
  - 5.3.3 Sugar solution
  - 5.3.4 Gasoline and similar solvents
  - 5.3.5 Cosmetics (see Chapter 8) (base coats, formaldehyde, false nails, depilatory products (Baran, 1980); nail polish removers (Milstein, 1982, Kechijian, 1991). Nickel derived from metal pellets in nail varnish
- 5.4 Physical – Chapter 7
  Thermal injury (accidental or occupational)
  Microwaves

Dermatol. **17**, 1012–1016.

Bazex J., Baran R., Monbrun F. *et al.* (1990) Hereditary distal onycholysis. *Clin. Exp. Dermatol.* **15**, 146–148.

Brueggmeyer C.D. & Ramirez G. (1984) Onycholysis associated with captopril. *Lancet* **1**, 1352–1353.

Heller J. (1927) Die Krankheiten der Nägel. In: *Handbuch der Haut-und Geschlechtskrankheiten*, ed. Jadassohn J., Bd VIII/2, Spezielle Dermatologie, pp. 150–172.

Kechijian P. (1991) Nail polish removers: are they harmful? *Seminars Dermatol.* **10**, 26–28.

Milstein H.G. (1982) Onycholysis due to nail polish remover. *The Schoch Letter* **32**, 51.

Ray L. (1963) Onycholysis. *Arch. Dermatol. Syphil.* **88**, 181.

Revuz J. & Pouget F. (1983) Photoonycholyse à l'apurone (flumequine). *Ann. Dermatol. Venereol.* **110**, 765.

Runne U., Goerz E. & Weese A. (1978) Lectitis purulenta et granulomatosa. *Z. Hautkr.* **53**, 625.

Schuppli R. (1963) Über eine mit Paradentose kombinierte Veränderung der Nägel. *Z. Haut Geschl. Kr.* **34**, 114–117.

Segal B.M. (1963) Photosensitivity, nail discoloration and onycholysis; side-effect of tetracycline therapy. *Arch. Int. Med.* **112**, 165.

Shewmake S.W. & Anderson B.G. (1979) Hydrofluoric acid burns. *Arch. Dermatol.* **115**, 593–596.

Taft F.H. (1968) Onycholysis. A clinical review. *Aust. J. Dermatol.* **2**, 345.

Torras H., Mascaro J.M. Jr & Mascaro J.M. (1989) Photo-onycholysis caused by clorazepate dipotassium. *J. Am. Acad. Dermatol.* **21**, 1304–1305.

Zaias N. (1990) *The Nail in Health and Disease*, 2nd edn. Lange & Appleton, Norwalk, CN.

Subungual hyperkeratosis

Besides congenital nail bed hyperplasia, epithelial hyperplasia of the subungual tissues results from exudative skin

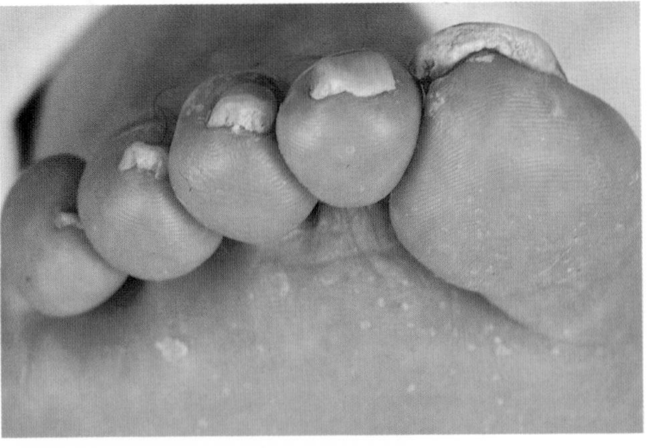

(a)

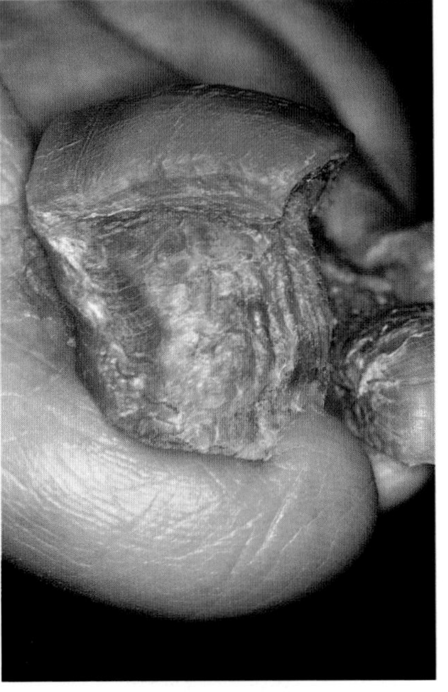

(b)

Fig. 2.40. Subungual hyperkeratosis: (a) mild; (b) severe.

diseases and may occur with any chronic inflammatory condition which involves this area. It is especially common in psoriasis, pityriasis rubra pilaris (Fig. 2.40) and chronic eczema, or it may be due to fungi. Histology reveals PAS-positive, homogeneous rounded or oval-shaped, amorphous masses surrounded by normal squamous cells usually separated from each other by empty spaces. These clumps, which coalesce and enlarge, have been described by Zaias (1990) in psoriasis of the nail. They are also found in some hyperkeratotic processes such as warts involving the subungual area. Subungual keratosis may also be seen in lichen planus, Reiter's disease, Sézary's syndrome, Darier's disease and in Norwegian scabies (Achten & Wanet-Rouard, 1970). The horny excrescences of the nail bed are not very marked but the ridged structure may become apparent if the nail plate is shortened.

In keratosis cristarum (Alkiewicz & Pfister, 1976) the keratinizing process is limited to the peripheral area of the nail bed (Fig. 2.41). It starts at its distal portion but may progress somewhat proximally. Scopulariopsis (acaulis) onychomycosis, which may present similar alterations, should be ruled out.

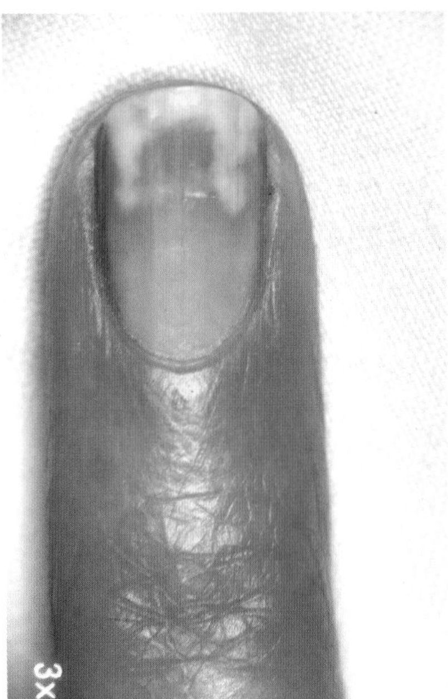

Fig. 2.41. Subungual hyperkeratosis of 'keratosis cristarum' type.

References

Achten G. & Wanet-Rouard J. (1970) Pachynonychia. *Br. J. Dermatol.* 83, 56.

Alkiewicz J. & Pfister R. (1976) *Atlas der Nagelkrankheiten.* Schattauer Verlag, Stuttgart.

Zaias N. (1990) *The Nail in Health and Disease*, 2nd edn. Lange & Appleton, Norwalk, CN.

Modifications in perionychial tissues

Paronychia, ingrowing nails, tumours of the nail folds and periungual telangiectasia are each described in the appropriate section. Thickened, hyperkeratotic, irregular ('ragged') cuticles have been reported, especially in dermatomyositis, but may be seen in normal individuals. Thickened cuticle composed of several layers and called 'polyeponychia bolboides' (onion-like) by Happle and Chang (1991) can be an unusual manifestation of factitious disorders.

Perionychial tissues are subject to trauma. There may be self-inflicted erosions of the nail folds in association with neurosis. The ulnar side of the nail is most vulnerable and there may be small, triangular tags of epidermis ('hang nail') which are painful and vulnerable to secondary infection.

Hang nails may also result from occupational injuries. With the hydration and dehydration caused by frequent

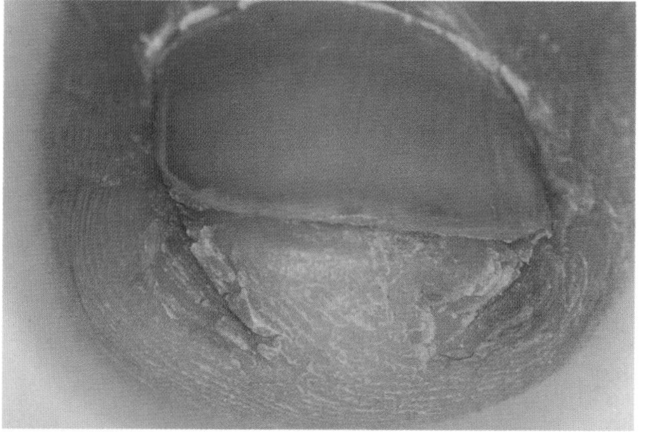

Fig. 2.42. Dorsolateral, distal fissures – may be painful.

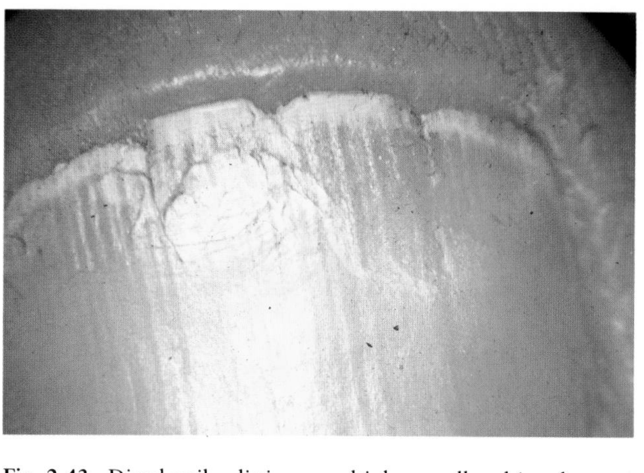

Fig. 2.43. Distal nail splitting – multiple crenellated 'castle battlement' appearance.

wetting, and in people with dry skin, particulary in winter, painful dorso-lateral fissures may be seen located distal to the lateral nail groove (Dawber & Baran, 1984) and converging to the tip of the finger (Fig. 2.42). They also can be observed in atopic patients and as occupational disorders in cement workers, for example. Hydrocolloid dressing (Epilyt) used by Baden (1989) markedly improved this condition.

References

Baden H.P. (1989) Management of fingertip cracking with Epilyt. *J. Am. Acad. Dermatol.* **20**, 1135–1136.

Dawber R.P.R. & Baran R. (1984) Painful dorso-lateral fissure of the fingertip – an extension of the lateral nail groove. *Clin. Exp. Dermatol.* **9**, 419–420.

Happle R. & Chang A. (1991) Polyeponychia bolboides: an unusual manifestation of factitious disorder. *Eur. J. Dermatol.* **1**, 35–37.

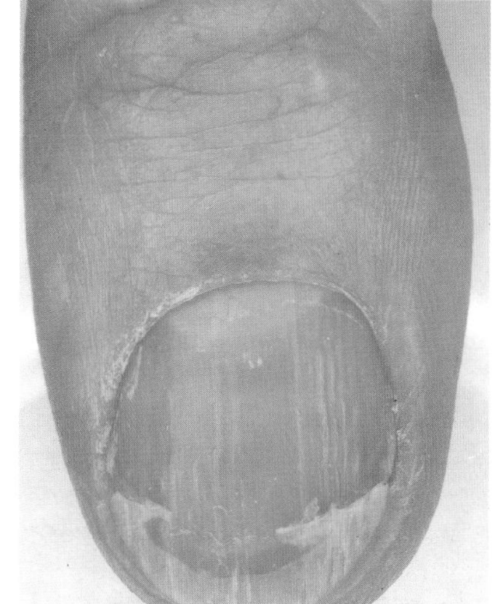

Fig. 2.44. Lateral transverse nail splitting.

Modifications in the consistency of the nail

The nail plate may be hard, soft, brittle or friable.

Hard nails are seen in pachyonychia congenita. They must be soaked for prolonged periods before they can be trimmed; large, 'professional' nail clippers are most suitable for this purpose. Jadassohn, who first described this syndrome, had to use a hammer and chisel on the hardened nails of his patient.

For very *soft nails* the term hapalonychia is used. Such nails may be thinner than usual (less than 0.5 mm) and bend easily and break or split at the free edge. In some cases the nails, which assume a semi-transparent, bluish-white hue, are referred to as 'egg-shell nails'. Hapalonychia has been noted in chronic arthritis, leprosy, myxoedema, acroasphyxia, peripheral neuritis, hemiplegia, cachexia, and other states. Occupational contact with chemicals is probably the most common cause. 'Soft nail disease' (Prandi & Caccialanza, 1977) is an unusual, congenital nail dystrophy with anatomical and functional defects of the nail matrix.

Brittle nails may be divided into four types (Baran, 1978).

1 An isolated split at the free edge which sometimes extends proximally. It may result from onychorrhexis with its shallow parallel furrows running in the superficial layer of the nail.

2 Multiple, crenellated splitting which resembles the battlements of a castle. Triangular pieces may easily be torn from the free margin (Fig. 2.43).

3 A lamellar splitting of the free edge of the nail into fine layers (see p. 53). It may occur in isolation or associated with the other types.

4 Transverse splitting and breaking of the lateral edge close to the distal margin (Fig. 2.44). The changes in brittle, friable nails are often confined to the surface of the nail

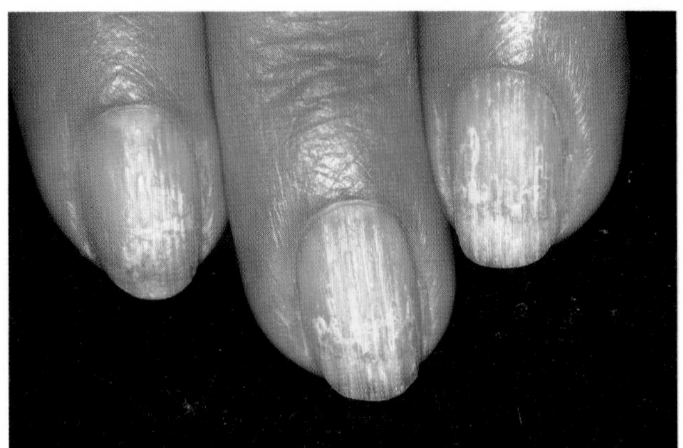

Fig. 2.45. Friability of the nail surface, here caused by nail cosmetic 'base coat'.

plate; friability occurs in superficial white onychomycosis and may be seen after application of nail polish or base coat which causes 'granulations' in the nail keratin (Fig. 2.45) (see Chapter 7). In advanced psoriasis and fungal infection the friability may extend throughout the entire nail.

The changes in nail consistency may be due to impairment of one or more of the factors on which the health of the nail depends, and include such elements as variations in the water content or the keratin constituent. Changes in the intercellular structures, cell membranes, and intracellular changes in the arrangement of keratin fibrils have been revealed by electron microscopy. Normal nails contain approximately 18% water. After prolonged immersion in water this percentage is increased and the nail becomes soft; this makes toenail trimming much easier. A low lipid content may decrease the nail's ability to retain water. If the water content is considerably reduced, the nail becomes brittle. Splitting, which results from this brittle quality, is probably partly due to repeated uptake of water and drying out.

The keratin content may be modified by chemical and physical insults, especially in occupational nail disorders (Chapter 7). Amino acid chains may be broken or distorted by alkalis, oxidizing agents and thioglycolates, such as chemicals employed in the permanent waving processes. These break or distort the multiple —S—S— bond linkages which join the protein chains to form the keratin fibrils. Keratin structure can also be changed in genetic disorders (Price *et al.*, 1980). In some congenital conditions, such as dyskeratosis congenita, the nail plate may be completely absent, or reduced to thin, dystrophic remnants.

The composition of the nail plate is sometimes related to generalized disease. High sulphur content is predominantly in the form of cystine, which contributes to the stability of the fibrous protein by the formation of disulphide bonds. A lack of iron can result in softening of the nail and koilonychia; conversely, the calcium content in the nail appears to contribute little towards its hardness. Calcium is mainly in the surface of the nail, in small absorbed quantities, and X-ray diffraction shows no evidence of calcite or apatite crystals. Damage to both the central and peripheral nervous system may result in nail fragility.

Causes of nail fragility

These may be local or, less frequently, systemic.

Local causes

The nail may be damaged by trauma or by chemical agents such as detergents, alkalis, various solvents and sugar solutions, and especially by hot water.

The nail plate requires 5–6 months in order to regenerate and therefore is vulnerable to daily insults. Those who carry out many domestic chores, particularly wet work, are very susceptible; particularly at risk are the first three fingers of the dominant hand. Anything which slows the rate of nail growth will increase the risk. Cosmetic causes are rare. Some varnishes will damage the superficial layers of the nail. Drying may be enhanced by some nail varnish removers and soaking fingers in a warm soapy solution, for removing the cuticle, is especially dangerous; this is common practice among manicurists. It has been shown that climatic and seasonal factors may affect the hydration of the nail plate.

Fragility, due to thinning of the nail plate, may be caused by a reduction in the length of the matrix. Diminution, or even complete arrest of nail formation over a variable width, may be the result of many dermatoses such as eczema, lichen planus, psoriasis (rare) and impairment of the peripheral circulation. The frequency of nail fragility in alopecia areata lends credence to the popular belief that nail and hair disorders are often associated.

Lubach and Beckers (1992) have shown that the bridges between nail corneocytes are possibly weaker in women than in men as a constitutional characteristic. Accordingly, frequent, alternating periods of hydration and drying increase the incidence of brittle nails, particularly in women.

General causes

Among these are included hypochromic anaemia, reduction in serum iron, arsenical intoxication, infection, diseases which produce severe, generalized effects, arthritic deformities of the distal joints, deficiencies in vitamins A, C and B_6, osteoporosis and osteomalacia: also, there are numerous inherited defects associated with atrophy of the nail. The diverse constituents of the nail plate, especially the enzymes necessary for the formation of keratin, are subject to genetic influences and changes in them are manifested in the form of hereditary disease.

Treatment of brittle nails

Moisture (excess hydration) and trauma must be avoided at all cost; routine household chores are particularly damaging. Protection with rubber gloves worn over light cotton glove liners should be used in order to avoid frequent direct contact with water.

Warm environment and hyperaemia may lead to faster growth. This could bring about a reduction in the time the nail plate is exposed to repeated minor chemical and physical actions which accentuate nail fragility.

There is no efficient barrier cream able to prevent oversoftening of the nails due to water and detergents. After hydration, the nail plate should be massaged with mineral oil or a lubricating cream to prevent the nail from drying out. Under experimental conditions hydration may be further enhanced by the addition of phospholipids which have been shown to be effective in increasing and maintaining the increased nail flexibility (Finlay *et al.*, 1980). This may result from an occlusive effect of the applications which may delay the evaporation of water. Base coat, nail polish and hard top coat act in a similar manner and also have a splint-like effect in strengthening the nail.

Soft nails may be hardened by painting them daily with 5% aluminium chloride in propylene glycol and water.

Systemic treatment may be helpful. Oral iron, even in the absence of demonstrable iron deficiency (given for 6 months), may be of some value. Campbell and McEwan (1980) suggested the following regime: evening primrose oil (Efamol G) two capsules t.i.d., pyridoxine 25–30 mg/day and ascorbic acid 2–3 g/day. Zaun (1981) demonstrated that brittle nails, tested with a standardized micrometric method, swell significantly less than normal nails: an increase of this 'swelling factor' was seen in 10 patients treated with Pantovigar (thiamin, calcium-D-panthothenate, L-cystine and *p*-aminobenzoic acid); gelatin has recently been advocated (Gehzing & Gloor, 1992). Biotin has been suggested for brittle nails (Colombo *et al.*, 1990; Hochman *et al.*, 1993).

References

Baran R. (1978) Fragilité des ongles. *Cutis* **2**, 457.

Campbell A.J. & McEwan G.C. (1980) Treatment of brittle nails and dry eyes. *Br. J. Dermatol.* **105**, 113.

Colombo V.E., Gerber F., Bronhofer M. *et al.* (1990) Treatment of brittle fingernails and onychoschizia with biotin: Scanning electron microscopy. *J. Am. Acad. Dermatol.* **23**, 1127–1132.

Finlay A.Y., Frost P., Keith A.D. *et al.* (1980) An assessment of factors influencing flexibility of human fingernails. *Br. J. Dermatol.* **103**, 357.

Gehzing W. & Gloor M. (1992) Vezbesserung der Nagelqualität durch gelatine. *Akt. Dermatol.* **18**, 364–366.

Hochman L.G., Scher R.K. & Meyerson M.S. (1993) Brittle nails: Response to daily biotin supplementation. *Cutis.* **51**, 303–305.

Lubach D. & Beckers P. (1992) Wet working conditions increase brittleness of nails, but do not cause it. *Dermatology* **185**, 120–122.

Prandi G. & Caccialanza M. (1977) An unusual congenital nail dystrophy (soft nail diseases) *Clin Exp. Dermatol.* **2**, 265.

Price V.H., Odom R.B., Ward W.H. & Jones F.T. (1980) Trichothiodystrophy: sulphur-deficient brittle hair as a marker for a neuroectodermal symptom complex. *Arch. Dermatol.* **116**, 1375.

Zaun H. (1981) Der Nagel-Quellfaktor als Kriterium für Wirksamkeit und aussichtsreichen Einsatz von Nageltherapeutika bei brüchigen und splitternden Nägeln. *Ärztl Kosmet.* **11**, 242.

Modification in colour: chromonychia or dyschromia

The term chromonychia indicates an abnormality in colour of the substance or the surface of the nail plate and/or subungual tissues.

Generally, abnormalities of colour depend on the transparency of the nail, its attachments and the character of the underlying tissues. Pigment may accumulate due to hyperproduction (of melanin) or storage (e.g. of copper, various drugs, exceptionally haemosiderin); or by surface deposition. Subungual haematoma leads to accumulation of blood which cannot be degraded to haemosiderin since it is located between the nail plate on top and the newly formed deeper nail plate portion from the more distal matrix. A narrow longitudinal haemosiderin band in the nail was described by Alkiewicz and Pfister (1976): a 24-year-old patient with adult prurigo developed a brownish-red stripe in his thumb nail from the matrix slowly reaching the free edge. It grew out after about 5 months. Haemosiderin granules were demonstrated by Prussian blue staining. Small granules were located intracellularly, large globules intercellularly.

Exposure to ferric chloride (10% solution) causes rapid oxidation and darkening of melanin, whereas the benzidine test is positive if haemoglobin is present (Pappert *et al.*, 1991).

The nails provide a long-sustained, historical record of profound temporary abnormalities of the control of skin pigment which otherwise might pass unnoticed. Colour is also affected by the state of the skin vessels and various intravascular factors such as anaemia and carbon monoxide poisoning.

Certain important points concerning the examination of abnormal nails are worthy of mention (Daniel, 1985). They should be studied with the fingers completely relaxed and not pressed against any surface. Failure to do this may alter the haemodynamics of the nail and change its appearance. The fingertip should then be blanched to see if the pigmented abnormality is grossly altered; this may help to differentiate between discoloration of the nail plate and of the vascular bed. If the discoloration is in the vascular bed, it will usually disappear. Further information may be gleaned by transillumination of the nail using a pen torch placed againt the pulp. If the discoloration is in the matrix or soft tissue, the exact position can more easily be identified. To determine if the colour is in the plate, a piece of nail should be cut off and examined while immersed in water. When nail specimens are allowed to dry, their true colour may be obscured by light scattering (Baden, 1987). Furthermore, if a topical agent is suspected (Cortese, 1981) as the cause, one can remove the discoloration by scraping or cleaning the nail plate with a solvent such as acetone. If the substance is impregnated more deeply into the nail or subungually, microscopic studies of potassium hydroxide preparations or biopsy specimens using special stains may be indicated. Wood's lamp examination is sometimes useful. Nail composition studies might be helpful in the future.

When there is nail contact with occupationally derived agents, or topical application of therapeutic agents the discoloration often follows the shape of the proximal nail fold. If the discoloration corresponds to the shape of the lunula, internal causes predominate (Zaias, 1990).

Causes of colour modification

The causes are summarized in the following list; the subtypes within these broad groups are described in the chapters indicated or in the tables which follow the main list.

1 **Exogenous causes** (see Chapters 6 and 7)
   (a) Contact with occupationally derived agents (see also Chapter 7).
   (b) Topical application of therapeutic agents (see Table 2.5).
   (c) Tobacco, cosmetics and miscellaneous (see Table 2.6).
   (d) Traumatic causes (see Table 2.7) (see also Chapter 10).
   (e) Physical agents (see Table 2.8).
   (f) Fungal and bacterial chromonychia (see also Chapter 4).

References (to Tables 2.5–2.8)

Alkiewicz J. & Pfister R. (1976) *Atlas der Nagelkrankheiten. Pathohistologie, Klinik und Differentialdiagnose*, pp. 28–29. Schattauer, Stuttgart.

Baden H.P. (1987) *Diseases of the Hair and Nails*, p. 21. Year Book Medical Publ., Chicago.

Baran R. (1987) Frictional longitudinal melanonychia: A new entity. *Dermatologica* **174**, 280–284.

Baran R. (1990) Nail biting and picking as a possible cause of longitudinal melanonychia. A study of 6 cases. *Dermatologica* **181**, 126–128.

Brodkin R.H. & Bleiberg J. (1973) Cutaneous microwave injury. A report of two cases. *Acta Derm. Venereol.* **53**, 50.

Cortese T.A. (1981) Capitrol shampoo, nail discoloration. *The Schoch Letter* **31**, 154.

Coulson I.H. (1993) 'Fade out' photochromonychia. *Clin. Exp. Dermatol.* **18**, 87–88.

Daniel C.R. (1985) Nail pigmentation abnormalities. *Dermatol. Clin.* **3**, 431–443.

Daniel C.R. & Osment L.S. (1982) Nail pigmentation abnormalities. *Cutis* **30**, 348.

Inalsingh A. (1972) Melanonychia after treatment of malignant disease with radiation and cyclophosphamide. *Arch. Dermatol.* **106**, 765.

Jeune R. & Ortonne J.P. (1979) Chromonychia following thermal injury. *Acta Derm. Venereol.* **59**, 91–92.

Lovemann A.B. & Fliegelman M.T. (1955) Discoloration of the nails. *Arch. Dermatol.* **72**, 153.

Mann R.J. & Hermann R.R.M. (1983) Nail staining due to hydroquinone skin-lightening creams. *Br. J. Dermatol.* **108**, 363–365.

Olsen T.G. & Jatlav P. (1984) Contact exposure to elemental iron causing chromonychia. *Arch. Dermatol.* **120**, 102.

Pappert A.S., Scher R.K. & Cohen J.L. (1991) Longitudinal pigmented nail bands. *Dermatol. Clin.* **9**, 703–716.

Platschek H. (1989) Brown hair and nail discoloration by water containing iron. *Hautazzt* **40**, 441–442.

Schauder S. (1990) Adverse reactions to sun screening agents in 58 patients. *Z. Hautkr.* **66**, 294–318.

Trevisan G. & Mlac M. (1979) Melanonychia post-irradiazone roentgen. *Min. Dermatol.* **114**, 165.

Verbov J. (1985) Topical tartrazine as an unusual cause of staining. *Br. J. Dermatol.* **101**, 729.

Zaias N. (1990) *The Nail in Health and Disease*, 2nd edn. Lange & Appleton, Norfalk, CN.

White discoloration of the nails is common with most fungal infections. The condition, superficial white onychomycosis (SWO), is an infection where the initial invasion occurs from the top surface of the nail plate. The disease normally presents with invasion of the superficial aspect of the nail plate together with a powdery discoloration which is chalky white. Fungal hyphae are present on the top surface of the nail. The main causes of this condition are *Trichophyton mentagrophytes*, *Microsporum persicolor*, *Fusarium*, *Aspergillus* and *Acremonium* spp. It has also been reported by Zaias (1990) that *Candida albicans* may produce this pattern of nail plate invasion in infants.

The colour of the nail in dermatophyte infections may also be yellow or brown, particularly in the case of *Trichophyton mentagrophytes* which may result in streaky pigmentation of the great toenails. *Scopulariopsis brevicaulis* causes an infection of the toenails in which the colour is a light cinnamon brown due to the pigmentation of the fungal spores in the nail matrix.

Acrothecium nigrum (Young, 1934) and *Fusarium oxysporum* (Ritchie & Pinkerton, 1959) are said to cause a black-green discoloration of the nail. There are a large number of brown pigmented fungi and some of these cause nail disease, although it is possible that in some reported cases fungi may simply have colonized areas of onycholysis.

Causes of fungal melanonychia are shown in Table 2.9. In fungal melanonychia the nail plate appears black but the pigment is often grouped into a cluster at the distal edge. The pigmentation has irregular density and is irregularly distributed.

In *Candida* infections of the nail there is often a greenish discoloration at the lateral margin and near the nail fold. This is particularly prominent in paronychia or where there is extensive onycholysis. The pigment is confined to the undersurface of the nail where there is onycholysis, and can be removed by scraping the area. In paronychia the pigment may involve the upper surface of the nail plate. In most cases this is due to the presence of *Pseudomonas* species, but it is not clear whether this is due to organisms within the nail plate or whether diffusible pigment is present. It is often difficult to exclude or prove in these cases whether Gram-negative bacteria are present as well (Moore & Marcus, 1951).

Pseudomonas species can colonize any area of the nail where there is onycholysis, as well as the nail fold. The pigmentation that follows this colonization varies both with the species involved and the composition of pigments produced. The colours vary from a light green to dark green/black. *Pseudomonas* species produce a number of different diffusible pigments such as pyocyanin (dark green) and fluorescein (yellow-green). These are soluble in water, the former in chloroform as well (Bauer & Cohen, 1957). This discoloration may involve the entire nail plate or only part of it. Green striped nails may result from repeated episodes of bacterial infection with deposition of organisms and pigment during each episode (Shellow & Koplon, 1963). Some help in the diagnosis can be obtained by soaking nail fragments in water or chloroform (Baran & Badillet, 1978). If these turn green it is likely that *Pseudomonas* has been or is present, and this is the most likely reason for the deposition of pigment in the nail. Black discoloration of the nails due to *Proteus mirabilis* has been reported (Zuehlke & Taylor, 1970; Higashi, 1990b).

Nail pigmentation due to fungi and possibly also to bacteria such as *Pseudomonas* spp. and *Proteus* spp. is usually readily identified also in histological nail sections. The nail plate exhibits a diffuse yellowish to brown discoloration that stands out in haematoxylin and eosin (H & E) stain and more clearly in PAS stains.

Pigmentation of the nail bed has been reported in pinta by Medina (1963).

Secondary syphilis may present with chromonychia (see Chapter 4).

References

Badillet G., Panagiotidou D. & Sené S. (1984) Etude rétrospective des *Trichophyton rubrum* a pigment noir diffusible isolés à Paris de 1971 à 1980. *Bull. Soc. Fr. Mycol. Méd.* **13**, 117–120.

Badillet G. (1988) Mélanonychies superficielles. *Bull. Soc. Fr. Mycol. Med.* **17**, 335–340.

Baran R. & Badillet G. (1978) Les ongles verts ou syndrome chloronychique. *Cutis (France)* **2**, 469–479.

Bauer M.F. & Cohen B.A. (1957) The role of *Pseudomonas aeruginosa* in infection about the nails. *Arch. Dermatol.* **75**, 394.

Daniel C.R. (1990) Pigmentation abnormalities. In: *Nails: Therapy, Diagnosis, Surgery*, eds Scher R.K. & Daniel C.R., Chap. 11. W.B. Saunders, Philadelphia.

Higashi N. (1990a) Melanonychia due to tinea unguium. *Hifu* **32**, 379–380.

Higashi N. (1990b) *Proteus mirabilis. Hifu* **32**, 245–249.

Matsumoto T., Matsuda T., Padhye A.A., Standard P.G. & Ajello L. (1992) Fungal melanonychia: an ungual phaeohyphomycosis caused by *Wangiella dermatitidis. Clin. Exp. Dermatol.* **17**, 83–86.

Medina R. (1963) El Carate en Venezuela. *Derm. Venez.* **3**, 160.

Moore M. & Marcus M.D. (1951) Green nails: role of *Candida* and *Pseudomonas aeruginosa. Arch. Dermatol.* **64**, 499.

Perrin C. & Baran R. (1994) Fungal melanonychia due to *Trichophyton rubrum*. In press.

Ritchie E.B. and Pinkerton M.E. (1959) Fusarium oxysporum infection of the nail. *Arch. Dermatol.* **79**, 705.

Shellow W.V.R. & Koplon B.S. (1963) Green striped nails: chromonychia due to *Pseudomonas aeruginosa.* Arch Dermatol. **97**, 149.

Young W.J. (1934) Pigmented mycotic growth beneath the nails. *Arch. Dermatol.* **30**, 186.

Zaias N. (1990) *The Nail in Health and Disease*, 2nd edn. Lange & Appleton, Norfalk, CN.

Zuehlke R.L. & Taylor W.B. (1970) Black nails with *Proteus mirabilis. Arch. Dermatol.* **102**, 154.

2 **Effects of systemic drugs and chemicals** (see also Chapter 6)

(a) Psoralens (see Table 2.10).

(b) Antimalarials (see Table 2.11).

(c) Cancer chemotherapeutic agents (see also Chapter 6).

(d) Antirheumatic drugs (see Table 2.12).

(e) Other systemic drugs and chemicals (see Table 2.13).

3 **Some dermatological conditions** (see Table 2.14; see also Chapters 9 and 15)

4 **Systemic infections** (see Table 2.15)

5 **Non-infectious systemic conditions** (see also Chapter 6)

(a) Alimentary tract disease (see Table 2.16).

(b) Cardiac failure and peripheral circulatory impairment (see Table 2.17).

(c) Blood dycrasias (see Table 2.18).

(d) Renal disease (see Table 2.19).

(e) Hormonal conditions (see Table 2.20).
(f) Malignancies (see Table 2.21).
(g) Miscellaneous (see Table 2.22).

6 Longitudinal melanonychia

Causes (see Table 2.23; see also Chapters 10 and 11).

References

Alkiewicz J. & Pfister R. (1976) *Atlas der Nagelkrankheiten*, pp. 28–29. F.K. Schattauer Verlag, *Stuttgart*.

Allenby C.F. & Snell P.H. (1966) Longitudinal pigmentation of the nails in Addison's disease. *Br. Med. J.* **1**, 1582–1583.

Aplas V. (1957) Hyperbilirubinämische Melanonychie. *Z. Hautkr.* **22**, 203–207.

Aratari E., Regesta G. & Rebora A. (1984) Carpal tunnel syndrome appearing with prominent skin symptoms. *Arch. Dermatol.* **120**, 517–519.

Baran R. (1979) Longitudinal melanotic streaks as a clue to Laugier–Hunziker syndrome. *Arch. Dermatol.* **115**, 1448–1449.

Baran R. (1987) Frictional longitudinal melanonychia: a new entity. *Dermatologica* **174**, 280–284.

Baran R., Jancovici E., Sayag J. *et al.* (1985) Longitudinal melanonychia in lichen planus. *Br. J. Dermatol.* **113**, 369–370.

Baran R. & Barrière H. (1986) Longitudinal melanonychia with spreading pigmentation in Laugier–Hunziker syndrome: a report of two cases. *Br. J. Dermatol.* **115**, 707–710.

Baran R. & Eichmann A. (1993) Longitudinal melanonychia associated with Bowen disease. Two new cases. *Dermatology* **186**, 159–160.

Table 2.5. Causes of nail colour modification: topical application of therapeutic agents

Aetiology	Colour	Location	Remarks
Ammoniated mercury	Brown	Nail	
Amphotericin B	Yellow	Nail	
Anthralin }		Nail	
Arning's tincture }	Orange	Nail	Cignoline
Chrysarobin }		Nail	
Chlorophyll derivatives	Green	Nail	Daniel & Osment (1982)
Cupric sulphate	Blue	Nail	
Dinitrochlorobenzene	Yellow	Nail	
Eosin	Red	Nail	
Fluorescein	Yellow	Nail	
5-Fluorouracil	Brown		
Formaldehyde	Grey	Nail	
Fuchsin	Purple	Nail	
Gentian violet	Purple	Nail	
Glutaraldehyde	Golden brown	Nail	
Hydroquinone	Grey	Nail	With light exposure
Iodine	Brown	Nail	
Iodochlorhydroxyquinolone	Orange-brown	Nail	Vioform
Mercurochrome	Red	Nail	
Mercury bichloride	Grey blue	Nail	After sun exposure
Methylene blue	Blue	Nail	
Methyl green	Green	Nail	
Nitric acid and derivatives	Yellow	Nail	
Picric acid	Yellow	Nail	
Potassium permanganate	Chestnut brown	Nail	Stain may be removed from nails with 3% hydrogen peroxide, sodium propionate
Prophyllin	Green	Nail	
Pyrogallol	Brown	Nail	
Resorcin	Brown	Nail	
Rivanol	Brown	Nail	Ethacridine lactate
Silver nitrate	Black	Nail	
Sodium hypochlorite	Leukonychia	Bed	Onycholysis
Sublimate	Brown	Nail	
Tars	Black/yellow	Nail	
Tartrazine	Yellow	Nail	Adhesive plaster pad (Verbov, 1985)
Tetracycline	Yellow	Nail	Treatment of acne

Table 2.6. Causes of nail colour modification: tobacco and cosmetics and miscellaneous (see Chapters 7 and 8)

Aetiology	Colour	Location	Remarks
Heavy smokers	Chestnut brown	Nail	Along the lateral nail fold and adjacent pulp 1st, 2nd and 3rd finger
Hair cosmetics			
Chloroxine	Spectrum of colours	Nail	Active ingredient in Capitrol shampoo (Cortese, 1981) Highly reactive to metals: aluminium + chloroxine → bright yellow; iron + chloroxine → green; nickel + chloroxine → deep green stainless steel + Capitrol → black
Hair dyes	Same as dye	Nail	
Henna	Chestnut brown	Nail	
Resorcinol	Yellow	Nail	Nail varnish (nitrocellulose) used with resorcinol containing products (Lovermann & Fliegelman, 1955)
Nail cosmetics			
False nails	Bluish, reddish	Nail	Subungual haemorrhage and its
Formaldehyde	then yellowish		resolution
Varnish	Spectrum of colours		
	Orange-brown	Nail	D & C reds especially
	Orange-green	Nail	Benzophenone (Schauder, 1990)
Bleaching agents			
Mercury	Greyish	Nail	Mercury intoxication (Chapter 7)
Hydroquinone	Orange brown	Nail	With light exposures (Mann & Hermann, 1983; Coulson, 1993)
Miscellaneous			
Dynap insecticide	Yellow	Nail	(Daniel & Osment, 1982)
Iron	Orange brown	Nail	Contact exposure to elemental iron (Olsen & Jatlav, 1984; Platschek, 1989)

Table 2.7. Traumatic causes of nail colour modification

Aetiology	Colour	Location	Remarks
Haematoma	Black Yellowish	Nail and bed	Depending on site of trauma Resolution of subungual haemorrhage
Splinter haemorrhage	Black	Bed	
Longitudinal melanonychia (after acute trauma)	Brown	Nail	Exeptional in Caucasians (Zehnder, 1970)
Frictional melanonychia	Brown	Nail	Baran (1987)
Nail biting and picking	Brown	Nail	Baran (1990)

Table 2.8. Physical agents contributing to nail colour modification

Aetiology	Colour	Location	Remarks
Radiotherapy of digits	Brown	Nail	Pigmented bands (Chapter 6)
Electron beam	Transverse pigmented band	Nail	Baran, personal observations
Radiotherapy for malignant disease elsewhere	Brown	Nail	Wide pigmented band (Inalsingh, 1972)
Cryotherapy	Transverse leuconychia	Nail	Transverse furrow
	Haemorrhage	Nail	
Thermal injury	Yellow-brown	Nail	Jeune & Ortonne (1979)
Microwaves	Whitish	Bed	Onycholysis Transverse dystrophic ridging (Brodkin & Bleiberg, 1973)

Table 2.9. Fungal causes of melanonychia

Proven	Possible
Alternaria spp.	*Aureobasidium pullulans*
Chaetomium perpulchrum	*Cladosporium sphaerospermum*
Cladosporium carrionii	*Phyllostictina sydowi*
Curvularia lunata	
Pyrenochaeta unguis-hominis	
Scytalidium dimidiatum (*Natrassia mangifera*, *Hendersonula toruloidea*)	
Trichophyton rubrum (Badillet *et al.*, 1984; Badillet, 1988; Higashi, 1990; Perrin & Baran, 1994)	
Wangiella dermatitidis (Matsumoto *et al.*, 1992)	

Baran R. & Simon C. (1988) Longitudinal melanonychia: a symptom of Bowen's disease. *J. Am. Acad. Dermatol.* **18**, 1359–1360.

Bisht D.B. & Singh S.S. (1962) Pigmented band on nails: a new sign in malnutrition. *Lancet* **1**, 507–508.

Bondy P.K. & Harwick H.J. (1969) Longitudinal banded pigmentation of nails following adrenalectomy for Cushing's syndrome. *N. Engl. J. Med.* **281**, 1056–1057.

Coskey R.J., Magnell T.D. & Bernacki E.G. Jr (1983) Congenital subungual nevus. *J. Am. Acad. Dermatol.* **9**, 747–751.

Daniel C.R. & Zaias N. (1988) Pigmentary abnormalities of the nails with emphasis on systemic diseases. *Dermatol. Clin.* **6**, 305–313.

Fisher B.K. & Warner L.C. (1987) Cutaneous manifestations of the acquired immunodeficiency syndrome: update 1987. *Int. J. Dermatol.* **26**, 615–630.

Freyer J.M. & Werth V.P. (1992) Pregnancy-associated hyperpigmentation: longitudinal melanonychia. *J. Am. Acad. Dermatol.* **26**, 493–494.

Table 2.10. Causes of nail colour modification: psoralens (see Chapter 6)

Aetiology	Colour	Location	Remark
8-Methoxypsoralen	Brown	Nail and/or bed	Pigmentation may be diffuse or present as longitudinal bands and haemorrhages may be seen in the nail bed with PUVA: photoonycholysis appears with PUVA or sunlight
5-Methoxypsoralen	Brown	Nail and/or bed	
Trimethylpsoralen	Brown	Nail and/or bed	

Table 2.11. Causes of nail colour modification: antimalarials (see Chapter 6)

Aetiology	Colour	Location	Remark
Camoquine	Blue-grey	Bed	
Chloroquine	Purplish-blue	Bed	
Quinacrine	Blue-green, slate grey White, yellow, grey	Bed Nail and/or bed	Green-yellow or whitish fluorescence under wood light

Table 2.12. Causes of nail colour modification: antirheumatic drugs (see Chapter 6)

Aetiology	Colour	Location	Remark
Benoxaprofen	White	Distal bed	Onycholysis and photoonycholysis
D-penicillamine	Yellow	Nail	Yellow nail syndrome
Gold salts	Black-brown	Nail	Latent onychomadesis

Table 2.13. Causes of nail colour modification: other sytemic drugs or chemicals (see Chapter 6)

Aetiology	Colour	Location	Remark
Acetanilide	Cyanosis	Bed	Methaemoglobinaemia
Acetyl salicyclic acid	Purpura	Bed	Aspirin
Acridine derivatives	Whitish	Distal bed	Acriflavine, trypaflavine photoonycholysis – onychoschizia
ACTH	Brown	Nail	Longitudinal streaks or diffuse pigmentation
Androgen	Half-and-half nail changes	Bed	
Aniline and nitrites derivatives of benzinic carbides	Purplish with cyanosis	Nail bed	Methaemoglobinaemia
Antimony	T. leuconychia		Poisoning
Arsenic	Brownish	Nail	Sometimes longitudinal bands (arsenicism)
	T. leuconychia	Nail	In acute intoxication (Mees' bands)
Betacarotene	Yellow–brown	Bed	
Brome	Haemorrhage	Bed	Acute poisoning
Canthaxantine	Yellow	Bed	
Carbon monoxide	Cherry red	Bed	Cochineal pink skin (Laugier, 1981)
Caustic soda	Yellow	Nail	High doses and
Chlorpromazine	Brown	Bed	prolonged treatment (psychiatric)
Chromium salts	Yellow ochre	Nail	
Phenytoin	Ochre brown	Nail	Fetal hydantoin syndrome
Dinitrophenol	Yellow	Bed	
Fluoride (fluorosis)	White patches, T. leuconychia	Nail	Brittleness, Beau's line, pits 'mottled nails'
	Longitudinal melanotic band		
5-Fluorouracil	Brown	Nail	When applied directly to periungual area
Heparin	T. red band	Bed	Acute poisoning (Alkiewicz & Pfister, 1976)
Iodine	Haemorrhage	Bed	
Ketoconazole	Brown	Nail and bed	Longitudinal bands; splinter haemorrhage
Lead	T. leuconychia	Nail	In acute poisoning; in chronic intoxication: onychomadesis, atrophy
Lithium carbonate	Rich golden	Distal bed	Great toenail, onychorrhexis, slow growth

continued on p. 70

Table 2.13. *Continued*

Aetiology	Colour	Location	Remark
MSH	Brown	Nail	Longitudinal streaks or diffuse pigmentation
Neosynephrine	Purpura	Bed	
Para amino salicylic acid	Cyanosis	Bed	Methaemoglobinaemia
PCB (polychlorinated biphenyls)	Brown to grey line	Nail and bed	Poisoning (Yusho) deformity of the nails
Phenindione	Orange	Nail	External cause due to trace amounts of the drug
Phenolphthalein	Dark grey	Lunula	
Picric acid	Yellow	Bed	Poisoning
Pilocarpine	T. leuconychia	Nail	Intoxication
Phosphorus	Haemorrhage	Bed	Poisoning
Practolol	Blotchy erythema	Bed	
Propanolol	Psoriasis like	Nail and bed Bed	
Santonin	Yellow		
Silver	Slate blue	Lunula and bed	Finger nails (due to UVA)
Sulfhydrilic acid	Cyanosis	Bed	Poisoning
Sulfonamide	T. leuconychia	Nail	
Sulfone	Cyanosis	Bed	Methaemoglobinaemia
Thallium	Brownish T. leuconychia	Nail	Mees' bands equivalent in acute intoxication
Thiazide diuretics	Whitish	Distal bed	Photoonycholysis
Tetryl	Yellow	Bed	Nitramine; yellow staining to skin and hair
Timolol maleate	Brown	Nail	Eye drops topically applied
TNT (absorption)	Red	Bed purpura	
Warfarin sodium	Purplish	Bed	

T., transverse.

Haneke E. (1991) Laugier–Hunziker–Baran Syndrom. *Hautarzt* **42**, 512–515.

Inalsingh C.H.A. (1972) Melanonychia after treatment of malignant disease with radiation and cyclophosphamide. *Arch. Dermatol.* **106**, 765–766.

Kolmsee I. & Schultka O. (1972) Keratoma palmare et plantare dissipatum hereditarium, Pachyonychia congenita und Hypotrichosis lanuginosa, malignes Melanom, Möller-Huntersche Glossitis, Vasculitis allergica superficialis (Bildberichte). *Hautarzt* **23**, 459–460.

Kopf A.W. & Waldo E. (1980) Melanonychia striata. *Aust. J. Dermatol.* **21**, 59–70.

Krutchik A.N., Taschina C.K., Buzdar A.U. *et al.* (1978) Longitudinal nail banding with breast carcinoma unrelated to chemotherapy. *Arch. Intern. Med.* **138**, 1302–1303.

Leyden J.J., Spott D.A. & Goldschmidt H. (1972) Diffuse and banded melanin pigmentation in nails. *Arch. Dermatol.* **105**, 548–550.

Monash S. (1932) Normal pigmentation in the nails of the Negro. *Arch. Dermatol.* **25**, 876–881.

Nixon D.W. & Samols E. (1970) Acral changes associated with thyroid disease. *JAMA* **212**, 1175–1181.

Pack G.T. & Oropeza R. (1967) Subungual melanoma. *Surg. Gynecol. Obstet.* **124**, 571–582.

Retsas S. & Samman P.D. (1983) Pigment streaks in the nail plate due to secondary malignant melanoma. *Br. J. Dermatol.* **108**, 367–370.

Ridley C.M. (1977) Pigmentation of fingertips and nails in vitamin B12 deficiency. *Br. J. Dermatol.* **97**, 105–107.

Rudolph R.E. (1987) Subungual basal cell carcinoma presenting as longitudinal melanonychia. *J. Am. Acad. Dermatol.* **16**, 229–233.

Rupp M., Khalluf E. & Toker C. (1987) Subungual fibrous histiocytoma mimicking melanoma. *J. Am. Pediatr. Med. Assoc.* **77**, 141–142.

Shelley W.B., Rawnsley H.M. & Pillsbury D.M. (1964) Postirradiation melanonychia. *Arch. Dermatol.* **90**, 174–176.

Valero A. & Sherf K. (1965) Pigmented nails in Peutz-Jeghers syndrome. *Am. J. Gastroenterol.* **43**, 56–58.

Zaias N. (1972) Onychomycosis. *Arch. Dermatol.* **105**, 263–274.

Zaias N. (1990) *The Nail in Health and Disease*, 2nd edn. Appleton & Lange, Norfalk, CN.

Zaun H. (1987) Krankhafte Veränderungen des Nagels. *Beitr. Dermatol.* 7. Erlangen: Perimed Fachbuch, 71.

Zehnder M.A. (1970) Post-traumatic nail (Letter). *N. Engl. J. Med.* **282**, 345.

Table 2.14. Some dermatological conditions affecting nail colour

Aetiology	Colour	Location	Remarks
Acanthosis nigricans	Leuconychia Greyish, brownish	Nail	See Chapter 6
Alopecia areata	Leuconychia, yellow, brown	Nail	See Chapter 5
Angioma	Reddish	Nail	See Chapter 11
Coat's syndrome	Red	Bed	See Chapter 9
Cronkhite–Canada syndrome	Grey or black	Nail	See Chapter 6
Dyshidrosis	T. leuconychia	Nail	
Enchondroma	Bluish	Bed	See Chapter 11
Erythema multiforme	T. leuconychia	Nail	See Chapter 5
Exostosis (subungual)	Brown	Bed	See Chapter 11
Fogo selvagem	Yellowish	Nail	See Chapter 5
Glomus tumor	Bluish	Bed	See Chapter 11
Keratosis lichenoides chronica	Variable	Nail/bed	See Chapter 5
Laugier–Hunziker's syndrome	Brown	Nail	LM, see Chapters 10 and 11
Lichen planus	Brownish	Plate/bed	LM, see Chapter 5
Lupus erythematosus discoides	Reddish	Bed	See Chapter 5
Melanocytic hyperplasia	Brown	Nail	LM, see Chapter 11
Melanocytic nevus	Brown	Nail	LM, see Chapter 11
Pityriasis rubra pilaris	Dark	Nail	See Chapter 5
Post-traumatic melanonychia	Brown	Nail	LM, see Chapter 10 and 11
Reiter's syndrome	Psoriasis-like	Nail/bed	See Chapter 5

LM, longitudinal melanonychia; T., transverse.

Table 2.15. Systemic infections causing modification of nail colour (see Chapters 5, 6 and 7)

Aetiology	Colour	Location	Remarks
Acute infection	T. leuconychia	Nail	
Jaundice	Yellow	Bed	Viral or spirochaetal
Leprosy	White	Bed	
Lymphogranuloma venereum	Red	Lunula	
Malaria	Grey, subungual haemorrhages, T. dark brown lines, T. leukonychia	Bed	
Pinta	Black	Bed	Medina, 1963
Pneumonia	T. leuconychia	Nail	
Rickettsiosis	T. leuconychia	Nail	
Subacute bacterial endocarditis	Splinter haemorrhages	Bed	
Syphilis	Brown	Bed	
Trichinosis	Splinter haemorrhages	Bed	
Visceral leishmaniasis	Diffuse grey	?	
Zoster	T. leuconychia	Bed	

T., transverse.

7 **Congenital and inherited disease** (see Chapter 10)

Leuconychia

White nails are the most common variant of nail dyschromia. They can be divided into three main types: (i) true leuconychia where nail plate involvement originates in the matrix; (ii) apparent leuconychia with involvement of the subungual tissue; and (iii) pseudo-leuconychia.

True leuconychia (Fig. 2.46) is produced by the nail matrix and results from a structural modification of the nail material itself, the nail appears opaque and white in colour owing to the diffraction of light in the parakeratotic cells; with polarized light, the nail structure appears

Table 2.16. Alimentary tract disease causing nail colour modification (see Chapter 6)

Aetiology	Colour	Location	Remarks
Cirrhosis	White	Bed	Terry's nails
Hyperbilirubinaemia	Brown	Nail	Aplas (1957)
Jaundice	Yellow	Bed	
Ulcerative colitis	T. leuconychia	Nail	
	Haemorrhages	Bed	

T., transverse.

Table 2.17. Cause of nail colour modification: cardiac failure and peripheral circulatory impairment (see Chapter 6)

Aetiology	Colour	Location
Cardiac insufficiency	Red	Lunula
Gangrene	Black	Bed
Myocardial infarction	T. leuconychia	Bed
Lupus erythematosus (acute)	Red	Bed
Venous stasis	Cyanotic	Bed
Yellow nail syndrome	Yellow brown	Nail

T., transverse.

disrupted due to disorganization of the keratin fibrils. The leuconychia may be complete, total leuconychia (rare), or incomplete, subtotal leuconychia. These forms can be temporary or permanent depending on the aetiology. Partial forms are divided into punctate leuconychia, which is common, transverse leuconychia, which is relatively common, and distal leuconychia, which is very rare.

Apparent leuconychia, sometimes called leukopathia, (Alkiewicz & Pfister, 1976) has a normal matrix and nail plate, and can be further subdivided into a white appearance of the nail due to: (a) underlying onycholysis and subungual hyperkeratosis; or (b) modification of the subungual tissue giving rise, for example, to an apparent macrolunula.

The term pseudo-leuconychia is used when the nail

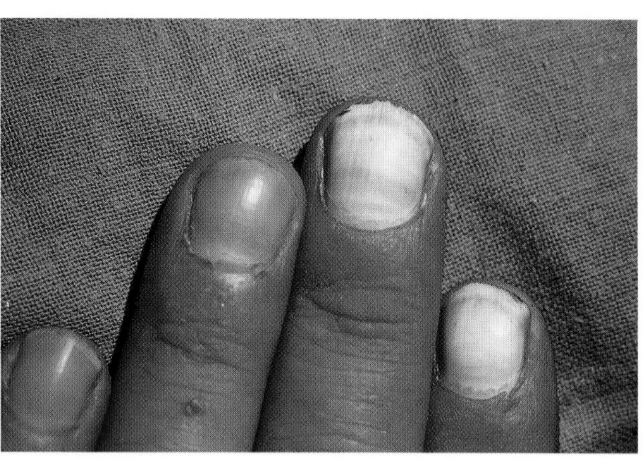
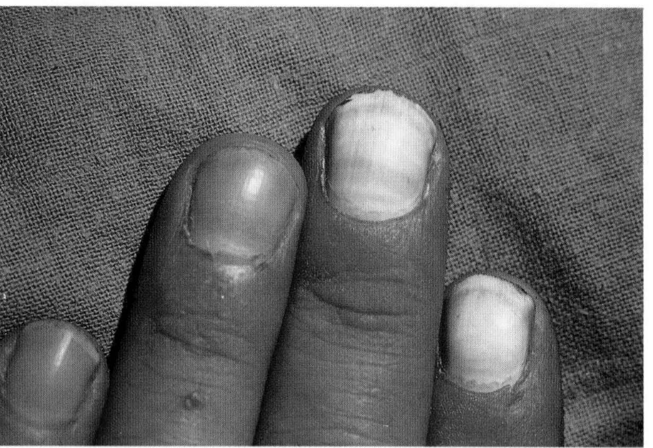

Fig. 2.46. True-leuconychia involving only two fingers.

plate alteration, has an external origin e.g. in onychomycosis (Fig. 2.49).

A different classification of leuconychia according to the location of the defect has also been suggested by Grossman and Scher (1990), who give other meanings to some of the terms that we and most dermatologists use.

Leuconychia is characterized on the morphological level by an alteration of the keratin fibres, and rarely by parakeratosis. This alteration can be the result of a disorder of the matrix keratinization or of a secondary disorder affecting the normally formed nail. This is the case with onychomycoses. With the exception of mycotic leuconychia, histological examination of the ungual keratin does not allow aetiological diagnosis of the lesion. It must none the less be remembered that the causes of leuconychia are very numerous. We have only dealt with a few of them which are among the most frequent.

True leuconychia

Total leuconychia (Fig. 2.47)

In this rare condition the nail may be milky, chalky, bluish, ivory or porcelain white in colour. The opacity of

Table 2.18. Cause of nail colour modification: blood dyscrasia (see Chapter 6)

Aetiology	Colour	Location	Remarks
Alkaline metabolic disease	Variable white	?	de Nichola *et al.* (1974)
Anaemia	Pallor	Bed	
Carbon monoxide	Cherry red	Bed	
Cryoglobulinaemia	Splinter haemorrhage	Bed	
Gout	T. leuconychia	Nail	
Hyperalbuminaemia	T. leuconychia	Nail	
Hypoalbuminaemia	White	Bed	Muehrcke's paired bands
Hypocalcaemia	T. leuconychia	Nail	
Methemoglobinaemia	Cyanotic	Bed	See Chapter 7
Polycythaemia	Dark red	Bed	
Protein deficiency	T. leuconychia	Nail	
Sickle cell anaemia	T. leuconychia	Nail	

T., transverse.

Table 2.19. Causes of nail colour modification: renal disease (see Chapter 6)

Aetiology	Colour	Location	Remarks
Kidney transplant	T. leuconychia	Nail	
Renal failure (acute or chronic)	T. leuconychia	Nail	
Uraemic onychopathia			
Lindsay's type (1967)	White	Bed	
	Pink, red or brown	Distal bed area	
Leyden's type (Leyden *et al.*, 1972)	White	Bed	
	Brown	Distal nail area	

T., transverse.

Table 2.20. Causes of nail colour modification: hormonal conditions (see Chapter 6)

Aetiology	Colour	Location	Remarks
Adrenal insufficiency	Brown	Nail	LM
Cushing's syndrome	Brown	Nail	LM
Diabetes mellitus	Yellow	Nail	
Menstrual cycle	T. leuconychia	Nail	
Parathyroid insufficiency	T. leuconychia	Nail	Fingernails (various onychodystrophies)
	Grey-brown	Nail	Toenails
Pregnancy	Brown	Nail	LM

LM, longitudinal melanonychia; T., transverse.

Table 2.21. Causes of nail colour modification: malignancies (see Chapter 6)

Aetiology	Colour	Location	Remarks
Acanthosis nigricans	Leuconychia	Nail	
Acrokeratosis paraneoplastica	Variable	Nail	
Breast carcinoma	Brown	Nail	LM
Carcinoid tumours of the bronchus	T. leuconychia	Nail	
Hodgkin's disease	T. leuconychia	Nail	
Intra-abdominal malignancies	T. leuconychia	Nail	
Lympho- or reticulosarcoma	Red	Lunula	de Nicola (1974)
Malignant melanoma	Brown	Nail/bed	Surrounding soft tissues
Melanocytic hyperplasia (atypical)	Brown	Nail	LM

LM, longitudinal melanonychia; T., transverse.

Table 2.22. Causes of nail colour modification: miscellaneous non-infectious systemic conditions (see Chapter 6)

Aetiology	Colour	Location	Remarks
Ageing	Yellow-grey	Nail	See Chapter 3
Cachectic state	T. leuconychia	Nail	
Familial amyloidosis with polyneuropathy	Yellow	Nail	
Fracture	T. leuconychia	Nail	
Malnutrition	Brown	Nail	LM
Occupational	Variable	Nail/nail bed	See Chapter 7
Pellagra	T. leuconychia	Nail	
Peripheral neuropathy	T. leuconychia	Nail	
Shock	T. leuconychia	Nail	
Surgery	T. leuconychia	Nail	
Sympathetic leuconychia	T. leuconychia	Nail	
Trauma	T. leuconychia	Nail	
Vitamin B_{12} deficiency	Brown	Nail	
Zinc deficiency	T. leuconychia	Nail	

LM, longitudinal melanonychia; T., transverse.

Table 2.23. Causes and simulators of longitudinal melanonychia

Single band		Multiple bands	
Non-neoplastic	Neoplastic	Non-neoplastic	Neoplastic
Carpal tunnel syndrome (Arateri *et al.*, 1984) Foreign body (subungual)* Haematoma (longitudinal) (Pack & Oropeza, 1967) Irradiation (local) (Shelley, 1984) Postinflammatory hyperpigmentation† Trauma (acute) (Zehnder, 1970) Trauma (chronic) (Baran, 1987, 1990)	*Melanocytic* Acquired melanocytic naevus (Kopf & Waldo, 1980) Congenital melanocytic naevus (Coskey *et al.*, 1983) Proliferation of normal melanocytes‡ Proliferation of atypical melanocytes‡ Post-operative recurrent/persistent melanocytosis Melanoma *in situ* (Kopf & Waldo, 1980) Metastatic melanoma (Kolmsee & Schultka, 1972) (Retsas & Samman, 1983) (Zaun, 1987) Subungual melanoma (Kopf & Waldo, 1980) (Feibleman, 1980) (Takahashi, 1983) (Nogaret, 1986) (Patterson, 1980) (Miura, 1985) *Non-melanocytic* Basal cell carcinoma (Rudolph, 1987) Bowen's disease (Baran & Simon, 1988, 1992) Mucous cyst (Daniel & Zaias, 1988) Subungual fibrous histiocytoma (Rupp *et al.*, 1987) Verruca vulgaris‡	*Dermatologic disorders* Laugier – Hunziker syndrome (Baran, 1979; Baran & Barrière, 1986; Haneke, 1991) Lichen planus (Baran *et al.*, 1985) Lichen striatus (Zaias, 1990) *Drugs and ingestants* (Jeanmougin, 1983; Daniel, 1985; Azon-Masoliver, 1988) Antimalarials, arsenic, bleomycin, busulfan, cyclophosphamide, diquat, daunorubicin, doxorubicin, fluoride, 5-fluorouracil, gold therapy, hydroxyurea, ketoconazole, melphalan, mepacrine, mercury, methotrexate, minocycline, nitrogen mustard, nitrosourea, phenothiazine, phenytoin, psoralen, sulfonamide, tetracycline, timolol, zidovudine *Microbial and fungal* (see Chapter 4) Acquired immunodeficiency syndrome (Fisher & Warner, 1987) Bacteria coexisting with onychomycosis (Zaias, 1972) *Exogenous/non-microbial* Irradiation (systemic) (Inalsingh, 1972) *Racial variation* African-American (Leyden *et al.*, 1972; Monash, 1932) Hispanic, Indian, and other dark-skinned races† Japanese *Systemic diseases and states* Addison's disease (Allenby & Snell, 1966) Adrenalectomy for Cushing's disease (Bondy & Harwick, 1969) Haemosiderosis (Alkiewicz & Pfister, 1976)	Breast carcinoma (Krutchik *et al.*, 1978)

* N. Goldfarb, personal communication.
† Personal observation.
‡ A.B. Ackerman, personal communication.

the whiteness varies. When faintly opaque, it may be possible to see transverse streaks of leuconychia (Fig. 2.47). Involvement of the medical or lateral half of the nail plate has been described in a patient presenting total leuconychia in some other digits.

Accelerated nail growth is associated with total leuconychia. Kates *et al.* (1986) presented the pedigree of a family with 28 affected members.

Subtotal leuconychia

In this form, there is a pink arc of about 2–4 mm width distal to the white area. This can be explained by the fact that the nucleated cells in the distal area mature, lose their keratohyalin granules and then produce healthy keratin several weeks after they have been formed. Juhlin (1963) discussed the possibility that there are parakeratotic cells along the whole length of the nail; these decrease in number as they approach the distal end, thus producing the normal pink colour up to the point of separation from the nail bed. There might, however, be enough left for the nail to acquire a whitish tint when it has lost contact with the nail bed. It has been suggested that subtotal leuconychia is a phase of total leuconychia based on the occurrence of both in different members of one family and the simultaneous occurrence in one person. In addition, either type may be found separately in some persons at different times.

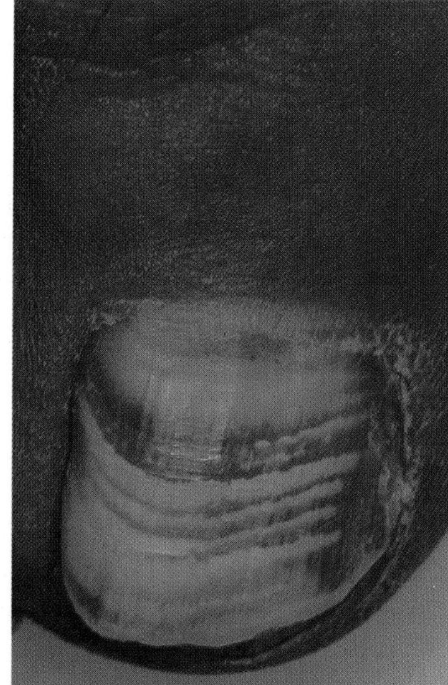

(a)

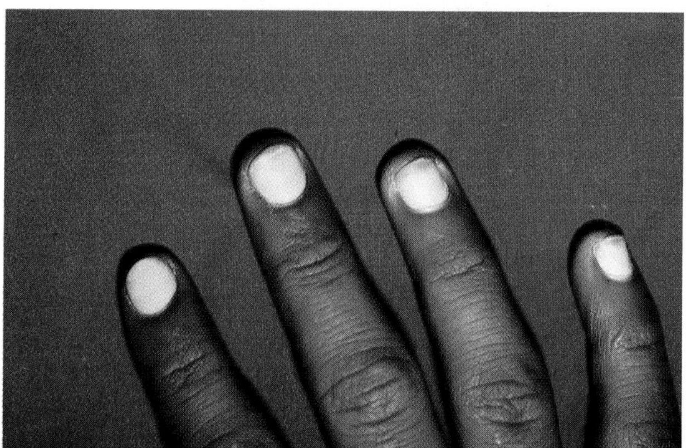

(b)

Fig. 2.47. True leuconychia. (a) Transverse striate; (b) complete varieties.

Albright and Wheeler (1964) saw also total or partial leuconychia in a single family. In Bettoli and Tosti's family (1986), in contrast, all the patients affected by total leuconychia at birth experienced a gradual improvement of the nail discoloration during the course of life.

Transverse leuconychia

In this condition one or several nails exhibit a band, usually transverse, 1 or 2 mm wide and often occurring at the same site in each nail, resulting, for example, from acute arsenic toxicity (Mees' lines), trauma or repeated microtrauma (Fig. 2.48) or acute rejection of renal allograft (Held *et al.*, 1989) (see Table 2.24). The condition may be inherited. Malher (1987) reported on a congenital type involving only the entire great toenail and half of the second toe of both feet.

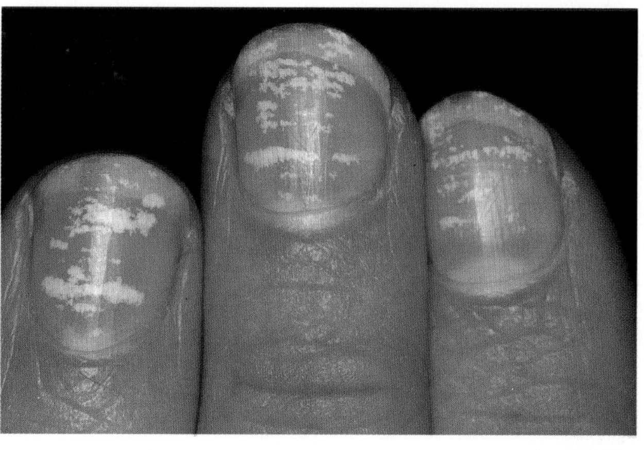

Fig. 2.48. Leuconychia variegata – irregular transverse streaks.

Punctate leuconychia

In this type, white spots of 1–3 mm in diameter occur singly or in groups; only rarely do they occur on toenails. Their appearance is usually due to repeated minor trauma to the matrix. The evolution of the spots is variable; appearing generally on contact with the cuticle, they grow distally with the nail but about half of them disappear in the course of their migration towards the free edge. This proves that parakeratotic cells are capable of maturing and losing their keratohyalin granules to produce keratin, even though they have been without vascularization for many months. Some white spots enlarge, while others appear at a distance from the lunula, suggesting that the nail bed is participating by incorporating groups of nucleated cells into the nail (Mitchell, 1953). A similar process could explain the exclusively distal leukonychia which is occasionally seen (Juhlin, 1963). A local or general fault in normal keratinization is not the only cause of punctate leuconychia. Infiltration of air, which is known to occur in cutaneous parakeratoses, may also play a part.

Leuconychia variegata (Alkiewicz & Pfister, 1976)

This consists of white, irregular, transverse, thread-like streaks (Fig. 2.48).

Longitudinal leuconychia

Longitudinal leuconychia is a typical example of a localized metaplasia (Alkiewicz & Pfister, 1976). It is characterized by a permanent greyish-white longitudinal streak, 1 mm wide, below the nail plate (Fig. 2.50). Histologically there is a mound of horny cells causing the white discoloration, which is due to a lack of transparency resulting in alteration in light diffraction.

Early stages of longitudinal splits and ridges of the nail may appear as white streaks. Two stripes in one nail may occur. Occasionally, two or three nails may be affected in

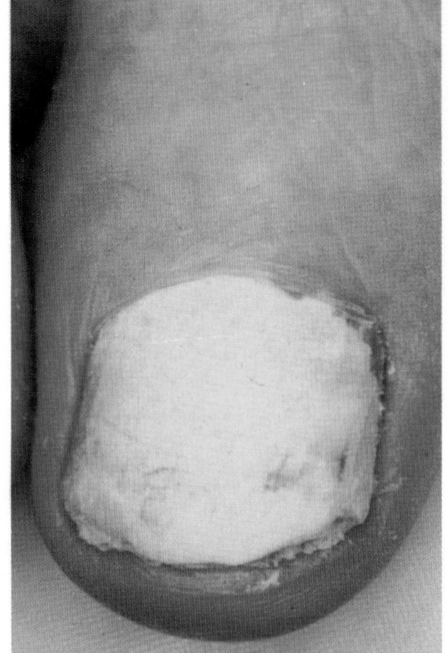

Fig. 2.49. Pseudo-leuconychia – caused by Scopulariopsis.

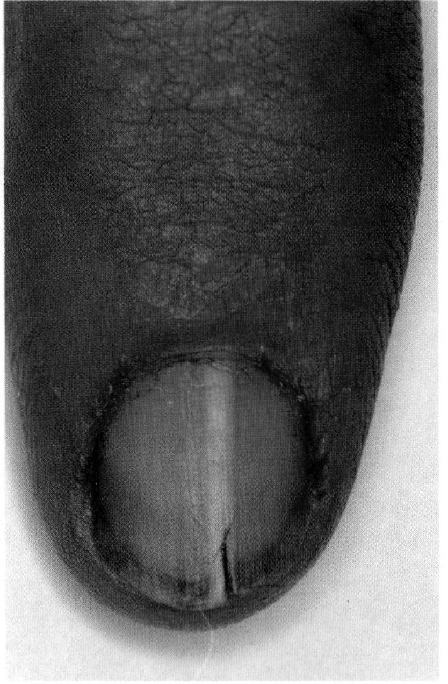

Fig. 2.50. Longitudinal leuconychia.

the same person (Zaun, 1991). Higashi *et al.* (1971) described longitudinal leuconychia resulting from parakeratotic hyperplasia of the nail bed epidermis, with or without abnormal keratinization of the deeper cells of the nail plate, due to naevoid matrix changes. According to Zaias (1990) this may represent Darier's disease, although it is debatable.

Aetiology of true leuconychia

Congenital forms are transmitted as autosomal dominant traits. They are usually total or subtotal and are rarely punctate or striate. These congenital forms can be associated with other malformations of the nail, skin or other tissue, or other disorders, e.g. deafness (see Chapter 8).

Acquired forms may be exogenous or endogenous. Overzealous manicuring is the main cause of punctate leuconychia. This can also produce transverse white striae. Traumatic transverse leuconychia lines are less homogeneous than endogenous ones, in which the borders are usually smoother. There are also occupational causes (see Chapter 6).

Endogenous leuconychia occurs after physiological phenomena such as birth (in neonates) (Becker, 1930), menstruation, severe stress, after acute diseases such as cardiac disease (myocardial infarction), diseases of the alimentary tract (ulcerative colitis) (Wolf, 1925), erythema multiforme, renal diseases and pellagra; it is also associated with shock, fractures and surgery and infectious diseases such as herpes zoster, measles, tuberculosis, syphilis and typhoid. It may be found in chronic diseases, such as autoimmune conditions (glomerulonephritis and vitiligo), neoplasia, Hodgkin's disease (Ronchese, 1951), intra-abdominal malignancies, breast cancer (Hortobagyi, 1983), chemotherapy (James & Odom, 1983), metabolic disorders (gout, autoimmunehaemolytic anaemia (Marino, 1990) and severe hyperalbuminaemia), peripheral neuropathy and also renal insufficiency. Hudson and Dennis (1966) noted that the size of the bands was an indication of the severity of the illness. Transverse leuconychia has been associated with acute rejection of renal allograft (Held *et al.*, 1989). Leuconychia has also been described after poisoning with thallium, arsenic, lead, sulphonamides and pilocarpine. In acute arsenic poisoning, Mees' bands, small transverse white lines occurring at the same site in each nail, are of medico-legal interest; such bands are quite distinctive, traversing the whole nail, and the proximal and distal borders are in parallel throughout their width (Krebs, 1983). In chronic arsenic poisoning, white diagonal striae are said to be equally characteristic. Acquired transverse leuconychia was also described in members of an expedition who were starved of protein for 1 month, but in whom no abnormality in serum protein was demonstrated.

Apparent leuconychia

Terry's nail

Terry (1954) was the first to describe a white opacity of the nails in patients with cirrhosis (Fig. 2.51). In the majority of cases the nails are of an opaque white colour, obscuring the lunula. This discoloration, which stops suddenly 1–2 mm from the distal edge of the nail, leaves a pink-brown area 0.5–3.0 mm wide not obscured by venous congestion and corresponding to the onychodermal band. It lies parallel to the distal part of the nail bed and may be irregular. The condition involves all nails uniformly.

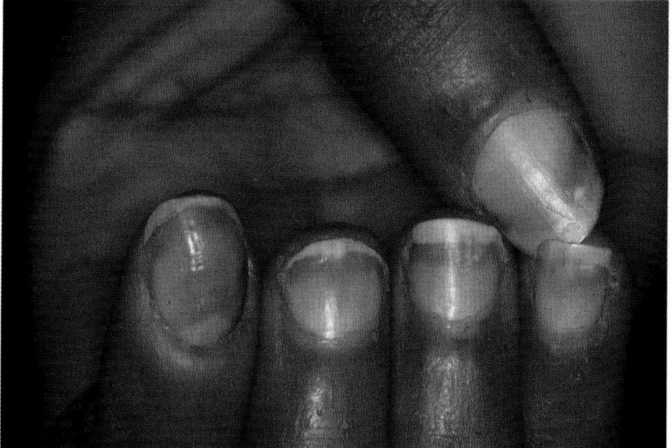

Fig. 2.51. Leuconychia – Terry's type associated with cirrhosis.

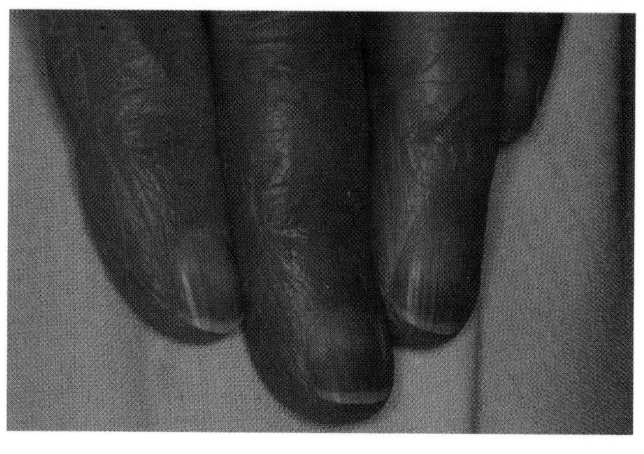

Fig. 2.52. Uraemic 'half-and-half' nail.

A revised definition and new correlations on Terry's nails have been advocated by Holzberg and Walker (1984). They found that a distal brown band was four times more frequent than the normal pink band described by Terry. The proximal nail beds of one-quarter of the patients were light pink, rather than white, with a ground-glass opacity. The nail abnormality is associated with cirrhosis, and associations have been demonstrated with chronic congestive heart failure, adult-onset diabetes mellitus, and age. The biochemical abnormalities associated with Terry's nails may be related to the underlying disease and not causally related to the nail disorder. The pathological findings from all three patients who underwent biopsy demonstrated an underlying change in vascularity. Telangiectasis was found in the dermis of the band.

Morey and Burke's nail

This is a variation of Terry's nail. The authors reported four cases in which the whitening of the nail extended to the central segment with a curved frontal edge; one of the cases had identical changes in the toes.

Uraemic half-and-half nail (Lindsay, 1967) *(Ongle équisegmenté hyperazotémique;* Baran & Gioanni, 1968)

In this disorder the nail consists of two parts separated longitudinally transverse by a well-defined line; the proximal area is dull white, resembling ground glass and obscuring the lunula; the distal area is pink, reddish or brown, and occupies 20–60% of the total length of the nail (average 33%) (Fig. 2.52). In typical cases diagnosis presents no difficulty, but in Terry's nail the pink, distal area may occupy up to 50% of the length of the nail, in which case the two types of nail may be confused. Half-and-half nail can display a normal proximal half portion and the colour of the distal part can be due to either an increase in the number of capillaries and thickening of their walls, or melanin in the nail bed. Sometimes the distinctly abnormal onychodermal band extends approximately 20–25% from the distal portion of the fingernail as a distal crescent of pigmentation with pigment throughout the brown arc of the nail plate (Daniel *et al.*, 1975). Half-and-half nails have occurred after chemotherapy, and in a breast cancer patient after androgen use; this patient had not required chemotherapy for her tumour (Nixon *et al.*, 1981).

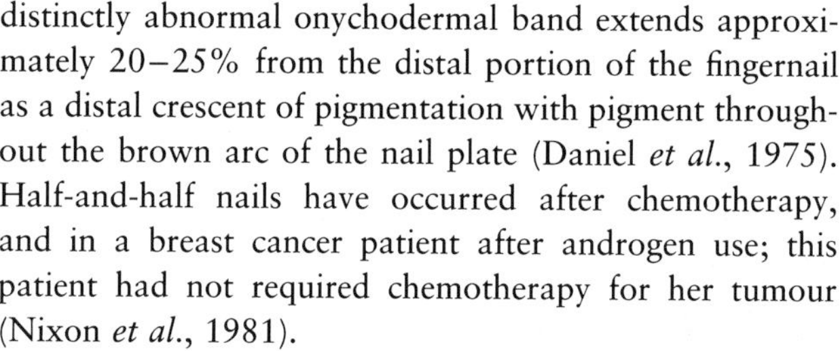

Nail changes similar to those reported by Terry (1954), Lindsay (1967) and Muehrcke (1956) have been termed 'Neapolitan nail' (Horan *et al.*, 1982); they are probably simply an age-related phenomenon.

Muehrcke's paired, narrow white bands (Muehrcke, 1956)

These bands, which are parallel to the lunula, are separated from one another and from the lunula by strips of pink nail. They usually disappear when the serum albumin level returns to normal and reappear if it falls again. It is possible that hypoalbuminaemia produces oedema of the connective tissue in front of the lunula just below the epidermis of the nail bed, changing the compact arrangement of the collagen in this area into a looser texture, resembling the structure of the lunula; hence the whitish colour. The correlation between the presence of the bands and the amount of serum albumin seems to confirm this hypothesis. However, white fingernails preceded by multiple transverse white bands have been reported with normal serum albumin levels. Nutritional deficiency such as zinc deficiency can present with Muehrcke's lines (Pfeiffer & Jenny, 1974) and low serum zinc levels may also be secondary to hypalbuminaemia. Cytotoxic drugs may produce Muehrcke's bands. Unilateral Muehrcke's lines may develop after trauma (Feldman & Gammon, 1989).

Apparent leuconychia may be preceded by multiple transverse white bands (Jensen, 1981). They disappear when blanching the fingertips. We have observed an identical case with vascular impairment. The white bands

Table 2.24. Classification of leuconychia (see appropriate chapters)

Congenital and/or hereditary
Isolated or associated with other conditions (Table 9.8)

Acquired
Pseudo-leuconychia
Onychomycosis
Keratin granulation (nail varnish, base coat)

Apparent leuconychia
Anaemia
Cancer chemotherapeutic agents
Cirrhosis
Fly tier's finger (MacAulay, 1990)
Half-and-half nail (renal diseases, androgen, 5-fluorouracil) and distal crescent pigmentation
Kawasaki's disease
Leprosy
Muehrcke's lines with normal albuminaemia or hypoalbuminaemia
Ulcerative colitis (Zaun, 1980)
Peptic ulcer disease and cholelithiasis (Ingegno & Yatto, 1982)

True leuconychia
Alkaline metabolic disease
Alopecia areata
Cachectic state
Carcinoid tumors of the bronchus
Cardiac insufficiency
Crow – Fukase syndrome (POEMS) (Shelley & Shelley, 1987)
Cytotoxic and other drugs (emetine, pilocarpine, sulphonamide, cortisone, quinacrine, trazodone (Longstreth & Hershman, 1985)
Dyshidrosis
Endemic typhus (Alkiewicz & Pfister, 1976)
Erythema multiforme (Bryer-Ash *et al.*, 1981)
Exfoliative dermatitis
Fasting periods in orthodox Jews
Fracture
Gout
Hodgkin's disease (Ronchese, 1951)
Hyperalbuminaemia
Hypocalcaemia
Infectious diseases and infectious fevers
Intra-abdominal malignancies
Kidney transplant (Linder, 1978)
Leuconycholysis paradentotica (Schuppli, 1963)
Leprosy
Lichen plano pilaris (Tosti *et al.*, 1988)
Malaria
Malnutrition and myoedema (Conn, 1965)
Menstrual cycle
Myocardial infarction (Urbach, 1945)
Nitric acid, nitrite solution (Zaun, 1991)
Occupational
Pellagra (Donald *et al.*, 1962)
Peripheral neuropathy
Pneumonia
Poisoning (antimony, arsenic, fluoride, lead, thallium) (see Chapter 6)
Protein deficiency
Psychotic episodes (acute)

continued

Table 2.24. *Continued*

Renal failure (acute or chronic) (Hudson & Dennis, 1966)
Rickettsiosis
Salt plant workers (Frenk & Leu, 1966)
Shock
Sickle cell anaemia
Surgery
Sympathetic leuconychia (Arnold, 1979)
Trauma
Trichinosis
Vascular impairment
Zinc deficiency
Zoster

transformed gradually into total apparent leuconychia each winter and reappeared each summer.

Anaemia

Anaemia produces a pallor with apparent leuconychia.

Dermatological forms of leuconychia

In psoriasis the nail may be affected by true leuconychia, due to involvement of the matrix, or apparent leuconychia, due to onycholysis, and/or to parakeratosis deposits in the nail bed. One of the earliest signs of leprosy is an apparent macrolunula, which may become total in dystrophic leprosy. Leuconychia may also occur in other acquired dermatoses, such as alopecia areata, dyshidrosis or inherited dermatoses (Darier's disease, Hailey–Hailey's disease, etc.) (see Chapter 9).

References

Albright S.D. & Wheeler C.E. (1964) Leuconychia: Total and partial leuconychia in a single family with review of the literature. *Arch. Dermatol.* **90**, 392–399.

Alkiewicz J. & Pfister R. (1976) *Atlas der Nagelkrankheiten.* Schattauer-Verlag, Stuttgart.

Arnold H.L. (1979) Sympathetic symmetric punctate leuconychia. *Arch. Dermatol.* **115**, 495.

Baran R. & Gioanni T. (1968) Half-and half nail (ongle équisegmenté hyperazotémique) *Bull. Soc. Fr. Dermatol. Syphil.* **75**, 399–400.

Becker S.W. (1930) Leuconychia striata. *Arch. Dermatol. Syphil.* **21**, 957–960.

Bettoli V. & Tosti A. (1986) Leuconychia totalis and partialis: a single family presenting a peculiar course of the disease. *J. Am. Acad. Dermatol.* **15**, 535.

Bryer-Ash M., Kennedy C. & Ridgway H. (1981) A case of leuconychia striata with severe erythema multiforme. *Clin. Exp. Dermatol.* **6**, 565.

Conn R.D. & Smith R.H. (1965) Malnutrition, myoedema and Muelizcke's lines. *Arch. Intern. Med.* **116**, 875–878.

Daniel C.R., Bower J.D. & Daniel C.R. Jr (1975) The half-and-half fingernail. The most significant onychopathological indicator of chronic renal failure. *J. Miss. St. Med. Assoc.* **16**, 367–370.

Donald G.F., Hunter G.A. & Gillman B.D. (1962) Transverse leuconychia due to pellagra. *Arch. Dermatol. Suppl.* 85–530.

Feldman S.R. & Gammon W.R. (1989) Unilateral Muehrcke's lines following trauma. *Arch. Dermatol.* **125**, 133–134.

Frenk E. & Leu F. (1966) Leukonychie durch beruflichen Kontakt mit gesalzenen Därmen. *Hautarzt* **17**, 233–235.

Grossman M. & Scher R.K. (1990) Leukonychia: review and classification. *Int. J. Dermatol.* **29**, 535–541.

Held J.L., Chew S., Grossman M.E. *et al.* (1989) Transverse striate leuconychia associated with rejection of renal allograft. *J. Am. Acad. Dermatol.* **20**, 513–514.

Higashi N., Sugai T. & Yamamoto T. (1971) Leuconychia striata longitudinalis. *Arch. Dermatol.* **104**, 192–196.

Holzberg M. & Walker H.K. (1984) Terry's nails: Revised definition and new correlations. *Lancet* **i**, 896–899.

Horan M.A., Puxty J.A. & Fox R.A. (1982) The white nails of old age (Neapolitan nails). *J. Am. Geriatr. Soc.* **30**, 734–737.

Hortobagyi G.N. (1983) Leukonychia striata associated with breast cancer. *J. Surg. Oncol.* **23**, 60–61.

Hudson J.B. & Dennis A.J. (1966) Transverse white lines in the fingernails after acute and chronic renal failure. *Arch. Intern. Med.* **117**, 276–279.

Table 2.25. Disorders in patients with red lunulae (from Cohen (1992) with permission)

Cardiovascular
(DeNicola *et al.*, 1974; Jorizzo *et al.*, 1983)
Angina pectoris
Atherosclerotic disease
Conduction abnormality
Congestive heart failure
Hypertension
Myocardial infarction
Rheumatic fever-induced heart disease

Dermatological
(Leider, 1955; Runne, 1980; Wilkerson & Wilkin, 1989)
Alopecia areata (Bergner *et al.*, 1992)
Chronic urticaria
Lichen sclerosus et atrophicus
Psoriasis vulgaris
Twenty-nail dystrophy
Vitiligo

Endocrine
(Terry, 1954; Wilkerson & Wilkin, 1989)
Diabetes mellitus
Thyroid disease
Hyperthyroidism
Not specified

Gastrointestinal
(Wilkerson & Wilkin, 1989)
Oesophageal strictures
Irritable bowel syndrome
Pyloric channel ulcer

Haematological
(Wilkerson & Wilkin, 1989)
Anaemia of chronic disease
Idiopathic transient leukopenia

Hepatic
(Terry, 1954; Wilkerson & Wilkin, 1989)
Cirrhosis

Infectious
(DeNicola *et al.*, 1974; Wilkerson & Wilkin, 1989)
Lymphogranuloma venereum
Pneumonia
Tuberculosis

Miscellaneous
(Terry, 1954; Leider, 1955; Misch, 1981; Daniel, 1985)
Alcohol abuse
Carbon monoxide poisoning
Chronic idiopathic lymphoedema
Corticosteroid therapy
Systemic
Topical
Hay fever pollen desensitization
Malnutrition
Tobacco abuse
Senile macular degeneration

Neoplastic
(Terry, 1954; DeNicola *et al.*, 1974)
Hodgkin's disease
Lymphoid follicular reticulosis
Lymphosarcoma
Myeloid leukaemia
Polycythaemia vera
Reticulosarcoma

Neurological
(Wilkerson & Wilkin, 1989)
Cerebrovascular accident

Pulmonary
(Terry, 1954; Wilkerson & Wilkin, 1989)
Chronic bronchitis
Chronic obstructive pulmonary disease
Emphysema

Renal (Wilkerson & Wilkin, 1989)
Proteinuria

Rheumatological
(Jorizzo *et al.*, 1983; Daniel, 1985; Wilkerson & Wilkin, 1989)
Baker's cyst
Dermatomyositis
Lupus erythematosus
Drug-induced (procainamide)
Systemic
Osteoarthritis
Polymyalgia rheumatica
Rheumatoid arthritis

Trauma
Repeated microtrauma (habit tic) (Baran, unpublished data)

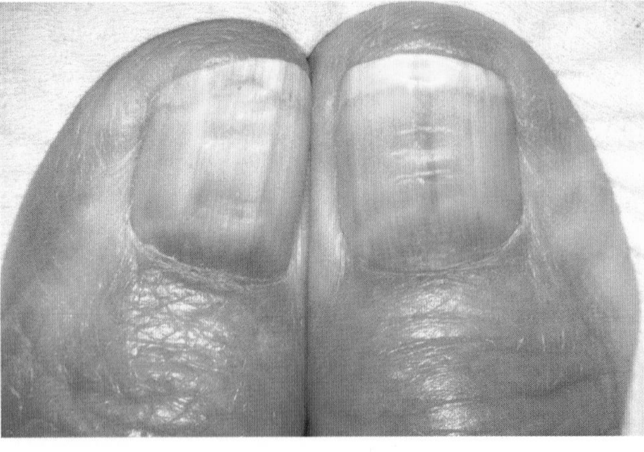

Fig. 2.53. Red lunulae.

Ingegno A.P. & Yatto R.P. (1982) Hereditary white nails, duodenal ulcer and gallstones. *NY State J. Med.* **13**, 1797.

James W.D. & Odom R.B. (1983) Chemotherapy induced transverse white lines in the finger nails. *Arch. Dermatol.* **119**, 334.

Jeanmougin M. & Civatte J. (1983) Nail dyschromia. *Int. J. Dermatol.* **22**, 279–290.

Jensen O. (1981) White fingernails preceded by multiple transverse white bands. *Acta Dermatol. Venereol.* **61**, 261–262.

Juhlin L. (1963) Hereditary leuconychia. *Acta Dermatol. Venereol.* **43**, 136.

Kates S.L., Harris G.D. & Nagle D.J. (1986) Leuconychia totalis. *J. Hand Surg.* **11B**, 465–466.

Krebs A. (1983) Veränderungen der Nägel durch Medikamente. *Aktuelle Dermat.* **9**, 53–59.

Laugier P. (1981) Dyschromies unguéales. *Schweiz Rund Med. (Praxis)* **70**, 1974.

Linder M. (1978) Striped nails after kidney transplant. *Ann. Intern. Med.* **88**, 809.

Lindsay P.G. (1967) The half-and-half nail. *Arch. Intern. Med.* **119**, 583.

Longstreth G.F. & Hershman J. (1985) Trazodone-induced hepatoxicity and leuconychia. *J. Am. Acad. Dermatol.* **13**, 149.

MacAulay J.C. (1990) Fly tyer's finger. *Can. J. Dermatol.* **2**, 67.

Malher R.H., Gerstein W. & Watters K. (1987) Congenital leuconychia striata. *Cutis* **39**, 453–454.

Marino M.T. (1990) Mees' lines. *Arch. Dermatol.* **126**, 827–828.

Mitchell J.C. (1953) A clinical study of leuconychia. *Br. J. Dermatol.* **65**, 121–130.

Muehrcke R.C. (1956) The fingernails in chronic hypoalbuminaemia. *Br. Med. J.* **1**, 1327.

Nixon D.W., Pirrozi D., York R.M. *et al.* (1981) Dermatologic changes after systemic cancer therapy. *Cutis* **27**, 181.

Pfeiffer C.C. & Jenney E.H. (1974) Fingernail white spots: Possible zinc deficiency. *JAMA* **228**, 157.

Ronchese F. (1951) Peculiar nail anomalies. *Arch. Dermatol. Syphil.* **63**, 565–580.

Schuppli R. (1963) Über eine mit Paradentose kombinierte Veränderung der Nägel. *Z. Haut-Geschlkr.* **34**, 114.

Shelley W.B. & Shelley E.D. (1987) The skin changes in the Crow–Fukase syndrome. *Arch. Dermatol.* **123**, 85–87.

Terry R.B. (1954) White nails in hepatic cirrhosis. *Lancet* **1**, 757.

Tosti A., De Padova M.P. & Fanti P. (1988) Nail involvement in lichen plano-pilaris. *Cutis* **42**, 213–214.

Urbach E. (1945) White cross striae of the fingernails following cardiac infarction. *Arch. Dermatol. Syphil.* **52**, 106–107.

Wolf M.S. (1925) Leuconychia striata. *Arch. Dermatol. Syphil.* **12**, 520–521.

Zaias N. (1990) Leuconychia. In: *The Nail in Health and Disease*, 2nd edn, pp. 183–185. Appleton & Lange, Norwalk, CN.

Zaun H. (1980) Milchglasnägel: Hinweis auf intestinale Erkrankungen. *Akt. Dermatol.* **6**, 107–108.

Zaun H. (1991) Leuconychias. *Sem. Dermatol.* **10**, 17–20.

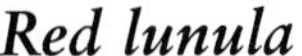

Red lunula

Red lunulae (Fig. 2.53) can be observed in patients with many cutaneous or systemic disorders (Table 2.25) (Cohen, 1992). They may also be idiopathic. The sharply circumscribed erythema of the lunulae can affect all fingers, and toenails, or only some fingernails, especially the thumb nails. Dark erythema may diffuse onto the proximal pink nail bed or a narrow white band may be present at the distal lunulae. The erythema of the fingernail lunulae migrated distally in a unique case of severe alopecia areata (Bergner *et al.*, 1992). The erythema disappears under pressure to the nail plate. The lunular erythema usually fades slowly even without therapy. The pathogenesis of red lunulae remains undetermined. A biopsy specimen taken from the red lunula of a thumb revealed neither an increased number nor size of capillaries (Wilkerson & Wilkin, 1989). 'Spotty', red lunulae may be seen in alopecia areata or psoriasis.

References

Bergner T., Donhauser G. & Ruzicka T. (1992) Red lunulae in severe alopecia areata. *Acta. Derm. Venereol. (Stockh.)* **72**, 203–205.

Cohen P.R. (1992) Red lunulae: Case report and literature review. *J. Am. Acad. Dermatol.* **26**, 292–294.

Daniel C.R. III (1985) Nail pigmentation abnormalities. *Dermatol. Clin.* **3**, 431–443.

DeNicola P., Morsiani M. & Zavagli G. (1974) *Nail Diseases in Internal Medicine*, p. 56. Charles C. Thomas, Springfield, IL.

Jorizzo J.L., Gonzalez E.B. & Daniels J.C. (1983) Red lunulae in a patient with rheumatoid arthritis. *J. Am. Acad. Dermatol.* **8**, 711–718.

Leider M. (1955) I. Progression of alopecia areata through alopecia totalis to alopecia generalizata. II. Peculiar nail changes (obliteration of the lunulae by erythema) while under cortisone therapy. III. Allergic eczematous contact dermatitis from the binding of a toupee or the adhesive used to hold it in position. *Arch. Dermatol.* **71**, 648–649.

Misch K.J. (1981) Red nails associated with alopecia areata. *Clin. Exp. Dermatol.* **6**, 561–563.

Runne V. (1980) Twenty-nail dystrophy 'mit knuckle pads' *Z. Hautkr.* **55**, 901–902.

Terry R. (1954) Red half-moon in cardiac failure. *Lancet* **2**, 842–844.

Wilkerson M.G. & Wilkin J.K. (1989) Red lunulae revisited: a clinical and histopathologic examination. *J. Am. Acad. Dermatol.* **20**, 453–457.

Chapter 3
The Nail in Childhood and Old Age

R. BARAN & R.P.R. DAWBER

Childhood
- Composition of the nail in childhood (see also Chapter 1)
- Newborn and early infancy
  - Transverse depressions
  - Self-inflicted bullous lesions
  - *Veillonella* infection of the newborn
  - Other bacterial infections
  - Fungal infection
  - Paronychia and finger sucking
  - Herpetic whitlow
  - Epidermolysis bullosa
- Infancy and childhood
  - Ingrowing toenail
  - Impetigo
  - Blistering distal dactylitis
  - Toxic shock syndrome
  - Parakeratosis pustulosa (Chapter 5)
  - Twenty-nail dystrophy
  - Atopic dermatitis (Chapter 5)

Old age
- Aetiology of senile changes
- Linear nail growth
- Variations in the contour
- Variations in the colour
- Variations in thickness and consistency
- Ingrowing toenail
- Tumours in the nail area
- Fungal infection

A classification of nail dystrophies according to age is rather arbitrary. Although some nail diseases have a predilection for certain age groups, the relationships to age are usually not clearly defined.

A variety of abnormalities occurring in any age group may be modified by the age of presentation, and underlying pathology may worsen or improve with advancing years. Activities such as habits, occupation and pastimes may have effects on the nail apparatus and are themselves influenced by the age of the patient.

Throughout this book in general nail pathology is dealt with in relation to its disease. There are, however, some conditions which are of special significance in the very young or the very old, and these are therefore given separate attention here.

Composition of the nail in childhood

X-ray microanalysis of the fingernails (Roomans *et al.*, 1978) showed a decrease in sulphur and aluminium, and a higher chlorine content in fullterm infants compared with preterm ones (Sirota *et al.*, 1988). The chloride and sodium content of nails of normal newborns is highest at birth and decreases by 50% within 3 days (Chapman *et al.*, 1985). The iron content of fingernails varies in the same individual through out the year (Harrison & Clemena, 1972). The iron status of an individual correlates with the iron content in nails (Sobolewski *et al.*, 1978).

Altered nail composition may be of some value in the diagnosis of certain metabolic disorders (see also Chapter 1). The elevated content of aluminium in preterm infants may be a clue to the osteopenia observed in these infants (Sirota *et al.*, 1988).

In cystic fibrosis, the sodium and potassium content of nail clippings were analysed by Kopito *et al.* (1965); their concentrations in both nails and hair were found to be elevated. Neutron activation analysis of sodium in nails (Roomans *et al.*, 1978) has proved to be a valuable diagnostic method in children over 1 year of age, showing increased concentration of sodium and potassium in the sweat of patients with mucoviscidosis; this is compatible with the suggestion that these elements are of extrinsic origin (Kollberg & Landström, 1974). The immediate attraction of nail sodium analysis lies in its potential as a postal screening service (Tarnoky *et al.*, 1976); however the sodium content of nail clippings is variable and depends on the subject's activities for some time before the nails are cut. A simple, unified set of instructions before obtaining samples from small children may be necessary.

The copper content in the hair and nails of patients with hepatolenticular degeneration (Wilson's disease) is higher than normal (Martin, 1964).

'Nail biopsies' in neonatal anabolic disorders have been advocated by Lockard *et al.* (1972). The fact that ill neonates have lower nail nitrogen and that it is significantly less than adult nail nitrogen suggests a pattern of nail protein accumulation which parallels that of muscle and the whole body in the developing fetus and neonate.

Hudson *et al.* (1988) measured index finger, nail and thumb dimensions in normal, fullterm infants within the first 3 days of life. In newborn infants the index fingernail length is 5.041 ± 0.703 mm and the width is 3.570 ± 0.354 mm. The thumb width is 9.800 ± 0.546 mm. These measurements will be helpful in describing any malformation syndromes, characterized by finger and nail dimension changes. In addition, measurements of the ratio of the distal phalangeal depth to the interphalangeal depth of the index finger have been used to quantitate digital clubbing in infants and children with cardiopulmonary disease.

Medically the length of the nails has been used as a morphological criterion for the assessment of gestational age in ill preterm babies (Lamberti *et al.*, 1981; Kolle *et al.*, 1985). Premature infants may have nail plates shorter than the distal digital pulp giving an ingrowing appearance (Silverman, 1990).

In healthy term infants, length, width and the calculated nail area are reliable measurements which enable qualitative comparisons to be made; approximately 75% of congenital syndromes are associated with dysplastic nails (Seaborg & Bordutha, 1989). The three most common findings in otherwise normal children are: (i) punctate leuconychia; (ii) onychophagia (nail biting); and (iii) pitting.

References

Chapman A.L., Fegley B. & Cho C.T. (1985) X-ray microanalysis of chloride in nails from cystic fibrosis and control patients. *Eur. J. Respir. Dis.* **66**, 218–223.

Harrison W.W. & Clemena G.G. (1972) Survey of the analysis of trace elements in human fingernails by spark source mass spectrometry. *Clin. Chim. Acta.* **36**, 485–492.

Hudson V.K., Flannery D.B., Karp W.B. *et al.* (1988) Finger and nail measurements in newborn infants. *Dysmorph. Clin. Gen.* **1**, 145–147.

Kollberg H. & Landström O. (1974) A methodological study of the diagnosis of cystic fibrosis by instrumental neutron activation analysis of sodium in nail clippings. *Acta Paed. Scand.* **63**, 405.

Kolle L.A.A., Leusin K.J. & Peer P.G.M. (1985) Assessment of gestational age: A simplified scoring system. *J. Perinat. Med.* **13**, 135–138.

Kopito L., Mahmoodian A., Townley R.R.W. *et al.* (1965) Studies in cystic fibrosis, analysis of nail clippings for sodium and potassium. *New. Engl. J. Med.* **272**, 504.

Lamberti G., Korner G. & Agorastos T. (1981) The role of skin and its appendages in the assessment of the newborns' maturity. *J. Perinat. Med.* **9** (suppl.), 147–148.

Lockard D., Pass R. & Cassady G. (1972) Fingernail nitrogen content in neonates. *Pediatrics* **49** 618.

Martin G.M. (1964) Copper content of hair and nails of normal individual and of patients with hepatolenticular degeneration. *Nature*, **202**, 903.

Roomans G.M., Afzelius B.A., Kollberg H. *et al.* (1978) Electrolytes in nails analysed by X-ray microanalysis in electron microscopy. *Acta Paed. Scand.* **67**, 89.

Seaborg B. & Bordurtha J. (1989) Nail size in normal infants. Establishing standards for healthy term infants. *Clin. Pediatr.* **28**, 142–145.

Silverman R.A. (1990) Pediatric diseases. In: *Nails, Therapy, Diagnosis, Surgery*, eds Scher R.K. and Daniel C.J. W.B. Saunders, Philadelphia.

Sirota L., Straussberg R. & Fishman P. (1988) X-ray microanalysis of the fingernails in term and preterm infants. *Pediatr. Dermatol.* **5**, 184–186.

Sobolewski S., Lawrence A.C.K. & Bagshaw I. (1978) Human nails and body iron. *J. Clin. Pathol.* **31**, 1068–1072.

Tarnoky A.L., Bayliss V.M. & Bowen H.J.M. (1976) The use of electrolyte measurement in the detection of cystic fibrosis. *Clin. Chim. Acta.* **69**, 505.

Newborn and early infancy

Koilonychia

At birth the nail curves over the tip of the digit towards the pulp; physiological clubbing may be seen in this age group. In childhood the nail is thin, flexible and transparent. Its surface is smooth, shiny and almost flat and the lunula is not visible on all digits. Occasionally the big toenail may show koilonychia which is deemed to be normal. There is however an increased prevalence of koilonychia due to minor trauma associated with barefoot walking and frequent water immersion (Yinnon & Matalon, 1988). These characteristics may be modified by disease. There is a significant correlation between koilonychia and iron deficiency in infants. This is a reliable clinical index of iron deficiency and may be seen before clinical and laboratory signs of anaemia develop (Hogan & Jones, 1970). Weak nails may result from selenium deficiency (Vinton *et al.*, 1987).

In early childhood, the nails often have oblique ridges which converge towards the centre distally (Fig. 3.1). These disappear by adult life (Pinkus, 1976).

References

Hogan G.R. & Jones B. (1970) The relationship of koilonychia and iron deficiency in infants. *J. Pediatr.* **77**, 1054–1057.

Pinkus H. (1976) In: *Cancer of the Skin*, eds Andrade R., Gumport S.L., Popkin G.L. & Rees T.D. W.B. Saunders, Philadelphia.

Vinton N.E., Dahlstrom K.A., Strobel C.T. *et al.* (1987) Selenium deficiency. *J. Pediatr.* **111**, 711–718.

Yinnon A.M. & Matalon A. (1988) Koilonychia of the toenails in children. *Int. J. Dermatol.* **27**, 685–687.

Nail fold capillaries

The nail fold capillary pattern matures quite rapidly during the first 3 months of life (Maricq, 1965); the loops appear in the neonatal period, subsequent evolution during the first 3 months depending on weight (i.e. neonatal maturity) (Syme & Riley, 1970).

References

Maricq H.R. (1965) Nailfold capillaries in normal children. *J. Nerv. Ment. Dis.* **141**, 197–203.

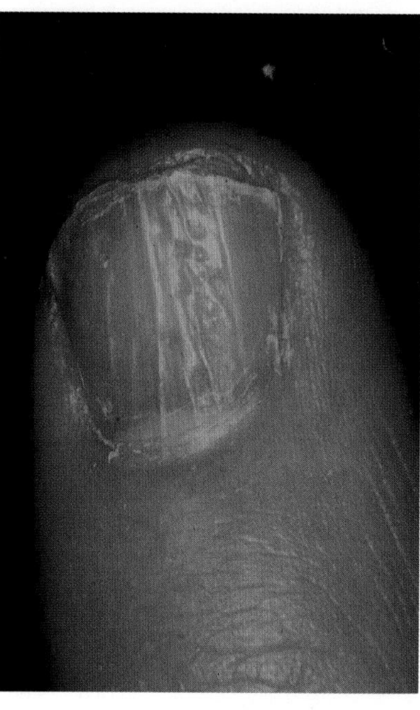

Fig. 3.1. Temporary, oblique ridges of early childhood – converging towards the centre distally here associated with pits.

Syme J. & Riley I.D. (1970) Nail fold capillary loop development in the infant of low birth weight. *Br. J. Dermatol.* **83**, 591.

Transverse depressions

In the studies by Turano (1968), 92% of normal infants between 8 and 9 weeks of age had a single transverse depression (Beau's line) of the fingernails; this first appeared at the proximal portion of the nail as early as 4 weeks of age and grew out to the distal edge by 14 weeks of age. Beau's lines of this type may be the result of malnutrition occurring during the transfer from intrauterine to extrauterine life. Wolf *et al.* (1982) reported Beau's lines in all 20 nails of a female infant soon after birth; the transverse linear depressions extended through the entire thickness of the nail which separated into two, giving rise to latent onychomadesis. The condition may have resulted from intrauterine distress. In childhood, cancer chemotherapy frequently produces Beau's lines or transverse leuconychia when antimitotic agents are administered; this is more common with intermittent 'bolus doses' of treatment.

References

Turano A.F. (1968) Transverse nail ridging in early infancy. *Pediatrics* **41**, 996.

Wolf D., Wolf R. & Golberg M.D. (1982) Beau's lines. A case report. *Cutis* **29**, 141.

Blistering diseases

Vesiculobullous lesions involving the nail apparatus are an infrequent occurrence and necessitate sterile puncture for Gram stain, Tzanck smear, bacterial and viral culture in order to rule out staphylococcal or herpetic infections. Both of these infections carry a high mortality during the neonatal period if left untreated (Silverman, 1990).

Reference

Silverman P.A. (1990) Diseases of the nails in infants and children. In: *Advances in Dermatology*, eds Callen J.P., Dahl M.V., Golitz L.E., Schachner L.A. & Stegman S.J., Vol. 5, pp. 153–171. Year Book Med. Publ., Chicago.

Self-inflicted bullous lesions

This bullous eruption in the newborn infant is always present from the time of birth, beginning *in utero* (Murphy & Langley, 1963). It may appear on the dorsum of the thumb or along the dorsal aspect of the index finger. The bullae measure from 0.5 to 1.5 cm in diameter. The fluid is typically clear and pale yellow in colour. Bacterial cultures show no growth. These lesions are presumed to be self-inflicted (*in utero*) as a consequence of vigorous reflex sucking in otherwise normal newborns.

The differential diagnosis (Murphy & Langley, 1963) includes epidermolysis bullosa, incontinentia pigmenti and congenital syphilis. Staphylococcal and streptococcal bullae generally do not occur before the fifth day of life; vesicular eruptions due to herpes simplex do not occur before the sixth day.

Reference

Murphy W.F. & Langley A.L. (1963) Common bullous lesion – presumably self inflicted – occurring in utero in the new infant. *Pediatrics* **32**, 1099.

Subungual infection in the newborn due to *Veillonella*

Forty-two epidemics of this subungual infection have been described by Sinniah *et al.* (1972) among infants in postnatal wards and special care baby units (Fig. 3.2). The number of fingers affected per patient ranged from one to 10; the thumbs were less frequently involved than other digits, the toenails usually being spared altogether. Three stages were found: firstly, a small amount of clear fluid appears under the centre of the nail, along with mild inflammation at the distal end of the finger. This initial vesicle lasts approximately 24 h; it occasionally enlarges but never to the edge of the nail. Some small lesions bypass the second, pustular stage, going directly into the third stage. As a rule the fluid becomes yellow within 24 h, the pus remaining for 24–48 h before gradually turning brown, and being absorbed. This colour fades progressively over a period of 2–6 weeks, leaving the nail

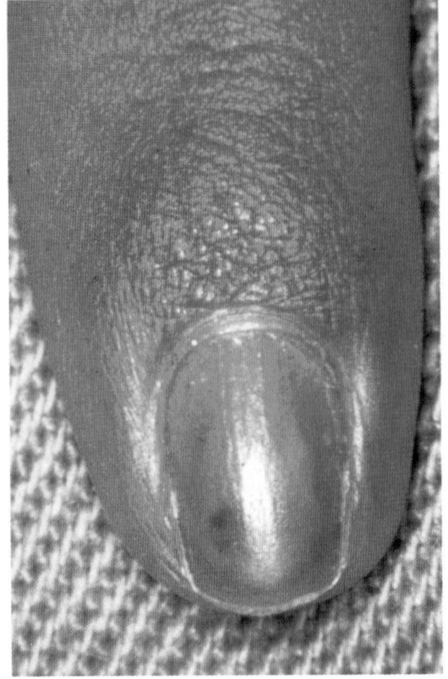

Fig. 3.2. *Veillonella* infection of the nail (courtesy D. Sinniah).

and nail bed apparently completely normal. Subungual pus obtained by aseptic puncture of the nails showed tiny, Gram-negative cocci about 0.4 um in diameter. These organisms resembled *Veillonella*, a group of anaerobes of dubious pathogenicity found as commensals in the saliva, vagina and respiratory tract. Systemic antibiotics did not change the clinical course of the nail lesions, which did not differ from those observed in other untreated and affected newborn infants.

Other bacterial infections

Anaerobic infections (*Bacteroides*, *Bacillus fragilis* and *Fusibacterium*) may affect many sites, including the fingers and nails beds (Hurwitz & Kahn, 1983). In the newborn, staphylococcal nursery epidemics produce cases of omphalitis, mammary abscess, dacryocystitis or paronychia. The localization is probably due to the presence of a locus minoris resistentiae, with trauma perhaps being a factor in paronychia (Koblenzer, 1978).

In Leiner's disease, recurrent paronychia infection (Fig. 3.3) and interdigital intertrigo (usually due to Gram-negative bacteria) may be only a fraction of the many infective episodes observed (Koblenzer, 1978). Topical clindamycin may be effective.

It is essential to remember that the nail matrix is very susceptible to infection in early life and may be irreversibly damaged within 48 h of the onset of acute infection.

References

Hurwitz S. & Kahn G. (1983) IXth postgraduate seminar in paediatric dermatology. *J. Am. Acad. Dermatol.* 8, 271.

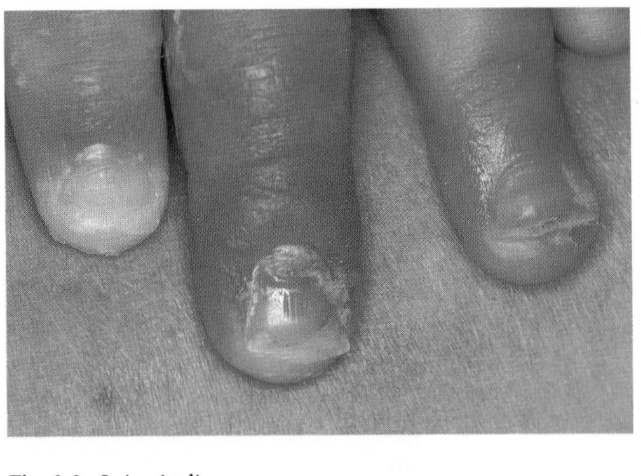

Fig. 3.3. Leiner's disease.

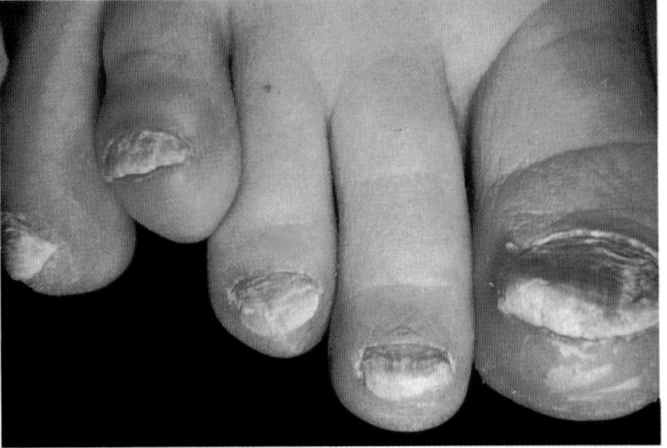

Fig. 3.4. Tinea unguium – uncommon in childhood, here due to *Trichophyton rubrum*.

Koblenzer P.J. (1978) Common bacterial infections of the skin in children. *Pediatr. Clin. N. Am.* **25**(**2**), 321.

Sinniah D., Sandiford B.R. & Dugdale A.E. (1972) Subungual infection in the newborn. An institutional outbreak of unknown etiology, possibly due to *Veillonella*. *Clin. Pediatr.* **11**, 690.

Fungal infection

Nail fungal infection in infancy is almost always due to *Candida*. It may be secondary to changes in nail composition, linear nail growth, local functional defects or a hormonal state. Onychomycosis caused by dermatophytes is uncommon (Fig. 3.4) (Philpot & Shuttleworth, 1989), unless associated with tinea of the scalp, namely *T. schoenleinii* or *T. violaceum*. The younger the child the more unusual is this infection. Cases reported in children under 2 are exceptional (Schmunes, 1976; Borbujo *et al.*, 1987). Both congenital and neonatal candidiasis have been reported (Chaland & Bouygues, 1986; Perel *et al.*, 1986; Kurgansky & Sweren, 1990) in the newborn, their limitation to the nails is unusual (Arbegast, 1990). In the case related by Plantin *et al.* (1992) neonatal candidiasis was restricted to paronychia of all the fingers of this 15-day-old child and was followed by onychomadesis and distolateral subungual onychomycosis affecting a minority of toes. *Candida* may be responsible for superficial white onychomycosis (see Chapter 4). Generalized chronic dermatophytosis in early childhood has also been observed.

In human immunodeficiency virus (HIV) infection in childhood, candidiasis presents with nail dystrophy identical to that seen in chronic mucocutaneous candidiasis, and dermatophytosis as severe onychomycosis may appear (Silverman, 1990).

References

Arbegast K.D., Lamberty L.F., Kyoung Kho J. *et al.* (1990) Congenital conditions limited to the nail plates. *Pediatr. Dermatol.* 7, 310–312.

Borbujo J.M., Fonseca E. & Gonzalez A. (1987) Onicomicosis por *Trichophyton rubrum* en un recién nacido. *Acta Dermo-Sif.* **78**, 207.

Chaland G. & Bouygues D. (1986) Candidose cutanée congénitale. Deux observations. *Pediatrie* **41**, 321–327.

Kurgansky D. & Sweren R. (1990) Onychomycosis in a 10-weeks-old infant. *Arch. Dermatol.* **126**, 1371 (letter).

Nolting S. (1990) Mykosen beim Adolessenten. *Z. Hautkr.* **65**, 334–336.

Perel Y., Taïeb A., Fonton J. *et al.* (1986) Candidose cutanée congénitale. Une observation avec revue de la littérature. *Ann. Dermatol. Venereol.* **113**, 125–130.

Philpot C.M. & Shuttleworth D. (1989) Dermatophyte onychomycosis in children. *Clin. Exp. Dermatol.* **14**, 203–205.

Plantin P., Jouan N., Calligaris C. *et al.* (1992) Onychomadese du nourrisson a *Candida albicans*. Contamination neonatale. *Ann. Dermatol. Venereol.* **119**, 213–215.

Schmunes E. (1976) Onychomycosis in a 14 month-old child. *S. Med. J.* **69**, 1097.

Silverman P.A. (1990) Diseases of the nails in infants and children. In: *Advances in Dermatology*, eds Callen J.P., Dahl M.V., Golitz L.E., Schachner L.A. & Stegman S.J., Vol. 5, pp. 153–171. Year Book Med. Publ., Chicago.

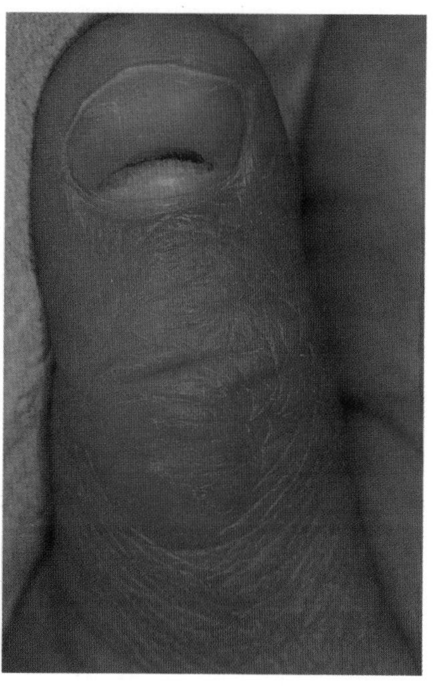

Fig. 3.5. Some nail apparatus and digital effects of thumb sucking.

Chronic paronychia and thumb sucking

Candida paronychia, usually in association with oral candidiasis, may arise as a result of chronic maceration due to thumb sucking, or it may occur without any obvious predisposing factors.

Chronic paronychia is not uncommon in children. It differs from the condition seen in adults in the source of the maceration, associated diseases (atopic dermatitis), the clinical appearance of the lesion, and the patients' responses to the symptoms (Stone & Mullins, 1968). In children the lesions are generally very prominent, with total involvement of the proximal nail fold. The skin is usually erythematous and glistening due to the wet environment produced by continuous thumb sucking. The quality of the nail substance is regularly altered, making its texture poor. The habit of sucking fingers or thumbs (Fig. 3.5) is the most important predisposing factor. Hyperglycaemia is not an associated finding. *Candida albicans* is usually present. With acute eczematous exacerbations the patient with atopic dermatitis experiences pruritus and discomfort in the proximal nail fold. Children respond to this by sucking, the symptoms of chronic paronychia perpetuating the habit which initiated the maceration. The lesions tend to be more severe in children than in adults, probably because exposure to saliva is more irritating than water in wet work (Stone & Mullins, 1968). The repeated minor trauma resulting from suction is capable of causing complete loss of the nail plate. However atopic dermatitis alone may also cause the dorsal aspect of the great toe to be abnormal (Hanifin, 1991).

Detection of candida in the mouth and gastrointestinal tract by cultures of saliva and stools may be important in the occasional patient with refractory paronychia. Multiple persistent and repeated paronychia in infancy suggests a more serious underlying disorder; such infants should be investigated for endocrine disease, immune deficiency syndromes (Solomon & Esterly, 1973) and systemic disease such as Langerhans cell histiocytosis, acrodermatitis enteropathica and Reiter's syndrome.

Thumb or finger sucking (Fig. 3.6(a)) is sometimes associated with herpes simplex (Fig. 3.6(b)). This may result in localized extension of the eruption producing viral stomatitis combined with involvement of the digit. Herpetic infection in patients who are less than 1 year old affects the index finger, the third finger and the thumb, whereas in adults the most commonly infected digits are the thumb and index finger. The incidence of involvement

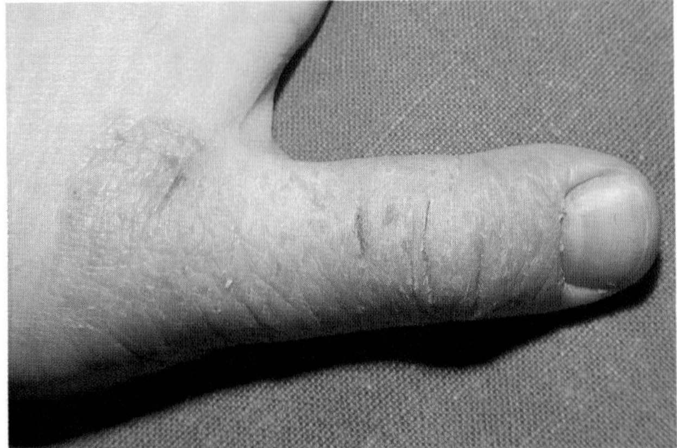

(a)

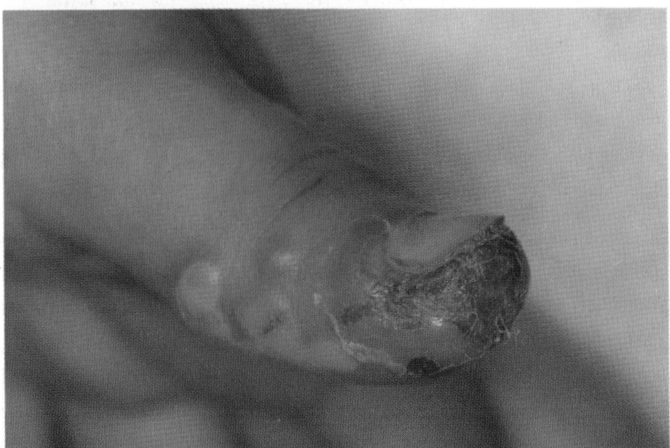

(b)

Fig. 3.6. (a) Thumb sucking. (b) Herpes simplex, sometimes associated with thumb or finger sucking.

of multiple digits is about twice the reported incidence of 10% in adults who have herpetic infection of the hand (Behr *et al.*, 1987). The report of herpetic whitlow of the great toe of a 3-year-old girl whose mother bit the child's nails is unique (Feder & Geller, 1992).

Herpetic whitlow

Herpetic whitlow is the major diagnostic consideration when a painful blister forms around the nail in children (Feder & Long, 1983; Feder & Geller, 1992). This condition presents with pain of the distal phalanx followed shortly by swelling and redness. A coalescent cluster of tapioca-like vesicles then develops. These lesions contain clear fluid that becomes turbid but rarely purulent over a 10-day period (in contrast to blistering distal dactylitis) (Silverman, 1990). The paronychial involvement may lead to onychomadesis, onycholysis and more rarely, permanent dystrophy.

Recurrent herpes labialis or gingivostomatis are frequently concurrent. Tzanck smear reveals multinucleated giant cells. 'Deroofing' of any large vesicles, and in the presence of paronychia, subungual decompression have been advocated for relieving severe pain. Topical and systemic antiviral agents are logical first-line therapy (Silverman, 1990).

Other similar infections in childhood may mimic herpetic whitlow, local trauma caused by onychophagia may result in the development of opportunistic infection by the normal oropharyngeal flora, amongst which are HB1 bacteria. Acute paronychia may be caused by BH1 organisms (*Eikenella corrodens*). It is uncommon in the absence of an immune deficiency (Barton & Anderson, 1974).

Therapy for childhood paronychia should first be directed at drying the affected digits. The near impossibility of preventing thumb sucking makes it difficult. Clotrimazole applied several times daily and topical clindamycin are nevertheless efficient. The latter kills bacteria, has a bitter taste to discourage further sucking, and has an alcohol propylene glycol vehicle that dries out residual moisture (Silverman, 1990).

References

Barton L.L. & Anderson L.E. (1974) Paronychia caused by HB1 organisms. *Pediatrics*, **54**, 372.

Behr J.T., Daluga D.J., Light T.R. *et al.* (1987) Herpetic infections in the fingers of infants. *J. Bone Joint Surg.* **69A**, 137–139.

Feder H.M. & Long S.S. (1983) Herpetic whitlow: epidemiology, clinical characteristics, diagnosis and treatment. Further observation. *Clin. Exp. Dermatol.* 7, 455–457.

Feder H.M. & Geller R.W. (1992) Herpetic whitlow of the great toe. *New Engl. J. Med.* **326**, 1295–1296.

Hanifin J.M. (1991) Atopic dermatitis in infants and children. *Pediatr. Clin. N. Am.* **38**, 763–790.

Silverman P.A. (1990) Diseases of the nails in infants and children. In: *Advances in Dermatology*, eds Callen J.P., Dahl M.V., Golitz L.E., Schachner L.A. & Stegman S.J., Vol. 5, pp. 153–171. Year Book Med. Publ., Chicago.

Solomon L.M. & Esterly N.B. (1973) *Neonatal Dermatology*. W.B. Saunders, Philadelphia.

Stone O.J. & Mullins F.J. (1968) Chronic paronychia in children. *Clin. Pediatr.* 7, 104.

Epidermolysis bullosa

The nail changes in epidermolysis bullosa are the consequence of trauma to the fragile nail apparatus (Fig. 3.7). Epidermolysis bullosa may however present at birth with periungual or subungual bullae resulting in onychomadesis or onycholysis with nail shedding. Nail dystrophy has been reported in all forms of dermolytic and junctional epidermolysis bullosa, as well in the simplex types other than the Weber–Cockayne and Koebner types (see Chapter 8). Recurrent bullae may result in nail thinning, pterygium formation and aplasia. Sometimes the nails become thickened and onychogryphotic. Meticulous hygiene, topical antibiotics (mupirocin) and synthetic dressing may optimize nail regrowth when possible. In these patients

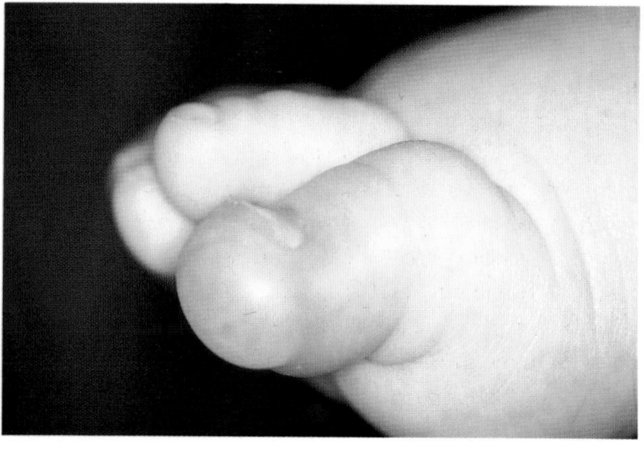

Fig. 3.7. Epidermolysis bullosa.

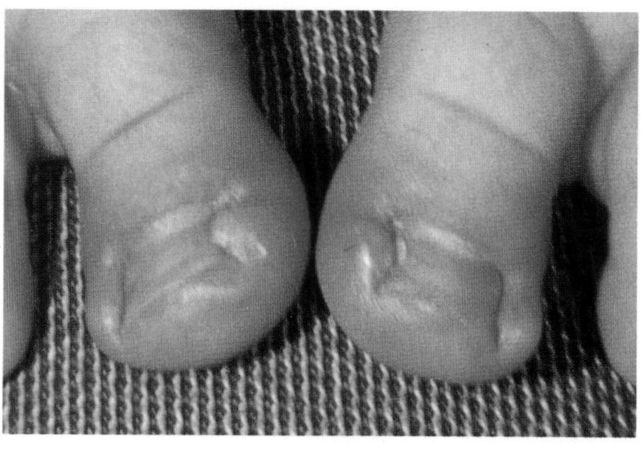

Fig. 3.8. Congenital bilateral hypertrophic lateral nail folds.

shoes with wide toe caps would also minimize loss of toenails from friction (Silverman, 1990).

Epidermolysis bullosa acquisita (EBA) may appear at any age (3 months in McCuaig *et al.*'s case, 1989) although no congenital cases have been reported. In McCuaig *et al.*'s patient most of the fingernails demonstrated distal onycholysis by 10 years of age. The right third fingernail was absent and replaced with firm, vertically striated and folded skin. A few of the toenails were opaque and thickened by subungual hyperkeratosis.

In this autoimmune disease, the autoantibodies are directed against type VII collagen. Differentiation of mechanobullous disease in children is critical in that significant clinical benefit may be achieved in EBA with prednisone and/or dapsone therapy.

References

McCuaig C.C., Chan L.S., Woodley D.T. *et al.* (1989) Epidermolysis bullosa acquisita in childhood. Differentiation from hereditary epidermolysis bullosa. *Arch. Dermatol.* **125**, 944–949.

Silverman P.A. (1990) Diseases of the nails in infants and children. In: *Advances in Dermatology*, eds Callen J.P., Dahl M.V., Golitz L.E., Schachner L.A. & Stegman S.J., Vol. 5, pp. 153–171. Year Book Med. Publ., Chicago.

Infancy and childhood

Ingrowing toenail in infancy

There are three kinds of ingrowing toenail in infancy (Baran, 1989): (i) congenital hypertrophic lip of the hallux; (ii) distal embedding with normally directed nail; and (iii) congenital malalignment of the big toenail.

Congenital hypertrophic lip of the hallux

When they appear at birth, hypertrophic lateral nail folds are generally bilateral and symmetrical, typically affecting the medial nail fold of the hallux (Fig. 3.8). They present as erythematous lateral pads, firm and tender on pressure, which enlarge progressively, sometimes covering one-third of the nail plate (Hammerton & Shrank, 1988). They may result from asynchrony between the growth of the soft tissue and the nail, the hypertrophic lateral lip growing faster than the nail plate, leading to ingrowing, with pain, which increases when walking begins (Martinet *et al.*, 1984). This condition, which resembles recurring digital fibrous tumour of childhood (and might be called pseudo-digital fibrous tumour of the hallux), usually disappears spontaneously after several months (Rufli *et al.*, 1992).

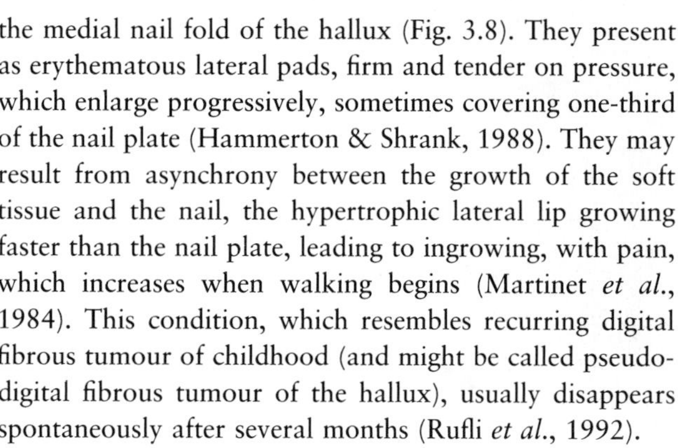

Distal embedding with normally directed nail

This condition should be distinguished from the ingrowing appearance of the nails of premature infants and some term infants which may be shorter than the distal digital pulp (Silverman, 1990).

The infantile type of ingrowing toenail presents a rim of tissue at the distal edge of the nail and some hypertrophy of the lateral nail fold. This prominent ridge of skin at the extremity of the big toe forms an anterior nail wall, which encourages ingrowing, and prevents the free margin of the nail growing normally (Fig. 3.9). The deformity produced by congenital hypertrophy of the distal soft tissue may sometimes be aggravated by acquired factors, such as the habit of sleeping prone in infancy (Bailie & Evans, 1978). The changes in the toenail occur at the time when the child starts kicking very actively and is subjected to tight-fitting clothing (jumpsuits of stretch able material) or to compression from tight shoes (Bird, 1978; Walker, 1979).

Careless cutting may leave a spicule of nail which penetrates the lateral nail fold as the nail grows forwards. In fact, if the big toenail is normally orientated, proper growth will be re-established by the age of 6 months in most cases, despite the previous barrier of distal tissue (Honig *et al.*, 1982).

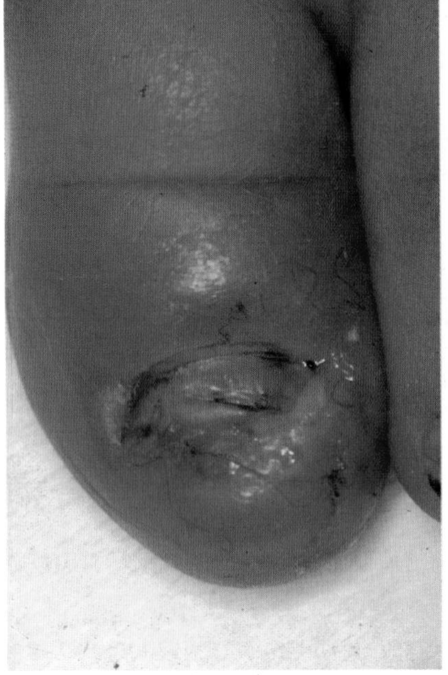

Fig. 3.9. Infantile ingrowing toenail, particularly prominent distally.

Paronychia must be treated conservatively. The infecting organisms should be cultured and tested for antibacterial sensitivity. Local treatment is by twice-daily application of antiseptics (Hibitane) or a combination of topical steroid and antiseptic, and shaving soap covered with non-adherent gauze, such as Telfa. Systemic antibiotics appropriate to the laboratory bacterial results can be added, if necessary.

If there is excess granulation tissue it is useful to alternate a topical steroid combined with antiseptic in the morning, and shaving soap in the evening, under occlusion (Blenderm tape). In resistant cases, after paring down granulation tissue, intralesional triamcinolone (5 mg/ml) may be injected into the swollen region, in addition to systemic antibiotic therapy. A chlorhexidine-soaked, cotton wool pledget introduced beneath the nail plate, under general anaesthesia, has been advocated (Connolly & Fitzgerald, 1988).

In the rare cases where permanent improvement has not been obtained by 10–12 months of age, or exceptionally earlier (Hendricks, 1979; Bentley-Phillips & Coll, 1983; Engels, 1985), a circular soft tissue resection should be performed, after X-ray has ruled out a subungual exostosis.

Congenital malalignment of the big toenail

In 1978, Samman described several cases of a 'dystrophy' limited to one or both great toenails. Baran *et al.* (1979) termed this 'congenital malalignment of the big toenail', placing emphasis on the main characteristic of this condition – the nail plate is deviated laterally with respect to the longitudinal axis of the distal phalanx (Fig. 3.10).

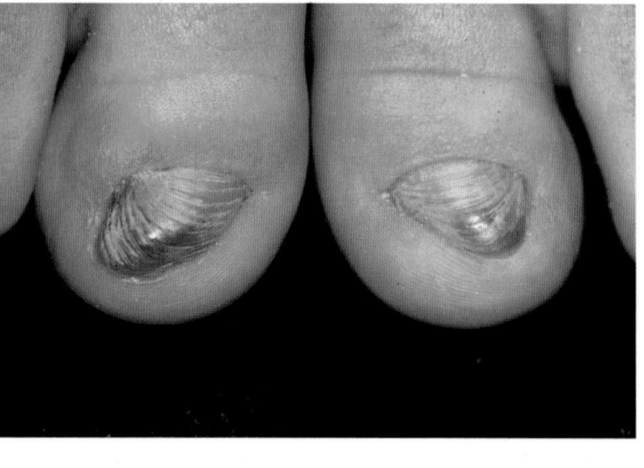

Fig. 3.10. Congenital malalignment of the great toenails.

Medial deviation is rare, but possible (Baran & Bureau, 1987).

Transverse ridging, single or more often multiple, is one of the earliest signs to appear and may develop over the entire surface of the nail plate (Baran, 1980; Baran, 1985). The ridges form regular waves when they are numerous. They seem to follow recurrent episodes of damage to the matrix, sometimes leading to latent onychomadesis or shedding of a large portion of the nail; the new nail is already well advanced before the old is lost.

The nail plate which may be thickened with gradual tapering of the distal portion does not adhere tightly to the nail bed. Sometimes there is associated onycholysis, whilst the nail may acquire a greyish tint, a brown discoloration (due to haemorrhage) or a greenish hue (which is due to *Pseudomonas*). This would be of minor importance if it were not for the complications that may arise both in infancy (ingrowing toenail) and in the elderly (hemionychogryphosis or nail dystrophy).

The most important complication is ingrowing toenail with painful inflammation of part of the perionychial area (Mackinnon, 1978; Cohen *et al.*, 1991). At this stage examination may show a nail which is short, pressing against a rim of skin at the extreme tip of the big toe and forming a lip. Primary malalignment of the nail appears then to be the main factor causing the 'nail embedding' with the resultant inability to grow to normal length. Because the main direction of nail growth in these patients occurs laterally, there is insufficient forward thrust to allow the nail plate to mount the heaped up tissue in front of it, even when physiological koilonychia exists (Baran *et al.*, 1979; Baran, 1980; Baran & Bureau, 1983). At this stage a simple surgical procedure successfully realigns the whole nail apparatus. The best results are obtained when the malalignment is corrected surgically before the age of 2 years. Spontaneous improvement, or even complete resolution occurs occasionally (Dawson, 1982; Handfield-Jones & Harman, 1988); in all patients in which the condition cleared this occurred before 10 years of age. However, it remains to be ascertained how frequently spontaneous realignment really does happen (Baran, 1989b; Dawson, 1989).

Management depends therefore on accurate assessment of the degree of malalignment and the associated changes (Baran, 1985).

1 If the nail deviation is mild, and in the absence of complications, the nail, as it hardens, may overcome the initial slight distal embedding, and sufficient normal nail may grow to the tip of the digit to prevent further secondary traumatic changes. Treatment should be conservative.

2 If the deviation is marked and the nail is buried in the soft tissues, the patient may be disabled later on, in childhood and in adult life. Surgical rotation of the misdirected matrix is then essential in order to prevent permanent nail dystrophy, despite the possibly favourable course of some cases. This anomaly is probably an inherited condition, as identical twins have been observed with similar changes in their great toes (Barth *et al.*, 1986; Harper & Beer, 1986).

The 'inherited nail dystrophy principally affecting the great toe nails over three generations' (Dawson, 1979) was definitely congenital malalignment of the great toenails. Guéro *et al.* (1994) have demonstrated the existence of a ligamentous structure type which corresponds to a dorsal expansion of the lateral ligament of the distal interphalangeal joint and is in very clear connexion with the nail matrix region.

References

Bailie F.B. & Evans D.M. (1978) Ingrowing toenails in infancy. *Br. Med. J.* **2**, 737–738.

Baran R. (1980) Congenital malalignment of toe nail. *Arch. Dermatol.* **116**, 1346.

Baran R. (1985) An inherited nail dystrophy principally affecting the great toenails. *Br. J. Dermatol.* **112**, 124 (letter).

Baran R. (1989a) The treatment of ingrowing toenails in infancy. *J. Dermatol. Treat.* **1**, 55–57.

Baran R. (1989b) Great toenail dystrophy. *Br. J. Dermatol.* **120**, 139–140.

Baran R. & Bureau H. (1983) Congenital malalignment of the big toenail as a cause of ingrowing toenail in infancy. Pathology and treatment (a study of thirty cases). *Clin. Exp. Dermatol.* **8**, 619–623.

Baran R. & Bureau H. (1987) Congenital malalignment of the big toenail. A new subtype. *Arch. Dermatol.* **123**, 437 (letter).

Baran R., Bureau H. & Sayag J. (1979) Congenital malalignment of the toe nail. *Clin. Exp. Dermatol.* **4**, 359–360.

Barth J.H., Dawber R.P.R., Ashton R.E. & Baran R. (1986) Congenital malalignment of great toenails in two sets of monozygotic twins. *Arch. Dermatol.* **122**, 379–380.

Bentley-Phillips B. & Coll I. (1983) Ingrowing toenail in infancy. *Int. J. Dermatol.* **22**, 115–116.

Bird S. (1978) Trouble with children's feet. *Br. Med. J.* **4**, 1297 (letter).

Cohen J.L., Scher R.K. & Pappert A.S. (1991) Congenital malalignment of the great toenails. *Pediatr. Dermatol.* **8**, 40–42.

Connolly B. & Fitzgerald R.J. (1988) Pledgets in ingrowing toe nails. *Arch. Dis. Child.* **63**, 71–72.

Dawson T.A.J. (1979) An inherited nail dystrophy principally affecting the great toenails. *Clin. Exp. Dermatol.* **4**, 309–313.

Dawson T.A.J. (1982) An inherited nail dystrophy principally affecting the great toe nails; further observations. *Clin. Exp. Dermatol.* **7**, 455–457.

Dawson T.A.J. (1989) Great toenail dystrophy. *Br. J. Dermatol.* **120**, 139 (letter).

Engels M. (1985) Nagelbettveränderungen im Neugeborenenalter. *Pädiat. Pädol.* **20**, 173–176.

Guéro *et al.* (1994) Ligamentary structure of the base of the nail. *Surg. Radiol. Anat.* (in press).

Hammerton M.D. & Shrank A.B. (1988) Congenital hypertrophy of the lateral nail folds of the hallux. *Pediatr. Dermatol.* **5**, 243–245.

Handfields-Jones S.E. & Harman R.R.M. (1988) Spontaneous improvement of the congenital malalignment of the great toe nails. *Br. J. Dermatol.* **118**, 305–306 (letter).

Hendricks W.M. (1979) Congenital ingrowing toenails. *Cutis* **24**, 393–394.

Honig P.J., Spitzer A., Bernstein R. *et al.* (1982) Congenital ingrown toenails. *Clin. Pediatr. (Phil.)* **21**, 424–426.

Mackinnon A.E. (1978) Trouble with childrens feet. *Br. Med. J.* **2**, 1297.

Martinet C., Pascal M., Civatte J. & Larrègue M. (1984) Bour relet latéro-unguéal du gros orteil du nourrisson. *Ann. Dermatol. Venereol.* **111**, 731–733.

Rufli T., von Schultess A. & Itin P. (1992) Congenital hypertrophy of the lateral nail folds of the hallux. *Dermatology* **184**, 296–297.

Samman P.D. (1978) Great toe nail dystrophy. *Clin. Exp. Dermatol.* **3**, 81–82.

Silverman R.A. (1990) Pediatric disease. In: *Nails: Therapy, Diagnosis, Surgery*, eds Scher R.K. & Daniel C.R. W.B. Saunders, Philadelphia.

Walker S. (1979) Paronychia of the great toe of infants. *Clin. Pediatr.* **18**, 247.

Impetigo

The dorsal aspect of the distal phalanx may be affected by impetigo. There are two types: (i) vesiculopustular with its familiar honey-crusted lesions (Jacobs, 1981), usually due to β-haemolytic streptococci; and (ii) bullous, usually due to phage type 71 staphylococci (Fig. 3.11). The latter is characterized by the appearance of large, localized, intraepidermal bullae, that persist for longer periods than the transient vesicles of streptococcal impetigo, and which subsequently rupture spontaneously to form very thin crusts. The lesions of bullous impetigo may mimic the non-infectious bullous diseases such as drug-induced bullae or bullous pemphigoid.

Oral therapy of bullous impetigo with a penicillinase-resistant penicillin should be instituted and continued until the lesions resolve. Cephalexin and erythromycin are acceptable alternatives (Stewardson-Krieger & Esterly, 1978). The lesions should be cleansed several times daily and topical mupirocin rubbed into all the affected areas.

Poorly trimmed nails may serve as a paronychial focus

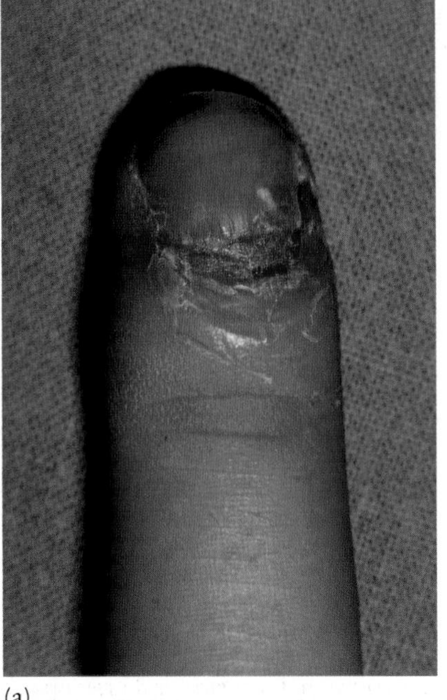

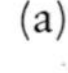

(a)

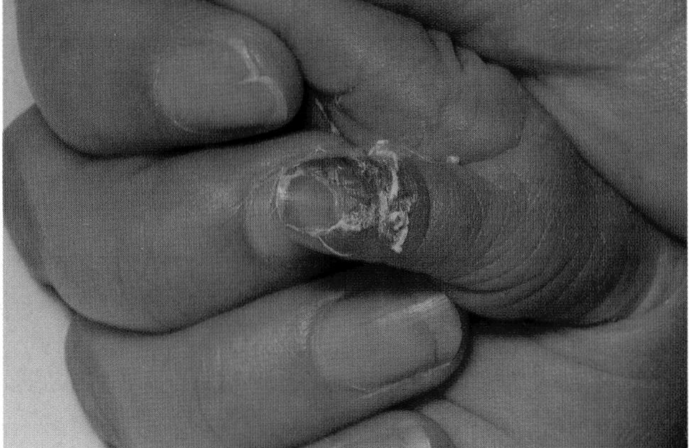

(b)

Fig. 3.11. (a & b) Impetigo of the nail apparatus.

for infection in children during remission induction treat ment for various malignant disorders (Gutjahr & Schmitt, 1984). Intense scratching of infected atopic dermatitis, coupled with minor trauma to the fingertips, creates distal subungual microabscesses that spread contiguously to the underlying bone (Boiko *et al.*, 1988).

References

Boiko S., Kaufman R.A. & Lucky A.W. (1988) Osteomyelitis of the distal phalanges in 3 children with severe atopic dermatitis. *Arch. Dermatol.* **124**, 418–423.

Gutjahr P. & Schmitt H.J. (1984) Caring of the nails and anti cancer treatment. *Eur. J. Pediatr.* **143**, 74.

Jacobs A.H. (1981) What's new in pediatric dermatology? *Acta Dermatol. Venereol. Suppl.* **95**, 91.

Stewardson-Krieger P.D. & Esterly N.B. (1978) Pyogenic infections. In: *Adolescent Dermatology*, eds Solomon L.M., Esterly N.B. & Loeffel E.D., p. 163. W.B. Saunders, Philadelphia.

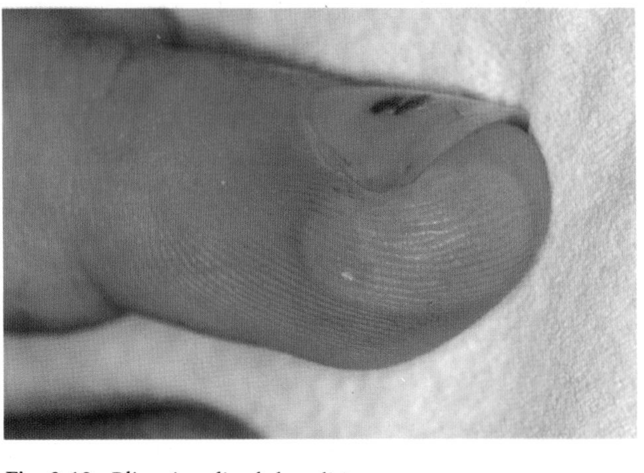

Fig. 3.12. Blistering distal dactylitis.

Blistering distal dactylitis (BDD)

BDD is a variant of streptococcal skin infection. This condition presents as a superficial, non-tender, blistering β-haemolytic streptococcal infection over the anterior fat pat of the distal phalanx of the finger (Hays & Mullard, 1975); *Staphylococcus aureus* and *S. epidermidis* are isolated less frequently. Multiple fingers affected might be a predictor of *Staph. aureus* (Norcross & Mitchell, 1993). The lesion may or may not have a paronychial extension and more than one digit is frequently involved (Schneider & Palette, 1982). The blister, which has an erythematous base, containing thin white pus, has a predilection for the tip of the digit (Fig. 3.12). It extends to the subungual area of the free edge of the nail plate. This area may provide a nidus for the β-haemolytic streptococcus and act as a focus of chronic infection (Baran, 1982), similar to rhinopharynx. Recurrent blistering dactylitis has also been reported with ingrowing toenail (Telfer *et al.*, 1989). The age range of affected patients is 2–16 years. The condition is exceptionally reported in adults: a healthy fishmonger (Palomo-Arellano *et al.*, 1985), an unusual case due to group B β-haemolytic streptococcus in a patient with insulin-dependent diabetes (Benson & Solivan, 1987); another case due to *Staphylococcus aureus* in an immunosuppressed patient (Zemtsov & Veitschegger, 1992); and a questionable publication (Parras *et al.*, 1988). For local care, incision (without pain), drainage (consisting of thin white pus) and soaking are indicated and facilitate a more rapid response to systemic antibiotic therapy: effective regimens include benzathine penicillin G in a single intramuscular dose, or a 10-day course of oral amoxycyllin or erythromycin ethyl succinate. This type of treatment decreases the reservoir of streptococci by preventing spread to family contacts (McCray & Esterly, 1981, 1982).

The differential diagnosis includes blisters resulting from friction, thermal and chemical burns, infectious states such as herpetic whitlow and staphylococcal bullous impetigo, and the Weber–Cockayne variant of epidermolysis bullosa (McCray & Esterly, 1981).

References

Baran R. (1982) Blistering distal dactylitis. *J. Am. Acad. Dermatol.* **6**, 948.

Benson P.M. & Solivan G. (1987) Group B streptococcal blistering distal dactylitis in an adult diabetic. *J. Am. Acad. Dermatol.* **17**, 310–311.

Hays G.C. & Mullard J.E. (1975) Blistering distal dactylitis: A clinically recognizable streptococcal infection. *Pediatrics* **56**, 129.

McCray M.K. & Esterly N.B. (1981) Blistering distal dactylitis. *J. Am. Acad. Dermatol.* **5**, 592.

McCray M.K. & Esterly N.B. (1982) Blistering distal dactylitis. *J. Am. Acad. Dermatol.* **6**, 949.

Norcross M.C. & Mitchell D.F. (1993) Blistering distal dactylitis caused by *Staphylococcus aureus*. *Cutis* **51**, 353–354.

Palamo-Arellano A., Jimenez-Reyes J., Martin-Moreno L. *et al.* (1985) Blistering distal dactylitis in an adult. *Arch. Dermatol.* **121**, 1242.

Parras F., Ezpelata C., Romero J. *et al.* (1988) Blistering distal dactylitis in an adult. *Cutis* **41**, 127–128.

Schneider J.A. & Palette H.L. (1982) Blistering distal dactylitis a manifestation of group A beta-hemolytic streptococcal infection. *Arch. Dermatol.* **118**, 879–880.

Telfer N.R., Barth J.H. & Dawber R.P.R. (1989) Recurrent blistering distal dactylitis of the great toe associated with an ingrowing toenail. *Clin. Exp. Dermatol.* **14**, 380–381.

Zemtsov A. & Veitschegger M. (1992) Staphylococcus aureus induced blistering distal dactylitis in adult immunosuppressed patient. *J. Am. Acad. Dermatol.* **26**, 784.

Toxic shock syndrome

In this *Staphylococcus aureus* infection with fever, hypotension, generalized erythema, diarrhoea, central nervous system and electrolyte abnormalities, hair and nails may shed about 2 months following the acute illness (Litt, 1983).

Reference

Litt I.F. (1983) Toxic shock syndrome: an adolescent disease. *J. Adolesc. Health Care* **4**, 270–274.

The twenty-nail dystrophy of childhood

The term 'twenty-nail dystrophy' was coined by Hazelrigg *et al.* (1977) to describe an entity already recognized by Samman (1965) as 'excess ridging' of childhood. This is an acquired, idiopathic nail dystrophy in which all 20 nails are uniformly and simultaneously affected with excess longitudinal ridging and loss of lustre. We have designated this condition 'vertical striated sand-paper twenty-nail dystrophy' (Baran & Dupré, 1977) (Fig. 3.13). Achten

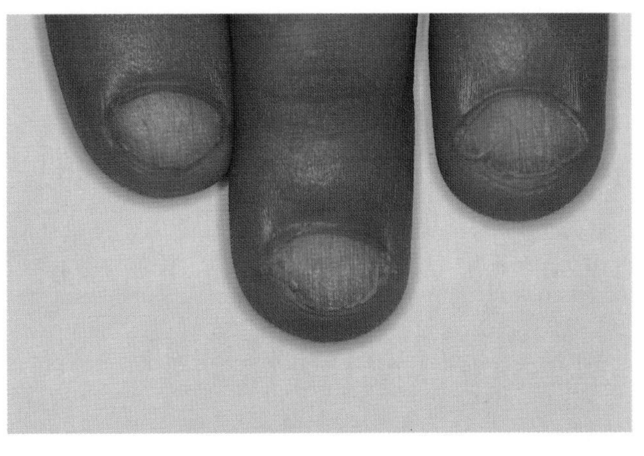

Fig. 3.13. Twenty-nail dystrophy of childhood – prominent longitudinal striations in this case.

and Wanet-Rouard (1974) used the term 'trachyonychia' after Alkiewicz (1950), who described a dystrophy characterized by roughness of the nail surface and grey opacity of the nail, which becomes brittle with terminal splitting. It begins insidiously in early childhood and resolves slowly with age. The pathogenesis is controversial (Wilkinson *et al.*, 1979). Alopecia areata (Baran *et al.*, 1978; Horn & Odom, 1980), less often lichen planus (Baran *et al.*, 1978; Scher *et al.*, 1978) or even both associated in the same patient (Fenton & Samman, 1988; Kanwar *et al.*, 1993) and rarely psoriasis (Baran *et al.*, 1978) have all been associated with the 'twenty-nail dystrophy'. Other possible causes include ichthyosis vulgaris, in association with atopic dermatitis (James *et al.*, 1981), selective IgA deficiency (Leong *et al.*, 1982), familial severe cases (Arias *et al.*, 1982; Pavone, 1982), dark red lunulae and knuckle pads (Runne, 1980) and rarely ectodermal dysplasias. This condition, reported in twins, may result from single localized tissue malformation (Commens, 1988). An autoimmune process may be involved in some cases (Person, 1984). We have presented a case of lichen planus-like graft-versus-host disease precipitated by an exchange transfusion in newborn (Brun *et al.*, 1984).

Congenital, familial and hereditary cases have occurred in both children and adults. Morphologically there are two main types (Baran, 1981). In the first type, 'vertical striated sandpapered twenty-nail dystrophy' or sandblasted nails is most frequently associated with alopecia areata. It is difficult to demonstrate the condition adequately on photographs. In the second type, all 20 nails are shiny, opalescent and have longitudinal ridging. This fine stippled appearance reflects light and is clearly seen on photographs (Baran, 1981).

Alopecia areata may occur in association with both types. In the descriptions by Hazelrigg *et al.* (1977) one case was of the second type; the majority were of the first type. Also the thumbnails and great toenails were yellow, thickened and rough, i.e. all nails were not uniformly affected despite the definition given by Hazelrigg *et al.* (1977).

Very few published reports include histological data. We have found, in children, either vacuolated cells with intercellular and intracellular oedema in the nail bed epidermis and squamous cells of the matrix presenting with homogeneous pale staining, or changes typical of lichen planus. Scher *et al.* (1978) reported one case that showed microscopic evidence of lichen planus. Silverman and Rhodes (1984) saw a child with oral lichen planus who had twenty-nail dystrophy. Donofrio and Ayala's (1984) patient showed psoriasiform epithelial hyperplasia with hypergranulosis. Wilkinson *et al.* (1979) presented histopathological findings that were incompatible with the definition of the condition as a variant of lichen planus; there was considerable distortion of the nail matrix with a fairly dense mononuclear inflammatory infiltrate below and within the matrix epithelium, together with marked spongiosis. No basal cell liquefaction was present. These changes suggested an eczematous picture. Alkiewicz (1950) described similar histological findings in two cases in which roughness of the nails had been induced by strong chemicals and in a third case involving all 20 nails with no obvious cause. Examination of nail biopsy specimens may therefore rule out lichen planus with its distinctive features and psoriasis restricted to the nails. Braun-Falco *et al.* (1981) reported spongiotic dermatitis of the nail matrix and the nail bed with column-like parakeratosis within the nail in trachyonychia, due to alopecia areata, atopic dermatitis and the idiopathic form. In those subjects with no obvious cause and histological evidence of eczematous changes, alopecia areata has occurred in some cases. Jerasutus *et al.* (1990) studied five cases, the youngest being 15 years old. All histological sections showed distinctive changes of spongiotic inflammation of the nail matrix suggesting that they represent a subgroup of allergic eczema or an autoimmunological response to the matrix. Tosti *et al.* (1991) found in 13 patients that a mild to moderate lymphocytic infiltration associated with exocytosis and spongiosis is the histological hallmark of trachyonychia due to alopecia areata.

We believe that the term 'twenty-nail dystrophy' has no specific significance. It is more useful clinically to describe the morphological appearance, such as roughness and ridging, and to examine nail biopsy specimens if possible to clarify the pathogenesis. Since the term has come to include such a wide variety of conditions and physical signs which affect all 20 nails, it has lost its diagnostic value and should therefore be discarded (Baran & Dawber, 1987). Treatment attempts have been unsuccessful. However, Halkier–Sørensen (1990) suggests that topical PUVA is worth trying, although regression occurs slowly and a maintenance dose is necessary for a long time to prevent recurrence.

References

Achten G. & Wanet-Rouard J. (1974) Atrophie unguéale et trachyonychie. *Arch. Belg. Dermatol.* **30**, 201.

Alkiewicz J. (1950) Trachyonychie. *Ann. Dermatol. Syphil.* **10**, 136.

Arias A.M., Yung C.W., Rendler S. *et al.* (1982) Familial severe twenty-nail dystrophy. *J. Am. Acad. Dermatol.* **7**, 349.

Baran R. (1981) Twenty nail dystrophy of alopecia areata. *Arch. Dermatol.* **117**, 1.

Baran R. & Dawber R.P.R. (1987) Twenty-nail dystrophy of childhood: A misnamed syndrome *Cutis* **39**, 481–482.

Baran R. & Dupré A. (1977) Vertical striated sand paper nails. *Arch. Dermatol.* **113**, 1613.

Baran R., Dupré A., Christol B. *et al.* (1978) L'ongle grésé peladique. *Ann. Dermatol. Venereol.* **105**, 387.

Braun-Falco O., Dorn M., Neubert U. *et al.* (1981) Trachyonychie: 20-Nägel-Dystrophie. *Hautarzt* **32**, 17.

Brun P., Baran R. & Czernielewski Y. (1984) Dystrophie lichénienne des 20 ongles. Manifestation possible d'une maladie du greffon contre l'hôte (MGCH) chronique par exsanguino-transfusion néo-natale? Presented at the annual 'Journées dermatologiques de Paris', March 1984.

Commens C.A. (1988) Twenty-nail dystrophy in identical twins. *Pediatr. Dermatol.* **5**, 117–119.

Donofrio P. & Ayala F. (1984) Twenty-nail dystrophy: report of a case and review of the literature. *Acta Derm. Venereol. (Stockh).* **64**, 180.

Fenton D.A. & Samman P.D. (1988) Twenty-nail dystrophy of childhood associated with alopecia areata and lichen planus. *Br. J. Dermatol.* **119**, suppl. 33, 63.

Halkier–Sørensen L., Cramers M. & Kragballe K. (1990) Twenty-nail dystrophy eated with topical PUVA. *Acta Derm. Venereol.* **70**, 510–511.

Hazelrigg D.E., Duncan W.C. & Jarrett M. (1977) Twenty nail dystrophy of childhood. *Arch. Dermatol.* **113**, 73.

Horn R.T. & Odom R.B. (1980) Twenty nail dystrophy of alopecia areata. *Arch. Dermatol.* **116**, 573.

James W.D., Odom R.B. & Horn R.T. (1981) Twenty nail dystrophy and *Ichythyosis vulgaris*. *Arch. Dermatol.* **117**, 316.

Jerasutus S., Suvanprakorn P. & Kitchawengkul O. (1990) Twenty-nail dystrophy. A clinical manifestation of spongiotic inflammation of the nail matrix. *Arch. Dermatol.* **126**, 1068–1070.

Kanwar A.J., Ghosh S., Thami G.P. *et al.* (1993) Twenty-nail dystrophy due to lichen planus in a patient with alopecia areata. *Clin. Exp. Dermatol.* **18**, 293–294.

Leong A.B., Gange R.W. & O'Connor R.D. (1982) Twenty nail dystrophy (trachyonychia) associated with selective IgA deficiency. *J. Pediatr.* **100**, 418.

Pavone L. (1982) Hereditary twenty nail dystrophy in a Sicilian family. *J. Med. Genet.* **19**, 131–135.

Person J.R. (1984) Twenty-nail dystrophy: a hypothesis. *Arch. Dermatol.* **120**, 437.

Runne U. (1980) Twenty-nail dystrophy mit 'Knuckle pads'. *Z. Hautkr.* **55**, 901.

Samman P.D. (1965) *The Nail in Disease*, p. 122. Heinemann, London.

Scher R.K., Fischbein R. & Ackerman A.B. (1978) Twenty-nail dystrophy. A variant of lichen planus. *Arch. Dermatol.* **114**, 612.

Silverman R.A. & Rhodes A.R. (1984) Twenty-nail dystrophy of childhood: a sign of localized lichen planus. *Pediatr. Dermatol.* **1**, 207–210.

Tosti A., Fanti P.A., Morelli R. *et al.* (1991) Trachyonychia associated with alopecia areata. A clinical and pathological study. *J. Am. Acad. Dermatol.* 25, 266–270.
Wilkinson J.D., Dawber R.P.R., Bowers R.P. *et al.* (1979) Twenty nail dystrophy of childhood. *Br. J. Dermatol.* 100, 217.

The nail in old age

The chemical composition of the nail plate is modified in older nails; calcium content is elevated and iron is decreased.

The elderly constitute a large and rapidly growing segment of the population. Some nail diseases exhibit a predilection for the aged or show a varying frequency of incidence with age. Some anomalies may persist from an earlier age but are modified by increasing years. Underlying pathology may worsen with the superimposition of degenerative changes and with increasing deformities. Chronic trauma to the toenail area can result from faulty biomechanics (Cohen & Scher, 1992).

In elderly people, distinctive changes may be noted in the nails (Baran, 1982). Most frequently the first and fifth digits are involved. The nail is heaped up as a result of pressure from each side. Excessive chronic pressure may cause loss of normal lateral nail grooves and matrix distortion, subungual keratosis, onychophosis (keratotic nail grooves) and ulceration (Helfand, 1989). These conditions, which can be extremely painful, may reduce stability and limit ambulation and require continuing management for relief. However, careful evaluation will often identify the cause as an anatomical or pathomechanical abnormality from changes in gait (Gilchrist, 1979).

Hallux valgus and overlapping toes for example, may require moulded shoes to provide adequate shoe fitting. This will relieve pressure and deformed joints, distribute pressure evenly over the foot and provide comfort (Gilchrist, 1979). The use of protective padding may be indicated.

Unfortunately in the elderly some subjects have difficulty reaching their feet, others find their nails too thick to cut, and finally they may be deterred by poor vision. Periodic treatment should be given to relieve pain.

Aetiology of senile changes

Old age nail changes may be attributed in part to arteriosclerosis even without gross evidence of obliteration of the vessel. The ability of an extremity to withstand trauma is severely limited when arterial insufficiency is present. Although a pulseless foot may have an adequate collateral circulation for ordinary metabolic demands, any break in the skin can lead to gangrene and amputation because the increased requirement for blood flow cannot be met (Bakow & Friedman, 1969). All these factors, associated with the dangers to the foot that they entail, combine to make chronic infection of the foot a major problem (Tarara, 1990). The histological study of Lewis and Montgomery (1955) bears out this concept since at least minimal thickening of the walls of the blood vessels was present in the nail generative areas. Alterations in elastic tissue are prominent and more diffuse in the dermis beneath the pink nail bed, and more pronounced than they are in the adjacent, glabrous perionychial skin. The change in elastic tissue, present to a lesser degree beneath the lunula, is absent from the dermis of the matrix area which is covered by the proximal nail fold. However, the whole subungual area may show thickening of the walls of blood vessels and reveal fragmentation of their elastic tissue. Parker and Diffey (1983) suggest that the nail plate acts as a very efficient sunscreen, with very low transmission in the damaging UVB range (280–315 nm). This term refers to the conspicuous cellular components forming a galaxy in the nail unit. They are retained shrunken nuclei with perinuclear eosinophilic material or vacuolization or both (Lewis & Montgomery, 1955). The nail plate contains an increased number of 'pertinax bodies' as compared with the younger adult nail (Fig. 3.14). They could be interpreted as remnants of nuclei of keratinocytes in the form of a galaxy.

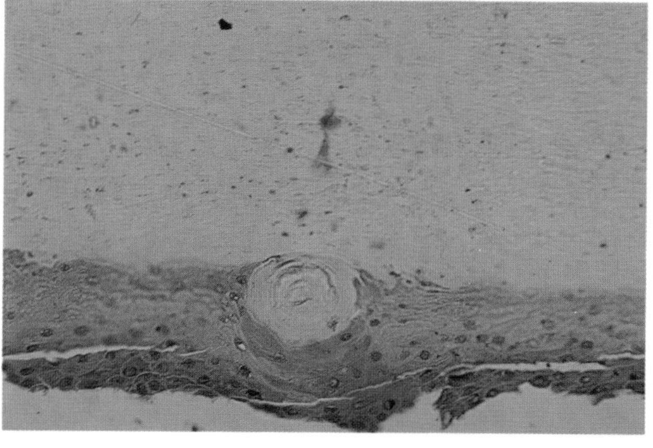

Fig. 3.14. Pertinax body of the nail apparatus.

Retarded nail plate growth results in larger corneocytes (Germann *et al.*, 1980).

Linear nail growth

Thumbnail growth measured by Orentreich and Scharp (1967) in 257 individuals decreased by an average of 38% from the third to the ninth decade. The decrease was greater in females up to the sixth decade. Subsequently, no further decrease occurred until the eighth decade, by which time the rate for males decreased more rapidly. Bean (1980) observed that the average daily growth of his left thumbnail decreased from 0.123 mm a day at 32 to 0.095 mm a day at 67 years of age. Alternating 7-year cycles of constant growth rate with 7-year periods of marked decline in nail growth have been suggested

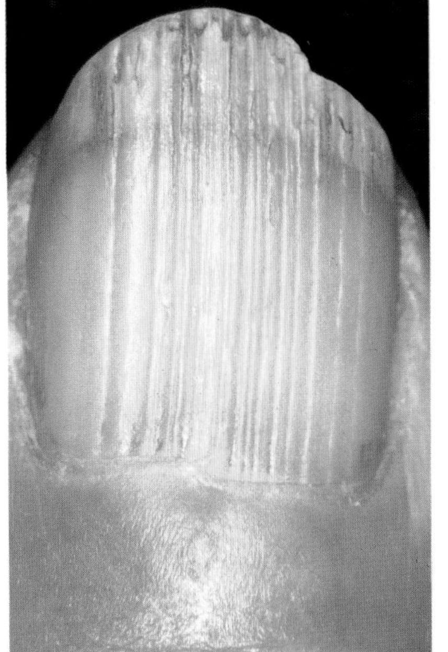

Fig. 3.15. Longitudinal ridges – age-related.

(Orentreich *et al.*, 1979). Underlying factors which may influence the rate of decline are actinic effects on the nail matrix, circulatory impairment, nutritional deficiency, hormonal changes, and local and systemic infections. Other factors may also be important (Chapter 1). According to Orentreich *et al.* (1979) the determination of the rate of linear nail growth may prove a useful measurement of physiological ageing.

Variations in the contour of the nail

The normal nail plate has a double curvature, longitudinal and transverse. Modifications of the contour in old age include platonychia (flattening) and koilonychia (spooning). Most typically the convexity is increased from side to side and decreased in the longitudinal axis. 'Watch-glass' nails and true clubbing are frequent in men affected by chronic pulmonary disease (Tammaro & Lampugnani, 1969). The longitudinal ridges become more pronounced and numerous (Fig. 3.15). This is possibly due to variation in the turnover rate of the matrix cells or may be related to whorls of generative cells in the most proximal region of the nail matrix.

Variations in colour

Distinctive changes are noted in the nails in elderly subjects. Macroscopically, the nails appear dull and opaque. The colour varies from shades of yellow to grey. Frequently, the lunula is not visible. The white nails of old age, similar to those reported in cirrhosis, uraemia and hypoalbuminaemia, have been termed 'Neapolitan nails' because of the three bands as in Neapolitan ice cream (Horan *et al.*, 1982). These white changes occur without detectable protein, liver or kidney abnormalities, differing from the leuconychia which may present as transverse white streaks of the nail plate (Helford, 1993) probably due to pressure or microtrauma which explains their lateral position on the nail.

Nail bed capillaries show frequent distortions in normal subjects over 70 years of age, including numerous short tortuous capillary loops, and the subpapillary venous plexus is ill-defined (Merlen *et al.*, 1972). This capillary distortion may explain the frequency, in the distal one-third, of splinter haemorrhages in the elderly, often caused by trauma to the nails such as through the use of walking aids and intake of multiple drugs beside anticoagulants. The latter are often responsible for subungual haematomas especially in the feet, but idiopathic subungual haemorrhage is also common in patients with diabetes mellitus, chronic renal disease or recent stroke (Helfand, 1989). Nevertheless, splinters appear less common in the elderly than in young people and they are a less useful physical sign in the elderly (Young & Mulley, 1987).

Acral arteriolar ectasia (Paslin & Heaton, 1972) is a distinct vascular malformation consisting of purple serpiginous vessels on the dorsa of the digits, first arising in the fifth decade of life. The vessels are ectatic arterioles and are believed to represent a rare vascular malformation.

Variations in thickness and consistency

The thickness of the plate may be normal, increased or decreased. The fingernail is often soft and fragile, a common finding in persons older than 60 years of age (Lubach *et al.*, 1986), prone to longitudinal fissuring and splitting into layers. Therefore, hands should be protected by cotton gloves during house work or other occupations. Gloves are more comfortable worn inside-out with the seams on the outside. The finger nail should never be used as a 'tool', crude traumatic tasks being done with 'finger pads' for 'finger chores'.

The toenail is usually thicker and harder with hyperkeratotic lesions in the toenail region. These are often present for several years before treatment is sought. The most common toenail deformities are hypertrophy, associated with chronic fungal infection, onychogryphosis and ingrowing toenail as residua of previous disease, trauma or deformity of adult life or childhood (Jahss, 1979). Ill-fitting shoes can be the cause of some foot disorders such as subungual heloma (Fig. 3.16) (see pp. 392–393), onychophosis (Fig. 3.17) (see p. 392) and onycholysis. Onychogryphosis (Fig. 3.18) may interfere with shoe comfort. Hemionychogryphosis with lateral deviation of the nail plate often results from congenital malalignment of the big toenail.

A hyperkeratotic heaping at the distal free edge of the toenails, irregular growth, and excess transverse over-curvature of the nails are characteristics of chronic arterial insufficiency (Kushner, 1992).

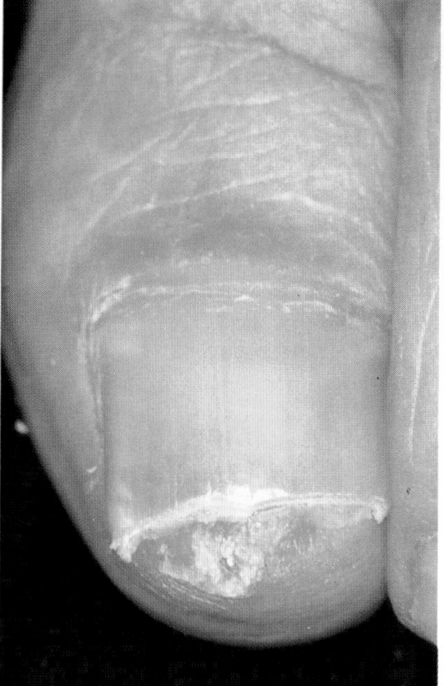

Fig. 3.16. Subungual heloma ('corn').

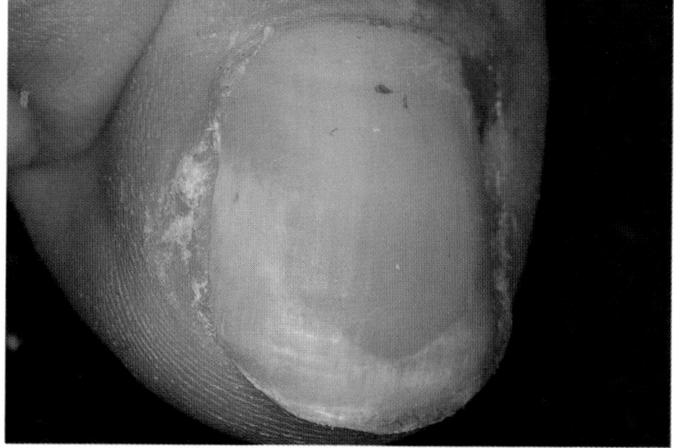

Fig. 3.17. Onychophosis.

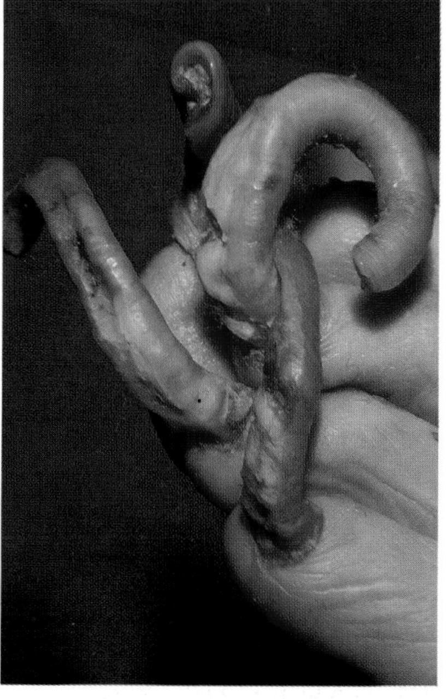

Fig. 3.18. Onychogryphosis.

Hallux valgus is seen predominantly in females. It is an acquired deformity, often secondary to ill-fitting shoes, but it can also be induced by congenital, anatomical factors. It is a medial laxity of the metatarso-sesamoido-phalangeal joint with lateral dislocation or subdislocation of the sesamoid bones. The latter is maintained by a lateral retraction which is aggravated by the motor muscles of the big toe, whose action is towards valgus, due to the natural angulation (Groulier, 1981).

The influence of hallux valgus on the corresponding big toenail has been stressed by Fabry (1983). Progressive lateral deviation of the big toenail appears with lateral overcurvature of the nail plate. Hyperkeratosis of the medial nail fold, and subungual hyperkeratosis in the distomedial nail area, are common. Relapsing ingrowing big toenail with granulation tissue in the lateral nail groove and adjacent nail bed is not exceptional in old age.

Ingrowing toenail (see Chapter 10)

Ingrowing toenail represents an inflammation of the lateral nail folds due to the intrusion of the adjacent margin of the nail plate. Improper cutting and pressure from ill-fitting footwear are probably the major factors in the elderly. In addition, blunt or sharp protuberance of the distal tuft, mainly associated to pincer nails, results from an abnormal positional relationship between the first metatarsal and hallux (Lemont & Christman, 1990). Although troublesome, ingrowing nail is usually only an inconvenience to the average sufferer. In an old person with impaired arterial circulation, ingrowing nail may become a serious problem since infection and gangrene may supervene.

Three major types characterize this common problem sometimes complicated by onychomycosis:

1 overcurvature of the nail plate (pincer nail, onychocryptosis);
2 subcutaneous ingrowing toenail;
3 hypertophy of the lateral nail fold.

Tumours in the nail area

The relative frequency of benign and malignant tumours in this area varies with age. Hyperostosis (sometimes called exostoses) is related to faulty pedal biomechanics in the elderly. Myxoid pseudocysts (mucous cysts, periungual ganglion) are probably the commonest benign tumour. They occur more commonly in women. The commonest site is on the proximal nail fold of the fingers, and they occur only rarely on the toes. The lesions are usually asymptomatic, varying from soft to firm, cystic to fluctuant. Longitudinal nail grooving may result from pressure on the matrix. Clinical signs of degenerative arthritis and Heberden's nodes are associated in about 15% of cases; radiologically the majority show terminal interphalangeal joint osteoarthritis – 'wear and tear' arthritis.

Carcinoma of the nail apparatus is not uncommon; about 150 cases have been reported in the literature. In a series of 58 cases of subungual epidermoid carcinoma, Attieh *et al.* (1979) reported 46 cases in the age range 50–79 years, peak incidence being in the seventh decade. The initial manifestations of Bowen's disease and squamous cell carcinoma are difficult to differentiate in this area; there may be localized pain, swelling and inflammation. Because of the many chronic conditions which affect this region, a high index of suspicion is required for the early detection of carcinoma. A biopsy is necessary in order to confirm the diagnosis.

Patterson and Helwig (1980) reported 66 cases of subungual melanomas; 53% were found on the foot, 98% occurring on the big toe. Of these patients 70% were aged between 50 and 80 years, peak incidence being in the eighth decade.

Although the majority of lesions in the nail area are inflammatory, infective or due to congenital or acquired deformity, neoplasia must be considered in the differential diagnosis of localized and chronic inflammatory conditions.

Nail fungal infection

Hyperkeratosis, especially beneath the nail, may occur primarily or secondarily to fungal infection of the skin. In either case, eventually several nails become infected, particularly toenails. Chronic paronychia is related to complicating factors, such as peripheral vascular insufficiency and diabetes mellitus. The toenails often become thickened to such a degree that the wearing of shoes may trigger pain.

English and Atkinson (1974) carried out fungal examinations for onychomycosis on the thickened toenail of 168 patients attending a chiropody clinic for old-age pensioners. The nails of 68 (41%) of the patients were microscopically positive. Cultures from 12% of these were negative. Of the remainder, 20 (12%) were infected by dermatophytes and 42 (25%) by moulds. Fungi and especially moulds (Achten *et al.*, 1979) have a predilection for the big toenail, especially after 60. Environmental conditions, peripheral vascular insufficiency (arterial, venous and lymphatic), orthopaedic defects (e.g. overriding of the toes) or onychogryphosis (Tanaka *et al.*, 1986) may be the cause of this site preference.

References

Achten G., Wanet-Rouard J., Wiame L. *et al.* (1979) Les onychomycoses à moisissures. *Dermatologica* **159**, suppl. 1, 128.

Attieh F.F., Shah J., Booher R.J. & Knapper W.H. (1979) Subungual squamous cell carcinoma. *J. Am. Med. Assoc.* **241**, 262–263.

Bakow R.B. & Friedman S.A. (1969) The significance of trophic foot changes in the aged. *Geriatrics* **11**, 135–139.

Baran R. (1982) Nail care in the 'golden years' of life. *Curr. Med. Res. Opin.* 7, suppl. 2, 96.

Baran R. & Dawber R.P.R. (1985) The ageing nail. In: *Skin Problems in the Elderly*, ed. Fry L. pp. 315–330. Churchill Livingstone, Edinburgh.

Bean W.B. (1980) Nail growth: thirty-five years of observations. *Arch. Intern. Med.* **140**, 73.

Cohen P.R. & Scher R.K. (1992) Geriatric nail disorders: Diagnosis and treatment. *J. Am. Acad. Dermatol.* **26**, 521–531.

English M.P. & Atkinson R. (1974) Onychomycosis in elderly chiropody patients. *Br. J. Dermatol.* **91**, 67.

Fabry H. (1983) Haut-und Nagelveränderungen bei Hallux valgus. *Akt. Dermatol.* **9**, 77–79.

Germann H., Barran W. & Plewig G. (1980) Morphology of corneocytes from human nail plates. *J. Invest. Dermatol.* **74**, 115–118.

Gilchrist A.K. (1979) Common foot problems in the elderly. *Geriatrics* **34**, 67–70.

Groulier P. (1981) Hallux valgus – hallux rigidus. *Rev. Prat.* **31**, 1031–1032.

Helfand A.E. (1989) Nail and hyperkeratotic problems in the elderly foot. *Am. Fam. Physica* **39**, 101–110.

Horan M.A., Puxly J.A. & Fox R.A. (1982) The white nails of old age (Neapolitan nails). *J. Am. Geriatr. Soc.* **30**, 734–737.

Jahss M.H. (1979) Geriatric aspects of the foot and ankle. In: *Clinical Geriatrics*, ed. Rossman I. Lippincott, Philadelplia.

Kushner D. (1992) Primary podiatric care of the vascularly compromised patient. *Clin. Podiatr. Med. Surg.* **9**, 109–123.

Lemont H. & Christman R.A. (1990) Subungual exostosis and nail disease and radiologic aspects. In: *Nails: Therapy, Diagnosis, Surgery*, eds Scher R.K. & Daniel C.R. III, pp. 250–257. W.B. Saunders, Philadelphia.

Lewis B. & Montgomery H. (1955) The senile nail. *J. Invest. Dermatol.* **24**, 11–18.

Merlen J.F., Coget J. & Vanderbeken J.P. (1972) Capillaroscopic patterns in functioning people aged 70 and over. *Bibliotheca Anatomica No. 11, 7th Eur. Conf. Microcirc*, Part I, eds Ditzel J. & Lewis D.H.S. Karger, Basel.

Orentreich N. & Scharp N.J. (1967) Keratin replacement as an ageing parameter. *J. Soc. Cosmet. Chem.* **18**, 537.

Orentreich N., Markowsky J. & Vegelman J.H. (1979) The effect of ageing on the rate of linear nail growth. *J. Invest. Dermatol.* **73**, 926.

Paslin D.A. & Heaton C.L. (1972) Acral arteriolar ectasia. *Arch. Dermatol.* **106**, 906–908.

Patterson G. & Helwig C. (1980) Subungual melanoma. *Cancer* **46**, 2074–2087.

Parker S.G. & Diffey B.L. (1983) The transmission of optical radiation through human nails. *Br. J. Dermatol.* **108**, 11.

Tammaro A.E. & Lampugnani P. (1969) Studio del complesso ungueale nell'eta senile. *Min. Med.* **60**, 3651–3655.

Tanaka T., Sohba S., Tanida Y. *et al.* (1986) Onychogryphosis due to *Tinea unguinum. Hifuka Rinsho.* **28**, 1336–1337.

Tarara E.L. (1970) Ingrown toenail: a problem among the aged. *Postgr. Med.* 199–202.

Young J. & Mulley G. (1987) Splinter haemorrhages in the elderly. *Age Ageing* **16**, 101–104.

Chapter 4
Fungal (Onychomycosis) and Other Infections Involving the Nail Apparatus

R.J. HAY, R. BARAN & E. HANEKE

Onychomycosis
- Distal and lateral subungual onychomycosis (DLSO)
- Superficial white onychomycosis (SWO)
- Superficial black onychomycosis (SBO)
- Proximal subungual onychomycosis (PSO)
  - Proximal white subungual onychomycosis (PWSO)
  - Proximal subungual onychomycosis from paronychia
- Total dystrophic onychomycosis (TDO)
- Laboratory investigations
  - Direct microscopy
  - Culture
  - Histopathology
- Differential diagnosis
- Chronic fungal paronychia
- Bacterial paronychia
- Other infective forms of paronychia
- Drug-induced paronychia
- Treatment of onychomycosis
  - Topical and oral agents
  - Nail removal
  - Urea chemical avulsion
  - Management of various sub-types
    - Non-dermatophyte moulds
    - Candida onychomycosis
    - Onycholysis with *Candida*
    - *Candida* chronic paronychia

Other fungal infections
- Sporotrichosis
- Chromoblastomycosis
- Coccidioidomycosis
- Blastomycosis (Chapter 5)

Other infections
- Herpes simplex
- Herpes zoster
- Gonorrhoea
- Syphilis
- Pinta
- Leprosy
- Leishmaniasis
- Trichinosis
- Scabies
- Pediculosis
- Tungiasis
- Larva migrans
- Subungual myasis

Infection in other chapters
- Chapter 3
  - Impetigo
  - *Veillonella*
  - Nursery staphylococcal infection
  - Blistering distal dactylitis
- Chapter 6
  - Malaria
  - Mucocutaneous lymph node syndrome
  - Acute febrile infection
  - Diphtheria
- Chapter 7
  - Tetanus
  - Erysipeloid
  - Prosector's wart (Tuberculosis verrucosa cutis)
  - *Mycobacterium marinum* infection
  - Tularaemia
  - Orf
  - Milker's nodule
- Chapter 10
  - Acute paronychia
  - Lectitis purulenta et granulomatosa

In this chapter the onychomycoses are considered in detail, together with a variety of infections occasionally seen in and around the nail apparatus; some infections are discussed, where appropriate, in other chapters.

Onychomycoses occur throughout the world but there are regional differences in incidence. Precise data as to their incidence are not available. Onychomycoses have increased enormously in the last 80 years, both absolutely and relatively. Sociocultural and occupational factors play an important part. In rural areas in Zaire, the incidence was found to be 0.89%, whereas in city dwellers it was 4% in men and 2.8% in women (Vanbreuseghem, 1977). Other authors have found an incidence of 2–13% (Seebacher, 1966; Walshe & English, 1966). Fungal infections of the nails have been reported in 6.5–27% of miners (Goetz, 1965; Tappeiner & Male, 1966). Some 1.5% of all patients attending dermatological centres have onychomycosis (Achten & Wanet-Rouard, 1981). Between 18% and 40% of all nail disorders are onychomycoses (Pardo-Castello & Pardo, 1960; Achten & Wanet-Rouard, 1978) and 30% of all dermatomycoses are nail infections (Langer, 1957).

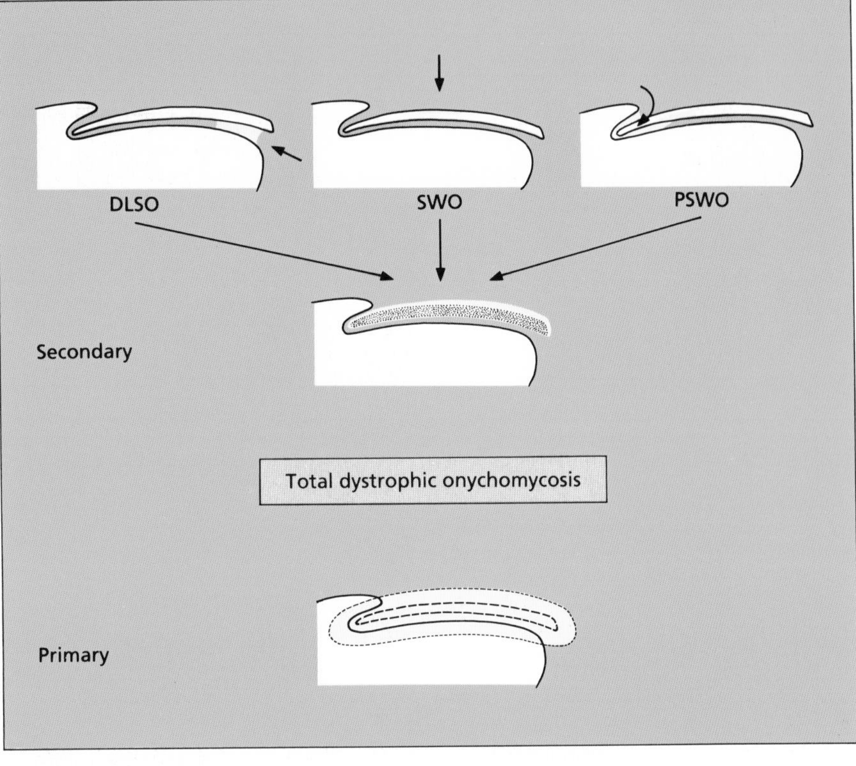

Fig. 4.1. Diagram to show site of invasion and types of onychomycosis. DLSO, distal and lateral subungual onychomycosis; SWO, superficial white onychomycosis; PSWO, proximal subungual white onychomycosis.

Onychomycosis

Fungal infections of the nail apparatus may be classified as superficial, distal or proximal according to the site of fungal invasion (Fig. 4.1). In this chapter, Zaias' classification (1972) has been expanded to include mycoses involving the whole nail apparatus. The appearance of the lesion may provide clues to the likely identity of the infecting organism, although it is seldom possible to identify the species on clinical grounds alone: for instance, irrespective of right or left handedness, involvement of one hand and both feet is a diagnostic feature of dermatophytosis caused by *Trichophyton rubrum*; in 90% of the cases, the rest being due to *Trichophyton mentagrophytes* (var. *interdigitale*) (Feldmann *et al.*, 1992) (Fig. 4.2(a) & (b)). Similarly onychomycosis confined to fingernails is more suggestive of a *Candida* infection, especially in paronychia and onycholysis, although infections caused by either *Hendersonula toruloidea* or *Scytalidium hyalinum* may both produce identical nail lesions. These observations contribute to the process of making the diagnosis but this will depend ultimately on the laboratory identification of the fungus. Invasive onychomycosis can also be proved convincingly by histology. A search for infections at other sites such as the hands, feet or groins, or the scalp in infants, should be instituted when there is a suspicion of onychomycosis. Dyschromic nail changes caused by fungi are considered in the section on chromonychia (Chapter 2).

Distal and lateral subungual onychomycosis (DLSO) (Figs 4.3–4.10)

Primary DLSO

In this pattern of infection the onychodermal band is disrupted by infection and the fungus reaches the underside of the nail via the hyponychium, the nail bed, or the lateral nail fold where the stratum corneum is invaded. The thickened horny layer raises the free edge of the nail plate with disruption of the normal nail plate–nail bed attachment. The disease spreads proximally and the nail becomes opaque. Fungal invasion leads to orthokeratosis of the nail bed epithelium. In advanced nail disease a more severe inflammatory reaction affects the nail bed with penetration of mononuclear cells and polymorphonuclear leucocytes into the subungual keratin, often mimicking Munro's microabscesses. Parakeratotic foci, often containing inspissated serum, may appear (Haneke, 1991). In time, tunnels produced by dermatophytes and containing air, described by Alkiewicz (1948) as a transverse net, appear as opaque streaks in the nail plate. Occasionally, this may be seen more clearly with the aid of a lens, after the nail plate has been treated with cedar oil to render it translucent. Where the network is sufficiently dense, it appears as an opaque white zone or streak, a clinical feature often seen in dermatophyte or mould infections. Often there is nail invasion in a longitudinal narrow band which follows the ridges of the nail bed. *Trichophyton*

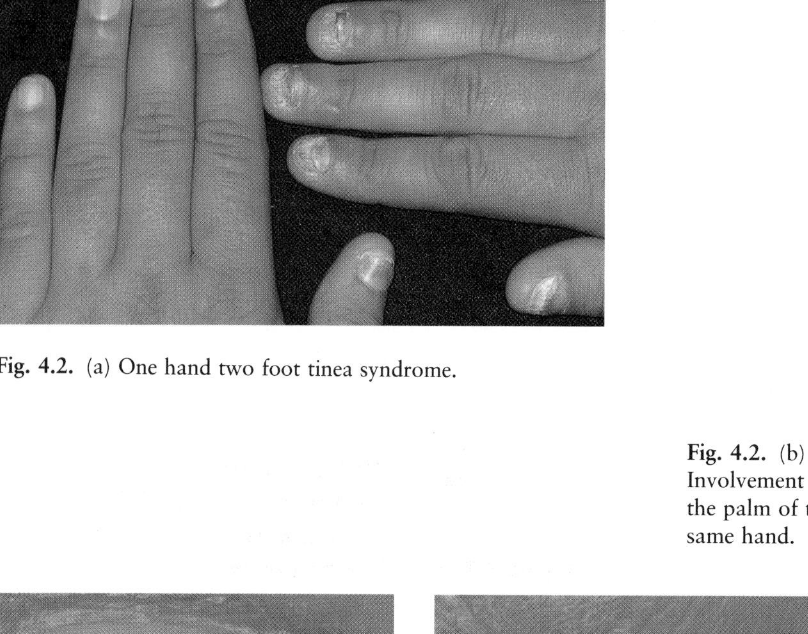

Fig. 4.2. (a) One hand two foot tinea syndrome.

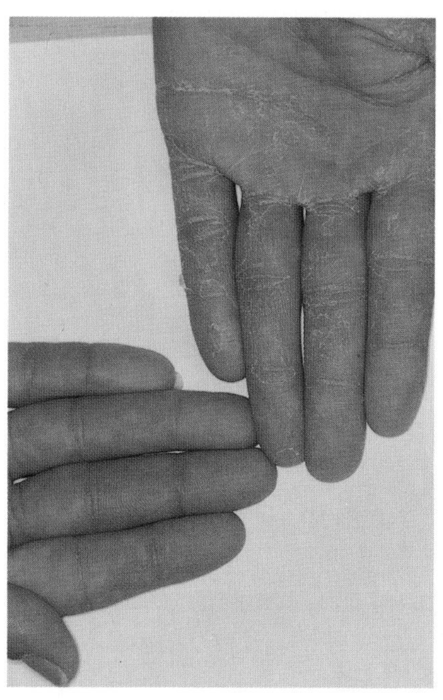

Fig. 4.2. (b) Involvement of the palm of the same hand.

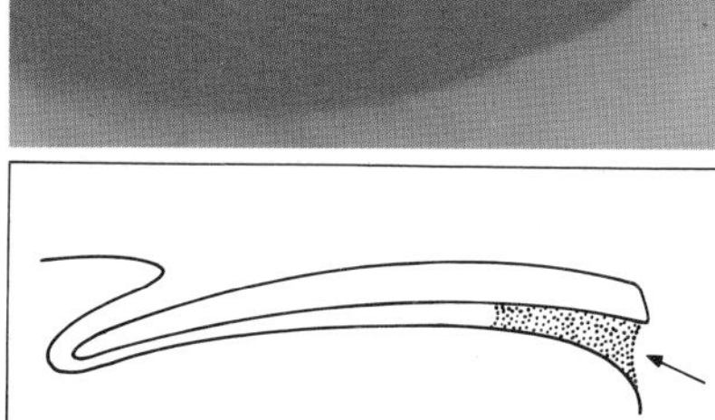

Fig. 4.3.

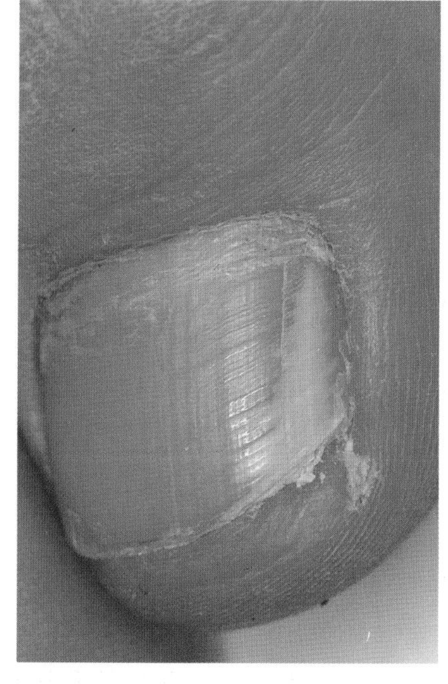

Fig. 4.4.

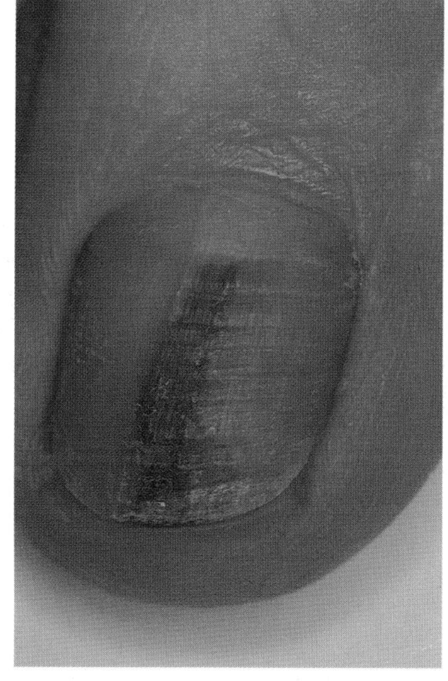

Fig. 4.5. DLSO due to *T. rubrum* presenting with longitudinal melanonychia.

Figs 4.2–4.10. Distal and lateral subungual onychomycosis – various degrees of invasion.

rubrum is the most common fungal organism. This usually invades the nail plate secondary to infection of the surrounding skin, chiefly either the sole or palm. Only in infants or young children is isolated nail disease without accompanying infection of the skin sometimes seen.

According to Zaias (1972), a variety of microorganisms may coexist in the ecological niche created by an area of onycholysis and these are responsible for colour changes

Fig. 4.6. Onycholysis due to *T. rubrum*.

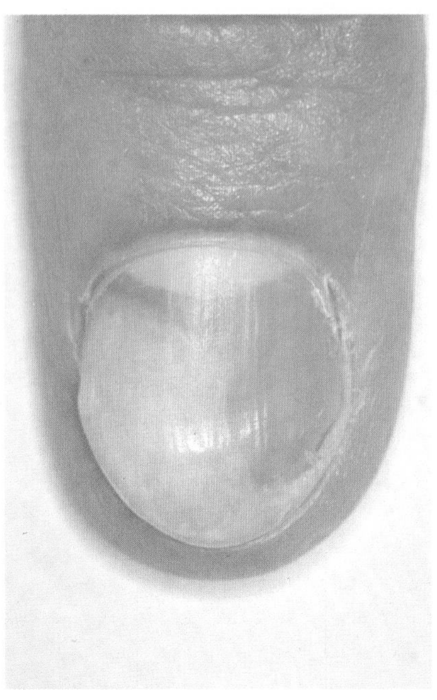
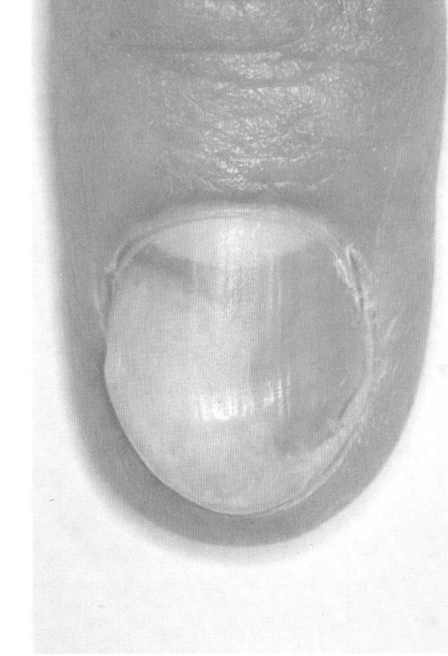

Fig. 4.7. Onycholysis due to *T. rubrum*.

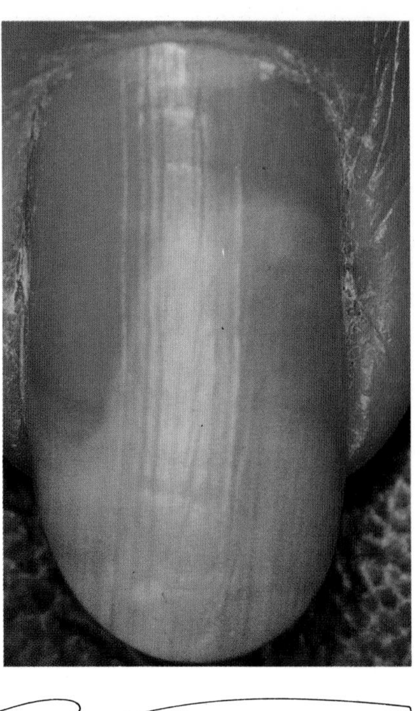
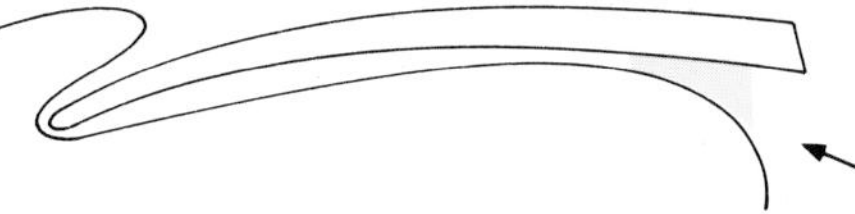

Fig. 4.8. Onycholysis due to *C. albicans*.

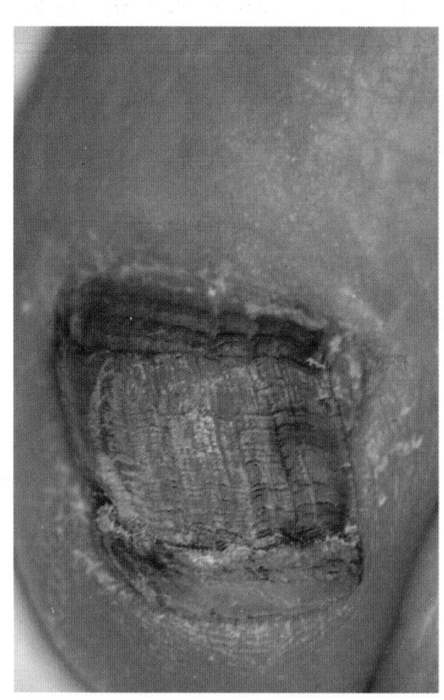

Fig. 4.9. DLSO due to *Hendersonula toluloidea* in a caucasian patient (courtesy of D. Jones, UK).

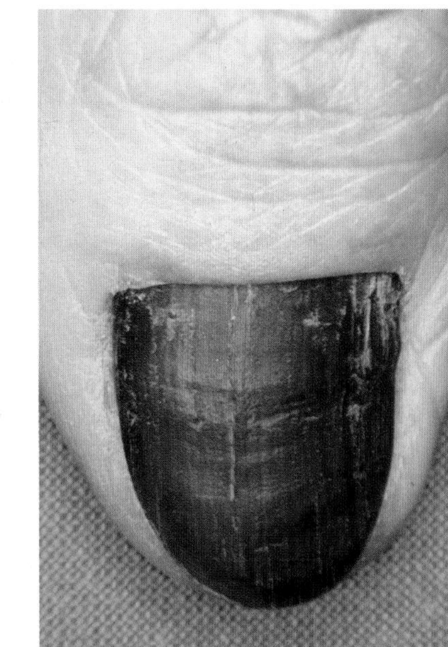

Fig. 4.10. Black nail due to *C. albicans* (courtesy of D. Binet, Paris, France).

Figs 4.2–4.10. (*continued*) Distal and lateral subungual onychomycosis – various degrees of invasion.

which vary from grey to chestnut brown. With progressive infection, the nail becomes friable and eroded at the lateral and distal borders.

The clinical appearances of nail dystrophies caused by different fungi are seldom diagnostic, but there may be some useful and potentially distinctive features apart from the differences in the overall pattern of nail involvement discussed previously. For example hyperkeratosis accompanying onycholysis is a common feature of dermatophyte infections which are the commonest causes of DLSO, whereas in *Candida* onychomycosis, gross hyperkeratosis is mainly seen as total nail plate involvement in patients with chronic mucocutaneous candidosis; in other cases of true *Candida* onychomycosis thickening of the nail plate may be minimal. There has been some debate about the role of *Candida* as a cause of DLSO. Except for *Candida albicans* which contains an acid peptidase capable of digesting keratin, *Candida* species are said not to have keratinases, therefore they cannot invade the healthy nail plate. There does appear to be a group of patients in whom there is genuine distal and lateral invasion of the nail plate with erosion, confirmed histologically, but without significant thickening. This is mainly seen in women, patients with endogenous or exogenous Cushing's syndrome or those with Raynaud's phenomenon (Hay *et al.*, 1988c). It may also occur in some tropical countries. While it is possible that some invasion is secondary to pre-existing onycholysis (see below), this is seldom possible to establish. There is often a distinctive brown or cinnamon coloured discoloration of nails, mainly toenails, affected by *Scopulariopsis brevicaulis*; it is caused by the presence of large numbers of pigmented conidia produced *in situ* (Belsan & Fragner, 1965). Likewise brown pigmentation appearing as an irregular streak in the nail plate, often at the lateral border of the great toenail, is also a feature of infections caused by *Trichophyton interdigitale* and *T. rubrum*, which may sometimes present with longitudinal melanonychia (Perrin & Baran, 1993). In this case the cause of the pigmentation is unknown. Infections of the fingernails due to dermatophytes which cause endothrix scalp infections may present with less nail plate thickening, but the plate is pitted and the distal margin covered with lamellar splits (Kalter & Hay, 1988). The nail dystrophies caused by *Hendersonula toruloidea (Scytalidium dimidiatum)* (Fig. 4.9) or *Scytalidium hyalinum* are similar to dermatophyte onychomycosis (Moore, 1978; Gugnani *et al.*, 1986). However, secondary paronychia appears to be commoner in fingernail infections and extensive onycholysis may also be a prominent feature of these infections. This may lead to a transverse fracture of the nail plate near the proximal nail fold and subsequent shedding of the distal plate.

DLSO secondary to onycholysis

On occasions dermatophytes may be isolated from nails, such as the big toenail, which show idiopathic or primary onycholysis. Davies (1968) reported on 3955 samples of nails infected with *Trichophyton rubrum*. Of those positive for fungi on direct microscopy, culture or both, 9% were from normal, healthy looking nails. This was confirmed by Baran and Badillet (1982) who examined 46 samples of normal nails from patients infected in other sites with *T. rubrum* (35 cases), *T. interdigitale* (10 cases, one patient having a mixed infection), and *Epidermophyton floccosum* (one case). *T. rubrum* was found in the nails of four of these patients, *T. interdigitale* in two and *E. floccosum* in one. A subsequent control study was carried out on 52 out-patients seeking medical advice for reasons other than big toenail dystrophy. Dermatophytes were isolated from clinically normal, big toenails in two patients, *T. rubrum* in one case and *E. floccosum* in the other. In these apparently healthy nails, the fungi were presumably acting as commensals rather than pathogens. However they are potentially invasive, particularly in nails showing onycholysis, and may be transmitted to a different host. On the fingers, primary onycholysis is more frequently associated with secondary invasion by *Candida* and/or *Pseudomonas*. It is most common in women in whom there is repeated contact with water, soap and detergents. Contrary to the classical pattern of DLSO, which usually starts with distal hyperkeratosis, there is a reversal of the usual order of evolution of each lesion in secondary onychomycosis. For example, in the fingernails onycholysis precedes any subsequent thickening of the distal subungual area, hence the name of DLSO associated with onycholysis. Repeated episodes of friction secondary to rubbing of the nails against shoes or the repeated episodic trauma incurred during running or jogging may also create an area of traumatic onycholysis where microorganisms are also potentially but not invariably pathogenic. A variety of fungi not normally considered pathogenic may be isolated from dystrophic nails, particularly in the elderly (English & Atkinson, 1974). The usual clinical pattern of nail involvement most closely resembles distal and lateral subungual onychomycosis. Hyperkeratosis and brown or green discoloration are common and the toenails are most commonly affected. The organisms isolated may include *Aspergillus* species such as *A. terreus* or *A. versicolor*, *Acremonium* spp., *Penicillium* spp. and *Pyrenochaeta unguium hominis* (Punithalingham & English, 1975). As these organisms do not appear to be able to break down keratin, it is assumed that they are colonists of dystrophic or abnormal nails. It is however difficult to be certain that they are not contributing to the nail dystrophy. There is some evidence that some of these species (e.g. *Acremonium* spp.) produce perforating organs, specialized hyphal structures usually associated with hair invasion, analogous to those seen in dermatophytosis. Other non-dermatophyte fungi invading nails, such as *S. brevicaulis*, can be demonstrated by electron microscopy inside keratinized cells (Achten *et al.*, 1979).

A variety of yeasts may also be isolated from the same site. These include *Candida* species such as *C. guilliermondii*. As with the moulds discussed above, it is assumed that they are secondary invaders. The distinction between nail pathogens and opportunistic organisms which inhabit nails under abnormal conditions is a tenuous one. As has been seen above, even the dermatophytes can be secondary invaders. Likewise, *S. brevicaulis* is often merely a colonist.

The clinical significance of nail invasion or colonization

by fungi, which are not normally pathogenic, needs to be carefully considered in the light of laboratory findings such as the results of nail biopsy. It is likely that organisms which colonize nails may play a more destructive role if the host's immune defences or the nail matrix is altered by disease or another infection.

Superficial white onychomycosis (SWO)

(Figs 4.11–4.13)

SWO is fairly rare and is normally confined to the toenails. Here the surface of the nail plate is the initial site of invasion. The causative organisms produce a clinical picture of small superficial white patches with distinct edges (Zaias, 1966). These later coalesce and may gradually cover the whole nail, hence the term leuconychia trichophytica (mycotica) (Jessner, 1922). The chalky white surface becomes roughened and the texture softer than normal. The appearance has been likened to 'paper-bark' (McAleer, 1981): the affected nail plate crumbles easily and old lesions acquire a yellowish colour. The upper surface of the nail plate is the primary site of fungal invasion. This type of nail invasion is caused by *T. interdigitale mentagrophytes* in more than 90% of the cases. Using epi-illumination microscopy the individual white flakes representing colonies of *T. interdigitale* can be observed clearly. Patches of SWO are not uncommonly seen in areas where the nail is occluded, for instance by an overlying adjacent toe. Infections caused by non-dermatophytes such as *Aspergillus terreus, Fusarium oxysporum* or *Acremonium* spp. are more often seen in patients in tropical or subtropical environments. *Candida albicans* has occasionally been isolated in infants. In human immunodeficiency virus (HIV) infected patients SWO is not rare in finger or toenails and is due to *Trichophyton rubrum*.

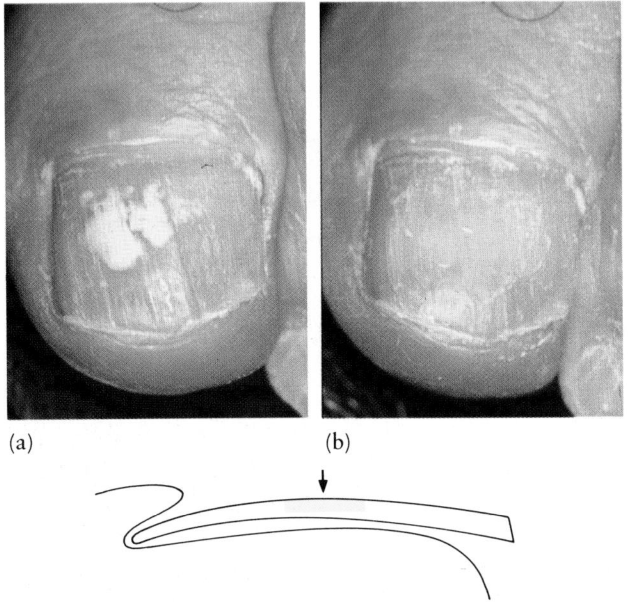

Fig. 4.11. SWO, (a) before scraping, (b) after superficial scraping.

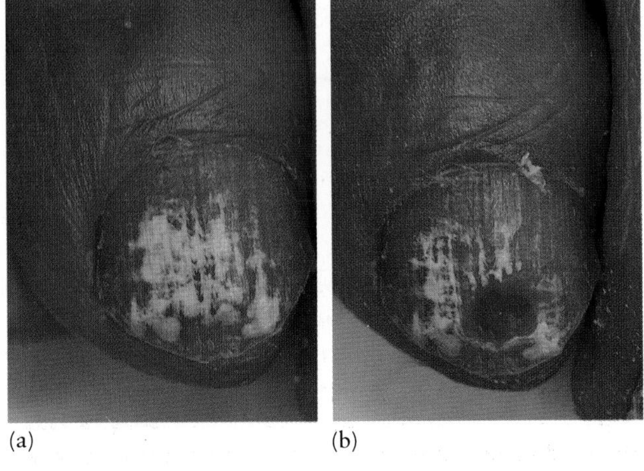

Fig. 4.12. (a) Before scraping, (b) after scraping.

Superficial black onychomycosis (SBO)

Exceptionally *Scytalium dimidiatum* may be responsible for SBO (Badillet, 1988; Miesel & Quadripur, 1992).

Proximal subungual onychomycosis (PSO)

Proximal white subungual onychomycosis (PWSO)

(Figs 4.14–4.18)

PWSO is rare and affects both finger and toenails. The clinical pattern of nail invasion is very rare. The causative organisms penetrate via the cuticle and the ventral aspect of the proximal nail fold, the stratum corneum being the primary site of the fungal invasion. When it reaches the

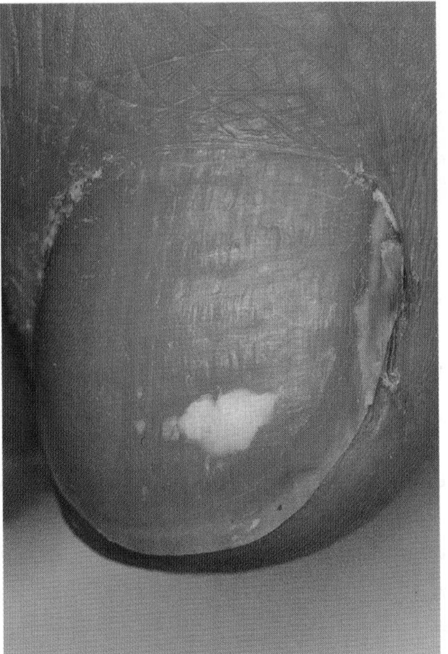

Fig. 4.13. Associated with DLSO.

Fig. 4.11–4.13. Superficial white onychomycosis.

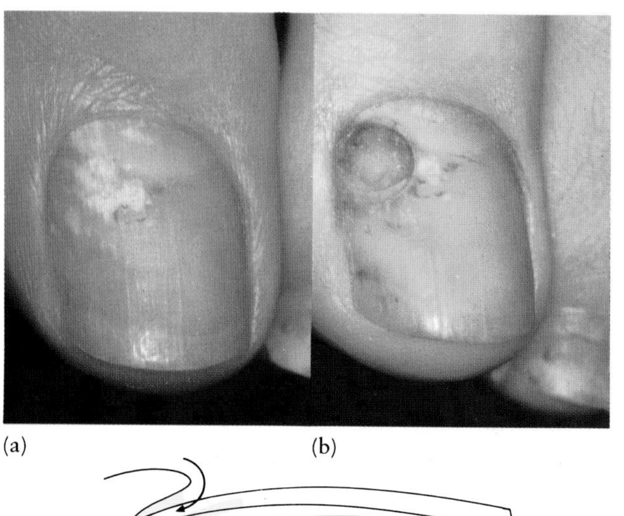

(a) (b)

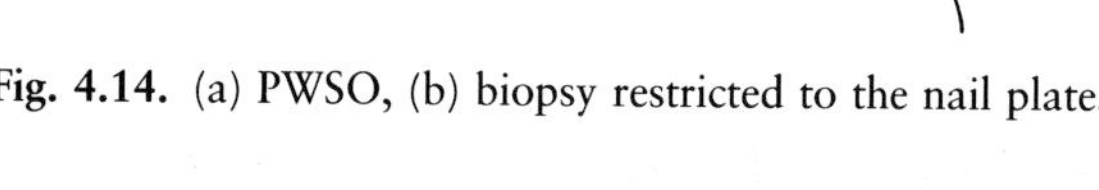

Fig. 4.14. (a) PWSO, (b) biopsy restricted to the nail plate.

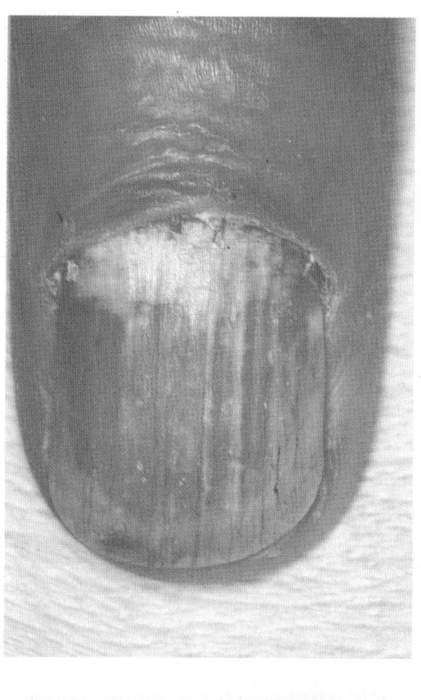

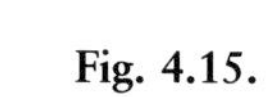

Fig. 4.15.

Fig. 4.16.

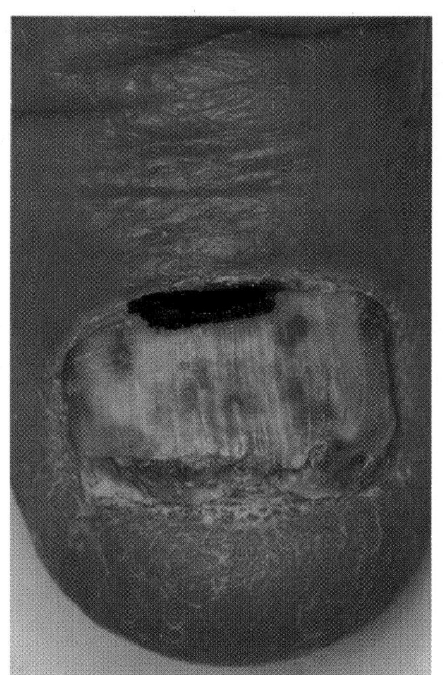

Fig. 4.17.

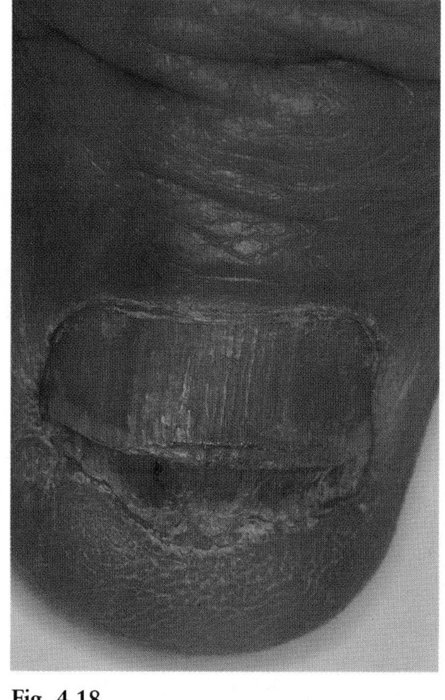

Fig. 4.18.

Fig. 4.14–4.18. Proximal white subungual onychomycosis (Figs 4.16–4.18 – treated by itraconazole).

matrix the fungus invades the dorsum of the nail plate. A white spot appears from beneath the proximal nail fold and, although it is confined initially to the lunula area, when the white spot moves distally, it still remains in the same layer of the nail plate. The fungus has to invade more distal parts of the matrix to get entrapped in the deeper layers of the nail plate. This is sometimes accompanied by slight discomfort. This pattern may also be seen where there is a recurrence of nail infection in an incompletely treated nail.

This type of nail invasion is usually caused by *T. rubrum,* but *T. megnini, T. schoenleinii* or *E. floccosum* may be seen.

Recently a rapidly developing form of PWSO has been recorded in patients with acquired immune deficiency syndrome (AIDS). Here the infection may spread rapidly under the nail from the proximal margin to all the finger and toenails (Dompmartin *et al.*, 1990). Histopathology shows that the entire nail plate is infiltrated with fungi, which are lying in a longitudinal parallel arrangement.

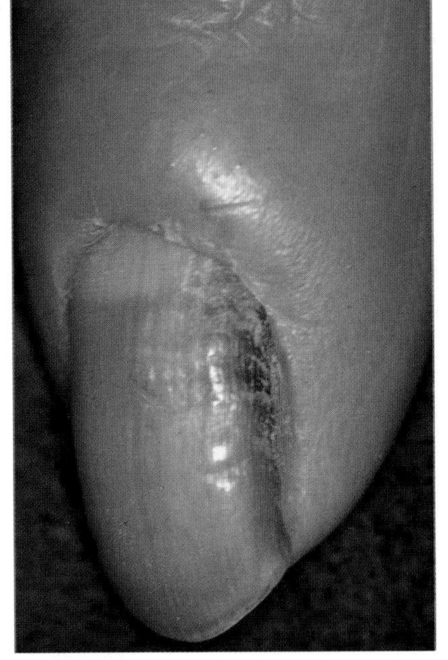

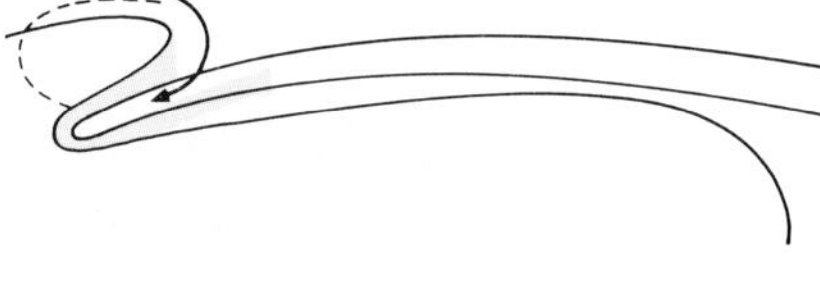

Fig. 4.19. Proximal subungual onychomycosis secondary to chronic paronychia.

However, the picture is complicated in that other surfaces such as the superior aspect of the plate and the distal or lateral margins may also be involved. Possibly because of the rapid spread these patients do not show much nail thickening (Weismann *et al.*, 1988).

PSO secondary to paronychia (Fig. 4.19) (see p. 112)

Paronychia is observed mainly in adults; women are affected three times more frequently than men. More than 75% of the cases occur on the hands, particularly on the index and/or middle fingers of the right hand in right-handed people. Frequent hand work with carbohydrate-containing foods, moisture, maceration, hyperhydration, occlusion, hyperhidrosis, acrocyanosis, diabetes mellitus, and other hormonal disturbances, medical treatment with corticosteroids, cytostatic drugs, and antibiotics promote *Candida* paronychia.

Trauma to the cuticle allows the yeasts to penetrate and to grow further. The nail fold, usually the lateral portion of the proximal nail fold or the junction between the proximal and lateral nail folds, becomes erythematous and swollen; consequently, the nail plate becomes detached from the eponychium. The thickened proximal free end of the nail fold becomes rounded and loses the ability to form a cuticle. This renders the proximal nail fold even more vulnerable and subject to inoculation with foreign material such as yeasts, bacteria and food debris. The disease tends to run a protracted course interrupted by subacute exacerbations. The nail fold inflammation will also affect the lateral portion of the matrix, eventually leading to nail plate deformity such as hyperconvexity, irregular transverse grooves and ridges, a rough surface, and some pits.

Proximal onychomycosis may develop secondary to *Candida* paronychia. The nail plate invasion is normally confined to a dark narrow strip down one or both lateral borders of the nail. In grossly infected fingers the whole nail plate may become involved. It is possible that invasion of the nails by *S. dimidiatum* or *S. hyalinum* as well as *Fusarium* infection may follow a similar pattern in some individuals.

Total dystrophic onychomycosis (TDO)

(Figs 4.20–4.26)

This represents the most advanced form of all the three types described above, especially DLSO. The nail crumbles and disappears leaving a thickened and abnormal nail bed which usually retains fragments of nail plate. All 20 nails may be involved in chronic generalized dermatophytosis (Hadida *et al.*, 1966; Boudghene-Stambouli & Merad-Boudia, 1991). Primary TDO is observed in patients suffering from chronic mucocutaneous candidiasis (CMC) or immunodeficiency states. Despite the fact that the initial site of *Candida* invasion is usually distal (DLSO), it spreads rapidly to involve all four nail structures (hyponychium, nail bed, matrix and proximal nail fold). This can be confirmed by histopathology. The whole nail plate is involved, and is thickened, opaque and yellow-brown in colour. The marked dermal inflammatory reaction with thickening of the soft tissues results in a swollen distal phalanx which is bulbous rather than clubbed. However, clubbing is also possible and may follow pulmonary disease such as bronchiectasis secondary to CMC. Hyperkeratosis secondary to *Candida* invasion may develop in

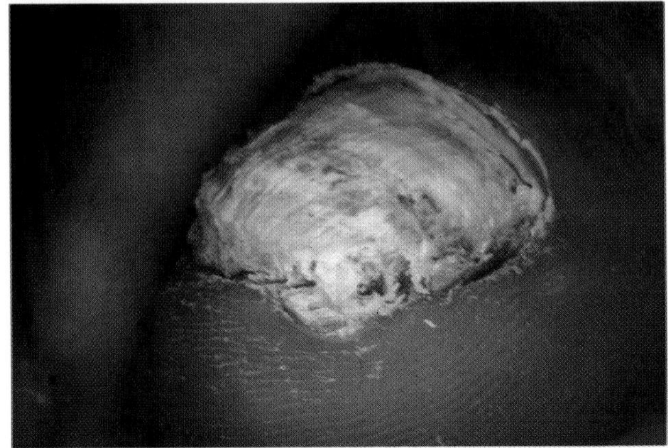

Fig. 4.20. Total dystrophic onychomycosis due to *Scopulariopsosis brevicaulis*.

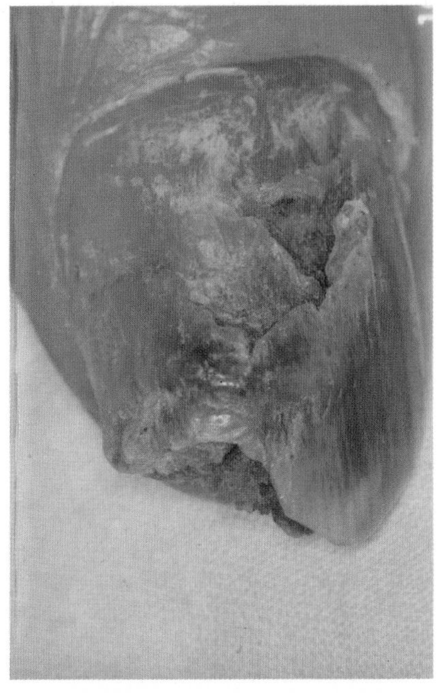

Fig. 4.21. Total dystrophic onychomycosis due to *T. rubrum*.

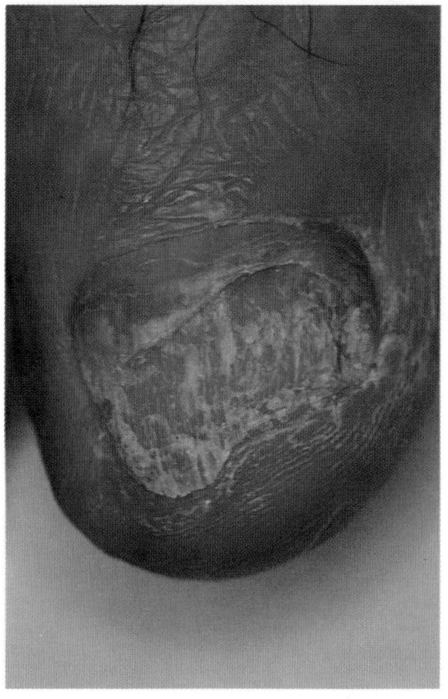

Fig. 4.22. Total dystrophic onychomycosis due to *T. rubrum*.

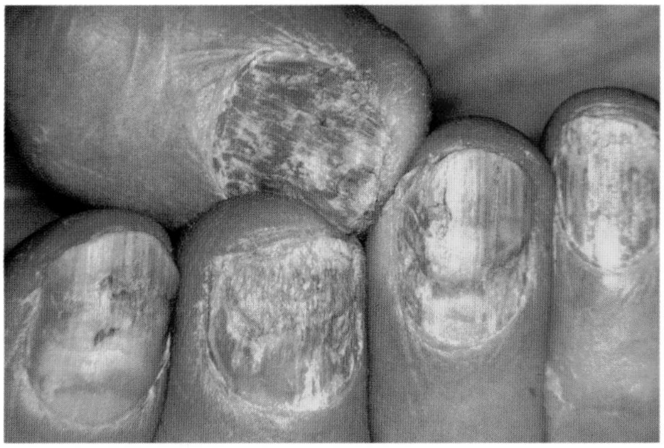

Fig. 4.23. Isolated candida dystrophy

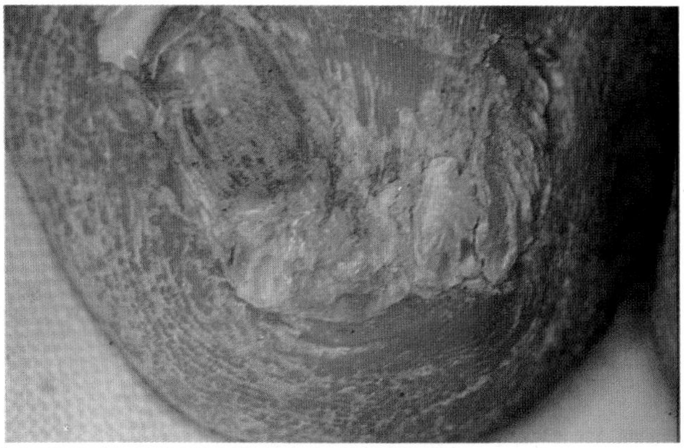

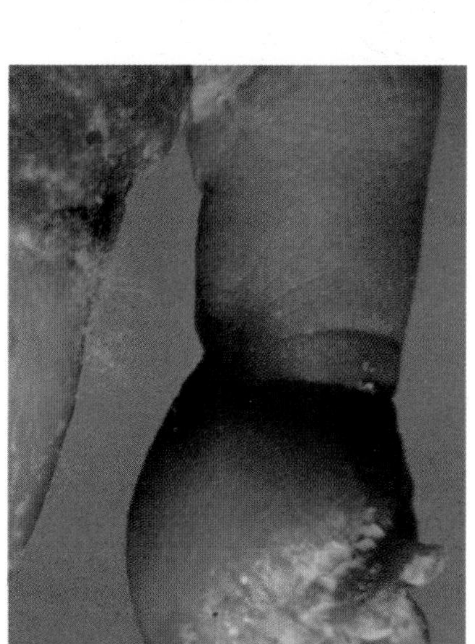

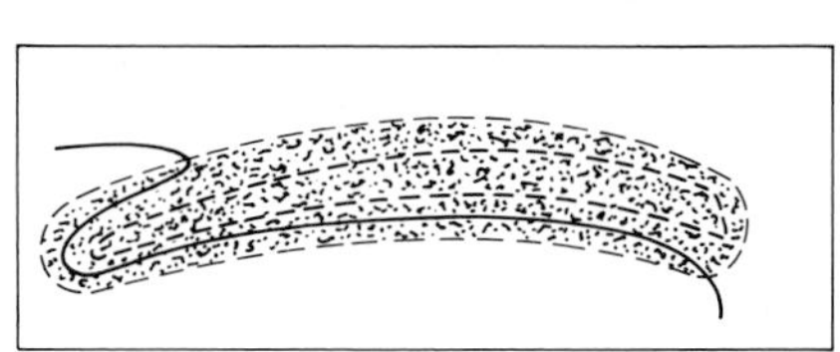

Fig. 4.25. Chronic mucocutaneous candidiasis, primary total dystrophic onychomycosis.

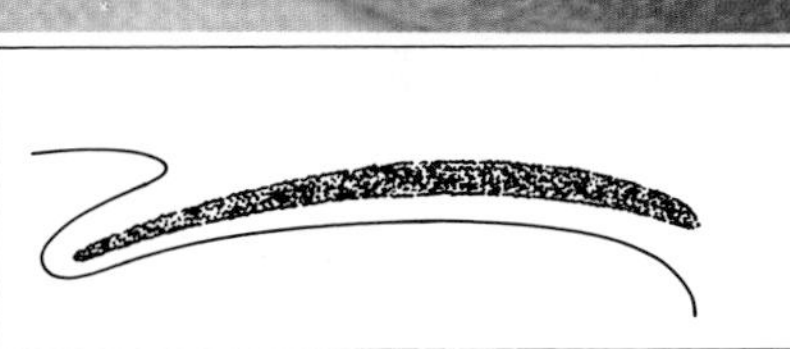

Fig. 4.24. *T. rubrum*, secondary total dystrophic onychomycosis.

Fig. 4.20–4.26. Total dystrophic onychomycosis (TDO).

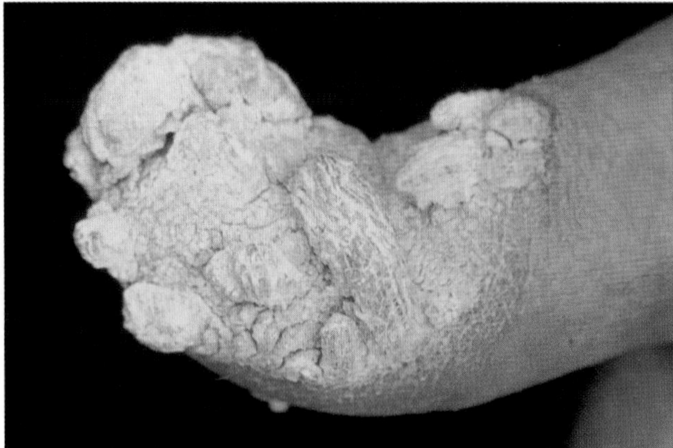

Fig. 4.26. Chronic mucocutaneous candidiasis (primary TDO).

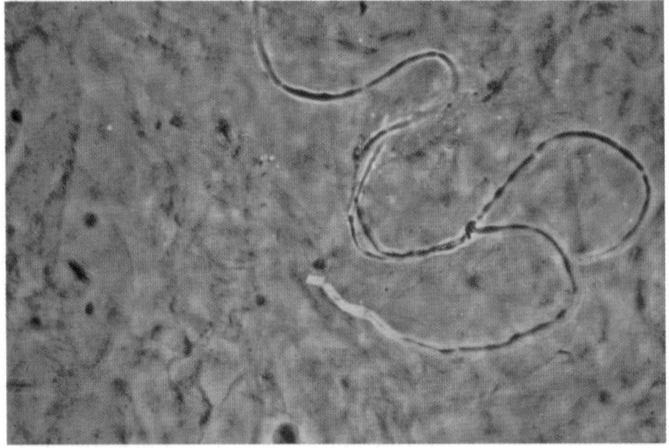

Fig. 4.27. Subungual nail scrapings mounted in KOH solution – mycelial strands are easily visible (*Hendersonula toruloidea*).

skin adjacent to the nail in these patients. Secondary infection with *T. rubrum* or *T. interdigitale* may occur (Haneke, 1988).

A new form of total nail dystrophy where the nail plate is only marginally thickened occurs in patients with AIDS and has been mentioned above (Weismann *et al.*, 1988). The characteristic features of this process are rapid spread over weeks to produce complete total whitening of the nail. Sometimes this infection appears to have spread from the posterior nail fold (PSO), but this has not been established in all cases. In addition the superficial aspect of the nail plate may also be involved. The name acute TDO might be appropriate.

Laboratory investigation

Direct microscopy

Small pieces taken from clinically infected areas of nail and particularly with subungual hyperkeratosis are treated with 10–30% potassium hydroxide. To hasten clearing of the nail the slide may be warmed over a Bunsen flame. The softened nail is flattened with gentle pressure applied to a cover slip. Zaias and Taplin (1966) recommended a formulation of potassium hydroxide and dimethylsulphoxide. Sixty millilitres of a 20% KOH solution is mixed with 40 ml pure DMSO. This technique is useful for preservation of specimens, but globular artefacts may sometimes be seen and these must be distinguished from yeasts. A further technique, useful in non-dermatophyte infections, is the use of an equivolume mixture of Parker Quink ink and potassium hydroxide (Milne, 1989). Spores of non-dermatophyte fungi and some mycelial elements are highlighted using this technique. Calcofluor white, a fluorescent whitening agent mixed with an equal volume of KOH, may also be used to highlight, non-specifically, the fungal elements in nail (Milne, 1989). Fluorescent whiteners specifically bind to structural carbohydrates of plants, e.g. chitin and lignin, but not to keratin and other animal proteins; the physicochemical process is called substrate binding.

The nail is examined for fungal hyphae or arthrospores. In *Candida* infections yeast forms are also present. In certain non-dermatophyte infections conidia may be formed *in situ*. This is characteristic of *Scopulariopsis* infections although it may also occur in onychomycosis caused by *Aspergillus* species. The hyphae of *S. dimidiatum* and *S. hyalinum* are very similar in appearance to those of dermatophytes although they may appear thinner, irregular and more sinuous. This is seen best with phase contrast illumination (Fig. 4.27).

Culture (Figs 4.28 & 4.29)

Scrapings from subungual keratosis and nails should be planted into Sabouraud's agar and incubated at 26°C. The different organisms can be recognized using morphological and/or biochemical criteria. The presence of chloramphenicol or streptomycin and penicillin in the medium prevents the growth of contaminant bacteria. Wherever possible nails should be plated on medium both with and without cycloheximide (actidione) as this inhibits non-dermatophyte moulds which may overgrow the slower growing dermatophytes.

It is sometimes difficult to isolate fungi, even from nails which are positive on direct microscopy. The problem is compounded if the patient has already received topical or systemic treatment and if the hyphae in the most accessible part of the nail plate are not viable (Gentles, 1971). In order to improve the isolation rate various methods have been devised. These include the use of a grinder (Zaias *et al.*, 1969; Daniel, 1985) or a dental drill fitted with a suction nozzle, which collects the nail dust for microscopy and culture (English & Atkinson, 1973). This latter instrument has raised the success rate of culture from microscopically positive nails from the usual 50–75%

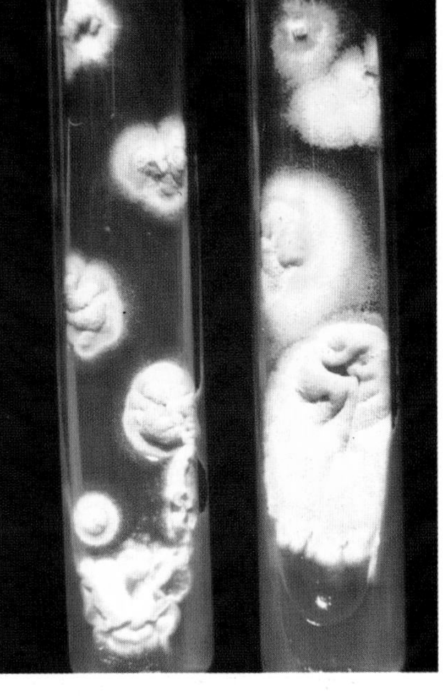

Fig. 4.28. Fungal culture (*Scopulariopsis brevicaulis*).

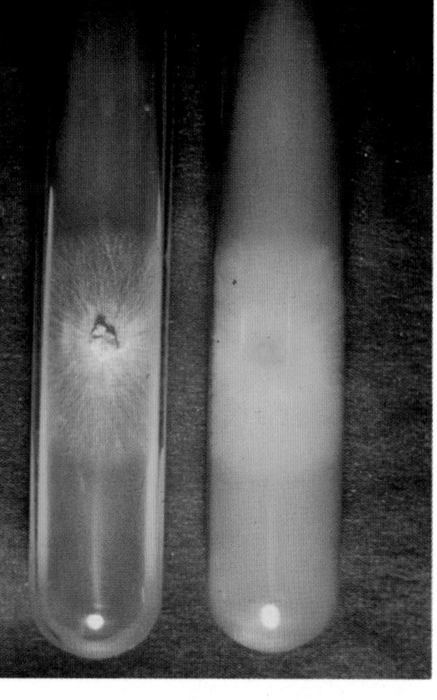

Fig. 4.29. Fungal culture (*Epidermophyton floccosum*).

rate to about 88%, but is not a practical procedure for the routine laboratory.

S. brevicaulis forms filaments as well as spores of characteristic size and morphology in nail. According to Ornsberg (1980), the demonstration of *S. brevicaulis* on direct microscopy and the presence of more than 10 colonies in culture is diagnostic of infections caused by this organism. If there are less than three colonies, and *S. brevicaulis* is not seen on direct microscopy, the organism is probably present as a commensal. *S. brevicaulis* is often found in toenails infected by dermatophytes, particularly *T. rubrum* or *T. interdigitale*. The dermatophyte responsible for the primary infection may eventually be isolated after repeated scrapings have been taken. *Aspergillus* spp. may also form conidia in nails *in vivo*.

English (1976) suggested that the following criteria are helpful in determining whether a fungus is merely a commensal or whether it is truly responsible for nail dystrophy.

1 If a dermatophyte is isolated, it is considered to be the likely pathogen.

2 If moulds or yeasts are isolated, they are thought to be significant only if mycelia, arthrospores or yeast cells are found on direct microscopic examination of the nail specimen.

3 Final confirmation of mould infection requires isolation of the mould on at least five out of 20 inocula, in addition to the absence of dermatophytes on either actidione-containing, or actidione-free media.

Most clinicians would find these criteria too stringent although they provide a useful guideline. They are also questionable since, in onycholysis of certain nails such as the big toenail, cultured dermatophytes may be present as commensals (Baran & Badillet, 1983). The clinical appearances of the nails, tortuous or 'atypical' hyphal elements in nail clippings and repeated isolations of a non-dermatophyte are all helpful clues to the possible involvement of an unusual organism. Likewise the presence of *Candida* species in material taken from under nails with onycholysis does not appear to be diagnostic of invasion of the nail plate, certainly if only yeast forms are seen on direct microscopy (Hay *et al.*, 1988a); the presence of *Candida* mycelium in nail material and the growth of *C. albicans* is more likely to imply a pathogenic role for these organisms in nail dystrophy.

Histological examination of the nail plate, with the underlying tissue, will not only demonstrate the fungal elements but also reveal the depth of their penetration into the nail plate. This may provide further evidence of the pathogenic role of fungi isolated in culture, particularly if they can be identified *in situ* on morphological grounds, or by immunofluorescent labelling using specific antisera.

Nail histopathology for demonstrating fungi

(Achten & Simonart, 1963, 1965; Achten & Wanet-Rouard, 1978; Achten *et al.*, 1979, Scher & Ackerman, 1980a; Haneke, 1985, 1991; Suarez *et al.*, 1991)

Histopathology reliably demonstrates whether a fungus is invasive or merely colonizing subungual debris (Figs 4.30–4.42).

According to the site of the pathology, nail clippings should be taken from the edge or the lateral part of the nail plate together with a shallow portion of subungual tissue (see Chapter 3). They are then embedded directly into paraffin without using a fixative. The specimens are

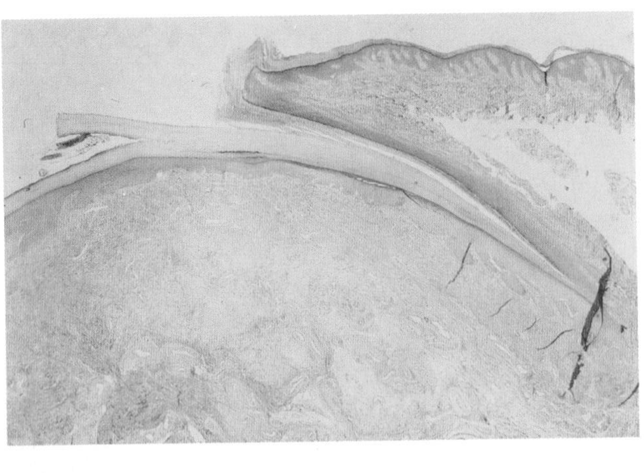

Fig. 4.30. Advanced DLSO (H&E stain, ×16).

Fig. 4.31. Advanced DLSO (H&E stain, ×100).

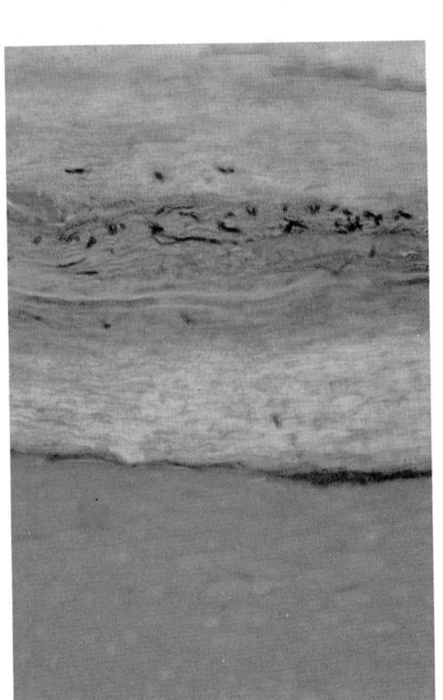

Fig. 4.32. Advanced DLSO (Grocott stain, ×250).

Figs 4.30–4.42. Nail histopathology for demonstrating fungi.

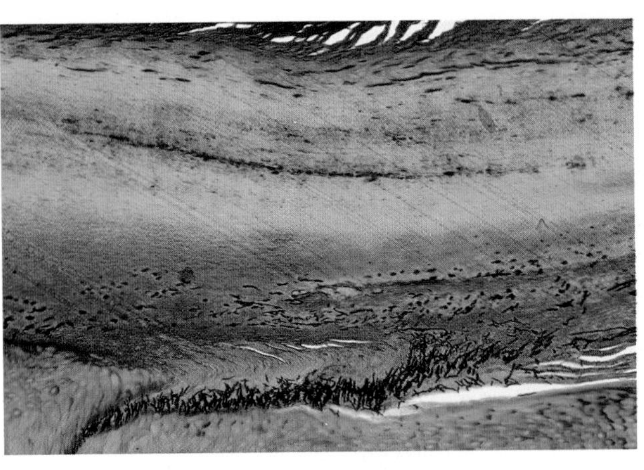

Fig. 4.33. DLSO (Grocott stain, ×100).

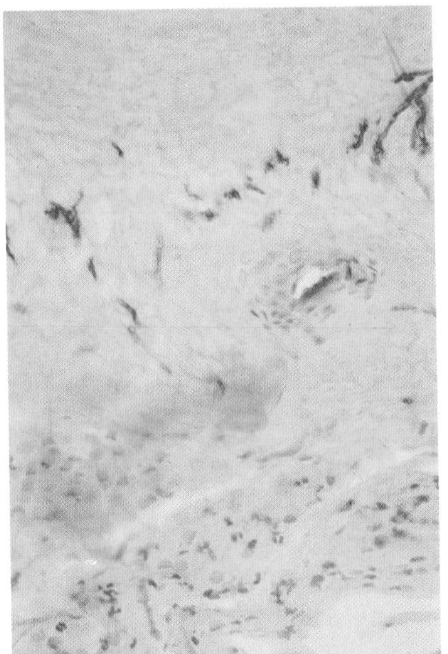

Fig. 4.34. DLSO (PAS stain, ×250).

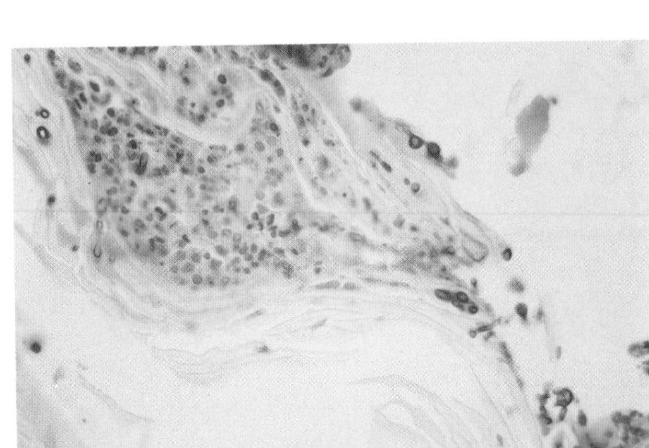

Fig. 4.35. DLSO (PAS stain, ×250).

Fig. 4.36. DLSO (PAS stain, ×250).

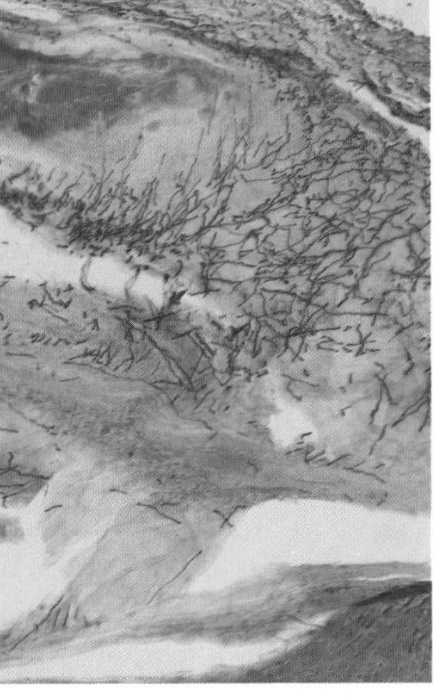

Fig. 4.37. TDO (PAS stain, ×100).

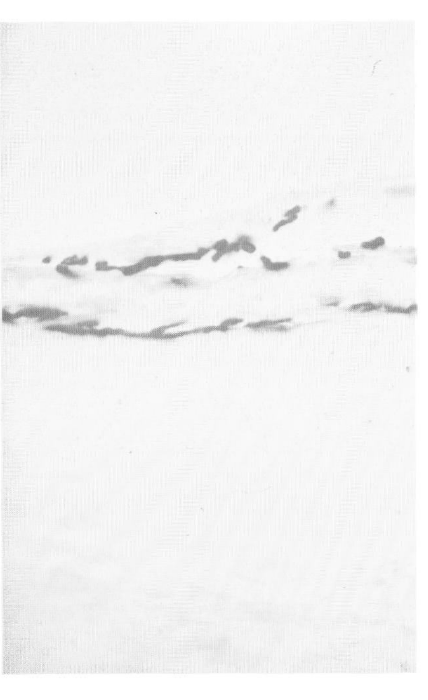

Fig. 4.38. SWO (PAS stain, ×100).

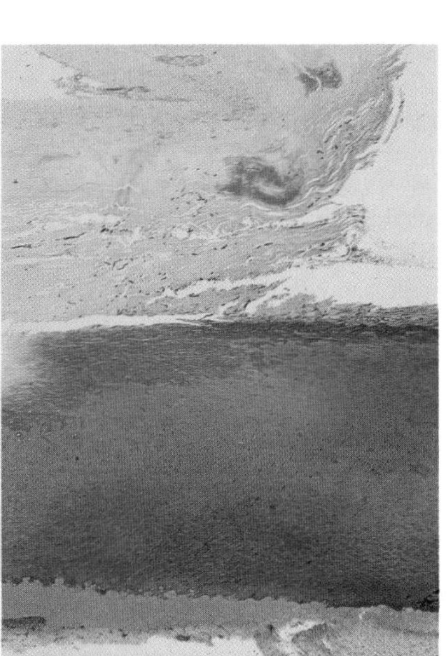
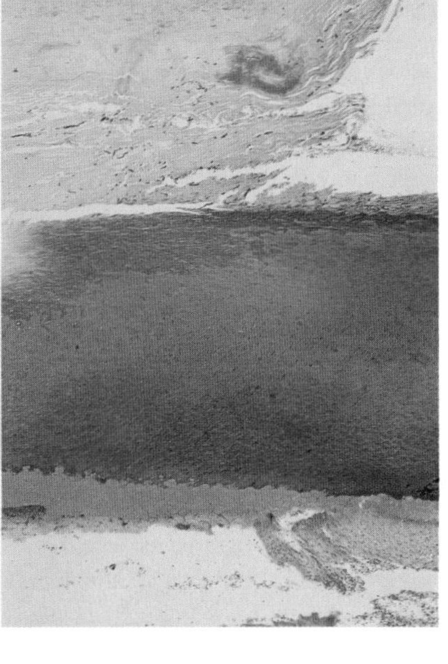

Fig. 4.39. Proximal subungual onychomycosis, showing fungal infection at the junction of the pale upper proximal nail fold (PNF) and the nail plate (red).

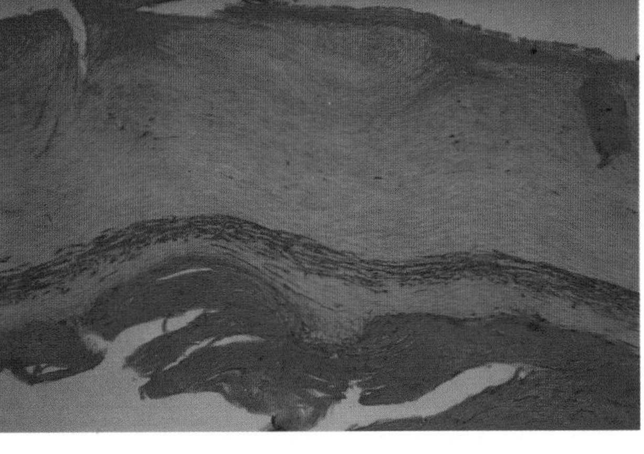

Fig. 4.40. PWSO.

stained with haematoxylin and eosin (H & E), periodic acid Schiff (PAS) and toluidine blue; calcofluor and Grocott's stain can also be used. The fungi can be seen in the subungual keratin and undersurface of the nail plate. Histopathological examination of nail clippings with subungual keratosis very often shows fungal elements even when cultures are repeatedly negative. However, some softening techniques may be applied beforehand to facilitate sectioning. Use of a keratin-softening solution containing mercuric chloride, chromic acid, acetic acid and 95% alcohol has been advocated as a means of enhancing the quality of the histological sections (Suarez *et al.*, 1991). PAS stain is usually sufficient to demonstrate fungi; however, small serum inclusions may be mistaken for fungi by the unexperienced since they are also PAS-positive (Haneke, 1985, 1988, 1991). Grocott stain and calcofluor are more selective (Haneke, 1985, 1991). The fungi are usually located in the subungual keratosis, but may have invaded the deepest parts of the nail plate. Histopathology shows whether the fungi are invasive or only contami-

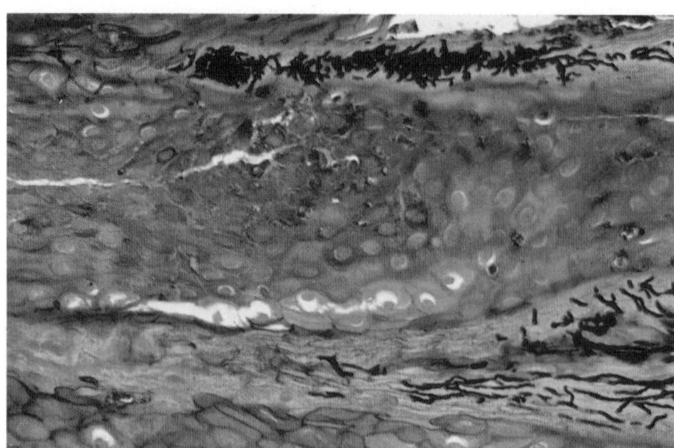

Fig. 4.41. TDO (Grocott stain, ×250).

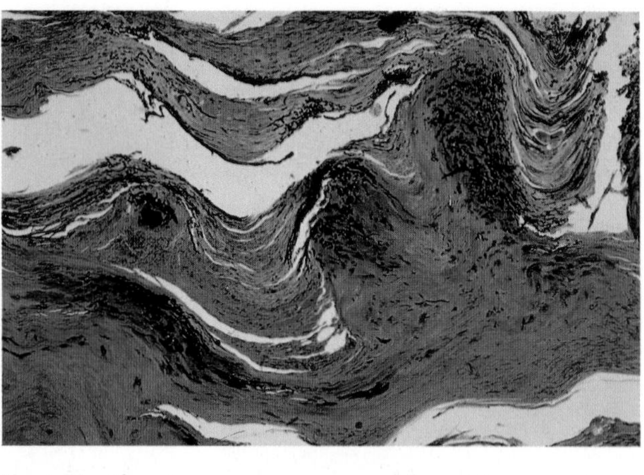

Fig. 4.42. Chronic mucocutaneous candidiasis (Grocott stain, ×100).

Table 4.1. Causes of DLSO

Dermatophytes	*Trichophyton rubrum, T. interdigitale, E. floccosum, T. schoenleinii, T. tonsurans, T. soudanense, T. erinacei, T. verrucosum, T. concentricum, T. violaceum, T. canis*
Yeasts	*Candida albicans, C. parapsilosis*
Moulds	*Scopulariopsis brevicaulis, Hendersonula toruloidea, Scytalidium hyalinum*

Table 4.2. Organisms found in DLSO with pre-existing onycholysis

Dermatophytes	*Trichophyton rubrum, T. interdigitale, E. floccosum*
Yeasts	*Candida albicans, C. parapsilosis, C. tropicalis*
Mould	Various species have been reported including *Aspergillus* and *Penicillium*
Bacterial invaders include *Pseudomonas* spp.	

Table 4.3. Causes of SWO

Dermatophytes	*Tricophyton interdigitale* (*M. persicolor, T. rubrum** and *T. equinum*)
Yeasts	*C. albicans* (only in infants; Zaias, 1980)
Moulds	*Acremonium* and *Fusarium* spp., *Aspergillus terreus*

* In this case fungal elements are found deep in the nail plate.

nants, e.g. spores in clefts of the subungual keratin. Fungi cannot be further indentified since both dermatophytes and moulds may produce hyphae and large, thick-walled arthrospores. Nail clippings often show abundant Munro-like abscesses in onychomycosis; since fungi may be sparse one cannot make the diagnosis of nail psoriasis from the presence of intracorneal abscesses in the absence of fungi alone. If the hyponychium is not affected, any non-

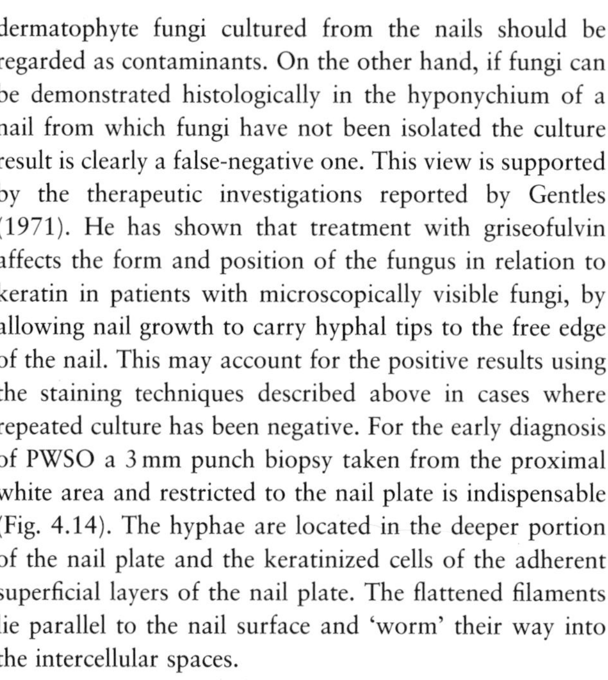

dermatophyte fungi cultured from the nails should be regarded as contaminants. On the other hand, if fungi can be demonstrated histologically in the hyponychium of a nail from which fungi have not been isolated the culture result is clearly a false-negative one. This view is supported by the therapeutic investigations reported by Gentles (1971). He has shown that treatment with griseofulvin affects the form and position of the fungus in relation to keratin in patients with microscopically visible fungi, by allowing nail growth to carry hyphal tips to the free edge of the nail. This may account for the positive results using the staining techniques described above in cases where repeated culture has been negative. For the early diagnosis of PWSO a 3 mm punch biopsy taken from the proximal white area and restricted to the nail plate is indispensable (Fig. 4.14). The hyphae are located in the deeper portion of the nail plate and the keratinized cells of the adherent superficial layers of the nail plate. The flattened filaments lie parallel to the nail surface and 'worm' their way into the intercellular spaces.

Another technique which can be used to highlight fungi in nail biopsy material is fluorescein-conjugated lectin stain (for instance concanavalin A) on nail biopsies softened with 10% KOH. Fungal elements are strongly stained with the lectin conjugate (Robles *et al.*, 1990).

Histopathology of nail biopsies has given considerable information concerning the pathogenesis of onychomycoses. It also allows one to subdivide the various clinical types of onychomycoses and provides convincing evidence of the different ways of infection and ports of entry.

Distal–lateral subungual onychomycosis develops from an infection of the hyponychium and almost invariably shows fungi in the hyperkeratosis of the distal nail bed. The fungi progress toward the matrix and induce mild inflammation. This causes an 'epidermization' of the nail bed with the formation of a pronounced granular layer and a thick, mainly orthokeratotic, horny layer. The latter is protected by the overlaying nail plate preventing its desquamation and keeping it moist and soft. This gives an ideal microenvironment for the fungi which are often present in very large amounts. The nail plate is invaded from its undersurface with the hyphae showing a parallel, often longitudinal arrangement. High power magnification frequently shows tunnels in the nail substance the diameters of which are considerably greater than those of the fungi; they are seen macroscopically as a transverse net (Alkiewicz, 1948). The subungual keratosis may be secondarily colonized by opportunistic bacteria and fungi which may produce discoloration, friability, and loss of lustre of the nail. Long-standing fungal infections may cause severe inflammatory changes with spongiosis, exocytosis of lymphocytes and polymorphonuclear leucocytes, and papillomatosis of the nail bed. The subungual keratosis then contains globules of serum and abundant microabscesses, but the keratosis is still mainly orthokeratotic. When the nail plate is destroyed the parallel longitudinal arrangement of the fungi gets lost and the fungi criss-cross the subungual keratin and nail plate remnants in an irregular arrangement.

Bacterial colonization may be seen, mostly as a line of small basophilic coccoid organisms. In onychomycosis nigricans, the nail plate and even a portion of the subungual keratosis is diffusely yellowish-brown to dark brown, and there is no specific pigmentary change (Haneke, 1986). Occasionally, a whitish-yellow longitudinal band is seen extending from the hyponychium towards the matrix; this is often left after an otherwise successful treatment of onychomycosis of the toenail and does not respond to further systemic antifungals. Histopathology reveals a PAS-positive globus consisting of a huge amount of densely packed fungal elements, mainly arthrospores but also hyphae.

Proximal subungual onychomycosis develops from infection of the proximal nail fold. Histopathology shows fungi in the cuticle, a hyperkeratotic eponychium with fungal invasion and usually a mild inflammatory infiltrate beneath the epidermis of the eponychium. The fungi may invade the nail plate surface; they are then again regularly arranged in a parallel longitudinal manner. They grow slowly toward the matrix and are then enclosed in the growing nail plate. Since the fungi are taken away from the matrix, there is only mild inflammation and progression of the pathogen from the proximal matrix to the nail bed takes a long time. Both hyphae and thick spores may be seen in different layers of the nail plate, often causing microscopic slits which may abruptly extend to a particular type of onycholysis with apparent leuconychia. In advanced PSO, there may be as severe changes as in DLSO (Haneke, 1985, 1988a).

In superficial white onychomycosis there are chains of round spores on the nail plate extending in between superficial splits of the nail. There is no inflammatory infiltrate in the nail bed beneath (Haneke, 1985, 1991).

Primary total dystrophic onychomycosis is a characteristic feature of chronic mucocutaneous candidiasis (Haneke, 1988b) and both DLSO and PSO may lead to secondary TDO.

TDO in chronic mucocutaneous candidiasis is characterized by a complete loss of the ordered nail structure. The proximal nail fold may have been reduced to a small rim of tissue, the cuticle is lost, matrix and nail bed are papillomatous and covered with a thick irregular keratosis and there is a heavy inflammatory infiltrate invading matrix and nail bed epithelium. Electron microscopic investigation shows composite keratohyalin granules in the matrix. Fungal elements are seen in variable amounts. When they form hyphae they are irregularly arranged since there is no orderly nail plate growth left (Haneke, 1988c).

Differential diagnosis

Subungual hyperkeratosis, onycholysis, leuconychia, splinter haemorrhages as well as dystrophy involving the whole nail plate may be seen both in dermatophytosis and in psoriasis, and it may be impossible to diagnose isolated psoriasis of the nails on clinical grounds unless there is extensive pitting and/or the oil drop sign. Nail clippings or, in total nail dystrophy, a shave biopsy from the hyperkeratotic zone of the affected nail bed, may be helpful in differentiating between psoriasis and dermatophytosis (Leyden *et al.*, 1972; Scher & Ackerman, 1980b); parakeratosis and neutrophils within this zone can be seen in both conditions. Koutselinis *et al.* (1982) suggested that in clinical practice, surface and subungual scrapings are satisfactory for the cytological diagnosis of psoriasis; the skin surface biopsy technique of Marks and Dawber (1971) may be used similarly (see Chapter 1).

In psoriasis neither hyphae nor spores are found in the cornified cells of the nail bed or in the lowest portion of the nail plate. However dual pathologies do occur and psoriatic nails, particularly toenails, may be associated with commensal fungi as secondary colonization invasion caused by *Candida* or more rarely a dermatophyte. Dermatophyte infections may involve the nails in Darier's disease, lichen planus and ichthyotic states such as the KID syndrome (keratosis, ichthyosis and deafness). The yellow nail syndrome may also be mistaken for a fungal infection. However the hardness of the nail plate, its increased longitudinal curvature and the light green/yellow discoloration are all typical. The irregularly buckled nail of eczema, and the ridged or dystrophic nail of lichen planus must be distinguished from onychomycosis (Roberts & MacKenzie, 1979).

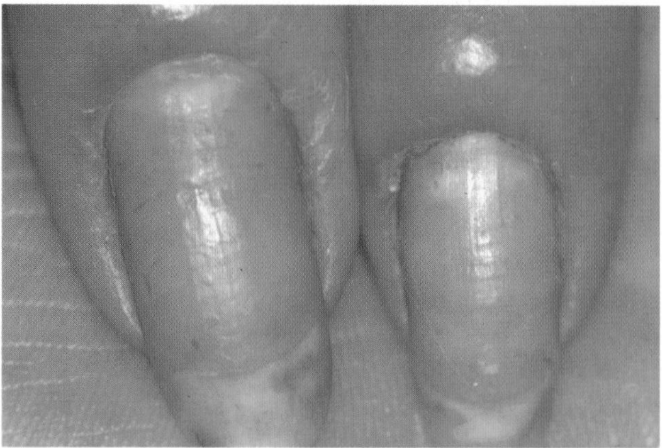

Fig. 4.43. Early stage – normal nails.

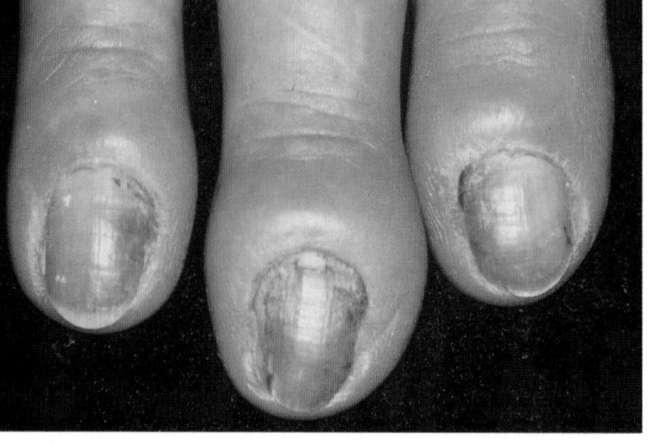

Fig. 4.44. Gross lateral periungual inflammation and swelling with early nail plate involvement.

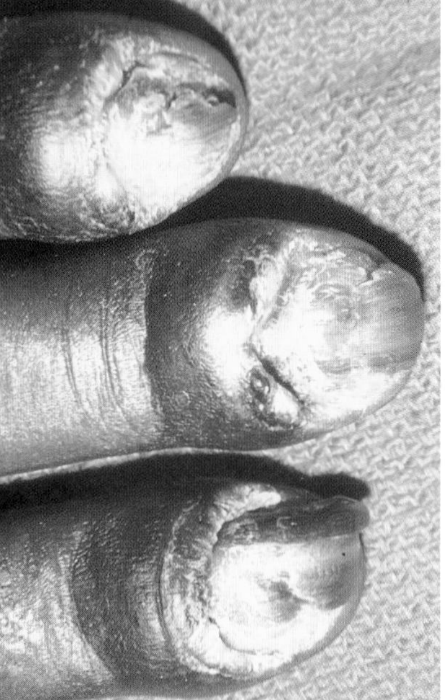

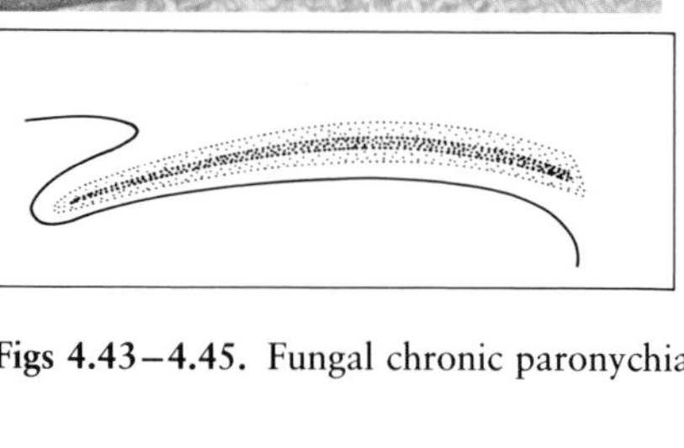

Fig. 4.45. Severe form with marked nail plate infection (TDO).

Figs 4.43–4.45. Fungal chronic paronychia.

Chronic fungal paronychia (Figs 4.43–4.45)

Candida species commonly cause infection of the proximal nail folds. A similar appearing lesion may also be caused by *Staphylococcus aureus*, particularly in patients with skin disease affecting this area, such as eczema or psoriasis. Hands which are repeatedly traumatized by immersion in water become vulnerable to chronic fungal paronychia. The condition is prevalent in people in contact with water, soap, detergents and other chemicals; women are affected three times more commonly than men. There is also a high incidence among chefs, barmen, confectioners and fishmongers.

Folds of the first and middle fingers of the right hand and the middle finger of the left hand are most often affected (Frain-Bell, 1957); these are the digits which are most subject to minor trauma, such as rubbing during hand-washing of clothes (Ganor & Pumpianski, 1974). The onset of infection is usually insidious. It starts with erythema and swelling, often in the vicinity of a lateral nail fold with loss of the adjacent cuticle. The lesion is usually tender. After several months or even years the perionychial tissue comes to resemble a semi-circular indurated cushion around the base of the nail plate, and it retracts and separates from the latter. Often a small bead of pus may be expressed from one corner of the nail fold for microscopy and culture. Rarely this procedure may be painful. The pus is formed within the pocket under the fold, and is not the product of an abscess within the perionychium. From time to time the persistent low-grade inflammation may be subject to subacute painful exacerbations which cause disturbance of the growth of the nail plate and a change in its colour, contour and surface. In the early stages the nail plate is unaffected, but one or both lateral edges may develop irregularities and yellow or brown or black discoloration which may subsequently extend over a large portion of the nail. Occasionally the whole nail becomes involved. This is believed to follow discoloration caused, in part, by dihydroxyacetone produced by the organisms in the nail fold (Stone *et al.*, 1964). By contrast *Pseudomonas* often produces a greenish discoloration. The lateral discoloured edges of the nail plate become cross-ridged when the disease is predominantly confined to the lateral nail fold. On the surface, which often becomes rough and friable, numerous irregular transverse ridges or waves appear as a result of subsequent repeated subacute exacerbations. After a time the size of the nail is considerably reduced, an effect which is exaggerated by the swelling of the surrounding soft tissues. After the paronychium has been treated successfully the onychia normally regresses, but sometimes it persists or may continue to increase. It is then difficult to distinguish between onychia caused by pyogenic bacteria or *Candida*. There is some disagreement as to the importance of the yeast in chronic *Candida* paronychia. The various factors which damage the area allow *Staph. aureus* and *Candida* spp. to attack the keratin and cause the detachment of the cuticle from the nail plate. The chronic inflammation of the proximal nail fold possibly in response to the presence of microorganisms causes it to swell and its free margin begins to round up, which essentially leads to loss of cuticle. *Candida* species may also act by simple colonization of the pocket under the proximal nail fold (Stone *et al.*, 1964). According to Barlow *et al.* (1970) a chronic paronychia is usually a mixed infection of *C. albicans* and intestinal bacteria (*Streptococcus faecalis*, coliforms, *Proteus*, *Pseudomonas* spp.). Stone and Mullins (1968) have also found streptococci in this site. The acute exacerbations are usually caused by secondary bacterial infection and may subside without treatment. *Candida* paronychia is frequently prolonged despite treatment. The organism may be derived from the mouth and the bowel (not usually the vagina) of the patient or family members, who may be sources of *C. albicans*, or from foreign material, including debris derived from the infective process. Persistence may also be due to continued exposure to predisposing conditions such as frequent immersion of the proximal nail fold, a response which tends to entrap debris and organisms, leading to chronicity of the condition. Foreign material such as wax (Stone *et al.*, 1964), hair (Stone, 1975) and foodstuffs may collect in the proximal nail fold. This may cause retraction of the nail fold and persistence of the paronychia. The development of immediate or delayed type hypersensivity to chemicals contained in food items may contribute to the pathogenesis of chronic paronychia and is probably the main factor (Zaias, 1990). Seven of 20 food handlers affected by chronic paronychia reacted positively to a 20-min open patch test with fresh foods applied on the proximal nail fold in a study by Tosti *et al.* (1991). Histology of the positive open patch test site showed acanthosis, exocytosis and spongiosis of the epidermis and lymphocytic infiltration in the dermis.

In children the most common predisposing factor to *Candida* paronychia is the habit of thumb sucking. This is potentially more harmful than occupational immersion as saliva is more irritating than water (Stone *et al.*, 1964).

Although infrequent, chronic paronychia of the toenails may develop in association with diabetes mellitus or peripheral vascular disease, both of which should be excluded unless an ingrowing nail is present.

Chronic fungal paronychia is usually due to yeasts, mainly *Candida* spp. When they get under the proximal nail fold they may cause a peculiar form of abscess between the nail plate and proximal nail fold. The latter shows a dense mixed inflammatory cell infiltrate and a spongiform pustule of the superficial zone of the epidermis. The proximal nail fold becomes swollen, the cuticle will be lost, the attachment of the eponychium and nail plate is lost. Secondary nail plate invasion may be seen in the late stage. Ridges in the lateral nail portion develop from extension of the inflammation to the nail plate (Haneke, 1991).

Differential diagnosis

Chronic paronychia may be associated with nail infections caused by *Hendersonula toruloidea* (Fig. 4.46), *Scytalidium hyalinum* or even *Fusarium* (Fig. 4.47). Brown discoloration starting at the lateral edges of the nail and spreading centrally into the nail has been seen in some cases. Rarely this is caused by a separate *Candida* infection, not directly related to the original *Scytalidium* infection (Roberts & MacKenzie, 1979). A syphilitic chancre on the perionychial area is usually painful. Pemphigus of the nail bed may produce considerable bolstering of the nail fold and closely resembles a chronic paronychia with accompanying onychomycosis. Parakeratosis pustulosa (Hjorth–Sabouraud's disease) may also mimic fungal paronychia. Psoriatic lesions, Reiter's disease and eczema sometimes involve the proximal nail fold.

Pure staphylococcal growth is more often found in patients with psoriasis or eczema affecting the nail fold. Secondary bacterial or yeast infections may develop in the area. Unusual causes of paronychia include digital enchondroma. Radiodermatitis may provoke paronychial inflammatory changes. One further disease which may be confused with fungal paronychia is a mucous pseudocyst affecting the nail fold. The characteristic groove down the nail plate, however, should allow the correct diagnosis to be made successfully.

Bacterial paronychia

Bacteria may play a role in the pathogenesis of paronychia associated with *Candida* (see above). In addition, *Staph. aureus* may cause an acute paronychia in an otherwise healthy patient. This generally arises as a results of an acute nail fold infection or whitlow and the nail fold may become swollen with subsequent discharge of pus via this area. Alternatively chronic paronychia caused by *Staph. aureus* is not infrequently seen in patients with skin disease affecting the nail fold such as psoriasis or eczema. Generally these are difficult to distinguish clinically from *Candida* infections. *Pseudomonas* infection of the proximal nail fold may produce transverse green stripes on the nail corresponding to exacerbations of the paronychia (Shellow & Koplon, 1968).

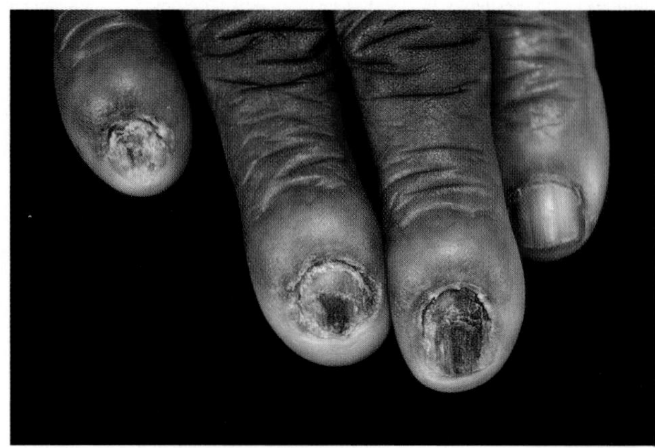

Fig. 4.46. Chronic paronychia – *Hendersonula toruloidea* infection.

Other infective forms of paronychia

On rare occasions other infections may involve the nail fold causing a form of paronychia. Amongst the fungi, the agents of sporotrichosis and, less commonly, chromoblastomycosis, coccidioidomycosis, blastomycosis and mycetoma may involve this area. Infections due to *Fusarium* species in neutropenic patients may affect the nail fold area either in the course of or prior to the onset of fungal septicaemia, suggesting that this may be a portal of entry for the organism in some cases.

Amongst the less common bacterial causes of paronychia, tuberculosis verrucosa cutis may affect the nail fold as the primary site of inoculation.

Drug-induced paronychia (see Chapter 6)

Tender paronychia may develop on the hands or feet during aromatic retinoid therapy. Methotrexate produced acute paronychia localized to all the toes (Wantzig & Thomsen, 1983) and cephalexin caused fixed drug eruption mimicking acute paronychia in fingernails (Baran & Perrin, 1991).

Treatment of onychomycosis

In the treatment of fungal nail disease the site of involvement and the identity of the organism are important factors. As the rate of growth of toenails is one-third to one-half that of fingernails, therapy of the former using the classical systemic drugs, such as griseofulvin or ketoconazole, must be continued for 12–18 months, whereas fingernail infection may be cured in 6 months. Drug effectiveness can be checked by Zaias and Drachman's method (1983) notching proximally the infected position of the nail plate. The age of the patient, and the cost and efficacy of treatment, particularly in toenail infections, must be considered before using systemic therapy (Korting & Schafer-Korting, 1992).

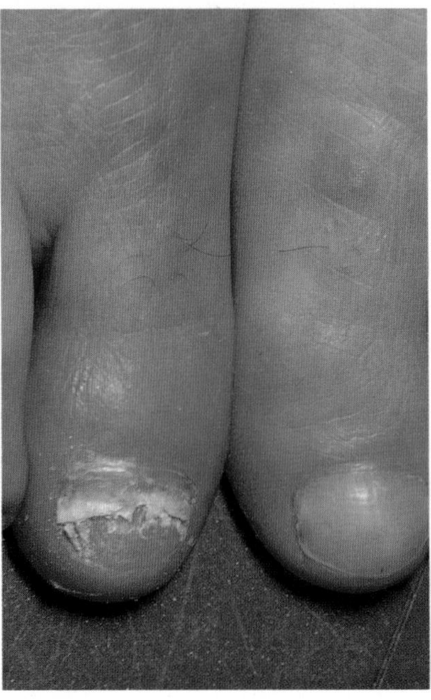

Fig. 4.47. Chronic paronychia – *Fusarium* infection.

Chemical removal or surgical avulsion of the nail plate may considerably shorten the duration of therapy but subsequent recurrence is common. The value of the older topical agents unaccompanied by nail ablation in onychomycosis is limited and cure is possible in a minority of cases. Most of the available antifungal agents, including the imidazoles, and other compounds, such as tolnaftate, can be applied directly to the nail with rather variable and generally disappointing results. Contact sensitivity to imidazoles has been reported (Marran & Powell 1992). The 28% formulation of tioconazole has been reported to work in some cases although the overall results have been disappointing, reported cure rates being no more than 20–22% (Hay *et al.*, 1985). It may also be used as an adjunct to oral antifungal drug therapy with griseofulvin and has been found to improve the recovery rates significantly (Hay *et al.*, 1987). It is safe to apply although it may cause a temporary glazed appearance of the nail plate.

New topical compounds with reported clinical efficacy in onychomycosis include 5% amorolfine and 8% ciclopirox. Amorolfine (Polak, 1988; Reinel *et al.*, 1990) and ciclopirox have both been reported to be effective in onychomycosis sparing the lunular area. They are used as nail lacquers acting as transungual delivery systems: 5% amorolfine nail lacquer, for instance, has been reported to produce mycological recoveries in up to 70% of patients with early nail plate infection sparing the lunula region. Fungicidal concentrations were found in nail after application of 8% ciclopirox nail lacquer (Ceschin-Roques *et al.*, 1991).

Finally, closer attention should be paid to preventive

local antifungal treatment following the cure of onychomycosis in previously affected nails, toewebs and soles.

Griseofulvin

Griseofulvin is an oral antifungal agent derived from certain *Penicillium* species such as *P. griseofulvum*. It is only active against dermatophytes. In nail infection, it is normally given in a daily dose of 500–1000 mg for adults, although this may be increased to 2 g in recalcitrant cases. Absorption of the drug is enhanced when it is given in microsize or ultramicrosize particle form and with food. In nail infections, griseofulvin is given until there is clinical and mycological recovery; the complete replacement of infected tissue with healthy nail depends upon the rate of growth, but some patients or some nails fail to improve even after treatment of apparently adequate dose and duration.

The results of treating toenail infections are usually not satisfactory, particularly in the elderly. The overall cure rate using griseofulvin for toenail infections is generally less than 40%. Treatment is the result of the interaction of a number of factors including penetration of the drug into nail keratin and leakage from the nail, the rate of nail growth and the sensitivity of the organism to the drug. Resistance to griseofulvin has been correlated with treatment failure by some investigators (Artis *et al.*, 1981), but not by others (Davies *et al.*, 1977). It is not clear whether the higher minimum inhibitory concentration (MIC) values seen in isolates from some clinically unresponsive cases are due to a permanent or reversible change in sensitivity. The latter has been demonstrated *in vitro* (Rosenthal & Wise, 1960) and this may explain why previously unresponsive cases sometimes clear after reintroduction of griseofulvin after a drug-free interval of 6–18 months. An alternative method of enhancing the effect of griseofulvin is the use of cimetidine as an adjunct to antifungal treatment (Presser & Blank, 1981). However the true value of this combined therapy in nail infections needs more objective assessment.

Allergic reactions such as urticaria may occur during griseofulvin therapy, but the most common reasons for discontinuing treatment are headache or gastrointestinal intolerance. Griseofulvin competes with some drugs including anticoagulants and contraceptives and there is interference with its absorption and metabolism by phenobarbitone (Davies, 1980). It may also be responsible for precipitating porphyria cutanea tarda in predisposed patients, as well as a lupus erythematosus-like eruption.

Ketoconazole

Ketoconazole, an imidazole drug, is an alternative to griseofulvin (Cox *et al.*, 1982). It works by blocking the cytochrome P450-dependent demethylation stage in the conversion of lanosterol into ergosterol in the formation of the fungal cell membrane. It is active against *Candida* as well as dermatophytes (Botter *et al.*, 1979; Baran, 1982), but has little effect on non-dermatophyte moulds such as *Scopulariopsis brevicaulis*. The daily adult dose is 200 mg given with food, but this may be increased to 400 or even 600 mg in some cases. Ketoconazole is effective in *Candida* onychomycosis including chronic mucocutaneous candidiasis (Figs 4.25 and 4.26) (Haneke, 1981; Hay & Clayton, 1992). It is also effective against chronic generalized dermatophyte onychomycosis. Side effects, including gastrointestinal intolerance, are less common than with griseofulvin. Ketoconazole also blocks human metabolic processes such as adrenal androgen biosynthesis dependent on cytochrome P450, causing symptoms such as gynaecomastia in males. These effects are mainly seen at higher doses (over 600 mg daily); drug interactions are known with cyclosporin A, warfarin, chloridiazepoxide astemizole, and antipyrine, and its efficacy is reduced by nifampicin and phenytoin. A sporadic drug-induced hepatitis has been associated with the drug on rare occasions (Heiberg & Svejgaard, 1981; Strauss, 1982; Tkach & Rinaldi, 1982); the risk of hepatitis has been assessed as 1 per 10 000 prescriptions, but appears to be slightly commoner in patients with onychomycosis (Fromtling, 1988), particularly when they had been treated previously with griseofulvin. The duration of therapy is similar to griseofulvin. Hepatic function has to be monitored regularly. Generally ketoconazole is now not much used for the management of onychomycosis in view of the risk, albeit rare, of hepatitis.

New oral antifungal agents

All three new systemic medications for treatment of onychomycosis have been shown to be effective not only when administered daily for several months but also when given for a short course of treatment (14 days to 3 months), or when used intermittently. The drugs reach the nail via incorporation into the matrix and by diffusion from the nail bed.

Itraconazole

Itraconazole is one of the new triazole antifungal drugs. Although its mode of action is similar to that of ketoconazole (Fromtling, 1988), it has not been reported to have serious side effects in man, since it binds more specifically to fungal cytochrome P450. The main adverse reactions are nausea, gastrointestinal fullness and headache. It has been used for a variety of mycoses including onychomycosis. In the latter, it has been found to have activity in patients with previously treatment-unresponsive dermatophytosis, as well as *Candida* nail infections (Hay *et al.*, 1988c). It does not appear to be effective in *Scytalidium* infections, but is very active against *Aspergillus* spp.

Studies of itraconazole have drawn attention to the mode of drug penetration and nail binding. Itraconazole is a lipid-soluble drug, and appears rapidly to penetrate into nails and is detectable within 2 weeks of the start of the therapy. It is detectable in this site for a considerable period thereafter, and in one study it was found in nail plate material 1 year after a 3 month period of therapy (Willemsen *et al.*, 1992). With a dose of 200 mg daily for 3 months significant recovery rates have been reported in both finger and toenail infection (Willemsen *et al.*, 1992). The recommended dose is now 200 mg of itraconazole daily resulting in mycological cure rates of over 90% in fingernails and over 70% in toenails. The recurrence rate was only 11% (compared with the high rates following griseofulvin therapy). Intraconazole 400 mg daily, in cycles of one week per month for four months could be a good alternative (Roseeuw & Doncker, 1993).

Fluconazole

Fluconazole, another azole antifungal drug of the triazole group, is mainly used (100 mg daily) in the management of systemic disease or superficial candidosis (Fromtling, 1988), especially in patients with AIDS and in other immunosuppressed subjects. There is however evidence that levels detectable by bioassay are found in nails within 48 h (Hay, 1988). This drug is unusual amongst the azole antifungals for its water solubility, which might account for its rapid penetration into nail (Grant & Clissold, 1990). It has a low frequency of mainly gastrointestinal side effects. It is considered to be less hepatotoxic than ketoconazole, but AIDS patients require careful monitoring of hepatic function because hepatotoxicity may develop (Munos *et al.*, 1991).

Montero-Gei *et al.* (1991) treated 10 patients with dermatophyte nail infection with a single 150 mg dose of fluconazole per week. Clinical and mycological cures were obtained in all patients receiving the drug for 19–21 weeks in fingernail infections, and 24–40 in toenail infections. This has recently been confirmed in more than 100 patients by several authors (Fraki *et al.*, 1993).

Terbinafine

Terbinafine is a member of the allylamine antifungal drug group which inhibit the epoxidation of squalene, a step in the formation of ergosterol in the fungal cell membrane (Petranyi *et al.*, 1987). This is a conversion stage which occurs earlier than that inhibited by the azoles. Terbinafine is active against a wide range of pathogenic fungi *in vitro*, but *in vivo* is only useful for dermatophytosis (250 mg daily).

One potential advantage of this drug is the fact that unlike the other antifungals it appears to be fungicidal *in vitro* at relatively low concentrations. In dermatophytosis of the dry type, rapid responses and low relapse rates have been recorded. In onychomycosis rather similar results have been seen with mycological remission of infected fingernails occurring within 3 months of starting therapy (Goodfield *et al.*, 1989). These results also suggest more rapid penetration into the nail, a fact now confirmed by studies of its distribution within nail. These drugs have a lower relapse rate than other compounds. This initial study has been extended to a placebo-controlled trial of terbinafine 250 mg daily in dermatophyte onychomycosis (Goodfield *et al.*, 1992). This has shown significant recovery rates of toenail infections at 3 months and fingernails at 6 weeks.

At present a 3-month treatment is recommended for fingernails and a 6-month course for toenails. Response rates are 90% for the former and nearly 80% for the latter. Recurrence rates are below 10%.

Nail removal (Figs 4.48–4.51)

It may be possible to enhance results of chemotherapy by various procedures.

1 Mechanical removal by cutting, filing or abrading.
2 Chemical removal by keratinolysis.
3 Surgical removal by total or partial nail ablation.

If removal of the nail plate is contemplated, it is advisable to commence systemic antifungal drugs 1 week before avulsion as griseofulvin must reach the nail through the matrix in order to be effective. There are a number of methods of chemical nail removal. For instance a 40% urea preparation was introduced by Farber and South (1978) and subsequently modified (South & Farber, 1980): it has been assessed by White and Clayton (1982). All these techniques may shorten the duration of therapy. However, there are problems with some of these methods; for instance with the urea technique only abnormal nail is removed (but the adjacent normal nail is also softened when the nail plate surface is roughened by filing) and there may be fungal elements present at the edge of the clinically normal section of the nail plate. With total surgical removal, the distal nail bed may shrink and become dislocated dorsally so that the regrowing nail then embeds itself by the free edge. This can be largely overcome by using partial nail removal (Baran & Hay, 1985) for onychomycosis of limited extent in lateral, distal or even proximal areas. (Figs 4.48–4.51).

Urea chemical treatment (Figs 4.52–4.54)

Urea ointment (Table 4.4) is applied to the nail plate after masking the surrounding skin with tape and the entire distal part of the digit is then covered with plastic or

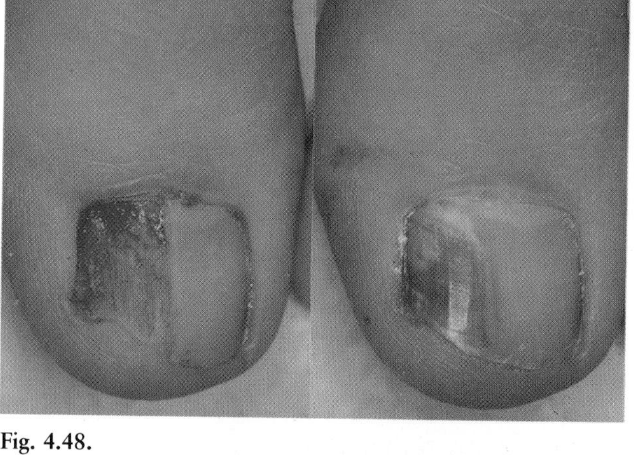

Fig. 4.48.

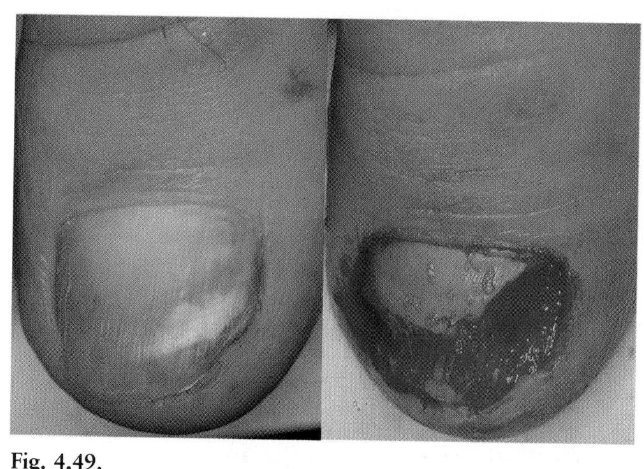

Fig. 4.49.

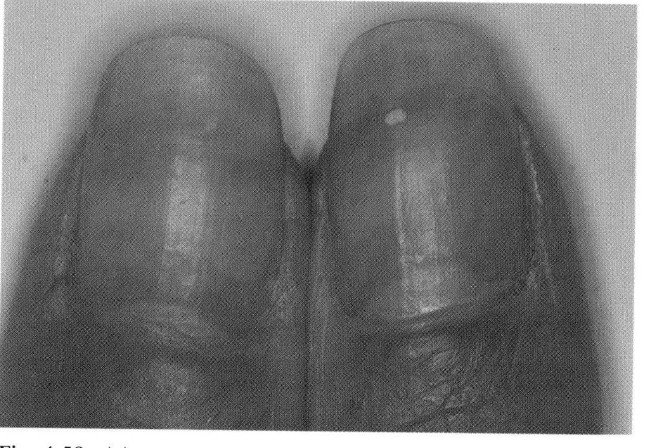

Fig. 4.50. (a)

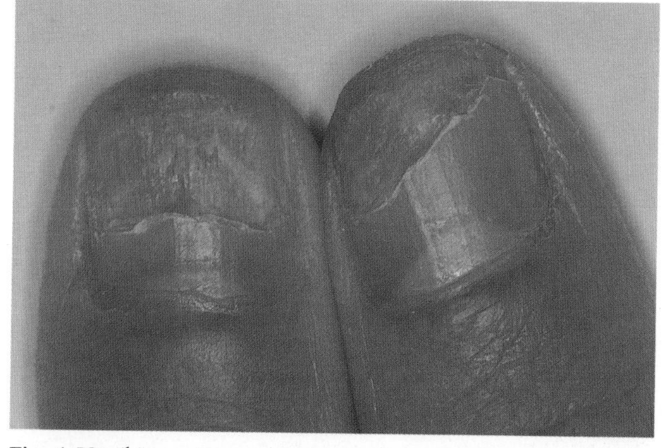

Fig. 4.50. (b)

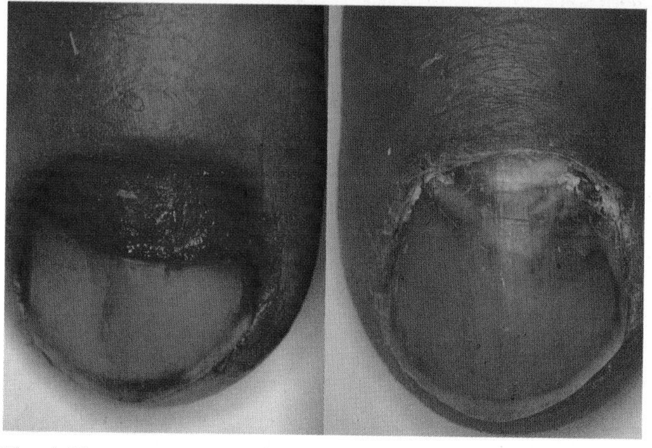

Fig. 4.51.

Figs 4.48–4.51. Various degrees of nail removal – may enhance subsequent topical (and systemic?) therapy which can be shortened.

cellophane wrap for 1 week. Urea ointment appears to act by dissolving the bond between the dystrophic nail plate and nail bed as well as softening the nail plate. Subsequent blunt dissection using a nail elevator and nail clipper will leave intact normal nail. Failure of 40% urea treatment, as well as with 50% potassium iodide ointment in anhydrous lanolin plus 0.5% iodochlorhydroxyquine (Dorn *et al.*, 1980), can sometimes be ascribed to gross thickening of the nail. Gentle abrasion of the nail surface may enhance penetration of these agents. One alternative is a combination of 20% urea (Onychomal) and 10% salicyclic acid ointment under occlusion for 2 weeks, a treatment which is useful for the removal of minimally dystrophic nails (Buselmeier, 1980). Following nail removal, topical antifungal agents (miconazole, clotrimazole, haloprogin, ciclopiroxolamine, etc.) are then applied and the patient may receive an oral antifungal agent until the new nail is formed. A further modification of this approach has been the incorporation of 1% bifonazole into the urea paste formulation (Hay *et al.*, 1988b). Results with this preparation have shown that responses are possible although the success rates claimed have varied from over 70 to 34%. It is possible to adapt this method for use by the patients themselves by applying the paste at night and removing

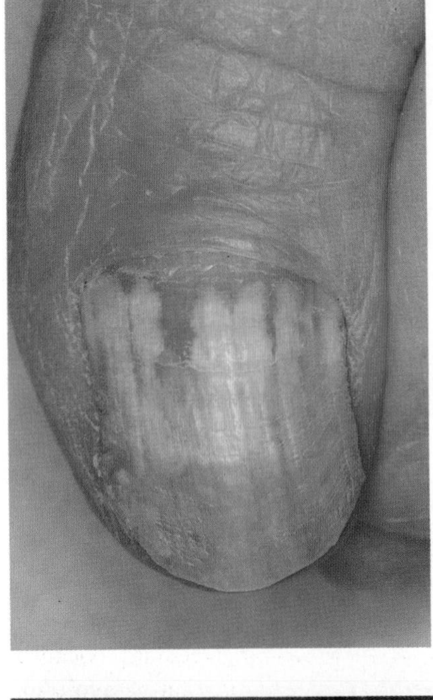

Fig. 4.52. DLSO caused by *S. brevicaulis*; may respond to urea treatment.

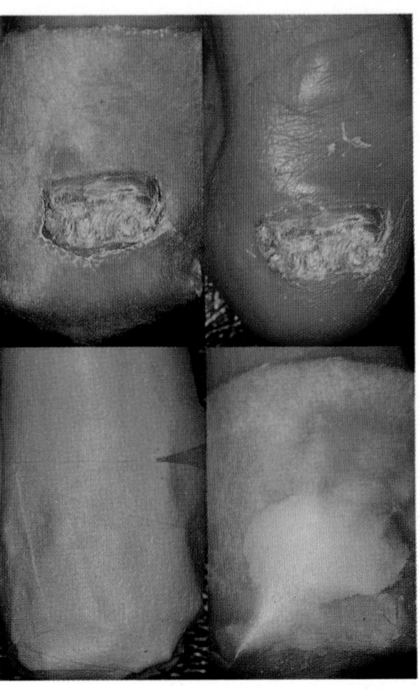

Fig. 4.53.

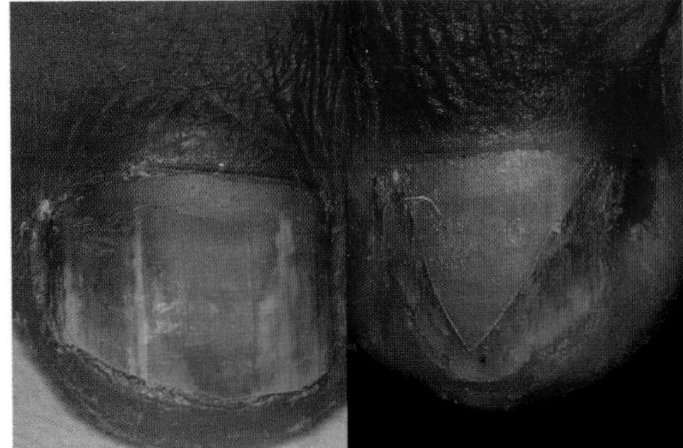

Fig. 4.54.

Figs 4.53–4.54. Urea chemical treatment.

Table 4.4. Urea ointment formulation

Urea	40%
White beeswax (or paraffin)	5%
Anhydrous lanolin	20%
White petrolatum	25%
Silica gel type H	10%

the softened nail and remaining paste using scissors or a modified scraper. The drug is available as a kit with nail remover and instruction sheet in some European countries. Generally the nail is soft enough for removal after about 8 h and becomes sequentially softer with each successive application. Clinical experience has shown that this topical treatment followed by daily application of bifonazole is successful when no more than three to five nails are affected and when infection does not extend beneath the primary nailfold.

A combination of systemic antifungal treatment and urea nail removal may be useful in some cases, particularly where localized areas of nail plate infection persist after a reasonable course of oral therapy. Sometimes an ivory to yellowish longitudinal stripe is resistant to any conservative treatment. Histopathology shows a huge amount of fungi compressed in this area. It is then wise to gently cut the nail away over the stripe using a sharp No. 15 scalpel blade, preferentially after prior nail softening with 40% urea ointment. An English nail splitter, or the double-action nail rongeur are good alternatives.

Management of various sub-types

In *primary onycholysis* of the big toenails, associated with dermatophyte invasion, measures should be taken to relieve the effects of pressure and trauma such as the provision of fitted shoes, padding or toe shields. Daily topical treatment with antifungal therapy and repeated trimming of the non-adherent portion of nails should be started.

Nails affected by *superficial white onychomycosis* (see Figs 4.11 & 4.12) should be abraded after confirming the diagnosis by taking scrapings. When the culture is negative a tangential piece of the nail plate, using the shave excision technique, is taken for histopathology. This will avoid unnecessary systemic therapy since topical treatments alone are effective. Alternatively a 10% glutaraldehyde solution (Cidex) which tints the nail bronze may be used for both dermatophytes and mould infections (Suringa, 1970). Coexistence of white superficial onychomycosis and distal and lateral subungual onychomycosis is an indication for oral therapy. In the elderly or those with isolated lesser toenail involvement, treatment may be unnecessary and control of nail thickening by chiropody may be the best alternative. The 40% urea–1% bifonazole ointment may be used combining the advantages of considerable nail softening with antimycotic action on the infectious keratotic debris from under the nail. It is wise to avoid salicylic acid in combination with urea if there is peripheral circulatory insufficiency.

Onychomycosis caused by non-dermatophyte moulds

Assuming that the pathogenic role of mould fungi isolated from the affected nails has been confirmed using the criteria discussed previously, three patterns of infection must be considered.

1 SWO caused by *Acremonium*, *Aspergillus* or *Fusarium* spp. (Fig. 4.11).

2 Distal and lateral subungual onychomycosis caused by *S. brevicaulis* (Fig. 4.52) and certain other moulds such as *Pyrenochaeta unguium-hominis* (Puntithalingham & English, 1975; English, 1980).

3 *Hendersonula toruloidea* (Gentles & Evans, 1970; Campbell *et al.*, 1973; Jones *et al.*, 1985) (Figs 4.9 & 4.46), renamed *Nattrassia mangiferae* (Sutton & Dyko, 1989), then *Scytalidium dimidiatum* or *S. hyalinum* infections (Campbell & Mulder, 1977; Elewski & Greer, 1991).

SWO caused by non-dermatophytes may respond to abrasion of the nail surface followed by topical therapy with imidazole agents, particularly those with better *in vitro* activity against mould fungi, such as econazole, clotrimazole or 28% tioconazole, amorolfine, ciclopiroxolamine, and 8% ciclopirox; 10% glutaraldehyde as seen above may also be effective. However, topical therapy is rarely useful for the other categories of infection. In these cases, repeated chemical removal of the nails followed by local applications of keratolytics and antifungal agents should be tried.

Candida onychomycosis

Nail dystrophy caused by *Candida* can be treated with oral itraconazole, ketoconazole, or chemical removal followed by local antifungal treatment. If these methods are unsuccessful, combined avulsion and chemotherapy should be used. In chronic mucocutaneous candidosis, the dose of ketoconazole may have to be increased to 400 or 600 mg daily. When remission is induced, treatment should be stopped. Resistance has been reported where low dose (200 mg daily) therapy is continued. Itraconazole is another effective alternative in this condition and resistance to this drug has not been recorded. Other antifungals such as low dose amphotericin B, intravenous miconazole or oral clotrimazole have been used in the past with limited success (Hay, 1981). In the near future lipid-associated amphotericin B may be another alternative offering less toxicity.

Onycholysis with Candida colonization

This variety often coexists with bacterial infection (*Pseudomonas* or *Proteus*). The patient should be advised to wear thin cotton gloves, which are regularly cleaned, under rubber gloves for all wet work, and to avoid excessive immersion in hot water, even when wearing protective gloves. After hand washing, the nail fold area must be dried carefully – in some cases the use of a hair dryer is recommended to keep the nail plate–nail bed space as dry as possible. The nail plate has to be trimmed as far back as possible: if the patient is anxious, local anaesthesia may be required. Scissors are used to separate the nail plate proximal to the onycholytic area; then the nail bed should be debrided with a piece of gauze wrapped around a stick. Four per cent thymol in chloroform or 15% sulphacetamide in 70% ethyl alcohol may be applied twice daily to the space to suppress growth of *Candida* and *Pseudomonas* (Samman, 1982). The specific antifungals (i.e. miconazole, clotrimazole) may supplement this treat ment. Thorough trimming should be repeated at intervals of 4 weeks until the nail reattaches. ‘Green nails’ deserve the same treatment, despite good but inconsistent results obtained by Zaias (1990) with Clorox, diluted 1:4, a few drops being applied three times a day. Polymyxin B is no longer used for *Pseudomonas* infections; brushing the nail area with 2% acetic acid is an alternative method. The patient should be warned against cleaning with a nail file or orange wood stick under an area of onycholysis as this may increase the split. Removal of organisms in patients with onycholysis may improve the appearance of the nails but will not produce healing of the split between nail plate and nail bed.

Chronic Candida paronychia

As in all varieties of paronychia, protection of the hands from water (as for onycholysis) is an indispensable part of management. Topical antifungal agents active against *Candida* must be applied to the groove between the nail

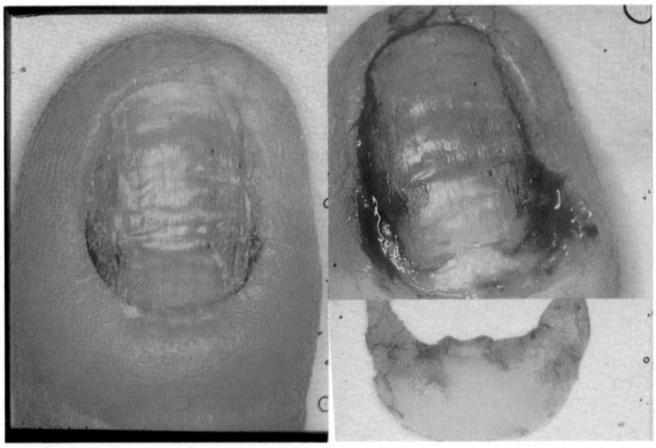

Fig. 4.55. Chronic paronychia – recalcitrant cases due to foreign bodies may resolve following removal of the indurated, chronically inflamed tissue as shown (right hand pictures showing section removed) (courtesy of G. Cannata, Italy).

plate and the proximal fold at least twice daily. Solution formulations of these drugs are much more effective than creams or ointments for paronychia. Treatment usually has to be continued for at least 3 months and until the nail fold lies flat against the nail plate. Systemic therapy, such as ketoconazole, works in this condition but is no more efficacious than topical treatment. Warm compresses with Burrow's solution (1:40 dilution) for 10 min three times a day may also decrease the inflammatory reaction. If there are frequent acute episodes, combined treatment using intralesional or systemic steroid therapy and systemic antibiotics such as erythromycin 1 g daily, or tetracycline 1 g daily for 1 week, may be useful. When the inflammation has disappeared, 15% sulphacetamide in 70% surgical spirit or 4% thymol in chloroform may both help to dry the nail fold.

Treatment should not be considered complete until the cuticle has regrown. Reattachment of the proximal nail fold to the nail can be encouraged by dabbing the groove with a toothpick dipped into 80% phenol. All the affected areas of the nail plate should be clipped away or abraded. An alternative is the use of azole antifungal lotions applied along the nail fold and allowed to seep under this area. Chemical removal is an alternative for completely dystrophic nails. Low-voltage X-ray therapy has been suggested using 100 R = 1 Gy given three times at weekly intervals with 50 kV, 1 mm Al filter and may produce good results on the paronychial inflammation. Surgical therapy is seldom necessary (Fig. 4.55) (Chapter 10).

In conclusion the future direction for treatment of onychomycosis will involve therapeutic combinations: systemic drugs with short duration regimens with antifungal nail lacquers.

References

Achten G. & Simonart J. (1963) L'ongle. Etude histologique et mycologique. *Ann. Dematol. Syphil.* **90**, 569–586.

Achten G. & Simonart J. (1965) Kératine unguéale et parasites fungiques: mycopathologie. *Mycologia* **27**, 193–199.

Achten G. & Wanet-Rouard J. (1978) Onychomycoses in the laboratory. *Mykosen* Suppl. 1, 125.

Achter G. & Wanet-Rouard J. (1981) Onychomycosis. *Mycology*, No. 5. Cilag Ltd., Brussels.

Achten G., Wanet-Rouard J., Wiame L. & Van Hoff F. (1979) Les onychomycoses à moisissures: champignons 'opportunistes'. *Dermatologica* **159** (suppl. 1), 128.

Alkiewicz J. (1948) Transverse net in the diagnosis of onychomycosis. *Arch. Dermatol. Syphil.* **58**, 385.

Artis W.M., Odle B.M. & Jones H.E. (1981) Griseofulvin-resistant dermatophytosis correlates with *in vitro* resistance. *Arch. Dermatol.* **117**, 16.

Badillet G. (1988) Mélanonychies superficielles. *Bull. Soc. Fr. Mycol. Med.* **17**, 335–340.

Baran R. (1982) Treatment of severe onychomycosis with ketoconazole. A new oral antifungal drug. *XVI Congressus Internationalis Dermatologiae*, Tokyo, p. 298.

Baran R. & Badillet G. (1982) Primary onycholysis of the big toenails; a review of 113 cases. *Br. J. Dermatol.* **106**, 529.

Baran R. & Badillet G. (1983) Un dermatophyte unguéal est-il nécessairement pathogéne? *Ann. Dermatol. Venereol.* **110**, 629–631.

Baran R. & Hay R. (1985) Partial surgical avulsion of the nail in onychomycosis. *Clin. Exp. Dermatol.* **10**, 413–418.

Baran R. & Perrin C. (1991) Fixed drug eruption presenting as acute paronychia. *Br. J. Dermatol.* **125**, 592–595.

Barlow A.J.E., Chattaway F.W., Holgate W.C. & Aldersley T.A. (1970) Chronic paronychia. *Br. J. Dermatol.*. **82**, 448.

Belsan I. & Fragner P. (1965) Onychomykosen, hervorgerufen durch *Scopulariopsis brevicaulis*. *Hautarzt* **16**, 258.

Botter A.A., Dethier F., Mertens R.L.J., Morias J. & Peremans W. (1979) Skin and nail mycoses: treatment with ketoconazole a new oral antimycotic agent. *Mykosen* **22**, 274.

Boudghene-Stambouli O. & Merad-Boudia A. (1991) La maladie dermatophytique en Algérie. Nouvelle observation et revue de la littérature. *Ann. Dermatol. Venereol.* **118**, 17–22.

Buselmeier F.J. (1980) Combination urea and salicylic acid ointment nail avulsion in non dystrophic nails: follow-up observation. *Cutis* **25**, 393.

Campbell C.K. & Mulder J.L. (1977) Skin and nail infection by *Scytalidium hyalium* sp. *Sabouraudia* **15**, 161–166.

Campbell C.K., Kurwa H., Abdel-Aziz A.H.M. & Hodgson C. (1973) Fungal infections of skin and nails by *Hendersonula toruloidea*. *Br. J. Dermatol.* **89**, 45.

Ceschin-Roques C.G., Hanel H., Pruja-Bougaret S.M. *et al.* (1991) Ciclopirox nail lacquer 8%: *in vivo* penetration into and through nails and *in vitro* effect on pig skin. *Skin Pharmacol.* **4**, 89–94.

Cox F.W., Stiller R.L. & South D.A. (1982) Oral ketoconazole for dermatophyte infections. *J. Am. Acad. Dermatol.* **6**, 455–462.

Daniel C.R. (1985) Nail micronizer. *Cutis* **36**, 118.

Davies R.R. (1968) Mycological test and onychomycosis. *J. Clin. Pathol.* **21**, 729.

Davies R.R. (1980) Griseofulvin. In: *Antifungual Chemotherapy*, ed. Speller D.C.E., pp. 149–182. John Wiley & Sons, Chichester.

Davies R.R., Everall J.D. & Hamilton E. (1977) Mycological and clinical evaluation of griseofulvin for chronic onychomycosis. *Br. Med. J.* **iii**, 464.

Dompmartin D., Dompmartin A., Deluol A.M. *et al.* (1990) Onychomycosis and AIDS. Clinical and laboratory findings in 62 patients. *Int. J. Dermatol.* 29, 337–339.

Dorn M., Kienity T. & Ryckmanns F. (1980) Onychomycosis: experience with non-traumatic nail avulsion. *Hautarzt* **31**, 30.

Elewski B.E. & Greer D.L. (1991) *Hendersonula toruloidea* and *Seytalidium hyalinum*. Review and update. *Arch. Dermatol.* **127**, 1041–1044.

English M.P. (1976) Nails and fungi. *Br. J. Dermatol.* **94**, 697.

English M.P. (1980) Infection of the finger-nail by *Pyrenochaeta unguis-ominis*. *Br. J. Dermatol.* **103**, 91–93.

English M. & Atkinson R. (1973) An improved method for the isolation of fungi in onychomycosis. *Br. J. Dermatol.* **88**, 273.

English M.P. & Atkinson R. (1974) Onychomycosis in elderly chiropody patients. *Br. J. Dermatol.* **91**, 67.

Farber E. & South D.A. (1978) Urea ointment in the nonsurgical avulsion of nail dystrophies. *Cutis* **22**, 689.

Feldmann R., Pupping D. & Harms M. (1992) Two feet-one-hand-Dermatophytose. *Z. Hautkz.* **67**, 680–681.

Frain-Bell W. (1957) Chronic paronychia. Short review of 590 cases. *Trans. St Johns Hosp. Dermatol. Soc.* 38, 29.

Fraki J. *et al.* (1993) Fluronazole in the treatment of onychomycosis: an open non-comparative multicenter study with oral 150 mg fluconazole once weekly. Poster No. 14. Dermatology 2000. Vienna. 18–21 May 1993.

Fromtling R.A. (1988) Overview of medically important anti fungal azole derivatives. *Clin. Microbiol. Rev.* **1**, 187–217.

Ganor S. & Pumpiasky R. (1974) Chronic *Candida albicans* paronychia in adult Israeli women. *Br. J. Dermatol.* **90**, 77.

Gentles J.C. (1971) Laboratory investigations of dermatophytes infections of nails. *J. Int. Soc. Hum. Anim. Mycol.* **9**, 149.

Gentles J.C. & Evans E.G.V. (1970) Infection of the feet and nails with *Hendersonula toruloidea*. *Sabouraudia*. **8**, 72–75.

Goetz H. & Hantschke D. (1965) Einblicke in du Epidemiologie der Dermatomykosen in Kohlenbezgbau. *Hautarzt* **16**, 543–548.

Gptz H. & Hantschke D. (1965) Einblicke in die Epidemiologie der Dermatomykosen im Kohlenbergbau. *Hautarzt* **16**, 543.

Goodfield M.J.D., Rowell N.R., Forster R.A. *et al.* (1989) Treatment of dermatophyte infections of the finger or toe nails with terbinafine (SFG 86–327, Lasimil) an orally active fungicidal agent. *Br. J. Dermatol.* **121**, 753–757.

Goodfield M.J.D., Andrew L. & Evans E.G.V. (1992) Short term treatment of dermatophyte onychomycosis with terbinafine. *Br. Med. J.* **304**, 1151–1154.

Grant S.M. & Clissold S.P. (1990) Fluconazole. A review of its pharmacodynamic and pharmacokinetic properties and therapeutic potential in superficial and systemic mycoses. *Drugs* **39**, 877–916.

Gugnani H.C., Nzelibe F.K. & Osunkwo I.C. (1986) Onychomycosis due to *Hendersonula toruloidea* in Nigeria. *J. Med. Vet. Mycol.* **24**, 23–241.

Hadida E., Schousboe A. & Sayag. J. (1966) Dermatophyties atypiques. *Bull. Soc. Fr. Dermatol. Syph.* 73, 917.

Haneke E. (1981) Ketoconazole treatment of dermatomycoses. In: *Current Chemotherapy and Immunotherapy*, eds Periti P. & Grass G.G., Vol. II, pp. 1012–1013. Am. Soc. Microbiol., Washington, DC.

Haneke E. (1985) Nail biopsies in onychomycosis. *Mykosen* **28**, 473–480.

Haneke E. (1986) Differential diagnosis of mycotic nail diseases. In: *Advances in Topical Antifungal Therapy*, ed. Hay R.J., pp. 94–101. Springer, New York.

Haneke E. (1988a) General aspects of onychomycoses. In: Proceedings X^th^ Congress of the International Society of Human and Animal Mycology, pp. 235–239. Pzous, Barcelona, Spain.

Haneke E. (1988b) The nails in chronic mucocutaneous can didosis. Presented at the 15th Annual Meeting, Soc. Cut. Ultrastructure Research. Nice, France (abstr.).

Haneke E. (1991) Fungal infections of the nail: nail disease. *Semin. Dermatol.* **10**, 41–51.

Hay R.J. (1981) Management of chronic mucocutaneous conditions. *Clin. Exp. Dermatol.* **6**, 515–519.

Hay R.J. (1988) New oral treatment for dermatophytosis. In: *Antifungal Drugs*, ed. St Georgiev V. *Ann. NY Acad. Sci.* **544**, 580–585.

Hay R.J. & Clayton Y.M. (1992) The treatment of patients with chronic mucocutaneous conditions and *Candida* onychomycosis with ketoconazole. *Clin. Exp. Dermatol.* **7**, 155–162.

Hay R.J., Mackie R.M. & Clayton Y.M. (1985) Tioconazole (28%) nail solution: an open study of its efficacy in onychomycosis. *Clin. Exp. Dermatol.* **10**, 152–157.

Hay R.J., Clayton Y.M. & Moore M.K. (1987) A comparison of tioconazole 28% nail solution versus base as an adjunct to oral griseofulvin in patients with onychomycosis. *Clin. Exp. Dermatol.* **12**, 175–177.

Hay R.J., Baran R., Moore M.K. & Wilkinson J.D. (1988a) *Candida* onychomycosis – an evaluation of the role of *Candida* in nail disease. *Br. J. Dermatol.* **118**, 47–58.

Hay R.J., Roberts D., Doherty V.R. *et al.* (1988b) The topical treatment of onychomycosis using a new combined urea/imidazole preparation. *Clin. Exp. Dermatol.* **17**, 164–167.

Hay R.J., Clayton Y.M., Moore M.K. *et al* (1988c) An evaluation of itraconazole in the management of onychomycosis. *Br. J. Dermatol.* **119**, 359–366.

Heiberg J.K. & Svejgaard E. (1981) Toxic hepatitis during ketoconazole treatment. *Br. Med. J.* **283**, 825.

Higashi N. (1990) Melanonychia due to *Tinea unguium*. *Hifu* **32**, 377–380.

Jessner M. (1992) Uber eine neue Form von Nagelmykosen (leukonychia trichophytica) *Arch. Dermatol. Syphil. (Berlin)* **141**, 1–8.

Jones S.K., White J.E., Jacobs P.H. *et al.* (1985) *Hendersonula toruloidea* infection of the nails in Caucasians. *Clin. Exp. Dermatol.* **10**, 444–447.

Kalter D.C. & Hay R.J. (1988) Onychomycosis due to *Trichophyton soudanense*. *Clin. Exp. Dermatol.* **13**, 221–227.

Korting H.C. & Schafer-Korting M. (1992) Is *Tinea unguium* still widely incurable? *Arch. Dermatol.* **128**, 243–248.

Koutselinis H., Aronis K. & Stratigos J. (1982) Cytology as an aid in the diagnosis of psoriasis of nails. *Acta Cytol.* **26**, 422.

Langer H (1957) Epidemiologische and klinische Untersuchungen bei Onychomykosen. *Arch. Klin. Exp. Dermatol.* **204**, 624.

Leyden J.J., Decherd J.W. & Goldschmidt H. (1972) Exfoliative cytology in the diagnosis of psoriasis of nails. *Cutis* **10**, 701.

McAleer R. (1981) Fungal infections of the nails in Western Australia. *Mycopathologica* **73**, 115.

Marks R. & Dawber R.P.R. (1971) Skin surface biospy – an improved technique for the examination of the horny layer. *Br. J. Dermatol.* **84**, 113.

Marren P. & Powell S. (1992) Contact sensitivity to triconazole and other imidazoles. *Contact Dermatitis* **27**, 129–130.

Meisel C.W. & Quadripur (1992) Onychomycosis due to *Hendersonula toruloidea*. *Hautnah* **6**, 232–234.

Milne L.J.R. (1989) Direct microscopy. In: *Medical Mycology – a Practical Approach*, eds Evans E.G.V. & Richardson M.D., pp. 17–45. IRL Press, Oxford.

Moore M.K. (1978) Skin and nail infections caused by non-dermatophyte filamentous fungi. *Mykosen* Suppl. 1, 128–132.

Munoz P., Moreno S., Berengues J. *et al.* (1991) Fluconazole-related hepatoxicity in patients with AIDS. *Arch. Intern. Med.* **151**, 1020–1021.

Negroni P. (1976) Erythrasma of the nails. *Med. Cut. I.G.A.* 5, 349.

Ornsberg P. (1980) *Scopulariopsis brevicaulis* in nails. *Dermatologica* **161**, 259.

Pardo-Castello V. & Pardo O.A. (1960) *Diseases of the Nails.* CC Thomas, Springfield, IL.

Petranyi G., Meingassner J.G. & Mieth H. (1987) Antifungal activity of the allylamine derivative, terbinafine, *in vitro. Antimicrob. Agents Chemother.* **31**, 1365–1368.

Polak A. (1988) Mode of action of morpholine derivatives. In: *Antifungal Drugs, ed.* St Georgiev V. *Ann. NY Acad. Sci.* **544**, 221–228.

Presser S.E. & Blank H. (1981) Cimetidine; adjunct in treatment of tinea capitis. *Lancet* **1**, 108.

Puntithalingham E. & English M.P. (1975) *Pyrenochaeta unguis-hominis* sp. *nov.* on human toenails. *Trans. Br. Mycol. Soc.* **64**, 539.

Reinel D., Reckers-Czaschka R. & Zaug M. (1990) Local therapy der Onychomykose mit Amorolfine 5%. *Nagellack. Zbl. Haut. Geschl. Kr.* **157**, 1004–1005.

Roberts S.O.B. & MacKenzie D.W.R. (1979) Mycology. In: *Textbook of Dermatology*, 3rd edn, eds Rook A., Wilkinson D.S. & Ebling F.J.G., Blackwell Scientific Publications, Oxford.

Robles Martinez W., Bhogal B., Morrell C.A. *et al.* (1990) The use of fluorescent lectin stains to identify fungi in clinical material from skin. *Br. J. Dermatol.* **123**, Suppl 37, 64.

Roseeuw D. & De Doncker P. (1993) New approaches to the treatment of onychomycosis. *J. Am. Acad. Dermatol.* **29**, 545–550.

Rosenthal S.N. & Wise R.S. (1960) Studies concerning the development of resistance to griseofulvin by dermatophytes. *Arch. Dermatol.* **81**, 684.

Samman P.D. (1982) Management of disorders of the nails. *Clin. Exp. Dermatol.* 7, 189.

Scher R.K. & Ackerman B.A. (1980a) The value of nail biopsy for demonstrating fungi not demonstrated by microbiologic techniques. *Am. J. Dermatopathol.* **2**, 55.

Scher R.K. & Ackerman B.A. (1980b) Histologic differential diagnosis of onychomycosis and psoriasis of the nail unit from cornified cells of the nail bed alone. *Am. J. Dermatopathol.* **21**, 255.

Seebacher J. (1966) Untersuchungen uber die Dilzflora kranker und gesunder zehennagel. *Mykosen* **11**, 893–902.

Shellow W.R. & Koplon B.S. (1968) Green striped nails: chromonychia due to *Pseudomonas aeruginosa. Arch. Dermatol.* 97, 149–153.

South D.A. & Farber E. (1980) Urea ointment in nonsurgical avulsion of nail dystrophies: reapraisal. *Cutis* **21**, 609.

Stone O.J. (1975) Chronic paronychia in which hair was a foreign body. *Int. J. Dermatol.* **19**, 661.

Stone O.J. & Mullins F.J. (1968) Chronic paronychia in children. *Clin. Pediatr.* 7, 104–107.

Stone O.J., Mullins J.F. & Head E.S. (1964) Chronic paronychia. Occupational material. *Arch. Environ. Health* **9**, 585–588.

Strauss J.S. (1982) Ketoconazole and the liver. *J. Am. Acad. Dermatol.* **6**, 546.

Suarez S.M., Silvers D.N., Scher R.K. *et al.* (1991) Histologic evaluation of nail clippings for diagnosing onychomycosis. *Arch. Dermatol.* **127**, 1517–1519.

Suringa D.W.R. (1970) Treatment of superficial onychomycosis with topically applied glutaraldehyde. *Arch. Dermatol.* **102**, 163.

Sutton B.C. & Dyko B.J. (1989) Revision of *Hendersonula. Mycol Res.* **93**, 466–488.

Tappeiner J. & Male O. (1966) Nagelveranderungen durch Schimmel pilze. *Dermatol. Int.* **5**, 145–148.

Tkach J.R. & Rinaldi M.G. (1982) Severe hepatitis associated with ketoconazole therapy for mucocutaneous candidosis. *Cutis* **29**, 482.

Tosti A., Guerra L., Mozelli R. *et al.* (1992) Role of foods in the pathogenesis of chronic paronychia. *J. Am. Acad. Dermatol.* **27**, 706–710.

Vanbreuseghem R. (1977) Prévalence des onychomycoses au Zaire particulièrement chez les coupeurs de canne à sucre. *Ann. Soc. Belg. Med. Trop.* **57**, 7.

Walshe M.M. & English M.P. (1966) Fungi in nails. *Br. J. Dermatol.* **78**, 198.

Wantzig G.L. & Thomsen K. (1983) Acute paronychia after high-dose methotrexate therapy. *Arch. Dermatol.* **119**, 623–624.

Weismann K., Knudsen E.A. & Pedersen C. (1988) White nails in AIDS/ARC due to *Trichophyton rubrum* infection. *Clin. Exp. Dermatol.* **13**, 24–25.

Willemsen M., de Doncker P. & Willems J. (1992) Post treatment itraconazole levels in the nail. *J. Am. Acad. Dermatol.* **26**, 731–735.

White N.I. & Clayton Y.M. (1982) The treatment of fungus and yeast infections of nails by the method of chemical removal. *Clin. Exp. Dermatol.* 7, 273.

Zaias N. (1966) Superficial white onychomycosis. *Sabouraudia* **5**, 99–103.

Zaias N. (1972) Onychomycosis. *Arch. Dermatol.* **105**, 263–274.

Zaias N. (1990) *The Nail in Health and Disease*, 2nd edn. Lange & Appleton, CN.

Zaias N. & Drachman D. (1983) A method for the determination of drug effectiveness in onychomycosis. *J. Am. Acad. Dermatol.* **9**, 912.

Zaias N. & Taplin D. (1966) Improved preparation for the diagnosis of mycologic diseases. *Arch. Dermatol.* **93**, 608.

Zaias N., Oertel I. & Elliot D.F. (1969) Fungi in toe-nails. *J. Invest. Dermatol.* **53**, 140.

Other fungal infections

Sporotrichosis (Figs 4.56 & 4.57)

Sporotrichosis is a subcutaneous fungal infection caused by the dimorphic yeast, *Sporothrix schenckii.* The infection follows implantation of the organism which is found in the environment in subtropical and tropical countries. The primary site of infection is commonly located on an exposed site and the nail fold is often involved (Figs 4.56 & 4.57). The area becomes oedematous and discharges pus and serous fluid. Secondary lesions along the course of draining lymphatics may develop subsequently. The

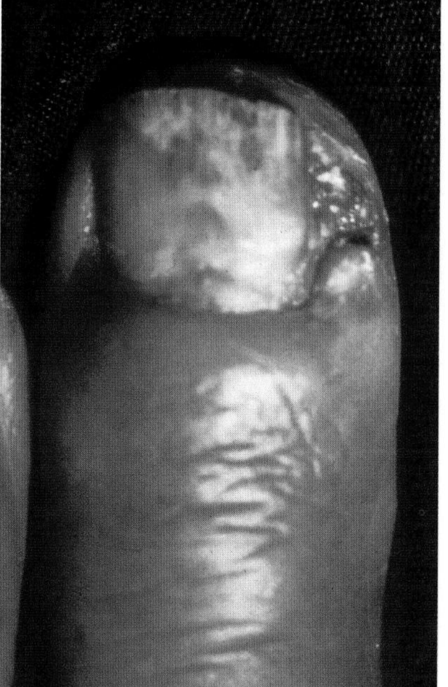

Fig. 4.56.

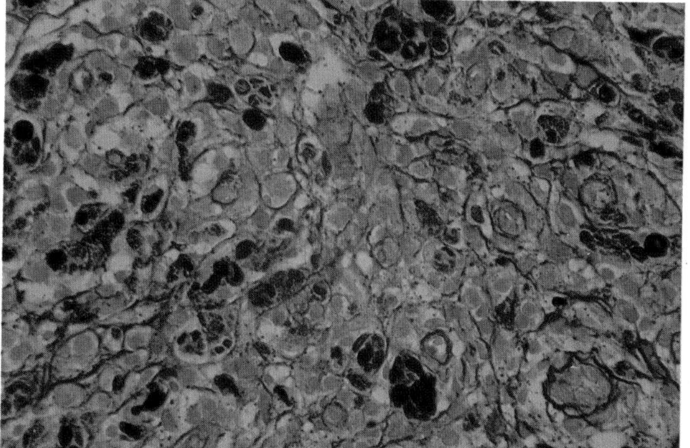

Fig. 4.57.

Figs 4.56 & 4.57. Sporotrichosis (*Sporothrix schenckii*).

best method of diagnosis is by culture although biopsy may reveal round or oval yeasts or asteroid bodies, yeast surrounded by a refractile eosinophilic halo. The usual treatment is a saturated solution of potassium iodide; oral itraconazole is an alternative.

Patients with chromoblastomycosis and coccidioidomycosis may present with a clinical picture of DLSO resulting from the invasion of the undersurface of the nail by the deep mycotic agent (Zaias, 1990).

Other infections

Herpes simplex (Figs 4.58–4.62)

Distal digital herpes simplex infections may affect the terminal phalanx as herpetic whitlows or start as an acute, intensely painful, paronychia. Recurrent forms are generally less severe and have a milder clinical course than the initial infection. Herpes simplex virus types I and II are found in equal frequency in digital herpes simplex.

After an incubation period of 3–7 days during which local tenderness, erythema and swelling may develop, a crop of vesicles appears at the portal of entry into the skin. The vesicles typically are distributed around the paronychium and on the volar digital skin and somewhat resemble a pyogenic infection of the fingertip. Close inspection, however, will reveal the classical pale, raised vesicles surrounded by an erythematous border. An acutely painful whitlow may develop and extend under the distal free edge of the nail and into the nail bed. A distinct predilection for the thumb and index finger was noted by La Rossa and Hamilton (1971) but any finger may be involved. Several fingers may be affected together. For 1–14 days the vesicles gradually increase in size, often coalescing into large, honeycomb-like bullae. New crops of lesions may appear during this time. Vesicular fluid is clear early in the disease but may become turbid, seropurulent or even haemorrhagic in the later stages. At times, the pale yellow colour of the vesicles will suggest pyogenic infection, yet frank pus is not usually obtained. Patients complain of tenderness and severe throbbing in the affected digit. Coexisting primary herpetic infections of the mouth and fingernails suggest autoinoculation of the virus into the nail tissues as a result of nailbiting or fingersucking (Muller & Hermann, 1970). We have seen coexisting primary herpetic infection of the penis and the thumb (Fig. 4.59).

Radiating pain along the C7 distribution is sometimes noted and may predict the onset of recurrent herpetic whitlows. Lymphangitis is almost always seen in periungual herpes simplex and may even precede the vesicles by 1 or 2 days. It usually starts from the wrist and extends to the axilla with enlarged and tender lymph nodes.

Numbness and hypoaesthesia following the acute episode has been observed (Chang & Gorbach, 1977). Persistent lymphoedema may also occur.

The diagnosis of herpetic infection can be made readily by examining the margin of the vesicles for the characteristic multinucleated 'balloon' giant cells, in stained smears. Characteristically, the nuclei of herpes simplex virus (HSV)-infected cells appear steel-blue and homogeneous. Viral culture is confirmatory and is usually positive within 24–48 h. Negative staining of blister fluid may show herpes viruses by electron microscopy. Monoclonal antibodies allow one to confirm the diagnosis by immunofluorescence and to differentiate type 1 from type 2 HSV.

Differential diagnosis

It is important to exclude primary or recurrent herpes simplex infection in the differential diagnosis of every

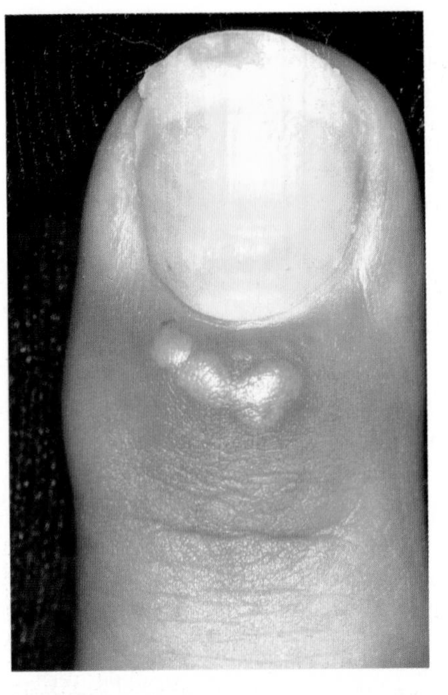
Fig. 4.58.

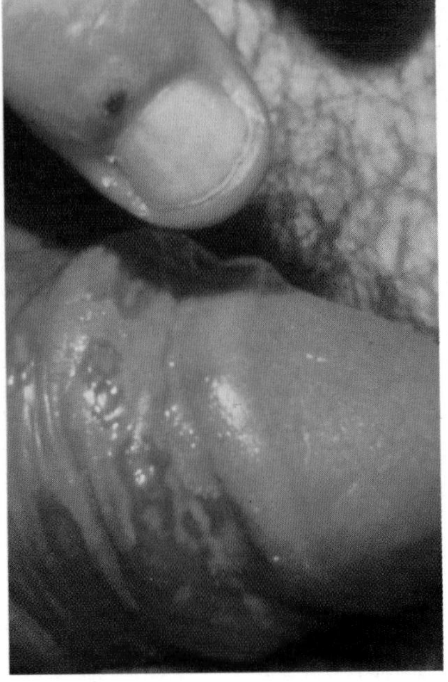
Fig. 4.59.

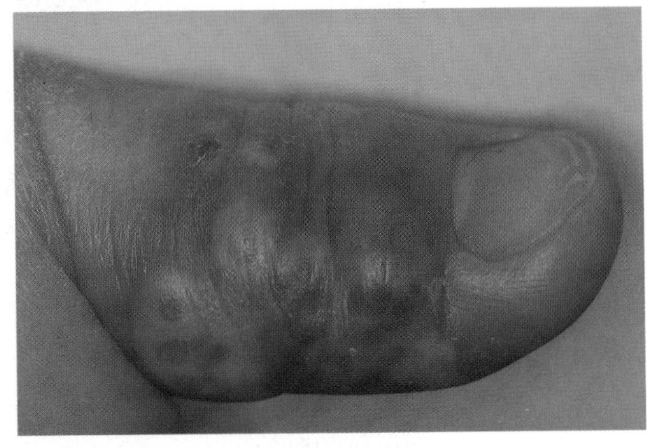
Fig. 4.60.

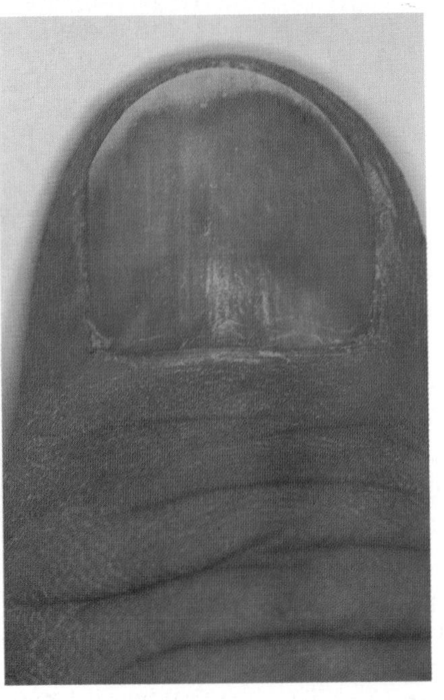
Fig. 4.61.

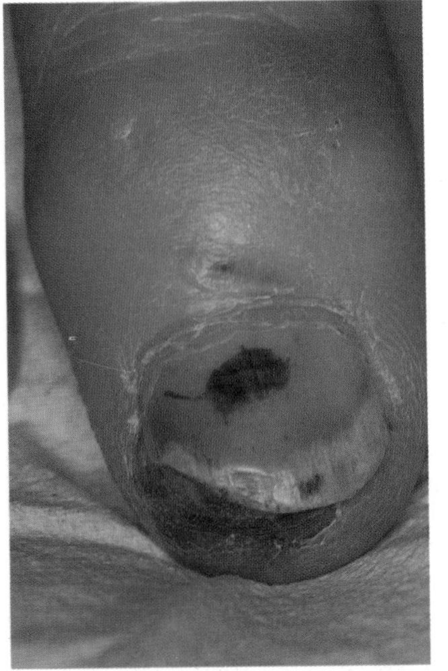
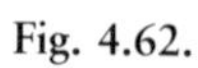
Fig. 4.62.

Figs 4.58–4.62. Herpes simplex infection affecting various components of the nail apparatus.

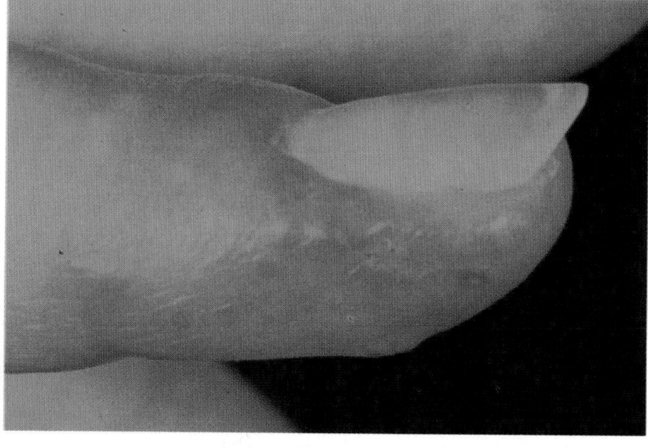

Fig. 4.63. *Mycobacterium marinum* infection mimicking herpes paronychia (J. Savoie, Canada).

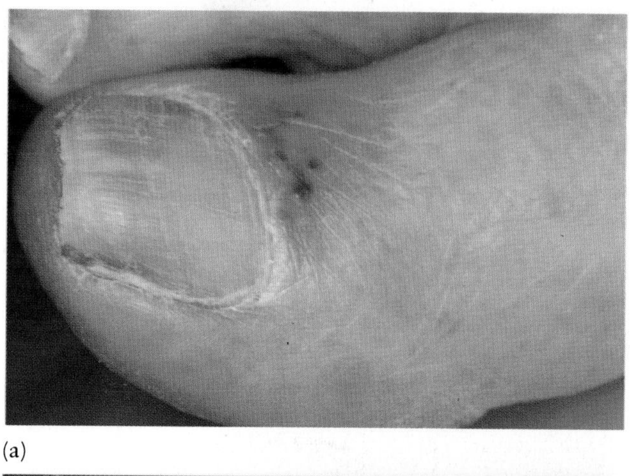

(a)

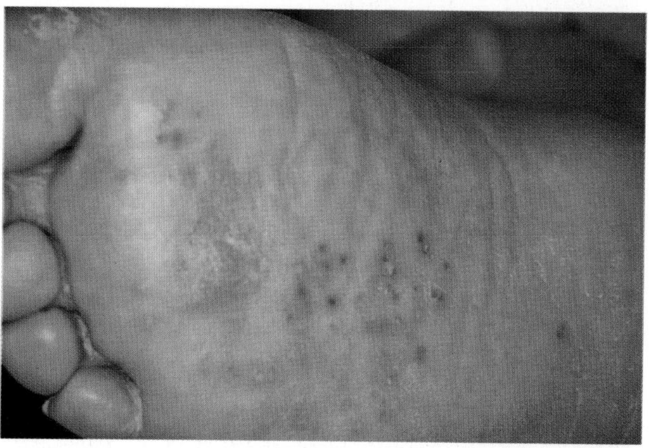

(b)

Fig. 4.64. (a & b) Herpes zoster.

finger infection. The typical appearance of the lesions with a disproportionate intensity of pain, the absence of pus in the confluent multiloculated vesiculopustular lesions and the lack of increased tension in the finger pulp aid in distinguishing this slow healing infection from a bacterial infection or paronychia (La Rossa & Hamilton, 1971).

Herpetic paronychia-like infection due to *Mycobacterium marinum* has been reported (Savoie, 1989) (Fig. 4.63).

Herpes zoster infections which may affect the proximal nail fold like herpes simplex, also involve the entire sensory dermatome (Fig. 4.64). The pustules of primary cutaneous *Neisseria gonorrhoeae* infection may resemble herpes simplex on the rare occasion when it occurs on the finger (Fig. 6.5). The diagnosis is established by Gram stain and bacteriological culture.

Treatment is primarily aimed at symptomatic relief and avoidance of secondary infection. Herpes simplex is a preventable infection. Gloves should always be worn on both hands for procedures such as intubation, removal of dentures or providing oral care (Hamory *et al.*, 1975) despite the additional costs involved (Orkin, 1975). While acycolvir may well ease the symptoms of the acute episode a single course will not affect the chances of relapse. Continuous oral acyclovir may prevent frequent relapses in patients with recurrent herpes simplex infections, but use of this regimen may be followed by drug resistance.

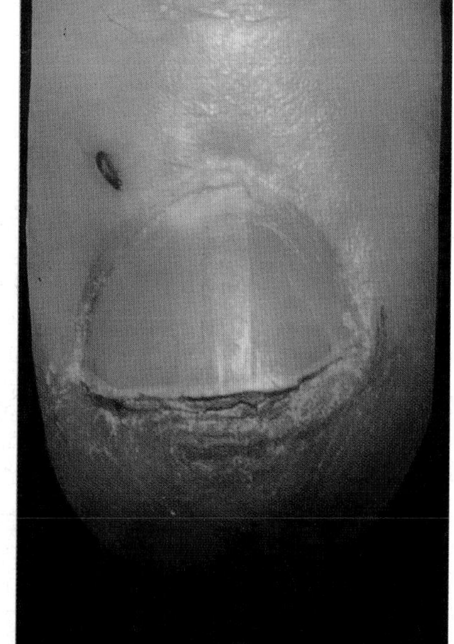

Fig. 4.65. Primary cutaneous gonorrhoea (courtesy of J.E. Fitzpatrick, USA).

References

Chang T. & Gorbach S.L. (1977) Primary and recurrent whitlow. *Int. J. Dermatol.* **16**, 752.

Hamory B.H., Osterman C.A. & Wenzel R.P. (1975) Herpetic whitlow. *New Engl. J. Med.* **292**, 268.

La Rossa D. & Hamilton R. (1971) Herpes simplex infections of the digits. *Arch. Surg.* **102**, 600.

Muller S.A. & Hermann E.C. (1970) Association of stomatitis and paronychias due to herpes simplex. *Arch. Dermatol.* **101**, 394.

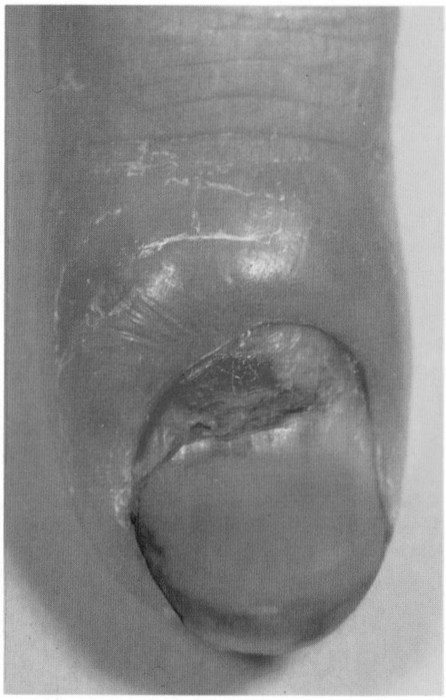

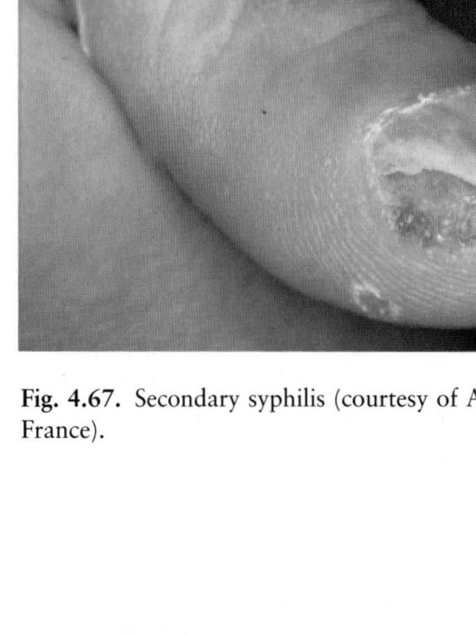

Fig. 4.66. Primary syphilis (courtesy of de Graciansky & Boulle, Paris, France).

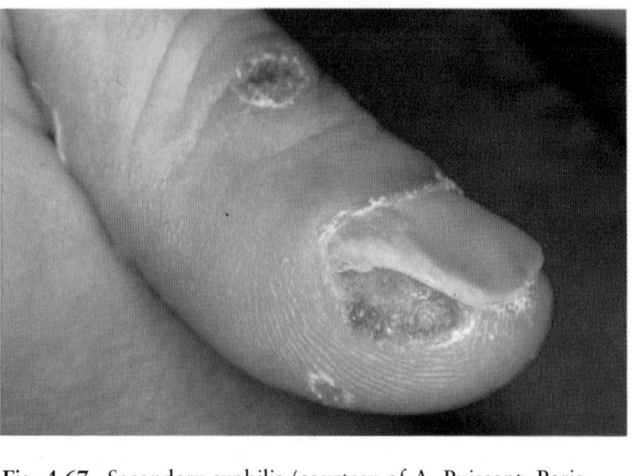

Fig. 4.67. Secondary syphilis (courtesy of A. Puissant, Paris, France).

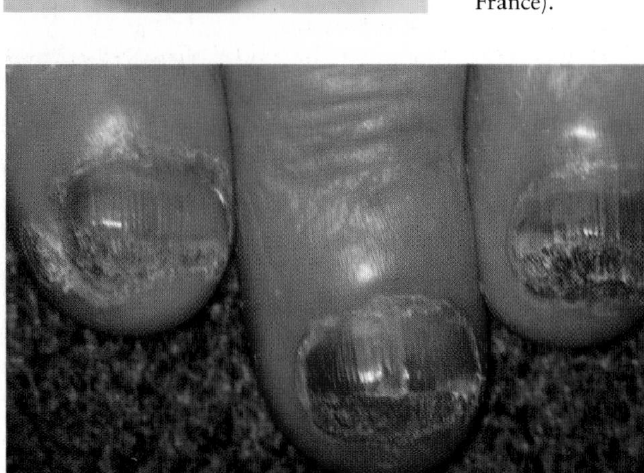

Fig. 4.68. Secondary syphilis (courtesy of M. Geniaux, Bordeaux, France).

Orkin F.K. (1975) Herpetic whitlow. *New Engl. J. Med.* **292**, 648–649.
Savoie J.M. (1989) Infection à *Mycobacterium marinum* (forme sporotrichoide). *Nouv. Dermatol.* **8**, 524–525.

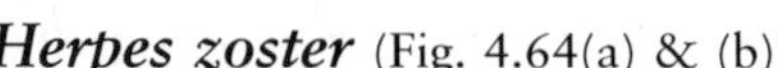

Herpes zoster (Fig. 4.64(a) & (b))

Herpes zoster is rarely seen around the nail. It may involve the proximal nail fold showing grouped vesicles. Nail bed involvement is particularly painful and leaves small subungual roundish haemorrhagic spots slowly growing out with the nail. Herpes zoster may produce transverse leuconychia by a uniform but temporary disturbance in the normal activity of each fingernail matrix, causing abnormal keratinization (Zigmor & Deluty, 1980).

Stained Tzanck smears reveal multinucleate epidermal cells which do not allow differentiation from herpes simplex.

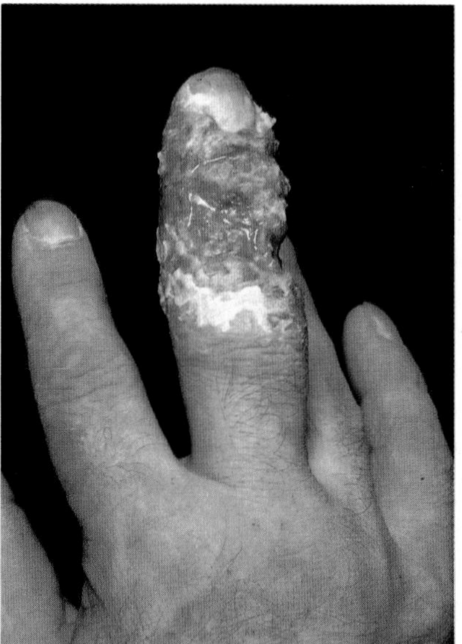

Fig. 4.69. Tertiary syphilis (courtesy of G.K. Steigleider, Cologne, Germany).

Figs 4.66–4.69. Syphilis of the nail apparatus.

Reference

Zigmor J. & Deluty S. (1980) Acquired leukonychia striata. *Int. J. Dermatol.* **19**, 49–50.

Gonorrhoea

The hallmark of disseminated gonococcaemia is the appearance of skin lesions (Silva & Wilson, 1979). The most common is a vesicopustule which occurs juxta-articularly over the extensor surfaces of the hands, dorsal surfaces of the toes and around the nails. Haemorrhagic bullae occur in smaller numbers but in the same area. The third dermatological manifestation is the appearance of focal petechiae over the digits or the medial aspects of the ankles.

Primary extragenital cutaneous gonorrhoea (Fig. 4.65) acquired sexually is extremely rare (Fitzpatrick *et al.*, 1981). It presents with a fingertip abscess extending under the nail plate with peripheral erythema from a pustular lesion. The diagnosis of gonococcal skin infection is often not entertained until unexpected findings on the Gram stain prompt further questions and culture.

Histopathology shows leucocytoclastic vasculitis with endothelial swelling, fibrinoid degeneration of vessel walls, extravasated erythrocytes and intraepidermal pustules which form from spongiform pustules.

References

Fitzpatrick J.E., Gramsted N.D. & Tyler H. (1981) Primary extragenital cutaneous gonorrhea. *Cutis* 27, 479–480.

Silva J. & Wilson K. (1979) Disseminated gonococcal infection. *Cutis* 24, 601–606.

Syphilis (Figs 4.66–4.69)

Chancres of the fingers (due to occupational infection or sexual contact) may present as periungual erosion or ulceration which may sometimes involve the nail bed, as in the syphilitic whitlow of Hutchinson, a paronychia, or it may resemble a pyogenic granuloma. A crusty ulceration covering the free edge of the nail in a half-moon shape or developing in one of the lateral nail folds has been reported. In this location chancres are usually painful and have a more chronic clinical course than elsewhere. Regional lymphadenopathy accompanies the primary lesion: chancres of the fingers are associated with painless unilateral, epitrochlear and/or axillary nodes. The affected lymph nodes are discretely enlarged, hard and non-suppurating.

Primary syphilis of the fingers accounted for 14% of extragenital chancres according to Starzycki (1983) who reported six cases. Of these, two had chancres on both their fingers and genitals resulting from sexual foreplay.

In the secondary stage, the nail changes may be divided into two main groups: in the first group the changes due to the involvement of the matrix seem to be confined to the nails themselves; in the second group the changes are those in which the nail abnormalities are a consequence of some inflammatory condition of the peri- and subungual tissues (Figs 4.67 & 4.68) and are without specific characteristics.

Various forms of 'dry' onychia have been described: unusual brittleness with a tendency to splitting and fissuring ('onyxis craquelé'), onycholysis, pitting with a linear arrangement of the pits from the root forwards and elkonyxis in the lunula region. Beau's lines may be seen, sometimes latent onychomadesis appears, and rarely, total nail loss. The whole nail plate may become dull, dry and thickened with a distinct line of demarcation between the affected and the distal portions which retain polish and colour, but a wedge-like thickening of the free end has been described.

Onychogryphosis may occur on the toenails. Dark or brownish pigmentation of the nail may involve the nail plate entirely or as longitudinal pigmented streaks (Vörner, 1907) (Fig. 4.68). The very rare amber-coloured nail plates resembling false nails were considered by Degos (1981) to be a characteristic change of late syphilis.

Pigmentation of the nail occurring over papules in the nail bed (Adamson & McDonagh, 1911) is seen in the second group of syphilitic nails which is more common than 'onychia sicca'. The nail lesions are secondary to local inflammatory disturbances.

Milian's (1936) lilac arch, located at the distal nail bed, is no longer considered to be a manifestation of syphilis. It probably corresponds to a prominent onychodermal band (Baran & Gioanni, 1968). The 'isolated papule of the nail bed' (Heller, 1927) occurs at the time of the exanthem. A pea- to bean-sized patch appears under the normally transparent nail. At first the patch is intensely red, later yellow. The nail plate becomes thinned and fractured at this spot. This condition was said to be always limited to one finger; in fact, nearly all the fingernails may be involved (Adamson & McDonagh, 1911).

In the 'moist' forms, several nails may be affected, but often only one is involved such as the thumb or the great toe. The lesion begins with erythema, swelling and pain in the proximal tissues surrounding the nail. Next the proximal and lateral nail folds separate from the nail plate allowing discharge of the entrapped inflammatory exudate (Kingsbury *et al.*, 1972). This results in a 'discharging horseshoe-shaped ulcer'. The nail blackens and falls, exposing an unhealthy looking ulcer (Adams & McDonagh, 1911) with permanent nail deformity or anonychia. This may be the end result of untreated syphilitic paronychia. Multiple inflammatory paronychia may also occur in congenital syphilis with active manifestations (Pardo-Castello & Pardo, 1960).

Danielyan and Mokrousov (1979) report an unusual delay of 3 years before the appearance of a normal nail following adequate treatment of early secondary syphilis with penicillin. The patient was a greengrocer; there may have been minor occupational trauma which could have resulted in the Koebner phenomenon causing oxychauxis.

The differential diagnosis includes acute septic paronychia which is generally more painful, and chronic par onychia (Fig. 4.69).

Tertiary syphilis (Fig. 4.69) very rarely affects the nail apparatus as gummata which result in secondary necrosis with permanent nail loss when the matrix has been destroyed (Fox, 1941). All individuals who have been exposed to infectious syphilis, occupationally or otherwise, within the preceding 3 months should be treated even if they show no evidence of having been infected (Felman *et al.*, 1982).

Pinta

See Chapter 2.

References

Adamson H.G. & McDonagh J.E.R. (1911) Two unusual forms of syphilitic nails: with some general remarks upon syphilis of the nails. *Br. J. Dermatol.* **23**, 68.

Baran R. & Gioanni T. (1968) Half-and-half nail. *Bull. Soc. Fr. Dermatol. Syph.* **75**, 399.

Danielyan E.E. & Mokrousov M.S. (1979) Involvement of nail plates in a patients with secondary early syphilis. *Vestn. Derm. Vener.* **12**, 59.

Degos R. (1981) *Precis de Dermatologie*, p. 1135. Flammarion, Paris.

Felman Y.M., Phil M. & Nikitas J.A. (1982) Primary syphilis. *Cutis* **29**, 122.

Fox H. (1941) Obstinate syphilitic onychia and gumma of the nose sucessfully treated by fever therapy. *Arch. Dermatol.* **44**, 1155.

Heller J. (1927) Die Krankheiten der Nagel. In: *Jadassohn's Handbuch Haut und Geschlechtskrankheiten*, Bd XIII/2. Springer, Berlin.

Kingsbury D.H., Chester E.C. & Jansen G.T. (1972) Syphilitic paronychia, an unusual complaint. *Arch. Dermatol.* **105**, 458.

Milian G. (1936) Les maladies des ongles. In: *Nouvelle Pratique Dermatologique*, 7, ed. Darier J. Masson, Paris.

Pardo-Castello V. & Pardo O. (1960) *Diseases of Nails*, 3rd edn. Charles C. Thomas, Springfield, IL.

Starzycki Z. (1983) Primary syphilis of the fingers. *Br. J. Vener. Dis.* **59**, 169–171.

Vörner H. (1907) *Ueber Nagelpigmentation bei sekundärer Syphilis*, p. 2483. Muenchener Medizinische Wochenschrift.

Leprosy (Figs 4.70–4.77)

Leprosy can cause many nail changes which have been observed in up to 64% of infected patients (Patki & Baran, 1991) (Table 4.5).

Leprosy is primarily an infection of the peripheral nervous system, caused by *Mycobacterium leprae.* Clinical presentations range from a total failure of cell-mediated resistance (lepromatous) to high but incomplete resistance (tuberculoid). The skin is involved as an integral part of the expression of this disease, and skin lesions are largely determined by the numbers of organisms present and the presence of effective immunological resistance. Tuberculoid or borderline tuberculoid forms where there are few organisms and multibacillary lepromatous and borderline lepromatous forms, are examples of this process.

Table 4.5. Classification of nail changes in leprosy (from Patki & Baran, 1991, with permission)

Neuropathy and trauma
Subungual haematoma
Onycholysis
Onychauxis
Onychogryphosis
Racket nail
Pterygium unguis (dorsal and ventral)
Ectopic nail
Spicule nail
Complete loss – anonychia
Vascular deficit
Thinning
Longitudinal splits
Onychauxis
Pterygium unguis (dorsal and ventral)
Atrophy
Infections
Bacterial
Fungal
Miscellaneous
Diffusion of lunula (pseudomacrolunula)
Leuconychia
Pallor
Hapalonychia
Beau's lines

Nail changes in leprosy can be caused by neuropathy and trauma, vascular impairment, infections and miscellaneous modifications. Often more than one factor will be important.

Trophic changes are responsible for modifications of the lunula in upper limbs; it becomes greyish and less sharply delineated from the rest of the subungual area resulting in an apparent leuconychia as a pseudomacrolunula.

In tuberculoid leprosy neurological involvement is usually asymmetrical and appears early in the course of the disease usually in areas of visible dermatological change. Nerve changes in lepromatous leprosy occur more slowly and are usually symmetrical producing a 'stocking-and-glove' anaesthesia, but paradoxically, nail changes in tuberculoid and lepromatous patients are similar, despite wide differences in pathology. Factors associated with only lepromatous disease are invasion of the bones of terminal phalanges by lepromatous granulomas and endarteritis occurring during type 2 lepra reactions. These may result in multiple Beau's lines (Patki, 1990b) and dorsal pterygium (Patki & Mehta, 1989).

The phalanges develop osteolysis (Fig. 4.72) and there is progressive telescoping of the digital bones (Queneau *et*

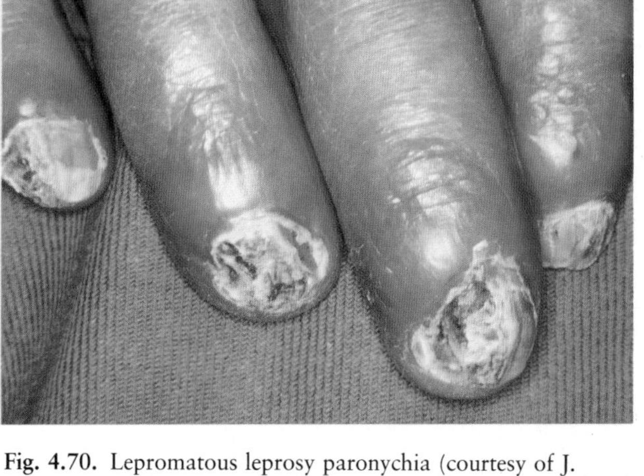

Fig. 4.70. Lepromatous leprosy paronychia (courtesy of J. Delacretaz, Lausanne).

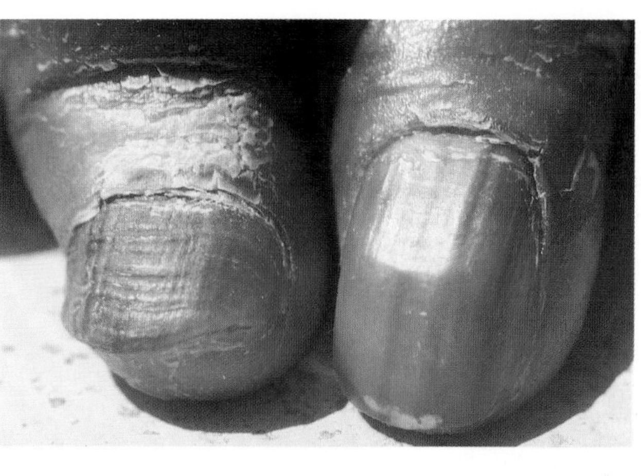
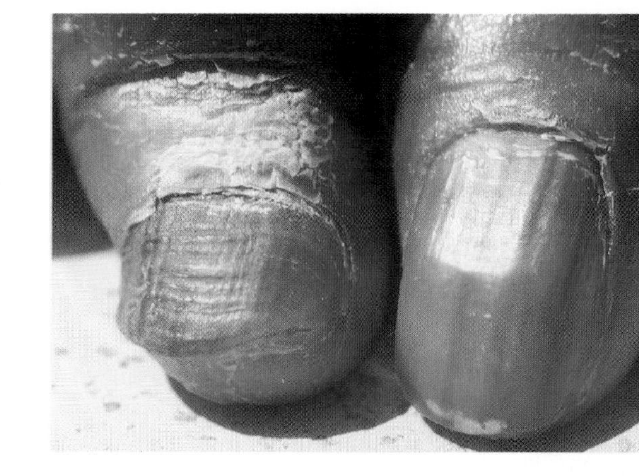

Fig. 4.71. Racket nail due to acroosteolysis (courtesy P. Saint-André, Bamako).

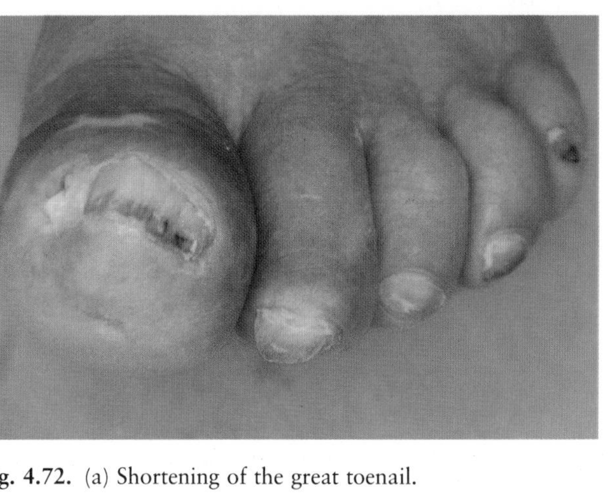

Fig. 4.72. (a) Shortening of the great toenail.

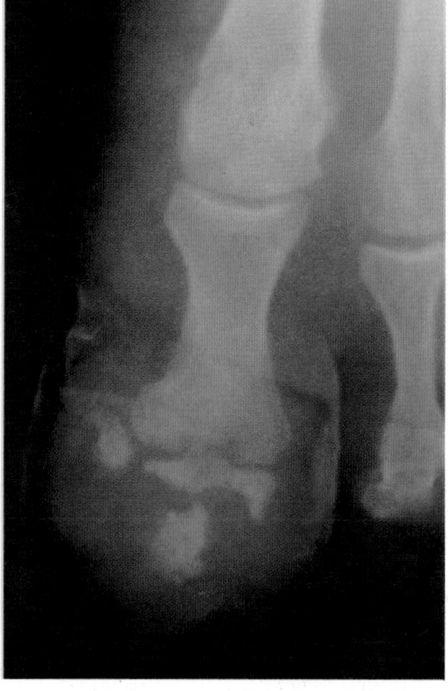

Fig. 4.72. (b) Same patient presenting with acroosteolysis.

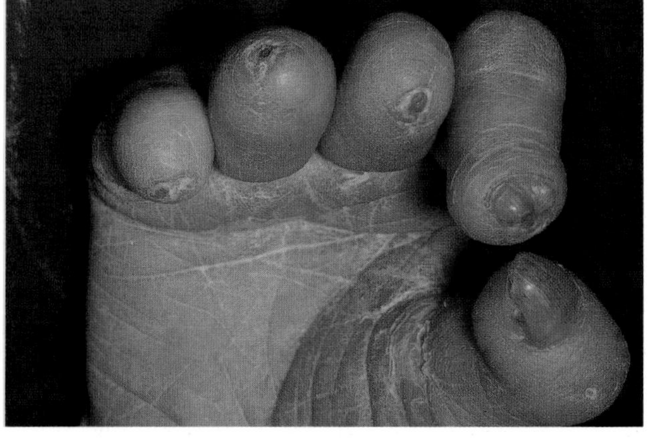

Fig. 4.73. Same patient presenting with acroosteolysis in the fingers (courtesy D. Wallach, Paris).

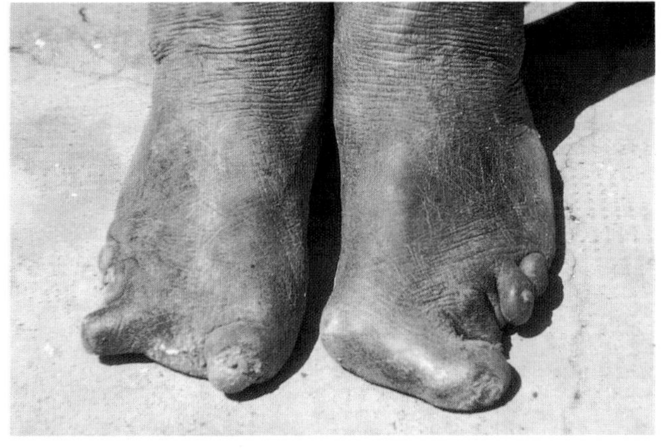

Fig. 4.74. (Courtesy P. Saint-André, Bamako).

Figs 4.70–4.77. Leprosy of varying degrees of severity in the nail apparatus and associated tissues.

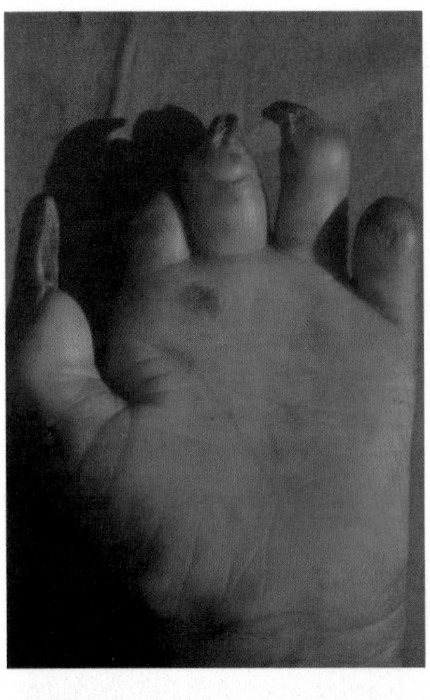

Fig. 4.75. Claw-like nails.

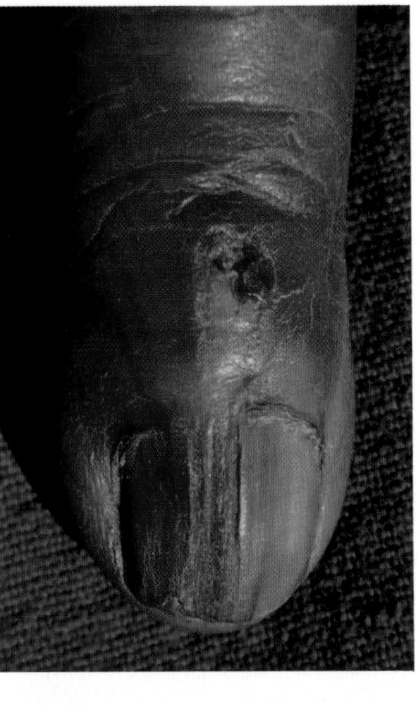

Fig. 4.76. Dorsal pterygion (courtesy of A.H. Patki).

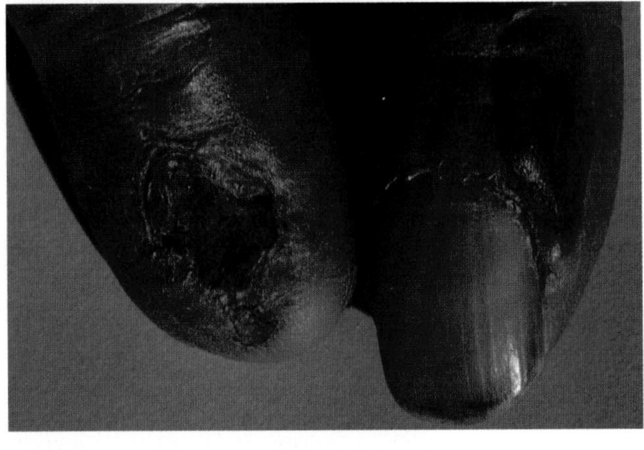

Fig. 4.77. (Courtesy of A.H. Patki).

Fig. 4.78. Leishmaniasis affecting dorsal aspect of the fingers and proximal nail fold of the index finger (courtesy of P.G. Butler).

al., 1982). When deformities such as 'preacher's hand' occur, clawnails (Fig. 4.73) and other unusual appearances are produced. Dystrophic changes may occur in the nails with progessive destruction leaving small fragments at the corner of the nail bed, dorsal or ventral pterygium (Patki, 1990a).

Painless abscesses may occur periungually with destruction of the nails. This appears more often in the upper than lower limbs. Delacrétaz (1980) presented a case of lepromatous leprosy paronychia demonstrating Hansen's bacilli in a cantharidin-induced blister on the distal part of the proximal nail fold and within the proximal nail debris.

The bare-foot state, the sitting position normally assumed and footwear, produce anatomical and physiological changes in the feet and legs. They lead to pathological processes or modify those that pre- or coexist.

Tachikawa (1941) studied 50 cases of nail leprosy histologically. The leprous infiltration in the nail bed was caused by changes in nodular leprosy, now called lepromatous leprosy, while atrophic changes followed injuries and infections in neural leprosy, presently termed tuberculoid leprosy.

References

Delacrétaz J. (1980) Les maladies infectieuses de l'ongle, *Jahresversammlung der Schweizerischen Gesellschaft für Dermatologie und Venerologie,* Zurich 3, 4 October 1980.

Patki A.H. (1990a) Pterygium inversum in a patient with leprosy. *Arch. Dermatolatol.* **126,** 110.

Patki A.H. (1990b) Multiple Beau's lines due to recurrent erythema nodosum leprosum. *Arch. Dermatol.* **126,** 110–111.

Patki A.H. & Baran R. (1991) Nail changes in leprosy. *Semin. Dermatol.* **10,** 77–81.

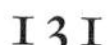

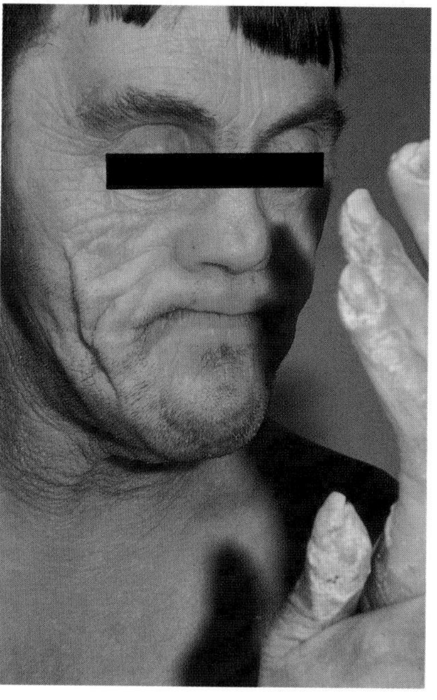

Fig. 4.79. (Courtesy J. Beurey, Nancy, France).

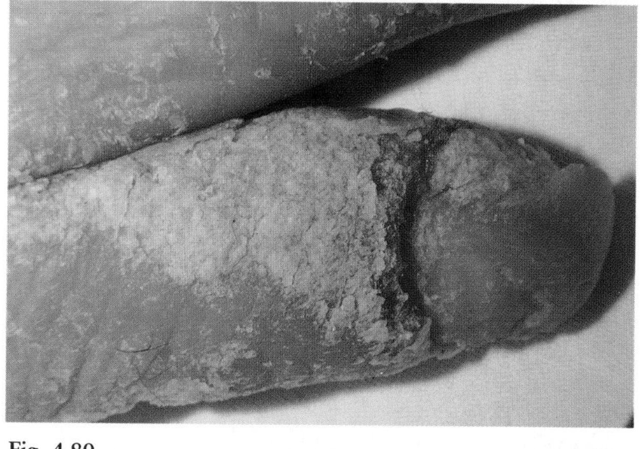

Fig. 4.80.

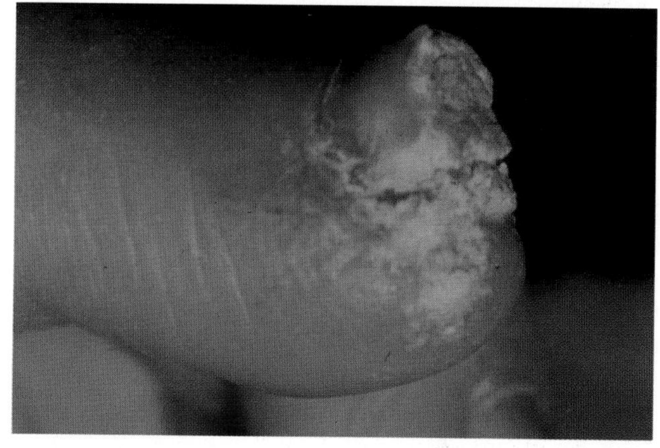

Fig. 4.81. Isolated subungual hyperkeratosis (courtesy of R. De Paoli and V. Marks, USA).

Fig. 4.79–4.81. Scabies affecting the nail apparatus – Norwegian variety in Down's syndrome.

Patki A.H. & Metha J.M. (1989) Pterygium unguis in a patient with recurrent type 2 lepra reaction. *Cutis* **44**, 311–312.

Queneau P., Gabbai A., Perpoint B. *et al.* (1982) Acro-ostéolyses au cours de la lèpre. A propos de 19 observations person nelles. *Rev. Rhum.* **49**(2), 111.

Tachikawa N. (1941) Leprosy of the nail. Pathological studies. *La Lepro* **12**, 111–182 (Jap).

Leishmaniasis (Fig. 4.78)

Cutaneous leishmaniasis lesions, with central granular ulceration and an elevated papular border, may involve the dorsal aspect of the distal phalanx. Levamisole has been successfully used therapeutically in 28 cases of chronic cutaneous leishmaniasis (Butler, 1982).

In post-Kalaazar dermal leishmaniasis, a characteristic greyish discoloration of the skin is most noticeable on the hands, the nails and other sites, and has resulted in the condition called the 'black disease' (Moschella, 1975).

References

Butler P.G. (1982) Levamisole and immune response phenomena in cutaneous leishmaniasis. *J. Am. Acad. Dermatol.* **6**, 1070–1077.

Moschella S.L. (1975) Leismaniasis. In: *Dermatology*, eds Moschella S.L., Pillsbury D.M. & Hurley H.J., p. 807. W.B. Saunders, Philadelphia.

Trichinosis

Splinter haemorrhages have been known to occur in all nails simultaneously in trichinosis (Fisher, 1957). Under these circumstances nail biopsy may be diagnostically useful (Groff, 1983).

References

Fisher A.A. (1957) Subungual splinter haemorrhages associated with trichinosis. *Arch. Dermatol.* **75**, 572–573.

Groff J.W. (1983) Organisms and associated disease. *J. Assoc. Milit. Dermatol.* **9**, 72–75.

Scabies (Figs 4.79–4.81)

Norwegian scabies is a rare variety of scabies infestation of the skin in which the entire body, even the scalp, is affected by *Sarcoptes scabiei*. The lesions of Norwegian scabies have a predilection for areas of pressure and are strikingly different in clinical appearance to ordinary scabies. The hyperkeratotic lesions are accompanied by large, psoriasis-like accumulations of scales under the nails of the fingers and toes (Schiff & Ronchese, 1964). This type of scabies is most often seen in the old and infirm, the mentally defective, and during therapeutic immunosuppresion, as well as in AIDS.

Chronic eczematoid dermatosis, atopic eczema, lichen simplex and psoriasis may be mimicked by this condition (Haydon & Caplan, 1971); topical use of corticosteroids may alter the clinical appearance of scabies.

One of the characteristic manifestations of this condition is the existence of dystrophic nail changes. Even after seemingly successful treatment of hyperkeratotic scabies, this dystrophy persists and may be the most important marker of the persistence of this type of infestation. The mites survive in these dystrophic nails and later colonize the skin, first around the nail plates. From there they extend proximally (Kocsard, 1984) and may be inoculated into all parts of the body by the scratching finger. The subungual material with abundant mites may not respond to topical therapy alone. Frequent trimming of nails and scrubbing twice daily with gamma benzene hexachloride is recommended. In resistant cases this should be supplemented by surgical scrubs using a scabicide and/or by 40% urea nail dissolution and partial nail avulsion (De Paoli & Marks, 1987).

In the ordinary forms of scabies, the clinically normal nails are not usually involved. However the distal subungual area may provide a nidus for mites, a source for small epidemics (Scher, 1983). A single case presenting with nail infestation alone has been reported, in which a big toenail was raised by large accumulations of hyperkeratotic debris, containing innumerable mites and eggs (Saruta & Nakamizo, 1978). In another case, an infant of 10 months has developed involvement of the multiple nail plates on hands and feet (Sokolova & Sizov, 1989).

Histopathology shows that the hyponychium may be infested with *Sarcoptes hominis* (*Acarus scabiei*) in elderly people. Tangential biopsies of the hyponychial keratosis with the overlying free edge of the nail plate may show mite burrows containing mites, eggs and faeces. In Norwegian scabies, the nail may be elevated by marked subungual hyperkeratosis with alternating parakeratosis and orthokeratosis. Abundant mites are usually present. A heavy mixed infiltrate often containing many eosinophils is seen in the dermis.

Reported associations of crusted scabies are listed in Table 4.6.

Table 4.6. Reported associations of crusted scabies (from De Paoli & Marks, 1987, with permission)

Neurological or mental disorders
Down's syndrome (Fig. 4.79)
Senile dementia
Syringomyelia
Tabes dorsalis
Parkinson's disease

Nutritional disorders
Vitamin A deficiency
Beriberi
Malnutrition

Infectious disease
Leprosy
Tuberculosis
Bacillary dysentery

Immunosuppression or impaired immunity
Genetic
  Bloom's syndrome
Acquired
  Topical and systemic corticosteroids
  Immunosuppressive drugs
  Radiotherapy
  Lymphoreticular malignancies
  Acquired immune deficiency syndrome

Miscellaneous
Diabetes
Rheumatoid arthritis
Poor hygiene

References

De Paoli R. & Marks V.J. (1987) Crusted (Norwegian) scabies: Treatment of nail involvement. *J. Am. Acad. Dermatol.* **17**, 136–138.

Haydon J.R. & Caplan R.M. (1971) Epidemic scabies. *Arch. Dermatolatol.* **103**, 168.

Kocsard E. (1984) The dystrophic nail of keratotic scabies. *Am. J. Dermatopathol.* **6**, 308–309.

Saruta T. & Nakamizo Y. (1978) Usual scabies with nail infestation. *Arch. Dermatol.* **114**, 956.

Scher R.K. (1983) Subungual scabies. *Am. J. Dermatopathol.* **5**, 187.

Schiff B.L. & Ronchese F. (1964) Norwegian scabies. *Arch. Dermatol.* **89**, 236.

Sokolova T.V. & Sizovie A. (1989) A case with nail plate involvement in an infant suffering from scabies. *Vestr. Dermatol. Venerol.* **2**, 68–69.

Pediculosis

Interestingly pediculosis of the foot limited to the hallux has also been reported (Diemer, 1985) in a patient with onychomycosis of all toenails, which were thickened. Debridement of the right great toenail exposed multiple cavities, housing approximately 10–12 body lice. The arthropods quickly dispersed upon being disturbed, returning to the nail within minutes, disappearing into the tunnels, which were present in the nail.

Fig. 4.82. (Courtesy Pradinaud, French Guyana).

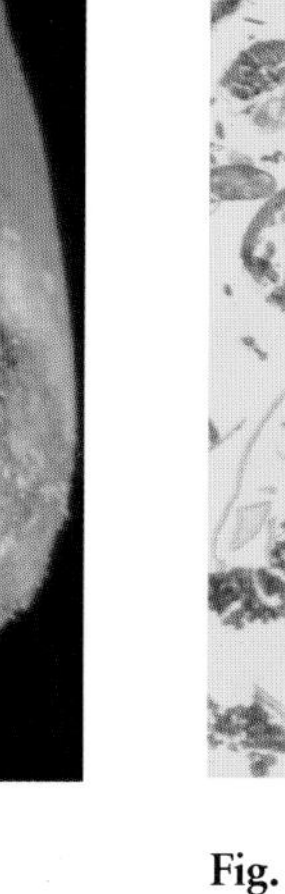

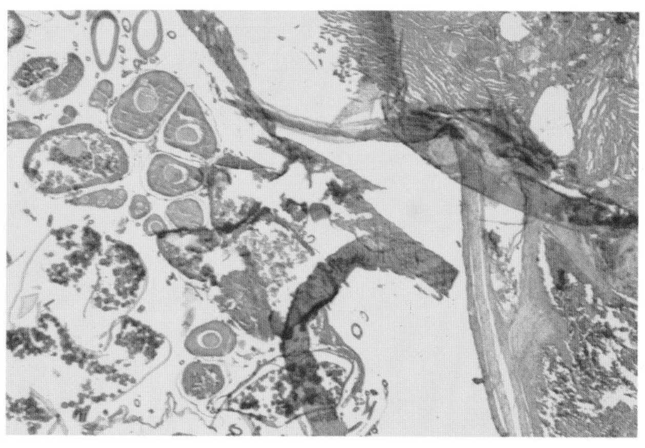

Fig. 4.84.

Fig. 4.83. (a) (Courtesy A. Basset, Strasbourg, France).

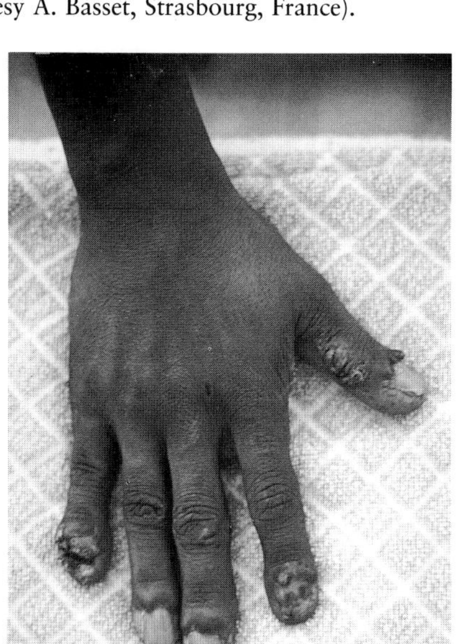

Figs 4.82–4.84. Tungiasis.

Fig. 4.83. (b)

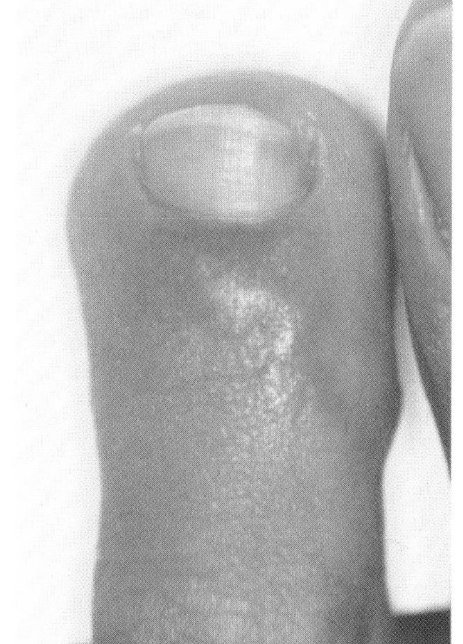

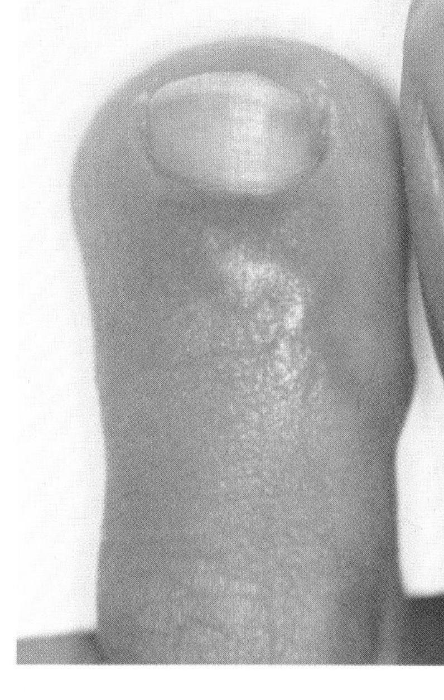

Fig. 4.85. Larva migrans (courtesy of G. Cannata, Italy).

Tungiasis (Figs 4.82–4.84)

Tungiasis is an inflammatory condition caused by the fertilized female sand flea *Tunga penetrans* and has been noted primarily in patients who have recently travelled to endemic areas.

Clinical features of tungiasis consist initially of a pruritic, tender, or painful small erythematous papule with central black dot produced by the posterior part of the flea's abdominal segments. The fully developed lesion is a white pea-sized nodule with a central black pit or plug located in the subungual and the periungual areas of the toes. Complications include cellulitis, gangrene, autoamputation of toes and tetanus (Sanusi *et al.*, 1989).

Clinical differential diagnosis of tungiasis includes fire ant bite, tick sting, scabies, creeping eruption (*Ancylostoma* sp.), cercarial dermatitis and myiasis. Definitive diagnosis rests upon demonstration of the flea using a mineral oil preparation or by examination of a biopsy

Reference

Diemer J.T. (1985) Isolated pediculosis. *J. Am. Pod. Med. Assoc.* 75, 99–101.

specimen. This reveals an intraepidermal cystic cavity lined by an eosinophilic cuticle. The cavity contains ring-shaped portions of the organism's respiratory and digestive tracts as well as multiple round to oval eggs that may contain a pale-staining round yolk sac (Wentzell, 1986; Basler *et al.*, 1988).

Treatment varies from physically removing the flea with a sterile needle to application of 4% formaldehyde solution, DDT, chloroform or turpentine. Systemic niridazole has been recommended if there are multiple sites of infection. Topical and sometimes systemic antibiotic treatment are advised. Tetanus prophylaxis should be given routinely. Wearing of shoes is the primary defence against tungiasis (Basler *et al.*, 1988).

References

Basler E.A., Stephens J.H. & Tschen J.A. (1988) *Tunga penetrans. Cutis* **42**, 47–48.

Sanusi D.J., Brown E.B., Shepard T.G. *et al.* (1989) Tungiasis: Report of one case and review of the 14 reported cases in the United States. *J. Am. Acad. Dermatol.* **20**, 941–944.

Wentzell J.M., Schwartz B.K. & Pesce J.R. (1986) Tungiasis. *J. Am. Acad. Dermatol.* **15**, 117–119.

Larva migrans (Fig. 4.85)

Intense pruritic migratory serpiginous burrows on the dorsum of the terminal phalanx may be observed with secondary dystrophic nail changes (Edelglass *et al.*, 1982). Thiabendazole or albendazole, orally and topically using a 10% suspension are effective.

Reference

Edelglass J.W., Douglass M.C. & Steifler R. (1982) Cutaneous larva migrans in northern climates. *J. Am. Acad. Dermatol.* **7**, 353.

Subungual myiasis

Infestation by larvae of *Musca domestica* is unusual in a subungual location. Three days after a traumatic event, Muñyon and Urbanc (1978) noted a subungual haematoma of the great toenail of a Caucasian female. The portion of the haematoma underneath the proximal nail fold was found to be teeming with larval forms identified as *Musca domestica*.

Reference

Muñyon T.G. & Urbanc A.N. (1978) Subungual myiasis. A case report and literature review. *J. Assoc. Milit. Dermatol.* **4**, 60–61.

Chapter 5
The Nail in Dermatological Diseases

R. BARAN & R.P.R. DAWBER

Psoriasis
- Acropustulosis
- Psoriatic arthritis
- Psoriatic onychopachydermoperiostitis
- Reiter's syndrome

Acrokeratosis paraneoplastic (Chapter 6)
Pityriasis rubra pilaris
Eczema, atopic dermatitis
Pityriasis rosea
Scabies (Chapter 4)
Parakeratosis pustulosa
Lichen planus
Lichen striatus
Lichen nitidus
Keratosis lichenoides chronica
Bullous pemphigoid
Pemphigus
Discoid lupus erythematosus
Alopecia areata
Darier's disease, Hailey–Hailey disease and acrokeratosis verruciformis (Hopf)
Porokeratosis of Mibelli
Stevens–Johnson syndrome (erythema multiforme)
Toxic epidermal necrolysis
Acroosteolysis
Acrokeratoelastoides
Pityriasis lichenoides acuta
Punctate keratoderma
Granuloma annulare
Erythema elevatum diutinum

Psoriasis

Psoriasis is an inherited hyperproliferative skin disease characterized by excessive cell proliferation, increased glycogen accumulation and incomplete differentiation in the cells of the epidermis (Maeda *et al.*, 1980). Up to 36% of psoriatic subjects have a family history of the disease; also, an association with HLA types BW17, BW16 and B13 has been established (Watson & Farber, 1977). The clinical signs of nail psoriasis can be correlated with the site of involvement of the epidermal structures of the nail. The histological changes in the nails are similar to those seen in the skin. Nail involvement in psoriasis is common and has been reported in up to 50% of cases (Zaias, 1969) but, over a lifetime, the incidence is probably nearer 80–90% (Samman, 1978). In children, nail involvement ranges from 7% (Puissant, 1970) and 13% (Asboe-Hansen, 1971) to 39% (Nanda *et al.*, 1990). Psoriasis may be restricted to the nails, but minimal changes should always be looked for in the scalp or on the genitalia. Severe nail involvement does not imply severe psoriasis of the skin and the type of nail change is not associated with any particular distribution of the skin lesions (Calvert *et al.*, 1963).

The psoriatic lesions seen in the nails are, in order of frequency: pits (Fig. 5.1), discoloration of the nail (Fig. 5.2), onycholysis (Fig. 5.3), subungual hyperkeratosis (Fig. 5.4), nail plate abnormalities and splinter haemorrhages (Fig. 5.5). There may be some soft tissue swelling accompanied by psoriatic involvement of the proximal nail fold (Fig. 5.6) and chronic paronychia is commonly found in association with nail psoriasis (Ganor, 1977a). The changes observed in the nail plate depend on the location of the lesion and the degree of involvement of the nail matrix by the parakeratotic process. The lesions may be transient, such as pits and transverse furrows (Fig. 5.7), or, in contrast, long lasting. The former originate from the proximal matrix. They are superficial, and sometimes extensive enough to produce gross abnormalities in colour and texture. The pits are usually small and shallow but can vary in size, depth and shape (Fig. 5.8); the presence, exclusively, of deep pits is characteristic of psoriasis (Zaias & Norton, 1980). Much larger pits and even punched out areas are seen occasionally. The pits are generally found scattered irregularly but may, as in alopecia areata, appear as regular lines in the transverse axis or at regular intervals in the long axis (Samman, 1978), or in a typical grid-like pattern. They grow out at the rate of the nail growth. Ganor (1977b) suggested that pitting of the nails in alopecia areata might, in reality, be an expression of psoriasis and less commonly of alopecia areata. Surprisingly, pitting is seldom observed in the toenails. Nail pits were present in 11 out of 14 infants with psoriasis (Farber & Jacobs, 1977); in one case the history suggested possible prenatal nail pitting. Fetal psoriasis has also been reported in a 1-week-old baby whose mother was affected by a widespread psoriasis (Stankler, 1988). Histologically the pits represent a defect in the superficial layers of the nail plate (Fig. 5.9). They are lined by parakeratotic cells loosely

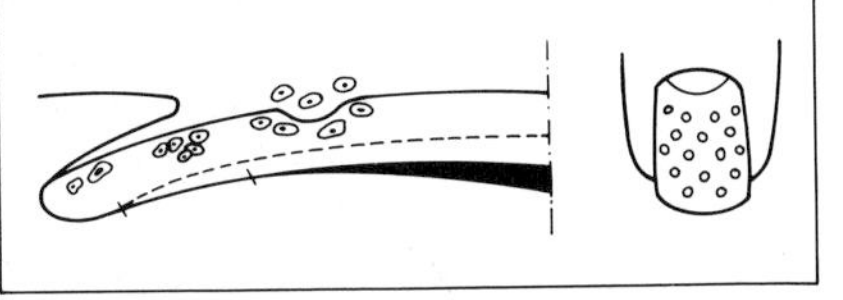
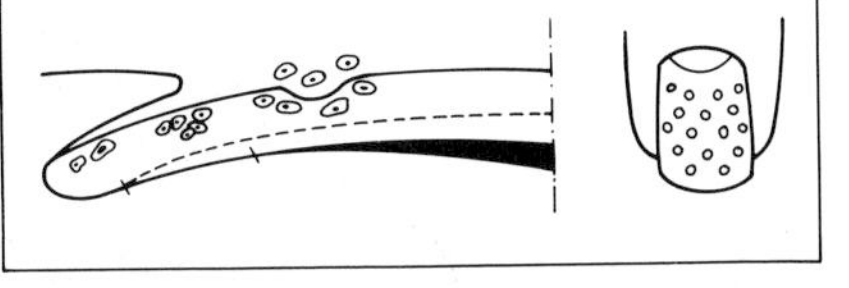
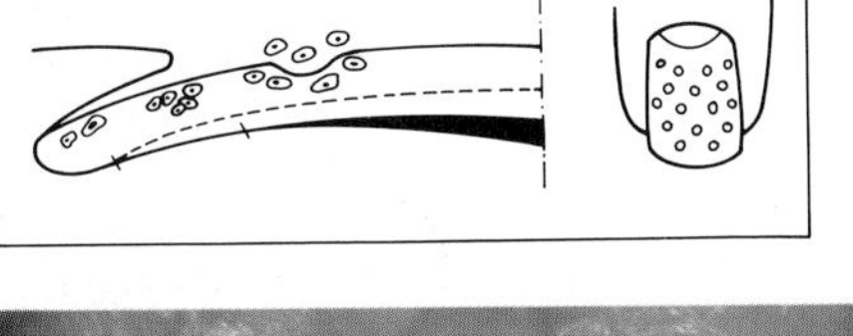

Fig. 5.1. Psoriasis – pitting.

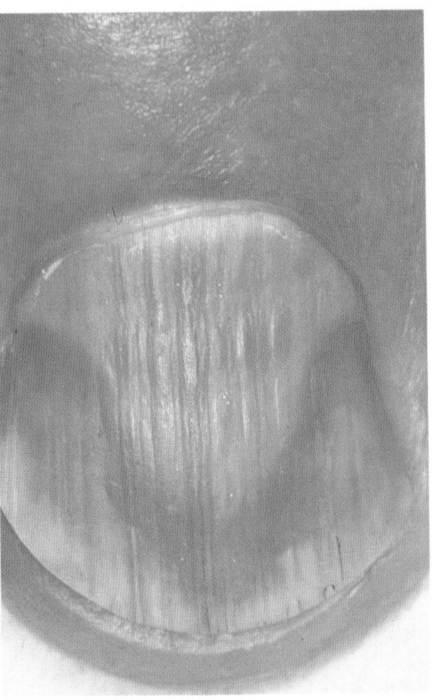
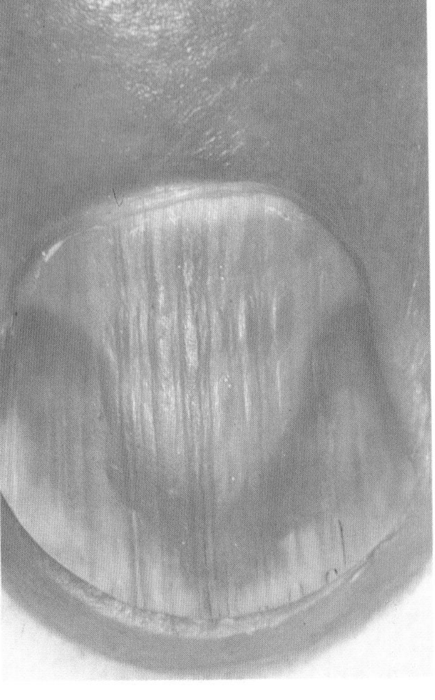

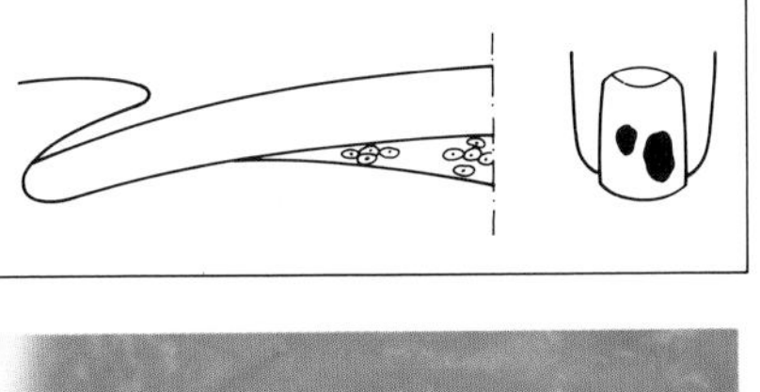

Fig. 5.3. Psoriasis – onycholysis with proximal brownish-red margin.

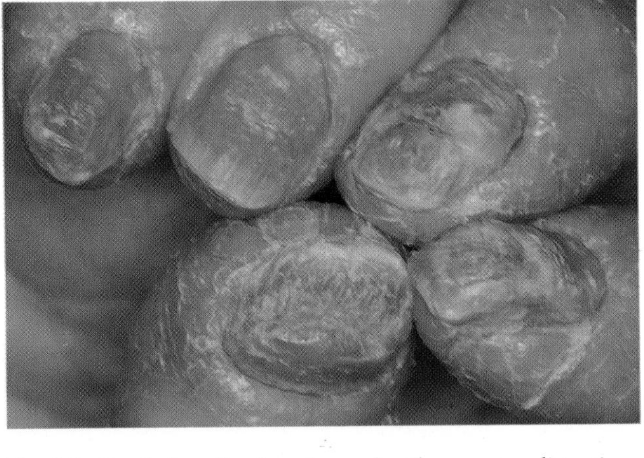

Fig. 5.2. Psoriasis – discoloration and nail apparatus distortion.

adherent to one another (Alkiewicz, 1948). These desquamate leaving a depression on the surface of the nail (Zaias, 1984). The proximal nail fold may also be responsible for pit formation. Parakeratotic and inflammatory cells in the stratum corneum adjacent to the matrix may be inlaid on the surface of the newly forming nail plate. Scanning electron microscopic studies of psoriatic nails (Mauro *et al.*, 1975; Pfister, 1981) have shown that the cells on the surface of pits are small and do not have an overlapping pattern. There are spaces between the poorly interdigitated cells. A striking feature is the presence of numerous micropits on the surface of the cells, analogous

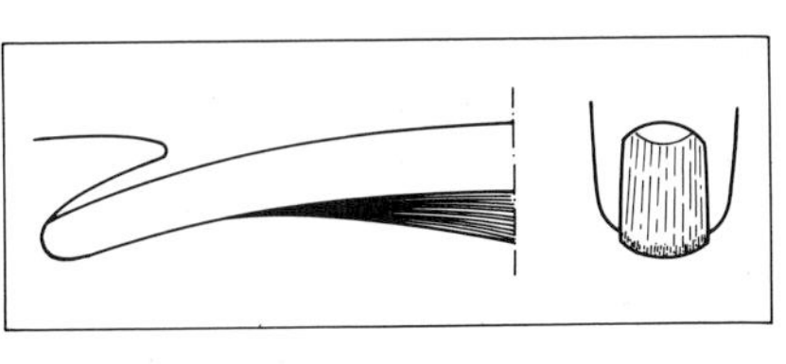

Fig. 5.4. Psoriasis – subungual hyperkeratosis.

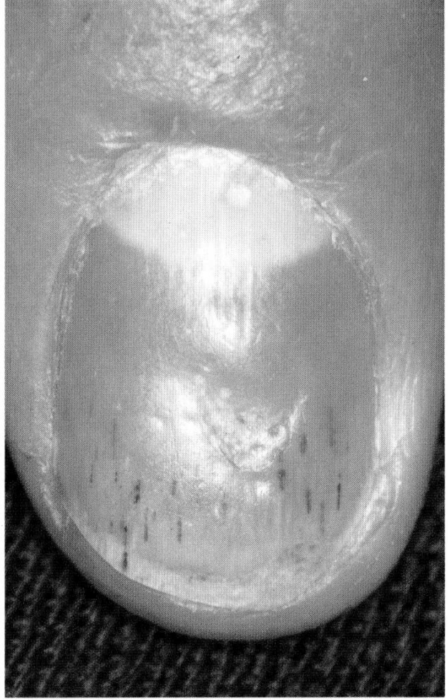

Fig. 5.5. Psoriasis – pitting and splinter haemorrhages.

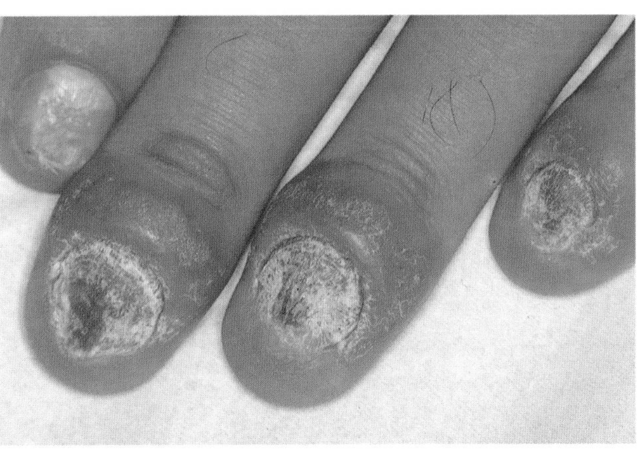

Fig. 5.6. Psoriasis – involvement of the proximal nail fold.

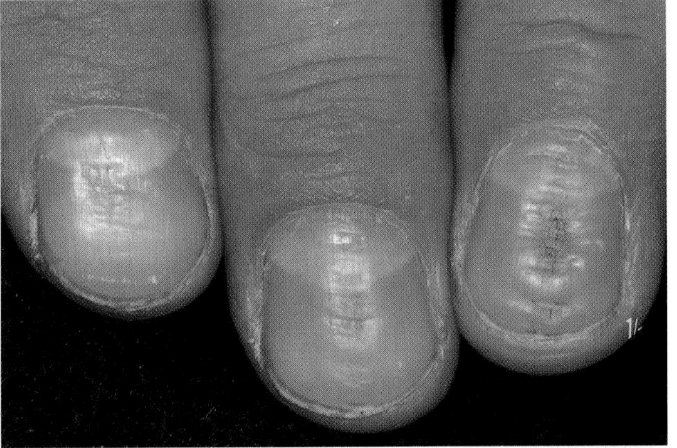

Fig. 5.7. Psoriasis – transverse furrows.

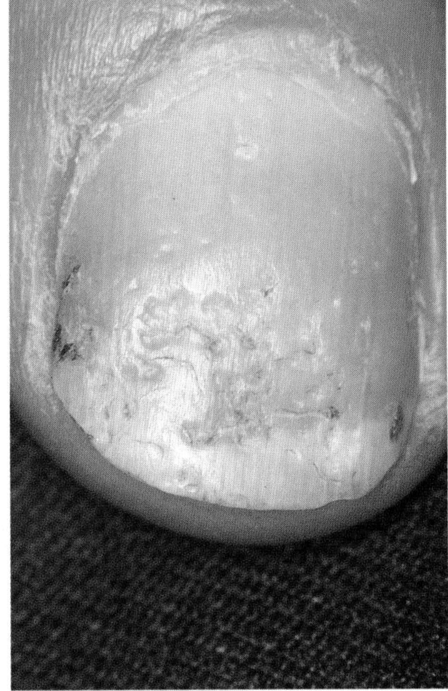

Fig. 5.8. Psoriasis – multiple pits.

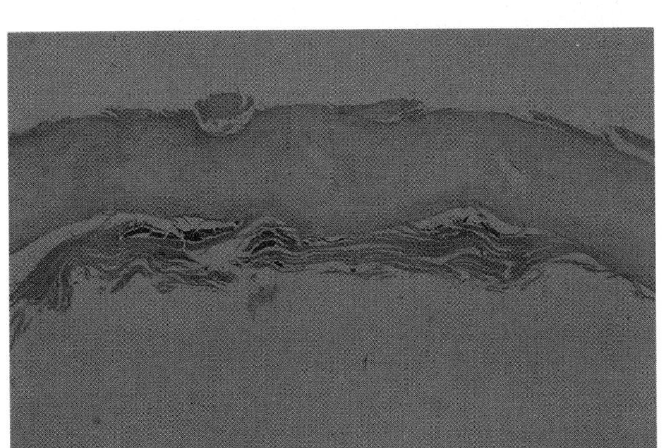

Fig. 5.9. Psoriasis – nail plate superficial pitting (H&E stain).

to the changes previously described in the stratum corneum (Dawber *et al*., 1972).

Several transverse depressions, an equivalent of expanded pitting, are common, especially on the thumbs where they may mimic 'washboard' nails, which result from the habit tic of pushing back the cuticle. They are due to lesions of the matrix of short duration.

In contrast to longitudinal furrows, which involve the whole nail plate and are produced by longer term pathology, longitudinal ridges of the nail with elevations that resemble drops of melted wax are considered as common changes by Baden (1987). Leuconychia results from abnormalities in the distal matrix (Fig. 5.10). The nail surface is absolutely smooth and intact (Alkiewicz, 1948). Concurrent proximal matrix involvement will lead to leuconychia with a rough surface (Zaias, 1969), or coarse nails (Samman, 1978). When the whole matrix is affected, the

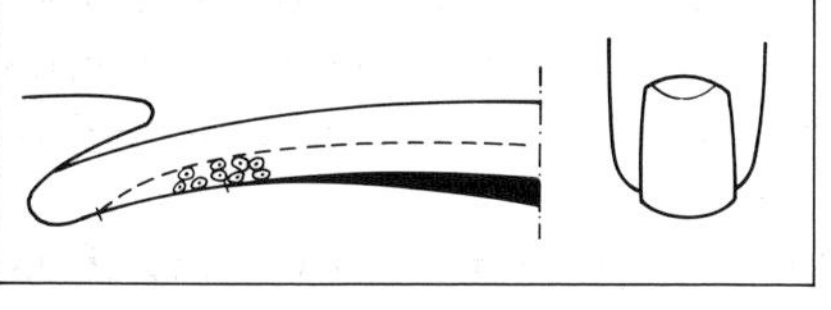

Fig. 5.10. Psoriasis – leuconychia.

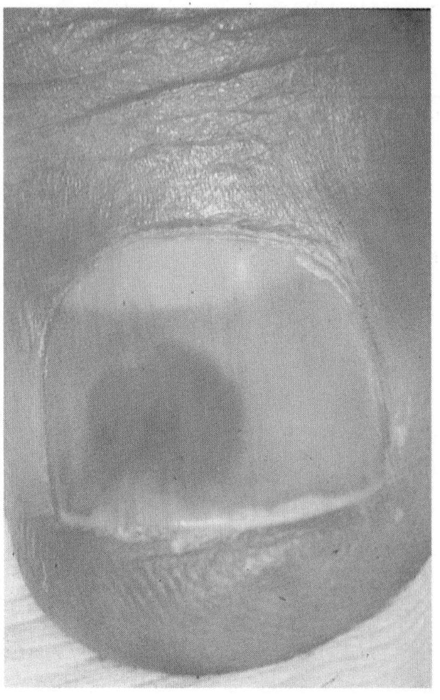

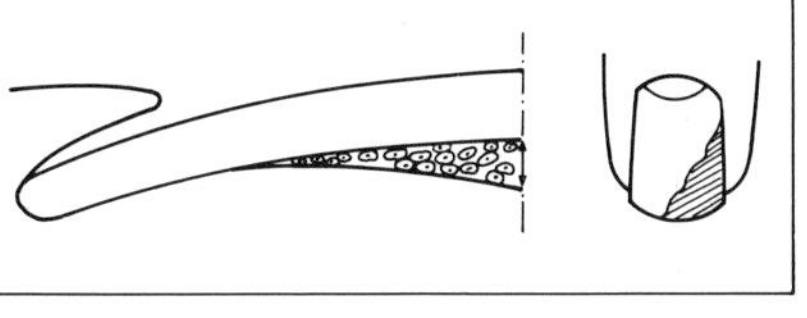

Fig. 5.12. Psoriasis – patch in the nail bed 'oil spot', brownish-red.

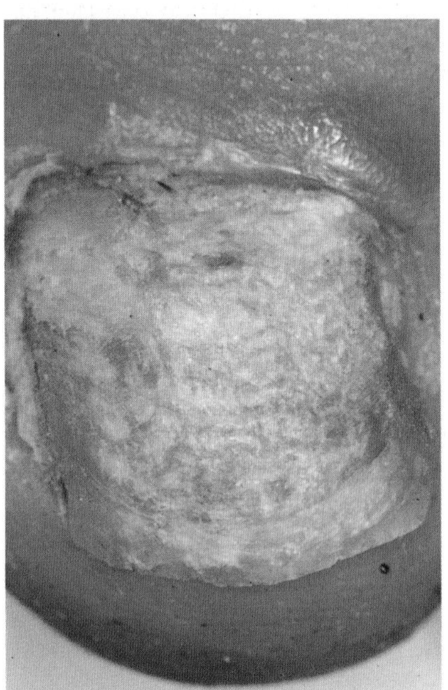

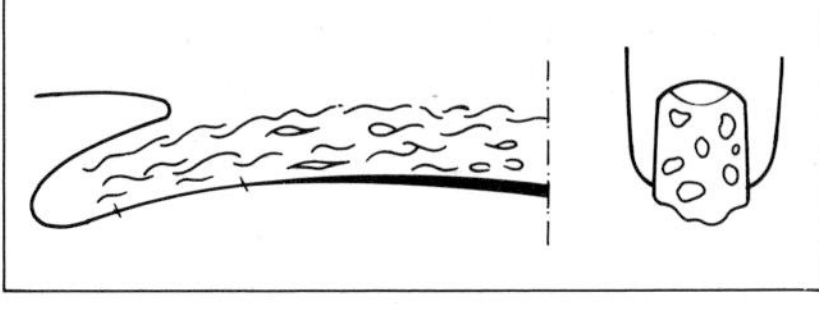

Fig. 5.11. Psoriasis – total matrix and nail plate involvement.

nail plate becomes whitish, crumbly and is poorly adherent (Zaias, 1969) (Fig. 5.11).

Radio-opaque lines within the nails in psoriasis (de Graciansky *et al.*, 1975) may be the result of topical substances applied to the keratin of the psoriatic nail. They differ from the subungual calcifications reported by Fischer (1982).

Nail bed and hyponychium involvement is common. Parakeratotic lesions located in the nail bed produce oval, 'oily' salmon-coloured spots of various sizes and variable duration (Fig. 5.12). When such patches affect the hyponychium medially or laterally, onycholysis occurs, the whitish colour resulting from air under the separated nail plate; the space then created serves as a favourable site for colonization by various microorganisms. Contamination with fungi, yeasts and *Pseudomonas* is common. Usually dermatophytes are not found in fingernails but they may occasionally be cultured in toenails (Zaias, 1984). In psoriatic nails the rate of dermatophytic infections is lower and the frequency of yeast infections higher than in primary onychomycosis (Szepes, 1986). Instead, Staberg *et al.* (1983) were not able to demonstrate any difference between the frequency of dermatophytic infections of involved psoriatic nails as compared with uninvolved psoriatic nails, or normal nails.

Splinter haemorrhages (Fig. 5.5) are seen in a high proportion of fingernails (42%) but much less often in toenails (6%) (Calvert *et al.*, 1963).

Subungual hyperkeratosis (Figs 5.2 and 5.4) is due to accumulated keratotic cells which have not lost their cohesion (cf. onycholysis). When the process involves the hyponychium, the nail plate becomes raised to a variable degree and may resemble pachyonychia congenita. Sometimes a horny mass may simulate loss of the nail plate (Zaias, 1969). Overcurvature of one or more nails may be seen occasionally (Samman, 1978). Special attention should be given to chromonychia due to psoriasis of the nail: we have seen that the matrix is responsible for leuconychia and subungual keratosis causes a silvery-white colour; the lunula may be red; a yellow-greenish tinge may be produced by the accumulation of large amounts of blood glycoprotein (Fig. 5.2), commonly seen when the hyponychium and the nail bed are involved in inflammatory processes (Zaias & Norton, 1980). Onycholysis surrounded by a reddish-brown margin visible between the pink normal nail bed and the whitish separated area is highly suggestive of psoriasis (Fig. 5.12). In all types of onycholysis, the deep surface of the nail plate retains nail bed cells (ventral matrix); Robbins *et al.* (1983) have re-emphasized this long known fact in relation to psoriatic onycholysis in which the place of separation is between the layers of neutrophil-containing parakeratotic horn of the nail bed. A greasy appearance of the nail plate, especially when it takes on a yellow-green hue, increases the probability of psoriasis if the presence of *Pseudomonas* has been ruled out (culture, Wood's lamp examination and chloroform solubility test). These 'oily' patches less commonly occur in acropustulosis and in systemic lupus erythematosus; very large oil patches have been observed in 'lectitis purulenta et granulomatosa' (Runne & Orfanos; 1981; see Chapter 4).

The nail abnormalities may be classified, on clinical criteria, into acute or chronic, depending on the degree of psoriatic activity (Lewin *et al.*, 1972). The acute psoriatic nail shows intense inflammation of the terminal phalanx and deformity or absence of the whole nail plate which is replaced by hyperkeratotic scales, firmly adherent to the underlying tissue or to a semi-translucent, keratinous crust. In psoriasis, the matrix and nail bed develop a granular layer, then taking on the appearance of the squamous epithelium of the skin. Mounds of parakeratosis containing neutrophils are seen. The neutrophils tend to be lodged in the summits of the mounds of parakeratosis (Ackerman, 1979). Foci of orthokeratotic cells are found interspersed between the mounds of parakeratotic horns which contain the neutrophils. The following factors may be of help when the diagnosis of psoriasis is difficult or equivocal.

1 When psoriasis is restricted to the nails the possibility of dermatophytosis and candidiasis presents a diagnostic problem. Potassium hydroxide preparations and cultures, coupled with cytological and histopathological examination (Leyden *et al.*, 1972; Scher & Ackerman, 1980; Haneke, 1991) (Chapter 4) showing the deeply sited organisms, are useful diagnostic aids. Secondary *Candida* infection is common.

2 The numerous non-psoriatic causes of onycholysis should be ruled out.

3 Considerable thickening of the nail occasionally occurs in pityriasis rubra pilaris, Darier's disease and in pachyonychia congenita.

4 Pits are found in eczema, but they are irregular in shape and size. They also occur in alopecia areata, exceptionally in lichen planus, or in type IV pityriasis rubra pilaris.

5 Isolated subungual hyperkeratosis does occur in which the clinical picture may be reminiscent of psoriasis or lichen planus of the nail bed and hyponychium. Badger *et al.* (1992) presented a case of unilateral subungual hyperkeratosis following a cerebrovascular incident in a patient with psoriasis.

6 The Koebner phenomenon, the development of isomorphic pathological lesions in the traumatized uninvolved skin of psoriatic patients, may affect the nail apparatus and raise difficult problems in occupational conditions (Fisher & Baran, 1992).

Psoriasis may affect any or all particular parts of the nail apparatus. The proximal nail fold is virtually always affected in psoriatic arthritis of the distal interphalangeal joints frequently also involving the proximal nail fold and the matrix. The surface of the proximal nail fold shows typical acanthosis with drop-shaped or rectangular rete ridges, suprapapillary thinning of the epidermis, lack of granular layer and parakeratosis with pycnotic polymorphonuclear leucocytes that may be grouped to Munro's microabscesses. Neutrophils also migrate through the epidermis but seldom form spongiform pustules. The capillaries of the papillary dermis are dilated and there is a nail fold inflammatory cell infiltrate around the vessels of the superficial dermis. When the distal free margin of the proximal nail fold is involved, the cuticle will be lost. Involvement of the undersurface of the proximal nail fold, the eponychium, induces similar changes, however there is usually less pronounced acanthosis, but some spongiosis.

Psoriasis of the most proximal portion of the matrix may cause pits. Histopathologically, a circumscribed area of matrix epithelium is affected resulting in a nidus of parakeratotic onychocytes; the width of the pit corresponds to the width of matrix involvement, its depth to the histopathological longitudinal diameter and the clinically visible length of the pit to the duration of the psoriatic lesion. In a longitudinal nail biopsy one may see, under the proximal nail fold, mounds of parakeratotic cells bulging into the surface of the nail plate. When they arrive at the free margin of the proximal nail fold they

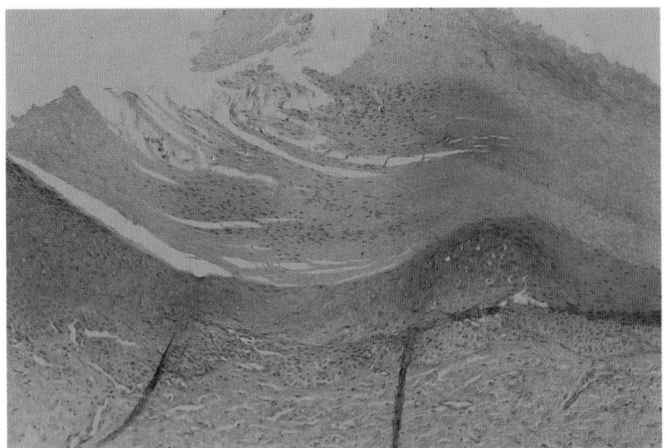

Fig. 5.13. Psoriasis – involvement of the nail bed and nail plate (PAS stain, ×100)

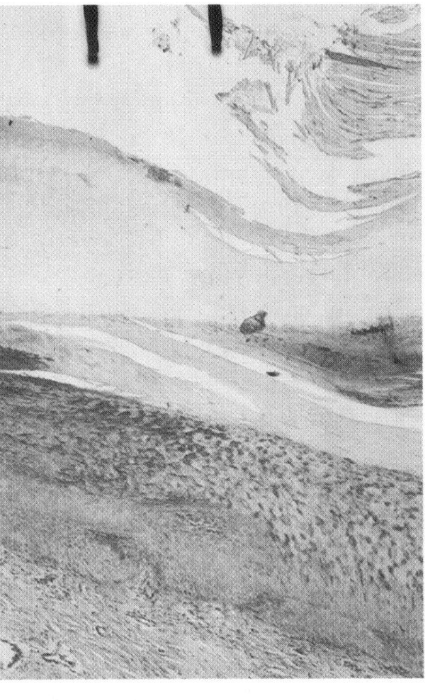

Fig. 5.14. Psoriasis – involvement of the nail matrix and nail plate (PAS stain, ×90).

easily break out from the nail plate leaving the characteristic cup-shaped depression clinically known as a pit.

Circumscribed psoriasis lesions of the middle and distal matrix produce parakeratotic foci within the nail plate which appear macroscopically as punctate leuconychia (Alkiewicz & Pfister, 1976).

Psoriasis of the matrix and nail bed is usually somewhat different from that of the epidermis elsewhere (Figs 5.13 & 5.14). In addition to classical features of acanthosis, neutrophils migrating into the matrix and nail bed epithelium, parakeratotic mounds with neutrophils in their summits (Ackerman, 1979), there is usually considerable spongiosis with some exocytosis of mononuclear cells as well as – paradoxically – a focal granular layer. There may be papillomatosis of matrix and nail bed epithelium often with spongiform pustules in the tips which then become necrotic. When this lesion involves the distal matrix and proximal nail bed, a salmon patch will be seen clinically; when it reaches the hyponychium it will lead to psoriatic onycholysis or, more rarely when the psoriatic parakeratosis remains cohesive, to subungual hyperkeratosis heaping up the nail plate.

The use of exfoliative cytological techniques provides, according to Leyden *et al.* (1972), a rapid test that can confirm an impression of psoriasis.

The severity of nail plate alteration depends on the extent of the psoriatic lesion: the more matrix is involved the more severe the alterations will be. This is easily seen in routine haematoxylin and eosin (H&E) sections, but the disorderly and irregular keratin structure is better visualized using Giemsa, Masson's trichrome stain or polarization microscopy. Small haemorrhages in the subungual keratin are demonstrated by the peroxidase reaction since they remain Prussian blue and Perl negative.

Scanning electron microscopy shows that the pits are small round depressions (Mauro *et al.*, 1975) with their surface cells being small, separated from each other and having minute surface depressions (Dawber *et al.*, 1972). Transmission electron microscopy of psoriatic leuconychia revealed a disorganization of keratin fibres in the onychocytes (André *et al.*, 1988).

Periodic acid Schiff (PAS) stain is necessary to rule out onychomycosis which may mimic nail psoriasis both clinically and histopathologically (Haneke, 1991). PAS stains fungi, neutrophils both with the epithelium and the keratoses, and glycoproteins which are mainly IgM positive and get in between the parakeratosis through the spongiosis. Although psoriatic nails may be secondarily infected or colonized by dermatophytes, yeasts and moulds, parakeratosis is usually more consistent and pronounced in psoriasis than in onychomycosis.

Treatment

Despite recent therapeutic advances, the management of nail psoriasis remains long, always tedious and sometimes unsatisfactory; indeed occasionally, many physicians justify a *laissez faire* or nihilistic stance.

Below are a few general remarks.

1 Discrete forms may be treated cosmetically which is easier for women who frequently use nail varnish.

2 Excessive manicuring is a source of aggravation as it activates a Koebner's isomorphic phenomenon.

3 The treatment should take into consideration the clinical variety, and cannot be the same in every case.

4 Avoid colouring treatments (tar, anthraline) as their effectiveness on the nail is still to be proved.

5 Refrain from treating children. However, avulsion with urea can be appreciated by parents who will have the possibility to repeat it upon request.

6 Good results can be obtained through an additional obstination by both the doctor and a motivated patient. The following may help in some cases.

1 Photochemotherapy will be of benefit in some cases within 6 months. For patients with severe nail involvement, it may be more practical, after the glabrous skin has been cleared, to continue more intensive treatment of nail and periungual region alone (Dobson & Thiers, 1981). Hofmann and Plewig (1977) have experimented with an apparatus designed to deliver high intensity UVA for the treatment of psoriatic nails. The technique is time-consuming and particularly valuable when only a few nails are affected since the nails are treated one by one. However one must state that the response of psoriatic nails to photochemotherapy is not impressive. Complete clearing has been obtained (Caccialanza & Frigerio, 1982) but is rare and pitting does not respond (Marx & Scher, 1980). Side effects such as subungual haemorrhage, photoonycholysis (Baran & Barthelemy, 1990) and pigmentation of the nail plate and the nail bed may be seen and these can be avoided by using protective nail varnish or sunscreen preparations. Parker and Diffey (1983) suggest that the mechanisms producing resolution of psoriatic nail changes are similar to those for psoriatic plaques: approximately 2.5 times the therapeutic dose for glabrous skin would have to be delivered to the surface of the nail plate (with appropriate protection for the surrounding skin) to achieve the same effect. This factor assumes a flat action spectrum for the regression of psoriatic lesions due to psoralen photo-chemotherapy. If wavelengths around 330 mm prove to be effective therapeutically the factor is likely to be closer to 5 because of the differing transmission characteristics of the epidermis and the nail plate. Müller *et al.* (1991) investigated the therapeutic effect of UV radiation with Hönle's dermalight Blue-Point on psoriasis patients with additional nail involvement. All the patients received a daily radiation of the nail matrix area for about 4 weeks (except on Sunday). The range of radiation time was 5–45 s per nail. More than 60% showed improvement with an average duration of about 10 months. Forty-two per cent of these reported a visible beginning of the restitution during their time in hospital which generally continued after discontinuation of the therapy. Twenty-eight per cent had complete nail restitution. Handfield-Jones *et al.* (1987) advocated local PUVA treatment using 1% 8-methoxypsoralen (Meladin) solution applied to the proximal nail fold of affected fingers up to the terminal phalanx. The backs of the hands are exposed to a UVA source producing 3 mW/cm^2 at a distance of 20 cm. The initial dosage needs to be low to avoid burning and 0.5 J increasing to a maximum of 2 J is used, two to three times a week.

2 After several years of use it is now possible to establish the indications for retinoids (Baran, 1982; Baran, 1990). Psoriasis vulgaris has been subject to controversial reports due to its variable response. Ellis and Voorhees (1987), reporting on more than 100 patients, found the results 'very good' with a 0.2–1.2 mg/kg/day dosage range. The authors' experience (Baran, 1990), however, suggests some caution in this evaluation. Since thinning of the nail is a common finding with etretinate it is apparent that good results will be obtained in psoriasis patients with thick nails. In contrast, disorders such as pitting or onycholysis can become worse due to the toxic action of the drug in the nail apparatus and to the possibility of an isomorphic response. Moreover, even though thinning of thick psoriatic nails is appreciated by some patients, others complain of increased sensitivity to external pressure and an inability to use the nails in a functional way. The side effects of the retinoids on the nail are described in Chapter 6.

3 Topical treatment: Fredriksson (1974) used 1% fluorouracil solution dissolved in propylene glycol applied twice daily for 6 months around the margin of the nail; it was gently massaged into the nail fold and allowed to dry. The treatment is only recommended for nails with pitting and hypertrophy as dominant symptoms and it should be avoided when there are signs of onycholysis. Success rates are not high. Twenty per cent urea plus 1% fluorouracil (Fritz, 1988) produced an improvement of more than 50% of the clinical signs such as oil spots, subungual hyperkeratosis and combined signs. Transient rhabdomyolysis connected with topical use of 5-fluorouracil is anecdotal (Schmied & Levy, 1986). High potency corticosteroids (i.e. flucinolone acetonide, triamcinolone acetonide, β-methasone, etc.) may be used under occlusive dressings such as non-porous tape or plastic gloves for short and repeated periods. Dermovate (clobetasol proprionate) can be used without occlusive dressing. Side effects such as distal phalangeal atrophy have been reported (Deffer & Goette, 1987; Requena *et al.*, 1990). A mixture of the topical steroid combined with 5–10% benzoyl peroxide or 0.1% retinoic acid cream may give better results. Intralesional injection of long-acting corticosteroids into the area of the nail matrix and/or bed is helpful especially when these structures are affected. For this procedure a suspension of triamcinolone acetonide is mixed with equal parts sterile saline and injected in quantities of 0.2–0.4 ml per nail (Norton, 1982). Haemorrhages, pain and reversible atrophy at the injection sites (Peachey *et al.*, 1976) as well as periungual hypopigmentation (Bedi, 1977) are the main side effects. Preliminary digital-block anaesthesia is advisable in those cases requiring multiple injections. Many authors have abandoned jet injectors because sterilization procedures for the apparatus do not prevent contamination with hepatitis viruses. This is because of the 'splash back' of small quantities of blood at the time of injection. Epidermoid implantation cysts, leading to amputation of a distal phalanx, were an unexpected complication

in a patient of J. Mascaro (personal communication).
4 Topical cyclosporin (Tosti *et al.*, 1990) has given excellent results in an anecdotal report. Calcipotriol ointment gently massaged into the nail folds twice daily resulted in excellent improvement in a patient with formerly recalcitrant psoriasis (Haneke, unpubl.).
5 Systemic treatment with methotrexate or cyclosporin has given good results in patients treated for psoriasis elsewhere. They should not be used for psoriasis restricted to the nails or exceptionally.

If onycholysis is present, the nail plate must be trimmed back to the point of separation if local medication is to be effective. Sometimes chemical avulsion may facilitate a more successful therapeutic response. Psoriasis and onychomycosis are two separate dermatological entities, which may combine to produce a wide spectrum of pathology. This may range from pure psoriasis at one end of the spectrum to onychomycosis at the other. In this spectrum of pathology, the Koebner phenomenon may result from the fungal element.

Direct microscopy, cultures and sometimes nail biopsy obtained from trimming the nail as far as possible should always be performed, even in typical cases. The resultant diagnosis may indicate that the treatment of the psoriatic nail should be supplemented with antifungal therapy, especially with the transungual delivery system lacquers.

In certain rare cases, in patients over 30 years old, low-voltage X-rays may be useful. Total dose per area, per lifetime, should not exceed 10 Gy (1000 R). Grenz rays (5 Gy) applied on 10 occasions at intervals of 1 week (Lindelöf, 1988) can be effective only when psoriatic nails are of normal thickness. This mode of treatment should not be rejected on safety grounds, since in a large-scale study of the incidence of malignant skin tumours in 14 140 patients who have received Grenz ray for benign skin disorders, the risk factor was small with regards to the development of non-melanoma skin tumours (Lindelöf & Eklund, 1986).

A double-blind study of superficial radiotherapy in psoriatic nail dystrophy has demonstrated a definite, albeit temporary benefit (Yu & King, 1992).

Unfortunately, irrespective of the type of treatment, recurrences do occur and concealing the lesions with nail varnish enables many women to tolerate this unsightly nail condition.

Psoriasis associated with other disorders

A number of conditions may produce clinical and/or histological nail changes similar to psoriasis or may be clinically and/or histologically related to psoriasis. Psoriasis associated with unilateral ectromelia and central nervous system anomalies has been reported by Shear *et al.* (1971), and probably belongs to the CHILD syndrome (Happle *et al.*, 1980) or CHILD naevus (Happle, 1987), which is a congenital homolateral epidermal hyperplasia and hypoplastic hemidysplasia (Laplanche *et al.*, 1980) with ptychotropism, a pronounced affinity for the body folds (Happle, 1990).

Psoriasis in acquired immune deficiency syndrome (AIDS) tends to be much more active and resistant to most forms of therapy (Lazar & Roenigk, 1988), as does Reiter's syndrome (Duvic *et al.*, 1987) but in some adult patients, a significant clearing of psoriasis is associated with the initiation of zidovudine therapy (Kaplan *et al.*, 1989).

Severe exacerbation of psoriasis may be due to drugs (Abel *et al.*, 1986; Nicolas *et al.*, 1987) the literature reports many cases of psoriasis aggravated by β-blockers and lithium. Psoriasis-like lesions involving the nail area can appear *de novo*; they disappear after the β-blockers are discontinued (Jensen *et al.*, 1976; Tegner, 1976). Lithium can aggravate and/or precipitate psoriasis (Sasaki *et al.*, 1989) and may even reveal isolated psoriasis nail changes (Rudolph, 1991) (Fig. 5.15) (Table 6.1).

Table 5.1. Drugs that may induce psoriasis

Amiodarone
Antimalarials (Luzza, 1982)
Aspirin, salicylates
Blockers (Neuman & van Jost, 1981)
Calcium channel blockers (Kitamura *et al.*, 1993)
Captopril (Gayrard *et al.*, 1990)
Clonidine
Corticoids
Digoxine
Gembifrozil (Fisher *et al.*, 1988)
Indometacine
Interferon alpha
Isotretinoine (Davis & Hayes, 1987)
Lithium (Sasaki *et al.*, 1989; Rudolph, 1991)
Mebhydrolin (McKenna & McMillan, 1993)
Meclofenamate (Meyerhoff, 1983)
Morphine
Oxyphenail bedutazone
Penicillins (Katz *et al.*, 1987)
Phenylbutazone
Potassium iodine
Procaine
Progesterone
Sulfonamides
Sulfapyridine
Terfenadine (Harrison & Stone, 1988; Navaratnam & Gebauer, 1990)
Timolol (ophtalmic sol., Coignet & Sayag, 1990)
Trazodone

Psoriatic mimicry in the nail apparatus

According to Zaias (1990) psoriasiform states of the nail apparatus share (i) a psoriasiform appearance; and (ii)

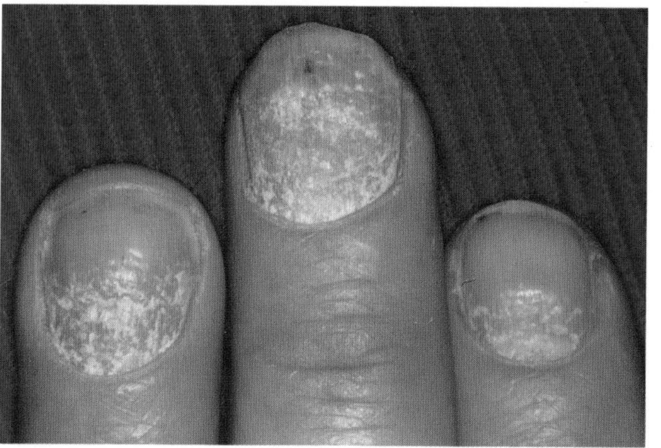

Fig. 5.15. Psoriasis – nail changes induced by lithium therapy (courtesy of R. Rudolph, USA).

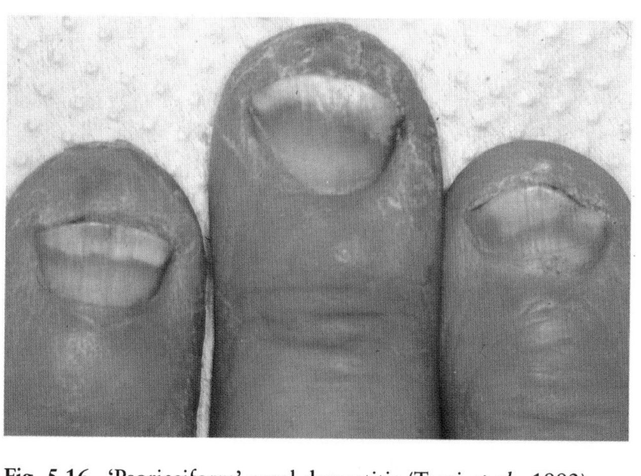

Fig. 5.16. 'Psoriasiform' acral dermatitis (Tosti *et al.*, 1992).

some histopathological similarities. They differ in their clinical courses, and sometimes their involvement with other organs and sites. We have expanded this definition by adding some diseases which may present a clinical psoriasiform appearance. These conditions include:

1 Reiter's syndrome;

2 pityriasis rubra pilaris;

3 acropustulosis – acrodermatitis continua of Hallopeau;

4 parakeratosis pustulosa (p. 152);

5 Norwegian scabies (see Chapter 4);

6 acral psoriasiform reaction to neoplasm – acrokeratosis paraneoplastica (see Chapter 6);

7 subungual hyperkeratosis, when the clinical picture is similar to psoriasis or lichen planus of the nail bed and hyponychium, but like hyperkeratosis histologically;

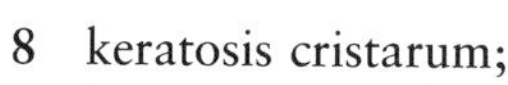

8 keratosis cristarum;

9 hyponychial dermatitis: contact dermatitis is suspected but all the tests are negative. Histologically an exudation of serum-like material, also seen in other nail diseases, is the characteristic feature; PAS stain is positive;

10 psoriasiform acral dermatitis (term coined by Zaias, 1990) looks clinically like psoriasis, but not histologically. The clinical presentation is distinctive since patients exhibit a chronic dermatitis of the terminal phalanges associated with marked shortening of the nail beds of the abnormal fingers. There is a leucocytic population involved in the skin. Tosti *et al.* (1992) reported the pathological and immunohistochemical study of three patients affected by this condition (Fig. 5.16). Histology shows exocytosis of lymphoid cells in the epidermis associated with marked spongiotic changes and pronounced parakeratosis with

Figs 5.17. & 5.18. Psoriasis – acropustulosis, before treatment and after 1 month on etretinate.

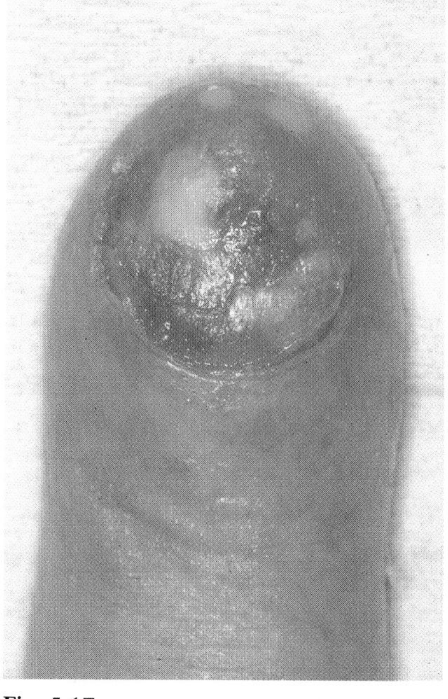

Fig. 5.17.

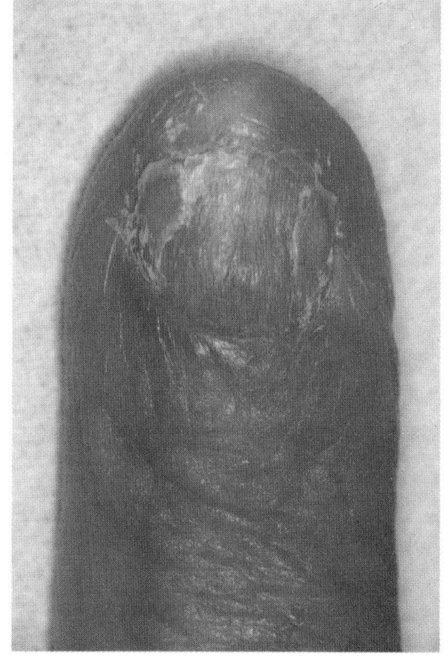

Fig. 5.18.

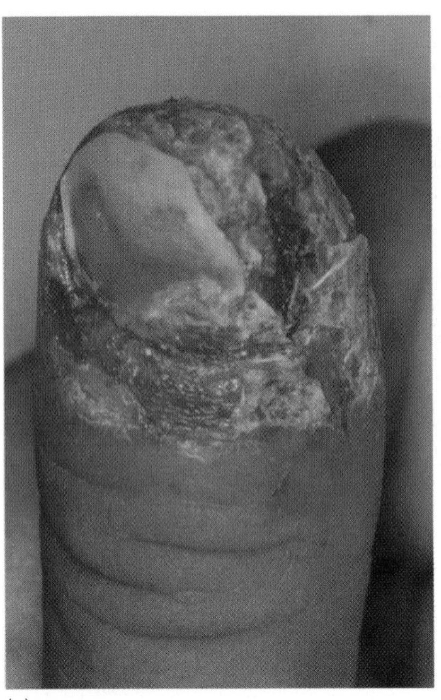

(a)

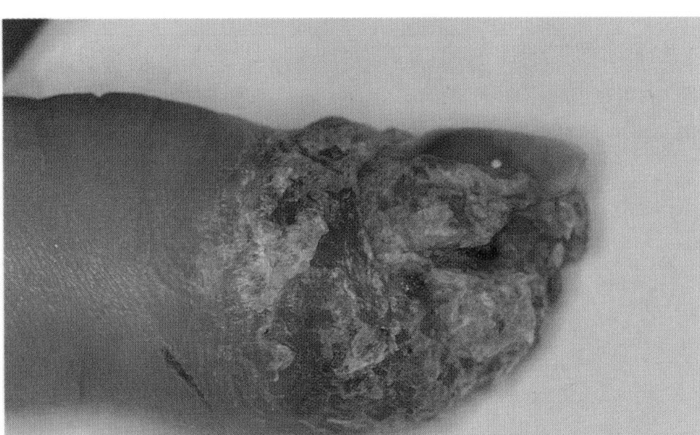

(b)

Fig. 5.19. (a & b) Psoriasis – very inflammatory acropustulosis in a 10-year-old child.

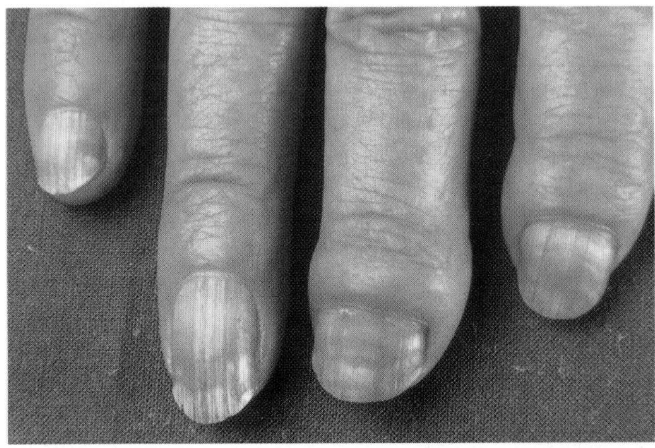

Fig. 5.20. Psoriasis – acral pustular psoriasis with acroosteolysis (see also Fig. 5.21) (courtesy of P. Combemale, Lyon, France).

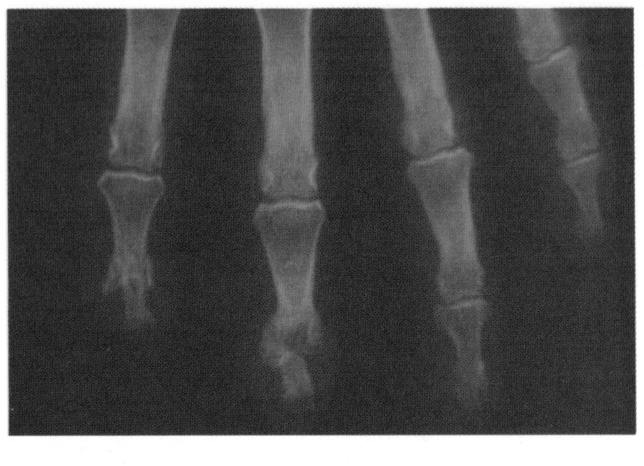

Fig. 5.21. Psoriasis – X-ray showing 'resorptive' osteolysis (see Fig. 5.20).

scale crust. There is an increased number of CD1a, CD4 and Langerhans' cells within the epidermis and the superficial dermis. Langerhans' cells are also present in the spongiotic vesicles. the mononuclear nail fold infiltrate consist of mature peripheral T-lymphocytes (CD2+, CD3+, CD5+) with a CD4/CD8 ratio of 1 : 1 in the epidermis and 3/1 in the dermis. Thirty per cent of the lymphocytes express the interleukin 2 receptor (CD25+).

Acropustulosis

In pustular psoriasis and acrodermatitis continua, involvement of a single digit is common (Figs 5.17 & 5.18). It is often misdiagnosed when the pustule appears beneath the nail plate with necrosis of tissue resulting in dessication and crust formation. New pustule formation may develop at the periphery or within the lesions (Fig. 5.19). The nail is lifted off by the crust and lakes of pus and new pustules may form on the denuded nail bed. Permanent loss is possible. Acral pustular psoriasis has been reported with resorptive osteolysis as a 'deep Koebner phenomenon' (Miller *et al.*, 1971; Combermale *et al.*, 1989) (Figs 5.20 & 5.21) and notable skin and subcutaneous tissue atrophy, but 'tuft' osteolysis may occur, independently of acropustuloses and arthritis in psoriasis (Cheesbrough, 1979). There may be progessive loss of entire digits in the feet and loss of fingertips and fingernails (Mahowald & Parrish, 1982). Histopathology may reveal Munro–Sabouraud 'microabscesses' (Fig. 5.22) or the spongiform pustule of Kogoj (Fig. 5.23). It may be the only means to confirm the true nature of a pustular and/or atrophying process of the tip of a digit, especially of a toe, even when no pustules can be seen macroscopically. There is extensive spongiform pustule formation in the epidermis either with merging of the neutrophils to typical, macroscopically visible pustules, or with necrosis of the superficial keratinocytes

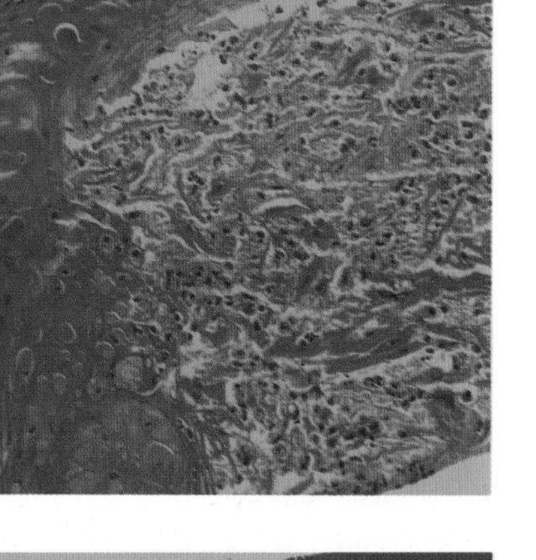

Fig. 5.22. Psoriasis – Munro microabscess formation histologically.

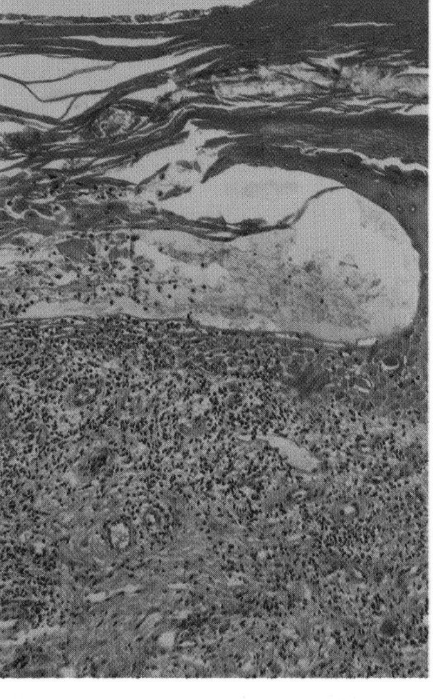

Fig. 5.23. Psoriasis – showing spongiform pustule of Kogoj.

and thick parakeratosis stuck with Munro's microabscesses, respectively. In the papillary dermis, there is usually some extravasation of erythrocytes which may get into the epidermis to eventually reach the paraketosis; this will add to the brownish colour of the scab.

Acute acral pustulosis

Acute palmoplantar pustulosis is a disorder distinguished from chronic palmoplantar pustulosis by the speed of onset and clinical signs. The large, unilocular pustules arise on normal skin and involve the dorsa of the hands,

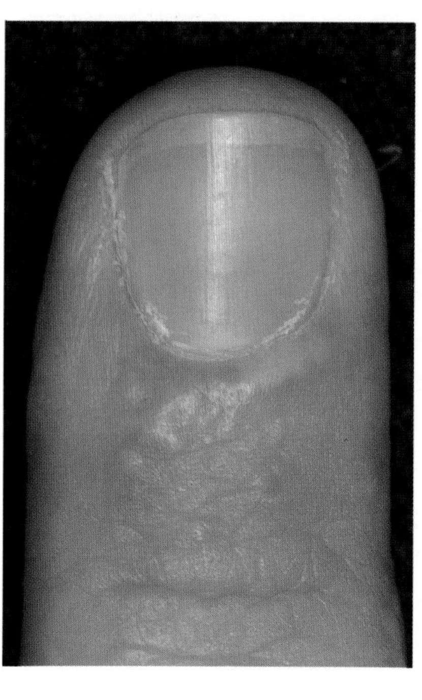

Fig. 5.24. Psoriasis – acute, acral pustulosis; proximal nail fold lesion.

fingers and feet (Fig. 5.24). This condition is precipitated by infection which should be treated, but as it is self-limiting, aggressive therapy is not indicated.

Localized PUVA can be of benefit. Aromatic retinoid therapy may give good short-term results (Deichmann & Spindeldreier, 1982), but recurrences appear 1–3 months after the treatment has been stopped (Baran, 1979, 1982). Combined retinoid and PUVA treatment delays and lowers the frequency of relapse, but recalcitrant cases can be observed (Brun *et al.*, 1985). Topical mechloretamine (Notowicz *et al.*, 1978) and 5% fluorouracil cream (Tsuji & Nishimura, 1991) have given some good results as has intramuscular triamcinolone acetonide (Arnold, 1978). Nimesulid has also been suggested (Piraccini *et al.*, 1993).

Differential diagnosis should rule out 'acral granulomatous dermatitis' (Miyagawa *et al.*, 1990), a condition which clinically resembles acrodermatitis continua of Hallopeau. In contrast to the latter, however, epidermis is normal histologically, above dermal and subcutaneous abscess formation with granuloma. The lesions respond to systemic corticosteroid therapy with residual atrophy and contractures of the fingers.

The differential diagnosis of acropustulosis may be controversial, particularly with regard to the subcorneal pustular dermatosis of Sneddon and Wilkinson. Chimenti and Ackerman (1981) have seen patients with pustular lesions described as subcorneal pustular dermatosis, but who had in addition stigmata suggestive of psoriasis. These included typical scaly plaques on the elbows and knees, pitted nails or arthropathy. It is, however, pointless to argue about Sneddon and Wilkinson's disease without applying the techniques available for identifying psoriatic behaviour, i.e. cell kinetics, complement activation in the stratum corneum, HLA/family studies and nail growth studies (Ryan, 1981).

Psoriatic arthritis (Fig. 5.25)

Nail lesions are present in greater frequency than in uncomplicated psoriasis. They begin at a later stage than the skin lesions, and commonly precede the development of arthritis.

Nail abnormalities may be of diagnostic usefulness in cases of digital inflammatory arthritis and also be helpful in family studies.

The work of Baker *et al.* (1964) showed that 83% of 53 patients with psoriatic arthritis had psoriatic involvement of finger- or toenails at some time during the period of study. All types of nail change were seen varying from mild pitting to gross distortion; these were not related to the distribution of the joint involvement. Patients with the more severe types of arthritis tended to have greater nail involvement whether or not there was significant terminal interphalangeal joint disease. No topographical relationship was found between arthritis of the distal joints and psoriatic change in the nail of the same digit. However Wright *et al.* (1979) found nail changes in all patients with distal arthritis and in 88% of patients with deforming arthritis and 67% of the patients with undiagnosed arthritis. The concept of psoriatic 'nail matrix arthropathy' is supported by the fact that the nail matrix and the terminal interphalangeal joint share the same blood supply (Abel & Farber, 1979). Onycholysis alone without previous nail injury suggests a psoriatic origin of nail dystrophy (Eastmond & Wright, 1979). A psoriatic origin is also favoured by the presence of other multiple nail abnormalities, such as horizontal ridging and pitting. The presence of more than 20 fingernail pits suggests a psoriatic cause of the nail dystrophy. More than 60 pits per person is unlikely to be found in the absence of psoriasis. In childhood, Sills (1980) noted a strong correlation between nail involvement and distal arthritis. Definite juvenile psoriatic arthritis was defined by Southwood *et al.* (1989) as arthritis associated with, but not necessarily coincident with, a typical psoriatic rash, or arthritis, plus at least three of four minor criteria: dactylitis, nail pitting, psoriasis-like rash or family history of psoriasis. It may however have more in common with juvenile rheumatoid arthritis than the seronegative spondylarthropathies with which it is traditionally associated. Young females with widespread plaque-type or suberythrodermic psoriasis, with also a strong family history of psoriasis and who have both nail changes and large joint arthropathy, may form a separate subgroup of patients with a strong family history of autoimmune disease (Harrison *et al.*, 1990).

The relationship between nail psoriasis and distal interphalangeal psoriatic joint involvement is not clear (Zaias & Norton, 1980). Using bone scintigraphy, Holzmann *et al.* (1992) demonstrated the involvement of the end phalanx as a deep Koebner phenomenon.

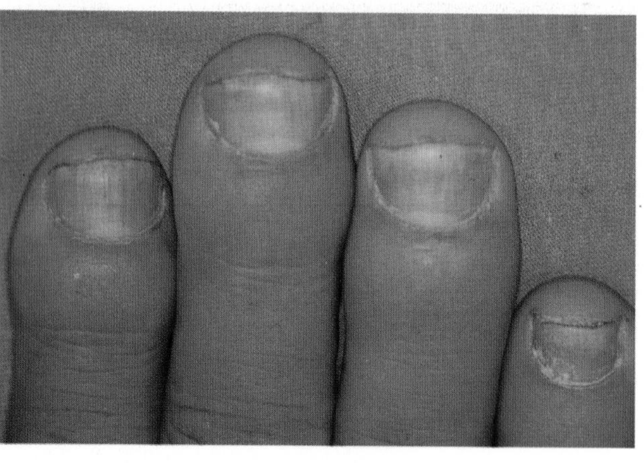

Fig. 5.25. Psoriasis – distal, interphalangeal joint arthropathy and periungual soft tissue inflammation (psoriatic acropachydermodactyly).

Biochemical analysis

The fingernails in psoriatic arthritis may be differentiated from those in rheumatoid arthritis by biochemical and statistical analysis of the fingernail amino acids (Greaves *et al.*, 1979); the amino acid content of clinically normal nails of patients with psoriatic and rheumatoid arthritis are significantly different with respect to threonine, proline and isoleucine. Rheumatoid normal nails differ from the dystrophic fingernails of patients with psoriatic arthritis with regard to threonine, proline and aspartic acid content. This may mean that the difference between psoriatic arthritis normal nail and psoriatic arthritis dystrophic nail resides in the presence of isoleucine in the former and aspartic acid in the latter. No difference has been found between normal nail and dystrophic nail in psoriatic arthritis.

Three abnormal metabolites in psoriatic nails have been detected (Maeda *et al.*, 1980): tetradecanoic acid octadecyl ester, hexadecanoic acid octadecyl ester and octadecanoic acid octadecyl ester. These esters could not be found in normal nails nor in ultrafiltrates of blood in cases of psoriasis. All these biochemical analyses are not routinely performed.

Psoriatic onychopachydermoperiostitis (psoriatic acropachydermodactyly)

In this variant of rheumatoid psoriasis, involvement of the great toe, psoriatic nail changes, and thickening of the distal soft tissues are associated with osteoperiostitis of

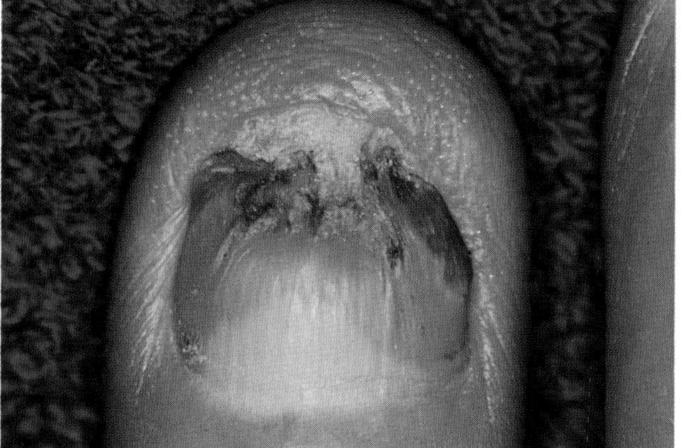

Fig. 5.26. Reiter's syndrome (courtesy J.L. Verret, Angers, France).

the distal phalanx, with normal interphalangeal joint (Fournié *et al.*, 1989). Other identical cases with involvement of all the digits has also been reported (Dompmartin *et al.*, 1992; de Pontville *et al.*, 1993). We have observed a similar case involving just the hands and accompanied by nail fold inflammation and a distal joint arthropathy (Marghéry *et al.*, 1991) (Fig. 5.25). Differential diagnosis includes osteoarthritis, pachydermoperiostitis, acromegaly and hypertrophic osteoarthropathy.

Reiter's syndrome

The clinical and histological features of the skin changes in patients with Reiter's syndrome may be indistinguishable from those of patients with psoriasis (Sturde, 1971). Skin changes resembling paronychia can accompany nail involvement suggesting inflammation of the proximal nail fold. Onycholysis, ridging, splitting, greenish-yellow or sometimes brownish-red discoloration and subungual hyperkeratosis may be present (Fig. 5.26). Small yellow pustules may develop and showly enlarge beneath the nail, often near the lunula. Their contents become dry and brown. The nails may be shed. Samman (1986) noted nail pitting in Reiter's syndrome, stating that deep pits and punched out lesions can occur. According to Lovy *et al.* (1980) nail pitting may reflect a predisposition to the development of psoriasis or psoriasiform lesions dependent on the HLA-A2 and B27 antigens, as suggested by previously reported HLA typing studies. HLA-A and B27 were present in a 6-year-old boy who had only the nail changes which were compatible with Reiter's syndrome; HLA-A and B27 were also present in his father, who had uveitis, arthritis and amyloidosis (Pajarre & Kero, 1977).

Antibiotics, steroids and non-steroidal anti-inflammatory drugs are without benefit. PUVA may be helpful. Aromatic retinoid therapy may clear the nails in Reiter's syndrome. Combined chemotherapy with methotrexate, aromatic retinoid and prednisolone has been suggested (Luderschmidt & Balda, 1982).

Histopathology cannot definitely differentiate psoriasis from Reiter's syndrome, however, nail changes in the latter tend to be more pustular than in psoriasis vulgaris and erythrocyte extravasation is usually more pronounced.

References

Psoriasis

Abel E.A., Dicicco L.M., Ozenberg E.K. *et al.* (1986) Drugs in exacerbation of psoriasis. *J. Am. Acad. Dermatol.* **15**, 1007–1022.

Ackerman B. (1979) Subtle clues to diagnosis by conventional microscopy. Neutrophils within the cornified layer as clues to infection by superficial fungi. *Am. J. Dermatol.* **1**, 69–75.

Alkiewicz J. (1948) Psoriasis of the nails. *Br. J. Dermatol.* **60**, 195–200.

Alkiewicz J. & Pfister R. (1976) *Atlas der Nagelkrankheiten: Pathohistologie, klinik und defferentialdiagnose.* FK Schattauer, Stuttgart.

André J., Achten G. & Laporte M. (1988) Normal and abnormal nails: light and electron microscopy. Dermatology in five continents. *Proceedings of XVII World Congress of Dermatology*, pp. 907–908. Springer, Berlin.

Asboe-Hansen G. (1971) Psoriasis in childhood. In: *Psoriasis. Proceedings of the International Symposium, Stanford University*, eds Farber E.M. & Cox A.J. Stanford University Press, Stanford, CA.

Baden H. (1987) *Diseases of the Hair and Nails*, p. 48. Year Book Med. Publishers, New York.

Badger J., Banerjee A.K. & McFadden J. (1992) Unilateral subungual hyperkeratosis following a cerebrovascular incident in a patient with psoriasis. *Clin. Exp. Dermatol.* **17**, 454–455.

Baran R. (1982) Action thérapeutique et complications du rétinoïde aromatique sur l'appareil unguéal. *Ann. Dermatol. Venereol.* **109**, 367.

Baran R. (1990) Retinoids and the nails. *J. Dermatol. Treat.* **1**, 151–154.

Baran R. & Barthelemy H. (1990) Photo-onycholyse induite par le 5-MOP (Psoraderm) et application de la méthode d'imputation des effets médicamenteux. *Ann. Dermatol. Venereol.* **117**, 367–369.

Bedi T.R. (1977) Intradermal triamcinolone treatment of psoriatic onychodystrophy. *Dermatologica* **155**, 24–27.

Caccialanza M. & Frigerio U. (1982) Risultati della fotochemioterapia orale nel trattamento della psoriasi ungueale. *G. Ital. Dermatol. Venereol.* **117**, 251–254.

Calvert H.T., Smith M.A. & Wells R.S. (1963) Psoriasis and the nails. *Br. J. Dermatol.* **75**, 415.

Coignet M. & Sayag J. (1990) Collyre béta-bloquant et psoriasis. *Nouv. Dermatol.* **9**, 552–553.

Davids T.L. & Hayes T.J. (1987) Isotretinoin-induced psoriasis: A case of Koebner's phenomenon. *J. Assoc. Milit. Dermatol.* **12**, 23–26.

Dawber R.P.R., Marks R. & Swift J.A. (1972) Scanning electron microscopy of the stratum corneum. *Br. J. Dermatol.* **86**, 272.

Deffer T.A. & Goette D.K. (1987) Distal phalangeal atrophy

secondary to topical steroid therapy. *Arch. Dermatol.* **123**, 571–572.

de Granciansky P., Larrègue M. & Katz M. (1975) Opacités linéaires intra-unguéales dans le psoriasis. *Ann. Dermatol. Syphil.* **102**, 121.

Duvic M., Johnson T., Rapini R.P. *et al.* (1987) AIDS associated psoriasis and Reiter's syndrome. *Arch. Dermatol.* **123**, 1622–1632.

Ellis C.N. & Voorhees J.J. (1987) Etretinate therapy. *J. Am. Acad. Dermatol.* **16**, 267–291.

Farber E.J. & Jacobs A.H. (1977) Nail infantile psoriasis. *Am. J. Dis. Child.* **131**, 1266.

Fischer E. (1982) Subunguale Kerkalkungen. *Frotsche. Röntgenstr.* **137**, 580–584.

Fisher A. & Baran R. (1992) Occupational nail disorders with reference to Koebner's phenomenon. *Am. J. Contact Dermatol.* **3**, 16–22.

Frederiksson T. (1974) Topically applied fluorouracil in the treatment of psoriatic nails. *Arch. Dermatol.* **110**, 735.

Fritz K. (1988) Psoriasis of the nail. Successful topical treatment with 5-fluorouracil. *Z. Hautkr.* **64**, 1083–1088.

Ganor S. (1977a) Diseases sometimes associated with psoriasis. I, Candidosis. *Dermatologica* **154**, 268.

Ganor S. (1977b) Diseases sometimes associated with psoriasis. II, Alopecia areata. *Dermatologica* **154**, 338.

Gayrard L., Nicolas J.F. & Thivolet J. (1990) Erythrodermies induites par le captopril chez une patiente porteuse d'un psoriasis vulgaire. *Nouv. Dermatol.* **9**, 28.

Handfield-Jones S.E., Boyle J. & Harman R.R.M. (1987) Local PUVA treatment for nail psoriasis. *Br. J. Dermatol.* **116**, 280.

Haneke E. (1991) Onychomycosis and psoriasis restricted to the nails. 50th Meeting AAD, Dallas.

Happle R. (1987) The lines of Blashko: a developmental pattern visualizing functional X-chromosome mosaicism. In: *Biology of Heritable Skin Diseases*, eds Wuepper K.D. & Gedde-Dahl T. *Curr. Prob. Dermatol.* **17**, 5–18.

Happle R. (1990) Ptychotropism as a cutaneous feature of the CHILD syndrome. *J. Am. Acad. Dermatol.* **23**, 763–766.

Happle R., Koch H. & Lenz W. (1980) CHILD syndrome: Congenital hemidysplasia with ichthyosiform erythroderma and limb defects. *Eur. J. Pediatr.* **134**, 27.

Harrison P.V. & Stone R.N. (1988) Severe exacerbation of psoriasis due to terfenadine. *Clin. Exp. Dermatol.* **13**, 275.

Hofmann C. & Plewig G. (1977) Photochemotherapie der Nagelpsoriasis. *Hautarzt* **28**, 408.

Jensen H.A., Mikkelsen H.I., Wadskov V. & Sondegaard J. (1976) Cutaneous reactions due to propanolol. *Acta Med. Scand.* **199**, 363.

Kaplan M., Sadick S., Wieder J. *et al.* (1989) Antipsoriatic effects of zidovudine in human immunodeficiency virus-associated psoriasis. *J. Am. Acad. Dermatol.* **20**, 76.

Katz M. & Weinrauch L. (1987) Penicillin-induced generalized pustular psoriasis. *J. Am. Acad. Dermatol.* **17**, 918–920.

Kitamura K., Kanasashi M., Suga C. *et al.* (1993) Cutaneous reactions induced by calcium channel blockers. High frequency of psoriasiform eruptions. *J. Dermatol.* **20**, 279–286.

Laplanche G., Grosshans E. & Gebriel-Robez O. (1980) Hyperplasie épidermique et hémidyplasie corporelle hypoplasique congénitale homolatérale. *Ann. Dermatol. Venereol.* **107**, 729.

Lazar A.P. & Roenigk H.H. (1988) AIDS can exacerbate psoriasis. *J. Am. Acad. Dermatol.* **18**, 144.

Lewin K., Dewit S. & Ferrington R.A. (1972) Pathology of the finger nail in psoriasis. A clinicopathological study. *Br. J. Dermatol.* **86**, 555.

Leyden J.L., Decherd J.W. & Goldschmidt H. (1972) Exfoliative cytology in the diagnosis of psoriasis of nails. *Cutis* **10**, 701–704.

Lindelöf B (1988) Psoriasis of the nails treated with Grenz rays: a double-blind bilateral trial. *Acta Dermatol. Venereol.* **69**, 80–82.

Lindelöf B. & Eklund G. (1986) Incidence of malignant skin tumours in 14 140 patients after Grenz-ray treatment for benign skin disorders. *Arch. Dermatol.* **122**, 1391–1395.

Luzza M.J. (1982) Hydrochloroquine in psoriatic arthropathy. Exacerbation of psoriatic skin lesions. *J. Rheumatol.* **9**, 462–464.

Maeda K., Kawaguchi S., Niwa T., Ohki T. & Kobayashi K. (1980) Identification of some abnormal metobolites in psoriasis nail using gas chromatography-mass spectrometry. *J. Chromatogr.* **221**, 199.

McKenna K.E. & McMillan J.C. (1993) Exacerbation of psoriasis, liver disfunction and thrombocytopenia associated with mebhydrolin. *Clin. Exp. Dermatol.* **18**, 131–132.

Marx L. & Scher R.K. (1980) Response of psoriatic nails to oral photochemotherapy. *Arch. Dermatol.* **116**, 1023.

Mauro J., Lumpkin L.R. & Dantzig P.I. (1975) Scanning electron microscopy of psoriatic nail pits. *NY J. Med.* **February**, 339.

Meyeroff J.O. (1983) Exacerbation of psoriasis with meclofenamate. *N. Engl. J. Med.* **309**, 496.

Müller J., Kordass D. & Boonen H.P.T. (1991) UV-Therapie der nagelpsoriasis. *Akt. Dermatol.* **17**, 166–169.

Nanda A., Kaur S., Kaur I. *et al.* (1990) Childhood psoriasis: an epidemiologic survey of 112 patients. *Pediatr. Dermatol.* **7**, 19–21.

Navaratnam A.E. & Gebauer K.A. (1990) Terfenadine-induced exacerbation of psoriasis. *Clin. Exp. Dermatol.* **15**, 78.

Neuman H.A.M. & Van Jous T. (1981) Adverse reaction of the skin to metaprolol and β-adrenergic blocking agents. *Dermatologica* **163**, 330–335.

Nicolas J.F., Maudit G., Larbre J.P. *et al.* (1987) Psoriasis aggravés ou induits par les médicaments. *Med. Hyg.* **45**, 1809–1814.

Norton L.A. (1982) Disease of the nails. In: *Current Therapy*, ed. Conn, p. 664. W.B. Saunders, Philadelphia.

Parker S.G. & Diffey B.L. (1983) The transmission of optical radiation through human nail. *Br. J. Dermatol.* **108**, 11.

Peachy R.D.G., Pye R.J. & Harman R.R. (1976) The treatment of psoriatic nail dystrophy with intradermal steroid injections. *Br. J. Dermatol.* **95**, 75.

Pfister R. (1981) Die Psoriasis des Nagels. *Schweiz Rund Med. (Praxis)* **70**, 1967–1973.

Puissant A. (1970) Psoriasis in children under the age of ten: a study of 100 observations. *Gazz Sanita* **19**, 191.

Requena L., Zamora E., Martin L. *et al.* (1990) Acroatrophy secondary to long-standing applications of topical steroids. *Arch. Dermatol.* **126**, 1013–1014.

Robbins T.D., Kouskoukis C.E. & Ackerman A.B. (1983) Onycholysis in psoriatic nails. *Am. J. Dermatopathol.* **5**, 39–41.

Rudolph R.I. (1991) Lithium induced psoriasis of the fingernails. *J. Am. Acad. Dermatol.* **26**, 135–136.

Runne U. & Orfanos C.E. (1981) *Curr. Prob. Dermatol.* **9**, 102., Karger, Basel.

Samman P. (1978) *The Nails in Disease*, 3rd edn. Heinemann, London.

Sasaki T., Saito S., Aihara M. *et al.* (1989) Exacerbation of psoriasis during lithium treatment. *J. Dermatol.* **16**, 59–63.

Scher R.K. & Ackerman A.B. (1980) Histologic differential diagnosis of onychomycosis and psoriasis of the nail unit from cornified cells of the nail bed alone. *Am. J. Dermatopathol.* **2**, 255.

Schmied E. & Levy P.M. (1986) Transient rhabdomyolysis connected with topical use of 5-FU in a patient with psoriasis of the nails. *Dermatologica* **173**, 257–258.

Shear C.S., Nyhan W.L., Frost P. & Weinstein G.D. (1971) Psoriasis associated with unilateral ectromelia and central nervous system anomalies: skin, hair and nails, birth defects. *Orig. Art. Ser.* **8**, 197.

Staberg B., Gammeltoft M. & Onsberg P. (1983) Onychomycosis in patients with psoriasis. *Acla. Derm. Venereol.* **63**, 436–438.

Stankler L. (1988) Foetal psoriasis. *Br. J. Dermatol.* **119**, 684.

Szepes E. (1986) Mycotic inail foldections of psoriatic nails. *Mykosen* **29**, 82–84.

Tegner E. (1976) Reversible overcurvature of the nails after treatment with practolol. *Acta Derm. Venereol.* **56**, 493.

Tosti A., Guerra L., Bardazzi F. *et al.* (1990) Topical ciclosporin in nail psoriasis. *Dermatologica* **180**, 110 (letter).

Tosti A., Fanti P.A., Morelli R. & Bardazzi F. (1992) Psoriasiform acral dermatitis: Report of three cases. *Acta Derm. Venereol.* **72**, 206–207.

Watson W. & Farber E.M. (1977) Controlling psoriasis. *Postgrad. Med.* **61**, 103.

White C.J. & Lapply T. (1952) Histopathology of nail diseases. *J. Invest. Derm.* **19**, 121–124.

Wolf R., Dorfman B. & Kzakowski A. (1987) Psorasiform eruption induced by captopril and chlorthalidone. *Cutis* **40**, 162–164.

Yu R.C.H. & King C.M. (1992) A double blind study of superficial radiotherapy in psoriatic nail dystrophy. *Acta Derm. Venereol.* **72**, 134–136.

Zaias N. (1969) Psoriasis of the nail. A clinical-pathology study. *Arch. Dermatol.* **99**, 567.

Zaias N. (1984) Psoriasis of the nail unit. *Dermatol. Clin.* **2**, 493–505.

Zaias N. (1990) *The Nail in Health and Disease*, 2nd edn. Appleton and Lange, Norwalk, CN.

Zaias N. & Norton L.A. (1980) In: *Clinical Dermatology*, eds Demis D.J., Dobson R.L. & McGuire J., Vol. 1, pp. 3–4.

Acropustulosis

Ackerman A.B. (1981) Is subcorneal pustular dermatosis of Sneddon and Wilkinson an entity sui generis? *Am. J. Dermatopathol.* **3**, 363.

Arnold H. (1978) Treatment of Hallopeau's acrodermatitis with Triamcinolone acetonide. *Arch. Dermatol.* **114**, 963.

Baran R. (1979) Hallopeau's acrodermatitis. *Arch. Dermatol.* **115**, 815.

Baran R. (1982) Action thérapeutique et complications du rétinoide aromatique sur l'appareil unguéal. *Ann. Derm. Venereol.* **109**, 367–371.

Brun P., Baran R. & Juhlin L. (1985) Acropustulose résistante à l'association étrétinate-PUVA thérapie. *Ann. Dermatol. Venereol.* **112**, 611–612.

Cheesbrough M.J. (1979) Osteolysis and psoriasis. *Clin. Exp. Dermatol.* **4**, 341.

Combemale P., Baran R., Flechaire A. *et al.* (1989) Acroosteolyse psoriasique. *Ann. Dermatol. Venereol.* **116**, 555–558.

Deichmann B. & Spindeldreier A. (1982) Aromatisches Retinoid zur Behandlung bie Psoriasis pustulosa an Händen und Füssen. *Z. Haut.* **57**, 425.

Mahowald M.L. & Parrish R.M. (1982) Severe osteolytic arthritis mutilans pustular psoriasis. *Arch. Dermatol.* **118**, 434.

Miller J.L., Soltani K. & Tourtellotte C.D. (1971) Psoriatic acro-osteolysis without arthritis. *J. Bone Joint Surg.* **53A**, 371–374.

Miyagawa S, Kitaoka M., Komatsu M. *et al.* (1990) Acral granulomatous dermatosis. *Br. J. Dermatol.* **122**, 709–713.

Notowicz A., Stolz E. & Heuvel N. (1978) Treatment of Hallopeau's acrodermatitis with topical mechlorethamine. *Arch. Dermatol.* **114**, 129.

Piraccini B.M., Fanti P.A., Morelli R. & Tosti A (1994) Hallopeau's acrodermatitis continua of the nail apparatus. *Acta. Dermato. Venerol.* (in press).

Ryan T.J. (1981) Sneddon and Wilkinson's pustular dermatosis does exist. *Am. J. Dermatopathol.* **3**, 383.

Tsuji T. & Nishimura M. (1991) Topically administrated fluorouracil in acrodermatitis continua of Hallopeau. *Arch. Dermatol.* **127**, 27–28.

Psoriatic arthritis

Abel E. & Farber E.M. (1979) Psoriasis. In: *Clinical Dermatology*, eds. Demis D.J., Dobson R.L. & McGuire J., Vol. 1, pp. 1–2.

Baker H., Golding D.N. & Thompson M. (1964) The nail in psoriatic arthritis. *Br. J. Dermatol.* **76**, 569.

Eastmond C.J. & Wright V. (1979) The nail dystrophy of psoriatic arthritis. *Ann. Rheum. Dis.* **38**, 226.

Greaves M.S., Fieller N.R.J. & Moll J.M.H. (1979) Differentiation between psoriatic arthritis and rheumatoid arthritis. A biochemical and statistical analysis of fingernails amino acids. *Scand. J. Rheum.* **8**, 33.

Harrison P.V., Khunti K. & Morris J.A. (1990) Psoriasis, nails, joints and autoimmunity. *Br. J. Dermatol.* **122**, 569 (letter).

Holzmann H., Werner R.J., Maul F.D. *et al.* (1992) Zur Kenntnis des Köbner–Phänomens am Skelett des Psoriatihers. *Hautarzt* **43**, 645–651.

Sills E.M. (1980) Psoriatic arthritis in childhood. *Johns Hopk. Med. J.* **146**, 49.

Southwood T.R., Petty R.E., Malleson P.N. *et al.* (1989) Psoriatic arthritis in children. *Arth. Rheum.* **32**, 1007–1013.

Wright V., Roberts M.C. & Hill A.G.S. (1979) Dermatological manifestations in psoriatic arthritis. A follow up study. *Acta Derm. Venereol.* **59**, 235.

Zaias N. & Norton L.A. (1980) Diseases of nails. In: *Clinical Dermatology*, eds Demis D.J., Dobson R.L. & McGuire J., Vol. 1, pp. 3–4.

Psoriatic onychopachydermoperiostitis

Bazex J., Marguery N.C., Baran R. & Pages M. (1993) Psoriatic alyropachydermodactyly. In: *Dermatology Progress and Perspective* (*18th World Congress of Dermatology*), eds Burgclorf W.H.C. & Katz S.I. The Parthenon Publishing Group, pp. 391–392.

Dompmartin A., De Ponville M., Remond B. *et al.* (1993) Onycho-pachydermopériostite psoriasique étendre ã tous les ongles (in press).

Fournié B., Viraben R., Durroux R. *et al.* (1989) L'onycho-pachydermo-périostite psoriasique du gros orteil. *Rev. Rhum.* **56**, 579–582.

Marghéry M.C., Baran R., Pages M. & Bazex J. (1991) Acropachydermie psoriasique. *Ann. Dermatol. Venereol.* **118**, 373–376.

de Pontville A., Dompmartin A., de Raucourt *et al.* (1993) Onycho-pachydermo-periostite psoriasique. *Ann. Derm. Venereol.* **120**, 229–232.

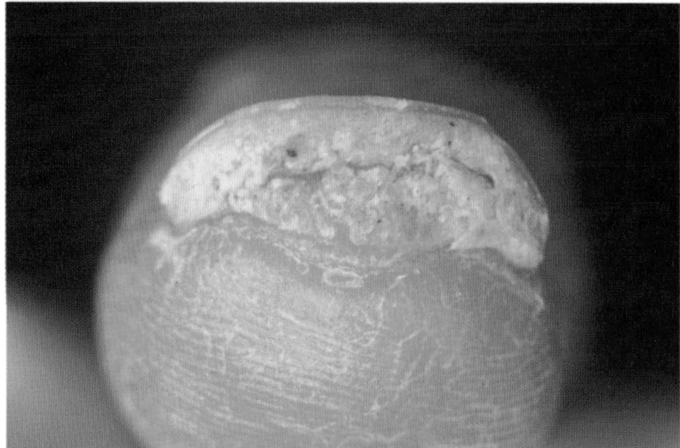

Fig. 5.27. (Type I) pityriasis rubra pilaris – prominent distal, subungual thickening.

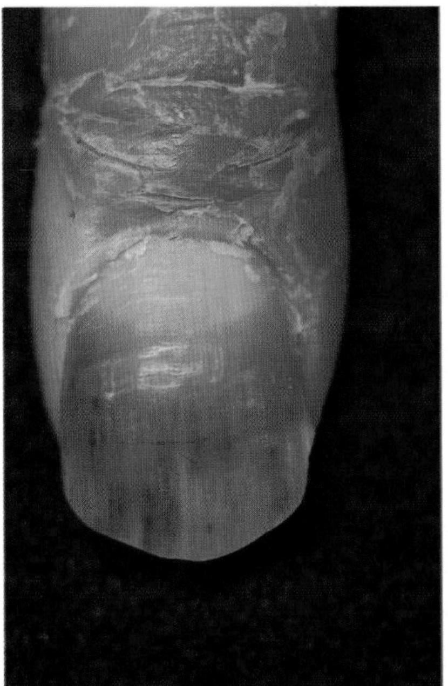

Fig. 5.28. (Type I) pityriasis rubra pilaris – mainly distal subungual changes.

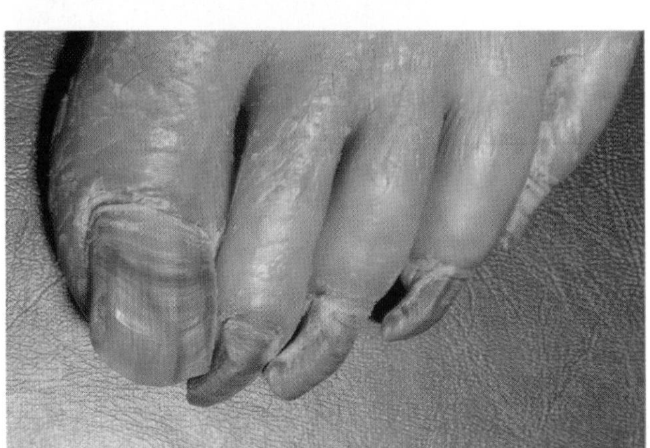

Fig. 5.29. (Type V) pityriasis rubra pilaris – onychogryphotic changes (courtesy of D. Lambert, Dijon, France).

Reiter's syndrome

Lovy M., Bluhm G. & Morales A. (1980) The occurence of pitting in Reiter's syndrome. *J. Am. Acad. Dermatol.* **2**, 66.

Luderschmidt C. & Balda B.R. (1982) Reiter's syndrome. Case presentations. In: *XVI Congressus Internationalis Dermatologiae, Tokyo*, p. 122.

Pajarre R. & Kero M. (1977) Nail changes as the first manifestation of the HLA-B27 inheritance. *Dermatologica* **154**, 350.

Samman P.D. (1986) In: *The Nails in Disease*, 4th edn, eds Samman P.D. & Fenton D. Heinemann, London.

Sturde H.C. (1971) Nagelveränderungen bei morbus Reiter. Hautarzt **22**, 353.

Pityriasis rubra pilaris (PRP)

When the palms and soles are affected, as in adult acute onset type I PRP (Griffiths, 1976; Cohen & Prystowsky, 1989), nail involvement is usual (Figs 5.27 & 5.28). The fingernails show well-marked changes, including terminal subungual hyperkeratosis with moderate thickening of the nail bed, splinter haemorrhages and longitudinal ridging. The condition is sometimes attended by a distal yellow-brown discoloration in the nails. Psorasiform pits in the nail plate are exceptionally noted, as well as onycholysis. 'Salmon patches' are not seen (Sonnex *et al.*, 1986). In the juvenile types nail changes are very much less common. Lambert and Dalac (1989) observed an unusual case with onychogryphosis of all 20 nails in a young girl afflicted by type V PRP (Fig. 5.29). In localized type IV PRP, psorasiform pitting may occur in the absence of any periungual abnormality (W.A.D. Griffiths, personal communication). Nail changes in chronic erythroderma due to Sézary syndrome are similar to those found in patients with type I PRP, suggesting a non-specific reaction to erythema (Sonnex *et al.*, 1986).

In adult type I PRP, there is patchy parakeratosis in the nail plate suggesting an 'onychization' disturbance in the matrix.

Parakeratotic areas are present over the nail bed epithelium which may be thickened and show focal basal liquefaction. Keratohyalin may be seen. An inflammatory infiltrate consisting of mononuclear cells may be present in the dermis of the nail fold. The hyponychium shows both orthokeratosis and parakeratosis (Sonnex *et al.*, 1986). Good responses have been obtained with etretinate (Lauharanta & Lassus, 1980) and with combined oral retinoid–PUVA therapy.

References

Cohen P.R. & Prystowsky J.H. (1989) PRP: a view of diagnosis and treatment. *J. Am. Acad. Dermatol.* **20**, 801–807.

Griffiths W.A.D. (1976) Pityriasis rubra pilaris: an historical approach. 2 – Clinical features. *Clin. Exp. Dermatol.* **1**, 37.

Lambert D.G. & Dalac S. (1989) Nail changes in type V PRP. *J. Am. Acad. Dermatol.* **21**, 811–812.

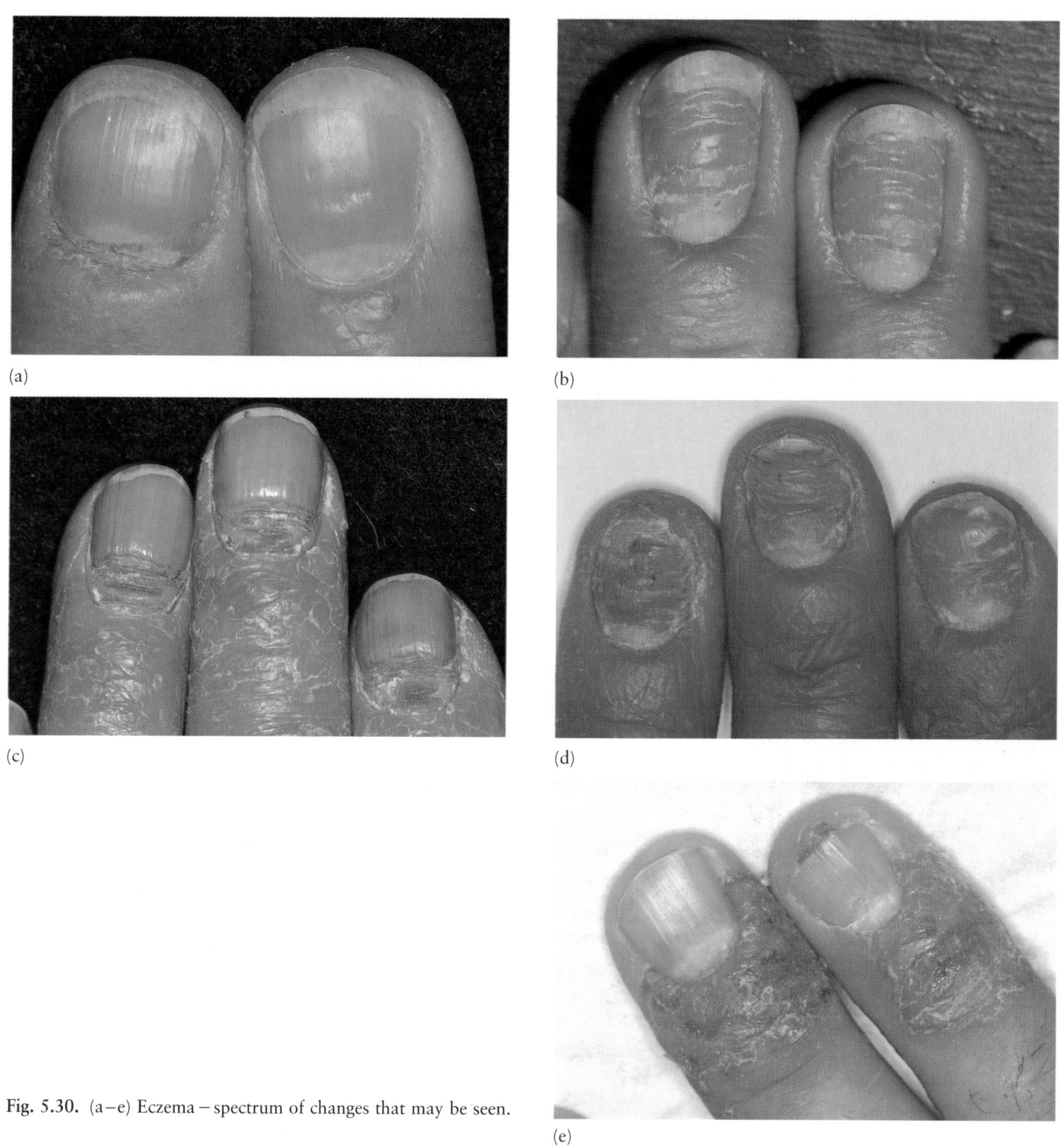

Fig. 5.30. (a–e) Eczema – spectrum of changes that may be seen.

Lauharanta J. & Lassus A. (1980) Treatment of PRP with an oral aromatic retinoid. *Acta Derm. Venereol.* **60**, 460–462.

Sonnex T.S., Dawber R.P.R., Zachary C.B. *et al.* (1986) The nails in adult type I pityriasis rubra pilaris. A comparison with Sézary syndrome and psoriasis. *J. Am. Acad. Dermatol.* **15**, 956–960.

Eczema

The nail apparatus is particularly vulnerable to eczematous involvement (Fig. 5.30) irrespective of the nature of the allergen or the route by which it reaches the nail apparatus. Many of the specific changes seen in non-constitutional eczema are described in Chapter 7.

The cause of the nail changes is obvious when the eczema of the fingers has a periungual distribution (Fig. 5.30(a)–(e)). However, the cause must be sought elsewhere if, as is frequently the case, the nail disorder is not associated with periungual eczema. General examination may reveal a specific type of eczema, e.g. atopic dermatitis, discoid eczema, pompholyx, etc. Modifications of the nail plate result from disturbances of the matrix. These may present as thickening, roughness, pitting and transverse ridging and furrowing, sometimes leading to shedding of the nail.

Eczema of the nail bed is seldom associated with cosmetic products such as nail varnish (Liden *et al.*, 1993) base coats, nail hardeners or hair setting lotions – the exception is prosthetic nails (see Chapter 8). The nail changes resulting from eczema at this site appear hours, days or even weeks later as splinter haemorrhages, soon followed by the development of subungual hyperkeratosis; sometimes onycholysis and paronychia may also be seen, resulting from formaldehyde application. Colour changes vary from a bluish-red appearance initially, to 'rust' and finally yellow. The affected areas may be intensely painful.

Common chemical sensitizers may show a wide range of clinical patterns in the nail area (see Chapter 9). Minimal damage may simply produce onycholysis. Subungual hyperkeratosis is frequent and may be accompanied by erythema, scaling and fissuring.

It has been suggested that parakeratosis pustulosa is a variant of atopic eczema, which may also be the basis of juvenile plantar dermatitis, where the periungual tissue resemble dry eczema, but pitting is not seen, except when it is associated with atopic eczema.

Constant rubbing and scratching of the skin, as in atopic dermatitis, causes the nails to be buffed; the surface of the nails becomes 'polished' and shiny.

It is therefore evident that the changes in the nail apparatus induced by eczematous processes depend on the cause, and site of involvement, and also the severity of the eczematous inflammation.

Eczema is histologically characterized by a spongiotic dermatitis. When it involves the proximal nail fold with the eponychium a severe intercellular oedema will be found with mononuclear cells migrating into the spongiotic epidermis. Since it will then also affect the tip of the matrix, surface irregularities such as ridges, furrows and pits will develop. The matrix, nail bed and particularly the hyponychium may be involved also. Histopathology reveals spongiosis, spongiotic vesicles, variable parakeratosis and granular layer with intermittent orthokeratotic foci. The dermis shows a predominantly superficial perivascular lymphocytic infiltrate. Giemsa stain usually exhibits severe alterations in the stain uptake of the nail plate. The latter may become disorderly and wavy. The pits usually do not contain parakeratotic onychocytes. PAS stain may show pronounced staining of the intercellular spaces probably due to trapping of serum glycoproteins inbetween the cells of the nail plate. They can get into the nail plate by the spongiosis of the matrix.

Treatment with topical corticosteroids to the proximal nail fold may be attempted though premature closure of underlying epiphyses is a risk. Corticosteroids may increase the risk of secondary nail infection such as osteomyelitis of the distal phalanges reported in three children (Boiko *et al.*, 1988).

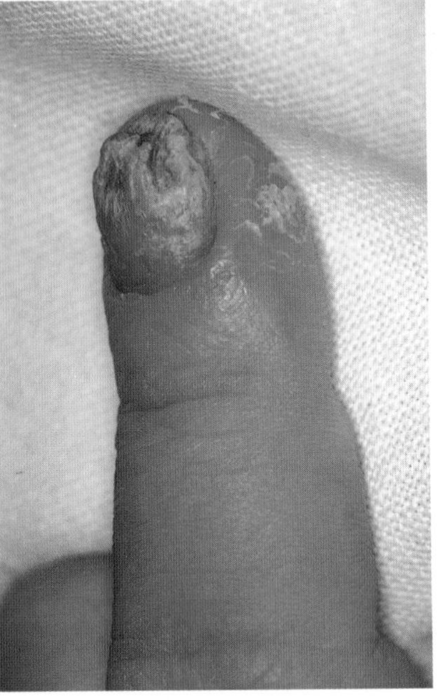

Fig. 5.31. Parakeratosis pustulosa.

Reference

Boiko S., Kaufman R.A. & Lucky A.W. (1988) Osteomyelitis of the distal phalanges in three children with severe atopic dermatitis. *Arch. Dermatol.* **124**, 418–423.

Liden C., Berg H., Faäzm G. *et al.* (1993) Nail varnish allergy with far-reaching consequences. *Br. J. Dermatol.* **123**, 57–62.

Pityriasis rosea

Sufficient damage may be done to the nail matrix in pityriasis rosea to produce multiple irregular indentations of the nails. These form rectangular areas of dystrophy observed in the middle third of each nail (Silvers & Glickman, 1964). We have seen pitting following the same condition, the pits being distributed in transverse lines.

Reference

Silver S.H. & Glickman F.S. (1964) Pityriasis rosea followed by nail dystrophy. *Arch. Dermatol.* **90**, 31.

Parakeratosis pustulosa (Hjorth–Sabouraud)

This parakeratotic condition of the fingertips has been well described by Sabouraud (1931) and Hjorth and Thomsen (1967). It usually occurs in girls of approximately 7 years of age. The lesions start close to the free margin of the nail of a finger or toe. In some cases, a few isolated pustules or vesicles may be observed in the initial phase; these usually disappear before the patient presents to the doctor. Confluent nail fold eczematoid changes cover the skin immediately adjacent to the distal edge of the nail (Fig. 5.31). The affected area is pink or of normal skin colour and densely studded with fine scales; there is a

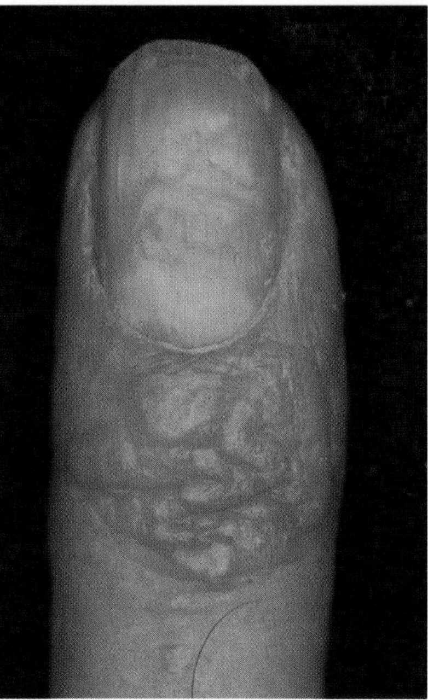

Fig. 5.32. Lichen planus.

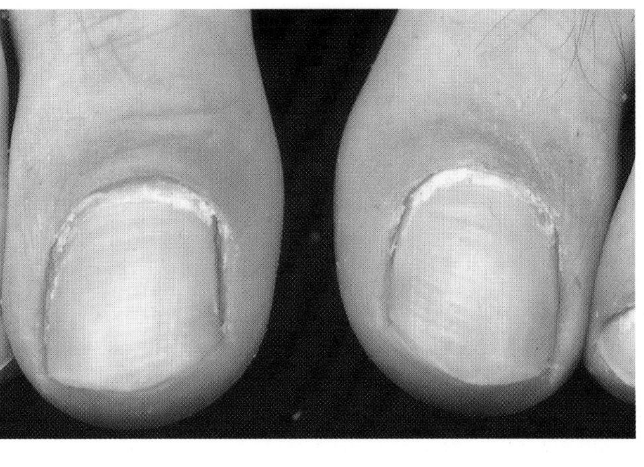

Fig. 5.33. Lichen planus – bluish colour in the dorsal nail fold.

clear margin between the normal and affected area. The skin changes may extend to the dorsal aspect of the finger or toe, but usually only the fingertip is affected. The most striking and characteristic change is the hyperkeratosis beneath the nail tip. The nail plate is lifted up, deformed, and often thickened. Commonly the deformity produced is asymmetrical and limited to one corner of the distal edge, or at least more pronounced at the corners of the nail. Pitting occurs; rarely transverse ridging of the nail plate is present. Most cases resolve within a few months but some cases persist for many years, even into adult life.

Histological findings (de Dulanto *et al.*, 1974) are of some value including hyperkeratosis and parakeratosis, pustulation and crusts, acanthosis and mild exocytosis, papillomatosis and heavy cellular infiltrates composed mainly of lymphocytes and fibroblasts around dilated capillary loops. According to Botella *et al.* (1973) the histology presents many of the features common to psoriasis and eczema. In the differential diagnosis of parakeratosis pustulosa, the following points are important:

1 pustules are very rare and only seen in the initial stage, as distinct from pustular psoriasis or Hallopeau's disease;

2 patients with psoriasis develop a coarse sheet of scales and not the fine type of scaling typically seen in parakeratosis pustulosa;

3 the age distribution differs from that found in atopic dermatitis which may cause transverse ridging due to the involvement of the proximal nail fold;

4 if nail changes predominate, especially on the feet, the disorder can be mistaken for tinea. Thumb sucking, which is a predisposing factor in chronic candidal paronychia, should be ruled out when a single thumb is affected.

No single treatment makes any difference to the frequency of recurrence or the overall duration of parakeratosis pustulosa (Hjorth & Thomsen, 1967). Topical steroids provide some symptomatic relief.

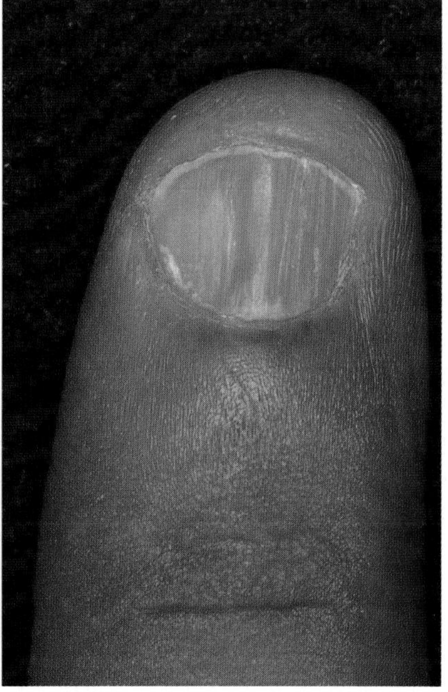

Fig. 5.34. Lichen planus (longitudinal bulge).

References

Botella R., Martinez C., Albero P. & Mascaro J.M. (1973) Parakeratosis pustulosa de Hjorth. Discussion nosologica a proposito de tres casos. *Acta Derm. Sifil.* **1–2**, 101.

de Dulanto F., Armijo-Moreno M. & Camacho-Martinez F. (1974) Parakeratosis pustulosa: histological findings. *Acta Derm. Venereol.* **54**, 365.

Hjorth N. & Thomsen K. (1967) Parakeratosis pustulosa. *Br. J. Dermatol.* **79**, 527.

Sabouraud R. (1931) Les parakeratoses microbiennes du bout des doigts. *Ann. Dermatol. Syphil.* **11**, 206.

Lichen planus

The etiology of lichen planus is still unknown. There is some evidence for a genetic susceptibility with increased

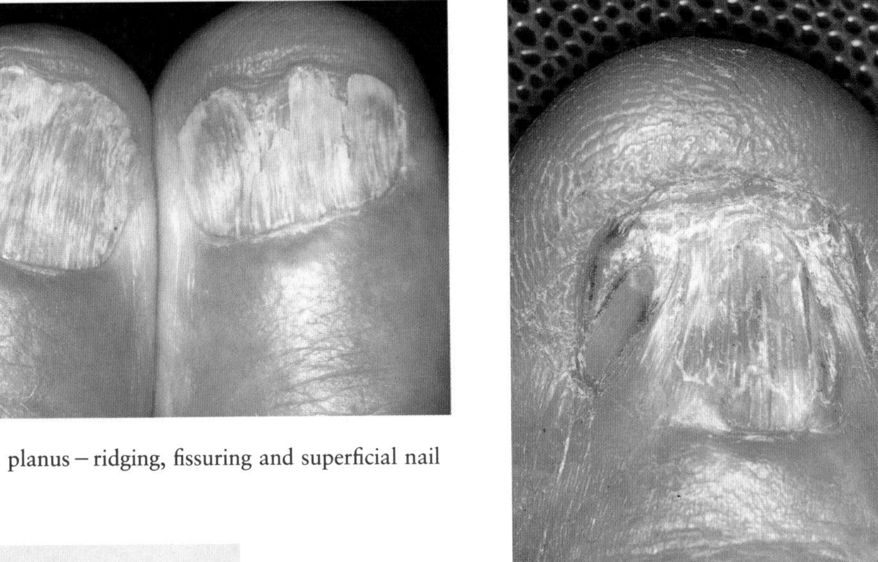

Fig. 5.35. Lichen planus – ridging, fissuring and superficial nail fragility.

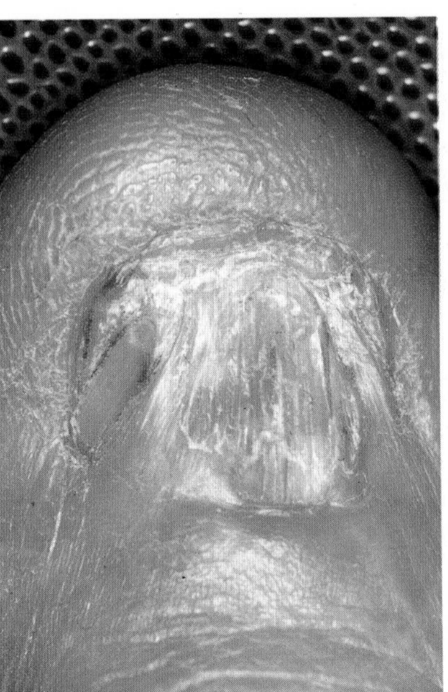

Fig. 5.36. Lichen planus – permanent atrophy and scarring.

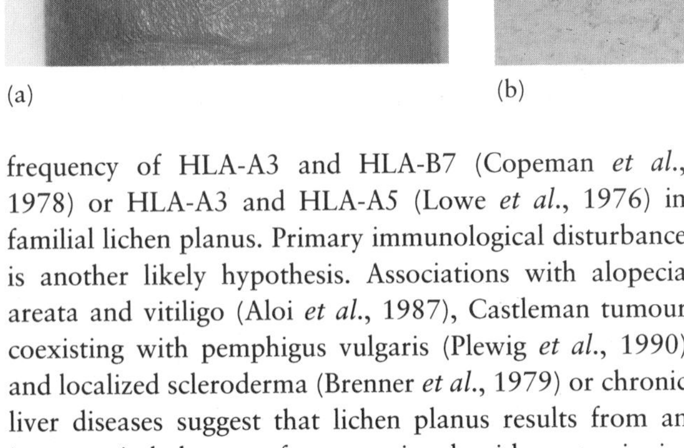

(a)

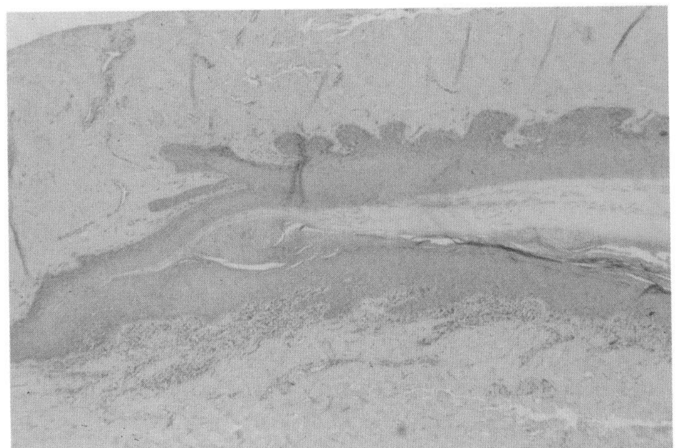

(b)

Fig. 5.37. Lichen planus. (a) Longitudinal melanonychia. (b) Matrix area – biopsy from nail in (a).

frequency of HLA-A3 and HLA-B7 (Copeman *et al.*, 1978) or HLA-A3 and HLA-A5 (Lowe *et al.*, 1976) in familial lichen planus. Primary immunological disturbance is another likely hypothesis. Associations with alopecia areata and vitiligo (Aloi *et al.*, 1987), Castleman tumour coexisting with pemphigus vulgaris (Plewig *et al.*, 1990) and localized scleroderma (Brenner *et al.*, 1979) or chronic liver diseases suggest that lichen planus results from an immune imbalance, often associated with systemic involvement (Cottoni *et al.*, 1988).

Nail involvement of one or all of the nail components occurs in 10% of patients with lichen planus (Fig. 5.32). Approximately 25% of patients with lichen planus of the nail have lichen planus in other sites before or after the onset of nail lesions (Tosti *et al.*, 1993). The clinical features observed depend upon the site affected by the pathological process. Sometimes there is a bluish or reddish colour in the dorsal nail fold, with or without swelling, which indicates that the proximal nail matrix is involved, and nail plate changes are likely to occur soon afterwards (Samman, 1961; Ronchese, 1965) (Fig. 5.33). A small lichen planus focus in the matrix may present clinically as a bulge under the proximal nail fold; instead of pitting, which occurs rarely, a depression may be visible on the nail (Fig. 5.34). Irregular longitudinal grooves, ridging with longitudinal fissuring (Fig. 5.35), distal splitting or notching, and progressive uniform thinning of the nail plate result from severe atrophy of the proximal portions of the matrix. Onychorrhexis, brittleness, crumbling or fragmentation of the nail plate may be present, as may onychoschizia, originating at the base of the nail, and onychomadesis leading to nail shedding.

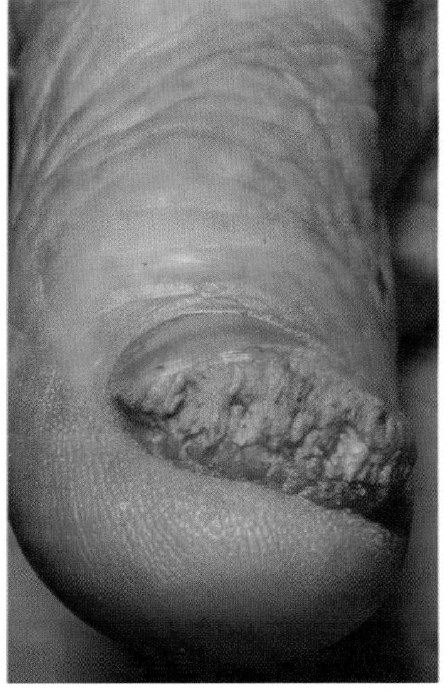

Fig. 5.38. Lichen planus – subungual hyperkeratosis.

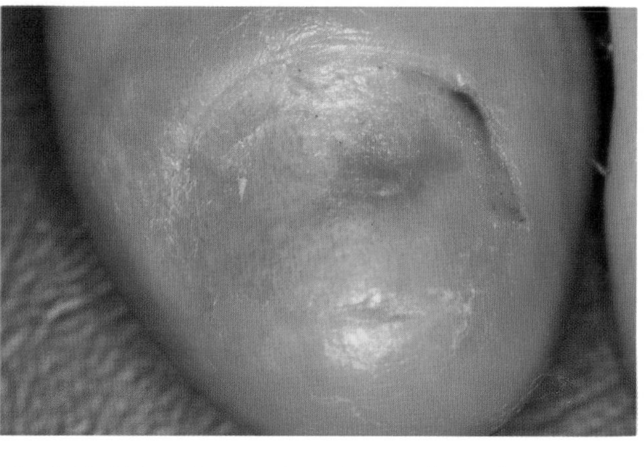

Fig. 5.40. Lichen planus – ulcerative, scarring variety.

The prognosis depends on the degree of matrix involvement, the intensity of inflammation and the scar produced. Pterygium formation is the hallmark of severe lichen planus. This is due to focal destruction of the matrix. Clinically a thin proximal epidermal nail fold adheres to the subungual epidermis with a loss of small areas of the nail plate. At this stage the overhanging proximal nail fold that attaches to the barren nail bed is flanked by a nail plate of normal thickness. Complete involvement of the matrix and nail bed will produce a total loss of the nail plate and permanent atrophy with scarring (Fig. 5.36). Red or violaceous lines or papules in the nail bed can be seen through the nail plate. They are different from longitudinal melanonychia involving the nail tissue in lichen planus (Fig. 5.37(a) & (b)), which can be seen even when lichen planus appears elsewhere. It has been reported in isolation (Baran *et al.*, 1985, 1988), and also after healing of the diseased nails, treated by intramuscular injections of Kenalog (Juhlin & Baran, 1989). This pigmentation is transitory and equivalent of that observed when skin lesions of lichen planus are healing (Juhlin & Baran, 1990). In black people, post-inflammatory subungual hyperpigmentation may appear (Zaias, 1970). In contrast, acquired leuconychia affecting all 20 nails was found in lichen planopilaris with a ventral involvement of the proximal nail fold by a papule of lichen planus as the only pathological change (Tosti *et al.*, 1988).

Lichen planus affecting the nail bed results in marked subungual hyperkeratosis which may lift the nail plate (Fig. 5.38). A keratotic tumour of the nail bed in a single finger is an unusual presentation (Lambert *et al.*, 1988) (Fig. 5.43). Subungual hyperkeratosis is sometimes associated with onycholysis (Kint & Vermander, 1982), but isolated onycholysis can also be seen (Fig. 5.39(a) & (b)). The 'pup tent' sign, in which the nail plate splits longitudinally and the lateral edges angle downward, is ap-

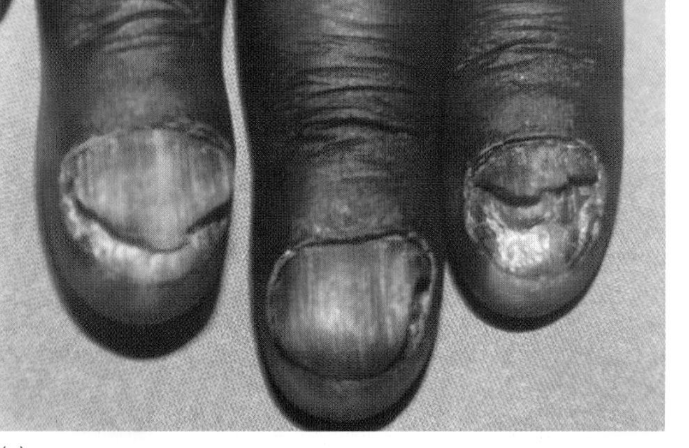

(a)

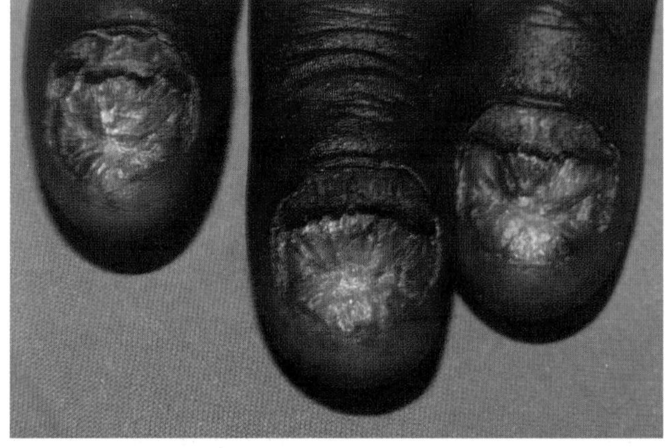

(b)

Fig. 5.39. (a & b) Lichen planus – severe progressive form with onycholysis (courtesy of J.L. Bonafé, Toulouse, France).

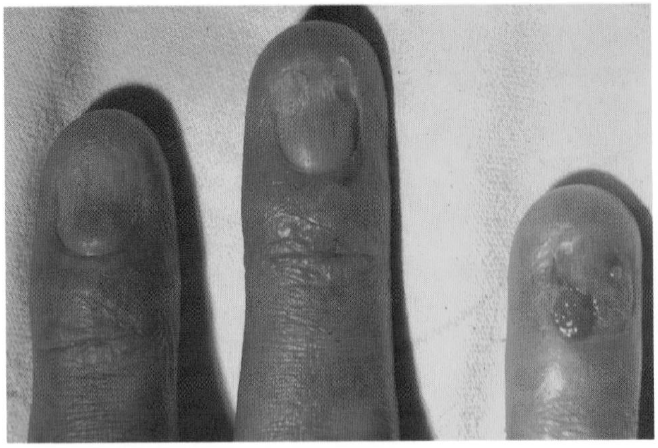

Fig. 5.41. Lichen planus-like ulcerative changes following bone marrow transplantation (graft-versus-host disease) (courtesy of J.H. Saurat, Geneva).

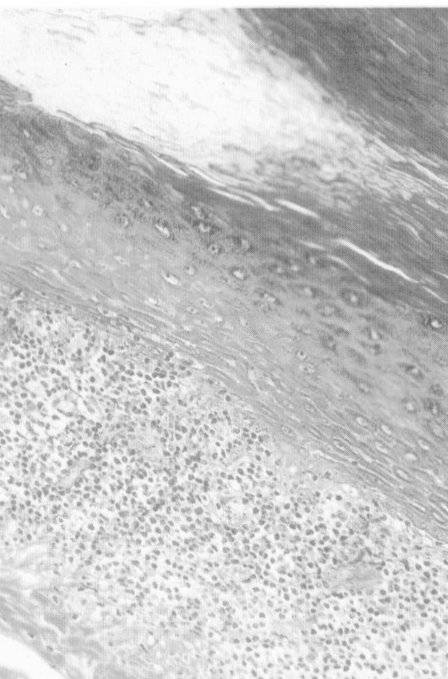

Fig. 5.42. Lichen planus – matrix area, showing prominent, dense dermal and dermo-epidermal inflammation and epidermal (matrix) spongiosis.

parent when viewing the nail on end (Boyd & Nelder, 1991). All these signs are reversible, except pterygium. Lichen planus nail involvement may be present in isolation or accompanied by typical skin, oral or genital lesions. Scalp lichen planus may be associated with severe forms, especially in women, and other atypical forms may occur. The nail changes are not pathognomonic for lichen planus but pterygium is highly suggestive; however dystrophic nail changes should be considered to be lichen planus when they improve approximately at the same time as the typical skin lesions. In familial lichen planus, the nails are frequently affected (Copeman, 1978), but there is no difference in the frequencies of nail lesions and palm and soles involvement (Kofoed & Wantzin, 1985). Lichen planus in children is rare (Jacyk, 1984; Milligan & Graham-Brown, 1990).

Ulcerative lichen planus (Perez *et al.*, 1982) is an entity characterized by chronic, painful bullae or erosions (Fabeiro *et al.*, 1989) (Fig. 5.40). They may be inflamed and occasionally haemorrhagic, leaving residual scarring (Cram *et al.*, 1966). Ulceration of the soles of the feet and toes and more rarely of the hands may occur. Often the mouth and other mucosa are involved and there may be associated cicatricial alopecia with the nail lesions. Often the eroded lesions appear on a surface that is already atrophic and the skin discoloured (Degos & Schnitzler, 1967). Healthy skin is rarely affected. This very incapacitating condition is aggravated by the spontaneous shedding of the nail, with atrophy of the matrix, leading to permanent anonychia (Oberste-Lehn & Kühl, 1954). Weidner and Ummenhofer (1979) have drawn clinical parallels between epidermolysis bullosa hereditaria dystrophica and dystrophica erosive lichen planus, stressing the different mode of blister formation.

When toenails are involved in ulcerative lichen planus, the lesions coexist with other manifestations of lichen planus. Lichen planus-like eruptions following bone marrow transplantation are a manifestation of graft-versus-host disease (Saurat & Gluckman, 1977). The nail changes are identical, in some cases, to those seen in typical lichen planus with fluting and onychatrophy, or there may be superficial ulceration in the lunula area similar to that found in ulcerative lichen planus (Fig. 5.41).

Disseminated lichenoid papular dermatosis has been observed in AIDS with a periungual distribution; progressively the nails become thinned with splinter haemorrhages and an irregular border of the distal margin of the lunula (Büchner *et al.*, 1989).

Drugs associated with a lichen planus-like reaction are numerous (Boyd & Nelder, 1991).

In addition to the classical pathological features of lichen planus of the skin and mucosae, such as a dense band-like lymphocytic infiltrate with epidermostropism, hydropic degeneration of basal cells, development of a stratum granulosum often consisting of several layers of cells with abundant keratohyalin granules, and a saw-tooth appearance of the epithelial rete ridges, there is often a marked spongiosis in the epithelium of the matrix and nail bed (Fig. 5.42), which may simulate allergic contact dermatitis. Due to the granular layer, the normal keratin which will be produced does not adhere to the nail plate thus giving rise to subungual (hyper-) keratosis and/or onycholysis. Foci with hypergranulosis in the matrix thus cannot produce nail keratin, and nail plate irregularities such as ridges or even nail atrophy will appear. Nail biopsies have shown that in lichen planus of the nails most commonly seen, that is with longitudinal ridges, depressions and superficial fragility, there is usually involvement of the eponychium, proximal tip and proximal part of the matrix – these structures are responsible for the surface of the nail plate. Unusually severe liquefaction degeneration of the basal layer of the nail bed has

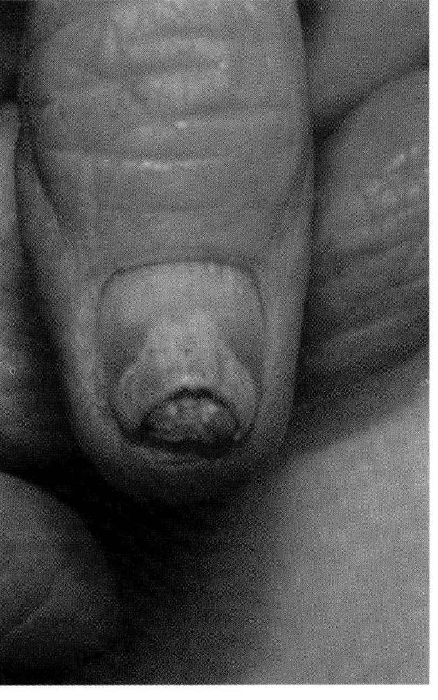

Fig. 5.43. Lichen planus – single digit involved; subungual keratotic variety (courtesy of V. Lambert, USA).

been shown to cause isolated bullous lichen planus of the nails (Haneke, 1983). Longitudinal melanonychia is a rare feature in ungual lichen planus (Baran *et al.*, 1985), probably due to activation of melanocytes by the inflammatory process and also the melanocyte destruction in the course of lichen planus (Fig. 5.37(a) & (b)). Fanti *et al.* (1992) suggest that in lichen planus the nail matrix loses its adult character and keratinizes through the formation of keratohyalin granules as is seen in the nail matrix primordium of embryos.

Isolated nail dystrophy due to lichen planus

It is uncommon for nail involvement to be the first and only or most important manifestation of the disease (Achten & Wanet-Rovarel, 1972; Marks & Samman, 1972; Scott & Scott, 1979; Tosti *et al.*, 1987). Nail lichen planus may appear in early childhood with no other signs (Burgoon & Kostrzewa, 1969; Bhargava & Goyal, 1975; Kanwar *et al.*, 1983; Kanwar *et al.*, 1993; Peluso *et al.*, 1993), or just with scalp involvement (de Berker & Dawber, 1991). Two main forms of nail dystrophy have been described: (i) a twenty-nail dystrophy; (ii) an atrophic cicatrizing form in which the nails are involved randomly with pterygion formation and progressive nail loss in black people and Asians. Only one child out of 17, in Kanwar *et al.*'s report (1991), had changes suggestive of lichen planus of the nails.

Some particular aspects deserve mention:

1 Permanent anonychia may be the only manifestation of ulcerative lichen planus (Cornelius & Shelley, 1967).

2 'Idiopathic atrophy of the nails' (Samman, 1969) was described at a time when nail biopsy was not performed routinely in such cases. Further reports in African and Asian children mentioning nail biopsies suggest that 'idiopathic atrophy' represents in fact a scarring atrophic variant of lichen planus of the nails (Marks & Samman, 1972; Colver & Dawber, 1987) in most of the cases. 'Idiopathic atrophy' with normal cuticle, relatively non-scarring disease and without characteristic abnormality on nail biopsy may however be a small group that does not pertain to lichen planus (Barth *et al.*, 1988). Congenital similar findings (Achten & Wanet-Rouard, 1974), even in siblings, have been reported (Suarez & Scher, 1990).

3 The monomorphic twenty-nail dystrophy is an idiopathic, acquired condition in which all 20 nails are uniformly and simultaneously affected with excessive longitudinal ridging. This condition is a clinical entity. It presents as the sole manifestation of epidermal pathology and can have several causes, which include a type of lichen planus (Scher *et al.*, 1978; Silverman & Rhodes, 1984) which has a relatively good prognosis (Fig. 5.44). Twenty-nail dystrophy does not therefore constitute a single pathological entity. Isolated lichen planus of the nails has been reported in association with primary biliary cirrhosis (Sowden *et al.*, 1989). Twenty-nail dystrophy due to lichen planus has been reported in a patient with alopecia areata (Kanwar *et al.*, in press).

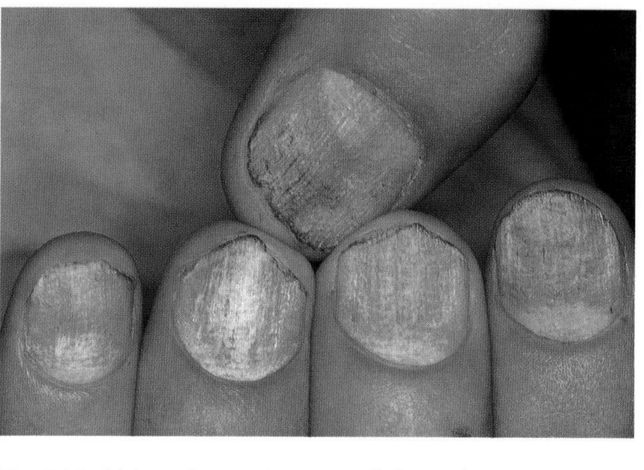

Fig. 5.44. Lichen planus – 'twenty-nail dystrophy' type.

When lichen planus is limited to the nails, accurate clinical diagnosis may be difficult. Because of its normally destructive nature, an early nail biopsy is necessary in order to establish the diagnosis and determine whether adequate treatment is possible. The characteristic histological features are hyperkeratosis and hypergranulosis; the basal layer has a 'sawtooth' appearance with small foci of basal cell degeneration, and band-like lymphocytic infiltrates hugging the epidermis. The differential diagnosis of lichen planus changes in the nail include dystrophy and onychatrophy following Stevens–Johnson syndrome sequelae of severe bacterial infection, genetic causes, impaired peripheral circulation, radiodermatitis, mechanical trauma to the matrix area and yellow nail syndrome (Scott & Scott, 1979; Norton, 1982; Haneke, 1983).

Treatment of lichen planus depends on the severity and the extension of the disease. However, long-term observation indicates that permanent damage to the nail is rare, even in patients with diffuse involvement of the matrix (Tosti *et al.*, 1993). Since there is no known specific cause, therapy is always symptomatic, e.g. anti-inflammatory. Since the common types of lichen planus generally resolve spontaneously within a few months of onset, very little treatment may be needed. Severe non-scarring types may be helped by potent topical or oral steroid therapy. Scarring and atrophic varieties may be temporarily arrested by oral steroids – up to 60 mg per day may be needed, so it is important that only particularly difficult cases, with no contraindications, should be so treated. Patients with ulcerative lichen planus may benefit from grafting (Crotty *et al.*, 1980). Aromatic retinoids are helpful in the treatment of lichen planus.

References

Achten G. & Wanet-Rouard J. (1972) Atrophie idiopathique des ongles et lichen plan. *Arch. Belges Dermatol.* **28**, 251.

Achten G. & Wanet-Rouard J. (1974) Atrophie unguéale et trachyonychi. *Arch. Belges Dermatol.* **30**, 201–207.

Aloi F.G., Colonna S.M. & Manzoni R. (1987) Associazone di lichen ruber planus, alopecia areata, vitiligine. *G. Ital. Dermatol. Venereol.* **122**, 197–200.

Baran R., Jancovici E., Sayag J. & Dawber R.P.R. (1985) Longitudinal melanonychia in lichen planus. *Br. J. Dermatol.* **113**, 369–374.

Baran R., Jancovici E., Sayag J., Dawber R.P.R. & Pinkus H. (1988) Lichen plan pigmentogène unguéal. *Rech. Dermatol.* **1**, 36–38.

Barth J.H., Millard P.R. & Dawber R.P.R. (1988) Idiopathic atrophy of the nails. A clinico-pathological study. *Am. J. Dermatopathol.* **10**, 514–517.

Bhargava R.K. & Goyal R.K. (1975) Involvement of nails in lichen planus. *Ind. J. Dermatol. Venereol.* **41**, 142.

Boyd A.S. & Neldner K.H. (1991) Lichen planus. *J. Am. Acad. Dermatol.* **25**, 593–619.

Brenner W., Diem E. & Gschnait F. (1979) Coincidence of vitiligo, alopecia areata, onychodystrophy, localized scleroderma and lichen planus. *Dermatologica* **159**, 356–360.

Büchner S.A., Itin P., Ruffi T. *et al.* (1989) Disseminated lichenoid papular dermatosis with nail changes in AIDS. *Dermatologica* **179**, 99–101.

Burgoon C.F. & Kostrzewa R.M. (1969) Lichen planus limited to the nails. *Arch. Dermatol.* **100**, 371.

Colver G.B. & Dawber R.P.R. (1987) Is childhood idiopathic atrophy of the nails due to lichen planus? *Br. J. Dermatol.* **116**, 709–712.

Copeman P.W.M., Tan R.S.H., Timlin D. & Samman P.D. (1978) Familial lichen planus. Another disease or a distinct people? *Br. J. Dermatol.* **98**, 573.

Cornelius C.E. & Shelley W.B. (1967) Permanent anonychia due to lichen planus. *Arch. Dermatol.* **96**, 434–435.

Cottoni F., Solinas A., Piga M.R. *et al.* (1988) Lichen planus, chronic liver diseases and immunologic involvement. *Arch. Dermatol. Res.* **280** (Suppl.), S55–60.

Cram D.L., Kierland R.R. & Winkelmann R.K. (1966) Ulcerative lichen planus of the feet. *Arch. Dermatol.* **93**, 692–701.

Crotty C.P., Su W.P.D. & Winkelmann R.K. (1980) Ulcerative lichen planus. *Arch. Dermatol.* **116**, 1252.

De Berker D. & Dawber R.P.R. (1991) Childhood lichen planus. *Clin. Exp. Dermatol.* **16**, 223.

Degos R. & Schnitzler L. (1967) Lichen érosif des orteils. *Ann. Dermatol. Syphil.* **94**, 241–253.

Fabiero J.M., Fernadez-Redondo V., Losada A. *et al.* (1989) Liquen ruber plano con afectación ungueal. *Actas Derm. Sif.* **80**(5), 319–321.

Fanti P.A., Tosti A., Peluso A.M. *et al.* (1992) Nail matrix lichen planus. *J. Cutan. Pathol.* **19**, 52.

Haneke E. (1983) isolated bullous lichen planus of the nails mimicking yellow nail syndrome. *Clin. Exp. Dermatol.* **8**, 425–428.

Juhlin L. & Baran R. (1989) Longitudinal melanonychia after healing of lichen planus. *Acta Derm. Venereol.* **69**, 338–339.

Juhlin L. & Baran R. (1990) On longitudinal melanonychia after healing of lichen planus. *Acta Derm. Venereol.* **70**, 183.

Kanwar A.J., Govil D.C. & Singh O.P. (1983) Lichen planus limited to the nails. *Cutis.* **32**, 163–168.

Kanwar A.J., Handa S., Ghosh S. *et al.* (1991) Lichen planus in childhood: A report of 17 patients. *Pediatr. Dermatol.* **8**, 288–291.

Kanwar A.J., Ghosh S., Kaur T. & Kaur S. (1993) Twenty nail dystrophy due to lichen planus in a patient with alopecia areata. *Clin. Exp. Dermatol.* **18**, 293–294.

Kint A. & Vermander F. (1982) Lichen ruber of the nails. *Dermatologica* **165**, 520–521.

Kofoed M.L. & Wantzin G.L. (1985) Familial lichen planus: more frequent than previously suggested? *J. Am. Acad. Dermatol.* **13**, 50–54.

Lambert D.R., Siegle R.J. & Camisa C. (1988) Lichen planus of the nail presenting as a tumor. Diagnosis by longitudinal nail bed biopsy. *J. Dermatol. Sur. Oncol.* **14**, 1245–1247.

Lowe N.J., Cudworth A.G. & Woodrow J.C. (1976) HL-A antigiens in lichen planus. *Br. J. Dermatol.* **95**, 169–171.

Marks R. & Samman P.D. (1972) Isolated nail dystrophy due to lichen phanus. *Trans. St Johns Hosp. Dermatol. Soc.* **58**, 93–97.

Milligan A. & Graham-Brown R.A.C. (1990) Lichen planus in childhood: a review of six cases. *Clin. Exp. Dermatol.* **15**, 340–342.

Norton L.A. (1982) *Disease of the Nails. Current Therapy*, ed. Conn H.F., p. 664. W.B. Saunders, Philadelphia.

Oberste-Lehn H. & Kühl M. (1954) Lichen planus pemphigoides mit ulcerationen und anonychie. *Haut-GeschlechtKr.* **17**, 195–199.

Peluzo A.M., Tosti A., Piraccini B.M. *et al.* (1993) Lichen planus limited to the nails in childhood. Case report and literature review. *Pediatr. Dermatol.* **10**, 36–39.

Perez A.G., Rodriguez Pichardo A.B. & Bueno Montes J. (1982) Liquer plano erosivo plantar con onicoatrofia. *Med. Cut. I.L.A.* **10**, 89.

Plewig G., Jansen T., Jungblut R.M. *et al.* (1990) Castelman-Tumor, lichen ruber und Pemphigus vulgaris eine immunologische Modellerkrankung? *Zentralblatt Haut Gschl Kr.* **157**, 975.

Ronchese F. (1965) Nail in lichen phanus. *Arch. Dermatol.* **91**, 347–350.

Samman P.D. (1961) The nails in lichen planus. *Br. J. Dermatol.* **73**, 288–292.

Samman P.D. (1969) Idiopathic atrophy of the nails. *Br. J. Dermatol.* **81**, 746–749.

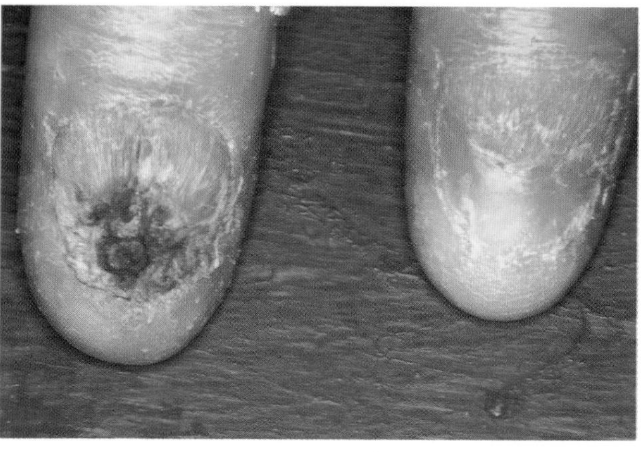

Fig. 5.45. Lichen planus – lupus erythematosus 'overlap' syndrome.

Saurat J.H. & Gluckman E. (1977) Lichen planus-like eruption following bone marrow transplanation: a manifestation of the graft-versus-host disease. *Clin. Exp. Dermatol.* **2**, 335.

Scher R.K., Fischbein R. & Ackerman A.B. (1978) Twenty-nail dystrophy. A variant of lichen planus. *Arch. Dermatol.* **114**, 612–613.

Scott M.J. Jr & Scott M.J. Sr (1979) Ungual lichen planus. *Arch. Dermatol.* **115**, 1197–1199.

Silverman R.A. & Rhodes A.R. (1984) Twenty-nail dystrophy of childhood: A sign of lichen planus. *Pediatr. Dermatol.* **1**, 207–210.

Sowden J.M., Cartwright P.H., Green J.R.B. *et al.* (1989) Isolated lichen planus of the nails associated with primary biliary cirrhosis. *Br. J. Dermatol.* **121**, 659–652.

Suarez S.M. & Scher R.K. (1990) Idiopathic atrophy of the nails: A possible hereditary association. *Pediatr. Dermatol.* **7**, 39–41.

Tosti A., De Padova M.P., Taffurelli M. *et al.* (1987) Lichen planus limited to the nails. *Cutis* **40**, 25–26.

Tosti A., De Padova M.P. & Fanti P. (1988) Nail involvement in lichen planopilaris. *Cutis* **42**, 213–214.

Tosti A., Peluso A.M., Fanti P.A. *et al.* (1993) Nail lichen planus. Clinical and pathological study of twenty-four patients. *J. Am. Acad. Dermatol.* **28**, 724–730.

Weidner F. & Ummenhofer B. (1979) Lichen ruber ulcerosus (dystrophicans). *Z. Haut.* **54**, 1088.

Zaias N. (1970) The nail in lichen planus. *Arch. Dermatol.* **101**, 264–271.

Lichen planus/lupus erythematosus overlap syndrome (Copeman *et al.*, 1970)

Despite extensive histological and immunopathological studies (Stary *et al.*, 1987) it is still not clear whether lichen planus and lupus erythematous can coexist or whether these cases represent an unusual variant of discoid lupus erythematosus (Romero *et al.*, 1977) (Fig. 5.45).

References

Copeman P.W.M., Schroeter K.L. & Kierland R.R. (1970) An unusual variant of lupus erythematosus or lichen planus. *Br. J. Dermatol.* **83**, 269–272.

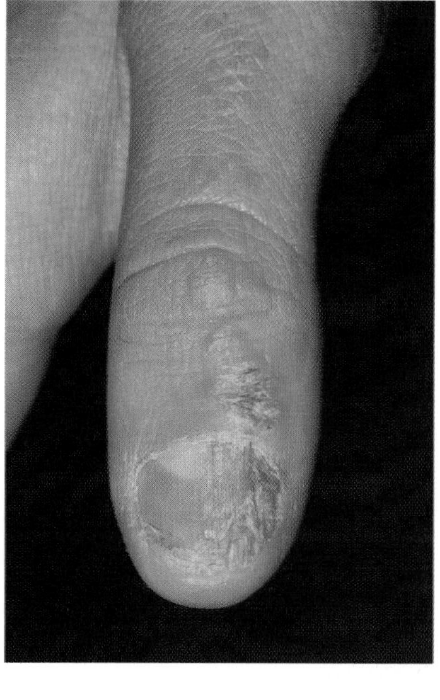

Fig. 5.46. Lichen striatus.

Romero R.W., Nesbitt L.T. & Reed R.J. (1977) Unusual variant of lupus erythematosus or lichen planus. *Arch. Dermatol.* **113**, 741–748.

Stary A., Schwarz T., Duschet P. *et al.* (1987) Das Lichen Ruber Planus – Lupus Erythematodes/Overlap-syndrom. *Z. Hautkr.* **62**, 381–394.

Lichen striatus

This is a linear dermatosis of unknown aetiology. It is characterized by the sudden appearance of erythematous, squamous or lichenoid papules arranged in a continuous or interrupted streak involving the entire length of an extremity. It may extend along a finger or a toe as far as the proximal nail fold and affect the nail plate. The reported cases (Senear & Caro, 1941; Samman, 1968; Kaufman, 1974; Owens, 1977; Meyers *et al.*, 1978; Vasili & Bhatia, 1981; Yaffee, 1981) illustrated several types of nail dystrophy including fraying, longitudinal splitting (Fig. 5.46), punctate or transverse leuconychia, shredding, onycholysis and total nail loss (Baran *et al.*, 1979). Zaias (1990) noted longitudinal dystrophy with hyperpigmentation on the lateral portion of the nail in two patients. All of these lesions are transient and can probably be explained by the pathological changes observed, particularly the transitory disruption of the basal layer. The presence of nail involvement in lichen striatus usually indicates a protracted course and the deformity of nail plate may persist for several years (Niren *et al.*, 1981). In such cases, lichen striatus may appear as a variant of inflammatory linear verrucous epidermal naevus (ILVEN) (Laugier & Olmos, 1976), therefore the differential diagnosis from ILVEN may be difficult when the linear lesion involves a digit, extends to the proximal nail fold and causes dystrophic linear ridging of the nail plate (Altman

& Mehregan, 1971; Landwehr & Starink, 1983). A periungual psoriasiform plaque, loss of cuticle and onycholysis but no pitting has also been reported in ILVEN (Chesbrough & Kilby, 1978). In linear epidermal naevus the affected nail is brown and dystrophic. Linear porokeratosis, a distinctive clinical variant of porokeratosis of Mibelli (Rahbari *et al.*, 1974), should be included in the list of differential diagnosis of linear keratotic cutaneous eruption in childhood.

References

Altman J. & Mehregan A.H. (1971) Inflammatory linear verrucose epidermal nevus. *Arch. Dermatol.* **104**, 385–389.

Baran R., Dupré A., Lauret P. & Puissant A. (1979) Le lichen striatus onychodystrophique. A propos de 4 cas avec revue de la littérature (4 cas). *Ann. Dermatol. Venereol.* **106**, 885–891.

Cheesbrough M.J. & Kilby P.E. (1978) The inflammatory linear verruous epidermal nevus. A case report. *Clin. Exp. Dermatol.* 3, 293–298.

Kaufman J.P. (1974) Lichen striatus with nail dystrophy. *Cutis.* **14**, 232–284.

Landwehr A.J. & Starink T.M. (1983) Inflammatory linear verrucous epidermal naevus: Report of case with bilateral distribution and nail involvement. *Dermatologica* **166**, 107–109.

Laugier P. & Olmos L. (1976) Naevus linéaire inflammatoire et lichen striatus. Deux aspects d'une même affection. *Bull. Soc. Fr. Dermatol. Syphil.* **83**, 48–53.

Meyers M., Storino W. & Barsky S. (1978) Lichen striatus with nail dystrophy. *Arch. Dermatol.* **114**, 964–965.

Niren N.M., Waldman G.D. & Barski S. (1981) Lichen striatus with onychodystrophy. *Cutis* **27**, 610–613.

Owens D.W. (1977) Lichen striatus with onychodystrophy. *Arch. Dermatol.* **105**, 457–458.

Rahbari H., Cordero A.A. & Mehregan A.H. (1974) Linear porokeratosis. *Arch. Dermatol.* **109**, 526–528.

Samman P.D. (1968) Nail dystrophy and lichen striatus. *Trans. St Johns Hosp. Dermatol. Soc.* **54**, 119.

Senear F.E. & Caro M. (1941) Lichen striatus. *Arch. Dermatol. Syphil.* **43**, 116.

Vasili D.B. & Bhatia S.G. (1981) Lichen striatus. *Cutis* 28, 442.

Yaffee H.S. (1981) Letter to the Editor. *Cutis* **28**, 650.

Zaias N. (1990) *The Nail in Health and Disease*, 2nd edn. Lange & Appleton, Norwalk, CN.

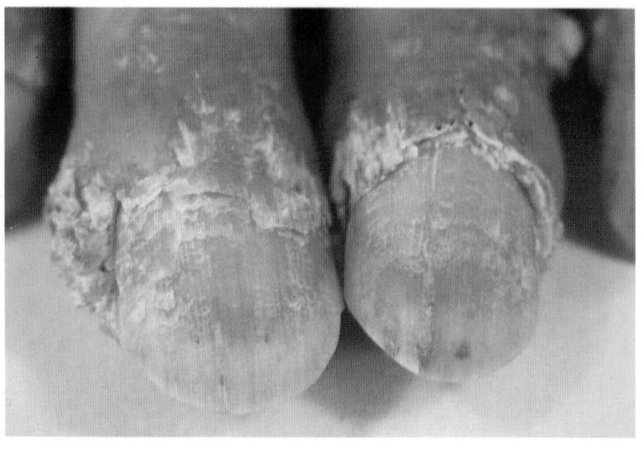

Fig. 5.47. (Courtesy L. Balus, Roma).

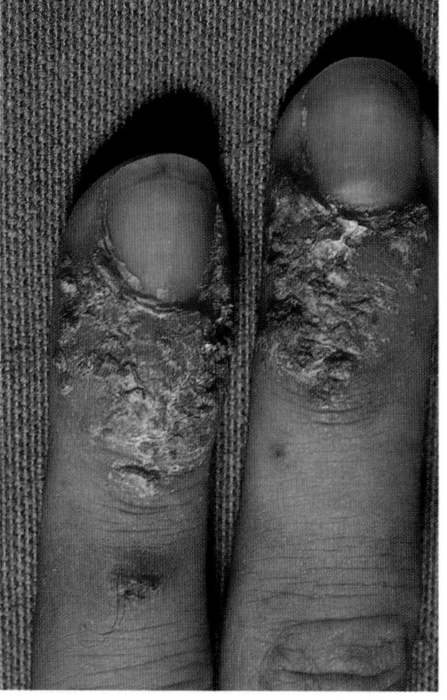

Figs 5.47. & 5.48. Keratosis lichenoides chronica. Hyperkeratotic hypertrophy of the periungual tissues.

Fig. 5.48. (Courtesy C. Grupper, Paris, France).

Lichen nitidus

Cases have been reported demonstrating nail changes (Zaias, 1990), especially as numerous pits (Fritsch, 1967) or fine pitting (Munro *et al.*, 1992), producing the effect of fine rippling towards the lateral border of some nails (Kellet & Beck, 1983). Some nails become brittle and ridged or have a beaded surface, while others show thickening and deep ridging (Barker, 1955). Rough nails with ridging and rippling were accompanied by swelling and violaceous discoloration of the posterior nail fold in a 15-year-old girl affected by lichen nitidus (Natarajan & Dick, 1986). Lichen planus restricted to the nails with giant cells was impossible to rule out in Fanti *et al.*'s (1991) case. Munro *et al.*'s (1993) finding of palmoplantar hyperkeratosis as well as nail dystrophy in lichen nitidus as in lichen planus might seem to support the hypothesis of a shared pathology.

References

Barker L.P. (1955) Lichen nitidus, generalized, with nail changes. *Arch. Dermatol. Syphil.* **72**, 487.

Fanti P.A., Tosti A., Morelli R. *et al.* (1991) Lichen planus of the nails with giant cells: Lichen nitidus? *Br. J. Dermatol.* **125**, 194–195.

Fritsch P. (1967) Der lichen Nitidus (Pinkus). *Z. Haut-Gesch Krankh.* **42(16)**, 649–666.

Kellet J.B. & Beck M. (1983) Lichen nitidus associated with distinctive nail changes. *Clin. Exp. Dermatol.* **9**, 201–204.

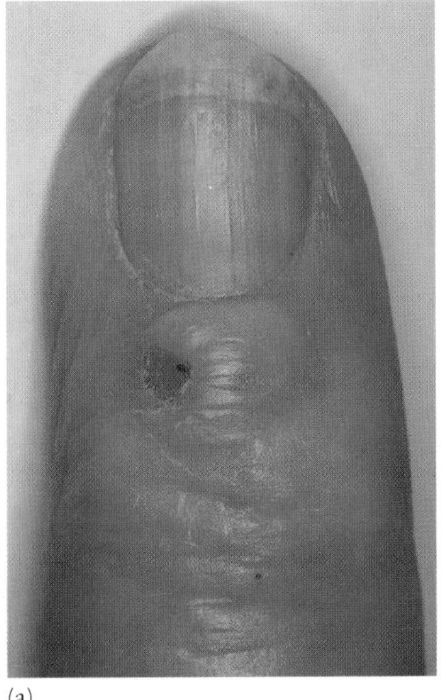
(a)

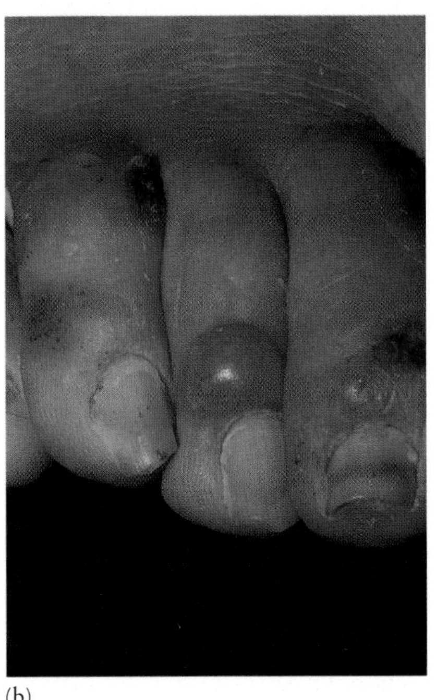
(b)

Fig. 5.49. (a & b) Bullous pemphigoid – mainly periungual involvement.

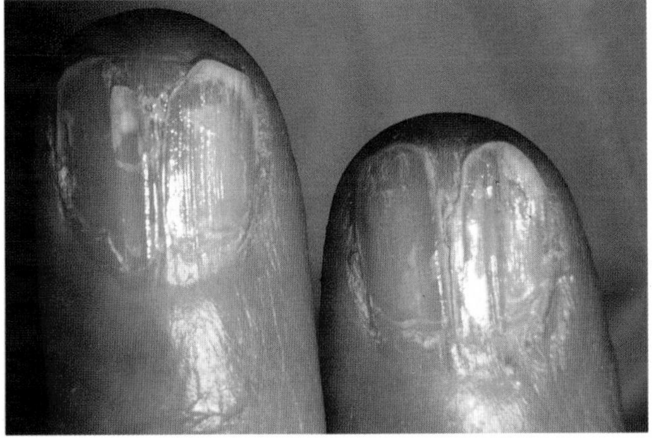
(a)

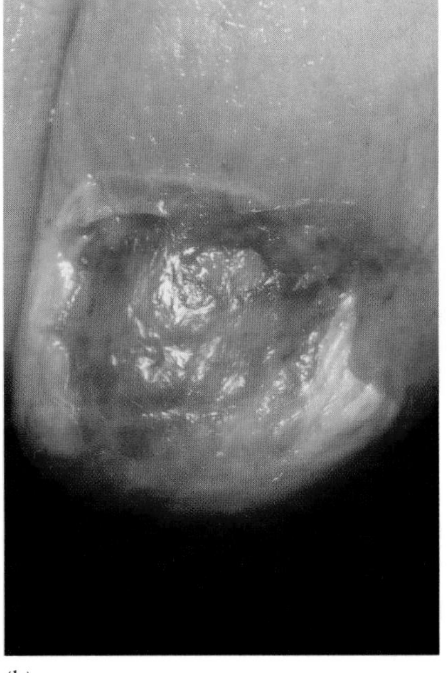
(b)

Fig. 5.50. (a & b) Bullous pemphigoid – nail plate and nail bed changes.

Munro C.S., Cox N.H., Marks J.M. *et al.* (1993) Lichen nitidus presenting as palmoplantar hyperkeratosis and nail dystrophy. *Clin. Exp. Derm.* **18**, 381–383.

Natarajan S. & Dick D. (1986) Lichen nitidus associated with nail changes. *Int. J. Dermatol.* **25**, 461–462.

Zaias N. (1990) *The Nail in Health and Disease*, 2nd edn. Lange & Appleton, Norwalk, CN.

Keratosis lichenoides chronica

The majority of patients affected by keratosis lichenoides chronica manifest three varieties of hyperkeratotic lesion: (i) linear, lichenoid and warty; (ii) yellowish keratotic patches; and (iii) raised papules with keratotic plugs – hence the name of lichenoid trikeratosis proposed by Pinol-Aguade *et al.* (1974).

Keratosis lichenoides chronica may appear clinically and even histologically to be a variant of lichen planus, but is a distinct entity (Braun-Falco *et al.*, 1989). About one-third of patients have nail involvement (Panizzon & Baran, 1981) with changes which may clinically resemble psoriasis, but pitting or pustulosis never occur. Hyperkeratotic hypertrophy of the periungual tissues is a distinc-

(a) (Courtesy, L. Juhlin, Uppsala, Sweden).

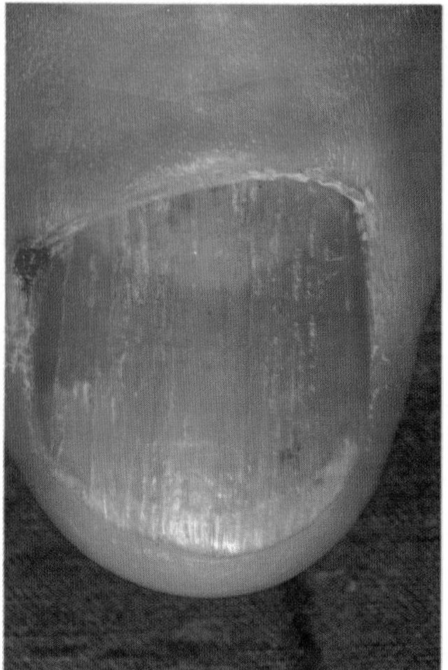

(b)

(c) (Courtesy A. Leroy, Caen, France).

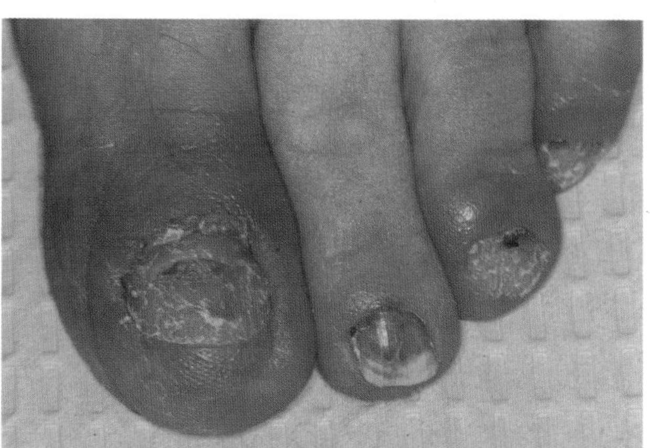

(d)

Fig. 5.51. (a–d) Pemphigus – degrees of nail apparatus involvement in permphigus vulgaris and vegetans (c).

tive sign (Figs 5.47 & 5.48) (Baran, 1983). PUVA therapy and etretinate (Schnitzler *et al.*, 1981; Baran *et al.*, 1984) have improved some cases.

References

Baran R. (1983) Nail changes in keratosis lichenoides chronica are not a variant of lichen planus. *Br. J. Dermatol.* (*Suppl.*) **109**, 43–46.

Baran R., Panizzon R. & Goldberg L.H. (1984) Nails in keratosis lichenoides chronica: characteristics and response to treatment. *Arch. Dermatol.* **120**, 1471–1474.

Braun-Falco O., Bieber T. & Heider L. (1989) Keratosis lichenoides chronica: Krankheitsvariante oder Krankheitsentität. *Hautarzt* **40**, 614–622.

Panizzon R. & Baran R. (1981) Keratosis lichenoides chronica. *Akt. Dermatol.* 7, 6–9.

Pinol-Aguade J., De Asprer J. & Ferrando J. (1974) Lichenoid trikeratosis (Kaposi-Bureau-Barrière-Grupper). *Dermatologica* **148**, 179–188.

Schnitzler L., Bouteiller G., Bechetoille A. *et al.* (1981) Keratose lichenoide chronique avec atteinte muqueuse synechiante sévère. Etude évolutive sur 18 ans. Thérapeutique par le rétinoïde aromatique. *Ann. Dermatol. Venereol.* **108**, 371–379.

Bullous pemphigoid (Figs 5.49(a) & (b) and 5.50(a) & (b))

In childhood, the finding of nail dystrophy consisting of hyperkeratosis, haemorrhage and horizontal ridging with a bullous eruption was against the diagnosis of childhood bullous pemphigoid and more in favour of epidermolysis bullosa (Fox *et al.*, 1982). However Esterly *et al.* (1973) reported a case of dystrophic nails in a 12-year-old girl who had unequivocal bullous pemphigoid. Miyagawa *et al.* (1981) reported dystrophic nails in a 59-year-old woman who had a chronic bullous disease with coexistent linear IgG and IgA at the basement membrane zone on direct immunofluorescence, and both IgG and IgA on indirect immunofluorescence. This case was thought to represent an overlap of bullous pemphigoid and dermatitis herpetiformis. Cases have been observed showing prominent Beau's lines (de Berker, personal observations, 1993).

Cicatricial pemphigoid with nail dystrophy consisting of atrophic, longitudinally ridged and split nails, resembling lichen planus, has been reported (Burge *et al.*, 1985). Cicatrizing nail dystrophy consisting of longitudinal splits and pterygium of several fingernails, in a patient with pemphigoid, revealed in the longitudinal nail biopsy, linear deposits of C3 and IgM at the basement membrane zone of the proximal nail fold and the nail bed (Barth *et al.*, 1987).

References

Barth J.H., Wojnarowska F., Millard P.R. & Dawber R.P.R. (1987) Immunofluorescence of the nail bed in pemphigoid. *Am. J. Dermatopathol.* **9**, 349–350.

Burge S.M., Powell S.M. & Ryan T.J. (1985) Cicatricial pemphigoid with nail dystrophy. *Clin. Exp. Dermatol.* **10**, 472–475.

Esterly N.B., Gotoff S.P., Lolekha S. *et al.* (1973) Bullous pemphigoid and membranous glomerulonephropathy in a child. *J. Pediatr.* **83**, 466.

Fox B.J., Odom R.B. & Findlay R.F. (1982) Erythromycin therapy in bullous pemphigoid: Possible anti-inflammatory effects. *J. Am. Acad. Dermatol.* **7**, 504.

Miyagawa S., Kiriyama Y. & Shirai T. *et al.* (1981) Chronic bullous disease with coexistent circulating IgG and IgA anti-basement membrane zone antibodies. *Arch. Dermatol.* **117**, 349.

Pemphigus

Nail involvement (Fig. 5.51(a)–(d)) is usually secondary to bullae that are adjacent to the fingernails and toenails. Dystrophic changes include discoloration, subungual and splinter haemorrhages (Böckers & Bork, 1987), chronic paronychia (Stone & Mullins, 1966) pitting, transverse grooves and onychomadesis (Parameswara & Naik, 1981). Beau's lines may appear on all 20 digits after each pemphigus flare (Lauber & Turk, 1990). The lateral and proximal nail folds of all 10 fingers (Dhawan *et al.*, 1990; Akiyama *et al.*, 1993) and even all 20 digits (Degos *et al.*, 1955) may present as an inflammatory paronychia, painful and tender, and sero-sanguineous fluid may be expressed (Fig. 5.51c). This is considered to be a hallmark of this condition. The nail fold disease resembles a pyogenic granuloma. Alterations of the nail surface appear as a secondary phenomenon. Primary involvement of the subungual region (Baumal & Robinson, 1973) is rare and results in nail shedding with a chronic, erosive process due to pemphigus. Nail bed biopsy showed suprabasal acantholysis and intercellular deposition of IgG and C3 in a single case (Fulton *et al.*, 1983).

In Brazilian pemphigus foliaceus, established cases show initially yellowish, and later dark discoloration of the nails (Vieira sign), onychorrhexis and onycholysis (Azulay, 1982). Nail shedding is not exceptional. Pterygium and subungual hyperkeratosis and even onychogryphosis have been recorded. The nails may be rough or, in constrast, shiny due to permanent rubbing and scratching (Costa, 1943).

In pemphigus vegetans of Hallopeau, the fingernails show pustules with onychatrophy. Sterile pus may be expressed from the nail folds (Leroy *et al.*, 1982). Histopathology of involved nail shows superbasal acantholytic clefts leading to intraepithelial blister formation in matrix (Fulton *et al.*, 1983) and nail bed (Baumal & Robinson, 1973). Immunoglobin G and C3 (Fulton *et al.*, 1983) are demonstrated in the intercellular spaces.

References

Akiyama C., Sou K., Furuya T. *et al.* (1993) Paronychia: A sign of heralding an exacerbation of pemphigus vulgaris. *J. Am. Acad. Dermatol.* **29**, 494–496.

Azulay R.D. (1982) Brazilian pemphigus foliaceus. *Int. J. Dermatol.* **21**, 122–124.

Baumal A. & Robinson M.J. (1973) Nail bed involvement in pemphigus vulgaris. *Arch. Dermatol.* **107**, 751.

Böckers M. & Bork K. (1987) Multiple gleichzeitige Hamatome der Finger – und Zehennägel mit nachfolgender Onychomadesis bei Pemphigus vulgaris. *Hautarzt* **38**, 477–478.

Costa O.G. (1943) Lesoes ungueais no penfigo foliaceo. *An. Brasil Derm. Sif.* **18**, 67–73.

Degos R., Carteaud A. & Delort J. (1955) Onyxis et perionyxis du pemphigus. *Bull. Soc. Fr. Dermatol. Syphil.* **62**, 475–476.

Dhawan S.S., Zaias N. & Pena N. (1990) The nail fold in pemphigus vulgaris. *Arch. Dermatol.* **126**, 1374–1375.

Fulton R.A., Campbell L., Carlyle D. & Simpson N.B. (1983) Nail bed immunofluorescence in pemphigus vulgaris. *Acta Derm. Venereol.* **63**, 170–172.

Lauber J. & Turk K. (1990) Beau's lines and pemphigus vulgaris. *Int. J. Dermatol.* **29**, 309.

Leroy D., Lebrun J., Maillard V. *et al.* (1982) Pemphigus végétant à type clinique de dermatite pustuleuse chronique de Hallopeau. *Ann. Dermatol. Venereol.* **109**, 549–555.

Parameswara Y.R. & Naik R.P.C. (1981) Onychomadesis associated with pemphigus vulgaris. *Arch. Dermatol.* **117**, 759.

Stone O.J. & Mullins J.F. (1966) Vegetative lesions in pemphigus. *Dermatol. Int.* **5**, 137.

Discoid lupus erythematosus

Discoid lupus erythematosus is seldom observed on the nail apparatus and never restricted to it. The nails (Fig. 5.52) present longitudinal ridging, which may be broken off in the distal part or partially split. The bluish-red colour of the nail bed may be diffuse (Kint & Van Herpe, 1976) or assume the aspect of minute spots through the atrophic nail plate (Sannicandro, 1960).

In 'lupus erythematosus unguium mutilans' (Heller, 1906) the nail area shows a cyanotic tinge, adherent scales

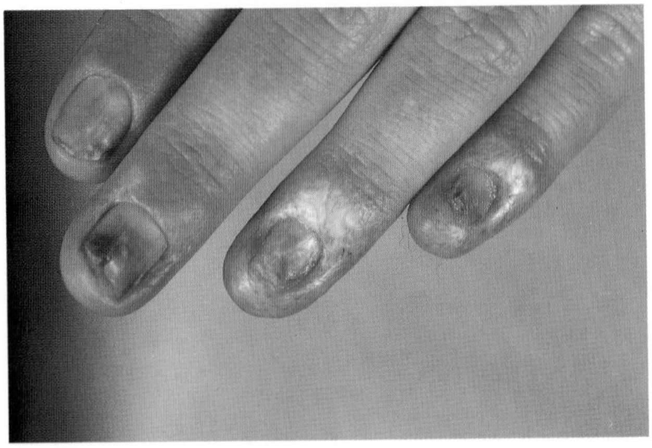

Fig. 5.52. Discoid lupus erythematosus (courtesy of P. Baptista, Coimbra, Portugal).

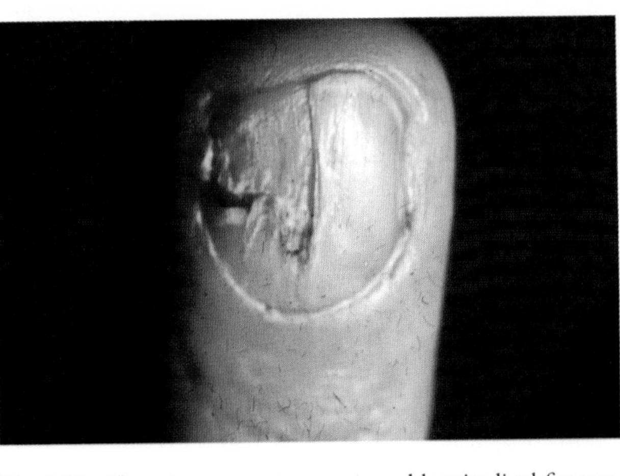

Fig. 5.53. Alopecia areata – transverse and longitudinal fissures, with onychorrhexis (courtesy of Prof. Achten, Belgium, Brussels).

and only the debris of the nail plate. Subungual friable yellowish-brown material may lift up the nail plate; some nails may be entirely destroyed leaving the nail bed exposed as a deep red, shiny area (McCarthy, 1930).

Horny growths on each finger, like birds' claws, have been observed. They are accompanied by lack of lustre, thickening of the nails and a dirty greyish discoloration with shallow longitudinal furrows (Yang, 1935).

The skin around the nails may be normal or reddish with brownish-grey adherent scales (Hekele & Mayer, 1959) and acral sclerosis of the nail apparatus (Sannicandro, 1960). In hypertrophic lupus erythematous gross hyperkeratosis of the palms and soles may extend onto the dorsa of toes to surround the nails which are longitudinally ridged with subungual hyperkeratosis (Buck *et al.*, 1988).

Although the clinical signs are not pathognomonic, the diagnosis may be suspected because of the combination of typical red-blue colouring of the nail bed and alterations in the nail plates which tend to crumble (Kint & Van Herpe, 1976). In chilblain lupus erythematosus, a chronic unremitting type seen predominantly in women, there is gross distortion of the fingertips and nail plates (Millard & Rowell, 1978). Lupus erythematosus has been associated with finger clubbing (Mackie, 1979).

Potent topical steroids under occlusion may lead to some improvement.

Lupus erythematous of the perionychium shows characteristic hyperkeratosis, liquefaction degeneration of basal cells, a predominantly lymphocytic infiltrate in the superficial dermis, and oedema with ectatic capillaries in the papillary dermis (Mackie, 1973). Lupus erythematosus of the nail bed causes hyperorthokeratosis with a corresponding granular layer, thinning of the spinous layer, and oedema of the basal cells which also exhibit ill-defined borders. Hyalin bodies are observed in the superficial der-

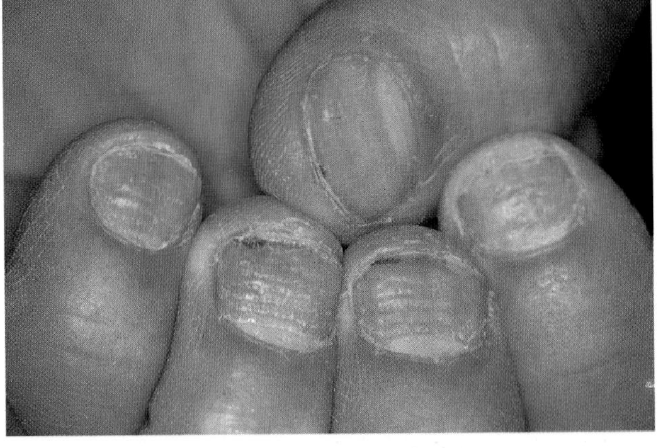

Fig. 5.54. Alopecia areata – multiple lines made of regular horizontal pits.

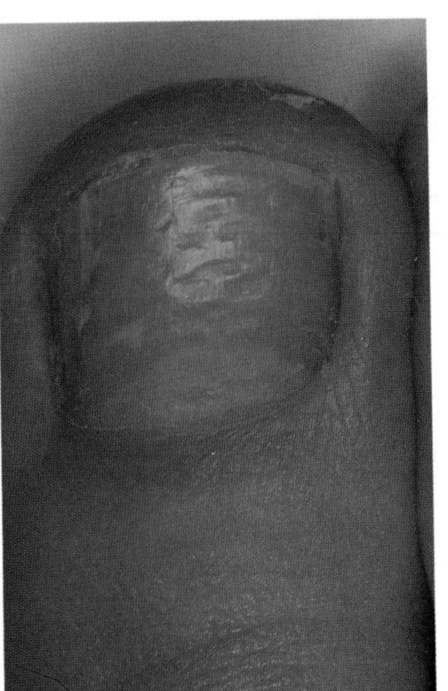

Fig. 5.55. Alopecia areata – irregular pitting.

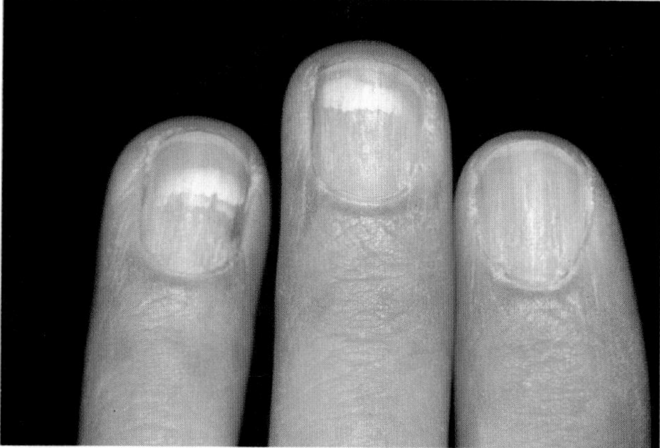

Fig. 5.56. Alopecia areata – leuconychia.

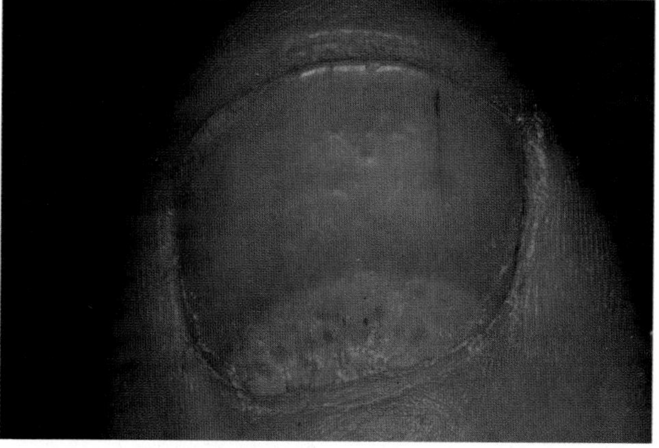

Fig. 5.57. Alopecia areata – 'spotty' lunula.

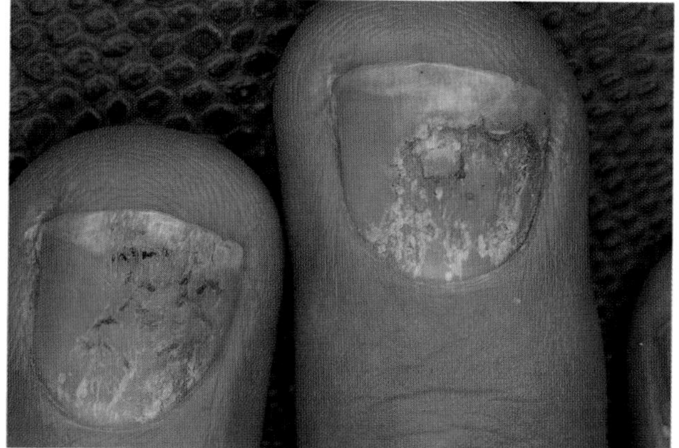

Fig. 5.58. Alopecia areata – dull, roughened, friable nails.

mis (Kint & Van Herpe, 1976). These features are consistent with, but not diagnostic of lupus erythematosus.

References

Buck D.C., Dodd H.J. & Sarkany I. (1988) Hypertophic lupus erythematosus. *Br. J. Dermatol.* **119** (Suppl. 33), 72–74.

Hekele K. & Mayer A. (1959) Seltene Lokalisation des Lupus erythematodes chronicus discoides. *Derm. Wschr.* **34**, 934.

Heller J. (1906) Lupus erythematosus der Nägel. *Derm. Z.* **13**, 613.

Kint A. & Van Herpe L. (1976) Ungual anomalies in lupus erythematosus discoides. *Dermatologica* **153**, 298.

Mackie R.M. (1973) Lupus erythematosus in associated with finger clubbing. *Br. J. Dermatol.* **89**, 533.

McCarthy L. (1930) Lupus erythematosus unguium mutilans treated with gold and sodium thiosulphate. *Arch. Dermatol. Syphil.* **22**, 647.

Millard L.G. & Rowell N.R. (1978) Chilblain lupus erythematosus (Hutchinson). *Br. J. Dermatol.* **98**, 497.

Sannicandro F. (1960) Contributo alla conoscenza clinica ed istologica del lupus eritematoso cronico disseminato del complesso ungueale. *Min. Dermatol.* **35**, 32–34.

Yang K.L. (1935) Lupus erythematosus with unusual changes in the finger tips and nails. *Acta Derm. Venereol.* **16**, 365.

Alopecia areata

Nail involvement in alopecia areata is relatively common but an exact frequency cannot be ascertained from the literature. Figures range from 7 to 66%. The nail involvement varies from marked alteration of the nails to diffuse fine pitting (Figs 5.53–5.58). The majority of the nails are sometimes involved but isolated nail involvement is probably more frequent than is generally believed. Gross nail dystrophy is said to be proportional to the degree of hair loss, especially in the early stages; in fact it is principally proportional to its suddenness. Onychodystrophy has been reported with minimal hair loss, and does not necessarily imply a poor prognosis for regrowth. Sometimes nail changes may precede the involvement of the hair but this has no bearing on the prognosis with regard to regrowth of hair. Onychodystrophy may persist or even develop subsequent to, and persist for some time after resolution of the alopecia areata. Modification in the configuration of the nail plate results in dystrophies such as koilonychia, friable stump-like nails or onychomadesis, which can be latent before leading to shedding of the nails. The nail plate may be thinned (most common) or thickened.

Surface alterations include ridging with frequent onychorrhexis, cross fissures (Fig. 5.53), Beau's lines or transverse lines of uniform, rather neatly arranged intermittent pits (Figs 5.54 & 5.55) which may be profuse. Pitting is the most frequent abnormality. This differs from trachyonychia and vertical sandpaper nail and from the large depressions seens in Sabouraud's faceted nails.

The appearance of the pits is subject to some controversy. Some authors described the pits as smaller and more regular than those found in psoriasis (Munro & Darley, 1979). Others, consider them larger and less deep than in psoriasis (Ebling & Rook, 1979). According to Samman (1978) the pits are small as in psoriasis. When they are uniformly distributed, they are arranged in lines, both transverse and longitudinal, giving rise to geometric patterning ('scotch-plaid' pattern).

The significance of the pitting is unknown. It appears to be more common in children than adults. In alopecia areata histologically two or three wave-like bands of hyperchromatic cells are seen running through the entire length of the nail. The pits are surrounded by a valley of hyperchromatic tissue which may be shed from the nail surface by washing and rubbing. The pits do not contain parakeratotic cells (Alkiewicz, 1964).

Chromonychia may be partial and appear as punctate or transverse leuconychia (Fig. 5.56), or more diffuse producing a variety of colour changes, opaque, asbestos nail (Van de Kerkhof, 1987), yellow, grey or brown. Red colour changes are rare but may be seen as dusky erythematous discoloration of the lunula or of proximal third of all the nails (Leider, 1955; Ringrose & Bahcall, 1957; Misch, 1981). Bergner *et al.* (1992) report two cases with red lunulae that developed a few weeks after the acute onset of hair loss, and disappeared slowly, leaving Beau's lines. Interestingly the erythema of the fingernail lunulae of their first patient migrated distally.

Mottled lunulae are frequently seen due to an irregular, spotty absence of whiteness (Shelley, 1980). The spots on the lunulae appear identical in colour with the regular nail bed (Fig. 5.57). These changes are reversible, coming and going for no definable reason. This phenomenon may also occur in association with psoriasis.

All the morphological changes observed may be explained by the different sites of damage within the nail apparatus, like in psoriasis.

Alopecia areata involves either some nails which may become dull, roughened fragile and friable (Fig. 5.58), or all the nails, in which case they present as a 'twenty-nail dystrophy.'

The following types can be distinguished.

1 The monomorphic twenty-nail dystrophy with sometimes thickened nails. Nails appear brown, irregular and the condition masquerades as an ectodermal dysplasia or longstanding onychomycosis. Multiple lines made of regular pits may be seen (Fig. 5.54).

2 The vertical, striated, sandpaper twenty-nail dystrophy. This belongs to the monomorphic group; the whole nail plate gives the appearance of having been sandpapered in a longitudinal direction. Because of this 'excessive ridging' the nail lustre disappears (Fig. 5.56).

3 The monomorphic, shiny twenty-nail dystrophy (Horn & Odom, 1980). In this type the opalescent nail plates present longitudinal ridging with a stippled appearance. They are thin and fragile.

4 The polymorphic twenty-nail dystrophy.

Any of the disorders mentioned above may be seen on different digits concurrently. Irrespective of the thickness of the nail plate, the nails appear fragile and friable.

Some diseases may be associated with alopecia aerata. In the triad 'alopecia universalis, onychodystrophy and total vitiligo' (Demis & Weiner, 1963), the nail dystrophy has the appearance of longstanding fungal infection. We believe that the pseudo-mycotic nail dystrophy observed in vitiligo (Milligan *et al.*, 1988) may well be due to alopecia areata restricted to the nails.

The coexistence of vitiligo, alopecia areata, onychodystrophy, localized scleroderma and lichen planus has been reported (Brenner *et al.*, 1979) with thickening of the nails, subungual hyperkeratoses and slight koilonychia. Lichen planus (Fenton & Samman, 1983; Kanwar *et al.*, 1993) or psoriasis may be associated with alopecia areata and it has been suggested that the pitting of the nails described in alopecia areata might be an expression of psoriasis (Ganor, 1977). This may explain Dotz *et al.*'s (1985) psoriasiform histological findings. However in alopecia areata the rate of growth of the nail plate is reduced compared with psoriatic nails. The differential diagnosis includes lichen planus, psoriasis and onychomycosis. Thorough clinical examination of the patient should rule out psoriasis. Involvement of the buccal and genital mucous membranes in lichen planus may be of some help in diagnosis. A nail biopsy is of great value when the disorder of the nail precedes the hair loss. When the condition is limited to the nails alone, it is impossible to determine the diagnosis with certainty. In such cases a nail biopsy may be useful to rule out conditions with a characteristic histology, such as lichen planus or psoriasis. It is interesting to note that, in some cases of 'idiopathic' twenty-nail dystrophy of childhood, the histological findings were reported as predominantly 'eczematous' (Baran *et al.*, 1978; Wilkinson *et al.*, 1979).

Nail biopsies in alopecia areata usually show a spongiotic dermatitis of the matrix, sometimes extending to the nail bed. There is a predominantly lymphocytic infiltrate with perivascular accentuation and epidermotropism. The epithelium is diffusely spongiotic and spongiotic vesicles are often seen. They extend up to the superficial epithelial layers and the proteinaceous exudate may be included in the nails; it is then visible as homogeneous eosinophilic, PAS-positive inclusions in the nail plate and subungual keratin. The nail plate keratin is wavy and irregularly arranged. Depressions are seen on the surface; however, in contrast to psoriatic pits, they do not contain parakeratotic cells (Alkiewicz, 1964; Laporte *et al.*, 1988; Achten *et al.*, 1991). It may be extremely difficult to differentiate alopecia areata of the nail, when there is marked spongiosis, from eczematous dermatitis; in the latter, there is usually spongiotic dermatitis of the eponychium and outer surface of the proximal nail fold. These features are not seen in alopecia areata (Haneke, 1984). Spongiotic inflammation of the nail matrix of patients with idiopathic trachyonychia suggests the possibility that it may sometimes represent a variety of alopecia areata limited to the nails (Tosti *et al.*, 1991).

Laporte *et al.* (1988) have studied light and electron microscopy of nail changes in alopecia areata. The upper part of the nail plate shows an architectural disorder of the corneocyte arrangement, sometimes little depressions, more often thin parallel pits giving a flaky aspect. Under electron microscopy, the cytoplasm is full of vacuoles of variable size (from 140 to 1600 nm) and electron-dense deposit material. Keratin fibres are rarefied. The intercellular spaces become larger while the number of 'ampullar dilatations' rises. The upper portion of the nail is more affected than the lower one.

Hair regrowth is generally accompanied by an improvement in the nail dystrophy which slowly clears within a few months. Therapy with intramatricial corticosteroids hastens resolution in some cases. Short courses of oral corticosteroids are also effective but should not be recommended for routine use. Squaric acid dibutyl ester treatment of the scalp alone also seems to bring some improvement in the nails, which is only temporary.

References

Achten G., André J. & Laporte M. (1991) Nails in light and electron microscopy. *Semin. Dermatol.* **10**, 54–64.

Alkiewicz J. (1964) Pathologische Reaktionen an den epithelialen Anhangsgebilden: Nägel. In: *Jadassohns Handbuch der Haut – une Geschlechtskrankheiten*, Ergänzungswerk 1/2, pp. 299–343. Springer, Berlin.

Baran R., Dupré A., Christol B. *et al.* (1978) L'ongle grésé peladique. *Ann. Dermatol. Venereol.* **105**, 387.

Bergner T., Donhauser G. & Ruzicka T. (1992) Red lunulae in severe alopecia areata. *Acta Derm. Venereol.* **72**, 203–205.

Brenner W., Diem E. & Gschnait F. (1979) Coincidence of vitiligo, alopecia areata, onychodystrophy, localized scleroderma and lichen planus. *Dermatologica.* **159**, 356.

Demis D.J. & Weiner M.A. (1963) Alopecia universalis, onychodystrophy, and total vitiligo. *Arch. Dermatol.* **88**, 195.

Dotz W.I., Lieber C.D. & Vogt P.J. (1985) Leukonychia punctata and pitted nails in alopecia areata. *Arch. Dermatol.* **121**, 1452–1454.

Ebling F.J. & Rook A. (1979) In: *Textbook of Dermatology*, 3rd edn, eds Rooks A., Wilkinson D.S. & Ebling F.J., p. 1781. Blackwell Scientific Publications, Oxford.

Fenton D.A. & Samman P.D. (1988) Twenty-nail dystrophy of childhood associated with alopecia areata and lichen planus. *Br. J. Dermatol.* **119** (Suppl. 33), 63.

Ganor S. (1977) Diseases sometimes associated with psoriasis: II, alopecia areata. *Dermatologica* **154**, 338.

Haneke E. (1984) Pathology of inflammatory nail diseases. *7th Colloquium of the Int. Soc. Dermatopathol.*, Graz/Austria.

Horn R.T. & Odom R.B. (1980) Twenty-nail dystrophy of alopecia areata. *Arch. Dermatol.* **116**, 573.

Kanwar A.J., Ghosh S., Thami G.P. *et al.* (1993) Twenty-nail dystrophy due to lichen planus in a patient with alopecia areata. *Clin. Exp. Dermatol.* **18**, 293–294.

Laporte M., André J., Stouffs-Vanhoof F. & Achten G. (1988) Nail changes in alopecia areata: light and electron microscopy. *Arch. Dermatol. Res.* **280** (Suppl.), 585–589.

Leider M. (1955) Progession of alopecia areata through alopecia totalis to alopecia generalizata. Peculiar nail changes (obliteration of the lunula by erythema) while under cortisone therapy. *Arch. Dermatol.* **71**, 648.

Milligan A., Barth J.H., Graham-Brown R.N.C. & Dawber R.P.R. (1988) Pseudo-mycotic nail dystrophy and vitiligo. *Clin. Exp. Dermatol.* **13**, 109–110.

Misch K.J. (1981) Red nails associated with alopecia areata. *Clin. Exp. Dermatol.* **6**, 561.

Munro D.D. & Darley C.R. (1979) In: *Dermatology in General Medicine*, eds Fitzpatrick T.B., Eisen A.Z., Wolff K., Freedberg I.M. & Austen K.F., p. 403. McGraw-Hill, New York.

Ringrose E.J. & Bahcall C.R. (1957) Alopecia areata symptomatica with nail base changes. *Arch. Dermatol.* **76**, 263.

Samman P.D. (1978) *The Nails in Disease.* Heinemann, London.

Shelley W.B. (1980) The spotted lunula. *J. Am. Acad. Dermatol.* **2**, 385.

Tosti A., Fanti P.A., Morelli R. *et al.* (1991) Trachyonychia associated with alopecia areata. A clinical and pathological study. *J. Am. Acad. Dermatol.* **25**, 266–270.

Van de Kerkhof P.C.M. (1987) Nail changes in alopecia areata. *Congressus Mondialae Dermatologiae. Berlin abstracts*, Part I WS 33, p. 288.

Wilkinson J.D., Dawber R.P.R., Bowers R.P. & Fleming K. (1979) Twenty-nail dystrophy of childhood. *Br. J. Dermatol.* **100**, 217.

Darier's disease, Hailey–Hailey disease and acrokeratosis verruciformis (Hopf)

The nail signs diagnostic of Darier–White disease or keratosis follicularis are very common. In a study on 145 patients, they were found in 92% by Burge and Wilkinson (1991). Ronchese (1965), Bingham and Burrow (1984) and Munro and MacLeod (1991) reported the occurrence of nail changes in the absence of other evidence of disease. The nail changes have been summarized by Zaias and Ackerman (1973) as longitudinal, subungual, red or white streaks, or both, associated with distal wedge-shaped subungual keratoses (Figs 5.59 & 5.60). The disease is inherited as an autosomal dominant. Penetrance of the gene is high. The nails lesions (54 out of 56 patients) and palmar pitting (49 out of 56 patients) are earlier and more consistent evidence of the presence of the gene than is the characteristic rash (Munro & McLeod, 1991).

The single or multiple red longitudinal streaks (Fig. 5.59(a)) may, with time, develop into white ones (Fig. 5.59(b)). Such changes extending through the nail and crossing the lunula are most characteristic. Where a streak meets the free edge of the nail a V-shaped notch is usually present originating from the distal nail bed and hyponychium. The wedge-shaped subungual keratosis may massively thicken the nail plate in severe cases (Fig. 5.60) (Savin & Samman, 1970). Less important signs are thinness, fragility and ridges appearing on the nails which tend to crack, splinter haemorrhages, and even subungual haemorrhages, true leuconychia resulting from epithelial hyperplasia of the matrix, and keratotic papules occurring on the proximal nail fold. Secondary invasion of the

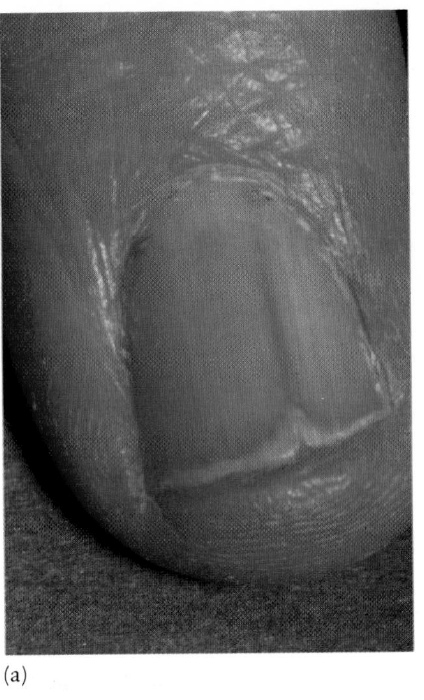
(a)

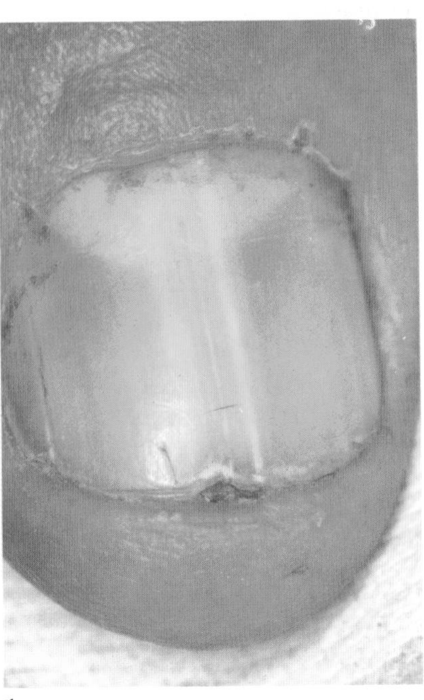
(b)

Fig. 5.59. Darier's disease – red line (a) and white line (b) with terminal notching of the nail (nail dystrophy).

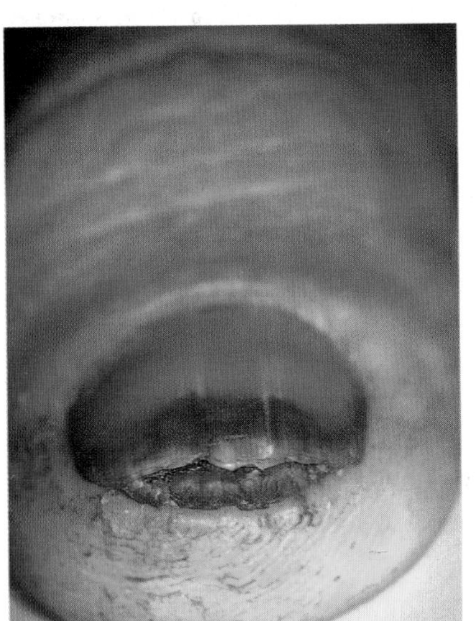

Fig. 5.60. Darier's disease – subungual hyperkeratosis.

Fig. 5.61. Hailey–Hailey disease – longitudinal white bands (Dr S. Burge, Stoke Mandeville Hospital, UK).

nails with dermatophytes, *Candida* and *Pseudomonas* is frequent. According to Zaias and Ackerman (1973), all constituents of the nail unit may be affected histologically in Darier's disease. The findings in the nail bed, however, differ in three respects from those in the skin by the absence of suprabasal clefts, the presence of multinucleated epithelial giant cells, and the absence of inflammatory infiltrate. These characteristic changes lead to the diagnosis in the rare cases where Darier's disease is limited to the nails, which rarely appears before the age of 5 years (Bingham & Burrow, 1984).

Differential diagnosis includes occupational marks in manual labourers, lichen planus, X-ray damage, epiloia and onychomycosis (Ronchese, 1965). Keratotic papules on the dorsal portion of the nail fold may resemble *acrokeratosis verruciformis (Hopf)* but, histologically, they demonstrate the features of Darier's disease (Zaias & Ackerman, 1973). The nails in the former are pearly white in childhood and become horny, brown and grooved later in life (Niedelman & McKusick, 1962). A probable linkage between both diseases has been recognized (Herndon & Wilson, 1966).

In *Hailey–Hailey disease*, Burge (1991) observed, in more than half of the 44 patients examined, longitudinal white bands (Fig. 5.61), but in contrast to Darier's disease, nail fragility was not a feature and the nail changes were asymptomatic (Fig. 5.61). Longitudinal leuconychia may be the first clue to the diagnosis of Hailey–Hailey disease (Kirtschig *et al.*, 1992).

Oral aromatic retinoids are effective on the keratotic papules of the proximal nail fold but the nail lesions are not improved by treatment (Burge *et al.*, 1981). In some cases Darier's disease seems to be a partially immunodeficient state (Jegasothy & Humeniuk, 1981) which could explain the recurrent pyoderma to which the nail area is particularly vulnerable.

The nail bed epithelium is hyperplastic giving rise to subungual parakeratosis which may be 10–30 cells thick. The nuclei of the nail bed epithelium vary in size and shape and abundant multinucleate keratinocytes are found throughout the nail bed. In contrast to epidermal dyskeratosis follicularis lesions there are usually neither suprabasilar acantholytic clefts nor multinucleate epithelial giant cells and the inflammatory infiltrate is nearly absent. The longitudinal red streaks are due to vasodilatation.

Matrix involvement results in parakeratotic layers in the nail plate and causes longitudinal white streaks. Multinucleate keratinocytes are included in the parakeratotic nail. The nail plate surface is altered when the most proximal part of the matrix is affected. Cleft formation may occur in the junction of the matrix and the undersurface of the proximal nail fold. Lesions on the proximal nail fold are identical to those of the epidermis.

References

Bingham E.A. & Burrow D. (1984) Darier's disease. *Br. J. Dermatol.* **111** (Suppl. 26), 88–89.

Burge S. (1991) Hailey–Hailey disease: A clinical study. *Br. J. Dermatol.* **125** (Suppl. 38), 13–14.

Burge S.M. & Wilkinson J.D. (1991) Darier's disease. A clinical study. *Br. J. Dermatol.* **125** (suppl. 38), 14–15.

Burge S.M., Wilkinson J.D., Miller A.J. & Ryan T.J. (1981) The efficacy on an aromatic retinoid in the treatment of Darier's disease. *Br. J. Dermatol.* **104**, 675–680.

Herndon J.H. & Wilson J.D. (1966) Acrokeratosis verruciformis (Hopf) and Darier's disease. *Arch. Dermatol.* **93**, 305.

Jegasothy B.V. & Humeniuk J.M. (1981) Darier's disease: a partially immunodeficient state. *J. Invest. Dermatol.* **76**, 129–132.

Kirtschig G., Effendy I. & Happle R. (1992) Leukonychia longitudinalis als ein Leitsymptom des Morbus Hailey–Hailey. *Hautarzt* **43**, 451–452.

Munro C.S. & MacLeod R.I. (1991) Variable expression of the Darier's disease gene. *Br. J. Dermatol.* **125** (Suppl. 38), 37.

Niedelman M.L. & McKusick V.A. (1962) Acrokeratosis verruciformis (Hopf): A follow-up study. *Arch. Dermatol.* **86**, 779–782.

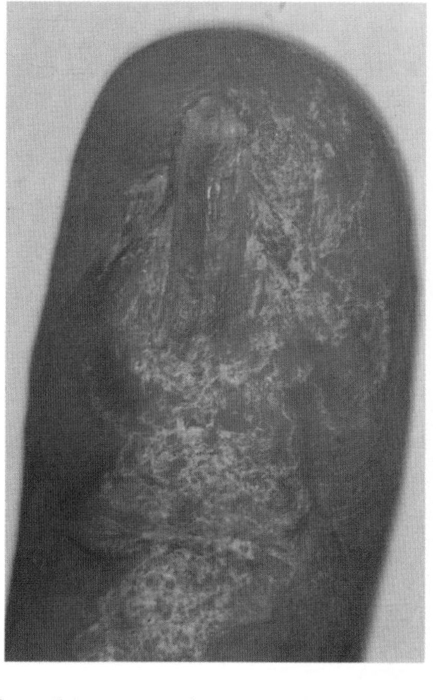

Fig. 5.62. Porokeratosis of Mibelli (courtesy J.L. Verret, Angers, France).

Ronchese F. (1965) The nail in Darier's disease. *Arch. Dermatol.* **91**, 617–618.

Savin J.A. & Samman P.D. (1970) The nail in Darier's disease. *Med. Biol. Ill.* **20**, 85–88.

Zaias N. & Ackerman A.B. (1973) The nail in Darier–White disease. *Arch. Dermatol.* **107**, 193–199.

Porokeratosis of Mibelli

The nails, only rarely affected in this condition, may be thickened, opaque, ridged, fissured or partially destroyed (Fig. 5.62). After nail loss the nail bed shows only warty debris. This appearance has been described by Respighi (1893) as 'hyperkeratosis eccentrica atrophicans'. The nail changes may also resemble those of impaired peripheral circulation (Samman & Fenton, 1986). Soft atrophic nails with pigmentation of the free edges were described by Franks and Davies (1943). Involvement of a toenail resembling an onychomycosis was accompanied by lesions of buccal mucosa in a case of generalized porokeratosis of Mibelli (Kobayasi, 1934).

Linear porokeratosis may involve the dorsal aspect of the digits (Rahbari *et al.*, 1974).

References

Franks A. & Davis J. (1943) Porokeratosis (Mibelli). *Arch. Dermatol.* **48**, 50.

Kobayasi G. (1934) Generalized porokeratosis of Mibelli with lesions of the buccal mucosa and of the nails. *Jpn. J. Dermatol. Urol.* **36**, 439.

Rahbari H., Cordero A.A. & Mehregan A.H. (1974) Linear porokeratosis, a distinctive clinical variant of porokeratosis of Mibelli. *Arch. Dermatol.* **109**, 526–528.

Respighi E. (1893) Di une ipercheratosi non ancora descritta. *G. Ital. Mal. Vener.* **28**, 356.

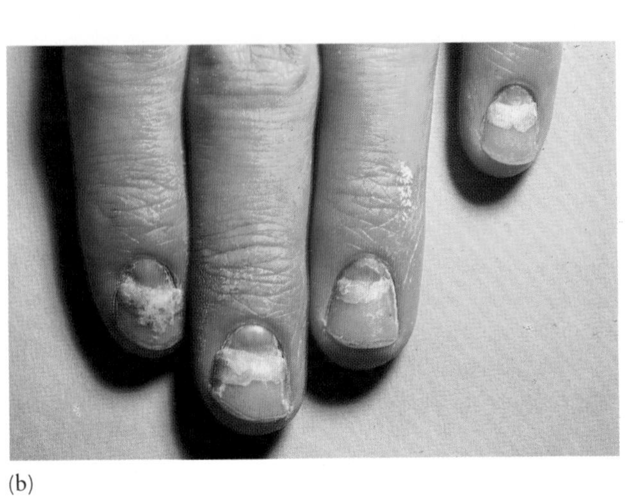

(a) (b)

Fig. 5.63. Erythema multiforme. (a) Peronychial changes; (b) nail shedding (courtesy of A. Krebs, Switzerland).

Samman P.D. & Fenton D. (1986) *The Nails in Disease*, 4th edn. Heinemann, London.

Stevens–Johnson syndrome (erythema multiforme)

Any drug that may induce bullae can cause nail changes or nail loss due to damage to the nail matrix. Erythema and oedema of the proximal nail often occur (Huff, 1985). In some cases sloughing of the whole nail is possible with eventual regrowth (Wentz & Seiple, 1946). In others, after discharge, all the nails are shed resulting in cicatricial anonychia and pterygium (Wanscher & Thomsen, 1977; Hansen, 1984).

In a review of 81 cases of erythema multiforme, Ashby and Lazar (1951) called attention to the fact that paronychia, as well as shedding of the nails (Fig. 5.63(a) & (b)), may be seen in cases of Stevens–Johnson syndrome. This was confirmed by Coursin (1966).

References

Ashby D.W. & Lazar T. (1951) Erythema multiforme exsudativum major (Stevens–Johnson syndrome). *Lancet* **19 May**, 1091.

Coursin D.B. (1966) Stevens-Johnson syndrome: nonspecific parasensitivity reaction. *JAMA* **198**, 133.

Hansen R.C. (1984) Blindness, anonychia and mucosal scarring as sequellae of the Stevens–Johnson syndrome. *Pediatr. Dermatol.* **1**, 298–300.

Huff J.C. (1985) Erythema multiforme. *Dermatol. Clin.* **3**, 141–152.

Wanscher B. & Thomsen K. (1977) Permanent anonychia after Stevens–Johnson syndrome. *Arch. Dermatol.* **113**, 970.

Wentz H.S. & Seiple H.H. (1947) Stevens–Johnson syndrome; a variation of erythema multiforme exsudativum (Hebra). A report of two cases. *Ann. Intern. Med.* **26**, 277.

Toxic epidermal necrolysis

In a case of junctional naevi following toxic epidermal necrolysis (Burns & Sarkany, 1978), finger- and toenails which had been shed during the acute episode failed to regrow; there was pterygium formation affecting most of the digits.

Reference

Burns D.A. & Sarkany I. (1978) Junctional naevi following toxic epidermal necrolysis. *Clin. Exp. Dermatol.* **3**, 323.

Acroosteolysis (Fig. 5.64(a) & (b))

The term acroosteolysis describes the occurrence of destructive changes of the distal phalangeal bone. The cutaneous signs of acroosteolysis range from bulbous fingertips with soft tissue tickening associated with pseudo-clubbing to severe destruction of the digits and metacarpal or metatarsal bones (Meyerson & Meier, 1972). Shortening of the distal phalanges causes the nails to appear abnormally broad (acquired racket-nails). Koilonychia may be observed. Pincer nail deformity has occurred after traumatic acroosteolysis. In severe cases the nail unit can be destroyed.

Toes are frequently affected in diseases that are characterized by neurosensory loss. Deformation and destruction of the digits is commonly accompanied by trophic changes in soft tissues and ulcerations (Phelip & Pras, 1975;

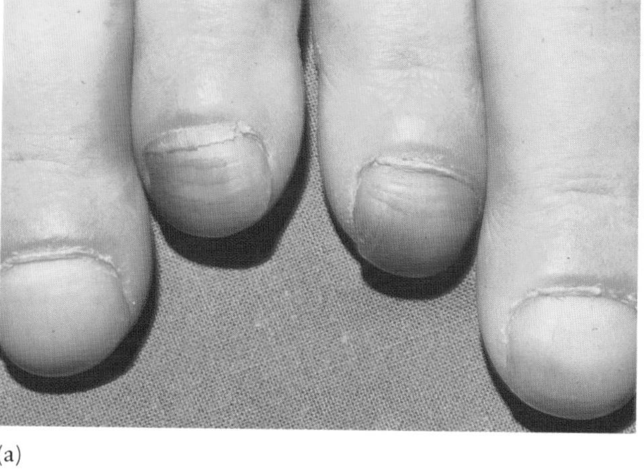
(a)

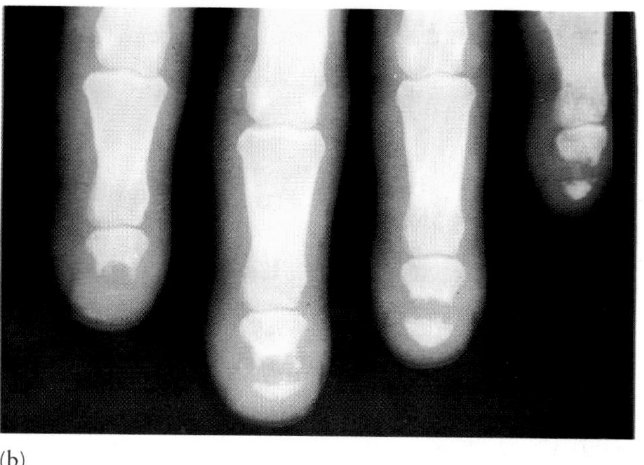
(b)

Fig. 5.64. (a) Acroosteolysis due to vinyl chloride disease; (b) radiological findings (courtesy of G. Moulin, Lyon, France).

Queneau *et al.*, 1982). Functional symptoms such as acroparaesthesia, dull pain or vasospastic changes of the digits can be early manifestations of acroosteolysis. In familial acroosteolysis, pain is a conspicuous symptom. On radiographic examination, two varieties of acroosteolysis, which may occur together or independently, may be seen: transverse acroosteolysis and longitudinal acroosteolysis (Destonet & Murphy, 1983; Kemp *et al.*, 1986). In transverse acroosteolysis the distal phalangeal shaft shows a transverse lytic band, while the tuft and base are preserved.

Fragmentation of the separated distal tuft can occur with near total loss of the tuft, i.e. radionecrosis. In longitudinal acroosteolysis, terminal resorption of the distal end of the phalanx progressively results in a 'licked candystick' appearance of phalangeal, metacarpal or metatarsal bones. The transverse radiological pattern is characteristic for vinyl chloride disease (Fig. 5.64), renal osteodystrophy, idopathic non-familial acroosteolysis and familial acroosteolysis. In longitudinal acroosteolysis, which may be observed in scleroderma, hyperparathyroidism, psoriasis, neurological disorders and frostbite, cystic changes and irregularity of the distal tufts can be followed by severe bone resorption resulting in pencilling of the phalanges. Progressive destruction of the bone produces peg-shaped phalanges.

Acroosteolysis can be idiopathic (familial or non-familial) or it can occur in association with a number of metabolic, neuropathic and collagen disorders (Table 5.2). It may also be a feature of several vascular disorders including atherosclerosis, Buerger's disease, ainhum and progeria.

Idiopathic acroosteolysis includes a number of different disorders which can be distinguished according to the presence or absence of genetic transmission and the association with familial renal disease, neuropathy and ulceratives skin lesion (Elias *et al.*, 1978). A large number of diseases which involve neurosensory loss can result in acroosteolysis. These include lepromatous leprosy, diabetic neuropathy, tabes dorsalis, syringomyelia, familial as well as non-familial mutilant ulcer acropathy (Thévenard's disease, Bureau–Barrière's disease) and congenital insensitivity to pain syndrome (Phelip & Pras, 1975; Queneau *et al.*, 1982). Acroosteolysis can also be observed in patients with infective, inflammatory, neoplastic or mechanical processes that involve the spine, Raynaud's phenomenon or scleroderma. Reversible occupational acroosteolysis that may be associated with Raynaud's phenomenon and sclerodermatous skin changes has been observed in 3–4% of the workers involved in the polymerization of vinyl chloride (Wilson *et al.*, 1967). A genetic susceptibility to vinyl choride disease has been suggested by HLA studies. In addition, acroosteolysis can complicate the course of some rheumatological disorders, such as rheumatoid arthritis or psoriatic arthropathy. Acromegaly and hyperparathyroidism also cause bone resorption leading to acroosteolysis (Phelip & Pras, 1975; Destouet & Murphy, 1983; Kemp *et al.*, 1986). The pathogenesis of acroosteolysis is still unknown. The occurrence of acroosteolysis after thermal or biomechanical injuries as well as in association with vascular or neurological disorders supports the view that different noxious events can induce the development of this condition. Vascular occlusion possibly plays a major role in the development of bone destruction. The hypothesis that vascular occlusion represents the common pathogenetic event for all the different varieties of acroosteolysis has been suggested (Elias *et al.*, 1978; Scher 1986).

References

Baran R. & Tosti A. (1993) Occupational acroosteolysis in a guitar player. *Acta. Derm. Venereol.* **73**, 64–65.

Destouet J.M. & Murphy W.A. (1983) Acquired acroosteolysis and acronecrosis. *Arth. Rheum.* **26**, 115–1151.

Elias A.N., Pinals R.S., Anderson H.C. *et al.* (1978) Hereditary

Table 5.2. Causes of acroosteolysis

Acrodermatitis continua Hallopeau
Acromegaly
Adjuvant of Freund
Bureau–Barrière's disease
Buerger's disease
Carpal tunnel syndrome
Collagen disease
  Mixed connective tissue disease
  Polymyositis
  Scleroderma
  Rheumatoid arthritis
  Sjögren's syndrome
Congenital insensitivity to pain syndrome
Diabetic neuropathy
Ehlers–Danlos syndrome
Epidermolysis bullosa
Gout
Hyperparathyroidism
Ichthyosiform erythroderma
Infection
Juvenile hyalin fibromatosis
Leprosy
Metastases
Mucopolysaccharidoses
Multicentric reticulohistiocytosis
Neoplasms
Nutritional deficiencies
Pachydermoperiostosis
Physical injuries
  Burns
  Frostbite
  Fulguration
  Mechanical stress (guitar players)
Pycnodysostosis
Porphyria
Pseudoxanthoma elasticum
Psoriatic arthritis
Progeria
Raynaud's disease
Renal osteodystrophy
Rothmund's syndrome
Sarcoidosis
Self-mutilation after spinal cord injury
Sézary syndrome
Spine tumours
Syringomyelia
Syphilis
Tabes dorsalis
Thévenard's disease
Vascular diseases
  Ainhum
  Atherosclerosis
  Burger's disease
Van Bogaert–Hazay syndrome
Vinyl chloride disease
Werner's syndrome

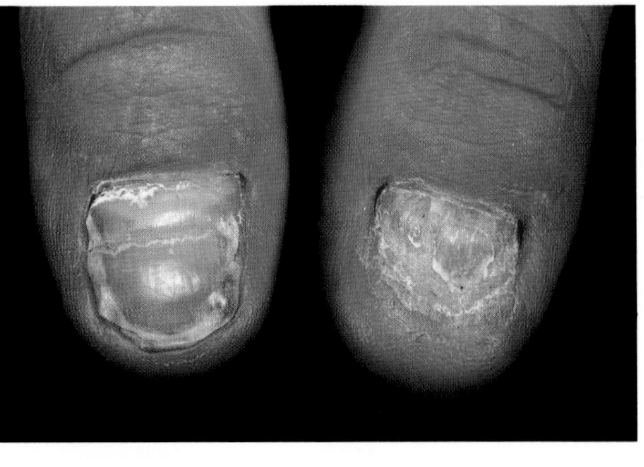

Fig. 5.65. Pityriasis lichenoides acuta (courtesy of R. Russel-Jones, London, UK).

osteodysplasia with acro-osteolysis (the Hajdu–Cheney syndrome) *Am. J. Med.* **65**, 627–636.

Kemp S.S., Dalinka M.K. & Schumacher H.R. (1986) Acro-osteolysis. Etiologic and radiological considerations. *JAMA* **255**, 2058–2061.

Meyerson L.B. & Meier G.C. (1972) Cutaneous lesions in acro-osteolysis. *Arch. Dermatol.* **106**, 224–227.

Phelip X. & Pras P. (1975) Les acro-ostéolyses. *Rheumatologie*, **49**, 325–333.

Queneau P., Gabbai A., Perpoint B. *et al.* (1982) Acro-ostéolyses au cours de la lèpre. *Rev. Rheum.* **49**, 111–119.

Scher R.K. (1986) Acroosteolysis and the nail unit. *Br. J. Dermatol.* **115**, 638–639.

Wilson R.H., McCormick W.E., Tatus C.F. *et al.* (1967) Occupational acroosteolysis. *JAMA* **201**, 83–87.

Acrokeratoelastoidosis

The keratotic lesions of this rare condition may be seen over the knuckles and the nail folds (Highet *et al.*, 1982).

Reference

Highet A.S., Rook A. & Anderson J.R. (1982) Acrokeratoelastoidosis. *Br. J Dermatol.* **106**, 337.

Pityriasis lichenoides acuta

In a case of acute 'vasculitic' and necrotic variety of pityriasis lichenoides acuta, permanent nail dystrophy occurred (Fig. 5.65).

Punctate keratoderma

Patients with palmoplantar keratoderma may exhibit nail changes that are commonly associated with diffuse palmoplantar keratoderma. Onychogryphosis, nail thickening, subungual hyperkeratosis, longitudinal fissures and onychomadesis have all been reported (Poppa & Santini, 1965; Stone & Mullins, 1965; Schirren & Dinger, 1966).

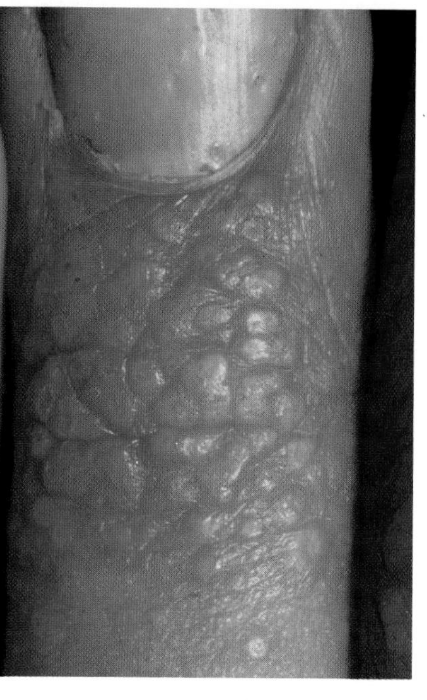

Fig. 5.66. Granuloma annulare – perforating variety (courtesy of C.P. Sanlaska, USA).

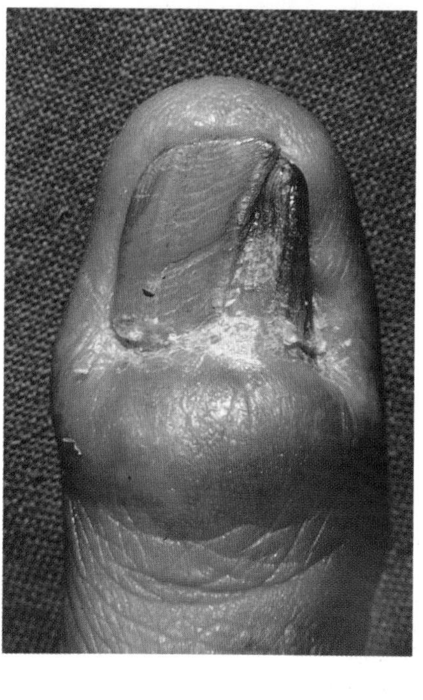

Fig. 5.67. Erythema elevatum diutinum (courtesy of G. Moulin, Lyon, France).

Tosti *et al.* (1993) have reported nail abnormalities which were suggestive of psoriasis in two patients. Subungual hyperkeratosis was a prominent feature, but onycholysis, splinter haemorrhages and pitting were also present. Pathological study of the nail bed and nail matrix revealed sharply limited columns of hyperkeratosis associated with hypergranulosis and depression of the underlying nail bed epidermis.

Etretinate therapy, which produced a significant improvement in the palmoplantar keratoderma, was of no apparent value in treating nail keratoderma.

References

Poppa A. & Santini R. (1965) Cheratodermia plamo-plantare punctata di Brauer-Buschke-Fischer. Keratoderma dissipatum hereditarium palmo-plantare di Brauer. *G. Ital. Dermatol. Venereol.* **125**, 527–558.

Schirren A. & Dinger R. (1966) Untersuchunen bei keratosis palmo-plantaris papulosa. *Arch. Klin. Exp. Dermatol.* **221**, 481.

Stone O.J. & Mullins J.F. (1965) Nail changes in keratosis punctata. *Arch. Dermatol.* **92**, 557–558.

Tosti A., Morelli R., Fanti P.A. *et al.* (1993) Nail changes of punctate keratoderma: a clinical and pathological study of two patients. *Acta. Derm. Venereol.* **75**, 66–68.

Granuloma annulare (Fig. 5.66)

The classical features of granuloma annulare include single or multiple flesh-coloured papules and expanding annular plaques that comprise small papules on the extremities.

Atypical changes such as pseudo chronic paronychia have been observed. Generalized perforating granuloma annulare (Samlaska *et al.*, 1992) is characterized by 1–4 mm umbilicated papules on the extremities, and is most commonly seen in children and young adults. Transepithelial elimination of mucinous, degenerating collagen fibres and surrounding palisading lymphohistiocytic granulomas are important histological features – perforating sarcoidosis may be difficult to rule out.

Reference

Samlaska C.P., Sandberg G.D., Maggio K.L. *et al.* (1992) Generalized perforating granuloma annulare. *J. Am. Acad. Dermatol.* **27**, 319–322.

Erythema elevatum diutinum

This rare condition consists of persistent symmetrical red or rust-coloured and purple plaques affecting the backs of the hands and other extensor surfaces overlying joints (Ryan, 1992). Smaller annular lesions on the extension aspects of the hands or lesions of the proximal nail fold have also been observed (Fig. 5.67).

Reference

Ryan T.J. (1992) Cutaneous vasculitis. In: *Rook/Wilkinson/Ebling Textbook of Dermatology*, 5th edn, eds Champion R.H., Burton J.L. & Ebling F.J.G. Blackwell Scientific Publications, Oxford.

Chapter 6
The Nail in Systemic Diseases and Drug-induced Changes

A. TOSTI, R. BARAN & R.P.R. DAWBER

Cardiac and circulatory disorders
- Cardiac
  - Clubbing (see also Chapter 2)
  - Cardiac failure
  - Bacterial endocarditis
- Circulatory
  - Raynaud's phenomenon and disease
  - Acrocyanosis
  - Cutaneous reactions to cold
  - Perniosis
  - Erythromelalgia
  - Venous ischaemia
  - Splinter haemorrhages (see also Chapter 2)
  - Gangrene
  - Ainhum

Respiratory disorders
- Hypertrophic pulmonary osteoarthropathy
- Yellow nail syndrome
- Shell nail syndrome
- Sarcoidosis
- Bronchial carcinoma
- Asthma

Renal disorders
- Muehrcke's lines
- Haemodialysis
- Leuconychia and renal failure
- Renal transplantation
- 'Half-and-half' nails
- Henoch–Schönlein purpura
- Nail–patella syndrome (see also Chapter 9)
- Acro-renal-ocular syndrome
- Yellow nail syndrome – nephrotic syndrome

Hepatic disorders
- Cirrhosis
- Wilson's disease
- Haemochromatosis
- Chronic active hepatitis

Gastrointestinal disorders
- Clubbing
- Ulcerative colitis
- Peutz–Jeghers–Touraine syndrome
- Cronkhite–Canada syndrome
- Plummer–Vinson syndrome
- Crohn's disease

Nutritional disorders and deficiencies
- Pellagra
- Vitamin A deficiency
- Vitamin C deficiency
- Vitamin B_{12} deficiency
- Zinc deficiency
- Selenium deficiency
- Fetal alcohol syndrome
- Iron deficiency
- Malnutrition

Endocrine disorders
- Hypogonadism
- Pituitary disease
- Adrenal disease
- Parathyroid disease
- Thyroid disease
- Pregnancy and menstrual factors

Metabolic disorders
- Diabetes
- Hyperoxaluria
- Cystic fibrosis
- Hartnup disease
- Histidinaemia
- Lipoid proteinosis
- Dyslipoproteinaemias
- Fabry's disease
- Gout
- Lesch–Nyhan syndrome
- Alkaptonuria
- Homocystinuria
- Fucosidosis
- Porphyria
- Amyloidosis

Nervous disorders
- Hereditary
- Phacomatoses
- Syringomyelia
- Hemiplegia
- Spinal cord injuries
- Congenital insensitivity to pain syndrome
- Peripheral neuropathies
- Causalgia
- Reflex sympathetic dystrophy (algodystrophy)
- Other CNS disorders

Psychological and psychiatric disorders

Connective tissue diseases
- Nail fold capillary microscopy
- Systemic sclerosis
- Systemic lupus erythematosus
- Dermatomyositis
- Rheumatoid arthritis
- Wegener's granulomatosis
- Periarteritis nodosa
- Microscopic polyarteritis
- Multicentric reticulohistiocytosis
- Follicular mucinosis (alopecia mucinosa)
- Fibroblastic rheumatism
- Osteoarthritis

Immunological disorders
- Primary deficiency syndromes
- Therapeutic immunosuppression
- Graft-versus-host disease

- Behçet's disease
- Vitiligo
- HIV and AIDS

Infectious diseases (see Chapters 4 & 7)
- Malaria
- Kawasaki syndrome
- Diphtheria

Haematological disorders
- Blood groups
- Polycythaemia
- Essential thrombocythaemia
- Haemoglobinopathies
- Anaemias
- Hereditary haemorrhagic telangiectasia
- Gamma heavy chain disease
- Cryoglobulinaemia

Neoplastic
- Histiocytosis
- Paraneoplastic disorders
- Acrokeratosis (Bazex & Dupré)
- Glucagonoma syndrome
- Lung neoplasm
- Acanthosis nigricans
- Digital ischaemia
- Papuloerythroderma
- Breast carcinoma
- Intestinal leiomyosarcoma
- Multicentric reticulohistiocytosis
- Nasopharyngeal carcinoma
- Castelman tumour
- Cowden's disease
- Metastases (see Chapter 11)
- Leukaemias
- Plasmocytoma
- Lymphoma
- HTLV-1 positive cutaneous T-cell lymphoma
- Hodgkin's disease

Systemic drugs
- Photoonycholysis
- Erythroderma
- Anticonvulsants
- Benzodiazepines
- Tricyclic antidepressants
- Phenothiazines
- Lithium
- Buspirone
- l-Dopa
- Cocaine
- Retinoids
- Psoralens
- Tetracyclines
- Cephalosporin
- Clofazimine
- Quinolones
- Sulphonamides
- Dapsone
- Emetine
- Azidothymidine (AZT, zidovudine)
- Acetanilid
- Aspirin
- Benoxaprofen
- Ibuprofen
- β-blockers
- Captopril
- Clonidine
- Calcium channel blockers
- Quinidine
- Amrinone
- Purgatives
- Intoxicants
  - Organic
  - Heavy metals
- Anticoagulants
- Antimalarials
- Oral contraceptive pill
- Androgens
- Parathyroid extracts
- Cortisone
- ACTH/MSH
- Cancer chemotherapeutic agents
- Radiation
- Pulse oximetry
  - Antihistamines
  - Carotene
  - Cyclosporin
  - Dimercaptosuccinic acid (DMSA)
  - Diuretics
  - Ergotamine
  - Fluorine
  - Gelatin, biotin, cystine, methionine
  - Hydroquinone
  - Ketoconazole
  - Peloprenoic acid
  - Penicillamine
  - Phenylephrine
  - Salbutamol
  - L-Tryptophan
  - Vitamin A

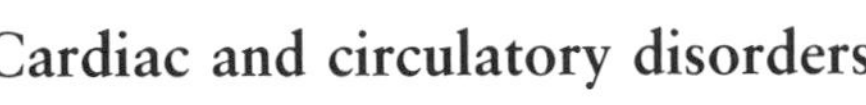

Cardiac and circulatory disorders

Cardiac disorders

Clubbing

In congenital cardiovascular diseases cyanosis and clubbing are common findings (Fig. 6.1). Regional distribution of clubbing and cyanosis (differential cyanosis) may give a clue to the identification of the specific abnormality

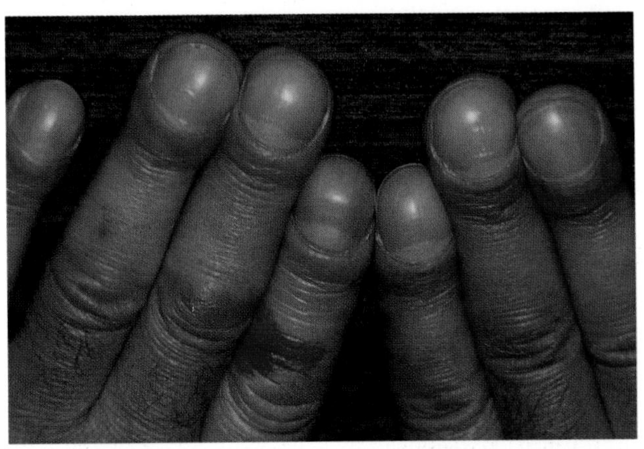

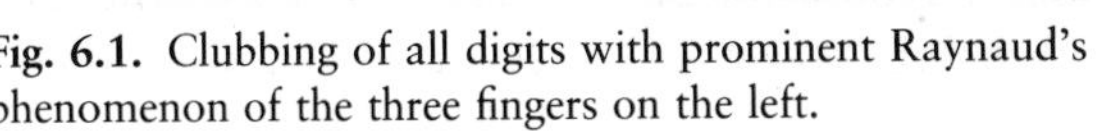

Fig. 6.1. Clubbing of all digits with prominent Raynaud's phenomenon of the three fingers on the left.

(Chesler *et al.*, 1968; Silverman & Hurst, 1968). Symmetrical clubbing and cyanosis of fingers and toes is diagnostic for congenital heart diseases with right to left shunt. Clubbing and cyanosis more evident on fingers than on toes (Fig. 6.4) suggests a complete transposition of the great vessels and a reversed shunt from the pulmonary artery into the aorta through a patent ductus arteriosus delivering oxygenated blood to the lower limbs. The anatomical proximity of the ductus to the left subclavian artery may result in differential cyanosis of the arms as well, since oxygenated blood from the pulmonary artery may enter the left subclavian artery through the ductus. The presence of coarctation or a complete interruption of the aortic arch may make the difference between upper and lower limbs more obvious. Unilateral clubbing has been reported in aneurysms of aortic arch, subclavian and innominate arteries.

Cyanosis and clubbing or hypertrophic osteoarthropathy of the lower extremities can occur secondary to a patent ductus arteriosus with reversal of blood flow. The left hand can also present minimal cyanosis, the left subclavian artery receiving an amount of unsaturated blood from the patent ductus; the right hand is, on the contrary, normal.

Hypertrophic osteoarthropathy limited to the lower extremities can be the initial symptom of an infected abdominal aortic graft associated with aortoenteric fistula (Dalinka *et al.*, 1982; Sorin *et al.*, 1990).

In aortic regurgitation distinctive peripheral signs are the flushing of the nail beds synchronized with the heart beat (Quincke pulsation) and the prominence of the proximal nail fold capillary loops.

Red fingertips (tuft erythema) can be a sign of small or intermittent right to left shunts which cause a minimal reduction of the arterial oxygen saturation.

References

Chesler E., Moller J.H. & Edwards J.E. (1968) Anatomic basis for delivery of right ventricular blood into localised segments of the systemic arterial system: Relation to differential cyanosis. *Am. J. Cardiol.* **21**, 72–80.

Dalinka M.K., Reginato A.J., Berkowitz H.D., Turner M.L., Freundlich B. & Steinberg M. (1982) Hypertrophic osteoarthropathy as indication of aortic graft infection and aortoenteric fistula. *Arch. Surg.* **117**, 1355–1359.

Silverman M.E. & Hurst J.W. (1968) The hand and the heart. *Am. J. Cardiol.* **22**, 718–728.

Sorin S.B., Askari A. & Rhodes R.S. (1990) Hypertrophic osteoarthropathy of the lower extremities as a manifestation of arterial graft sepsis. *Arth. Rheum.* **23**, 768–770.

Cardiac failure

Suffusion or redness of the proximal portion of the half moons has been associated with cardiac failure (Terry, 1954). Red lunulae however can also be observed in many other diseases, such as rheumatoid arthritis, systemic lupus erythematosus, alopecia areata, hepatic cirrhosis, lymphogranuloma venereum, psoriasis, carbon monoxide poisoning, as well as reticulosarcoma and chronic obstructive pulmonary disease (Wilkerson & Wilkin, 1989).

References

Terry R. (1954) Red half-moons in cardiac failure. *Lancet* **ii**, 842–844.

Wilkerson M.G. & Wilkin J.K. (1989) Red lunulae revisited: a clinical and histopathologic examination. *J. Am. Acad. Dermatol.* **20**, 453–457.

Bacterial endocarditis

Petechiae are the most frequent manifestation of subacute bacterial endocarditis. Subungual splinter haemorrhages are a common symptom as well, even though they are frequently observed in a wide variety of unrelated diseases (Chapter 10). Although splinter haemorrhages in subacute bacterial endocarditis are referred to be painful and proximally located, sufficient data to confirm this are not available.

Osler's nodes (Fig. 6.2) can be an important clinical clue for the diagnosis of subacute bacterial endocarditis. These small red tender nodules precisely localized in the finger pulp or around the nails may develop over a period of anything from hours to days. Non-tender haemorrhagic or nodular lesions on the palms and soles (Janeway lesions) are also suggestive of subacute bacterial endocarditis (Sahn & Bluestein, 1992). Although the pathogenesis of Osler's nodes and Janeway lesions is still under discussion, septic microemboli are possibly the cause.

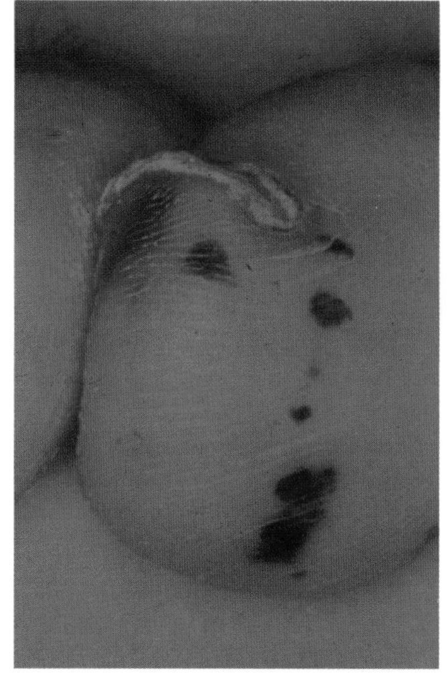

Fig. 6.2. Bacterial endocarditis – Osler's nodes.

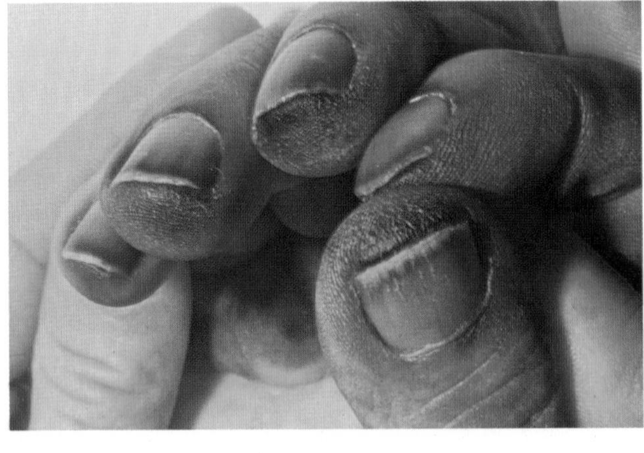

Fig. 6.3. Acral cyanosis associated with disseminated intravascular coagulation (courtesy of Cl. Beylot, Bordeaux, France).

Gram-positive coccobacilli have been detected in the dermal abscesses of a typical Janeway lesion from a patient with bacterial endocarditis (Cardullo *et al.*, 1990). Finger clubbing may occur in 7–52% of patients. It is usually a late sign (Lerner & Weinstein, 1966). Acral cyanosis (Fig. 6.3) evolving towards purpura and even necrosis has been reported during widespread intravascular coagulation complicating acute bacterial endocarditis (Beylot *et al.*, 1974).

References

Beylot C., Castaing R., Poisot D., Bioulac P. & Cazaugade M. (1974) 'Acral cyanosis' manifestation d'une coagulation intravasculaire disséminée au cours d'une endocardite bactérienne aigue. *Ann. Dermatol. Syphil.* **101**, 375–382.

Cardullo A.C., Silvers D.N. & Grossman M.E. (1990) Janeway lesions and Osler's nodes: a revue of histopathologic findings. *J. Am. Acad. Dermatol.* **22**, 1088–1090.

Lerner P.I. & Weinstein L. (1966) Infective endocarditis in the antibiotic era. *N. Engl. Med. J.* **274**, 259–266.

Sahn E.E. & Bluestein E. (1992) Purpuric palmar macule in a child with fever of unknown origin. *Arch. Dermatol.* **128**, 681–686.

Circulation disorders

In peripheral functional or organic arterial diseases the nail plates can present late dystrophic changes as a consequence of the reduced vascular supply to the fingers. Nails may become thin, brittle, longitudinally ridged and distally split. Onycholysis can be an additional feature. Platonychia or a tendency to koilonychia as well as apparent leuconychia affect generally the proximal three-quarters of the nail plate. Beau's lines or even complete shedding of one or more nails (onychomadesis) can be observed. Thickening and distortion of the nail growth (onychogryphosis) may be a sign of impaired peripheral circulation in elderly persons (Samman & Strickland, 1962; Sarteel *et al.*, 1985).

In vasospastic conditions severe peripheral ischaemia may give rise to dorsal or ventral pterygium. Pterygium more frequently affects fingernails than toenails (Edwards, 1948). In arterial obliteration periungual tissues are frequently involved with recurrent paronychia, fingertip ulceration or infection and pulp atrophy or gangrene. When gangrene sets in, nails usually become distorted and may finally be destroyed and replaced by scar tissue.

Digital ischaemia is encountered in a large number of diseases. Many disorders give rise to digital ischaemia through vasospasm, others that organically occlude the vessels often cause considerable secondary vasospasm (Edwards, 1954).

In arterial major obstruction such as in arteriosclerosis, thromboangiitis obliterans (Buerger's disease), Volkmann's contracture, neurovascular compression at the root of the upper limb (thoracic outlet or cervical rib, scalenus, costoclavicular, hyperabduction syndrome), and neurovascular compression of the lower limb (popliteal artery entrapment syndrome), digital ischaemia and gangrene usually affect a single limb (Dorazio & Ezzet, 1979; Ferrero *et al.*, 1980; De Palma & Broadbent, 1981; Kerdel, 1984). In Buerger's disease, ulceration and gangrene can develop at the sides of the nails or the tips of the digits, especially after trauma. In early phases of the disease, pulp of digits may present painful vesicles with intense hyperaemia and hypersensitivity of the surrounding skin (Quenneville *et al.*, 1981). Pseudo-whitlow resulting from finger arteritis can occur (Thiebot *et al.*, 1990). Growth abnormalities of the nails are common (Giblin *et al.*, 1989). Subungual splinter haemorrhages have been reported as an early symptom of Buerger's disease (Quenneville *et al.*, 1981). Intermittent blue discoloration of the left extremity was the initial symptom of thoracic outlet syndrome in a 26-year-old woman (Oriba & Lo, 1990).

Ischaemia affecting a single hand, especially the left, after acute coronary ischaemia, suggests a diagnosis of shoulder–hand syndrome due to reflex vasospasm. Diffusion of the lunulae limits (pseudomacrolunulae) can be a sign of hand ischaemia.

In chronic digital ischaemia of the lower limbs the nail plate can be distorted, thickened, rough and darkened. Nail growth is frequently reduced and onychogryphosis may occur. Periungual hyperaesthesia which can accompany severe digital ischaemia should be differentiated from an ingrown toenail. Improvement of the circulation is usually followed by a nearly normal growth of the nail plate (Samman & Strickland, 1962).

Microembolization to the digital arteries from aortoiliac or femoropopliteal atheromatous plaques can cause an acute digital ischaemia (blue digit syndrome) which requires immediate surgical treatment in order to prevent limb gangrene (Lee *et al.*, 1984; Sperandio & McCarthy, 1988). Cyanosis and digital gangrene due to

Table 6.1. Mechanism and conditions leading to symmetrical peripheral gangrene

Hypotension	Shock
	Cardiac failure of different origin
	Treatment with β-blocking agents
Vasoconstriction	Shock
	Frostbite
	Treatment with vasoactive agents, ergotamine, vasopressin, dopamine *and* chloroquine
	Secondary Raynaud's phenomenon
Endothelial damage	Treatment with bleomycin
	Bacterial sepsis
	Rickettsiosis
	Viral diseases: hepatitis, measles, chickenpox
	Vasculitis of different origin
	Arterial calcification: uraemia, oxalosis
	Carbon monoxide poisoning
	Kaposi's sarcoma
	Black foot disease
Obliteration	Thromboembolic occlusion
	Disseminated intravascular coagulation
	Cholesterol embolism
	Septic embolism
	Malaria
	Sickle cell anaemia
	Essential thrombocythaemia
	Heparin-induced thrombosis
	Cold haemagglutinin disease
	Polycythaemia vera
	Chronic myelogeneous leukaemia
	Hyperviscosity states
	Primary hyperoxaluria
	Cryoglobulinaemia
	Paraproteinaemia
	Hypernatraemic dehydration
	Venous thrombosis

Modified from Itin *et al.*, 1986.

cholesterol microemboli may occur in patients with advanced arteriosclerosis of the abdominal aorta (Calhoun, 1975).

Ischaemic necrosis affecting simultaneously the distal parts of two or more limbs without obstruction of the great arteries (symmetrical peripheral gangrene) can be observed in a large number of diseases (Table 6.1) (Itin *et al.*, 1986). Disseminated intravascular coagulation due to bacterial septicaemia and dehydration due to acute gastrointestinal fluid loss are the most common causes of peripheral gangrene in children (Bass & Cywes, 1989). Hypotension, vasoconstriction, endothelial damage and vascular obstruction are possible pathogenetic mechanisms of symmetrical peripheral gangrene. Agglutination should be suspected when distal cyanosis is difficult to relieve by elevation or stroking. Symmetrical peripheral gangrene has also been described during the blast crisis in chronic myelogenous leukaemia, small blood vessels being occluded by large non-deformable myeloblasts (Frankel *et al.*, 1987). Patients with cold haemagglutinin disease develop acrocyanosis or even symmetrical peripheral gangrene on exposure to cold as a consequence of vascular occlusion due to agglutinated red cells (Shelley & Shelley, 1984). Thirty-six per cent of primary hyperoxaluria patients at European dialysis centres develop distal ischaemia and gangrene (Baethge *et al.*, 1988).

Extensive venous thrombosis of almost the entire venous system of an extremity can cause reversible tissue ischaemia or real gangrene without arterial or capillary occlusion (Hirschmann, 1987). Blood flow within the arteries is arrested as a result of the high venous and intramuscular pressure.

The association of severe pain, extensive oedema, cyanosis and prominence of the superficial veins of a single limb are diagnostic for ischaemic acute venous thrombosis. When gangrene occurs, petechiae, purpura, bullae and finally blackened skin develop (Duschet *et al.*, 1993). Persistent digital ischaemia is an uncommon paraneoplastic syndrome. Gangrene can occasionally develop (Albin *et al.*, 1986).

Digital gangrene has been occasionally described after ergotamine or β-blocker administration, as well as after injection of large volumes of local anaesthetic, especially when epinephrine is used. It can also occur as a postoperative complication of digital cyanosis secondary to poor tissue handling or bandaging technique.

In pseudoxanthoma elasticum ischaemic symptoms as well as ischaemic resorption of the terminal phalanges (acroosteolysis) can occur (Reed & Sugarman, 1974).

References

Albin G., Lapeyre A.C., Click R.L. & Callahan M.J. (1986) Paraneoplastic digital thrombosis: a case report. *Angiology* 37, 203–206.

Baethge B.A., Sanusi I.D., Landreneau M.D., Rohr M.S. & McDonald J.C. (1988) Livedo reticularis and peripheral gangrene associated with primary hyperoxaluria. *Arth. Rheum.* **31**, 1199–1203.

Bass D.H. & Cywes S. (1989) Peripheral gangrene in children. *Pediatr. Surg. Int.* **4**, 408.

Calhoun P. (1975) Cholesterol emboli causing gangrene of the extremities. *Arch. Dermatol.* **111**, 1373–1375.

De Palma R.G. & Broadbent R.W. (1981) Management of occlusive disease of the subclavian and innominate arteries. *Am. J. Surg.* **142**, 197–202.

Dorazio R.A. & Ezzet F. (1979) Arterial complications of the thoracic outlet syndrome. *Am. J. Surg.* **138**, 246–250.

Duschet P., Seifert W., Halbmayer W.M. *et al.* (1993) Ischemic venous thrombosis caused by a distinct disturbance of the extrinsic clotting system. *J. Am. Acad. Dermatol.* **28**, 831–835.

Edwards E.A. (1948) Nail changes in functional and organic arterial disease. *New Engl. J. Med.* **239**, 362–365.

Edwards E.A. (1954) Varieties of digital ischemia and their management. *New Engl. J. Med.* **250**, 709–717.

Ferrero R., Barile C., Bretto P., Buzzacchino A. & Ponzio F.

(1980) Popliteal artery entrapment syndrome. *J. Cardiovasc. Surg.* **21**, 45–52.
Frankel D.H., Larson R.A. & Lorincz A.L. (1987) Acral lividosis: a sign of myeloproliferative diseases. *Arch. Dermatol.* **123**, 921–924.
Giblin W.S., James W.D. & Benson P.M. (1989) Buerger's disease. *Int. J. Dermatol.* **28**, 638–642.
Hirschmann J.V. (1987) Ischemic forms of acute venous thrombosis. *Arch. Dermatol.* **123**, 933–936.
Itin P., Stalder H. & Vischer W. (1986) Symmetrical peripheral gangrene in disseminated tuberculosis. *Dermatologica* **173**, 189–195.
Kerdel F.A. (1984) Subclavian occlusive disease presenting a painful nail. *J. Am. Acad. Dermatol.* **10**, 523–525.
Lee B.Y., Brancato R.F., Thoden W.R. & Madden J.L. (1984) Blue digit syndrome: urgent indication for digital salvage. *Am. J. Surg.* **147**, 418–422.
Oriba H.A. & Lo J.S. (1990) Blue extremity: a cutaneous manifestation of thoracic outlet syndrome. *Int. J. Dermatol.* **29**, 385–386.
Quenneville J.G., Prat A. & Gossard D. (1981) Subungual-splinter haemorrhage an early sign of thromboangiitis obliterans. *Angiology* **32**, 424–432.
Reed W.B. & Sugarman G.I. (1974) Thermography in the study of pseudoxanthoma elasticum. *Cutis* **13**, 423–424.
Samman P.D. & Strickland B. (1962) Abnormalities of the finger nails associated with impaired peripheral blood supply. *Br. J. Dermatol.* **74**, 165–173.
Sarteel A.M., Merlen J.F. & Larere J. (1985) L'ongle en pathologie vasculaire. *J. Mal. Vasc.* **10**, 199–206.
Shelley W.B. & Shelley E.D. (1984) Acrocyanosis of cold agglutinin disease successfully treated with antibiotics. *Cutis* **33**, 556–557.
Sperandio C.P. & McCarthy D.J. (1988) Digital arterial embolism – blue toe syndrome. A histopathologic analysis. *J. Am. Pod. Med. Assoc.* **78**, 593–598.
Thiebot B., Lecrocq C., Balguerie X. *et al.* (1990) Neuf aspects de la pathologie du doigt. *Nouv. Dermatol.* **9(4)**, 340–345.

Raynaud's phenomenon and Raynaud's disease
(Figs 6.5–6.9)

In Raynaud's disease bilateral symmetrical involvement of multiple digits is usually observed. The classic triphasic colour changes which characterize Raynaud's phenomenon consist of pallor – 'white finger syndrome' (due to acute vasoconstriction) – followed by cyanosis and finally hyperaemia. Permanent cyanosis may be present in advanced cases. The nails are frequently thin, brittle, longitudinally ridged and split at the free edge. Koilonychia can be observed. Unilateral splinter haemorrhages have been reported in two patients affected by unilateral Raynaud's phenomenon (Ramelet *et al.*, 1982).

Dorsal or ventral pterygium, chronic paronychia, painful puckered ulcers of the fingertips and rarely gangrene are symptoms of severe Raynaud's disease. Massive digital necrosis resulting from severe Raynaud's phenomenon may be the first manifestation of a collagen disease (Saban *et al.*, 1991). The most useful signs for predicting the development of a collagen disease in patients with Raynaud's phenomenon are digital pitting scars, puffy fingers, the presence of antinuclear antibodies and capillaroscopy changes.

Physical examination, screening for antinuclear antibodies, capillaroscopy and radiography of the hands and chest are useful in distinguishing Raynaud's disease from the early stage of systemic scleroderma. Asymmetric in-

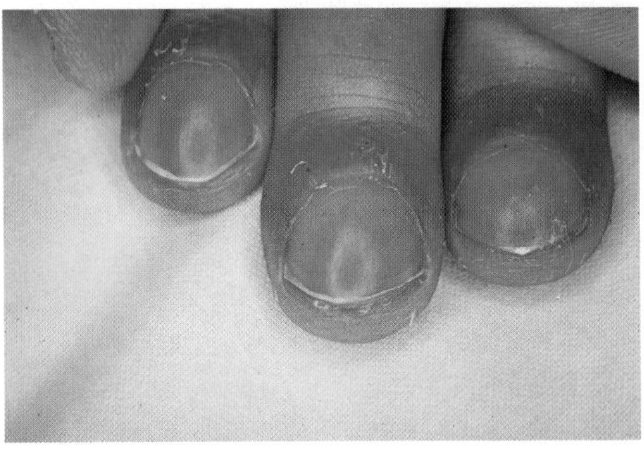

Fig. 6.4. Congenital heart disease – clubbing with cyanosis.

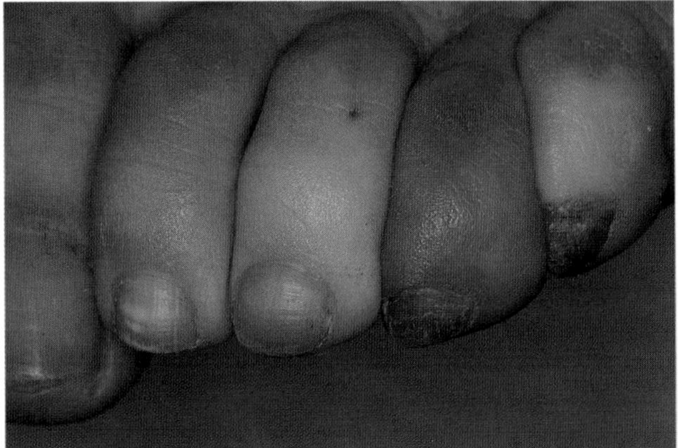

Fig. 6.5. Raynaud's phenomenon.

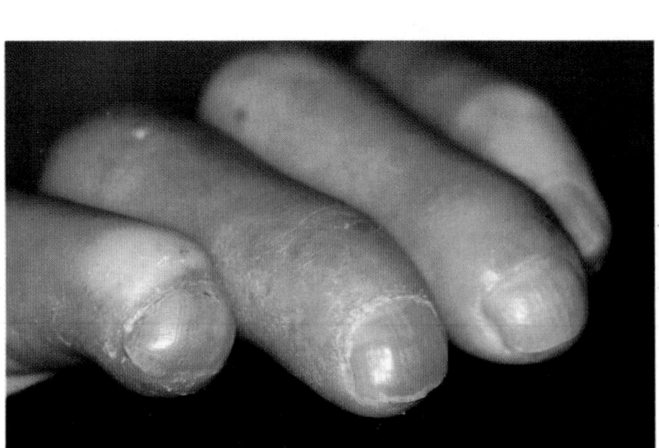

Fig. 6.6. Raynaud's disease and acrosclerosis.

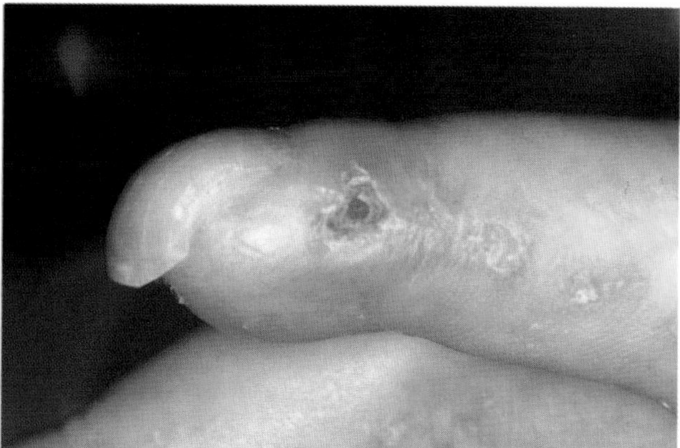

Fig. 6.7. Raynaud's disease and acrosclerosis.

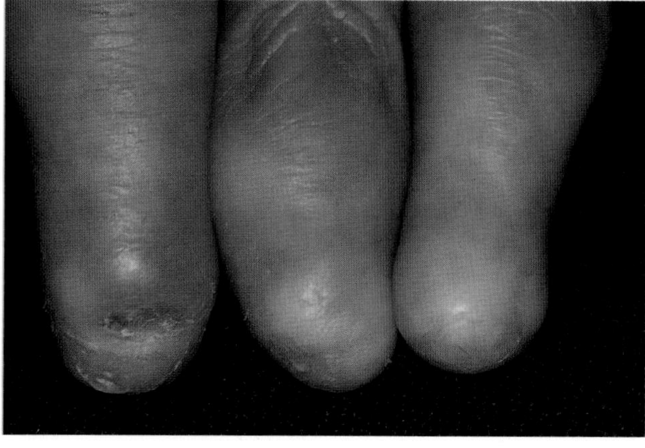

Fig. 6.8. Severe acrosclerosis.

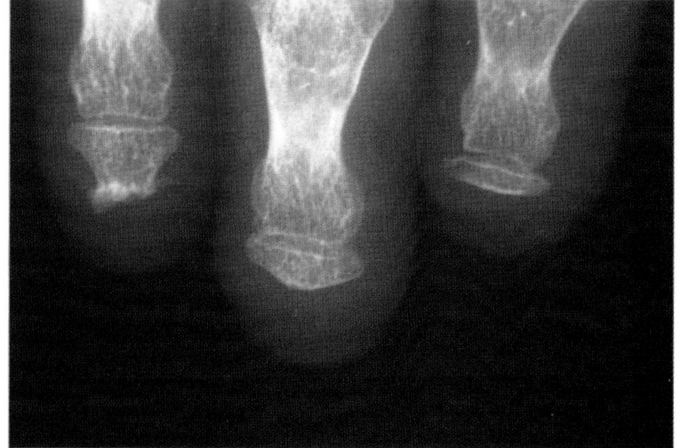

Fig. 6.9. X-ray showing loss of terminal phalangeal bone in acrosclerosis.

volvement of a few digits suggests Raynaud's phenomenon secondary to arterial diseases. Other possible causes of Raynaud's phenomenon include drugs, occupation, haematological diseases, hepatitis B virus infection, neurovascular compression and tumours (Kleinsmith, 1985; Escudier *et al.*, 1982).

Management of Raynaud's disease includes avoidance of excessive exposure to cold, chemical and mechanical trauma, tobacco and consumption of some drugs such as β-blockers, ergotamine or oestrogen/progestogenic that can decrease cutaneous blood flow. So far no perfect treatment for Raynaud's disease has been developed. Biofeedback training and Pavlovian conditioning can be useful therapeutic tools (Jobe *et al.*, 1985). Vasodilators such as nifedipine, prazosin, methyldopa and topical nitroglycerine can be prescribed when vasospastic phenomena are very frequent and prevent the patient from pursuing normal activities. More invasive treatments such as intra-arterial or intravenous reserpine, intravenous infusion of prostaglandin PGE_1 and PGE_2 or low molecular weight dextran, plasmapheresis, and cervicothoracic sympathectomy are still controversial. Ketanserine, a selective antagonist of 5-hydroxytryptamine (5-HT, serotonin) is still experimental but might represent a hope for the future (Dowd, 1986).

References

Dowd P.M. (1986) The treatment of Raynaud's phenomenon. *Br. J. Dermatol.* **114**, 527–533.

Escudier B., Barrier J., Bletry O., Malinsky M., Cabane J. & Godeau P. (1982) Une cause rare d'artérite digitale avec phénomène de Raynaud et nécroses pulpaires: le virus B de l'hépatite. *Ann. Med. Int.* **133**, 600–603.

Jobe J.B., Beetham W.P., Roberts D.E. *et al.* (1985) Induced vasodilation as a home treatment for Raynaud's disease. *J. Rheumatol.* **12**, 953–956.

Kleinsmith D.A.M. (1985) Raynaud's syndrome: an overview. *Semin. Dermatol.* **4**, 104–113.

Ramelet A.A., Tscholl R. & Monti M. (1982) Association d'hématomes filiformes des ongles et d'un syndrome de Raynaud. *Ann. Dermatol. Venereol.* **109**, 655–659.

Saban J., Rodriguez-Garcia J.L., Pais J.R., Mellado N. & Munoz E. (1991) Raynaud's phenomenon with digital necrosis as the first manifestation of undifferentiated connective tissue syndrome. *Dermatologica* **182**, 121–123.

Acrocyanosis (Figs 6.10 & 6.11)

In acrocyanosis persistent blue or reddish discoloration of the digits of the hands and/or feet is present. The nail bed reveals permanent cyanosis. Chronic paronychia and dystrophic changes of the nail plate can be observed. Nail fold capillary microscopy (Figs 6.10 & 6.11) shows dilated, tortuous and often thrombosed capillaries. Brittleness, roughness and transverse grooving may be present. Increased sweating favours the development of onycholysis. Subungual hyperkeratosis, which is painful at slight trauma, is an additional symptom (Sarteel *et al.*, 1985).

Reference

Sarteel A.M., Merlen J.F. & Larere J. (1985) L'ongle en pathologie vasculaire. *J. Mal. Vasc.* **10**, 199–206.

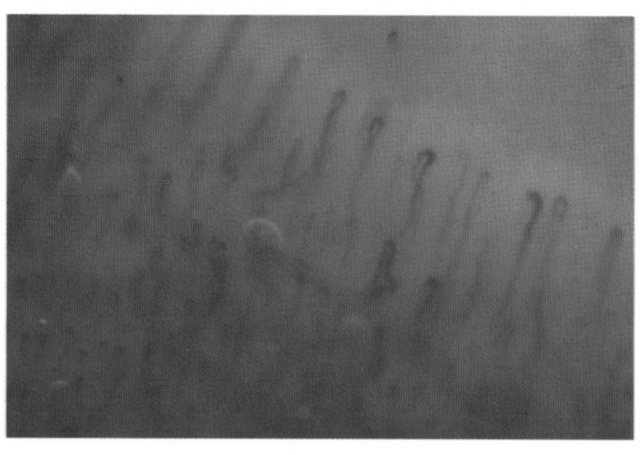

Fig. 6.10. Acrocyanosis. Nail fold capillary microscopy – elongated, tortuous capillary loops.

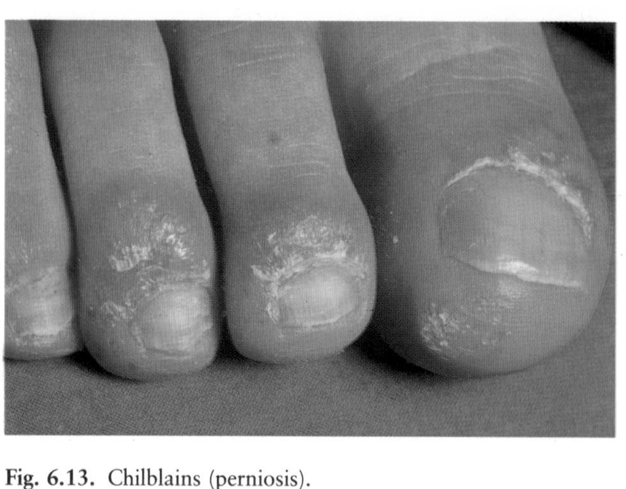

Fig. 6.13. Chilblains (perniosis).

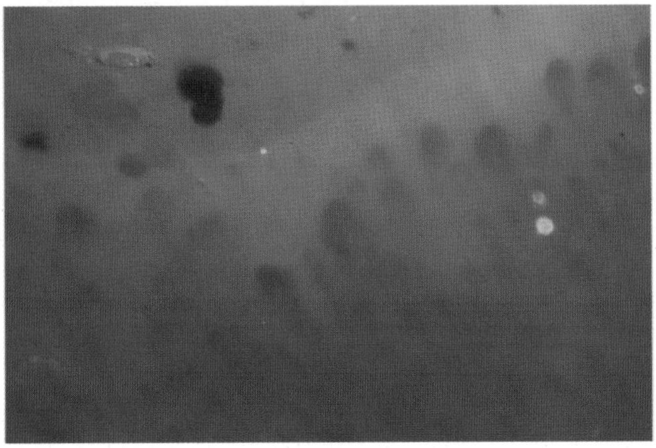

Fig. 6.11. Acrocyanosis. Nail fold capillaries show dilatation, stasis and thrombosis of many vessels.

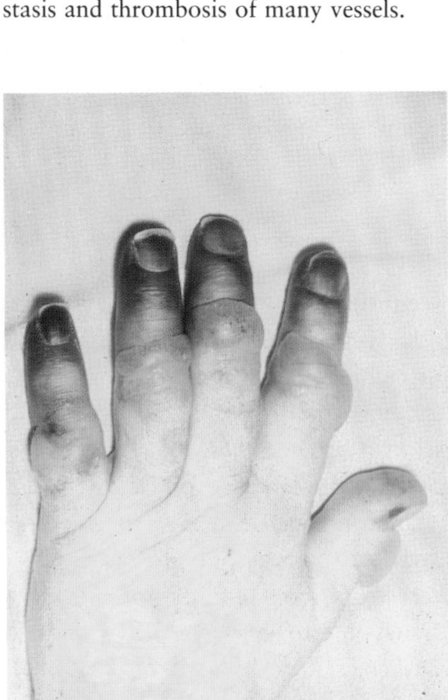

Fig. 6.12. Gangrene due to frostbite (courtesy of Dr Webster, USA).

Cutaneous reactions to cold

Exposure to abnormal cold can damage the nail apparatus. Beau's lines and onychomadesis result from injury to the nail matrix. In severe frostbite, gangrene of the fingertips and toes may be seen (Corbett, 1982) (Fig. 6.12). Epiphyseal destruction causing stunted growth and mild flexion deformity of the fingers has been described after frostbite in children (Nakazato & Ogino, 1986).

References

Corbett D.W. (1982) Cold injuries. *J. Assoc. Mil. Dermatol.* **8**, 34–40.

Nakazato T. & Ogino T. (1986) Epiphyseal destruction of children's hands after frostbite: a report of two cases. *J. Hand Surg.* **11A**, 289–292.

Perniosis (chilblains)

Perniosis represents an abnormal reaction to cold exposure. In acute perniosis, the lesions that are usually bilateral, symmetrical and self-limiting are associated with an itching and burning sensation. Erythema, cyanosis and oedematous patches that change into tender blue nodules are seen on the extremities (Fig. 6.13). Vesicles, bullae, petechiae, haemorrhages and ulcers can occasionally occur in severe cases. In chronic perniosis the lesions begin as burning erythematous blue patches that develop into tender nodules and then into haemorrhagic bullae that rupture leaving shallow, slow-to-heal ulcers. Clinical variants of perniosis include annular, papular or pustular lesions. Herman *et al.* (1981) described painful red–purple macules, papules and plaques on the digits, predominantly on the toes, in nine women. They considered this disorder, which was histologically characterized by a lymphocytic vasculitis, as a distinct variant of perniosis.

Reference

Herman E.W., Kezis J.S. & Silvers D.N. (1981) A distinctive variant of perniosis. *Arch. Dermatol.* **117**, 26–28.

Erythromelalgia

Erythromelalgia is a rare condition characterized by burning pain in the extremities associated with local erythema and warmth. Clinical symptoms are usually aggravated by exercise or warming. Acrocyanosis and gangrene of the digits can occasionally occur (Lorette & Machet, 1991). Erythromelalgia may be apparently idiopathic or secondary to other conditions, most commonly myeloproliferative disorders. In secondary erythromelalgia, asymmetrical involvement of the extremities can be seen (Healsmith *et al.*, 1991).

References

Healsmith M.F., Graham-Brown R.A.C. & Burns D.A. (1991) Erythromelalgia. *Clin. Exp. Dermatol.* **16**, 46–48.

Lorette G. & Machet L. (1991) Erithromélalgie. *Ann. Dermatol. Venereol.* **118**, 739–742.

Venous ischaemia

In chronic venous stasis and in postphlebitic venous stasis clubbing of the toenails can be observed. Nails are thickened, darkened and present a hyperplastic nail bed. Onychogryphosis frequently occurs. Nails are commonly infected by dermatophytes and more often by moulds (Sarteel, 1985).

Reference

Sarteel A.M., Merlen J.F. & Larere J. (1985) L'ongle en pathologie vasculaire. *J. Mal. Vasc.* **10**, 199–206.

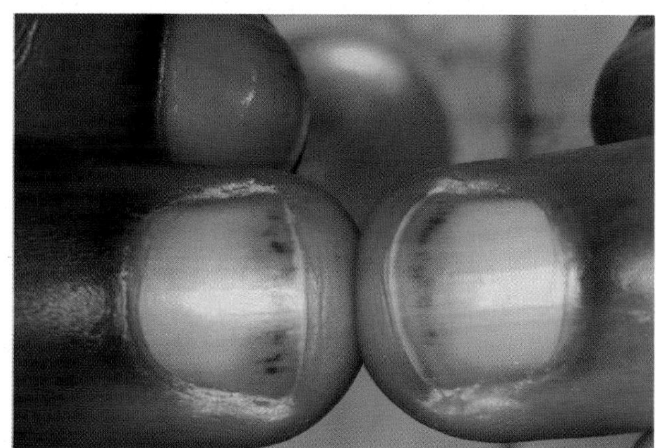

Fig. 6.14. Splinter haemorrhages in systemic lupus erythematosus (courtesy of A. Pons, Paris).

Splinter haemorrhages (SH) (Fig. 6.14)

The longitudinal orientation of the capillary vessels in the nail bed explains the linear pattern of nail bed haemorrhages. The nature of SH is not clearly known (Wood, 1956). They may result from emboli in the terminal vessels of the nail bed (Platts & Greaves, 1958), which may be unilateral (Tobi & Kobrin, 1981; Ramelet *et al.*, 1982). The emboli may be septic (Fanning & Aronson, 1977), or due to trauma of various types. They are more common in the first three fingers of both hands.

The majority of SH originate within the distal third of the nail where the nail plate separates from the nail bed. In this region, special delicate 'spirally wound' capillaries produce the pink line normally seen through the nail, about 4 mm proximal to the tip of the finger. The rupture of these superficially located thinwalled vessels gives rise to linear haemorrhages looking like wood splinters under the nails (Martin & Platts, 1959). SH are contained in the basal layer of the nail plate and move superficially and distally with the growth of the nail; at this stage they can be scraped from the under-surface of the nail plate.

Proximal SH are rare. Although proximal splinters have been reported as a characteristic physical sign of subacute bacterial endocarditis there are no published data to confirm this (Young *et al.*, 1988).

SH involving the whole nail bed have been described in chronic mountain sickness, in cyanotic congenital heart diseases, in congenital arterovenous fistula of the lung and in a patient affected by a rectal cancer with hepatic metastasis (Alkiewicz & Paluszynski, 1962; Heath *et al.*, 1981).

When first formed, SH appear as plum-coloured long thin linear structures but darken to brown and then black in 1–2 days. SH have been observed in 26–56% of healthy subjects and trauma is the most common cause of this nail symptom. However, chronic persistence of SH independent of disease or trauma has been described (Miller & Vaziri, 1979). Traumatic SH affect almost exclusively the fingernails (most commonly the right thumb) and are distally located and symptomless (Heath & William, 1978; Monk, 1980). The 'pen push' manoeuvre used in assessing pain responses was responsible for proximal nail bed haemorrhages in a comatose patient (Pierson *et al.*, 1993).

There is a statistically greater incidence of SH in male patients compared with female patients, and in black people compared with white people (Kilpatrick *et al.*, 1965). Although trauma is the most common cause, increased capillary fragility, microemboli and capillaritis have also been considered as possible mechanisms of SH formation (Young *et al.*, 1988). The simultaneous appearance of SH in several nails, especially in females, should raise the suspicion of an underlying pathological disorder.

Table 6.2. Conditions associated with splinter haemorrhages

Altitude (high)
Amyloidosis
Antiphospholipid syndrome (Ames *et al.*, 1992)
Arterial emboli
Arthritis (notably rheumatoid arthritis and rheumatic fever)
Behçet's disease
Blood dyscrasias (severe anaemia, thrombocytopaenia)
Buerger's disease
Cirrhosis
Collagen diseases
Cryoglobulinaemia (with purpura)
Cystic fibrosis
Darier's disease
Diabetes mellitus
Drug reactions (especially with tetracyclines)
Eczema
Exfoliative dermatitis
Severe illness
Heart disease (notably uncomplicated mitral stenosis and subacute bacterial endocarditis)
Haemochromatosis
Haemodialysis and peritoneal dialysis
Hepatitis
Histiocytosis X
HIV infection
Hypertension
Hypoparathyroidism
Indwelling brachial artery cannula
Irradiation
Keratosis lichenoides chronica
Leukaemia
Malignant neoplasia
Mitral stenosis
Mycosis fungoides
Occupational hazards
Onychomycosis
Pemphigus
Peptic ulcer
Porphyria
Pityriasis rubra pilaris
Psittacosis
Psoriasis
Pterygium
Pulmonary disease
Radial artery puncture
Radiodermatitis
Raynaud's disease
Renal disease (chronic glomerulonephritis)
Osler–Rendu–Weber disease
Sarcoidosis
Scurvy
Septicaemia
Thyrotoxicosis
Trauma
Trichinosis
Vasculitis

Many conditions have been associated with the presence of SH (Table 6.2). In patients with subacute bacterial endocarditis, trichinosis or indwelling arterial catheters, SH can be associated with pain (Young *et al.*, 1988). Ten–thirty per cent of patients affected by trichinosis develop SH during the larval migrating phase of the infestation. Splinters which are 2 mm wide and 4–5 mm long appear initially red, then plum-coloured and finally black (Fisher, 1957). SH may result from emboli in the terminal vessels of the nail bed, e.g. in patients with major arterial embolus or mitral stenosis. Unilateral splinters may follow the insertion of catheters into the radial or brachial arteries even in the absence of catheter infection. Mountain climbers at high altitude can develop multiple SH which are probably a result of raised haemoglobin levels associated with repeated finger trauma (Heath & Williams, 1978; Heath *et al.*, 1981).

References

Alkiewicz J. & Paluszynski J. (1962) Hématomes multiples filiformes intra-unguéaux. *Ann. Dermatol. Syphil.* **89**, 47–51.

Ames D.E., Asherson R.A., Aynes B. *et al.* (1992) Bilateral adrenal infarction, hypoadrenalism and splinter haemorrhages in the primary antiphospholipid syndrome. *Br. J. Rheumatol.* **31**, 117–120.

Fanning W.L. & Aronson M. (1977) Osler node, Janeway lesions and splinter hemorrhages. *Arch. Dermatol.* **113**, 648–649.

Fisher A.A. (1957) Subungual splinter hemorrhages associated with trichinosis. *Arch. Dermatol.* **75**, 752–754.

Heath D. & Williams D.R. (1978) Nail haemorrhages. *Br. Heart J.* **40**, 1300–1305.

Heath D., Harris P., Williams D. & Kruger H. (1981) Nail haemorrhages in native highlanders of the Peruvian Andes. *Thorax* **36**, 764–766.

Kilpatrick Z.M., Greenberg P.A. & Sanford J.P. (1965) Splinter haemorrhages, their clinical significance. *Arch. Int. Med.* **115**, 730–735.

Martin B.F. & Platts M.M. (1959) A histological study of the nail region in normal human subjects and in those showing splinter hemorrhages of the nails. *J. Anat.* **93**, 323–330.

Miller A. & Vaziri N.D. (1979) Recurrent traumatic subungual splinter hemorrhages in healthy individuals. *South. Med. J.* **72**, 1418–1420.

Monk B.E. (1980) The prevalence of splinter haemorrhages. *Br. J. Dermatol.* **103**, 183–185.

Pierson J.C., Lawlor K.B. & Steck W.D. (1993) Pen push purpura: iatrogenic nail bed hemorrhages in the intensive care unit. *Cutis* **51**, 422–423.

Platts M.M. & Greaves M.S. (1958) Splinter hemorrhages. *Br. Med. J.* **19**, 143–144.

Ramelet A.A., Tscholl R. & Monti M. (1982) Association d'hématomes filiformes des ongles et d'un syndrome de Raynaud. *Ann. Dermatol. Venereol.* **109**, 655–659.

Tobi M. & Kobrin I. (1981) Splinter hemorrhages associated with an indwelling brachial artery cannula. *Chest* **80**, 767.

Wood P.H. (1956) *Disease of Heart and Circulation*, Eyre and Spottiswood, London. 2nd edn, p. 648

Young J.B., Will E.J. & Mulley G.P. (1988) Splinter haemorrhages: facts and fiction. *J. R. Coll. Phys. London* **22**, 240–243.

Gangrene

Table 6.1 shows the various mechanisms and conditions associated with symmetrical peripheral gangrene.

Ainhum

Ainhum affects the black population on subtropical regions of America, Africa and Asia. A painful constricting band encircles the fifth toe with eventual spontaneous amputation. The condition is often secondary to an abnormality in the foot vessels producing an abnormal blood supply (Dent *et al.*, 1981).

Reference

Dent D.M., Fataer S. & Rose A.G. (1981) Ainhum and angiodysplasia. *Lancet* **ii**, 396–397.

Respiratory disorders

Nail clippings from patients with cystic fibrosis show an elevated sodium and chloride content (Runne & Orfanos, 1981; Chapman *et al.*, 1985).

References

Chapman A.L., Fegeley B. & Cho C.T. (1985) X-ray microanalysis of chloride in nails from cystic fibrosis and control patients. *Eur. J. Respir. Dis.* **66**, 218–223.
Runne U. & Orfanos C.E. (1981) The human nail. *Curr. Prob. Dermatol.* **9**, 102–149.

Hypertrophic pulmonary osteoarthropathy

Hypertrophic osteoarthropathy (HO) is a syndrome consisting of digital clubbing, joint effusion and periosteal new bone formation. HO is frequently associated with intrathoracic neoplasms, either primary or metastatic, and occurs in 0.7–12% of patients with bronchogenic carcinoma (Firooznia *et al.*, 1975). Lung cancer (primary or metastatic) accounts for 80% of the cases, pleural tumours for 10% and other intrathoracic tumours for 5% (Coury, 1960). It can also be observed in patients with chronic intrathoracic suppurative diseases, such as bronchiectasis empyema, lung abscesses, pulmonary blastomycosis, pulmonary aspergillosis and rarely pulmonary tuberculosis.

HO can also occur in association with a variety of extrapulmonary abnormalities including inflammatory bowel disease, chronic methaemoglobinemia, liver disorders, gastrointestinal neoplasms and cyanotic congenital heart diseases. Occasionally it is idiopathic or hereditary.

HO limited to the lower limbs can be the initial symptom of an infected abdominal graft associated with aortoenteric fistula.

The complete clinical manifestations of HO include:

1 digital clubbing accompained by acromegalic features of the upper and lower extremities;

2 painful swelling and tenderness of the distal third of the arms and legs and adjacent joints;

3 joint effusions;

4 bilateral proliferative periostitis of the long bones of the extremities at X-ray and scintigraphic examinations.

Mechanisms involved in the pathogenesis of HO are still unknown. A neural reflex initiated by the lung and mediated by the vagus nerve has been suggested by the fact that the symptoms are dramatically relieved by intrathoracic or cervical vagotomy (Holling, 1967).

HO can be either an early or a late symptom of pulmonary tumours and removal of the malignant neoplasm usually results in the resolution of clinical manifestations (Stenseth *et al.*, 1967).

Clubbing of the fingers is discussed more fully in the section on modifications of the normal nail form (Chapter 2).

References

Coury C. (1960) Hippocratic fingers and hypertrophic osteoarthropathy: Study of 350 cases. *Br. J. Dis. Chest.* **54**, 202–209.
Firooznia H., Seliger G., Genieser N.B. & Barasch E. (1975) Hypertrophic pulmonary osteoarthropathy in pulmonary metastases *Radiology* **115**, 269–274.
Holling H.E. (1967) Pulmonary hypertrophic osteoarthropathy *Ann. Int. Med.* **66**, 232–234.
Stenseth J.H., Clagett O.T. & Woolner L.B. (1967) Hypertrophic pulmonary osteoarthropathy. *Dis. Chest* **52**, 62–68.

Yellow nail syndrome (YNS) (Figs 6.15 & 6.16)

YNS is an uncommon disorder of unknown aetiology characterized by the triad of yellow nails, lymphoedema and respiratory tract involvement. The term (Samman & White, 1964) was originally used to describe the association of slowly growing yellow nails with primary lymphoedema. Pleural effusion (Emerson, 1966) was later recognized as an additional sign of the syndrome. Since then other respiratory conditions such as bronchiectasis, sinusitis, bronchitis and chronic respiratory infections have been associated with the disorder. Although all the three signs which classically characterize the triad of YNS

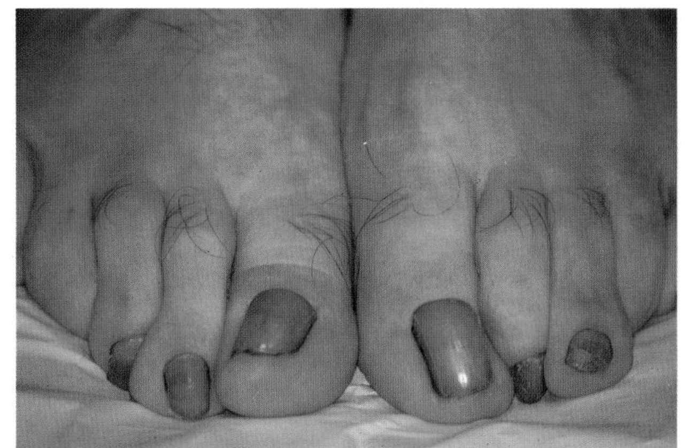

Fig. 6.15. Yellow nail syndrome.

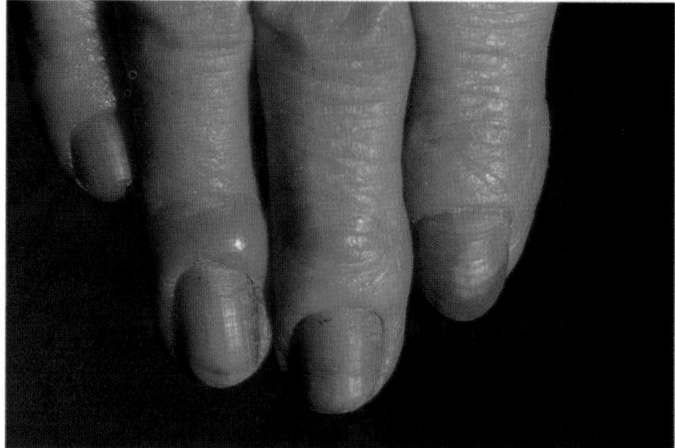

Fig. 6.16. Yellow nail syndrome with paronychia.

do not occur in every patient, the presence of typical nail alterations should be considered an absolute requirement for the diagnosis.

The time between the development of the various manifestations may range from months to years.

YNS is more common in adults but can also occur in children (Magid *et al.*, 1987), males and females being equally affected.

Nail changes are characteristic, usually affecting both finger- and toenails, and are associated with a very slow growth rate (less than 0.2 mm week) (Samman & White, 1964). Nails are thickened and excessively curved from side to side (Fig. 6.15) so that coverage of the lateral ridges by the surrounding soft tissues is less than normal and the cuticles are deficient. Hardness of the nails (scleronychia) makes it difficult to take a biopsy through the nail plate. Erythema and oedema of the proximal nail fold can be present. Chronic paronychia can occasionally be observed (Fig. 6.16). The entire nail plate shows a diffuse pale yellow to dark yellow-green discoloration. The edges of the nails are occasionally darker than the remainder and the proximal part of the nail plate can sometimes maintain a normal colour. Nails are frequently opaque so that the lunulae are no longer visible. The nail surface is usually smooth but transverse ridging due to periodical variations in the growth rate can be present. Onycholysis may occur and extend far enough toward the matrix to cause complete shedding, the nails being replaced extremely slowly. Partially separated nails sometimes show a distinctive hump.

The pathogenesis of nail and systemic manifestations of YNS is still being discussed. Impaired lymphatic drainage is thought to be the underlying defect responsible for the various clinical findings in patients with YNS. While lymphangiograms have shown abnormal findings such as atresia, hypoplasia and varicose abnormalities of peripheral lymphatics in some patients, this has not been a consistent finding. It has been suggested that a widespread lymphatic abnormality that is adequate early in life becomes deficient following inflammation or stress.

A defective lymph drainage in the nail regions can be responsible for the slow nail growth and for the thickened yellow nails that characterize the syndrome. Lymphatic obstruction resulting from the sclerosing process in the subungual stroma has been recently postulated (De Coste *et al.*, 1990). The appearance of the nails probably depends on the slow growth rate. The resolution of the nail changes is, in fact, always associated with resumption of normal nail growth. Abnormal nail keratinization has been suggested by the presence of keratohyalin granules in the nail plate (Pavlidakey *et al.*, 1984). Deposition of an acetone-soluble yellow substance (Ohkuma, 1982) has not been confirmed (Reynes *et al.*, 1984). Accumulation of lipofuscin pigments may be the source of the nail colour (Norton, 1985).

Evidence of lymphoedema or respiratory manifestations may not become evident for years after the nails have become involved. Lymphoedema is usually more obvious in the ankles and legs but hands or even the face can be affected. It can rarely be generalized. Congenital lymphoedema has also been reported in association with YNS.

Respiratory manifestations of YNS include pleural effusion or other signs of upper and lower respiratory disease such as sinusitis, bronchitis and bronchiectasis (Hiller *et al.*, 1972).

YNS has been reported to occur on several occasions in patients with thyroiditis, rheumatoid arthritis, nephrotic syndrome, underlying malignancies and immune deficiencies (Malliet *et al.*, 1985; Nordkild *et al.*, 1986). Occasional reports indicate that YNS has occurred along with a large variety of disorders including mental retardation, sleep apnoea, connective tissue diseases, breasts of unequal size, hypoplastic kidney, myocardial infarction, increased susceptibility to skin and soft tissue infections, chronic pulmonary and hepatic tubercolosis, chylothorax, D-penicillamine therapy and even extremely hard ear wax. A case of reversible YNS in association with chronic graft-versus-host reaction has been reported (Mascaro & Martin-Ortega, 1993).

The term YNS has been improperly used to describe yellow discoloration of the nails in patients with human immunodeficiency virus (HIV) infection (Chernosky & Finley, 1985). These patients did not present the characteristic nail changes of YNS (Daniel, 1986; Haas & Dover, 1986; Scher, 1988).

Improvement or clearing of nail changes concomitant with the resolution of systemic manifestations has been reported in a number of cases of YNS. Spontaneous improvement of the nails can also occur (Samman, 1973; Venencie & Dicken, 1984). Intradermal triamcinolone injections in the proximal nail matrix have been reported to be useful. Vitamin E at dosages ranging from 600 to 1200 IU daily can induce a complete clearing of the nail changes

(Ayres & Mihan, 1973; Norton, 1985; Rommel *et al.*, 1985). Although the mechanism of action of vitamin E in YNS is still unknown, antioxidant properties of α-tocopherol may account for its efficacy.

In the patient reported by Arroyo and Cohen (1993) total resolution of yellow nails and lymphoedema was observed following oral zinc supplementation for 2 years. A 'brownish black nail syndrome' in a Nigerian patient has been described as the equivalent of YNS in Caucasians (Somorin & Adesugba, 1978).

References

Arroyo J.F. & Cohen M.L. (1993) YNS cured by zinc supplementation. *Clin. Exp. Dermatol.* **18**, 62–64.

Ayres S. & Mihan R. (1973) Yellow nail syndrome. Response to vitamin E. *Arch. Dermatol.* **108**, 267–268.

Chernosky M.E. & Finley V.K. (1985) Yellow nail syndrome in patients with acquired immunodeficiency disease. *J. Am. Acad. Dermatol.* **13**, 731–736.

Daniel C.R. (1986) Yellow nail syndrome and acquired immunodeficiency disease. *J. Am. Acad. Dermatol.* **14**, 844–845.

De Coste S., Imber M.J. & Baden H.P. (1990) Yellow nail syndrome. *J. Am. Acad. Dermatol.* **22**, 608–611.

Emerson P.A. (1966) Yellow nails, lymphoedema and pleural effusions. *Thorax* **21**, 247–253.

Haas A. & Dover J.S. (1986) Yellow nail syndrome and acquired immunodeficiency disease. *J. Am. Acad. Dermatol.* **14**, 845.

Hiller E., Rosenow E.C. & Olsen A.M. (1972) Pulmonary manifestations of the yellow nail syndrome. *Chest* **61**, 452–458.

Magid M., Esterly N.B., Prendiville J. & Fujisaki C. (1987) The yellow nail syndrome in an 8-year-old girl. *Pediatr. Dermatol.* **4**, 90–93.

Malliet C., Marcucilli A., Aubin B. & Lefebvre G. (1985) Syndrome des ongles jaunes. *Sem. Hop. Paris* **61**, 2871–2876.

Mascaro J.M. & Martin-Ortega E. (1993) Nail alterations in graft-versus-host disease and other immunological disorders. In: *Dermatology Progress and Perspectives*. The Parthenon Publishing Group, New York, pp. 393–394.

Nordkild P., Kromann-Andersen H. & Struve-Christensen E. (1986) Yellow nail syndrome – the triad of yellow nails, lymphedema and pleural effusions, *Acta Med. Scand.* **219**, 221–227.

Norton L. (1985) Further observations on the yellow nail syndrome with therapeutic effects of oral alpha-tocopherol. *Cutis* **6**, 457–462.

Ohkuma M. (1982) Studies on yellow nails. In: *Proc. of XVIth Int. Congr. Derm.*, eds Kukita A. & Seiji M. Tokyo Univ. Press, Tokyo.

Pavlidakey G.P. & Hashimoto K. & Blum D. (1984) Yellow nail syndrome. *J. Am. Acad. Dermatol.* **11**, 509–512.

Reynes J., Bernard E., Dellamonica P., El Baze P. & Ortonne J.P. (1984) Un cas de syndrome des ongles jaunes. *Ann. Dermatol. Venereol.* **111**, 273–275.

Rommel A., Havet M., Ball M., Geniaux M. & Texier L. (1985) Syndrome des ongles jaunes: réponse a la vitamine E. *Ann. Dermatol. Venereol.* **112**, 625–627.

Samman P.D. (1973) The yellow nail syndrome (report on 55 cases). *Trans. St Johns Hosp. Dermatol. Soc.* **59**, 37–38.

Samman P.D. & White W.F. (1964) The yellow nail syndrome. *Br. J. Dermatol.* **76**, 153–157.

Scher R.K. (1988) Acquired immunodeficiency syndrome and yellow nails *J. Am. Acad Dermatol.* **18**, 758–759.

Somorin A.O. & Adesugba A.J. (1978) The yellow nail syndrome associated with sinusitis, bronchiectasis and transitory lymphoedema in a Nigerian patient. *Clin. Exp. Dermatol.* **3**, 31–33.

Venencie P.Y. & Dicken C.H. (1984) Yellow nail syndrome: report of five cases. *J. Am. Acad. Dermatol.* **10**, 187–192.

Shell nail syndrome

This term was coined to describe a peculiar nail deformity which occurred in a 37-year-old woman affected by bronchiectasis (Cornelius & Shelley, 1967). All fingernails and big toenails showed a similar dystrophy characterized by excessive longitudinal curvature of the nail plate associated with atrophy of the distal nail bed. A small shell-like space was present between the curved thickened nail plate and the atrophic nail bed. X-rays of fingers showed thinning of the distal phalanges with complete loss of tufting. These changes seem to be the reverse of clubbing. There is atrophy of the nail bed instead of bulbous soft tissue proliferation and bony atrophy instead of new bone formation and chronic periostitis as found in clubbing.

Reference

Cornelius C.E. & Shelley W.B. (1967) Shell nail syndrome associated with bronchiectasis. *Arch. Dermatol.* **96**, 694–695.

Sarcoidosis

Nail involvement in sarcoidosis is rare and is usually associated with bone involvement and other features of chronic sarcoidosis. Although nail involvement is more commonly associated with lupus pernio of the digits or with sarcoidal dactylitis, it can also occur without apparent involvement of the adjacent soft tissue. Sarcoid dactylitis occurs in 0.2% of patients with sarcoidosis. Fusiform swelling can involve single or numerous digits and it is usually painful (Fig. 6.17). Digital swelling and pain can precede changes in routine X-rays (Lovy, 1981; Pitt *et al.*, 1983). A necrotizing variety of sarcoid dactylitis characterized by finger ulcerations and dystrophic nails has been reported in South African black people (Leibowitz *et al.*, 1985). All except one of the patients with sarcoidal nail dystrophy reported in the literature had bone changes.

Nail plate alterations include thickening, brittleness, fragility, longitudinal ridging, cracking, layering and pitting. Clearing of the nail changes after treatment with oral prednisone and chloroquine phosphate has been reported (Patel & Sharma, 1983). Convexity of nail plates has been observed. Partial or complete atrophy of the nails can also occur (Cox & Gawkrodger, 1988). The nail biopsy can reveal the presence of sarcoid granulomas (Saada & Elbez, 1990). Nail pterygium due to sarcoidosis of the nail matrix

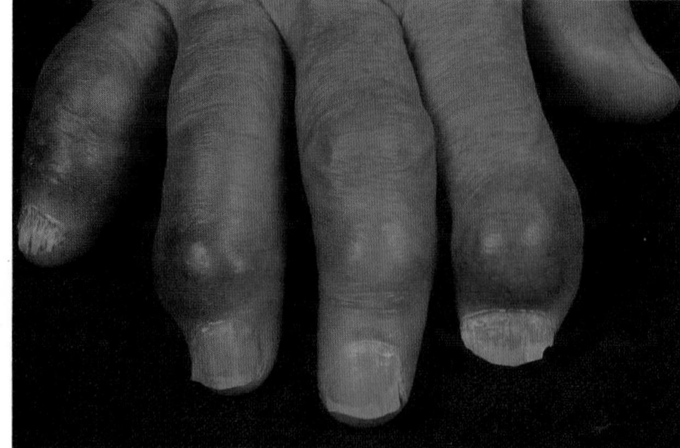

Fig. 6.17. Sarcoidosis.

has been described in a patient who did not present any other cutaneous sign of sarcoidosis (Kalb & Grossman, 1985). SH and red or brown discoloration of the nail bed may also occur. Finger clubbing is very rarely associated with pulmonary sarcoidosis (Yancey, 1972). It may be unidigital or asymmetric (Hashmi & Kaplan, 1992).

Acquired painful clubbing of all fingers and toes without evidence of cyanosis has been reported in a patient with diffuse chronic sarcoidosis (West *et al.*, 1981). Subungual and periungual plaques and nodules of big toenails due to sarcoid granuloma have been observed in a 46-year-old patient (Guillet *et al.*, 1984). The presence of a nail dystrophy in a patient with sarcoidosis is an indication for a X-ray examination of the fingers to detect the lytic, or destructive radiological features of the disease.

References

Cox H.N. & Gawkrodger D.J. (1988) Nail dystrophy in chronic sarcoidosis. *Br. J. Dermatol.* **118**, 697–701.

Guillet G., Labouche F., Guillet J., Morin P.P. & Massé R. (1984) La scintigraphie au citrate de Gallium (67 Ga) dans la Sarcoidose *Ann. Dermatol. Venereol.* **111**, 1023–1027.

Hashmi S. & Kaplan D. (1992) Asymmetric clubbing as a manifestation of sarcoid bone disease. *Am. J. Med.* **93**, 471.

Kalb R.E. & Grossman M.E. (1985) Pterygium formation due to sarcoidosis. *Arch. Dermatol.* **121**, 276–277.

Leibowitz M.R., Essop A.R., Schamroth C.L., Blumsohn D. & Smith E.H. (1985) Sarcoid dactylitis in Black South African patients. *Sem. Arth. Rheum.* **14**, 232–237.

Lovy M.R. (1981) Sarcoidosis presenting as subacute polydactylitis. *J. Rheum.* **8**, 350–352.

Patel K.B. & Sharma O.P. (1983) Nails in sarcoidosis: response to treatment. *Arch. Dermatol.* **119**, 277–278.

Pitt P., Hamilton E.B.D., Innes E.H., Morley K.D., Monk B.E. & Hughes G.R.V. (1983) Sarcoid dactylitis. *Ann. Rheum. Dis.* **42**, 634–639.

Saada V. & Elbez P. (1990) Sarcoidose unguéale. A propos d'un cas. *Rev. Eur. Dermatol. MST* **2**, 157–160.

Yancey J. (1972) Clubbing of the fingers in sarcoidosis. *J. Am. Med. Assoc.* **222**, 582.

West S.G., Gilbreath R.E. & Lawless O.J. (1981) Painful clubbing and sarcoidosis. *J. Am. Med. Assoc.* **246**, 1338–1339.

Bronchial carcinoma

Onycholysis involving all the fingernails has been described in a patient affected by squamous cell carcinoma of the lung (Hickmann, 1977).

Reference

Hickmann J.W. (1977) Onycholysis associated with carcinoma of the lung. *J. Am. Med. Assoc.* **238**, 1246–1247.

Asthma

Minimal digital clubbing may rarely occur in children with uncomplicated asthma (Sly *et al.*, 1972). Significant clubbing has also been seen in children with severe asthma requiring long-term corticosteroids. In addition, all cases had atopic eczema. Complete disappearance of the clubbing followed improvement of the asthma (Rao *et al.*, 1981).

References

Rao M., Victoria M.S., Maraya R., Jabbar H. & Steiner P. (1981) Digital clubbing in children with chronic asthma – a clinical experience at Kings County Hospital. *J. Asthma* **18**, 49–56.

Sly R.M., Faqua G, Matta E.G. & Waring W.W. (1972) Objective assessment familial of minimal digital clubbing in asthmatic children. *Ann. Allergy* **30**, 575–578.

Renal disorders

Nail clippings from patients with chronic renal failure can reveal elevated levels of creatinine (Levitt, 1966). Uraemic patients can present thickening and yellow or grey discoloration of fingernails and toenails. Onycholysis has also been reported (Bencini *et al.*, 1987).

Acral necrosis due to calciphylaxis may involve several digits (Scheinman *et al.*, 1991). Calciphylaxis has also occurred in patients undergoing renal transplantation (Fox *et al.*, 1983) and in patients undergoing long-term peritoneal dialysis and haemodialysis (Gibstein *et al.*, 1976).

References

Bencini P.L., Valeriani D.E., Bianchini F.E., Sala F., Graziani G. & Crosti C. (1987) Alterazioni cutanee nell'uremia. *G. Ital. Dermatol. Venereol.* **122**, 407–412.

Fox R., Banowsky L.H. & Cruz K.B. (1983) Post-renal transplant calciphylaxis. *J. Urol.* **129**, 362–363.

Gibstein R.M., Cobrun J.W. & Adams D.A. (1976) Calciphylaxis in man: a syndrome of tissue necrosis and vascular calcification in 11 patients with chronic renal failure. *Arch. Int. Med.* **136**, 1273–1280.

Levitt, J.I. (1966) Creatine concentration of human fingernail and toenail clippings. *Ann. Intern. Med.* **64**, 312–327.

Scheinman I.L., Helm K.F. & Fairley J.A. (1991) Acral necrosis in a patient with chronic renal failure. *Arch. Dermatol.* **127**, 247–252.

Muehrcke's lines

Muehrcke's lines of the fingernails represent an important cutaneous sign of chronic severe hypoalbuminaemia (Muehrcke, 1956). Muerhrcke's lines, that belong to the group of apparent leuconychia, appear as paired narrow white transverse bands in the nail bed. The two bands that run parallel to the lunula are non-palpable and separated from the lunula and from each other by normal pink nail. Bands do not move distally with the growth of the nails and compression of the fingertips will cause the lines to disappear temporarily.

Muehrcke's lines are more commonly observed on the second, third and fourth fingers. They are rarely seen on the thumbs. The distal white band may be slightly wider than the proximal band.

Muehrcke reported these lines in the nail beds of patients with persistent severe hypoalbuminaemia (below 2.2 g/100 ml). Muehrcke's lines appear to be more pronounced in patients who have had serum albumin levels of under 1.8 g/100 ml for at least 4 months. It was especially noted that the lines disappeared when serum albumin levels were above 2.2 g/100 ml. Although Muehrcke's lines are most frequently observed in patients with nephrotic syndrome, they can also occur in association with other diseases causing hypoalbuminaemia. Conn and Smith (1965) found myoedema and Muehrcke's line useful 'bedside' indicators of the serum albumin level.

The pathogenesis of Muehrcke's lines is still uncertain. Oedematous changes in the nail bed connective tissue (Lewin, 1965) or alteration of the nail plate–nail bed attachment have been offered as possible explanations for the nail discoloration. Muehrcke's lines have also been described in patients submitted to combination chemotherapy for malignant neoplasms in the absence of decreased albumin levels (Schwartz & Vickerman, 1979).

References

Conn R.D. & Smith R.H. (1965) Malnutrition, myoedema and Muehrcke's lines. *Arch. Intern. Med.* **116**, 875–878.

Lewin K. (1965) The finger nail in general disease. *Br. J. Dermatol.* 77, 431–438.

Muehrcke R.C. (1956) The finger-nails in chronic hypoalbuminemia. *Br. Med. J.* **1**, 1327–1328.

Schwartz R.A. & Vickerman C.E. (1979) Muehrcke's lines of the fingernails. *Arch. Intern. Med.* **139**, 242.

Haemodialysis

Splinter haemorrhages can be observed in patients receiving regular haemodialysis (Blum & Aviram, 1978) or peritoneal dialysis (Kilpatrick *et al.*, 1965). Brittle nails, platonychia and koilonychia have also been reported. Half-and-half nails frequently occur in chronic haemodialysis patients (Lubach *et al.*, 1982).

Sixteen per cent of patients undergoing chronic dialysis develop self-limited bullous lesions that resemble porphyria cutanea tarda (pseudoporphyria) on the dorsal side of the hands and other sun-exposed areas. Foot involvement can rarely occur (Black & Frenske, 1982). A black patient who developed severe photoonycholysis followed by loss of the nail plates and ulceration of the nail beds has been described (Guillaud *et al.*, 1990) (Fig. 6.18). Deep-seated, thick-walled burn-like blisters of the volar fingertips have been described in a patient after haemodialysis. The condition has been referred to as a variant of bullous dermatosis of haemodialysis (Shelley & Shelley, 1989).

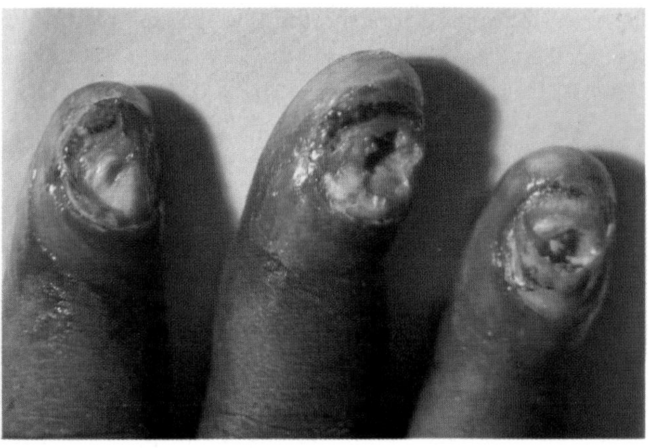

Fig. 6.18. Haemodialysis pseudoporphyria – erosive nail changes.

References

Black J.R. & Frenske N.A. (1982) Bullous dermatosis of haemodialysis in the foot and hand. *J. Am. Pediatr. Assoc.* **72**, 399–401.

Blum M. & Aviram A. (1978) Splinter haemorrhages in patients receiving regular haemodialysis. *J. Am. Med. Assoc.* **239**, 47.

Guillaud V., Moulin G., Bonnefoy M., Cognat T., Balme B. & Barrut D. (1990) Photo-onycholyse bulleuse au course d'une pseudoporphyrie des hémodialysés. *Ann. Dermatol. Venereol.* **117**, 723–725.

Kilpatrick Z.M., Greenberg P.A. & Sanford J.P. (1965) Splinter haemorrhages: their clinical significance. *Arch. Intern. Med.* **115**, 730–735.

Lubach D., Strubbe J. & Schmidt J. (1982) The half and half nail phenomenon in chronic haemodialysis. *Dermatologica* **164**, 350–353.

Shelley W.B. & Shelley D. (1989) Blisters of the fingertips: a variant of bullous dermatosis of haemodialysis. *J. Am. Acad. Dermatol.* **21**, 1049–1051.

Leuconychia and renal failure

After the treatment of acute or chronic renal failure, six patients developed a single 1–2-mm-wide transverse white band affecting all fingernails. The white bands which presented regular borders and a colour similar to the lunula completely crossed the nail. White lines were more prominent in the patients who had been most ill and their distance from the proximal nail fold reflected the approximate time of renal failure. The transverse true leuconychia disappeared with outward growth of the nails (Hudson & Dennis, 1966).

Reference

Hudson J.B. & Dennis A.J. (1966) Transverse white lines in the fingernails after acute and chronic renal failure. *Arch. Intern. Med.* **117**, 276–279.

Renal transplantation

Onychoschizia lamellina was observed in 11 of 32 children who had a kidney transplant. Onychoschizia involved the toenails (from two to 10 nails) in all patients. The fingernails were affected in only one case. No apparent relationship was present between onychoschizia and immunosuppressive treatment. Two of the 32 children presented pigmented transverse striae of the toenails. These were probably related to uraemia (Menni *et al.*, 1991).

Transverse true leuconychia has been associated with acute rejection of renal transplants (Linder, 1978; Held *et al.*, 1989). Leuconychia was observed in one of 67 kidney transplant recipients treated with cyclosporin and methylprednisolone (Bencini *et al.*, 1986). Lugo-Janer *et al.* (1991) found a high prevalence of onychomycosis, including *Candida* onychomycosis and chronic or subacute paronychia, in a group of 82 kidney transplant recipients. Skin cancers have been reported as the predominant malignant neoplasm in immunosuppressed patients after kidney transplantation. A patient developed a verrucous non-pigmented malignant melanoma of the nail bed 7 years after kidney transplantation (Merkle *et al.*, 1991).

References

Bencini P.L., Montagnino G., Sala F., De Vecchi A., Crosti C. & Tarantino A. (1986) Cutaneous lesions in 67 cyclosporin-treated renal transplant recipients. *Dermatologica* **172**, 24–30.

Held J.L., Chew S., Grossman M.E. & Kohn S.R. (1989) Transverse striate leuconychia associated with acute rejection of renal allograft. *J. Am. Acad. Dermatol.* **20**, 513–514.

Linder M. (1978) Striped nails after kidney transplant. *Ann. Intern. Med.* **88**, 809.

Lugo-Janer G., Sanchéz J.L. & Santiago-Delpin E. (1991) Prevalence and clinical spectrum of skin diseases in kidney transplant recipients. *J. Am. Acad. Dermatol.* **24**, 410–414.

Menni S., Beretta D., Piccinno R. & Ghio L. (1991) Cutaneous and oral lesions in 32 children after renal transplantation. *Pediatr. Dermatol.* **8**, 194–198.

Merkle T., Landthaler M., Eckert F. & Braun-Falco O. (1991) Acral verrucous melanoma in an immunosuppressed patient after kidney transplantation. *J. Am. Acad. Dermatol.* **24**, 505–506.

Half-and-half nails

A reddish discoloration of the distal nail was first reported by Bean (1963) in two patients with azotaemia. Lindsay (1967) introduced the term 'half-and-half nails' to describe the same condition that he believed to be a distinctive uraemic onychopathy.

Half-and-half nails are characterized by a red, pink or brown discoloration of the distal nail bed occupying 20–60% of the nail length. Half-and-half nails can be observed both in fingernails and toenails (Stewart & Raffle, 1972; Lubach *et al.*, 1982).

The proximal portion of the nails can either have a dull whitish ground glass appearance or present a normal colour. Distal and proximal portions of each nail are always sharply demarcated. The longitudinal length of the distal band is not correlated with the severity of azotaemia (Lindsay, 1967; Lubach *et al.*, 1982). Although the distal arc does not disappear with nail growth, when pressure is applied the discoloration does not fade completely. A slow rate of nail growth has been recorded (Leyden & Wood, 1972). The reported occurrence of half-and-half nails in patients with established chronic renal diseases is 9–50% (Stewart & Raffle, 1972; Daniel *et al.*, 1985). They were not seen in patients with acute renal failure and are very rarely detected in other disease states. A precise clinical differentiation between half-and-half nails and Terry's nails (in cirrhosis) can at times be difficult. Occasional overlap of the width of the distal discoloured zone in half-and-half nails and Terry's nails is unquestioned. The term erythematous crescent has been coined to describe a reddish discoloration of the distal nail involving less than 40% of the nail bed (Daniel *et al.*, 1985).

Erythematous crescents have been reported in healthy subjects and occur frequently in patients with chronic medical illnesses including renal failure. There is no correlation between the presence or absence of pigmented nail arcs and the degree of renal function impairment or serum creatinine levels. Once present, half-and-half nails usually persist unchanged and are not influenced by haemodialysis (Lubach *et al.*, 1982).

The complete disappearance of nail discoloration has been observed after successful kidney transplantation (Lubach *et al.*, 1982; Daniel *et al.*, 1985; Bencini *et al.*, 1986).

The pathogenesis of half-and-half nails is still unknown. Stimulation of nail melanocytes by increased levels of plasma melanotrophic hormone has been suggested. Substantially high levels of circulating melanotrophic hormone have been found in patients treated by maintenance dialysis for chronic renal failure (Gilkes *et al.*, 1975). Melanin granules in the basal layer of the nail bed epidermis (Stewart & Raffle, 1972) or in the distal portion of the nail plate (Leyden & Wood, 1972) have been detected on the nail biopsies of three patients. Kint *et al.*, who found an increase in the number of capillaries and a distinct thickening of their walls in the nail bed of two deceased patients, did not confirm the presence of pigment

(Kint *et al.*, 1974). Deposition of lipochrome in the nail plate has also been suggested (Stewart & Raffle, 1972).

References

Bean W.B. (1963) A discourse on nail growth and unusual fingernails. *Trans. Am. Clin. Climat. Assoc.* **74**, 132–167.

Bencini P.L., Montagnino G., Sala F., De Vecchi A., Crosti C. & Tarantino A. (1986) Cutaneous lesions in 67 cyclosporin-treated renal transplant recipients. *Dermatologica* **172**, 24–30.

Daniel C.R., Sams W.M. & Scher R.K. (1985) Nails in systemic disease. *Dermatol. Clin.* **3**, 465–483.

Gilkes J.J.H., Eady R.A.J., Rees L.H., Munro D.D. & Moorhead J.F. (1975) Plasma immunoreactive melanotrophic hormones in patients on maintenance haemodialysis. *Br. Med. J.* **1**, 656–658.

Kint A., Bussels L., Fernandes M. & Ringoir S. (1974) Skin and nail disorders in relation to chronic renal failure. *Acta Derm. Venereol.* **54**, 137–140.

Leyden J.J. & Wood M.G. (1972) The half-and-half nail. *Arch. Dermatol.* **105**, 591–592.

Lindsay P.G. (1967) The half-and-half nail. *Arch. Intern. Med.* **119**, 583–587.

Lubach D., Strubbe J. & Schmidt J. (1982) The half and half nail phenomenon in chronic haemodialysis. *Dermatologica* **164**, 350–353.

Stewart W.K. & Raffle E.J. (1972) Brown nail-bed arcs and chronic renal disease. *Br. Med. J.* **1**, 784–786.

Henoch–Schönlein purpura

Dilated nailfold capillary loops have been reported in Henoch–Schönlein purpura (Greenberg, 1983).

Reference

Greenberg L.W. (1983) Nailfold capillary abnormalities in Henoch–Schönlein purpura. *J. Pediatr.* **103**, 665–666.

Nail–patella syndrome

Forty per cent of all cases of nail–patella syndrome develops a nephropathy. Asymptomatic proteinuria is found in about 60% of patients with nail–patella syndrome. In 5.5–8% of cases the disease leads to the necessity of haemodialysis because of renal insufficiency.

Electron microscopy studies have revealed characteristic electronlucent areas and collagen fibril-like deposits in the glomerular basement membrane (Browning *et al.*, 1988). Similar changes have been found in the nail matrix vessels (Bonner & Keeling, 1991).

References

Bonner M.V. & Keeling J.H. (1991) Nail patella syndrome. Presented at the 50th Annual Meeting of the Am. Acad. of Dermatol., Dallas, 1991.

Browning M.C., Weidner N. & Lorentz W.B. (1988) Renal histopathology of the nail patella syndrome in a two-year-old boy. *Clin. Nephrol.* **29**, 210–213.

Acro-renal-ocular syndrome

Seven individuals from three generations of a French–Canadian family presented mild to severe thumb hypoplasia in association with renal and ocular defects (Halal *et al.*, 1984).

Reference

Halal F., Homsy M. & Perreault G. (1984) Acro-renal-ocular syndrome. Autosomal dominant thumb hypoplasia, renal ectopia and eye defect. *Am. J. Med. Genet.* **17**, 753–762.

YNS and nephrotic syndrome

YNS has been reported in association with nephrotic syndrome. Treatment of the nephrotic oedema coincided with return of normal nail growth in one patient (Cockram & Richards, 1979).

Reference

Cockram C.S. & Richards P. (1979) Yellow nails and nephrotic syndrome. *Br. J. Dermatol.* **101**, 707–709.

Hepatic disorders

Erythema at the base of the nails can be observed in hepatic diseases (Sarkany, 1987). Multiple pigmented bands of the nail plate have been reported in patients with hyperbilirubinaemia (Aplas, 1957). A yellow colour of the nail bed is a clinical sign of jaundice.

Cirrhosis

Nail clippings from patients with liver cirrhosis present increased Na, Mg and P content and decreased S and Cl content (Djaldetti *et al.*, 1987).

Curved nails with or without clubbing and cyanosis of the fingers have been reported in cirrhotics (Ratnoff & Patek, 1942; Djaldetti *et al.*, 1987; Berman & Lamkin, 1989). Hypertrophic osteoarthropathy has been described in biliary as well as portal cirrhosis (Buchan & Mitchell, 1967; Han & Collins, 1968). Flattening of the fingernails can also be observed. Nails lose their curvature and become flat; the nail beds are usually whitish or light pink, possibly due to anaemia (Kleeberg, 1951). Longitudinal ridging and nail thickening have been reported as well (Terry, 1954). Splinter haemorrhages can occur.

Terry's nails have been described as a common sign of liver cirrhosis which has been found in 82% of patients (Terry, 1954). Terry's nails were originally reported as white fingernails exhibiting a ground-glass-like opacity of almost the entire nail bed except for a 1–2 mm distal band of normal pink colour. The distal pink band that corresponds to the onychodermal band (Terry, 1955) can occasionally be wider (Holzeberg & Walker, 1984). The distal margin of the white nail bed can present a central or lateral peaking (Morey & Burke, 1955). The lunula may or may not be distinguishable.

Symmetrical distribution of nail bed whiteness is characteristic and thumbs and forefingers frequently present more marked changes. Nail discoloration does not vary with nail growth. Compression of the middle phalanx accentuates the contrast between the white nail bed and the distal pink zone that becomes congested. The presence or absence of Terry's nails has no correlation to severity of cirrhosis. Terry's nails are not specific to hepatic cirrhosis and they have been observed in a variety of other diseases that include chronic congestive heart failure, adult-onset diabetes mellitus, thyrotoxicosis, rheumatoid arthritis, malignancies, disseminated sclerosis, pulmonary tuberculosis, pulmonary eosinophilia, malnutrition and keratosis. They have also been frequently detected in young children and adolescent females.

In normal adults the frequency of Terry's nails has been reported to increase with ageing. The possibility of an increased risk of systemic diseases in young patients with Terry's nails has been suggested (Holzberg & Walker, 1984).

Multiple transverse white bands preceded the development of white nails in one patient (Jensen, 1981).

The following have been forwarded as explanations for clinical changes observed in Terry's nails: abnormal steroid metabolism, abnormal ratio of oestrogens to androgens, increased digital blood flow (Holzberg & Walker, 1984), alteration of the nail bed–nail plate attachment (Terry, 1954) and overgrowth of the connective tissue between the nail and bone (Sarkany, 1987). The pathological findings of three patients showed the presence of telangiectases in the upper dermis of the distal band (Holzberg & Walker, 1984). The association between primary biliary cirrhosis and the CREST variant of systemic sclerosis was first described by Reynolds *et al.* (1971). A 20% prevalence of biliary cirrhosis among patients with CREST syndrome has been reported (Dubois *et al.*, 1978). Lichen planus confined to the nails occurred in a patient with primary biliary cirrhosis (Sowden *et al.*, 1989).

Wilson's disease

The nails of patients with hepatolenticular degeneration can present an increased copper content (Djaldetti *et al.*, 1987). Bluish discoloration of the lunulae has been reported in the fingernails of patients with Wilson's disease. The azure-blue discoloration can fade proximally and be more intense at the distal margins of the lunulae (Bearn & McKusick, 1958). The differential diagnosis includes blue discoloration of the lunulae due to argyria, phenolphthalein, busulfan and antimalarial drugs (Koplon, 1966).

Haemochromatosis

Diffuse grey or brown nail plate pigmentation can be observed in haemochromatosis (Daniel, 1985). Abnormal greyish or bronze-brown hyperpigmentation of the periungual area is very frequent. Black-coal pigmentation of the lower extremities occurred in an ethylic patient with haemochromatosis (Pierard & Reginster, 1986).

Koilonychia has been observed in 49% of patients, mainly involving the thumb, index and middle fingers. Longitudinal striations, brittleness and true or apparent leuconychia have also been described (Chevrant-Breton *et al.*, 1977). Similar physical signs may be evident in Kashin–Beck disease, a poorly understood disorder seen in Asia that has been attributed to excessive amounts of iron in the water supply (Fairbanks & Fairbanks, 1971).

Chronic active hepatitis

Clubbing as well as white nails and splinter haemorrhages can occur in patients with chronic active hepatitis (Sarkany, 1987).

References

Aplas V. (1957) Hyperbilirubinamische melanonychia. *Z. Haut. Krankh.* **22**, 303.

Bearn A.G. & McKusick V.A. (1958) An unusual change in the fingernails in two patients with hepatolenticular degeneration (Wilson's disease) 'azure lunulae'. *J. Am. Med. Assoc.* **166**, 904–906.

Berman J.E. & Lamkin B.C. (1989) Hepatic disease and the skin. *Dermatol. Clin.* **7**, 435–447.

Buchan D.J. & Mitchell D.M. (1967) Hypertrophic osteoarthropathy in portal cirrhosis. *Ann. Intern. Med.* **66**, 130–135.

Chevrant-Breton J., Simon M., Bourel M. & Ferrand B. (1977) Cutaneous manifestations of idiopathic hemochromatosis. *Arch. Dermatol.* **113**, 161–165.

Daniel C.R. (1985) Nail pigmentation abnormalities. *Dermatol. Clin.* **3**, 431–443.

Djaldetti M., Fishman P., Harpaz D. & Lurie B. (1987) X-ray microanalysis of the fingernails in cirrhotic patients. *Dermatologica* **174**, 114–116.

Dubois A., Jourdan J., Blotman F. *et al.* (1978) L'association calcinose souscutanée, syndrome de Raynaud, scérodactylie et téleangiectasies (CREST syndrome): intéret en hépatologie. *Gastroenterol. Clin. Biol.* **2**, 805–809.

Fairbanks V.F. & Fairbanks G.E. (1971) Haemosiderosis and haemochromatosis. In: *Clinical Disorders of Iron Metabolism*, ed. Beutter E., p. 399. Grune & Stratton, New York.

Han S.Y. & Collins L.C. (1968) Hypertrophic osteoarthropathy in cirrhosis of the liver: report of two cases. *Radiology* **91**, 795–796.

Holzeberg M. & Walker H.K. (1984) Terry's nails: revised definition and new correlations. *Lancet* **i**, 896–899.

Jensen O. (1981) White fingernails preceded by multiple transverse white bands *Acta Derm. Venereol.* **61**, 261–262.

Kleeberg J. (1951) Flat finger-nails in cirrhosis of the liver. *Lancet* **ii**, 248–249.

Koplon B.S. (1966) Azure lunulae due to argyria. *Arch. Dermatol.* **94**, 333–334.

Morey D.A.J. & Burke J.O. (1955) Distinctive nail changes in advanced hepatic cirrhosis. *Gastroenterology* **29**, 258–261.
Pierard G.E. & Reginster M. (1986) Hémochromatose et mélanose mouchetée noire. *Nouv. Dermatol.* **5**, 423.
Ratnoff O.D. & Patek A.J. (1942) The natural history of Laennec's cirrhosis of the liver: Analysis of 387 cases. *Medicine* **21**, 207.
Reynolds T.B., Denison E.K., Frankl M.D., Lieberman F. & Peters R.L. (1971) Primary biliary cirrhosis with scleroderma, Raynaud's phenomena and telangiectasia. *Am. J. Med.* **50**, 301–312.
Sarkany I. (1987) Cutaneous manifestations of hepatobiliary disease. In: *Dermatology in General Medicine*, eds Fitzpatrick T.B., Eisen A.Z., Wolff K., Freedberg I.M. & Austen K.F., pp. 1947–1964. McGraw Hill Book Company, New York.
Sowden J.M., Cartwright P.H., Green J.R.B. & Leonard J.N. (1989) Isolated lichen planus of the nails associated with primary biliary cirrhosis. *Br. J. Dermatol.* **121**, 659–662.
Terry R.B. (1954) White nails in hepatic cirrhosis. *Lancet* **i**, 757–759.
Terry R.B. (1955) The onychodermal band in health and disease. *Lancet* **i**, 179–181.

Gastrointestinal disorders

Splinter haemorrhages have occurred in peptic ulcer. They can be painful in trichinosis (De Nicola *et al.*, 1974). Nail brittleness has been described in coeliac disease. Patients with steatorrhoea commonly exhibit thin, brittle and deformed nails. Beau's lines have also been reported (Simpson, 1954). Hereditary leuconychia can be associated with duodenal ulcer and gallstones (Ingegno & Yatto, 1982).

References

De Nicola P., Morsiani M. & Zavagli G. (1974) *Nail Diseases in Internal Medicine.* p. 54. Charles C. Thomas, Springfield, IL.
Ingegno A.D. & Yatto R.P. (1982) Hereditary white nails (leukonychia totalis) duodenal ulcer and gallstones: genetic implications. *NY State J. Med.* **82**, 1797–1800.
Simpson J.A. (1954) Dermatological changes in hypocalcemia. *Br. J. Dermatol.* **66**, 1–15.

Clubbing

Finger clubbing or hypertrophic osteoarthropathy have been observed in association with a large number of diseases that involve tissues with a vagus nerve supply. Finger clubbing has been described in ulcerative colitis (14% of the cases), multiple polyposis, chronic bacillary dysentery, amoebic dysentery, Crohn's disease (30% of the cases), tuberculosis, Hodgkin's disease, intestinal lymphoma, carcinoma, coeliac disease, ascariasis, whipworm infestation, duodenal ulcer with pyloric stenosis, gastrooesophageal reflux with protein-losing enteropathy and idiopathic steatorrhoea (Young, 1966; Bowie *et al.*, 1978; Kitis *et al.*, 1979). Clubbing of the fingers and toes has been reported in children affected by Crohn's disease of the jejunum (Chrispin & Tempany, 1967). Hypertrophic osteoarthropathy has occurred in association with chronic ulcerative colitis, Crohn's disease, multiple polyposis and upper gastrointestinal neoplasms (Singh *et al.*, 1960; Farnan *et al.*, 1971; Ullal, 1972). Regression of clubbing has been reported after eradication of ascariasis or whipworm infestation (Bowie *et al.*, 1978). Reversible clubbing of the fingers and toes has been described in association with purgative abuse (Silk *et al.*, 1975; Levine *et al.*, 1981). Finger clubbing was present in 77% of patients with kwashiorkor and may have been related to diarrhoea (Amla & Marayan, 1968). Diffuse thickening of the gastric mucosal folds has been reported in patients with pachydermoperiostosis (Venencie *et al.*, 1988).

References

Amla I. & Marayan J.V. (1968) Finger nail clubbing in kwashiorkor. *Ind. J. Pediatr.* **35(240)**, 19–22.
Bowie M.D., Morrison A., Ireland J.D. & Duys P.J. (1978) Clubbing and whipworm infestation. *Arch. Dis. Child.* **53**, 411–413.
Chrispin A.R. & Tempany E. (1967) Crohn's disease of the jejunum in children. *Arch. Dis. Child.* **42**, 631–635.
Farman J., Effman E.L. & Grnja V. (1971) Crohn's disease and periostal new bone formation. *Gastroenterology* **61**, 513–522.
Hollis W.C. (1967) Hypertrophic osteoarthropathy secondary to upper-gastrointestinal-tract neoplasm. *Ann. Intern. Med.* **66**, 125–130.
Kitis G., Thompson H. & Allan R.N. (1979) Finger clubbing in inflammatory bowel disease its prevalence and pathogenesis. *Br. Med. J.* **2**, 825–828.
Levine D., Goode A.W. & Wingate D.L. (1981) Purgative abuse associated with reversible cachexia, hypogammaglobulinaemia, and finger clubbing. *Lancet* **i**, 919–920.
Silk D.B.A., Gibson J.A. & Murray C.R.H. (1975) Reversible finger clubbing in a case of purgative abuse. *Gastroenterology* **68**, 790–794.
Singh A., Jolly S.S. & Bansal B.B. (1960) Hypertrophic osteoarthropathy associated with carcinoma of the stomach. *Br. Med. J.* **2**, 581–582.
Ullal S.R. (1972) Hypertrophic osteoarthropathy and leiomyoma of the esophagus. *Am. J. Surg.* **123**, 356–358.
Venencie P.Y., Boffa G.A., Delmas P.D. *et al.* (1988) Pachydermoperiostosis with gastric hypertrophy, anemia and increased serum bone Gla-protein levels. *Arch. Dermatol.* **124**, 1831–1834.
Young J.R. (1966) Ulcerative colitis and finger-clubbing. *Br. Med. J.* **1**, 278–279.

Ulcerative colitis

Patients with ulcerative colitis occasionally experience painful haemorrhages in the nail bed. Rarely, this is followed by a liquefaction and necrosis at the site. Vesicular, tender erythematous areas developing at the base of the volar surface of the digits have also been reported (Kelly, 1968; Daniel, 1985).

Finger clubbing has been detected in seven of 77 patients affected by ulcerative colitis with involvement in that part of the colon innervated by the vagus nerve (the proximal two-thirds of the transverse colon). Clubbing did not occur in patients who had disease limited to the distal colon (Young, 1966).

Hypertrophic osteoarthropathy has also been associated with ulcerative colitis. Zaun (1980) described Terry's nails in a young man with ulcerative colitis. A patient with ulcerative colitis, sclerosing cholangitis and pyoderma gangrenosum involving the tip of the great toe has been reported (Shelley & Shelley, 1988).

References

Daniel C.R. (1985) Nail pigmentation abnormalities. *Dermatol. Clin.* 3, 431–443.

Kelly M.L. (1968) Purulent mucocutaneous lesions associated with ulcerative colitis. *Med. Radiogr. Photogr.* **44**(2), 39–41.

Shelley E.D. & Shelley W.B. (1988) Cyclosporine therapy for pyoderma gangrenosum associated with sclerosing cholangitis and ulcerative colitis. *J. Am. Acad. Dermatol.* **18**, 1084–1088.

Young J.R. (1966) Ulcerative colitis and finger-clubbing. *Br. Med. J.* **1**, 278–279.

Zaun H. (1980) Milchglasnagel: hinweis auf intestinale erkrankungen. *Akt. Dermatol.* **6**, 107–108.

Peutz–Jeghers–Touraine syndrome

Pigmented macules on the fingers and toes are a distinctive sign of Peutz–Jeghers–Touraine syndrome. Longitudinal pigmented bands of fingernails and toenails due to melanin deposits in the nail plate have been reported (Valero & Sherf, 1965). Punctate brown pigmentation of the nail has also been described (Daniel, 1985). Differential diagnosis should rule out Laugier–Hunziker syndrome (Baran & Barrière, 1986).

References

Baran R. & Barrière H. (1986) Longitudinal melanonychia with spreading pigmentation in Laugier–Hunziker syndrome: a report of two cases. *Br. J. Dermatol.* **115**, 707–710.

Daniel C.R. (1985) Nail pigmentation abnormalities. *Dermatol. Clin.* 3, 431–443.

Valero A. & Sherf K. (1965) Pigmented nails in Peutz–Jeghers syndrome. *Am. J. Gastroenterol.* **43**, 56–58.

Cronkhite–Canada syndrome

This rare syndrome is characterized by non-familial generalized gastrointestinal polyposis associated with skin hyperpigmentation, hair loss and nail dystrophy (Cronkhite & Canada, 1955). Changes in the fingernails and toenails were noted in 51 of 55 patients and may precede gastrointestinal symptoms. Nail thinning, splitting and discoloration are commonly observed. The nails become fragile, brittle and soft and the nail plate surface can be scaled, ridged or spoon-like. Nail colour can vary from white to yellow to brown-black. Proximal or distal onycholysis can also occur. Complete loss of all fingernails and toenails is not rare (Daniel *et al.*, 1982; Freeman *et al.*, 1985; Aanestad *et al.*, 1987). Partial or total regeneration of nails can occur spontaneously or during remissions (Daniel *et al.*, 1982; Peart *et al.*, 1984). Patients exhibiting a thin and soft triangular nail plate in the proximal half of several fingernails and toenails have been reported. Distal nail plates were hard, thick, ridged and brown in colour (Cunliffe & Anderson, 1967; Daniel *et al.*, 1982; Peart *et al.*, 1984).

References

Aanestad O., Raknerud N., Aase S.T. & Narverud G. (1987) The Cronkhite–Canada syndrome. Case report. *Acta Chir. Scand.* **153**, 143–145.

Cronkhite L.W. & Canada W.J. (1955) Generalized gastrointestinal polyposis: an unusual syndrome of polyposis, pigmentation, alopecia and onychotrophia. *N. Engl. J. Med.* **252**, 1011–1015.

Cunliffe W.J. & Anderson J. (1967) Case of Cronkhite–Canada syndrome with associated jejunal diverticulosis. *Br. Med. J.* **4**, 601–602.

Daniel E.S., Ludwig S.L., Lewin K.J., Ruprecht R.M., Rajacich G.M. & Schwabe A.D. (1982) The Cronkhite–Canada syndrome. An analysis of clinical and pathological features and therapy in 55 patients. *Medicine* **61**, 293–309.

Freeman K., Anthony P.P., Miller D.S. & Warin A.P. (1985) Cronkhite–Canada syndrome: a new hypothesis. *Gut* **26**, 531–536.

Peart A.G., Sivak M.V., Rankin G.B., Kish S. & Steck W.D. (1984) Spontaneous improvement of Cronkhite–Canada syndrome in a postpartum female. *Digest. Dis. Sci.* **29**, 470.

Plummer–Vinson (Patterson–Kelly–Brown) syndrome

This syndrome describes the association of chronic dysphagia with atrophic changes in the oral mucosa and hypochromic anaemia. Koilonychia occurs in 40–50% of patients and usually involves the first three digits of the hands but spares the toenails. Nail brittleness is also frequent. Nail changes as well as the other clinical manifestations of Plummer–Vinson syndrome are reversible with iron therapy (Archard, 1987).

Reference

Archard H.O. (1987) Disorders of mucocutaneous integument. In: *Dermatology in General Medicine*, eds Fitzpatrick T.B., Eisen A.Z., Wolff K., Freedberg I.M. & Austen K.F., pp. 1152–1239. McGraw Hill, New York.

Crohn's disease

Nail fold capillary microscopy of patients with Crohn's disease may reveal microcirculatory abnormalities (Gasser

& Affolter, 1990). An increased occurrence of psoriasis in patients with Crohn's disease has been reported (Lee *et al.*, 1990).

References

Gasser P. & Affolter H. (1990) Pathogenesis of Crohn's disease. *Lancet* **335**, 551.

Lee F.I., Bellary S.V. & Francis C. (1990) Increased occurrence of psoriasis in patients with Crohn's disease and their relatives. *Am. J. Gastroenterol.* **85**, 962–963.

Nutritional disorders and deficiencies

Pellagra

Transverse leuconychia is described in pellagra and may be associated with a general loss of nail translucency (Brownson, 1915). Poikilodermatous skin and onycholysis can also be observed (Zaias, 1990).

References

Brownson W.C. (1915) An unusual condition of the nails in pellagra. *South. Med. J.* **8**, 672–675.

Zaias N. (1990) *The Nail in Health and Disease*, 2nd edn pp. 189–199. Appleton & Lange, Norwalk, CT.

Vitamin A deficiency

The presence of 'eggshell' nail changes in vitamin A deficiency has been observed (Bereston, 1950).

Reference

Bereston E.S. (1950) Diseases of the nails. *Clin. Med.*, 238–240.

Vitamin C deficiency

Subungual haemorrhages can occur in scurvy (Miller, 1989).

Reference

Miller S.J. (1989) Nutritional deficiency and the skin. *J. Am. Acad. Dermatol.* **21**, 1–30.

Vitamin B_{12} deficiency

Reversible hyperpigmentation of the skin can be observed in patients with megaloblastic anaemia due to vitamin B_{12} or folate deficiency. Skin hyperpigmentation is particularly pronounced over the knuckles and terminal phalanges. Bluish-black discoloration of fingernails and toenails can rarely occur. Uniform nail hyperpigmentation as well as longitudinal or transverse pigmented bands have been reported. Pigment changes are reversible with vitamin B_{12} administration (Baker *et al.*, 1963; Ridley, 1977; Carmel, 1985; Marks *et al.*, 1985). It has been suggested that vitamin B_{12} deficiency results in a decreased amount of intracellular-reduced glutathione, which normally inhibits tyrosinase activity in melanogenesis (Marks *et al.*, 1985; Noppakun & Swasdikul, 1986).

References

Baker S.S., Ignatius M., Johnson S. & Vaish S.K. (1963) Hyperpigmentation of skin. A sign of vitamin B_{12} deficiency. *Br. Med. J.* **1**, 1713–1715.

Carmel R. (1985) Hair and fingernail changes in acquired congenital pernicious anemia. *Arch. Intern. Med.* **145**, 484–485.

Marks V.J., Briggaman R.A. & Wheeler C.E. (1985) Hyperpigmentation in megaloblastic anemia. *J. Am. Acad. Dermatol.* **12**, 914–917.

Noppakun N. & Swasdikul D. (1986) Reversible hyperpigmentation of skin and nails with white hair due to vitamin B_{12} deficiency. *Arch. Dermatol.* **122**, 896–899.

Ridley C.M. (1977) Pigmentation of fingertips and nails in vitamin B_{12} deficiency. *Br. J. Dermatol.* **97**, 105–107.

Zinc deficiency

Acrodermatitis enteropathica is a rare and inherited disease due to a specific deficit of zinc absorption. Diarrhoea, alopecia and acral dermatitis are the characteristic manifestations of the disorder. Nail involvement such as longitudinal ridging, striations, brittleness and grey discoloration of the nails has been reported in 96% of patients. Chronic paronychia as well as vesicobullous and erosive or psoriasiform lesions on the dorsal aspect of the terminal phalanges are distinctive symptoms of the disease. The lesions have an increased occurrence around the nails and between the fingers and toes. Beau's lines can occasionally be observed after recurrences (Wells & Winkelmann, 1961; Weismann, 1977; Miranda *et al.*, 1986). A transient symptomatic zinc deficiency may occasionally occur in breast-fed premature infants. Clinical symptoms closely resemble acrodermatitis enteropathica and include chronic paronychia. A low breast-milk zinc content has been detected in some cases (Munro *et al.*, 1989).

An acute zinc deficiency associated with an acrodermatitis enteropathica-like syndrome can occur in patients submitted to total parenteral nutrition for inflammatory or neoplastic gastrointestinal disorders. Paronychia (Nurnberger, 1987) and purpuric blisters of the proximal nail fold have been described (Zaias, 1990). Histologically the bullous lesions were characterized by intraepidermal vacuolar changes with massive ballooning, leading to intraepidermal vesiculation and blistering, with prominent epidermal necrosis and without acantholysis (Borroni *et al.*, 1992). Transverse paired white bands, which resemble Muerhrcke's lines of chronic hypoalbuminaemia or Beau's lines can be observed after recovery from acute zinc deficiency (Weismann, 1977; Brazin *et al.*, 1979; Ferràndez *et al.*, 1981; Nurnberger, 1987). Since 85% of serum zinc is bound to albumin, the hypothesis that Muerhrcke's lines may actually represent a marker for zinc deficiency has been put forward (Pfeiffer & Jenney, 1974; Ferràndez *et al.*, 1981). Periungual brown discoloration and thickened irregular cuticles have been observed in a patient with acute zinc deficiency due to total parenteral nutrition (Brazin *et al.*, 1979).

References

Brazin S.A., Johnson W.T. & Abramson L.J. (1979) The acrodermatitis enteropathica-like syndrome. *Arch. Dermatol.* **115**, 597–599.
Borroni G., Brazzelli V., Vignati G., Zaccone C., Vignoli G.P. & Rabbiosi G. (1992) Bullous lesions in acrodermatitis enteropathica. Histopathologic findings regarding two patients. *Am. J. Dermatopath.* **14**, 304–309.
Ferràndez C., Henkes J., Peyri J. & Sarmiento J. (1981) Acquired zinc deficiency syndrome during total parenteral alimentation. *Dermatologica* **163**, 255–266.
Miranda M., Polanco I., Fonseca E., Alzate C., Rodriguez J.L. & Contreras F. (1986) Acrodermatitis enteropatica y dermatitis hipozinquémica en la infancia. *Acta Derm. Sif.* **77(1)**, 655–668.
Munro C.S., Lazaro C. & Lawrence C.M. (1989) Symptomatic zinc deficiency in breast-fed premature infants. *Br. J. Dermatol.* **121**, 773–778.
Nurnberger F. (1987) Zinkmangel bei Kunstlicher ernahrung. *Z. Hautkr.* **62** (Suppl. 1), 104–110.
Pfeiffer C.C. & Jenney E.H. (1974) Fingernail white spots: possible zinc deficiency. *J. Am. Med. Assoc.* **228**, 157.
Weismann K. (1977) Lines of Beau: possible markers of zinc deficiency. *Acta Dermatol. Venereol.* **57**, 88–90.
Wells B.T. & Winkelmann R.K. (1961) Acrodermatitis enteropathica. *Arch. Dermatol.* **84**, 90–102.
Zaias N. (1990) *The Nail in Health and Disease*, 2nd edn, pp. 189–199. Appleton & Lange, Norwalk, CT.

Selenium deficiency

Four children receiving long-term total parenteral nutrition developed macrocytosis, loss of hair and skin pigmentation, elevated transaminase and creatine kinase activities as well as profound muscle weakness. Selenium levels were low. Nail strengthening was observed after selenium supplementation (Vinton *et al.*, 1987).

Reference

Vinton N.E., Dahlstrom K.A., Strobel C.T. & Ament M.E. (1987) Macrocytosis and pseudoalbinism: manifestations of selenium deficiency. *J. Pediatr.* **111**, 711–717.

Fetal alcohol syndrome

Absence or dysplasia of the fingernails and toenails was found in more than 20% of patients (Crain *et al.*, 1983).

Reference

Crain L.S., Fitzmaurice N.E. & Mondry C. (1983) Nail dysplasia and fetal alcohol syndrome. Case report of a heteropaternal sibship. *Am. J. Dis. Child.* **137**, 1069–1072.

Iron deficiency

Brittle nails, koilonychia and longitudinal ridging can be observed in iron deficiency anaemia. The iron content of the fingernails is not an indication of the iron levels in iron-deficient patients (Djaldetti *et al.*, 1987).

Reference

Djaldetti M., Fishman P. & Hart J. (1987) The iron content of finger-nails in iron deficient patients. *Clin. Sci.* **72**, 669–672.

Malnutrition

Abnormal nail growth (Daniel *et al.*, 1985) and multiple pigmented bands (Bisht & Singh, 1962) have been described in malnutrition. Soft and brittle nails are frequently observed in cachexia (Runne & Orfanos, 1981). Persons with marasmus often exhibit fissured nails (Miller, 1989). Finger- and toenails are severely dystrophic in kwashiorkor (Albers *et al.*, 1993).

References

Albers S.E., Brozena S.J. & Fenske N.E. (1993) A case of kwashiorkor. *Cutis* **51**, 445–446.
Bisht D.B. & Singh S.S. (1962) Pigmented bands on nails: a new sign in malnutrition. *Lancet* **i**, 507–508.
Daniel C.R., Sams W.M. & Scher R.K. (1985) Nails in systemic disease. *Dermatol. Clin.* **3**, 465–483.
Miller S.J. (1989) Nutritional deficiency and the skin. *J. Am. Acad. Dermatol.* **21**, 1–30.
Runne U. & Orfanos C.E. (1981) The human nail. *Curr. Probl. Dermatol.* **9**, 102–149.

Endocrine disorders

Hypogonadism

Reversible onychauxis of the fingernails has been reported in a eunuchoid (Lisser, 1924). Infantile, longitudinally striated, small nails have been described in adipose genital syndrome (De Nicola *et al.*, 1974).

References

De Nicola P., Morsiani M. & Zavagli G. (1974) *Nail Diseases in Internal Medicine*, pp. 67–70. Charles C. Thomas, Springfield, IL.

Lisser H. (1924) Onychauxis in a eunuchoid. *Arch. Dermatol. Syphil.* **10**, 180–182.

Pituitary disease

The hypertrophy of the soft tissues of the fingers that characterizes acromegaly causes the nails to appear short and broad (Haneke, 1989). Lunulae can be absent. Nail brittleness, koilonychia and macronychia have been described. Generalized hyperpigmentation of nails and digits is occasionally seen. Nail thickening and hardening can also occur (Freinkel & Freinkel, 1987). Chronic paronychia and ingrowing fingernails have been described in a patient affected by acromegaly (Keefe *et al.*, 1987). Thin and brittle nails have been noted in three adolescent patients affected by cerebral gigantism (Sotos syndrome) (Wit *et al.*, 1985). Disappearance of the lunulae, brown spots, as well as long and thin nails have been described in hypopituitarism (De Nicola *et al.*, 1974). Nail thickening, fragility and striation along with Beau's lines of the thumbnails occurred in a patient with Sheehan's syndrome (Biava, 1974). Thickening of the nail plates was reported in a patient with hypopituitarism and feminine genotype (Hollander, 1920).

References

Biava L. (1974) Le alterazioni ungueali nel morbo di Sheehan. *Chron. Derm.* **3–4**, 814–818.

De Nicola P., Morsiani M. & Zavagli G. (1974) *Nail Disease in Internal Medicine.* Charles C. Thomas, Springfield, IL.

Freinkel R.K. & Freinkel N. (1987) In: *Dermatology in General Medicine* eds Fitzpatrick T.B., Eisen A.Z., Wolff K., Freedberg I.M. & Austen K.F., pp. 2063–2081. McGraw Hill, New York.

Haneke E. (1989) Nagelveranderungen bei hormonellen Storungen. *Med. Mo. Pharm.* **12**(6), 173–178.

Hollander L. (1920) Onychauxis due to hypopituitarism. *Arch. Dermatol. Syphil.* **2**, 35–43.

Keefe M., Chapman R.S. & Peden N.R. (1987) Ingrowing fingernails: an unusual complication of acromegaly successfully treated by conservative means. *Clin. Exp. Dermatol.* **12**, 343–344.

Wit J.M., Beemer F.A., Barth P.G. *et al.* (1985) Cerebral gigantism (Sotos syndrome). Complied data of 22 cases. Analysis of clinical features, growth and plasma somatomedin. *Eur. J. Pediatr.* **144**, 131–140.

Adrenal disease

Cutaneous and mucosal hyperpigmentation is one of the most characteristic signs of chronic adrenal insufficiency. Longitudinal pigmented bands in fingernails and toenails are occasionally observed. Nail hyperpigmentation progressively disappears after replacement therapy (Allenby & Snell, 1966; Bissel *et al.*, 1971). Cutaneous hyperpigmentation due to a pituitary tumour (Nelson's syndrome) occurs in about 10% of patients submitted to bilateral adrenalectomy for Cushing's syndrome. Longitudinal pigmented bands in fingernails and toenails have been described (Bondy & Harwick, 1969). Primary distal and lateral onycholysis as well as chronic paronychia due to *Candida* have been described in association with Cushing's syndrome (Hay *et al.*, 1988; Haneke, 1989).

References

Allenby C.F. & Snell P.H. (1966) Longitudinal pigmentation of the nails in Addison's disease. *Br. Med. J.* **1**, 1582–1583.

Bissel G.W., Surakomol K. & Greenslet F. (1971) Longitudinal banded pigmentation of nails in primary adrenal insufficiency. *J. Am. Med. Assoc.* **215**(**10**), 1666–1667.

Bondy P.K. & Harwick H.J. (1969) Longitudinal banded pigmentation of nails following adrenalectomy for Cushing's syndrome. *New Engl. J. Med.* **281**, 1056–1057.

Haneke E. (1989) Nagelveranderungen bei hormonellen Storungen. *Med. Mo. Pharm.* **12**(**6**), 173–178.

Hay R.S., Baran R., Moore M.K. & Wilkinson J.D. (1988) *Candida* onychomycosis – an evaluation of the role of *Candida* species in nail diseases. *Br. J. Dermatol.* **118**, 45–58.

Parathyroid disease

Nail and hair changes can precede other clinical manifestations of hypocalcaemia. Characteristic nail changes have been described in hypoparathyroidism. The distal half of the nail plate becomes brittle and then crumbles. The proximal nail plate is covered with irregular longitudinal grooves. Thinning, fragility, and splitting at the distal free edge of the nails is commonly observed. Nail changes usually disappear when serum calcium is restored to normal levels (Simpson, 1954). All 20 nails can occasionally appear opalescent, thin and brittle with fine longitudinal ridges (Yuzuk *et al.*, 1986). Splinter haemorrhages have also been reported.

Secondary *Candida* infection of the nails is frequently observed. A defect in cell-mediated immunity, combined with the nail changes that favour yeast invasion, is a possible explanation for the increased susceptibility to *Candida* infection.

Shortening and thickening of the fingernails and toenails along with overgrowth of the periungual tissues have been reported in a patient suffering from idiopathic hypoparathyroidism (Emerson *et al.*, 1941). Nail brittleness and Beau's lines can occur 4–6 weeks after a severe attack of acute hypocalcaemia. Shedding of the nails and necrosis of the nail beds have also been described (Simpson, 1954). Impaired circulation caused by spasm in the nail bed capillary loops has been detected in latent tetany. Calcium administration can prevent angiospasm (Simpson, 1954).

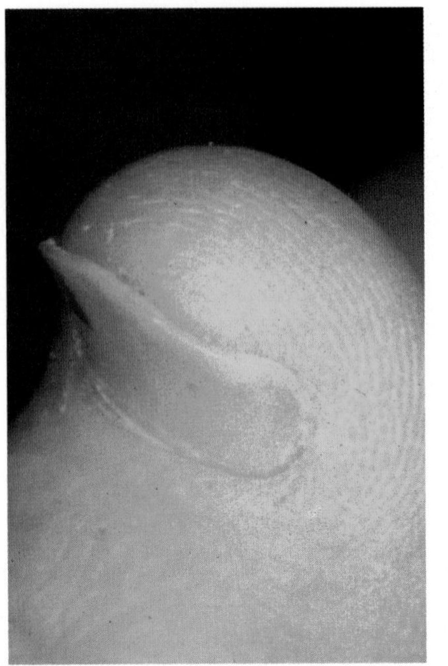

Fig. 6.19. Hyperparathyroidism – acquired racket-nails and koilonychia (courtesy of B. Schubert, Mulhouse, France).

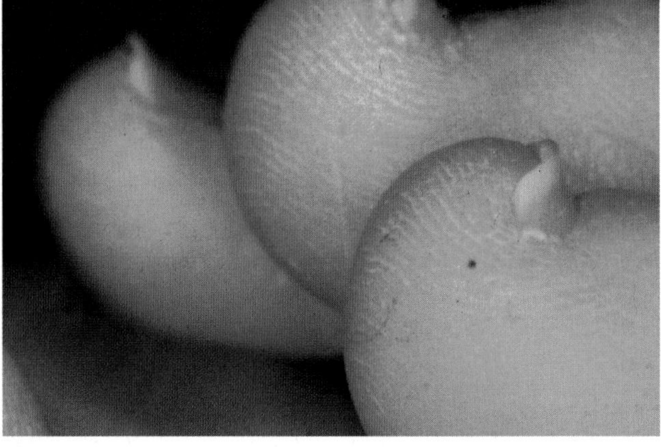

Fig. 6.20. Hyperparathyroidism – acquired racket-nails (courtesy of B. Schubert, Mulhouse, France).

In polyglandular type I autoimmunity syndromes, chronic mucocutaneous candidiasis is associated with hypoparathyroidism and adrenal insufficiency (Ahonen *et al.*, 1990). An inherited defect in cell-mediated immunity has been recognized.

Brachydactyly is a common feature of pseudohypoparathyroidism. In hyperparathyroidism, acroosteolysis due to calcium mobilization can occur. Shortening of distal phalanges causes the nails to appear abnormally broad (acquired racket-nails) (Fairris & Rowell, 1984) (Figs 6.19 & 6.20). Nail shedding has been reported after treatment with parathyroid extracts (Perrot *et al.*, 1973).

References

Ahonen P., Myllarniemi S., Sipila I. & Perheentupa J. (1990) Clinical variation of autoimmune polyendocrinopathy–candidiasis–ectodermal dystrophy (APECED) in a series of 68 patients. *N. Engl. J. Med*, **322**, 1829–1836.

Emerson K., Walsh F.B. & Howard J.F. (1941) Idiopathic hypoparathyroidism; a report of two cases. *Ann. Intern. Med.* **14**, 1256–1270.

Fairris G.M. & Rowell N.R. (1984) Acquired racket nails. *Clin. Exp. Dermatol.* **9**, 267.

Perrot H., Tourniere J. & Fournier M. (1973) Onychopathie induite par la parathormone. *Bull. Soc. Fr. Dermatol. Syphil.* **80**, 313.

Simpson J.A. (1954) Dermatological changes in hypocalcemia. *Br. J. Dermatol.* **66**, 1–15.

Yuzuk S., Keren G., Lobel D., Kahana M. & Schewach-Millet M. (1986) Primary cutaneous manifestation in a child with idiopathic hypoparathyroidism. *Int. J. Dermatol.* **25**, 531–532.

Thyroid disease

Nail changes are seen in approximately 5% of hyperthyroid patients. Brittle nails and onycholysis are common signs of hyperthyroidism. Koilonychia is occasionally observed (Mullin & Eastern, 1986). A variable brown colour can be present in the nail plate (Daniel, 1985).

In thyrotoxicosis, a characteristic onycholysis occurs in which the free edge of the nail is undulated and curved upward (Plummer's nails). The fourth digits of the hands are initially involved but the alteration may affect any or all of the finger and toenails. Plummer's nails are reversible with treatment of the hyperthyroidism (Luria & Asper, 1958).

Diamond syndrome, which is a rare manifestation of Graves' disease, describes the association of finger clubbing (thyroid acropathy) with ophthalmopathy and pretibial myxoedema.

In hypothyroidism, the nails can appear dry, flat, brittle and longitudinally ridged. Onycholysis is occasionally observed (Keipert & Kelly, 1978; Baran, 1986). Thick, hard and lustreless nails have also been described (Haneke, 1989; Zaias, 1990).

References

Baran R. (1986) Les onycholyses. *Ann. Dermatol. Venereol.* **113**, 159–170.

Daniel C.R. (1985) Nail pigmentation abnormalities. *Dermatol. Clin.* **3**, 431–443.

Haneke E. (1989) Nagelveranderungen bei hormonellen Storungen. *Med. Mo. Pharm.* **12**(6), 173–178.

Keipert J.A. & Kelly R. (1978) Acquired juvenile hypothyroidism presenting with nail changes. *Aust. J. Dermatol.* **19**, 89–90.

Luria M. & Asper S. (1958) Onycholysis in hyperthyroidism. *Ann. Intern. Med.* **49**, 102–108.

Mullin G.E. & Eastern J.S. (1986) Cutaneous consequences of accelerated thyroid function. *Cutis* **37/2**, 109–114.

Zaias N. (1990) *The Nail in Health and Disease*, 2nd edn, pp. 189–199. Appleton & Lange, Norwalk, CN.

Pregnancy and menstrual factors

Nail growth is accelerated in pregnancy and slowed during lactation (Runne & Orfanos, 1981). Although Beau's lines, increased brittleness and softening as well as subungual keratosis and onycholysis can occur in pregnancy, they are probably not related to hormonal factors (Wong & Ellis, 1984). Hyperpigmentation is very common in pregnancy and can be associated with longitudinal melanonychia (Texier, 1980; Freyer & Werth, 1992). Beau's lines have been associated with dysmenorrhoea but they can also occur physiologically with each menstrual cycle (Colver & Dawber, 1984). Transverse leuconychia has also been associated with menstruation (Daniel *et al.*, 1985).

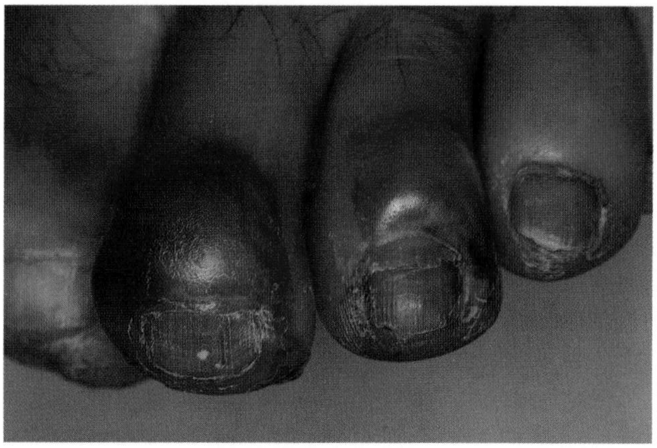

Fig. 6.21. Diabetic foot – periungual blisters.

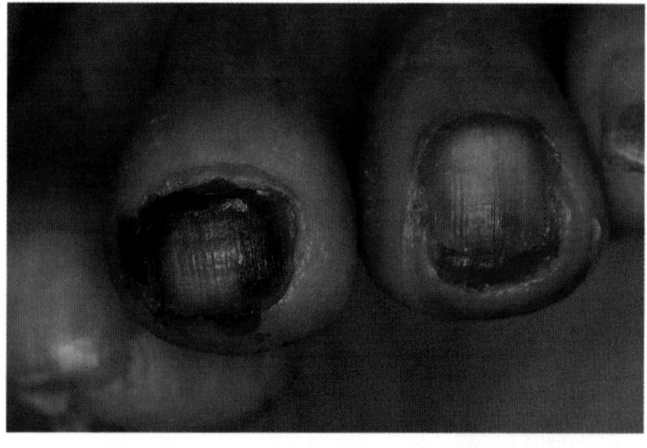

Fig. 6.22. Diabetic foot – nail thickening, periungual haemorrhage and early ulceration.

References

Colver G.B. & Dawber R.P.R. (1984) Multiple Beau's lines due to dysmenorrhoea? *Br. J. Dermatol.* **111**, 111–113.

Daniel C.R. (1985) Nail pigmentation abnormalities. *Dermatol. Clin.* **3**, 431–443.

Freyer J.M. & Werth V.P. (1992) Pregnancy-associated hyperpigmentation longitudinal melanonychia. *J. Am. Acad. Dermatol.* **26**, 493–494.

Runne U. & Orfanos C.E. (1981) The human nail. *Curr. Prob. Dermatol.* **9**, 102–149.

Texier L. (1980) Chromonychie en bandes longitudinales de la grossesse. Presented at the meeting of the Société Française de Dermatologie. Filiale du sud-ouest, Bordeaux, France, 21 June.

Wong R.C. & Ellis C.N. (1984) Physiologic skin changes in pregnancy. *J. Am. Acad. Dermatol.* **10**, 929–940.

Metabolic disorders

Diabetes

Furosine and fructose–lysine values in the nails are indicators of non-enzymatic glycosylation associated with diabetic hyperglycaemia. A significant correlation exists between nail glycosylation and glycosylated haemoglobin as well as fasting blood glucose levels in diabetics (Bakan & Bakan, 1985). Furosine and fructose–lysine levels in the nails reflect the blood glucose levels within 3–5 months before nail clipping (Oimomi *et al.*, 1986). No correlations have been detected between furosine values of stratum corneum, nails and the prevalence of cutaneous manifestations in diabetics (Nozaki *et al.*, 1988).

Periungual erythema and telangiectasia can be a very early manifestation of diabetes mellitus. Proximal nail fold capillaroscopy can reveal venous dilatation and tortuosity. The former has been suggested to be an indicator of functional microangiopathy and of long-term blood glucose control. Venous tortuosity, on the contrary, has been related to long-term microangiopathy (Huntley, 1989). Haemorrhages and ischaemic areas can also be present.

Scleroderma-like skin changes involving the fingers and dorsum of the hands occur in 20–30% of diabetic patients. Thickening of the skin on the dorsum of the fingers causes the skin on the periungual regions and knuckles to have a pebbled or rough appearance (Huntley, 1989). Chronic paronychia and onycholysis due to *Candida* are frequently observed in diabetics. Onychomycoses are common as well. A positive correlation has been detected between blood glucose levels and the percentage of positive fungal cultures in toenails (Greene & Scher, 1987).

Smooth thickened toenails of yellow or yellowish-green colour have been described in diabetics. The great toes usually present prominent changes and the yellow discoloration is most often evident on the distal aspect of the nails (Lithner, 1976). Clear, non-scarring blisters on the tips of the toes or fingers can occasionally be observed. (Fig. 6.21). Toenail thickening (Fig. 6.22) or onychogryphosis can result from diabetic angiopathy and neuropathy. Neuropathic ulcers, ischaemic ulcerations of the nail bed and gangrene are major complications of diabetic foot.

Infections are frequent and are also the most likely cause of foot amputation (Brodsky & Schneidler, 1991).

Large hands and feet and clubbing have been described in congenital lipodystrophic diabetes with acanthosis nigricans (Seip–Lawrence syndrome) (Reed *et al.*, 1965).

References

Bakan E. & Bakan N. (1985) Glycosylation of nail in diabetics: possible marker of long-term hyperglycemia *Clin. Chim. Acta* **147**, 1–5.

Brodsky J.W. & Schneidler C. (1991) Diabetic foot infections. *Orth. Clin. North Am.* **22**, 473–489.

Greene R.A. & Scher R.K. (1987) Nail changes associated with diabetes mellitus. *J. Am. Acad. Dermatol.* **16**, 1015–1021.

Huntley A.C. (1989) Cutaneous manifestations of diabetes mellitus. *Dermatol. Clin.* **7**, 531–546.

Lithner F. (1976) Purpura, pigmentation and yellow nails of the lower extremities in diabetics. *Acta Med. Scand.* **199**, 203–208.

Nozaki S., Sueki H., Fujisawa R., Aoki K. & Kuroiwa Y. (1988) Glycosylated proteins of stratum corneum, nail and hair in diabetes mellitus: correlation with cutaneous manifestations. *J. Dermatol.* **15**, 320–324.

Oimomi M., Nishimoto S., Kitamura Y., Matsumoto S., Hatanaka H. & Baba S. (1986) Increased fructose-lysine of nail protein and blood glucose control in diabetic patients. *Horm. Metabol. Res.* **18**, 827–829.

Reed W.B., Dexter R., Corley C. & Fish C. (1965) Congenital lipodystrophic diabetes with acanthosis nigricans. *Arch. Dermatol.* **91**, 326–334.

Hyperoxaluria

Primary hyperoxaluria is a rare genetic disorder of glyoxalate metabolism characterized by hyperoxaluria, recurrent calcium oxalate nephrolithiasis, chronic renal failure and early death from uraemia. Ungual oxalate granuloma has been reported (Sina & Lutz, 1990). Acrocyanosis and Raynaud's phenomenon, livedo reticularis, loss of distal pulses, peripheral gangrene and cutaneous calcifications of the digits have also been reported (Baethge *et al.*, 1988; Villada *et al.*, 1990).

References

Baethge B.A., Sanusi I.D., Landreneau M.D., Rohr M.S. & McDonald J.C. (1988) Livedo reticularis and peripheral gangrene associated with primary hyperoxaluria. *Arthr. Rheum.* **31**, 1199–1202.

Sina B. & Lutz L.L. (1990) Cutaneous oxalate granuloma. *J. Am. Acad. Dermatol.* **22**, 316–317.

Villada G., Bressieux J.M., Schillinger F. *et al.* (1990) Manifestations cutanées d'une oxalose par hyperoxalurie primitive. *Ann. Dermatol. Venereol.* **117**, 844–846.

Cystic fibrosis

Periungual telangiectasia and splinter haemorrhages can occur in cystic fibrosis (Zaias, 1990).

Reference

Zaias N. (1990) *The Nail in Health and Disease*, 2nd edn. Appleton & Lange, Norwalk, CN.

Hartnup disease

Nail 'streaks' have been described in Hartnup diseae (Daniel *et al.*, 1985).

Reference

Daniel C.R. Sams W.M. & Scher R.K. (1985) Nails in systemic disease. *Dermatol. Clin.* **3**, 465–483.

Histidinaemia

Pachyonychia, indistinct lunulae, onychoschizia and Beau's lines have been reported in a patient affected by histidinaemia (Pravatà *et al.*, 1987).

References

Pravatà G., Amato S. & Corrao A. (1987) Ipotricosi, onicopatia distrofica, anomalie dentarie in un caso di istidinemia. *G. Ital. Dermatol. Venereol.* **122**, 361–366.

Lipoid proteinosis (Urbach–Wiethe disease)

In patients with lipoid proteinosis nail growth can be arrested (Konstantinov *et al.*, 1992).

References

Konstantinov K., Kabakchiev P., Karchev T. *et al.* (1992) Lipoid proteinosis. *J. Am. Acad. Dermatol.* **27**, 293–297.

Dyslipoproteinaemias

Nail clippings from patients with type IV and V hyperlipoproteinaemia present significant amounts of Sudan IV positive substances. A relationship between the lipids found in the nail plate and the status of circulating triglycerides has been suggested (Salamon *et al.*, 1988).

Plane xanthomas on the tips of the fingers can occur in patients with type III and IV hyperlipoproteinaemia (Fine & Moschella, 1985). Extensive tuberous xanthomas on the fingers have been described in a patient with type III hyperlipoproteinaemia (Brewer & Fredrickson, 1987). Tendon xanthomas of extensor tendons of the fingers occur in cerebrotendinous xanthomatosis (Rodman, 1981), in sitosterolaemia and familial hypercholesterolaemia.

Periungual pseudo-Koenen's tumours of the second and the third toes have been reported in a patient affected by familial hypercholesterolaemia (Keller, 1960).

References

Brewer H.B. & Fredrickson D.S. (1987) Dyslipoproteinemias and xanthomatoses. In: *Dermatology in General Medicine*, eds Fitzpatrick T.B., Eisen A.Z., Wolff K., Freedberg I.M. & Austen K.F., pp. 1722–1738. McGraw Hill, New York.

Fine J.D. & Moschella S.L. (1985) Diseases of nutrition and metabolism. In: *Dermatology*, eds Moschella S.L. & Hurley H.J., pp. 1422–1532. W.B. Saunders, Philadelphia.

Keller P.H. (1960) Hypercholesterinamische xanthomatose. *Derm. Wschr.* **141**, 336.

Rodman O. (1981) The spectrum of cerebrotendinous xanthomatosis. *J. Assoc. Mil. Dermatol.* 7, 8–11.

Salamon T., Nikuln A., Grujic M. & Plavsic B. (1988) Sudan IV-positive material of the nail plate related to plasma triglycerides. *Dermatologica* **176**, 52–54.

Fabry's disease (Fig. 6.23)

Telangiectatic hyperkeratotic papules can be localized on the pulp of the fingernails and toenails. A 'turtle-back' configuration of the fingernails has been reported (Fine & Moschella, 1985), and a distal purpuric-like border has been observed in the fingernails of a patient with Fabry's disease (Carsuzaa *et al.*, 1985).

References

Carsuzaa F., Rommel A., Geniaux M., Texier L., Bobin P. & Surlève-Bazeille J.E. (1985) Maladie de Fabry. *Ann. Dermatol. Venereol.* **112**, 635–638.

Fine J.D. & Moschella S.L. (1985) Diseases of nutrition and metabolism. In: *Dermatology*, eds Moschella S.L. & Hurley H.J., pp. 1422–1532. W.B. Saunders, Philadelphia.

Gout

Tophi can occasionally have a periungual location and cause distortion of the nail apparatus (Fig. 6.24). Longitudinal striations, brittleness and crumbling of the nails have been described (Rail, 1969). These nail changes, which closely resemble nail psoriasis, can be of diagnostic importance in atypical joint diseases (Runne & Orfanos, 1981). Onychogryphosis has been reported as a common manifestation of hyperuricaemia occurring in 45–73% of hyperuricaemic patients (Harvàth & Vecék, 1986). In hereditary hyperuricaemia, the nails can show thickening, splitting and dystrophic changes (Gospos, 1976).

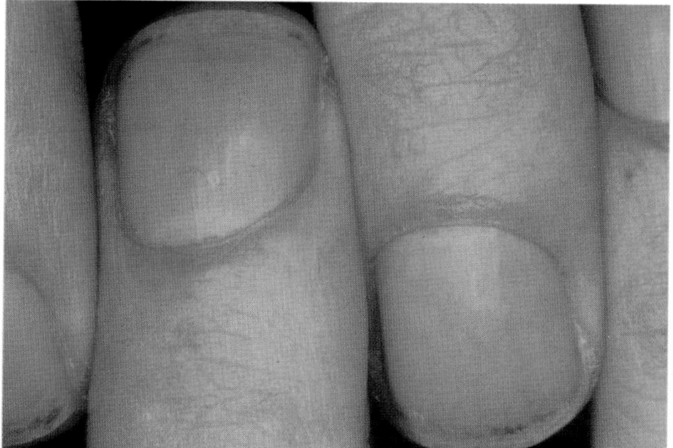

Fig. 6.23. Fabry's disease – subtle, purpuric border in the distal nail bed (courtesy L. Texier, Bordeaux, France).

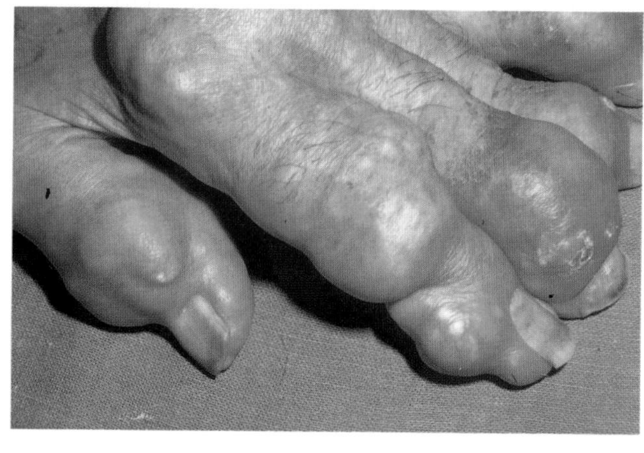

Fig. 6.24. Gout.

References

Gospos C. (1976) Gicht. Subacute periarticulare knotige hautgicht der endphalangen mit nageldystrophie. *Z. Haut.* **51**, 29

Harvàth G. & Vecék F. (1986) Uricaemia and onychogryphosis. *Cesk. Dermatol.* **61**, 388–390.

Rail G.A. (1969) Nail changes in gout. *Br. Med. J.* **ii**, 782–783.

Runne U. & Orfanos C.E. (1981) The human nail. *Curr. Prob. Dermatol.* **9**, 102–149.

Lesch–Nyhan syndrome

Lesch–Nyhan syndrome, an X-linked inborn error of metabolism, is characterized by hyperuricaemia, mental retardation, spastic cerebral palsy, choreoathetosis and compulsive self-biting of the lips, fingers and hands. The enzyme defect has been identified as a deficiency in hypoxanthine-guanine phosphoribosyl-transferase.

Alkaptonuria

Alkaptonuria is a rare autosomal recessive metabolic disorder caused by the deficiency of homogentisic acid oxidase. This leads to deposition of oxidized homogentisic acid pigment in connective tissues. The clinical manifestations of alkaptonuria include a distinctive skin pigmentation (ochronosis), arthritis and dark urine. Extensor tendons of the hands and finger nail beds can present a bluish-grey, bluish-black or brown pigmentation (Goldsmith, 1987).

Reference

Goldsmith L.A. (1987) Cutaneous changes in errors of aminoacid metabolism: alkaptonuria In: *Dermatology in General Medicine*, eds Fitzpatrick T., Eisen A.Z., Freedberg I.M. & Ansten K.F., pp. 1642–1646. McGraw Hill, New York.

Homocystinuria

Periungual telangiectasia can be observed in homocystinuria. Longitudinal ridging in the absence of nail fragility has also been reported (Baden & Zaias, 1987).

Reference

Baden H.P. & Zaias N. (1987) Nails. In: *Dermatology in General Medicine*, eds Fitzpatrick T., Eisen A.Z., Freeberg I.M. & Ansten K.F., pp. 651–666. McGraw Hill, New York.

Fucosidosis

Purple nail bands can be a feature of type III fucosidosis, an autosomal recessive metabolic disorder, which mimics Fabry's disease (Epinette *et al.*, 1983). The disease is caused by deficiency of the lysosomial enzyme α-L-fucosidase.

Reference

Epinette W.W., Norins A.L. & Drew A.L. (1973) Angiokeratoma corporis diffusum with alpha-L-fucosidase deficiency. *Arch. Dermatol.* 107, 754–757.

Porphyria

Increased levels of porphyrins in hair and fingernails have been detected in patients with porphyria cutanea tarda (Alberdi Y Jeronimo *et al.*, 1991). In congenital erythropoietic porphyria (Gunther's disease), severe mutilating deformities of the fingers result from repeated episodes of blistering. Photoonycholysis can also occur (Duterque *et al.*, 1983). In two patients with lateonset congenital erythropoietic porphyria, koilonychia preceded the onset of the skin manifestation (Deybach *et al.*, 1981). Red fluorescence of the nail plate with Wood's light has been described in erythropoietic porphyria (Daniel, 1985). Acute nail changes can occur during attacks of erythropoietic protoporphyria. Local pain, tenderness and sensation of fluid accumulation beneath the nail plate is followed by onycholysis that can result in loss of the fingernail (Schmitd *et al.*, 1974; Marsden & Dawber, 1977). Nail involvement can be a prominent symptom of the disease in black people (Bovenmyer, 1976). Total leuconychia and opaque blue-grey or brownish fingernails with absent lunulae have also been reported (Redeker & Bronow, 1964; Thivolet *et al.*, 1968).

Photoonycholysis is a possible manifestation of porphyria cutanea tarda (Figs 6.25 & 6.26), variegate porphyria and Bantu porphyria. It has also been reported in porphyria cutanea tarda-like syndrome of haemodialysis (Guillaud *et al.*, 1990). Digital and subungual bullae are observed. Nail discoloration due to a fungal or *Pseudomonas* infection can occur. Onycholysis was the presenting sign of contraceptive pill-induced porphyria cutanea tarda in a patient (Byrne *et al.*, 1976).

Yellow, black or brown discoloration of the nail, finger clubbing and loss of the lunula have been reported in porphyria cutanea tarda. Splinter haemorrhages, koilonychia and longitudinal pigmented bands or distal hemitorsion of the nail plate can also occur (Puissant *et al.*, 1971; Baran,

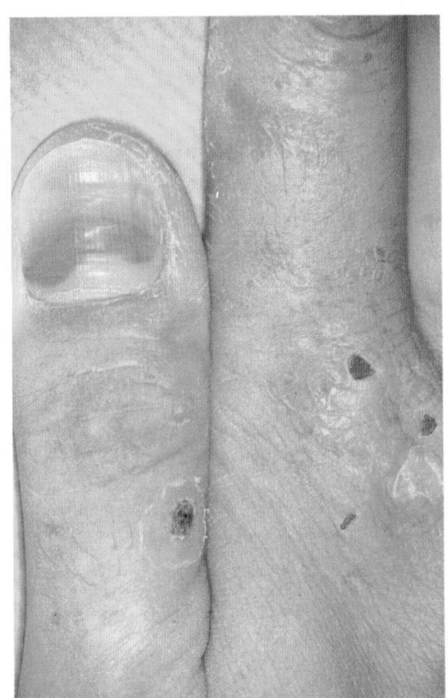

Fig. 6.25. Porphyria cutanea tarda – onycholysis and blistering.

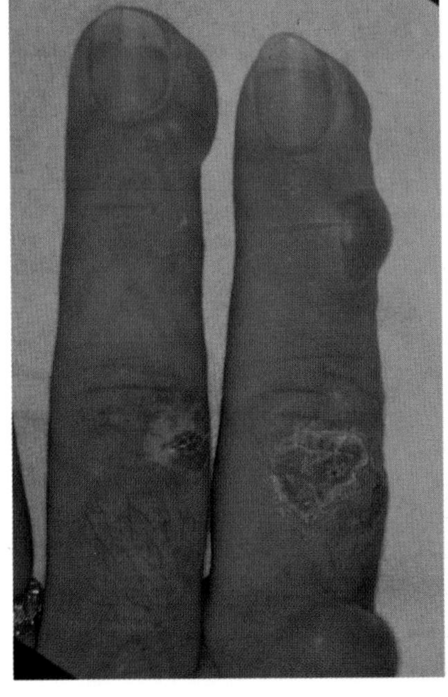

Fig. 6.26. Porphyria cutanea tarda – digital blistering.

1981; Pizzino *et al.*, 1988). Mutilating scarring deformities of fingers are seen in hepatoerythropoietic porphyria.

References

Alberdi Y., Jeronimo E., Stella A.M., Melito V. *et al.* (1991) Porfirinas en pelos y unas de pacientes con porfiria cutanea tardia en tratamiento con cloroquina y de ratas intoxicadas con hexachlorobenceno. *Rev. Arg. Dermatol.* 72, 70–79.

Baran R. (1981) The nail in dermatological disease. In: *The Nail*, ed. Pierre M., pp. 46–53. Churchill Livingstone, Edinburgh.

Bovenmyer D.A. (1976) Erythropoietic protoporphyria: first report of cases in the American Negro. *Cutis* **18**, 277–280.

Byrne J.P.H., Boss J.M. & Dawber R.P.R. (1976) Contraceptive pill-induced porphyria cutanea tarda presenting with onycholysis of the fingernails. *Postgrad. Med. J.* **52**, 535–538.

Daniel C.R. (1985) Nail pigmentation abnormalities. *Dermatol. Clin.* **3**, 431–443.

Deybach J.C., De Verneuil H., Phung N., Nordmann Y, Puissant A. & Boffety B. (1981) Congenital erythropoietic porphyria (Gunther's disease): enzymatic studies on two cases of late onset. *J. Lab. Clin. Med.* **97**, 551–558.

Duterque M., Civatte J., Jeaumougin M. & Nordmann Y. (1983) Porphyrie érythropoiétique de Gunther de revelation tardive. *Ann. Dermatol. Venereol.* **110**, 709–710.

Guilland V., Moulin G., Bonnefoy M., Cognat T., Balme B. & Barrut D. (1990) Photo-onycholyse bulleuse au cours d'une pseudoporphyrie des hémodialysés. *Ann. Dermatol. Venereol.* **117**, 723–725.

Marsden R.A. & Dawber R.P.R. (1977) Erythropoietic protoporphyria with onycholysis. *Proc. Roy. Soc. Med.* **70**, 572–574.

Pizzino D., De Padova M., Labanca M. & Varotti C. (1988) Patologia degli annessi cutanei nella porfiria cutanea tarda. *G. Ital. Dermatol. Venereol.* **123**, 607–608.

Puissant A., David V., Lachiver D. & Aitken G. (1971) Formes clinique atypiques de la porphyrie cutanée tardive. *Boll. Ist Derm. San Gallicano* 7, 19.

Redeker A.G. & Bronow R.S. (1964) Erythropoietic protoporphyria presenting as hydroa aestivale. *Arch. Dermatol.* **89**, 104–109.

Schmitd H., Snitker G., Thomsen K. & Lintrup J. (1974) Erythropoietic protoporphyria. *Arch. Dermatol.* **110**, 58–64.

Thivolet J., Freycon J., Perrot H., Guibaud P. & Beyvin A.J. (1968) Protoporphyrie érythropoiétique. *Bull. Soc. Fr. Dermatol. Syphil.* 75, 829–841.

Amyloidosis (Figs 6.27–6.31)

Dystrophic nail changes are a possible early manifestation both of primary and myeloma-associated systemic amyloidosis (Breathnach & Black, 1979; Breathnach *et al.*, 1979; Wheeler & Barrows, 1981; Blanc *et al.*, 1982). Nail abnormalities can closely mimic nail lichen planus. The nails appear uniformly thinned, brittle, longitudinally ridged and distally split (Fig. 6.27) (Fanti *et al.*, 1991). Nail flattening, cracking, crumbling and even partial or complete anonychia can occur (Jones *et al.*, 1972; Breathnach, 1988). Narrow pink longitudinal subungual striations as well as splinter haemorrhages have occasionally been reported (Desirello *et al.*, 1988). Yellow discoloration

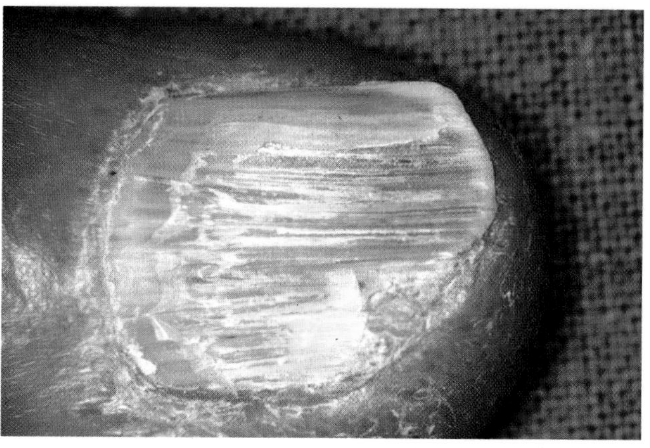

Fig. 6.27. Systemic amyloidosis – longitudinal ridging and brittleness.

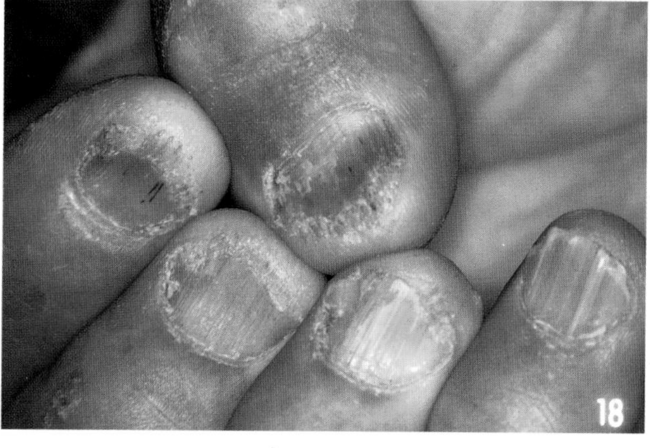

Fig. 6.28. Systemic amyloidosis – atrophic nail changes.

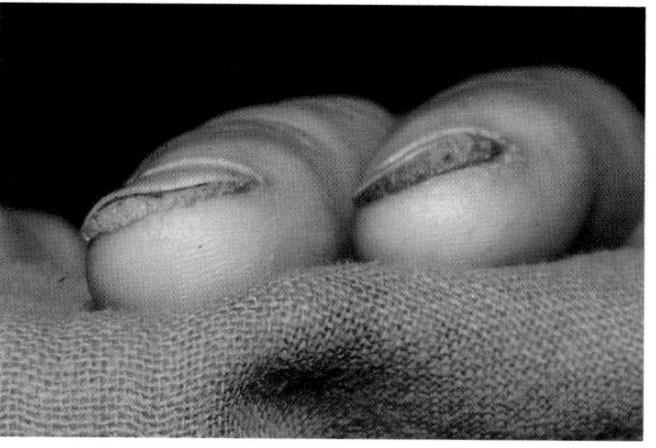

Fig. 6.29. Systemic amyloidosis – subungual papillomatous thickening.

of the nail plate, subungual papillomatosis (Fig. 6.29) and onycholysis have also been described. Scleroderma-like diffuse infiltration of the hands and fingertip ulcerations can occur (Brownstein & Helwig, 1970). At nail biopsy typical amyloid deposits are detectable (Figs 6.30 & 6.31)

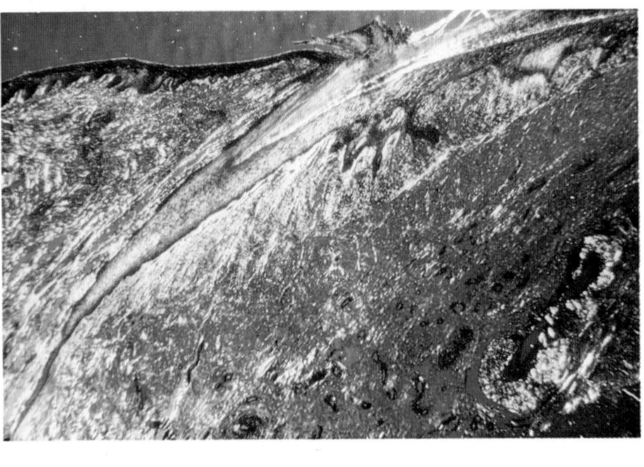
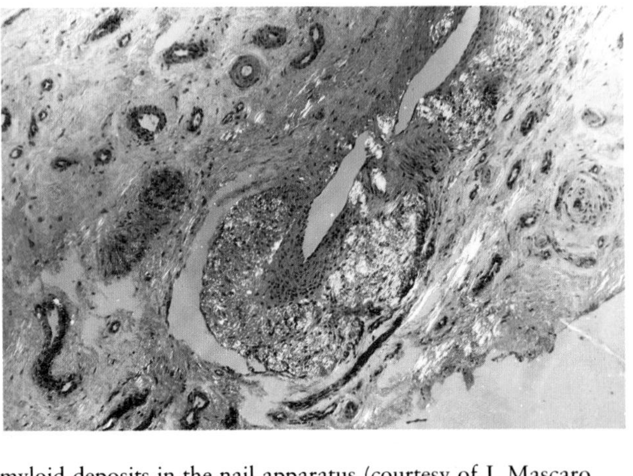

Figs 6.30 & 6.31. Systemic amyloidosis – stain to show perivascular amyloid deposits in the nail apparatus (courtesy of J. Mascaro, Barcelona, Spain).

in the superficial dermis and around blood vessels (Pineda *et al.*, 1988; Fanti *et al.*, 1991). Chronic ulcerations of distal extremities due to neuropathic changes can be observed in heredofamilial amyloid polyneuropathy (Brownstein & Helwig, 1970). Smooth, thickened yellow toenails and black nail beds have also been described (Lithner, 1976).

Shaw *et al.* (1983) described a case of macular cutaneous amyloidosis with autosomal dominant nail changes consisting of marked thickening and yellow discoloration. These nail changes resolved during the third and fourth decades of life.

References

Blanc D., Kienzler J.L., Faivre R. *et al.* (1982) Amylose systématisée primitive avec alopécie et onychodystrophie généralisées. *Ann. Dermatol. Venereol.* **109**, 877–880.

Breathnach S.M. (1988) Amyloid and amyloidosis. *J. Am. Acad. Dermatol.* **18**, 1–16.

Breathnach S.M. & Black M.M. (1979) Systemic amyloidosis and the skin: a review with special emphasis on clinical features and therapy. *Clin. Exp. Dermatol.* **4**, 517–536.

Breathnach S.M., Wilkinson J.D. & Black M.M. (1979) Systemic amyloidosis with underlying lymphoproliferative disorder. Report of a case in which nail involvement was a presenting feature. *Clin. Exp. Dermatol.* **4**, 495–599.

Brownstein M.H. & Helwig E.B. (1970) The cutaneous amyloidosis. *Arch. Dermatol.* **102**, 20–28.

Desirello G., Nazzari G., Stradini D., Fusco F. & Crovato F. (1988) Amiloidosi primaria. *G. Ital. Dermatol. Venereol.* **123**, 99–101.

Fanti P.A., Tosti A., Morelli R. & Galbiati G. (1991) Nail changes as the first sign of systemic amyloidosis. *Dermatologica* **183**, 44–46.

Jones N.F., Hilton P.J., Tighe J.R. & Hobbs J.R. (1972) Treatment of 'primary' renal amyloidosis with melphalan. *Lancet* **ii**, 616–619.

Lithner L. (1976) Skin lesions of the legs and feet and skeletal lesions of the feet in familial amyloidosis with polyneuropathy. *Acta Med. Scand.* **199**, 197–202.

Pineda M.S., Herrero C., Palou J., Vilalta A. & Mascarò J.M. (1988) Nail alterations in systemic amyloidosis: report of one case, with histologic study *J. Am. Acad. Dermatol.* **18**, 1357–1359.

Shaw M., Jurecka W., Beack M.M. & Kurwa A.R. (1983) Macular amyloidosis associated with familial nail dystrophy. *Clin. Exp. Dermatol.* **2**, 363–368.

Wheeler G.E. & Barrows G.H. (1981) Alopecia universalis. A manifestation of occult amyloidosis and multiple myeloma. *Arch. Dermatol.* **117**, 815–816.

Nervous disorders

Hauser (1983) believes that localization of nail diseases only to certain nails may be caused by visceral-cutaneous reflexes that produce alterations in the terminal vascular system.

Reference

Hauser W. (1983) Zur lokalization und pathogenese von nagelkrankugen. *Akt. Dermatol.* **9**, 70–74.

Hereditary

Thick, hard nails with onychogryphosis occur in Morgagni–Stewart–Morel syndrome (Kup, 1958). Onychomadesis is seen in Bogaert–Scherer–Epstein syndrome (cerebrotendinous xanthomatosis) and nail plate disorders are a feature of Divry–Van Bogaert syndrome (meningeal angiomatosis). Polydactyly and polyonychia occur as part of the Lawrence–Moon–Bield syndrome. Self-mutilation occurs in the Lesh–Nyhan syndrome.

Reference

Kup J. (1958) Beiträge zu dem hypothalamischen Zentralregulie rung sorgan des Nagelsystems. *Zentralb. Allg. Pathol. Anat.* **98**, 290–293.

Phacomatoses

Supernumerary digits and congenital enlargement of limbs or digits can occur in neurofibromatosis (Chao, 1961). Plexiform neurofibroma can produce hypertrophic fingers or toes with dislocation of the nails. Macrodactyly of the foot associated with plexiform neurofibroma of the digital branches of the medial plantar nerve was the sole manifestation of von Recklinghausen's neurofibromatosis in one patient (Turra *et al.*, 1986). A patient with pterygium inversum unguis-like changes has also been reported (Patterson, 1977).

Periungual fibromas (Koenen's tumours) are a pathognomonic sign of tuberous sclerosis (see Chapter 11). They occur in approximately 50% of patients and are usually noticed after puberty but continue to develop with age. They appear as pedunculated, smooth, firm, flesh-coloured, pointed, grain-shaped growths that originate in the periungual groove and usually extend outward over the nail plate. The nail plate frequently shows longitudinal ridging and grooving resulting from pressure on the matrix. Partial or complete atrophy of the nail plate can also occur. Pachyonychia may be observed in toenails. Cuticular hyperkeratosis, which may indicate a subclinical Koenen tumour, has been observed in some cases (Colomb *et al.*, 1976). Nail plate abnormalities can also occasionally be seen in digits without a Koenen tumour. Histologically, Koenen's tumours can be considered fibrokeratomas that originate from the proximal nail fold or the surrounding connective tissue (Kint & Baran, 1988). Extensive subungual fibromas that disrupt the entire nail bed have been reported (Nickel & Reed, 1962). Cyst-like lesions and periosteal thickening of the phalanges are frequently observed. Macrodactyly can also occur.

References

Chao D.H.C. (1961) Congenital neurocutaneous syndromes in childhood. *J. Pediatr.* 189–199.

Colomb D., Racouchot J. & Jeunne R. (1976) Les lésions des ongles dans la sclérose tubéreuse de Bourneville isolées ou associées aux tumeurs de Koenen. *Ann. Dermatol. Venereol.* **103**, 431–437.

Kint A. & Baran R. (1988) Histopathologic study of Koenen tumours. *J. Am. Acad. Dermatol.* **18**, 369–372.

Nickel W.R. & Reed W.B. (1962) Tuberous sclerosis. *Arch. Dermatol.* **85**, 209–226.

Patterson J.W. (1977) Pterygium inversum unguis-like changes in scleroderma. *Arch. Dermatol.* **113**, 1429–1430.

Turra S., Frizziero P., Cagnoni G. & Jacopetti T. (1986) Macrodactyly of the foot associated with plexiform neurofibroma of the medial plantar nerve. *J. Pediatr. Orthop.* **6**, 489–492.

Syringomyelia

Segmental loss of pain and temperature sensation in the hands and arms is the principal clinical feature of syringomyelia. Thickening and callosities of the skin on the fingers and knuckles result from repeated minor trauma. Swelling and oedema of the hands are frequent. Macrodactyly of either or both the index and medium fingers can be present (Ambrosetto, 1965). Nails can be deformed and present a reduced growth rate. Longitudinal striations can occur. Painless ulceration of the fingers, painless ulceration and crusting of periungual tissue resembling chronic paronychia as well as painless whitlows are commonly observed (Adams, 1987). Resorption or spontaneous amputation of the terminal phalanges can also occur (Tosti *et al.*, 1994). Asymmetric anonychia has been reported in one patient (Leopold & Wassilew, 1988) (Fig. 6.32). Many of these changes correspond to the syndrome of Morvan, in which an analgesic whitlow with dermal changes of these types affect the upper extremities.

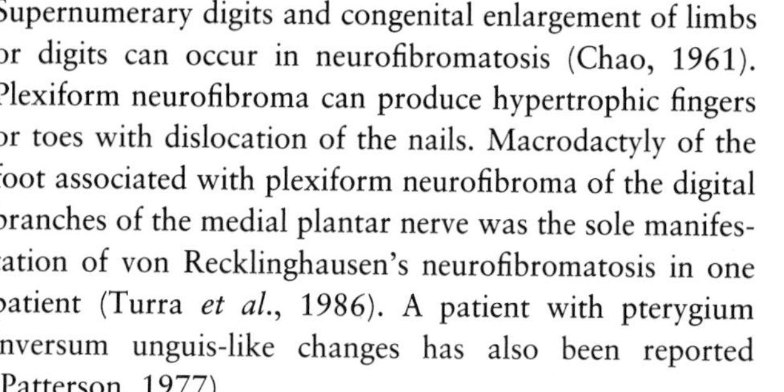

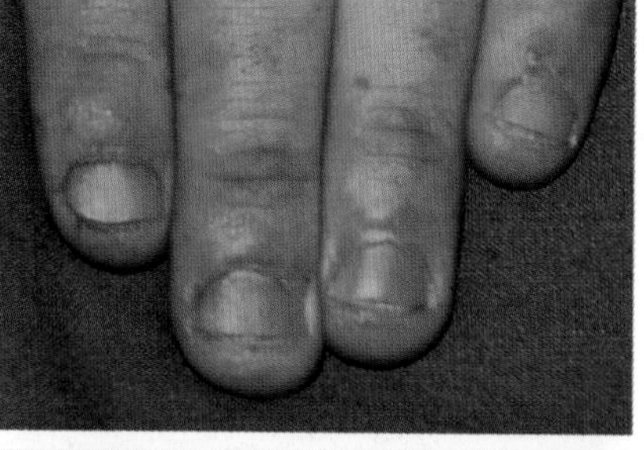

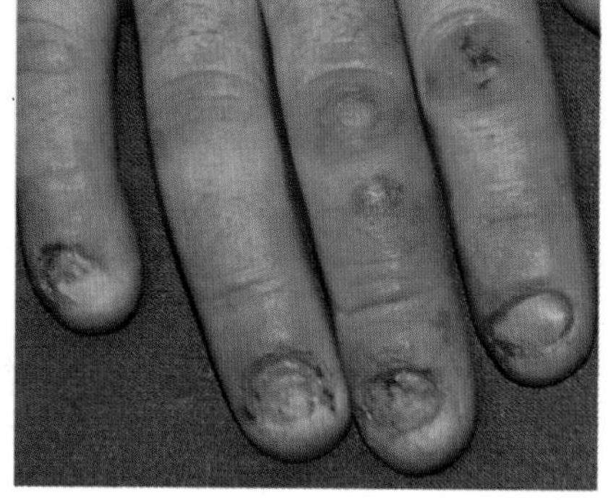

Fig. 6.32. Unilateral syringomyelia showing affected digits on the bottom.

Differential diagnosis includes leprosy and hereditary sensory neuropathy.

References

Adams R.D. (1987) Neurocutaneous diseases. In: *Dermatology in General Medicine*, eds Fitzpatrick T.B., Eisen A.Z., Wolff K., Freedberg J.N. & Austen F.D., p. 2053. McGraw Hill, New York.

Ambrosetto C. (1965) La patologia della mano in neurologia, II parte. *Relazioni. Clin. Sci.* **90**, XVII, 10–17.

Leopold A. & Wassilew S.W. (1988) Cutaneous changes in syringomyelia. *Z. Hautkr.* **6**, 494–496.

Tosti A., Peluso A.M., Morelli R. *et al.* (1994) Cutaneous amputation of the terminal phalanges in syringomyelia. *Dermatology* (in press).

Hemiplegia

The nail growth rate is retarded on the affected side in hemiplegia. Overcurvature and narrowing of the nails have been reported (Lewis & Pickering, 1935). Longitudinal and transverse striations or onychomadesis can occur. Unilateral pterygium inversum unguis involving the right fingers and toes has been described in a patient affected by a paresis of the entire right side after a cerebrovascular accident. Mild subungual hyperkeratosis was also present (Morimoto & Gurevitch, 1988). Neapolitan nails only occurred unilaterally on the hemiparetic side in some patients who previously had had strokes (Horan *et al.*, 1982). A patient with a longstanding history of psoriasis developed progressive nail changes consisting of subungual hyperkeratosis and accelerated nail growth confined to his left hand 2 years after a mild left side hemiparesis due to a cerebrovascular event (Badger *et al.*, 1992).

References

Badger J., Banerjle A.K. & McFadden J. (1992) Unilateral subungual hyperkeratosis following a cerebrovascular incident in a patient with psoriasis. *Clin. Exp. Dermatol.* **17**, 454–455.

Horan M.A., Puxty J.A. & Fox R.A. (1982) The white nails of old age (Neapolitan nails). *J. Am. Geriatr. Soc.* **30**, 734–737.

Lewis T. & Pickering G.W. (1935) Circulatory changes in the fingers in some diseases of the nervous system, with special reference to the digital atrophy of peripheral nerve lesions. *Clin. Sci.* **2**, 149–183.

Morimoto S.S. & Gurevitch A.W. (1988) Unilateral pterygium inversum unguis. *Int. J. Dermatol.* **27**, 491–494.

Spinal cord injuries

Ingrowing toenails, which usually occur after the initial period of bed rest, are very common in patients with a spinal cord injury. Tetraplegics appear to be more frequently affected than paraplegics. Nail brittleness, atrophic skin changes and toe flexor spasms have been considered the main predisposing factors in the development of ingrowing toenails in patients with spinal injuries (Jaffray & El Masri, 1985).

Progressive self-biting of the fingers and hands resulting in multiple finger amputations has been described in two patients following C4 complete spinal cord injury. Stress, isolation and loss of sensation were responsible for this self-abusive behaviour (Dahlin *et al.*, 1985). Acroosteolysis of the fingers as the result of self-mutilation has been observed in a quadriplegic patient after a spinal cord injury at the C5–C6 level (Marmolya *et al.*, 1989).

References

Dahlin P.A., Van Buskirk N.E., Novotny R.W., Hollis I.R. & George J. (1985) Self-biting with multiple finger amputations following spinal cord injury. *Paraplegia* **23**, 306–318.

Jaffray D. & El Masri W. (1985) Ingrowing toenails and tetraplegia. *Paraplegia* **23**, 176–181.

Marmolya G., Yagan R. & Freehafer A. (1989) Acro-osteolysis of the fingers in a spinal cord injury patient. *Spine* **14**, 137–139.

Congenital insensitivity to pain syndrome

This is another syndrome in which self-mutilative acts occur. This rare syndrome is present at birth, but destructive lesions of the skin, nails and mouth do not appear until the teeth have erupted (Thompson *et al.*, 1980). Chewing of nails leads to nail thickening, loss and deformity. Lack of pain sensation can result in severe finger mutilation. Compulsive self-biting of the lips, fingers and hands in the absence of sensory deficits is a typical symptom of Lesch–Nyhan syndrome. X-ray studies of the fingers may show partial resorption of the terminal phal-anges (Ozbarlas *et al.*, 1993).

References

Ozbarlas N., Sarikayalar F. & Kale G. (1993) Congenital insensitivity to pain with anhidrosis. *Cutis* **51**, 373–374.

Thompson C.C., Park R.I. & Prescott G.H. (1980) Oral manifestations of the congenital insensitivity-to-pain syndrome. *Oral. Surg. Oral. Med. Oral. Pathol.* **50**, 220–225.

Peripheral neuropathies

Congenital and acquired sensory neuropathies that produce analgesia are frequently associated with recurrent painless acral skin ulcers. Spontaneous amputation of the digits can occasionally occur.

In Bureau–Barriere's non-familial mutilant ulcer acropathy (Fig. 6.33) annular constriction (pseudo-ainhum) leading to spontaneous loss of fingers is one of the most frequent symptoms (Torres Cortijo, 1973, 1982; Eichorn

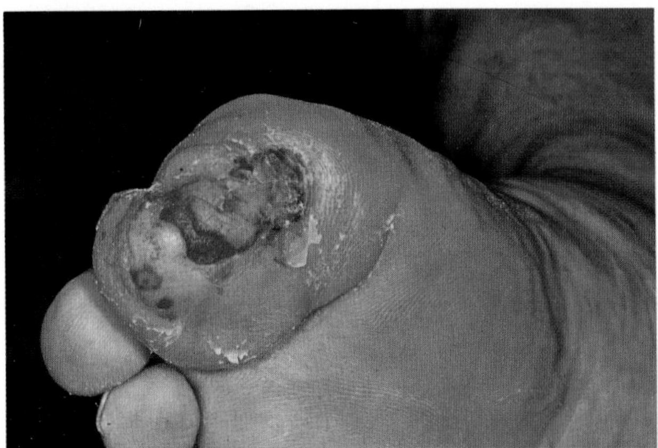

Fig. 6.33. Mutilating (non-familial) ulcerated acropathy (Bureau-Barriere).

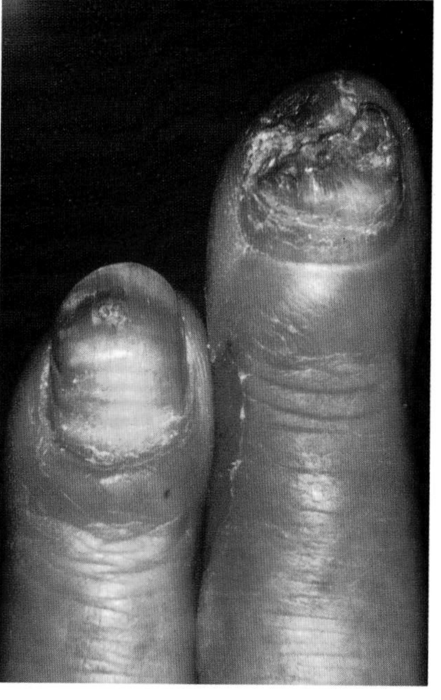

Fig. 6.34. Carpal tunnel syndrome nail dystrophy.

& Schauder, 1989). In leprosy neurological involvement can produce severe dystrophic changes and acroosteolysis of the fingers (De Las Agnas, 1973).

In cervical rib syndrome, compression of subclavian vessels and brachial plexus can produce cutaneous changes of the affected limb. Deficient vascular supply can cause fingertip ulceration, cyanosis and gangrene. Nail grooving, pachyonychia and onycholysis can also be present. Thinning, discoloration, ridging and shortening of the nails have been reported in the absence of peripheral ischaemia symptoms (Rubin & Cipollaro, 1939). In Volkmann syndrome, thinning and tapering of the fingers as well as overcurvature of the nails can occur (Ambrosetto, 1965).

In carpal tunnel syndrome, either or both index and medium fingers can present torpid ulcerations of both the fingertip and subungual regions as well as dystrophic nail changes (Fig. 6.34). Gangrene, spontaneous amputation and acral osteolysis of the terminal phalanges have been described seldom (Bouvier *et al.*, 1979; Treves *et al.*, 1980; Adoue *et al.*, 1984; Geffray *et al.*, 1984; Tosti *et al.*, 1993). In a case of carpal tunnel syndrome, the skin changes included anhydrosis, alopecia, nail dystrophy and episodes of acute necrosis. The nail alterations involved the left third finger that presented a longitudinal black streak in the nail plate along with hyperkeratotic cuticles and transverse grooving. Moreover, the same finger presented an escharotic bulla on the dorsal aspect of the distal phalanx (Aratari *et al.*, 1984). A 70-year-old man affected by squamous cell carcinoma developed carpal tunnel syndrome and acrokeratosis paraneoplastica of Bazex. Both conditions improved after treatment of the tumour. This suggests that carpal tunnel syndrome was a paraneoplastic phenomenon (Poskitt & Duffie, 1992).

Koilonychia limited to the second and third fingernails of both hands has also been reported; nail changes completely regressed after surgical treatment (Beurey *et al.*, 1984).

Retarded growth of the fingernails usually follows damage to median or ulnar nerves. However, increased nail growth has also been reported after median nerve injuries (Ambrosetto, 1965). Fingerpads become atrophic and nails can appear narrowed and clawlike. The bones of the affected fingers become rarefied and in longstanding cases can decrease in size (Lewis & Pickering, 1935). Continued immobility without change in the nervous system can produce similar nail changes. Unidigital clubbing has been described with trauma to the digit or median nerve (Stoll & Beetham, 1954).

Marked nail changes following median nerve injury have been reported (Ross & Ward, 1987). A bilateral ulnar neuropathy produced shortening, fragility and yellow discoloration of the nails on the ring and little finger of both hands in a diabetic patient affected by mononeuritis multiplex (Mann & Burton, 1982). Onycholysis occurred after collateral palmar nerve injury (Waintraub *et al.*, 1937). Symptomatic pterygium inversum unguis has been associated with lesions of the peripheral nerves in the fingers and toes (Runne & Orfanos, 1981). Three patients developed onychomadesis and focal haemorrhages at multiple proximal nail folds after major peripheral or major peripheral and central neurologic deficits (Baran & Goettmann, 1993).

In POEMS syndrome (Crow–Fukase syndrome) the acronym indicates the association of polyneuropathy with organomegaly, endocrinopathy, M proteins and skin changes. The skin changes of POEMS syndrome include hyperpigmentation, hypertrichosis, haemangioma and skin thickening that resembles scleroderma. Clubbing of the fingers occurs in 44% of cases. Apparent leuconychia (Terry's nails) (Fig. 6.35), acrocyanosis and Raynaud's phenomenon have also been reported (Tang *et al.*, 1983;

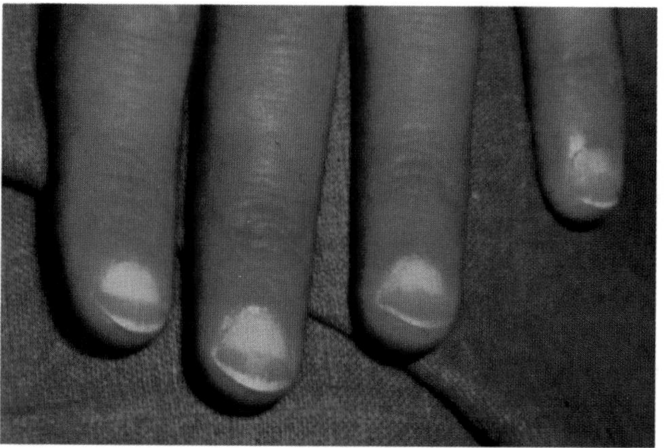

Fig. 6.35. POEMS syndrome – white nails (courtesy of J.J. Gilhou, Montpellier, France).

Shelley & Shelley, 1987; Dereure *et al.*, 1990). This multisystem disease is generally associated with a plasmacytoma or with an osteosclerotic myeloma.

Arnold (1979) described sympathetic leuconychia in nails adjacent and controlateral to an injured nail.

References

Adoue D., Arlet P., Giraud P., Giraud M., Bories P. & Bonafé J.L. (1984) Syndrome du canal carpien avec ulcérations digitales chez un insuffisant rénal en hémodialyse périodique. *Ann. Dermatol. Venereol.* **111**, 1019–1021.

Ambrosetto C. (1965) La patologia della mano in neurologia, II parte. *Relazioni Clin. Sci.* **90**, XVII, 10–17.

Aratari E., Regesta G. & Rebora A. (1984) Carpal tunnel syndrome appearing with prominent skin symptoms. *Arch. Dermatol.* **120**, 517–519.

Arnold H.L. (1979) Sympathetic symmetric punctate leuconychia. *Arch. Dermatol.* **115**, 495–496.

Baran R. & Goettmann S. (1993) Nail bleeding in neurological deficits. *Dermatology* **187**, 197–199.

Beurey J., Weber M., Barthelme D., Eich D. & Schmutz J.L. (1984) Koilonychie et syndrome du canal carpien. *Ann. Dermatol. Venereol.* **111**, 49–52.

Bouvier M., Lejeune E., Rouillat M. & Marionnet J. (1979) Les formes ulcéro-mutilantes du syndrome du canal carpien. *Rev. Rhum.* **46**, 169–176.

De Las Agnas J.T. (1973) Lecciones de Leprologia, Fontille, Spain, p. 251.

Dereure O., Guillot B., Dandurand M. *et al.* (1990) Les signes cutanés du syndrome POEMS. A propos de 3 observations et revue de la littérature. *Ann. Dermatol. Venereol.* **117**, 283–290.

Eichhorn K. & Schauder S. (1989) Nicht familiare Akroosteopathia ulcero-mutilans der Fuße. *Hautarzt* **40**, 316–318.

Geffray L., Leman C., Dehais J. & David-Chaussé J. (1984) Deux cas de syndrome du canal carpien avec ulcérations digitales et acroostéolyse. *Rev. Rhum.* **51**, 45–47.

Lewis T. & Pickering G.W. (1935) Circulatory changes in the fingers in some diseases of the nervous system, with special reference to the digital atrophy of peripheral nerve lesions. *Clin. Sci.* **2**, 149–183.

Mann R.J. & Burton J.L. (1982) Nail dystrophy due to diabetic neuropathy. *Br. Med. J.* **284**, 1445.

Poskitt B.L. & Duffie M.B. (1992) Acrokeratosis paraneoplastica of Basex presenting with carpal tunnel syndrome. *Br. J. Dermatol.* **127**, 544–545.

Ross J.K. & Ward C.M. (1987) An abnormality of nail growth associated with median nerve damage. *J. Hand Surg. Br.* **12**, 11–13.

Rubin L.C. & Cipollaro A.C. (1939) Onychodystrophy caused by cervical rib. *Arch. Dermatol.* **39**, 430–433.

Runne U. & Orfanos C.E. (1981) The human nail. *Curr. Prob. Dermatol.* **9**, 102–149.

Shelley W.B. & Shelley E.D. (1987) The skin changes in the Crow–Fukase (POEMS) syndrome. *Arch. Dermatol.* **123**, 85–87.

Stoll B.A. & Beetham W.R. (1954) Unidigital clubbing with report of a case. *Med. J. Aust.* **825**, 5.

Tang L.M., Hsi M.S., Ryu S.J. & Minauchi Y. (1983) Syndrome of polyneuropathy, skin hyperpigmentation, oedema and hepatosplenomegaly. *J. Neurol. Neurosurg. Psychiat.* **46**, 1108–1114.

Torres Cortijo A. (1973) Constricturas anulares ainhum y seudoainhum *Med. Cut.* **2**, 95–102.

Torres Cortijo A.V. (1982) Annular constriction (pseudo-ainhum) as first symptom of Bureau–Barriere's mutilant ulcer acropathy. Case presentation, *XVI Congressus Internat. Dermatol.*, Tokyo, pp. 58–59.

Tosti A., Morelli R., D'Alessandro R. & Bassi F. (1993) Carpal tunnel syndrome presenting with ischemic skin lesions, acroosteolysis and nail changes. *J. Am. Acad. Dermatol.* **29**, 287–290.

Treves R., Arnaud J.P., Benabbou M. & Desproges-Gotteron R. (1980) Ulcerations digitales an cours d'un syndrome du canal carpien avec Syndrome de Raynaud. *Rev. Rhum.* **47**, 578–579.

Waintraub L.C., Charaf E. & Laudan M. (1937) Un cas de troubles trophique unguéal d'origine traumatique. *Rev. Fr. Dermatol. Venereol.* **13**, 14–16.

Causalgia

Causalgia is characterized by a burning pain that makes manicuring intolerable. Convexity and ridging of the nails can be observed. Unilateral clubbing of the fingers has been reported in a patient affected by causalgic syndrome that occurred after a closed injury to the right forearm (Saunders & Hanna, 1988).

Reference

Saunders P.R. & Hanna M. (1988) Unilateral clubbing of fingers associated with causalgia. *Br. Med. J.* **297**, 1635.

Reflex sympathetic dystrophy (algodystrophy)

In this condition painful inflammatory changes of the extremities are followed by joint dystrophy and cutaneous involvement. Scleroatrophy of the skin that is commonly associated with nail brittleness can be a permanent consequence of the condition. The pathogenesis of algodystrophy is possibly related to microcirculation troubles secondary to abnormal excitation and stimulation of the sympathetic fibres. Predisposing causes include nervous system, cardiac, respiratory and metabolic diseases, drugs, as well as traumatic, infective and vascular disorders of the limbs (Cony & Gerniaux, 1990). Two cases of sympathetic dystrophy after a fingernail biopsy have been reported (Ingram *et al.*, 1987; Haneke, 1992). We observed a patient whose reflex sympathetic dystrophy appeared with acute inflammatory nail changes that resembled bacterial whitlows (Tosti *et al.*, 1993).

References

Cony M. & Gerniaux M. (1990) Signes cutanés de l'algodystrophie. *Rev. Eur. Dermatol. MST* **2**, 281–288.

Haneke E. (1992) Sympathische Reflexdystrophie (Sudeck-Dystrophie) nach Nagelbiopsie. *Zbl. Haut. Geschl. Kr.* **160**, 263.
Ingram G.J., Scher R.K. & Lally E.V. (1987) Reflex sympathetic dystrophy following nail biopsy. *J. Am. Acad. Dermatol.* **16**, 253–256.
Tosti A., Baran R., Peluso A.M. *et al.* (1993) Reflex sympathetic dystrophy with prominent involvement of the nail apparatus. *J. Am. Acad. Dermatol.* **29**, 865–868.

Other central nervous system disorders

The paralysed limbs of patients with anterior poliomyelitis can exhibit toes or fingers that are considerably diminished in size and have retarded nail growth (Lewis & Pickering, 1935). Hyponychial haemorrhages, horizontal ridging, onycholysis and onychomadesis have also been described.

Multiple sclerosis can produce longitudinal striations.

An increased nail growth rate as well as hyponychial haemorrhages have been reported in Parkinson's disease. Onycholysis and onychomadesis have been described in tabes dorsalis; the latter also occurs in patients with rabies encephalomyelitis and epilepsy. Beau's lines may follow a severe epileptic convulsion.

Multiple paronychia has been recorded in epidemic encephalitis (Schirmer, 1924).

References

Lewis T. & Pickering G.W. (1935) Circulatory changes in the fingers in some diseases of the nervous system, with special reference to the digital atrophy of peripheral nerve lesions. *Clin. Sci.* **2**, 149–183.
Schirmer O. (1924) Ueber trophische Nagelveranderungen (multiple Panaritien) bie einem Fall von encephalitis epidemica. *Schwerz. Med. Wod.* **54**, 984–985.

Psychological and psychiatric disorders

Nail biting is an extremely common habit in childhood and affects up to 60% of children. The reported occurrence in teenagers is 45% (Odenrick & Brattstrom, 1985), but the incidence in adulthood is much less.

Whether nail biting in adults should be categorized as a psychological or psychiatric disease-associated sign is controversial. Although nail biting has been associated with sociopathy, anxious and obsessional symptoms, as well as aggressive needs, no evidence indicates a direct relationship between this habit and an underlying mental disorder. The patterns of nail biting vary among patients and may involve one, many or all nails (Singer & Gibson, 1988).

Nail biting, which makes nails short and irregular, frequently induces secondary bacterial infections of periungual tissues. Longitudinal melanonychia due to matrix melanocyte stimulation can be a further consequence of this habit (Baran, 1990). Picking, breaking or chewing of the skin over the posterior nail fold is frequently associated with nail biting. The terms perionychophagia and perionychomania have been coined for describing this autodestructive habit. According to Hirsch (1991) the symptom is not only a tension reducing measure but a protosymbolically created surrogate of the early mother–child unit in which skin, hand and mouth play a dominant role.

Periungual warts commonly afflict nail biters. Apical root resorption (Odenrick & Brattstrom, 1985) or nail pterygium are uncommon complications of this habit. Osteomyelitis has also been reported as a complication of nail biting (Waldman & Frieden, 1990; Tosti *et al.*, 1993).

When nail biting persists in adult life it is usually severe and associated with a poor prognosis.

Self-induced trauma to the nails commonly causes nail deformities. The tic habit of grinding or horizontally stroking the edge of the second or third nail plate across both or either the proximal thumb nail plate and nail fold produces the characteristic deformity of multiple transverse lines associated with central nail depression on the thumbnails (Samman, 1963). Although onychotillomania is usually a sign of an underlying psychological or psychiatric illness, self-induced nail changes are occasionally claimed to be due to occupational exposure (Norton, 1987). Compulsive rubbing, picking or tearing of the nails can result in their gradual destruction or mutilation (Sait & Garg, 1985). Instruments such as scissors, knives, pliers and razor blades have been used by patients for causing self-inflicted damage (Colver, 1987).

The clinical presentation of onychotillomania can mimic other nail disorders or have bizarre features. Preservation of the nail folds is usual. Self-inflicted onycholysis, splinter haemorrhages and subungual haematoma can be confused with other more common nail diseases. Traumatic picking or cutting of the corners of the nail plate can lead to ingrown toenails or fingernails. Nail plate depressions, scratches and even hollows may result from gouging nails with an instrument. Nail pterygium is the result of severe destruction and scarring. Picking and tearing of the exposed nail bed can follow nail plate destruction with pustular infection of the nail bed and proximal nail fold and produce nail bed destruction (Corraze, 1965).

Although most patients deny manipulating their own nails, some patients do admit their habit but give an unreliable explanation for it. Parasitophobia has been reported in some patients (Sait & Garg, 1985; Colver, 1987). Treatment of the underlying psychological disorders and occlusive dressings should be performed in order to prevent irreversible changes.

A double-edged nail can be observed in patients with psychoses (Daniel *et al.*, 1985). An acute psychotic episode may be accompanied by broad white banding in the nails (Pfeiffer & Jenney, 1974).

The subpapillary plexus of the proximal nail fold is clearly visible and extensive in many schizophrenic patients. A significant correlation has been reported between the visibility of the subpapillary plexus and the family history, duration and severity of schizophrenia. Patients with nail fold changes frequently present glossy, smooth, thin-looking skin on the terminal phalanges. Capillary haemorrhages as well as long and straight sweat ducts in the nail fold area have also been commonly detected (Maricq, 1969).

Transverse leuconychia has been described in patients with manic depressive illness. Brittle hair and nails are frequently observed in anorexia nervosa. They may be due to the hypothyroid state that results from starvation. Finger clubbing associated with laxative abuse has also been reported (Gupta *et al.*, 1987).

References

Baran R. (1990) Nail biting and picking as a possible cause of longitudinal melanonychia. *Dermatologica* **181**, 126–128.

Colver G.B. (1987) Onychotillomania. *Br. J. Dermatol.* **117**, 397–402.

Corraze M.J. (1965) Un cas de pathomimie inhabituel: périonyxis pustuleux. *Bull. Soc. Fr. Dermatol.* **72**, 191–192.

Daniel R.C., Sams W.M. & Scher R.K. (1985) Nails in systemic disease. *Dermatol. Clin.* **3**, 465–483.

Gupta M.A., Gupta A.K. & Haberman H.F. (1987) Dermatologic signs in anorexia nervosa and bulimia nervosa. *Arch. Dermatol.* **123**, 1386–1390.

Hirsch M. (1991) Perionychomanie und perionychophagie oder habituelles nagelbettreiben. *Forum Psychoanal.* **7**, 127–135.

Maricq H.R. (1969) Association of a clearly visible subpapillary plexus with other peculiarities of the nailfold skin in some schizophrenic patients. *Dermatologica* **138**, 148–154.

Norton L.A. (1987) Self induced trauma to the nails. *Cutis* **40**, 223–227.

Odenrick L. & Brattstrom V. (1985) Nailbiting: frequency and association with root resorption during orthodontic treatment. *Br. J. Orthod.* **12**, 78–81.

Pfeiffer C.C. & Jenney E.H. (1974) Fingernail white spots: possible zinc deficiency. *J. Am. Med. Assoc.* **228**, 157.

Sait M.A. & Garg R.B.R. (1985) Onychotillomania. *Dermatologica* **171**, 200–202.

Samman P.D. (1963) A traumatic nail dystrophy produced by habit tic. *Arch. Dermatol.* **88**, 895–899.

Singer P. & Gibson G.H. (1988) Unilateral onychodystrophy secondary to nail biting. *Cutis* **42**, 191–192.

Tosti A., Peluso A.M., Bardazzi F., Morelli R. & Bassi F. (1993) Phalangeal osteomyelitis due to nail biting. *Acta. Derm. Venereol.* (in press).

Waldman B.A. & Frieden I.J. (1990) Osteomyelitis caused by nail biting. *Pediatr. Dermatol.* **7**, 189–190.

Connective tissue diseases

In collagen diseases, the proximal nail fold is the most important site of alterations. Periungual ischaemic lesions resulting from small vessel necrotizing vasculitis reflect the underlying vasculopathy of collagen diseases and may be a cutaneous manifestation of several disorders including rheumatoid arthritis, systemic lupus erythematosus, dermatomyositis, periarteritis nodosa and Wegener's granulomatosis.

Nail fold erythema and telangiectasia are common features of patients affected by dermatomyositis, systemic lupus erythematosus or systemic sclerosis. In these patients irregular capillary loops are frequently visible even without a lens. Massive digital necrosis resulting from Raynaud's phenomenon can be the first manifestation of a collagen disease (Saban *et al.*, 1991).

Reference

Saban J., Rodriguez-Garcia J.L., Pais J.R., Mellado N. & Munoz E. (1991) Raynaud's phenomenon with digital necrosis as the first manifestation of undifferentiated connective tissue syndrome. *Dermatologica* **182**, 121–123.

Nail fold capillary microscopy (Table 6.3)

Nail fold capillary microscopy is a simple, non-invasive technique which can give useful information for early diagnosis of collagen diseases. Several instruments have been successfully used for the *in vivo* examination of the nail fold capillary bed. Portable capillaroscopes (Panasonic light scope or Micro Mike) and common ophthalmoscopes can be used in ordinary screening (Goldman, 1981; Minkin & Rabhan, 1982; Studer *et al.*, 1991). Stereomicroscopes that permit higher magnifications (×40) and photographic documentation of the nail fold capillary bed are advisable

Table 6.3. Nail fold capillary pattern in connective tissue diseases

	Capillary density	Morphological changes
Scleroderma	Paucity of visible capillaries, avascular areas	Enlarged capillary loops
SLE, DLE	Normal	Tortuous capillary loops, meandering loops
MCTD and dermatomyositis	Paucity of visible capillaries	Enlarged capillary loops, tortuous capillary loops
Rheumatoid arthritis	Normal, paucity of visible capillaries	Normal, irregular capillary loops

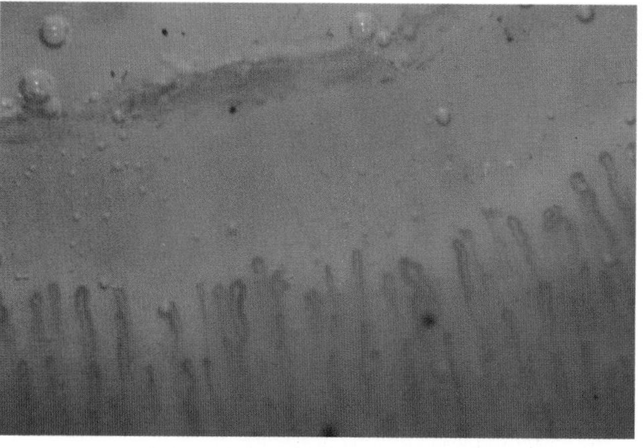

Fig. 6.36. Capillary microscopy – normal nail fold capillary loops (×60).

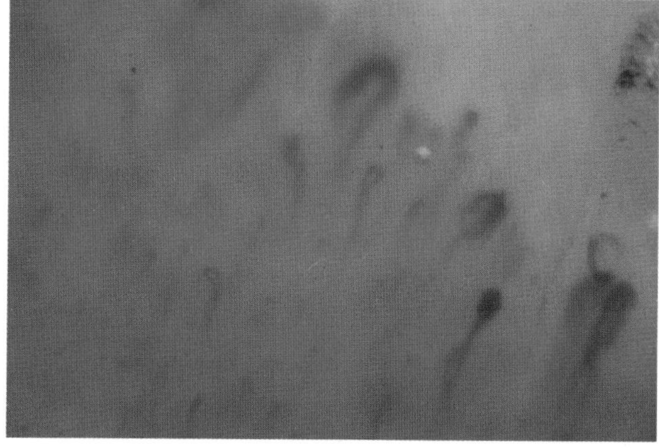

Fig. 6.37. Nail fold capillaries in systemic sclerosis – dilated, tortuous and many obstructed and thrombosed capillaries (×60).

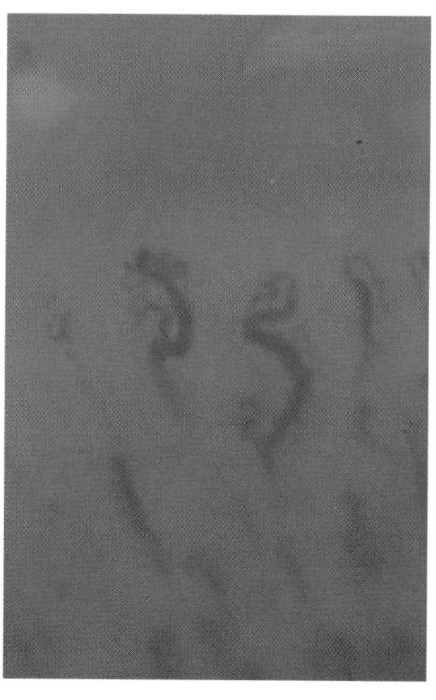

Fig. 6.38. Dilated capillary loops in lupus erythematosus (×60).

for a long-term follow-up of the microangiopathic alterations. Capillary microscopy of the proximal nail fold requires the application of a thin layer of oil to the skin in order to increase its transparency. The orientation of proximal nail fold capillaries parallel to the surface of the skin permits the observation of both the arterial and the venous limbs of the capillary.

In normal subjects (Fig. 6.36) nail fold capillaries are arranged in parallel rows and appear as fine regular loops with a small space between the afferent and efferent limbs. In collagen disorders, the morphology of the vascular nail bed loops may be grossly altered (Table 6.3).

An examination of the proximal nail fold in patients with scleroderma (Fig. 6.37) characteristically reveals capillary enlargement and loss. These capillary changes, consisting of enlarged loops and avascular areas, are present in most patients affected by systemic sclerosis and by its CREST variant, but not in morphoea (Minkin & Rabhan, 1982; Studer *et al.*, 1991) or in eosinophilic fasciitis (Herson *et al.*, 1989). When patients with localized scleroderma show typical nail fold capillary abnormalities a possible association with systemic sclerosis should be ruled out (Maricq, 1992). The severity of the proximal nail fold changes has been proposed as an index of the degree of systemic involvement and it has been suggested that it reflects the state of the total vascular system (Maricq *et al.*, 1976; Schmidt & Mensing, 1988). The prognostic value of capillary changes in scleroderma is, however, still being discussed (Lovy *et al.*, 1985) and quantitative morphological studies have failed to confirm this evidence (Lefford & Edwards, 1986; Statham & Rowell, 1986). Nail bed capillary microscopy may permit the differentiation of early scleroderma from idiopathic Raynaud's phenomenon (Carpentier *et al.*, 1983), which is not generally associated with microvascular changes in the nail fold. Capillaroscopy may also be useful in distinguishing the CREST variant of systemic sclerosis from hereditary haemorrhagic telangiectasia which is characterized by the presence of giant capillaries (Maire *et al.*, 1986). The aetiology of reduced capillary numbers in scleroderma is unknown, but may be related to the frequent capillary thromboses observed in the nail fold in this condition. Such thromboses lead to microinfarcts that heal by scarring.

In systemic lupus erythematosus (Fig. 6.38) the nail fold examination shows a normal density of capillary loops but a marked deformation of the individual capillaries. The vessel dilatation is minimal although the arrangement of the capillary loops is tortuous and can be corkscrew shaped (Redisch *et al.*, 1970; Minkin & Rabhan, 1982; Granier *et al.*, 1986). Meandering loops that may resemble glomerular tufts can occasionally be observed. Similar proximal nail fold abnormalities have been described in discoid lupus erythematosus (Rowell, 1986). In

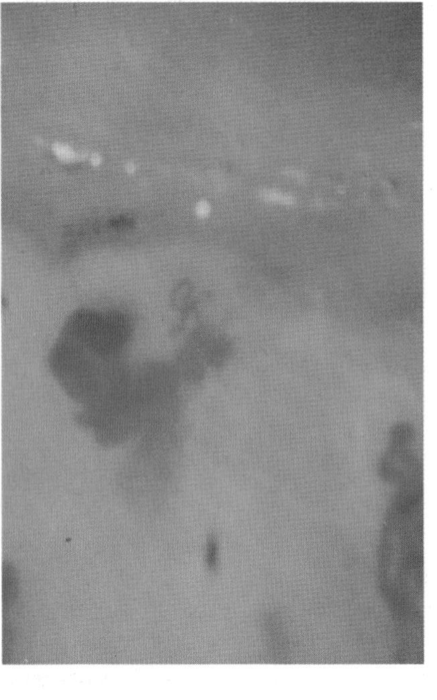

Fig. 6.39. Dermatomyositis – thrombosed nail fold capillaries.

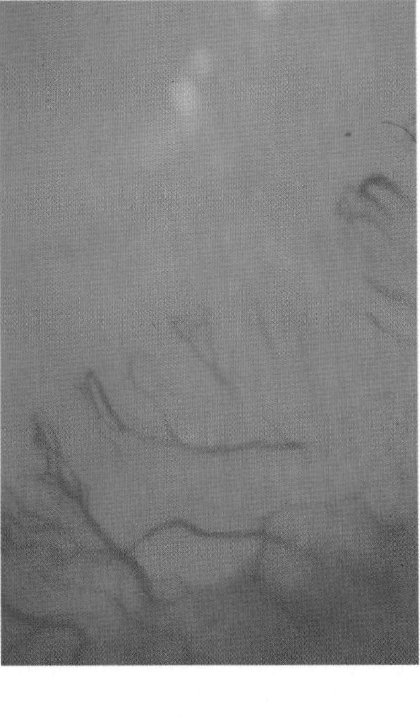

Fig. 6.40. Rheumatoid arthritis – rather elongated capillary loops.

systemic lupus erythematosus direct immunofluorescence of the proximal nail fold shows the typical lupus band test (Schnitzler *et al.*, 1980).

In patients with polymyositis, dermatomyositis and mixed connective tissue disease, the capillaroscopy changes resemble those described in patients with scleroderma. Capillary dilatation and drop out are the most common findings (Fig. 6.39). Tortuosity, deformation and bushy appearance of the individual capillaries are frequently associated features (Granier *et al.*, 1986; Wong *et al.*, 1988). The severity of the microvascular abnormalities has been observed to lessen with prolonged disease remission (Ganczarczyk *et al.*, 1988). A recent study of 85 cases of dermatomyositis showed severe disturbances of microcirculation including vasodilatation with megacapillaries, irregular and tortuous capillary loops, a decrease in the number of loops, an aggregation of erythrocytes, a granular and slow blood stream, a stasis in the transitional portion of the loops, a cloudy microscopic field as well as marked exudation, haemorrhages and invisibility of subpapillary blood plexus (Liu *et al.*, 1991). These changes were more marked in patients with visceral disorders and when the disease was in an active stage. In childhood dermatomyositis, the presence of enlarged capillaries and avascularity correlated with more severe and persistent forms of the disease (Spencer-Green *et al.*, 1983; Silver & Maricq, 1989).

Patients affected by rheumathoid arthritis (Fig. 6.40) generally do not present any alterations in the nail fold capillaries (Lefford & Edwards, 1986). Tortuosity, elongation of loops, paucity of visible capillaries and increased plasma skimming have been occasionally described, however (Redisch *et al.*, 1970). Although capillary microscopy is a useful complementary investigation for the evaluation of patients with collagen disorders, it should not be used as a diagnostic criterion in individual patients. In fact, some of the capillary microscopy abnormalities which are observed in patients with collagen diseases may even occur in normal controls.

The clinical signs in the nail apparatus associated with connective tissue diseases are outlined in Table 6.4.

References

Carpentier P., Franco A., Beani J.C., Reymond J.L. & Amblard P. (1983) Intéret de la capillaroscopie périunguéale dans le diagnostic précoce de la sclérodermie systemique. *Ann. Dermatol. Venereol.* **110**, 11–20.

Ganczarczyk M.L., Lee P. & Armstrong S.K. (1988) Nailfold capillary microscopy in polymyositis and dermatomyositis. *Arth. Rheum.* **31**, 116–119.

Goldman L. (1981) A simple portable capillaroscope. *Arch. Dermatol.* **117**, 605–606.

Granier F., Vayssairat M., Priollet P. & Housset E. (1986) Nailfold capillary microscopy in mixed connective tissue disease. *Arth. Rheum.* **29**, 189–195.

Herson S., Brechignac S., Piette, J.C. *et al.* (1989) Capillaroscopie unguéale au cours de la fasciite avec éosinophilie: un élément distinctif d'avec la sclérodermie systémique. *Ann. Med. Intern.* **140**, 440–443.

Lefford F. & Edwards J.C.W. (1986) Nailfold capillary microscopy in connective tissue disease: a quantitative morphological analysis. *Ann. Rheum. Dis.* **45**, 741–749.

Liu C., Su W. & Luo Y. (1991) Changes in cutaneous microcirculation, hemorrheology and platelet aggregation function in dermatomyositis. *J. Dermatol. Sci.* **2**, 346–352.

Lovy M., Mac Carter D. & Steigerwald J.C. (1985) Relationship between nailfold capillary abnormalities and organ involvement in systemic sclerosis. *Arth. Rheum.* **28**, 496–501.

Maire R., Schnewlin G. & Bollinger A. (1986) Videomikroskopische Untersuchungen von Teleangiektasien bei Morbus Osler und Sklerodermie. *Schweiz Med. Wschr.* **116**, 335–338.

Maricq H.R., Spencer Green G. & Le Roy E.C. (1976) Skin capillary abnormalities as indicators of organ involvement in scleroderma (systemic sclerosis), Raynaud's syndrome and dermatomyositis. *Am. J. Med.* **61**, 862–870.

Maricq H.R. (1992) Capillary abnormalities, Raynaud's phenomenon, and systemic sclerosis in patients with localized scleroderma. *Arch. Dermatol.* **128**, 630–632.

Minkin W. & Rabhan N.B. (1982) Office nail fold capillary microscopy using ophthalmoscope. *J. Am. Acad. Dermatol.* 7, 190–193.

Redisch W., Messina E.J., Hughes G. & McEven C. (1970) Capillaroscopic observations in rheumatic diseases. *Ann. Rheum. Dis.* **29**, 244–253.

Rowell N.R. (1986) Lupus erythematosus, scleroderma and dermatomyositis. The 'collagen' or 'connective-tissue' diseases. In: *Textbook of Dermatology*, eds Rook A., Wilkinson D.S., Ebling F.J.G., Champion R.H. & Burton J.L., pp. 1281–1392. Blackwell Scientific Publications, Oxford.

Schmidt K.U. & Mensing H. (1988) Are nailfold capillary changes indicators of organ involvement in progressive systemic sclerosis? *Dermatologica* **176**, 18–21.

Schnitzler L., Baran R. & Verret J.L. (1980) La biopsie du repli sus-ungueal dans les maladies dites du collagéne. Etude histologique, ultrastructurale et en immunofluorescence de 26 cas. *Ann. Dermatol. Venereol.* **107**, 777–785.

Silver R.M. & Maricq H.R. (1989) Childhood dermatomyositis: serial microvascular studies. *Pediatrics* **83**, 278–283.

Spencer-Green G., Schlesinger M., Bove K.E. *et al.* (1983) Nailfold capillary abnormalities in childhood rheumatic diseases. *J. Pediatr.* **102**, 341–346.

Statham B.N. & Rowell N.R. (1986) Quantification of the nail fold capillary abnormalities in systemic sclerosis and Raynaud's syndrome. *Acta Derm. Venereol.* **66**, 139–143.

Studer A., Hunziker T., Lutolf O., Schmidli J., Chen D. & Mahler F. (1991) Quantitative nailfold capillary microscopy in cutaneous and systemic lupus erythematosus and localized and systemic scleroderma. *J. Am. Acad. Dermatol.* **24**, 941–945.

Wong M.L., Highton J. & Palmer D.G. (1988) Sequential nail fold capillary microscopy in scleroderma and related disorders. *Ann. Rheum. Dis.* **47**, 53–61.

Systemic sclerosis (see also Figs 6.5–6.9)

Raynaud's phenomenon usually precedes the development of the other cutaneous signs of scleroderma. Swelling of the fingers can be an early symptom of systemic sclerosis. The round fingerpad sign has been described recently as a useful clinical diagnostic sign of scleroderma. This sign describes the disappearance of the peaked contour on the fingerpads and its replacement by a hemisphere-like fingerpad contour. The round fingerpad sign is most commonly found on the ring fingers. A positive sign has been observed not only in patients with scleroderma but also in patients with Raynaud's phenomenon or mixed connective tissue disease (Mizutami *et al.*, 1991).

In well-developed cases of scleroderma, the fingers have a tapered appearance due to sclerosis of the overlying skin and frequently exhibit flexion contractures. Patients with hereditary sclerodactyly may resemble systemic sclerosis but there is no Raynaud's phenomenon (Eubel *et al.*, 1985).

Periungual ischaemic lesions and ulcers are frequent in systemic scleroderma (Fig. 6.41). Digital gangrene is occasionally seen even in the absence of severe systemic involvement (Fig. 6.42). A patient has been reported in whom digital gangrene was the sole cutaneous evidence of systemic sclerosis (Barr & Robinson, 1988).

Chronic paronychia and onycholysis are common complaints and discoloration of the nail plate may be symptomatic of a secondary mycotic or bacterial infection. The nail folds can present ragged cuticles (Rowell, 1986). Impaired peripheral circulation can lead to nail thinning

Table 6.4. Nail alterations in connective tissue diseases

	Periungual tissues	Nail unit
Scleroderma	Ischaemic lesions, ulcers, gangrene, dissolution of the terminal phalanges	Chronic paronychia, onycholysis, onychogryphosis, pterygium inversum unguis*, parrot's beak nail*
SLE	Digital ulcers, gangrene	Nail fold telangiectasia, cuticolar haemorrhages, leuconychia, pitting, ridging, onycholysis, onychomadesis, nail bed hyperkeratosis
DLE		Nail bed hyperkeratosis
Dermatomyositis		Nail fold telangiectasia, cuticolar haemorrhages, cuticolar hyperkeratosis
Rheumatoid arthritis	Ischaemic lesions	Nail fold infarcts*, beading, ridging, yellow nail syndrome, red lunulae*
Wegener's granulomatosis	Necrotic lesions	Linear infarcts of the proximal nail fold
Periarteritis nodosa	Necrotic lesions	Nail fold infarcts

* Distinctive changes.

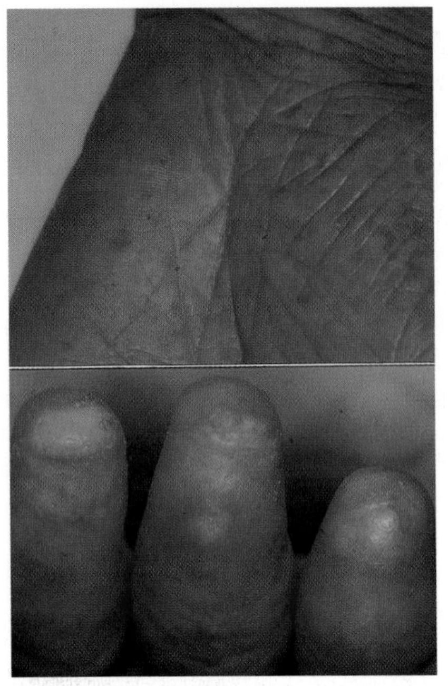

Fig. 6.41. Systemic sclerosis – telangiectasia and acrosclerosis.

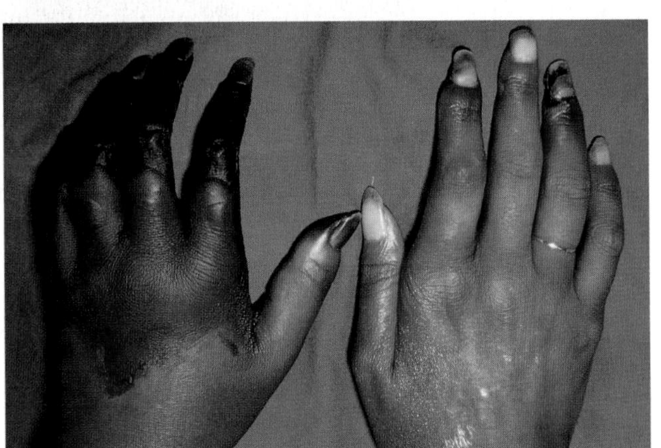

Fig. 6.42. Systemic sclerosis – gangrenous appearance of the left hand (courtesy of N.R. Rowell, UK).

and ridging. When atrophy of the terminal phalanges occurs, the nails become small and brittle. Onychogryphosis can also be observed.

Pterygium inversum unguis and parrot's beak nail are the only distinctive nail changes of systemic scleroderma (see Chapter 2). Pterygium inversum unguis was first linked to scleroderma by Patterson (1977). Although more frequently observed in patients with acrosclerosis and fingertip ulcerations, it can aid diagnosis of the disease (Zaias, 1990). Pterygium inversum unguis consists of the obliteration of the normal distal separation between the ventral surface of the nail plate and the skin of the hyponychium. The resulting adhesion between the nail plate and the fingertip skin leads to pain when the nails are clipped. Pterygium inversum associated with scleroderma is probably a consequence of the fingertip ulcerations and scarring. No form of treatment for this condition has been effective.

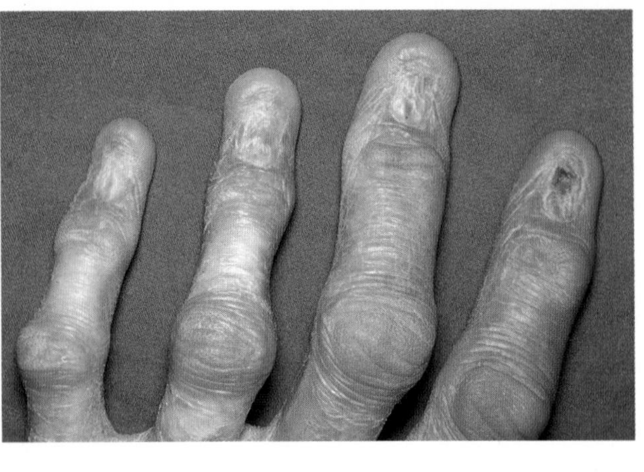

Fig. 6.43. Acral pansclerotic morphoea (courtesy of N.R. Rowell, UK).

Parrot's beak nail, otherwise known as nail beaking (Chapter 2), is a nail change that occurs as a consequence of the atrophy of the fingertip soft tissues which characterizes severe acrosclerosis. The nail plate bends around the shortened fingertip. Complete destruction of the nail apparatus is the final consequence of the dissolution of the terminal phalanges which occurs in the most severely affected patients.

Systemic sclerosis-like disorders have been reported to develop following exposure to vinyl chloride, aliphatic and aromatic hydrocarbons, epoxy resins, silicon, bleomycin, L-tryptophan and toxic oil as well as after silicone 'breast implants' (Bélangé *et al.*, 1989; Connolly *et al.*, 1990; Rustin *et al.*, 1990). A syndrome resembling systemic sclerosis characterizes the chronic phase of graft-versus-host disease.

Although localized scleroderma is not usually associated with nail changes, complete loss of both finger- and toenails has been reported (Fig. 6.43) in a patient affected by acral pansclerotic morphoea (Rowell, 1987).

References

Barr W.G. & Robinson J.A. (1988) Systemic sclerosis and digital gangrene without scleroderma. *J. Rheumatol.* **15**, 875–877.

Bélangé G., Chaouat D. & Chauoat Y. (1989) Les connectivities induites non médicamenteuses. *Rev. Med. Intern.* **10**, 135–141.

Connolly S.M., Quimby S.R., Griffing W.L. & Winkelmann R.K. (1990) Scleroderma and L-tryptophan: a possible explanation of the eosinophilia myalgia syndrome. *J. Am. Acad. Dermatol* **23**, 451–457.

Eubel R., Klose L. & Mahrle G. (1985) Hereditare sklerodaktylie und syndactylie. *Hautarzt* **36**, 302–304.

Mizutami H., Mizutami T., Okada H., Kupper T.S. & Shimizu M. (1991) Round fingerpad sign: an early sign of scleroderma. *J. Am. Acad. Dermatol.* **24**, 67–69.

Patterson J.W. (1977) Pterygium inversum unguis-like changes in scleroderma. *Arch. Dermatol.* **113**, 1429–1430.
Rowell N.R. (1986) Lupus erythematosus, scleroderma and dermatomyositis. The 'collagen' or 'connective-tissue' diseases. In: *Textbook of Dermatology*, eds Rook A., Wilkinson D.S., Ebling F.J.G., Champion R.H. & Burton J.L., pp. 1281–1392. Blackwell Scientific Publications, Oxford.
Rowell N.R. (1987) Acral pansclerotic morphea with intractable pain. CVII Congressus Mundi Dermatologiae Berlin. *Clin. Dermatol.* 178–180.
Rustin M.H.A., Bull H.A., Ziegler V. *et al.* (1990) Silica associated systemic sclerosis is clinically, serologically and immunologically indistinguishable from idiopathic systemic sclerosis. *Br. J. Dermatol.* **123**, 725–734.
Zaias N. (1990) *The Nail in Health and Disease*, pp. 189–199. Appleton & Lange, Norwalk, CN.

Systemic lupus erythematosus (Figs 6.44–6.46)

Blood vessel infarction leading to focal necrosis of the nail fold and cuticular haemorrhages are common features of systemic lupus erythematosus. Digital ulcers and/or gangrene may represent a clinical manifestation of cutaneous vasculitis but are not necessarily related to systemic involvement (Hashimoto *et al.*, 1983). Although a wide spectrum of nail abnormalities has been described in systemic lupus erythematosus, none is sufficiently distinctive to be useful in the diagnosis of the disease (Figs 6.4–6.11; 6.44–6.46). Patients may, in fact, present an altered keratinization of the nail matrix leading to punctate or striate leuconychia as well as nail pitting or ridging. Onycholysis or onychomadesis can occur. Onycholysis has been reported as the most frequent nail abnormality in systemic lupus erythematosus (Urowitz *et al.*, 1978). Red lunulae (Jorizzo *et al.*, 1983; Wilkerson & Wilkin, 1989) as well as oil patches of the nail bed (Runne & Orfanos, 1981) have been described. Nail fold hyperkeratosis, ragged cuticles and splinter haemorrhages can also be observed (Rowell, 1986) (Fig. 6.44). In patients with antiphospholipid antibodies the formation of platelet thrombi in the smaller vessels may result in splinter haemorrhages and acral microlivedo digital ischaemia (Asherson, 1990; Ames *et al.*, 1992; Wolf *et al.*, 1992). Finger clubbing has been occasionally reported (Mackie, 1973; Menkes *et al.*, 1980). A diffuse, dark blue–black pattern of hyperpigmentation intermixed with longitudinal pigmented bands was present in 52% of 33 black patients with systemic lupus erythematosus (Vaughn *et al.*, 1990). Nail bed hyperkeratosis may be seen both in discoid and in systemic lupus erythematosus. In the latter, it has been described in association with periungual and palmoplantar hyperkeratosis (Buck *et al.*, 1988).

The term lupus erythematosus ungium mutilans describes a rare destructive involvement of the nails associated with decalcification and atrophy of the distal phalanges (McCarthy, 1931).

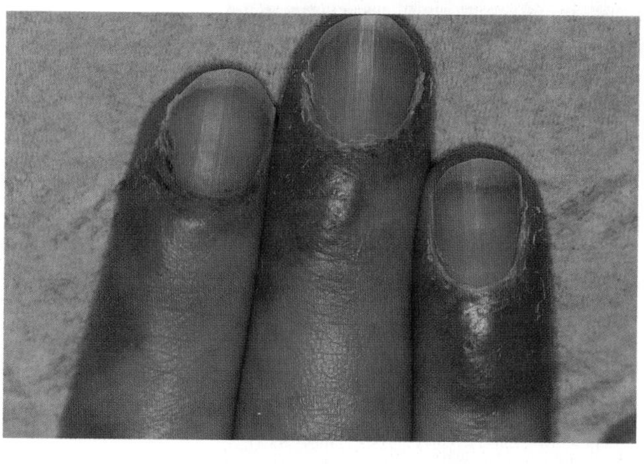

Fig. 6.44. Systemic lupus erythematosus.

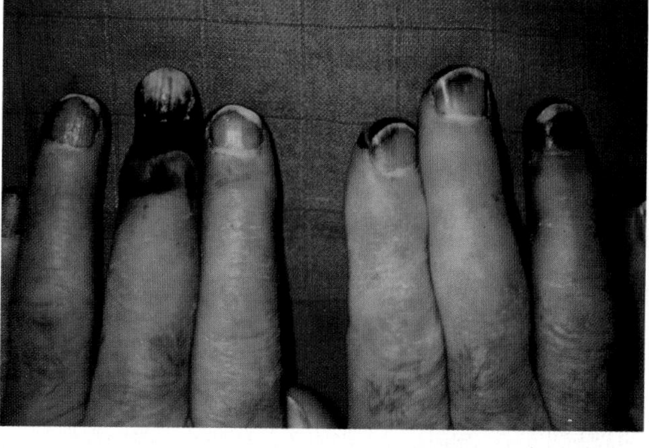

Fig. 6.45. Systemic lupus erythematosus with gangrenous digits.

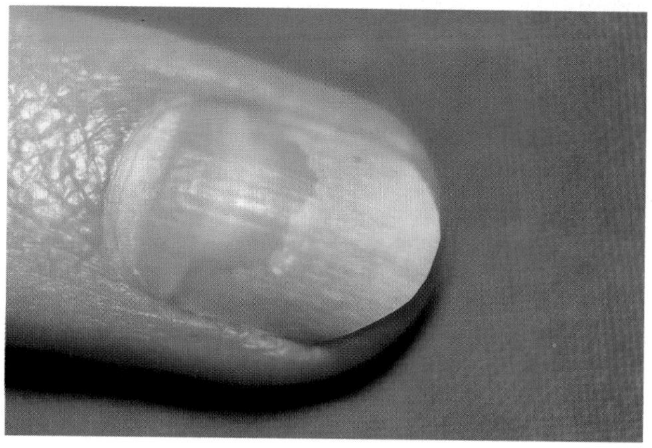

Fig. 6.46. Lupus erythematosus – vasculitic nail lesion.

References

Ames D.E., Asherson R.A., Ayres D. *et al.* (1992) Bilateral adrenal infarction hypoadrenalism, and splinter haemorrhages in the 'primary' antiphospholipid syndrome. *Br. J. Rheumatol.* **31**, 117–120.

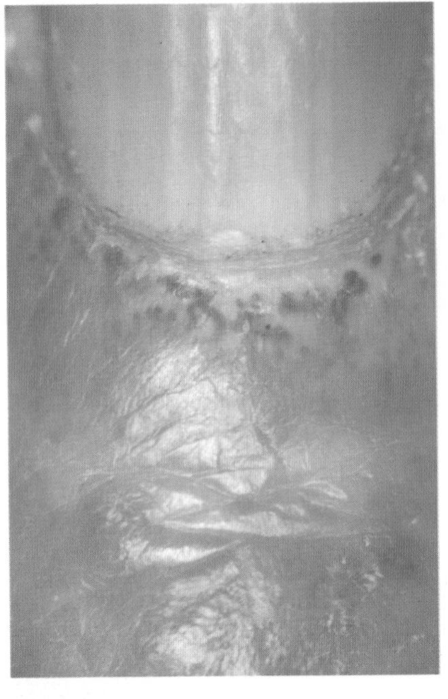

Fig. 6.47. Dermatomyositis – ragged cuticles and dilated nail fold capillaries.

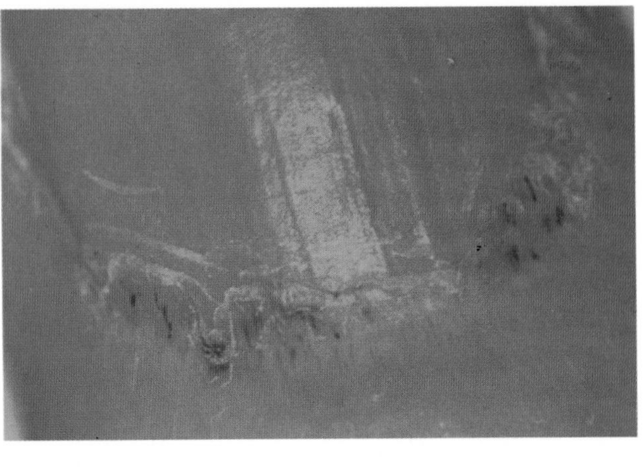

Fig. 6.48. Dermatomyositis – close-up of Fig. 6.47.

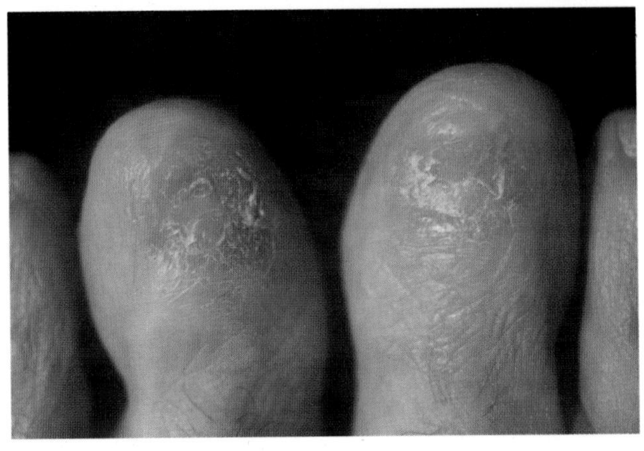

Fig. 6.49. Dermatomyositis – loss of toenails.

Asherson R.A. (1990) Subungual splinter haemorrhages: a new sign of the antiphospholipid coagulopathy? *Ann. Rheum. Dis.* **49**, 268–271.

Buck D.C., Dodd H.J. & Sarkany I. (1988) Hypertrophic lupus erythematosus. *Br. J. Dermatol. Suppl.* **33**, 72–74.

Hashimoto H., Tsuda H., Takasaki Y., Fujimaki N., Suzuki M. & Shiokawa Y. (1983) Digital ulcers/gangrene and immunoglobulin classes/complement fixation of Anti-dsDNA in systemic lupus erythematosus patients. *J. Rheumatol.* **10**, 727–732.

Jorizzo J.L., Gonzalez E.B. & Daniels J.C. (1983) Red lunulae in a patient with rheumatoid arthritis. *J. Am. Acad. Dermatol.* **8**, 711–714.

Mackie R.M. (1973) Lupus erythematosus in association with finger-clubbing. *Br. J. Dermatol.* **89**, 533–535.

McCarthy L. (1931) Lupus erythematosus ungium mutilans treated with gold and sodium thiosulphate. *Arch. Dermatol. Syphil.* **24**, 647–654.

Menkes C.S., Marin A. & Delbarre F. (1980) Rupture de tendons et hippocratisme digital an cours du lupus érythémateux disséminé. *Rhumathisme* **50**(5), 333–335.

Rowell N.R. (1986) Lupus erythematosus, scleroderma and dermatomyositis. The 'collagen' or 'connective-tissue' diseases. In: *Textbook of Dermatology*, eds Rook A., Wilkinson D.S., Ebling F.J.G., Champion R.H. & Burton J.L., pp. 1281–1392. Blackwell Scientific Publications, Oxford.

Runne U. & Orfanos C.E. (1981) The human nail. *Curr. Prob. Dermatol.* **9**, 102–149.

Urowitz M.B., Gladman D.D., Chalmers A. & Ogryzlo M.A. (1978) Nail lesions in systemic lupus erythematosus. *J. Rheumatol.* **5**, 441–447.

Vaughn R.Y., Bailey J.P., Field R.S. *et al.* (1990) Diffuse nail dyschromia in black patients with systemic lupus erythematosus. *J. Rheumatol.* **17**, 640–643.

Wilkerson M.G. & Wilkin J.K. (1989) Red lunulae revisited: a clinical and histopathologic examination. *J. Am. Acad. Dermatol.* **20**, 453–457.

Wolf P., Soyer H.P., Aver-Greumbach P. & Kerl H. (1992) Acral microlivedo – a clinical manifestation of the antiphospholipid syndrome. *Z. Hautke* **67**, 714–717.

Dermatomyositis

Erythema and telangiectasia of the proximal nail fold are typical features of dermatomyositis (Figs 6.48 & 6.49). Thickness, hardness, roughness and hyperkeratosis of the cuticles are common in patients with dermatomyositis even in the absence of nail fold abnormalities (Fig. 6.47) (Samitz, 1974). Cuticular haemorrhages are frequent. Pitting of the fingernails may be seen occasionally (Rowell, 1986; Dupré *et al.*, 1981). Presence of periungual ischaemic lesions can be a predictive sign of malignancy in adult dermatomyositis (Basset-Seguin *et al.*, 1990).

We have described complete loss of several toenails (Fig. 6.49) in a patient with dermatomyositis (Tosti *et al.*, 1987). Erythema and scaling of the nail bed along with nail fold erythema and telangiectasia were prominent features. Thickening of the nail cuticles was also evident. Red lunulae have been reported in a patient with dermatomyositis (Jorizzo *et al.*, 1983). Gottron's papules may be seen at the proximal area of the dorsal aspect of the terminal phalanx (Fig. 6.50).

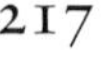

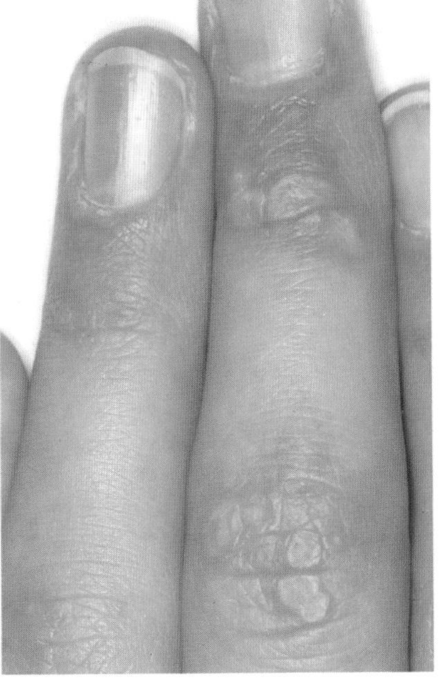

Fig. 6.50. Dermatomyositis – Gottron's lichenoid papules on the knuckles.

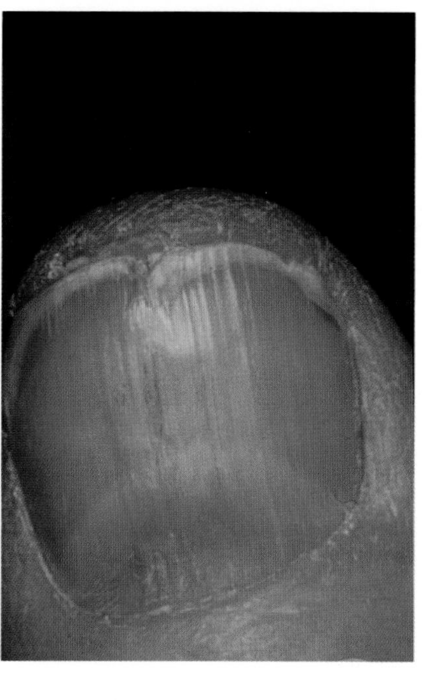

Fig. 6.51. Rheumatoid arthritis – red lunula.

References

Basset-Seguin N., Roujeau J.C., Gheradi R. *et al.* (1990) Prognostic factors and predictive signs of malignancy in adult dermatomyositis. *Arch. Dermatol.* **126**, 633–637.

Dupré A., Viraben R., Bonafe J.L., Touron P. & Lamon P. (1981) Zebra-like dermatomyositis. *Arch. Dermatol.* **117**, 63–64.

Jorizzo J.L., Gonzalez E.B. & Daniels J.C. (1983) Red lunulae in a patient with rheumatoid arthritis. *J. Am. Acad. Dermatol.* **8**, 711–714.

Rowell N.R. (1986) Lupus erythematosus, scleroderma and dermatomyositis. The 'collagen' or 'connective-tissue' diseases. In: *Textbook of Dermatology*, eds Rook A., Wilkinson D.S., Ebling F.J.G., Champion R.H. & Burton J.L., pp. 1281–1392. Blackwell Scientific Publications, Oxford.

Samitz M.H. (1974) Cuticular changes in dermatomyositis. *Arch. Dermatol.* **110**, 866–867.

Tosti A., De Padova M.P., Fanti P., Bonelli U. & Taffurelli M. (1987) Unusual severe nail involvement in dermatomyositis. *Cutis* **40**, 261–262.

Rheumatoid arthritis (Figs 6.51–6.55)

Palmar erythema and nail fold telangiectasia are well-known features of rheumatoid arthritis. The nail growth rate may be reduced in severe generalized rheumatoid disease (De Nicola *et al.*, 1974). Longitudinal ridging with beading of the nails is commonly observed (Hamilton, 1960). Thumb and great toenails are more frequently affected. A global pattern of beading on the surface of at least six fingernails or four toenails has been reported to be highly specific for rheumatoid arthritis (predictive value of about 95%). Since nail beading is not frequent in the early phase of the disease, the diagnostic value of this nail abnormality is limited. It has been suggested that nail beading results from microvascular changes in the nail bed (Grant *et al.*, 1985). Hapalonychia, subungual hyperkeratosis, onychorrhexis and toenail onychogryphosis (Figs 6.53 & 6.54) have been reported to be common in rheumatoid patients (De Nicola *et al.*, 1974). Nail thickening and discoloration as well as splinter haemorrhages can also occur (Daniel *et al.*, 1985).

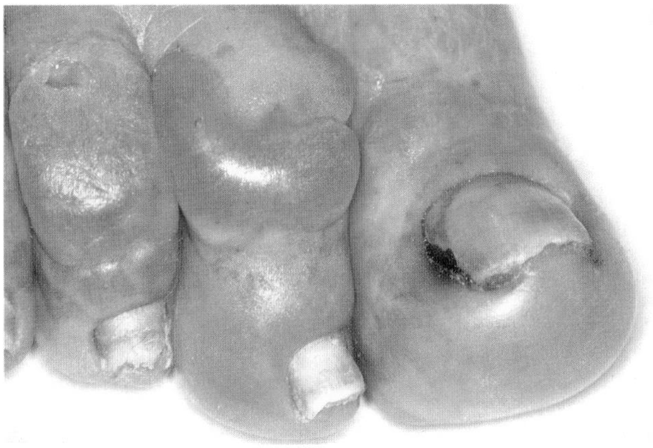

Fig. 6.52. Rheumatoid arthritis – peripheral blisters and lateral periungual infarction.

Yellow nail syndrome has been occasionally associated with rheumatoid arthritis or with penicillamine therapy in the latter condition. A pink or dusky red homogeneous discoloration of the proximal part of the lunula is quite characteristic of rheumatoid arthritis (Fig. 6.51). The prevalence of this alteration in rheumatoid arthritis has never been studied but red lunulae, which are more commonly observed in thumbs and big toes, are possibly more frequent than the literature suggests (Jorizzo *et al.*, 1983).

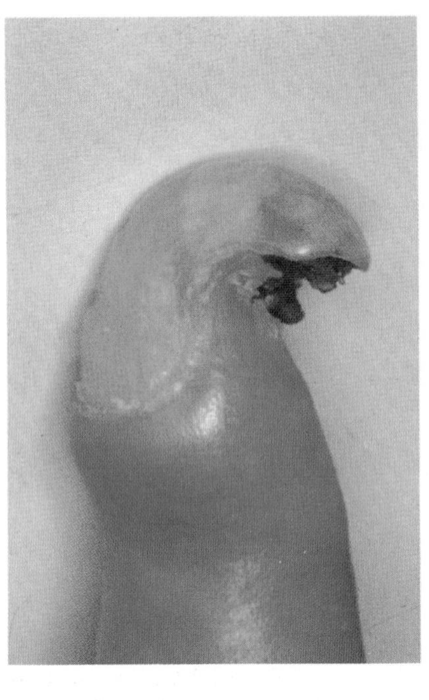

Fig. 6.53. Rheumatoid arthritis – onychogryphosis.

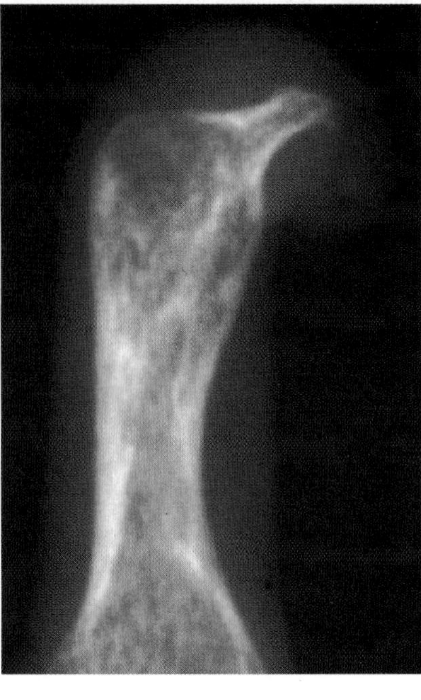

Fig. 6.54. Rheumatoid arthritis – onychogryphosis (same patient as Fig. 6.53).

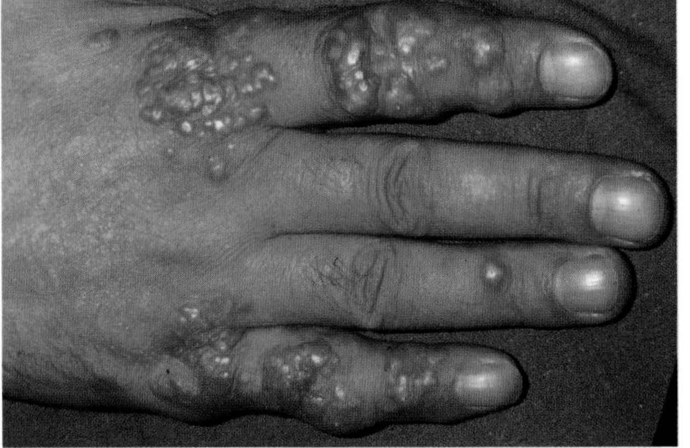

Fig. 6.55. Rheumatoid nodules – 'benign' adult type (courtesy of A. Rebora, Italy).

Red lunulae have also occasionally been described in systemic lupus erythematosus, dermatomyositis, obstructive pulmonary disease and congestive heart failure (Wilkerson & Wilkin, 1989).

Occasionally a 0.5–1 mm sharply demarcated deep violet area that runs parallel to the lunula at 4–5 mm from the free edge of the nails can be seen. This can also occur in some infectious diseases such as syphilis and leprosy (De Nicola *et al.*, 1974).

Rheumatoid nodules (Fig. 6.55) can be localized on the terminal pads of the fingers and at the free edge of the nails. The histopathology of rheumatoid nodules shows fibrinoid necrosis surrounded by a palisade of lymphohistiocytic cells. They can also occur in the absence of signs or symptoms of rheumatic disease (Rongioletti *et al.*, 1990). Nail fold and pulp lesions due to necrotizing vasculitis are not uncommon in patients with rheumatoid arthritis. Small painless infarcts of the nail fold are a characteristic feature of rheumatoid patients. The chronological evolution of these lesions has been clearly described by Bywaters and Scott (1963). Periungual swelling precedes the appearance of skin haemorrhages and necrosis; eschars usually disappear within a few days without scarring and this eventually results in grooving of the nail. Trauma may favour the occurrence of small ischaemic periungual lesions (Koebner phenomenon). Ischaemic areas on the nail fold (Fig. 6.52) can resemble an area of superficial paronychia (Bywaters, 1957; O'Quinn *et al.*, 1965). These lesions may heal with scarring and the appearance of scars over the joints, in the nail fold areas and on the ends of the digits is frequent.

Large haemorrhages and bullae of digital pulps as well as digital gangrene are clinical signs of the most severe form of rheumatoid vasculitis (Fig. 6.52).

References

Bywaters E.G.L. (1957) Peripheral vascular obstruction in rheumatoid arthritis and its relationship to other vascular lesions. *Ann. Rheum. Dis.* **16**, 84–103.

Bywaters E.G.L. & Scott J.T. (1963) The natural history of vascular lesions in rheumatoid arthritis. *J. Chron. Dis.* **16**, 905–914.

Daniel R.C., Sams W.M. & Scher R.K. (1985) Nails in systemic disease. *Dermatol. Clin.* **3**, 465–483.

De Nicola P.D., Morsiani M. & Zavagli G. (1974) *Nail Diseases in Internal Medicine*. Charles C. Thomas, Springfield, IL.

Grant E.N., Bellamy N., Buchanan W.W., Grace E.M. & O'Leary S. (1985) Statistical reappraisal of the clinical significance of nail beading in rheumatoid arthritis. *Ann. Rheum. Dis.* **44**, 671–675.

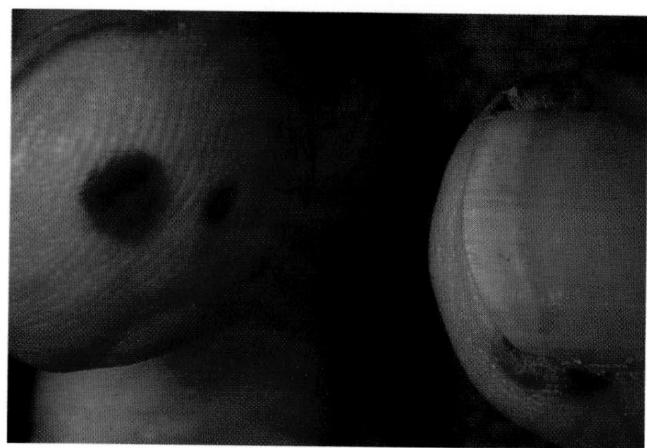

Fig. 6.56. Wegener's granulomatosis (courtesy G.T. Spigel).

Hamilton E.B.D. (1960) Nail studies in rheumatoid arthritis. *Ann. Rheum. Dis.* **19**, 167–173.
Jorizzo J.L., Gonzalez E.B. & Daniels J.C. (1983) Red lunulae in a patient with rheumatoid arthritis. *J. Am. Acad. Dermatol.* **8**, 711–714.
O'Quinn S.E., Kennedy B.C. & Baker D.T. (1965) Peripheral vascular lesions in rheumatoid arthritis. *Arch. Dermatol.* **92**, 489–494.
Rongioletti F., Cestari R., Cozzani E. & Rebora A. (1990) Nodules rhumatoides bénins chez un adulte (evaluant depuis 16 années). *Nouv. Dermatol.* **9**, 655–656.
Wilkerson M.G. & Wilkin J.K. (1989) Red lunulae revisited: a clinical and histopathologic examination. *J. Am. Acad. Dermatol.* **20**, 453–457.

Wegener's granulomatosis

Papular, pustular and necrotic lesions of the periungual tissues may be observed in Wegener's granulomatosis. Linear small infarcts around the nail fold have been reported in a patient affected by limited Wegener's granulomatosis (Spigel *et al.*, 1983) (Fig. 6.56).

Reference

Spigel G.T., Krall R.A. & Hilal A. (1983) Limited Wegener's granulomatosis: unusual cutaneous, radiographic and pathologic manifestations. *Cutis* **32**, 41–51.

Periarteritis nodosa (Fig. 6.57)

Small infarcts of the nail fold and of the distal aspects of fingers and toes may be a feature of periarteritis nodosa. Digital gangrene can rarely occur (Broussard & Baethge, 1990). Thinning, splitting and ridging of the fingernails and toenails associated with a blue–red rash on finger and toe tips have been reported in a patient affected by benign cutaneous periarteritis nodosa (Kassis *et al.*, 1985).

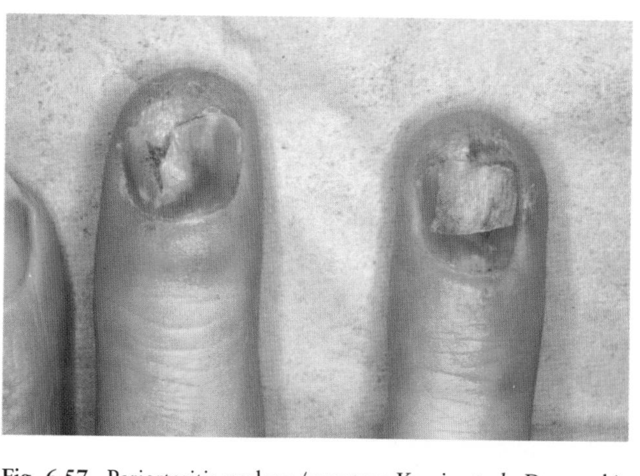

Fig. 6.57. Periarteritis nodosa (courtesy Kassis *et al.*, Denmark).

References

Broussard R.K. & Baethge B.A. (1990) Peripheral gangrene in polyarteritis nodosa. *Cutis* **46**, 53–55.
Kassis V., Kassis E. & Thomsen H.K. (1985) Benign cutaneous periarteritis nodosa with nail defects. *J. Am. Acad. Dermatol.* **13**, 661–663.

Microscopic polyarteritis

Microscopic polyarteritis is a systemic small vessels vasculitis that primarily involves the kidneys. Lung, nervous system and skin can also be affected. Ecchymotic lesions and haemorrhagic crusted macules and papules may affect periungual tissues (Homas *et al.*, 1992).

References

Homas P.B., Bajar D.K.M., Fitzpatrick J.E. *et al.* (1992) Microscopic polyarteritis. *Arch. Dermatol.* **128**, 1223–1228.

Multicentric reticulohistiocytosis

(Figs 6.58 & 6.59)

Multicentric reticulohistiocytosis is a rare disorder characterized by papulonodular skin lesions, a disabling polyarthritis and a typical dermal infiltration of histiocytes and multinucleated giant cells. Wart-like dark red to flesh-coloured nodules arranged around the nail folds of fingers in a 'coral bead' configuration occur in about half of the patients (Fig. 6.58) (Lesher & Allen, 1984). Hard and painful nodules on the fingertips have been reported. Joint destruction leads to shortening of the distal phalanges, and racket nails are characteristic (Barrow, 1967). Nail brittleness, longitudinal ridging, hyperpigmentation and atrophy have also been described. Although approximately one-fourth of patients have associated malignancies, the possibility that multicentric reticulohistiocytosis is a paraneoplastic syndrome is still under discussion (Aldridge

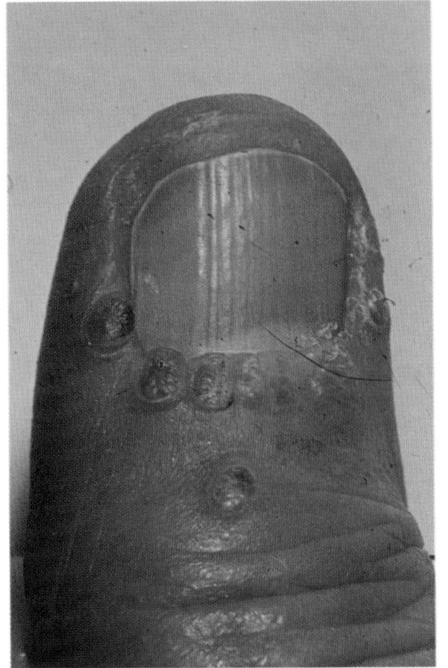

Fig. 6.58. Multicentric reticulohistio-cytosis.

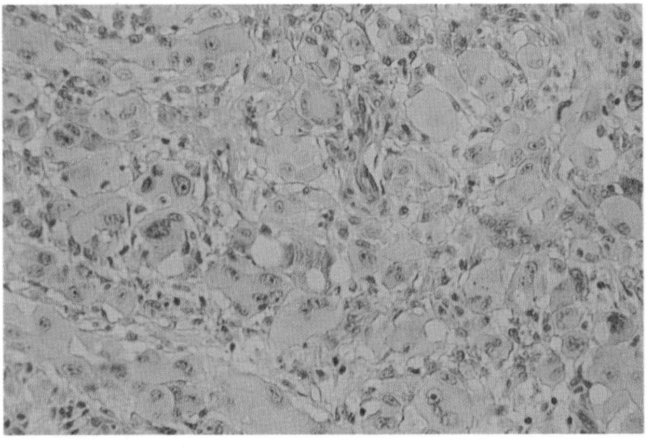

Fig. 6.59. Multicentric reticulohistiocytosis – cellular infiltrate from an affected area.

et al., 1984; Lesher & Allen, 1984; Nunnink *et al.*, 1985; Oliver *et al.*, 1990).

References

Aldridge R.D., Main R.A. & Daly B.M. (1984) Multicentric reticulohistiocytosis and cancer. *J. Am. Acad. Dermatol.* **10**, 296–297.

Barrow M.V. (1967) The nails in multicentric reticulohistiocytosis. *Arch. Dermatol.* **95**, 200–201.

Lesher J.L. & Allen B.S. (1984) Multicentric reticulohistiocytosis. *J. Am. Acad. Dermatol.* **11**, 713–723.

Nunnink J.C., Krusinski P.A. & Yates J.W. (1985) Multicentric reticulohistiocytosis and cancer: a case report and review of the literature. *Med. Pediatr. Oncol.* **13**, 273–279.

Oliver G.F., Umbert I., Winkelmann R.K. & Muller S.A. (1990) Reticulohistiocytoma cutis – review of 15 cases and an association with systemic vasculitis in two cases. *Clin. Exp. Dermatol.* **15**, 1–6.

Follicular mucinosis (alopecia mucinosa)

Lapiere *et al.* (1972) reported a case of follicular mucinosis with nail involvement. All fingernails and toenails were thickened, brittle and ridged. Periungual tissues were normal. At biopsy, the nail was hollowed out by cavities running parallel to the surface and filled with amorphous material stained by mucicarminian and PAS. In the nail bed a dense histiolymphocytic cell infiltrate that resembled the perifollicular infiltration separated the basal layer from the overlying keratinocytes.

Reference

Lapiere S., Castermans-Elias S. & Pierard G. (1972) Mucinose folliculaire et unguéale généralisée. *Bull. Soc. Fr. Dermatol. Syphil.* 79, 235–238.

Fibroblastic rheumatism

This entity, first reported in 1980 by Chaouat *et al.*, is characterized by the association of symmetric polyarthritis

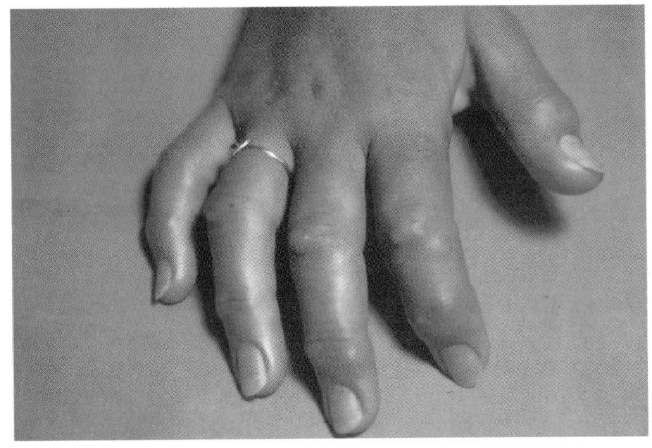

Fig. 6.60. Fibroblastic rheumatism – clinical appearance (courtesy of A.L. Claudy, Lyon, France).

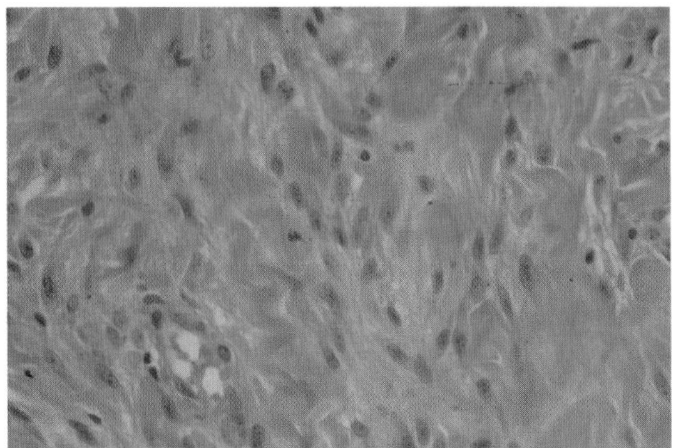

Fig. 6.61. Fibroblastic rheumatism – fibroblastic proliferation and collagen bundles in 'whorl-like' pattern (same patient as in Fig. 6.60).

and skin nodules. The histological picture of the skin nodules is specific, revealing fibroblastic proliferation and fibrosis with thickened collagen bundles that are arranged in a 'whorl-like pattern' (Vignon-Pennamen *et al.*, 1986) (Figs 6.60 & 6.61). Cutaneous nodules are located mostly over the extensor aspect of the fingers. The nodules are firm, flesh-coloured or yellowish, measuring from 0.5 to 1 cm in diameter. Sclerodactyly and Raynaud's phenomenon can also occur (Lévigne *et al.*, 1990).

References

Chaouat Y., Aron-Brunietiere R., Faures B., Binet O., Ginet C. & Aubard D. (1980) Une nouvelle entité: Le rheumatisme fibroblastique. A propos d'une observation. *Rev. Rheumatol.* **47**, 345–351.

Lévigne V., Perrot J.L., Faisant M., Deville V. & Claudy A.L. (1990) Rheumatisme fibroblastique. *Ann. Dermatol. Venereol.* **117**, 199–202.

Vignon-Pennamen M.D., Navran B., Foldes C. *et al.* (1986) Fibroblastic rheumatism. *J. Am. Acad. Dermatol.* **14**, 1086–1088.

Osteoarthritis

Leuconychia, longitudinal grooves and nail ridging have been reported in patients with primary interphalangeal osteoarthritis of the hand. Osteoarthritic changes of the distal interphalangeal joints may cause nail lesions by exerting direct pressure on the nail matrix or by interfering with local blood flow. Inflammation of Heberden's nodes seems to participate in the development of the nail alterations. Mucinous (myxoid) cysts are frequently observed (Cutolo *et al.*, 1990).

Reference

Cutolo M., Cimmino M.A. & Accardo S. (1990) Nail involvement in osteoarthritis. *Clin. Rheum.* **9**, 242–245.

Immunological disorders

Primary immunological deficiency syndromes

Susceptibility to infections is a typical feature of congenital hypogammaglobulinaemias. Pyoderma can affect periungual tissues causing acute paronychia. A 10-month-old boy affected by trachyonychia involving all fingernails and toenails (twenty-nail dystrophy) and selective IgA deficiency has been reported (Leong *et al.*, 1982). Chronic mucocutaneous candidiasis and pyoderma are frequently found in severe combined immunodeficiency (Roberts & Weismann, 1986). Dystrophic nails are a feature of Zinsser–Engman–Cole syndrome and koilonychia has been described in the Nezelof syndrome (Roberts & Weismann, 1986). In biotine-responsive multiple carboxylase deficiencies candidal paronychia and onychodystrophy may occur. Patients with immunodeficiency and short-limbed dwarfism exhibit short, stubby hands and extremities (Ammann, 1987). In Wiskott–Aldrich syndrome, characterized by the triad of thrombocytopaenia, atopic eczema and recurrent infections, acute paronychia as well as nail pitting and transverse ridging due to atopic eczema can occur. Intense scratching results in a polished shiny surface of the nails.

Persistent *Candida* infections of the skin, nails and mucous membranes occur in chronic mucocutaneous candidiasis, and nail involvement can occasionally be the sole manifestation of the condition (Ammann, 1987). Chronic paronychia is commonly observed. *Candida* invasion of the nail plate produces thickening, distortion and fragmentation of the nail keratin (Palestine *et al.*, 1983). A combination of dermatophyte and *Candida* infection may be seen. Fingertips can show a bulbous appearance (Goslen & Kobayashi, 1987).

Elevated levels of IgE, eczematoid skin lesions and recurrent cold staphylococcal abscesses are the characteristic features of Job's syndrome (hyper-IgE syndrome), where acute paronychia, atrophic changes, mild clubbing and chronic candidal infection of the fingernails can occur (Davis *et al.*, 1966).

Osteomyelitis of the distal phalanges has been reported in three children with severe atopic dermatitis. The insidious onset of distal wedge-shaped subungual black macules was followed by oedema, erythema and pain in the involved fingers (Boiko *et al.*, 1988). The occurrence of osteomyelitis can be a consequence of the decreased cutaneous resistance to bacteria in atopic dermatitis coupled with repetitive scratching of infected skin that collected necrotic keratin and bacteria beneath the distal nail plate.

References

Ammann A.J. (1987) Cutaneous manifestations of immunodeficiency disorders. In: *Dermatology in General Medicine*, eds Fitzpatrick T.B., Eisen A.Z., Wolff K., Freedberg I.M. & Austen K.F., pp. 2507–2522. McGraw Hill, New York.

Boiko S., Kaufman R.A. & Lucky A.W. (1988) Osteomyelitis of the distal phalanges in three children with severe atopic dermatitis. *Arch. Dermatol.* **124**, 418–423.

Davis S.D., Schaller J. & Wedgwood R.J. (1966) Job's syndrome. *Lancet* **i**, 1013–1015.

Goslen J.B. & Kobayashi G.S. (1987) Fungal diseases with cutaneous involvement. In: *Dermatology in General Medicine*, eds Fitzpatrick T.B., Eisen A.Z., Wolff K., Freedberg I.M. & Austen K.F., pp. 2193–2248. McGraw Hill, New York.

Leong A.B., Gange R.W. & O'Connor R.D. (1982) Twenty-nail dystrophy (trachyonychia) associated with selective Ig-A deficiency. *J. Pediatr.* **100**, 418–419.

Palestine R.F., Su W.P.D. & Liesegang T.J. (1983) Late-onset chronic mucocutaneous and ocular candidiasis and malignant thymoma. *Arch. Dermatol.* **119**, 580–586.

Roberts S.O.B. & Weismann K. (1986) The skin in systemic disease. In: *Textbook of Dermatology*, eds Rook A., Wilkinson D.S., Ebling F.J.G., Champion R.H. & Burton J.L., pp. 2343–2347. Blackwell Scientific Publications, Oxford.

Therapeutical immunosuppression

Paronychia and onychomycosis can be seen in patients undergoing therapeutic immunosuppression. Norwegian scabies can also occur. Blistering distal dactylitis due to haemolytic *Staphylococcus aureus* has been described in an adult patient taking high doses of systemic steroids for the treatment of Crohn's disease (Zemtsov & Veitschegger, 1992).

Reference

Zemtsov A. & Veitschegger M. (1992) *Staphylococcus aureus* induced blistering distal dactylitis in adult immunosuppressed patient. *J. Am. Acad. Dermatol.* **26**, 784–785.

Graft-versus-host disease (GVHD)

(see Table 6.5)

Acral erythema is a frequent manifestation of acute cutaneous GVHD and may first appear as reddening of the tips of the fingers and periungual skin (Horwitz & Dreizen, 1990). A violaceous hue of periungual tissues has also been described (Farmer & Hood, 1987). Onychomadesis is possible.

In chronic GVHD, nail changes can closely resemble nail lichen planus. Longitudinal ridging, brittleness, roughness and even partial or complete atrophy of the nails may be observed as well as pterygium formation (Liddle & Cowan, 1990). Superficial ulcerations of the lunula (elkonyxis) have been described. Periungual erythema with swelling, nail plate opacification, thickening and onycholysis can also occur (James & Odom, 1983). Cuticular telangiectasia may be seen in the scleroderma-like changes resulting from GVHD. Secondary fungal infections are not uncommon. Mascaro and Martin-Ortega (1993) reported a series of 40 patients who presented nail alterations in relation to GVHD (Table 6.5). Nail changes were more frequent in chronic lichenoid phase and were associated with cutaneous lesions of GVHD or only with oral manifestation. Onychomycosis and nail infection were uncommon. Immunophenotyping of inflammatory cells performed on the nail biopsy of a child who developed a severe lichen planus-like onychodystrophy after transfusion of non-irradiated blood, showed a prevalence of T-suppressor lymphocytes and epidermal expression of HLA-Dr (Ia) antigens (Brun *et al.*, 1985).

White superficial onychomycosis due to *Trichophyton rubrum* was the initial cutaneous presentation of chronic GVHD in Basuk and Scher's patient (1987). Differential diagnosis of cutaneous and nail manifestations of chronic GVHD includes dyskeratosis congenita, a rare genodermatosis that frequently requires bone marrow transplantation because of pancytopaenia (Ling *et al.*, 1985; Esterly, 1986).

Table 6.5. Nail alterations in GVHD (courtesy of J. Mascaro, Barcelona)

Nail alteration	Acute GVHD N/N (total 12)	Chronic GVHD N/N (total 28)
Leuconychia	3/12	3/28
Melanonychia	2/12	2/28
Yellow nail syndrome	0/12	1/28
Loss of brightness	0/12	13/28
Bed haemorrhages	1/12	3/28
Cuticular haemorrhages	0/12	2/28
Bed erythema	6/12	6/28
Periungual erythema	11/12	22/28
Fingertip erythema	7/12	8/28
Dorsal pterygium	0/12	4/28
Subungual hyperkeratosis	0/12	6/28
Cuticular hyperkeratosis	6/12	3/28
Onychomadesis	2/12	5/28
Onycholysis	5/12	13/28
Nail atrophy	0/12	4/28
Pachyonychia	0/12	3/28
Trachyonychia	2/12	19/28
Onychorrhexis	3/12	15/28
Onychoschizia	0/12	5/28
V-shaped onychoschizia	0/12	1/28
Longitudinal ridges	7/12	28/28
Transversal ridges	2/12	6/28
Beau's lines	0/12	4/28
Pitting	0/12	1/28
Bed erosions	0/12	3/28
Onychomycosis (*C. albicans*)	0/12	1/28

References

Basuk P.J. & Scher R.K. (1987) Onychomycosis in graft versus host disease. *Cutis* **40**, 237–241.

Brun P., Baran R., Desbas C. & Czernielewski J. (1985) Dystrophie lichénienne isolée des 20 ongles. Etude en immunofluorescence par les anticorps monoclonaux. Conséquences pathologiques. *Ann. Dermatol. Venereol.* **112**, 215.

Esterly N.B. (1986) Nail dystrophy in dyskeratosis congenita and chronic graft-versus-host disease. *Arch. Dermatol.* **12**, 506–507.

Farmer E.R. & Hood A.F. (1987) Graft-versus-host disease. In: *Dermatology in General Medicine*, eds Fitzpatrick T.B., Eisen A.Z., Wolff K., Freedberg I.M. & Austen K.F., pp. 1344–1352. McGraw Hill, New York.

Horwitz L.J. & Dreizen J. (1990) Acral erythema induced by chemotherapy and graft-versus-host disease in adults with hematogenous malignancies. *Cutis* **46**, 397–404.

James W.D. & Odom R.B. (1983) Graft-versus-host disease. *Arch. Dermatol.* **119**, 683–689.

Liddle B.J. & Cowan M.A. (1990) Lichen planus-like eruption and nail changes in a patient with graft-versus-host disease. *Br. J. Dermatol.* **122**, 841–843.

Ling N.S., Fenske N.A., Julius R.L., Espinoza C.G. & Drake L.A. (1985) Dyskeratosis congenita in a girl simulating chronic graft-versus-host disease. *Arch. Dermatol.* **121**, 1424–1428.

Mascaro J.M. & Martin-Ortega E. (1993) Nail alterations in graft versus host disease and other immunological disorders. In: *Dermatology Progress and Perspectives*. The Parthenon Publishing Group, New York.

Behçet's disease

Proximal nail fold capillaroscopy of patients with Behçet's disease frequently reveals non-specific abnormalities (Wechsler *et al.*, 1984). Subungual flame-shaped haemorrhagic lesions that are probably due to nail bed vasculitis have also been described (O'Duffy *et al.*, 1971; Casanova *et al.*, 1986; Cornelis *et al.*, 1989). Sabin *et al.* (1990) reported a patient who had Behçet's disease and half-and-half nails.

References

Casanova J.M., Delgado S., Menéndez F., Bueno C. & Làzaro P. (1986) Hemorragias subungueales en el curso de la enfermedad de Behçet. *Acta Derm. Sif.* 77, 137–141.

Cornelis F., Sigal-Nahum M., Gaulier A., Bleichner G. & Sigal S. (1989) Behçet's disease with severe cutaneous necrotizing vasculitis: response to plasma exchange. Report of a case. *J. Am. Acad. Dermatol.* **21**, 576–579.

O'Duffy J.D., Carney J.A. & Deodhar S. (1971) Behçet's disease. Report of 10 cases, 3 with new manifestations. *Ann. Intern. Med.* 75, 561–570.

Sabin A.A., Kalyoncu A.F., Toros Z., Coplu L., Celebi C. & Baris Y.I. (1990) Behçhet's disease with half-and-half nail and pulmonary artery aneurysm. *Chest* **97**, 1277.

Wechsler B., Huong Du L.T., Mouthon J.M., Cabane J. & Godeau P. (1984) Aspects capillaroscopiques péri-unguéaux au cours de la maladie de Behçet. *Ann. Dermatol. Venereol.* **111**, 543–550.

Vitiligo

Nail changes similar to many of those seen with alopecia areata (see Chapter 5) may occur, but only rarely.

HIV diseases and acquired immune deficiency syndrome (AIDS)

Fungal, viral and bacterial infections may affect the nails either primarily or secondarily in patients with AIDS (Daniel *et al.*, 1992). Mucocutaneous candidiasis is a common manifestation of HIV infection. Acute and chronic paronychia as well as total dystrophic onychomycosis due to *Candida albicans* are frequently observed (Kaplan *et al.*, 1987). Onychomycosis due to dermatophytes is also frequent and *T. rubrum* is the most common isolated organism, which may even involve periungual tissues (Fischer & Warner, 1987; Kaplan et al., 1987; Torssander *et al.*, 1988; Prose, 1990). Proximal white subungual onychomycosis due to *T. rubrum* is common in AIDS (Dompmartin *et al.*, 1990). This clinical form of onychomycosis, which is rarely encountered in HIV-negative patients, starts as an irregular white patch that appears from beneath the proximal nail fold and progressively extends distally to involve the whole nail plate (Noppakun & Head, 1986; Weismann *et al.*, 1988). *Pityrosporum ovale* was the only microorganism isolated in two patients with AIDS who presented a total dystrophic onychomycosis of all fingernails (Dompmartin *et al.*, 1990). It is interesting how changes in the immune response can modify the pathogenic effect of the invading organism. For example, *T. rubrum*, which does not often produce superficial white onychomycosis (a clinical pattern of infection resulting usually from *T. mentagrophytes* var. *interdigitale* and some moulds), is now responsible for most such cases in HIV-positive individuals. Moreover, another feature of the altered immune response is characterized by the finding of multiple involvement of several digits with proximal subungual onychomycosis of rapid onset. *Scopulariopsis brevicaulis* infection leading to destruction of fingernails and toenails has been reported in AIDS.

Periungual warts are common and frequently recur after removal. A severe herpetic whitlow may also be the first sign of the disease (Cockerell, 1990). This has also been described in children with AIDS (Prose, 1990). Herpes simplex infections frequently produce atypical cutaneous manifestations in patients with AIDS. Baden *et al.* (1991) described a 35-year-old man with AIDS who exhibited gangrenous lesions of the fingers due to herpes simplex virus. Dramatic improvement was seen after intravenous acyclovir treatment. Norwegian scabies can occur in patients with HIV infection and cause dystrophic nails with subungual crusting (Jucowics *et al.*, 1989; Inserra & Bickley, 1990; Aricó *et al.*, 1992).

Typical nail changes of Reiter's syndrome and psoriasis can be observed in patients with HIV infection (Fischer & Warner, 1987; Cockerell, 1990). Splinter haemorrhages have also been seen (Kaplan *et al.*, 1987). Digital clubbing has been reported in infants with AIDS (Scott *et al.*, 1984). Yellow discoloration of the distal portion of some nails is a frequent finding in HIV-infected patients. Although originally described under the diagnosis of yellow nail syndrome (Chernosky & Finley, 1985), the yellow discoloration of the nails observed in patients with HIV infection is a different condition. Typical nail changes of YNS such as reduced nail growth, nail plate overcurvature, scleronychia and loss of cuticles are not observed. Colour changes can be preceded by opacification and decreased size or loss of the lunulae. Onycholysis at the distal part of the lateral nail folds as well as transverse and/or longitudinal ridging can be present. Great toenails are most commonly involved whereas fingernails are only rarely affected. Asymmetrical involvement of several nails is usual. Yellow toenail changes have been considered together with seborrhoeic dermatitis, hairy leukoplakia and oral candidiasis as possible indicators of progression to established AIDS in HIV-positive patients (Morfeld-Manson *et al.*, 1989). Although dermatophytes have been suggested as a contributing factor in the development of

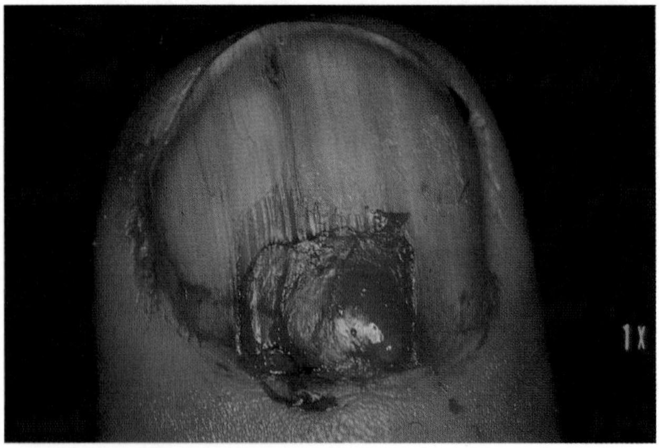

Fig. 6.62. AIDS – Kaposi's sarcoma.

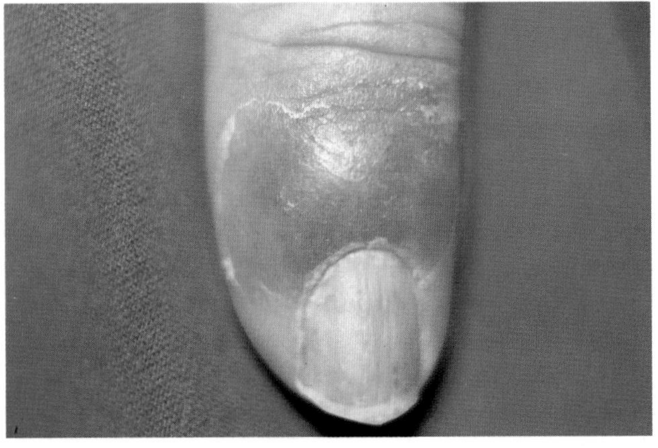

Fig. 6.63. AIDS – Kaposi's sarcoma.

yellow nails, bacterial and mycological cultures usually fail to reveal any infectious microorganisms.

A lichenoid dermatitis associated with nail changes has been described in a 39-year-old man with AIDS. The nail plates were thinned and the distal margin of the lunula presented an irregular border and longitudinal bands. Splinter haemorrhages and periungual lichenoid papules were also present (Buchner *et al.*, 1989).

Generalized lichen spinulosus was accompanied by extensive onychodystrophy in a HIV-positive male (Cohen & Dicken, 1991).

Patients with AIDS or AIDS-related complex may develop Beau's lines following episodes of severe illness (Prose *et al.*, 1992).

Diffuse nail pigmentation as well as longitudinal or transverse hyperpigmented bands are frequently seen in HIV-positive patients receiving AZT (zidovudine). Multiple longitudinal melanonychia as well as hyperpigmented macules on the palms, soles and mucous membranes unrelated to AZT treatment have also been described in AIDS. The serum levels of α-MSH were significantly increased in one patient (Fisher & Warner, 1987; Gallais *et al.*, 1992). Mild bluish pigmentation of fingernails and toenails has been observed in two black patients with newly diagnosed HIV infection (Chandrasekar, 1989).

Kaposi's sarcoma can involve the nail area (Friedman-Kien & Saltzman, 1990; Dompmartin *et al.*, 1990). A periungual Kaposi's sarcoma resembling a chronic paronychia has been reported in a patient with AIDS (Fischer & Warner, 1987) (Fig. 6.63).

Subungual squamous cell carcinoma has also been described (Daniel, 1993), and it is usually associated with HPV 16 infection. Onychophagia and onychotillomania are not uncommon (Valenzano *et al.*, 1988).

References

Aricò M., Noto G., La Rocca E. *et al.* (1992) Localized crusted scabies in the acquired immunodeficiency syndrome. *Clin. Exp. Dermatol.* **17**, 339–341.

Baden L.A., Bigby M. & Kwan T. (1991) Persistent necrotic digits in a patient with the acquired immunodeficiency syndrome. *Arch. Dermatol.* **127**, 113–114.

Buchner S.A., Itin P., Rufli T. & Hungerbuhler U. (1989) Disseminated lichenoid papular dermatosis with nail changes in acquired immunodeficiency syndrome: clinical, histological and immunohistochemical considerations. *Dermatologica* **179**, 99–101.

Chandrasekar P.H. (1989) Nail discoloration and human immunodeficiency virus infection. *Am. J. Med.* **86**, 506–507.

Chernosky M.E. & Finley V.K. (1985) Yellow nail syndrome in patients with acquired immunodeficiency disease. *J. Am. Acad. Dermatol.* **13**, 731–736.

Cockerell C.J. (1990) Cutaneous manifestations of HIV infection other than Kaposi's sarcoma: clinical and histologic aspects. *J. Am. Acad. Dermatol.* **22**, 1260–1269.

Cohen S.J. & Dicken C.H. (1991) Generalized lichen spinulosus in a HIV-positive man. *J. Am. Acad. Dermatol.* **25**, 116–118.

Daniel C.R. (1993) Nail disease in patients with HIV infection. In: *Dermatology Progress and Perspectives, 18th World Congress*, eds Burgdorf W.H.C. & Katz S.I., pp. 382–385. Parthenon Publishing Group, New York.

Daniel C.R., Norton L.A. & Scher R.K. (1992) The spectrum of nail disease in patients with HIV infection. *J. Am. Acad. Dermatol.* **27**, 93–97.

Dompmartin D., Dompmartin A., Deluol A.M., Grosshans E. & Conland J.P. (1990) Onychomycosis and AIDS. Clinical and laboratory findings in 62 patients. *Int. J. Dermatol.* **29**, 337–339.

Feital de Carvalho M.T., Fischman O., Mota de Avelar Alchorne M. *et al.* Onychomycosis in patients who are bearers of AIDS. *An. Bras. Dermatol.* **66**, 113–116.

Fischer B.K. & Warner L.C. (1987) Cutaneous manifestations of the acquired immunodeficiency syndrome. *Int. J. Dermatol.* **276**, 615–630.

Friedman-Kien A.E. & Saltzman B.R. (1990) Clinical manifestations of classical, endemic African and epidemic AIDS-associated Kaposi's sarcoma. *J. Am. Acad. Dermatol.* **22**, 1237–1250.

Gallais V., Lacour J.P., Perrin C. *et al.* (1992) Acral hyperpigmented macules and longitudinal melanonychia in AIDS. *Br. J. Dermatol.* **126**, 387–391.

Inserra D.W. & Bickley L.K. (1990) Crusted scabies in acquired immunodeficiency syndrome. *Int. J. Dermatol.* **29**, 287–289.

Jucowics P., Ramon M.E., Don P.C., Stone R.K. & Bamji M. (1989) Norwegian scabies in an infant with acquired immunodeficiency syndrome *Arch. Dermatol.* **125**, 1670–1671.

Kaplan M.H., Sadick N., McNutt S., Meltzer M., Sarngadharan M.G. & Pahwa S. (1987) Dermatologic findings and manifestations of acquired immunodeficiency syndrome *J. Am. Acad. Dermatol.* **16**, 485–506.

Lacour J.P., Gallais V., Bodokh I., Ghanem G. & Ortonne J.P. (1991) Hyperpigmentations cutaneo-muqueuses au cours du SIDA. *IIeme Journéee Franco-Italienne de Dermatologie de la Riviera*, p. 45.

Morfeld-Manson L., Julander I. & Nillson B. (1989) Dermatitis of the face, yellow toe nail changes, hairy leukoplakia and oral candidiasis are clinical indicators of progression to AIDS opportunistic infection in patients with HIV infection. *Scand. J. Infect. Dis.* **21**, 497–505.

Noppakun N. & Head E. (1986) Proximal white subungual onychomycosis in a patient with acquired immune deficiency syndrome. *Int. J. Dermatol.* **25**, 586–587.

Prose N.S. (1990) HIV infection in children. *J. Am. Acad Dermatol.* **22**, 1223–1231.

Prose N.S., Abran K.G. & Scher (1992) Disorders of the nail and hair associated with human immunodeficiency infection. *Int. J. Dermatol.* **31**, 453–457.

Scott G.B., Buck B.E., Laterman J.G., Bloom F.L. & Parks W.P. (1984) Acquired immunodeficiency syndrome in infants. *New Engl. J. Med.* **310**, 76–81.

Torssander J., Karlsson A., Morfeld-Manson L., Putkamen P.O. & Wasserman J. (1988) Dermatophytosis and HIV infection. *Acta Dermatol. Venereol.* **68**, 53–56.

Valenzano L., Giacalone B., Grillo L.R. *et al.* (1988) Compromis sione ungueale in corps di AIDS. *G. Ital. Derm. Venereol.* **123**, 527–528.

Weismann K., Knudsen E.A. & Pedersen C. (1988) White nails in AIDS/ARC due to *Trichophyton rubrum* infection. *Clin. Exp. Dermatol.* **13**, 24–25.

Infectious diseases (see also Chapters 4 and 7)

Acute febrile illness and some systemic diseases may produce transverse linear grooves (Beau's lines) with slightly elevated proximal ridging resulting from matrix damage. All nails of the fingers and toes are usually involved but this change may occasionally be restricted to the thumbs and great toes. In severe cases the nail becomes detached (Figs 6.64 & 6.65(a) & (b)) but usually the grooves are superficial. The lines appear from under the cuticle at about 1 month after the acute illness and grow forward as the nail grows, thereby giving a way of assessing the date at which the illness began. Transverse leukonychia may have the same significance as Beau's lines.

Malaria

Changes in nail colour occur during acute episodes. Immediately prior to the fever, the nails become pale grey and this is maintained throughout the pyrexia. Subungual haemorrhages, striate leuconychia and koilonychia are described in quartan malaria as are multiple transverse, dark brown lines and furrows. Beau's lines may occur following infection with *Plasmodium vivax malaria* (Glew & Howard, 1973).

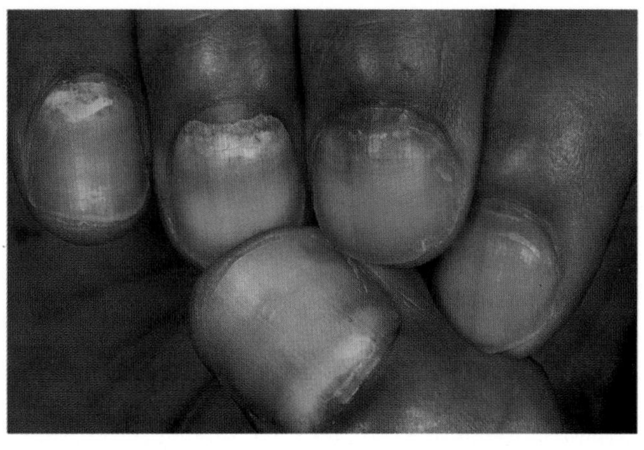

Fig. 6.64. Toxic epidermal necrolysis (bacterial type) – early nail sheddings.

Reference

Glew R.H. & Howard W.A. (1973) Transverse furrows of the nails associated with *Plasmodium vivax malaria. J. Hopkins Med. J.* **132**, 61–64.

Kawasaki disease (mucocutaneous lymph node syndrome – MCLS)

In this disease, affecting children from 6 months to 10 years of age, rarely adults (Butler *et al.*, 1987; Beau's lines may develop in the nail plate 1 or 2 months after onset of the illness in 94% of patients, and complete shedding of the nails and telogen effluvium can be seen (Traedwell, 1987). Transient apparent leuconychia reported by Iosub and Gromish (1984) in three patients with involvement of most fingernails and toes characteristically occurs 14 days after the onset of symptoms at the skin–nail junctions. This sign is the major feature used to distinguish MCLS from other similar entities (Kawasaki *et al.*, 1974). Late changes include fissuring of the nail beds and peeling of fingernails (Levin & Dillon, 1992). Ischemic necrosis of the extremities is a rare complication (Ames *et al.*, 1985).

References

Ames E.L., Jones J.S., Van Dommelen B. *et al.* (1985) Bilateral hand necrosis in Kawasaki syndrome. *J. Hand Surg.* **10A**, 391–395.

Butler D.F., Hough D.R., Friedman S.J. *et al.* (1987) Adult Kawasaki syndrome. *Arch. Dermatol.* **123**, 1356–1361.

Iosub S. & Gromish D.S. (1984) Leuconychia partialis in Kawasaki disease. *J. Infect. Dis.* **150**, 617–618.

Kawasaki T., Kosaki F. & Okawa S. (1974) A new infantile acute febrile mucocutaneous lymph node syndrome prevailing in Japan. *Paediatrics* **54**, 271–276.

Levin M. & Dillon M.J. (1992) Kawasaki disease. In: *Recent Advances in Dermatology*, eds Champion R. & Pye R.J. Churchill Livingstone, Edinburgh.

Treadwell P.A. (1987) Kawasaki disease. In: *Advances in Der-*

matology, eds Callen J.P., Dahl H.V., Golitz L.E., Rasmussen J.E. & Stegman S.J., Vol. 2, pp. 112–116. Year Book Medical Publishers, Chicago.

Cutaneous diphtheria

Cutaneous diphtheria has become a rare disease following widespread immunization; however cases of cutaneous diphtheria have recently been reported in travellers to endemic areas (Antos *et al.*, 1992) and in a patient with AIDS (Haliova *et al.*, 1992).

From a clinical aspect, cutaneous diphtheria typically begins looking like a pustule, and then becomes a slightly depressed round-shaped ulceration varying in size from 0.5 cm to a few centimetres in diameter, with inflammatory edges covered with a false membrane which bleeds after being scraped off. The natural anaesthetic, even hypoaesthetic nature of the lesion is emphasized by most of the authors. Within 1–3 weeks, the false membrane becomes a blackish scab, which rapidly falls off giving way to an atrophic scar. Cutaneous diphtheria is usually found on the lower and upper limbs. Differential diagnosis includes impetigo, echthyma and even eczema (Livingood *et al.*, 1946; Bixby, 1948).

Thus, cutaneous diphtheria most often appears on pre-existing dermatological lesions, such as traumatic wounds, burns and dermatosis (impetigo, pyodermites, insects bites).

References

Antos H., Mollison L.C., Richards M.J., Boquest A.L. & Tosolini F.A. (1992) Diphtheria: another risk of travel. *J. Infection* **25**, 307–310.

Bixby E.W. (1948) Cutaneous diphtheria. *Arch. Derm. Syph.* **58**, 381–384.

Haliova B., Patey O., Casciani D. *et al.* (1992) Diphtérie cutanée chez un patient infecté par le virus de l'immunodeficience humaine (VIH). *Ann. Dermatol. Venereol.* **119**, 874–877.

Livingood C.S., Perry D.J. & Forrest J.S. (1946) Cutaneous diphtheria: a report of 140 cases. *J. Invest. Dermatol.* **7**, 341–364.

Haematological disorders

Blood groups

Determination of blood groups can be performed on nail clippings (Garg, 1983; Wegener & Bulnheim, 1990).

References

Garg R.K. (1983) Determination of ABO (H) blood specific substances from fingernails. *Am. J. Forens. Med. Pathol.* **4**, 143–144.

Wegener R. & Bulnheim U. (1990) Determination of ABO antigens in fingernails using the APAAP (immunoalkaline phosphatase) technique. *Forens. Sci. Int.* **46**, 11–14.

Polycythaemia

Red nail beds are seen in polycythaemia. Ischaemic acral necrosis and/or ulcers can be caused by peripheral arterial occlusions (Fagrell & Mellstedt, 1978). A lamellar dystrophy of the nails has been reported in two patients affected by polycythaemia rubra vera. In one of them, improvement of the dystrophy was noticed after treatment of polycythaemia (Graham-Brown & Holmes, 1980). Erythromelalgia can occur in association with polycythaemia. Koilonychia has been reported by De Nicola *et al.* (1974).

References

De Nicola P., Morsiani M. & Zavagli G. (1974) *Nail Diseases in Internal Medicine*, p. 79. Charles C. Thomas, Springfield, IL.

Fagrell B. & Mellstedt H. (1978) Polycythaemia vera as a cause of ischemic digital necrosis. *Acta Chir. Scand.* **144**, 129–132.

Graham-Brown R.A.C. & Holmes R. (1980) Polycythaemia rubra vera with lamellar dystrophy of the nails: a report of two cases. *Clin. Exp. Dermatol.* **5**, 209–212.

Essential thrombocythaemia

Cutaneous manifestations of essential thrombocythaemia include erythromelalgia, livedo reticularis and microvascular occlusive events that may lead to gangrene of toes and fingers (Itin & Winkelmann, 1991). Painful ulcerated and necrotic lesions are especially observed on the distal parts of limbs, in particular the toes (Velasco *et al.*, 1991). Acrocyanosis and Raynaud's phenomenon have also been reported (Itin & Wilkelmann, 1991).

References

Itin P.H. & Winkelmann R.K. (1991) Cutaneous manifestations in patients with essential thrombocythemia. *J. Am. Acad. Dermatol.* **24**, 59–63.

Velasco J.A., Santos J.C., Bravo J. & Santana J. (1991) Ulceronecrotic lesions in a patient with essential thrombocythaemia. *Clin. Exp. Dermatol.* **16**, 53–54.

Haemoglobinopathies

Symmetrical peripheral gangrene can be observed in patients with sickle cell anaemia. Phalangeal osteomyelitis has also been described (Haltalin & Nelson, 1965). Mee's lines have been reported by Hudson and Dennis (1966). Cyanosis of the lunulae is a typical sign of nigraemia, a rare hereditary disease that is associated with the presence of an abnormal haemoglobin (haemoglobin M) (Tamura, 1964).

References

Haltalin K.C. & Nelson J.D. (1965) Hand–foot syndrome due to streptococcal infections. *Dermatol. Clin.* **109**, 156–159.

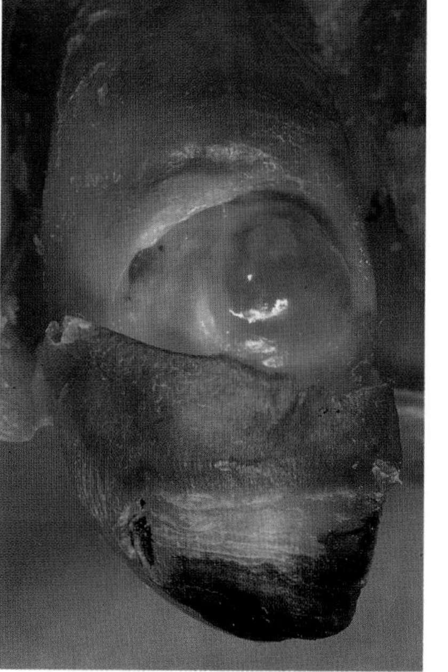

(a)

(b)

Fig. 6.65. Toxic epidermal necrolysis: (a) nail shedding; (b) after healing.

Hudson J.B. & Dennis A.J. (1966) Transverse white lines in the fingernails after acute and chronic renal failure. *Arch. Intern. Med.* **117**, 276–279.

Tamura A (1964) Nigremia. *Jap. J. Human Gen.* 9, 183–192.

Anaemias

Pallor of the nail bed and reduction or absence of the lunula are frequently observed in anaemias, with decrease of linear nail growth rate (De Nicola *et al.*, 1974). Splinter haemorrhages can occur. Nail brittleness, ridging and koilonychia are commonly reported in hypochromic anaemia (see also p. 196). Reversible shedding of fingernails and toenails has been described in one patient (Handfield-Jones & Kennedy, 1988). Bluish-black discoloration of fingernails and toenails rarely appears in patients with megaloblastic anaemia (Carmel, 1985) (see p. 195). Transverse leuconychia of fingernails and toenails has been reported in a patient with immunohaemolytic anaemia associated with warm-reacting antibodies (Marino, 1990).

References

Carmel R. (1985) Hair and fingernail changes in acquired and congenital pernicious anemia. *Arch. Intern. Med.* **145**, 484–485.

De Nicola P., Morsiani M. & Zavagli G. (1974) *Nail Diseases in Internal Medicine*, pp. 79–80. Charles C. Thomas, Springfield, IL.

Handfield-Jones S.E. & Kennedy C.T.C. (1988) Nail dystrophy associated with iron deficiency anemia. *Clin. Exp. Dermatol.* **13**, 54.

Marino M.T. (1990) Mees' lines. *Arch. Dermatol.* **126**, 827–828.

Hereditary haemorrhagic telangiectasia (Osler–Rendu–Weber syndrome)

Subungual telangiectasia and haemorrhages occur in patients with Osler–Rendu–Weber syndrome (De Nicola *et al.*, 1974) (Fig. 6.66). Capillaroscopy of the proximal nail fold can reveal the presence of giant capillaries (Maire *et al.*, 1986).

References

De Nicola P., Morsiani M., Zavagli G. (1974) *Nail Diseases in Internal Medicine*, pp. 79–80. Charles C. Thomas, Springfield, IL.

Maire R., Schnewlin G. & Bollinger A. (1986) Videomikroskopische Untersuchungen von Teleangiektasien bei Morbus Osler und Sklerodermie. *Schweiz Med. Wschr.* **116**, 335–338.

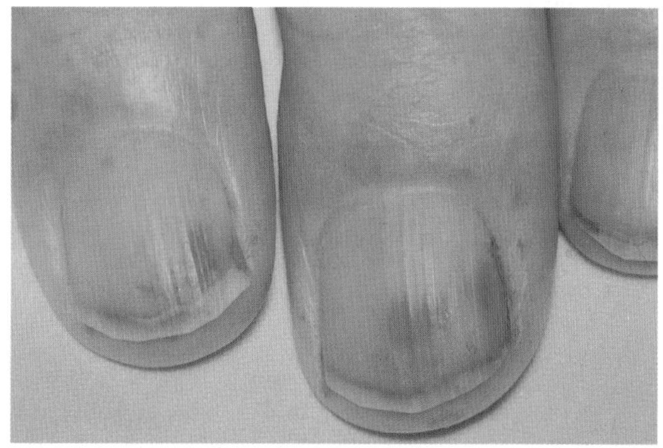

Fig. 6.66. Hereditary haemorrhagic telangiectasia (Osler–Rendu–Weber) (courtesy of L. Juhlin, Uppsala, Sweden).

Leukaemias

See p. 234.

Plasmocytoma

See p. 235.

Lymphoma

See p. 235.

Hodgkin's disease

See p. 237.

Gamma heavy chain disease

This condition, which mainly occurs in association with lymphoproliferative and autoimmune disorders, is characterized by the presence in serum and urine of a structurally abnormal heavy chain devoid of light chains. Cutaneous lesions are the most frequent extrahaematopoietic manifestations of the disease. A patient with gamma heavy chain disease developed cutaneous nodules, livedo reticularis and digital necrosis caused by necrotizing vasculitis (Lassoned *et al.*, 1990).

Reference

Lassoned K., Picard C., Danon F. *et al.* (1990) Cutaneous manifestations associated with gamma heavy chain disease. *J. Am. Acad. Dermatol.* **23**, 988–991.

Cryoglobulinaemia (Fig. 6.67)

Livedo reticularis, Raynaud's phenomenon and painful digital necrosis can be observed in cryoglobulinaemia, particularly in patients with type 1 or type 2 cryoglobulinaemia (Garceau *et al.*, 1990).

Reference

Garceau S., Gilbert M., Marceau D. & Cloutier R. (1990) A propos d'un cas de nécrose d'un doigt. *Rev. Eur. Dermatol. MTS* **2**, 590–593.

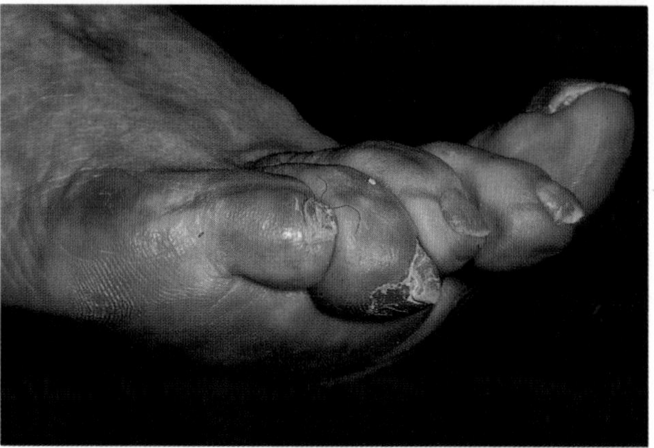

Fig. 6.67. Cryoglobulinaemia.

Neoplastic disorders

Langerhans' cell histiocytosis

Nail involvement in histiocytosis X (Langerhans' cell histiocytosis) is rare (Esterly *et al.*, 1985) and has been considered to represent an unfavourable prognostic sign (Timpatanapong *et al.*, 1984). It has been reported both in patients with Letterer–Siwe disease and in those with Hand–Schuller–Christian disease, but not in patients with eosinophilic granuloma of the bone. Nail changes can be observed in both fingernails and toenails.

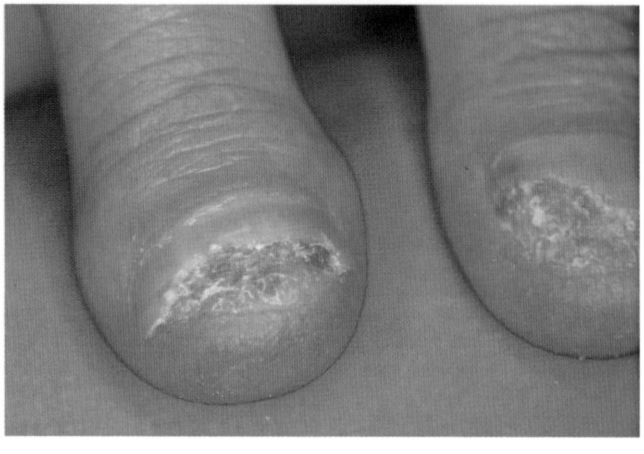

Fig. 6.68. Langerhans' cell histiocytosis – nail lesions.

Erythema and swelling of periungual tissues resembling chronic paronychia along with subungual hyperkeratosis and onycholysis are the most frequent findings (Fig. 6.68). Small pustules of the nail bed and subungual haemorrhages or purpuric macules can occur (Harper & Staughton, 1983). Paronychia with subungual purpura is quite specific for histiocytosis X. Nail pitting, longitudinal grooving, distal splitting as well as nail plate thickening, elkonyxis and onychomadesis have also been reported (de Berbler *et al.*, 1993). Specific infiltration by CD1+ histiocyte-like cells produced persistent and progressive destruction of the thumb nail plates in a patient with Hand–Schuller–Christian disease (Alsina *et al.*, 1991).

Histology

Involvement of the nails is histologically characterized by subepithelial infiltrate of atypical histiocytes with reniform

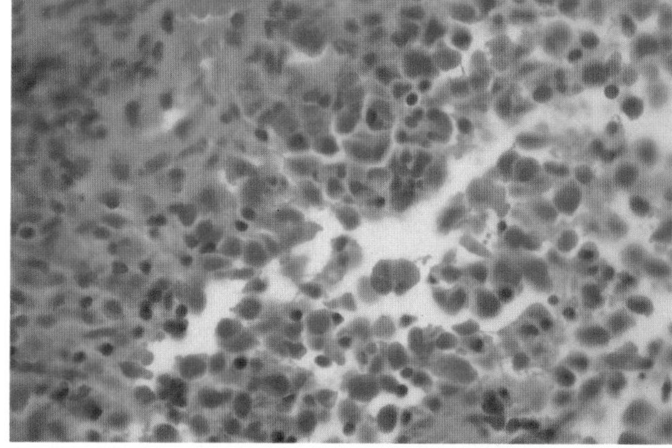

Fig. 6.69. Infiltrate in biopsy from nail lesion.

nuclei and usually abundant cytoplasm. These cells migrate into the epidermis causing slight spongiosis and some intraepithelial cell accumulations. There is usually subepidermal oedema and admixture of lymphocytes and a variable number of eosinophils. The atypical histiocytes express the CD1-antigen (OKT6), protein S-100 and are stained with peanut agglutinin. Electron microscopy usually reveals abundant Langerhans' cells (Birbeck) granules which sometimes are in continuity with the cell membrane.

Focal collections of atypical histiocytes with large hyperchromatic and pleomorphic nuclei were detected in the proximal nail fold, matrix and nail bed (Fig. 6.69) of a 21-month-old child affected by Letterer–Siwe disease. Electron microscopy and S100 protein staining confirmed that the infiltration was formed by Langerhans' cells (Holzberg *et al.*, 1985).

Nail changes occasionally respond to antineoplastic therapy but usually recur when the disease progresses (Timpatanapong *et al.*, 1984). A child is reported who, despite severe nail involvement, showed spontaneous remission of her disease (Ellis, 1985).

Juvenile xanthogranuloma can rarely affect the fingers (Sonoda *et al.*, 1985; Yamashita *et al.*, 1990). A solitary xanthogranuloma of the second left toenail has been reported in a 1.5-year-old boy. The nail appearance resembled onychogryphosis (Frumkin *et al.*, 1987).

References

Alsina M.M., Zamora E., Ferrando J., Mascaro J. & Conget J.I. (1991) Nail changes in histiocytosis X. *Arch. Dermatol.* **127**, 1741.

de Berker D., Lever L.R. & Windebank (1994) Nail features in Langerhans' cell histiocytosis. *Br. J. Dermatol.* (in press).

Ellis J.P. (1985) Histiocytosis X – unusual presentation with nail involvement. *J. Roy. Soc. Med.* **78** (Suppl.), 11, 3–5.

Esterly N.B., Maurer H.S. & Gonzalez-Crussi (1985) Histiocytosis X: a seven-year experience at a children's hospital. *J. Am. Acad. Dematol.* **13**, 481–496.

Frumkin A., Roytman M. & Johnson S.F. (1987) Juvenile xanthogranuloma underneath a toenail. *Cutis* **40**, 244–245.

Harper J.I. & Staughton R. (1983) Letter to the editor. *Cutis* **31**, 493–494.

Holzberg M., Wade T.R., Buchanan I.D. & Spraker M.K. (1985) Nail pathology in histiocytosis X. *J. Am. Acad. Dermatol.* **13**, 522–523.

Sonoda T., Hashimoto H. & Enjoji M. (1985) Juvenile xanthogranuloma. Clinico-pathologic analysis and immunohistochemical study of 57 patients. *Cancer* **56**, 2280–2286.

Timpatanapong P., Hathirat P. & Isarangkura P. (1984) Nail involvement in histiocytosis X. A 12-year retrospective study. *Arch. Dermatol.* **120**, 1052–1056.

Yamashita J.T., Rotta O., Michalany N.S. & Filho S.T. (1990) Xanthogranulome juvénile du majeur chez un nourrisson. *Ann. Dermatol. Venereol.* **117**, 295–296.

Nail changes and paraneoplastic disorders

(see Fig. 6.70(a), (b) and (c))

Nail abnormalities can occur in association with numerous paraneoplastic syndromes such as glucagonoma syndrome, malignant acanthosis nigricans, Bazex syndrome, pachydermoperiostosis, palmoplantar keratoderma pemphigus and dermatomyositis (Fig. 6.70(a)). Finger clubbing and pachydermoperiostosis are well-known signs of primary or metastatic intrathoracic neoplasms.

Yellow nail syndrome and shell nail syndrome have been described in patients with bronchial tumours. Koilonychia due to hypochromic anaemia can be a sign of haemorrhagic gastrointestinal neoplasms. Terry's nails have been described in pancreas carcinoma with hepatic metastases. White banding of the nails has been observed in patients with carcinoid tumours.

Acrokeratosis paraneoplastica of Bazex and Dupré

(see Fig. 6.70(b) and (c))

Acrokeratosis paraneoplastica has now been observed in numerous countries: US, eight cases (Pecora *et al.*, 1983; Witkowski & Parish, 1982); Canada, (Richard & Giroux, 1987); Germany, nine cases (von Hintzenstern *et al.*, 1990); UK, five cases (Wishart, 1986; Douglas *et al.*, 1991; Handfield-Jones *et al.*, 1992); Italy, (Scarpa *et al.*, 1971); Denmark, (Jacobsen *et al.*, 1984). However, most of the patients are French; about 65 cases, mostly in white men over 40, with two cases in blacks (Boudoulas & Camisa, 1986) and only three cases in women (Scarpa *et al.*, 1971; Grimwood & Lekan, 1987; Martin *et al.*, 1989) have been reported.

Acrokeratosis paraneoplastica (Bazex *et al.*, 1965, 1973) occurs in association with malignant epitheliomata of the upper respiratory or digestive tract. It has been reported in malignancy of the pharyngolaryngeal area-pyriform fossa, tonsillar area, epiglottis, hard and soft

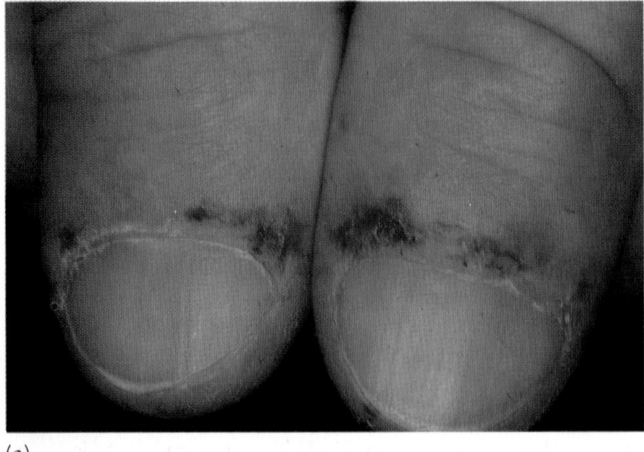

(a)

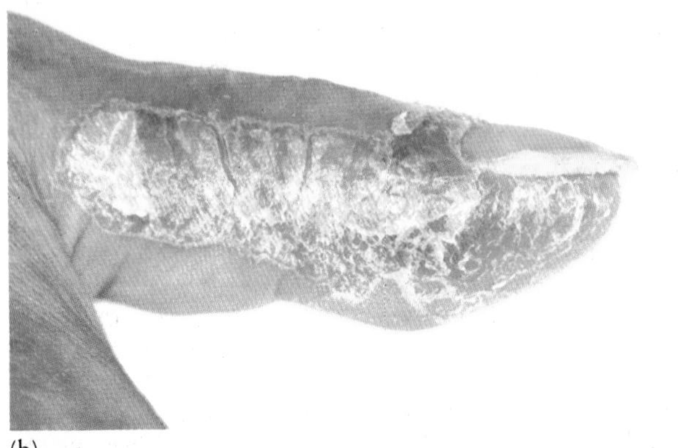

(b)

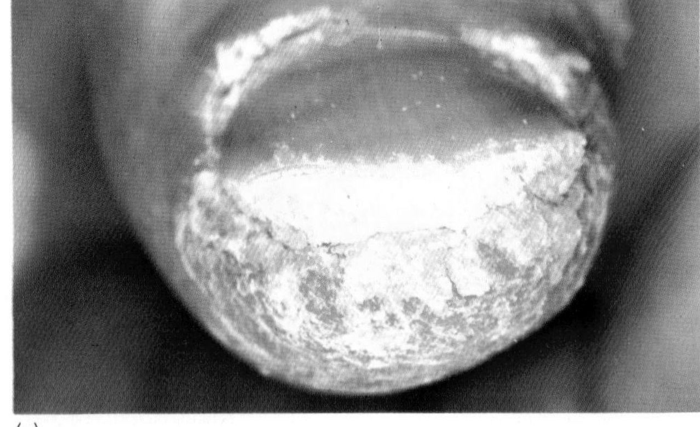

(c)

Fig. 6.70. (a) Dermatomyositis—paraneoplastic type (courtesy of C. Beylot, Bordeaux, France); (b) and (c) acrokeratosis paraneoplastica.

palate, vocal cords, tongue, lower lip, oesophagus and the upper third of the lungs. It also occurs with metastases to the cervical and upper mediastinal lymph nodes. This 'paraneoplasia' may precede the signs of the associated malignancy (several months), disappear when the tumour is removed or reappear with its recurrence. However, the nail involvement does not always benefit from total recovery, in contrast to the other lesions (Cahuzac *et al.*, 1981). This condition almost exclusively occurs in men over 40 years of age. The lesions are erythematous, violaceous, keratotic and have ill-defined borders. They are symmetrically distributed, affecting hands, feet, ears and occasionally the nose. The toenails suffer more severely than the fingernails. Roughened, irregular, keratotic, fissured and warty excrescences are found equally on the terminal phalanges of both fingers and toes.

The nails are invariably involved and are typically the earliest manifestation of the disease (Baran, 1977). In mild forms, the nail involvement is discrete; the affected nails are thin, soft and may become fragile and crumble. In more established disease, the nails are flaky, irregular, whitened and the free edge is raised by subungual hyperkeratosis. In severe forms, the lesions resemble advanced psoriatic nail dystrophy and may progress to complete loss of the diseased nails. The nail bed is eventually replaced by a smooth epidermis to which the irregular horny vestiges of the nail still adhere. The periungual skin shows an erythemato-squamous eruption, predominantly on the dorsum of the terminal phalanges. This may be associated with chronic paronychia with occasional, acute suppurative exacerbations (Bureau *et al.*, 1971). Skin and nail hyperpigmentation preceded the onset of typical skin lesions in the patient reported by Espasandin and Vignale (1990). Hyperkeratosis or warty thickening of the nail folds with ridging of the nails were observed in Handfield-Jones *et al.*'s cases (1992).

The two extremes of the disease may coexist. In these cases, the proximal third of the nail is atrophic and the distal two-thirds exhibit hypertrophic changes (Thiers *et al.*, 1973). The histopathological changes are non-specific. They show an ill-defined lymphocytic infiltrate around the upper dermal vessels which does not reach the dermo-epidermal junction. There is mild acanthosis and hyperkeratosis with scattered parakeratotic foci. In some cases fibrinoid degeneration in the superficial capillaries is seen. The infiltrate usually contains a few pycnotic neutrophils resembling allergic vasculitis. Other changes reported include eosinophilic hyalinization of individual prickle cells and scattered vacuolar degeneration (Bazex & Griffiths, 1980). We have found, in amino acid analysis of the hyperkeratotic and friable nails, that they differed from normal and other investigated diseased nails by an increase in the per cent residues of lysine, methionine and glycine, accompanied by a decrease of arginine, threonine, proline and cysteine (Juhlin & Baran, 1984). Differential diagnosis includes psoriasis, Reiter's disease, onychomycosis, acrodermatitis continua, secondary syphilis, keratoderma palmaris and plantaris. Whether the paraneoplastic syndrome of Nazzaro *et al.* (1974) is a different entity from Bazex' is debatable. It resembles pityriasis rubra, keratosis pilaris, Kyrle's disease and acrokeratosis paraneoplastica. All the nails are thickened and show multiple Beau's lines.

Topical steroids (Bazex & Griffiths, 1980), systemic steroids (Martin *et al.*, 1989) and etretinate (Wishart, 1986), have been reported to improve the eruption.

References

Baran R. (1977) Paraneoplastic acrokeratosis of Bazex. *Arch. Dermatol.* **113**, 2613.

Bazex A. & Griffiths A. (1980) Acrokeratosis paraneoplastica. A new cutaneous marker of malignancy. *Br. J. Dermatol.* **102**, 304.

Bazex A., Salvator R., Dupré A. & Christol B. (1965) Syndrome paranéoplasique à type d'hyperkératose des extrémités. Guérison aprés traitement de l'épithélioma laryngé. *Bull. Soc. Fr. Dermatol. Syphil.* **72**, 182.

Bazex A., Dupré A., Christol B. & Combes P. (1973) Onychose paranéoplasique, forme localisée d'acrokératose paranéoplasique. *Bull. Soc. Fr. Dermatol. Syphil.* **82**, 117.

Boudoulas O. & Camisa C. (1986) Paraneoplastic acrokeratosis. Bazex syndrome. *Cutis* **37**, 449–453.

Bureau Y., Barriére H., Litoux P. & Bureau B. (1971) Acrokeratose paranéoplasique de Bazex. Importance des lésions unguéales. A propos de 2 observations. *Bull. Soc. Fr. Dermatol. Syphil.* **78**, 79.

Cahuzac P., Faure M. & Thivolet J. (1981) Onychoartrophie résiduelle au cours d'une acrokératose paranéoplasique de Bazex. *Ann. Dermatol. Vénereol.* **108**, 773.

Douglas W.S., Bisland D.J. & Howatson R. (1991) Acrokeratosis paraneoplastica of Bazex. A case in the U.K. *Clin. Exp. Dermatol.*, **16**, 297–299.

Espasandin J. & Vignale R.A. (1990) Acroqueratosis paraneoplàsica de Barex. Un eano clinico con hyperpigmentaciòn. *Med. Cut. I.L.A* **18**, 257–262.

Grimwood R.E. & Lekan C. (1987) Acrokeratosis paraneoplastica with esophageal squamous cell carcinoma. *J. Am. Acad. Dermatol.* **17**, 685–686.

Handfield-Jones S.E., Matthews C.N.A., Ellis J.P. *et al.* (1992) Acrokeratosis paraneoplastica of Bazex. *J. Royal Soc. Med.* **85**, 548–550.

Jacobsen F.K., Abildtrup N. & Laursen S.O. (1984) Acrokeratosis neoplastica (Bazex syndrome). *Arch. Dermatol.* **120**, 502–504.

Juhlin L. & Baran R. (1984) Abnormal aminoacid composition of nails in Bazex' paraneoplastic acrokeratosis. *Acta. Derm. Venereol.* **64**, 31–34.

Martin R.W., Cornitiu T.G., Naylor M.F. *et al.* (1989) Bazex' syndrome in a woman with pulmonary adenocarcinoma. *Arch. Dermatol.* **125**, 847–848.

Nazzaro P., Argentieri R., Balus L. *et al.* (1974) Syndrome paranéoplasique avec lésions papulo-kératosiques des extremités et kératose pilaire spinulosique diffuse. *Ann. Dermatol. Venereol.* **101**, 411–413.

Pecora A.L. *et al* (1983) Acrokeratosis paraneoplastic (Bazex syndrome). *Arch. Dermatol.* **119**, 820–826.

Richard M. & Giroux J.M. (1987) Acrokeratosis paraneoplastica (Bazex' syndrome). *J. Am. Acad. Dermatol.* **16**, 178–183.

Scarpa C., Nini G., Pasqua M.C. *et al.* (1971) Singolare osservazione di eritro-acrocheratosi paraneoplastica. *G. Ital. Dermatol.* **46**, 17–25.

Thiers H., Moulin G., Haguenauer J.P. & Poupon P. (1973) Acrokeratose paraneoplastique. *Bull. Soc. Fr. Dermatol. Syphil.* **80**, 129.

Von Hintzenstern J., Kiesewetter F., Simon M. *et al.* (1990) Paraneoplastische Akrokeratose Bazex-verlang under palliativer therapie eines Zungengrund Karzinoms. *Hautarzt* **41**, 490–493.

Wishart J.M. (1986) Bazex paraneoplastic acrokeratosis, a case report and response to Tigason. *Br. J. Dermatol.* **115**, 595–596.

Witkowski J.A. & Parish L.C. (1982) Bazex syndrome. *J. Am. Med. Assoc.* **248**, 2883–2884.

Glucagonoma syndrome (Fig. 6.71)

Necrolytic migratory erythema, stomatitis, weight loss and diabetes are the characteristic signs of this syndrome. In the first report the nails were distorted, with pitting, longitudinal striae and deposits of yellowish-white subungual material (Becker *et al.*, 1942). Erythema, fissuring and swelling of periungual tissues resembling chronic paronychia are frequently observed (Guillausseau *et al.*, 1982; Rappersberger *et al.*, 1987). Fingertips can also be affected. Paronychia and pyogenic granulomas of the first and third left toes have been reported by Picard *et al.* (1988). Soft friable nails with flaking and crumbling may be seen (Mallinson *et al.*, 1974).

References

Becker S.W., Kahn D. & Rothman S. (1942) Cutaneous manifestations of internal malignant tumours. *Arch. Dermatol. Syph.* **45**, 1069–1080.

Guillausseau P.J., Guillausseau C., Villet R. *et al.* (1982) Les glucagonomes. *Gastroenterol. Clin. Biol.* **6**, 1029–1041.

Mallinson C.N., Bloom S.R., Warin A.P., Salmon P.R. & Cox B. (1974) A glucagonoma syndrome. *Lancet* **ii**, 1–5.

Picard C., Mazer J.M., Bilet S. *et al.* (1988) Syndrome du glucagonome. *Ann. Dermatol. Venereol.* **115**, 1142–1145.

Rappersberger K., Wolff-Schreiner E., Konrad K. & Wolff K. (1987) Das glukagonom-syndrom. *Hautarzt* **38**, 589–598.

Lung neoplasm

Hypertrophic pulmonary osteoarthropathy and finger clubbing are commonly seen in patients with primitive or secondary pulmonary neoplasms. Onycholysis of the fingernails has been observed in a 45-year-old man affected by a poorly differentiated squamous cell carcinoma of the lung who had received radiotherapy (Hickman, 1977).

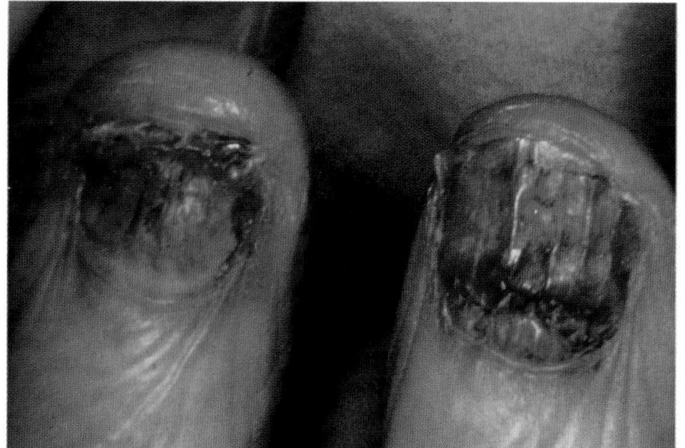

Fig. 6.71. Glucagonoma syndrome (courtesy of J. Hewitt, Paris).

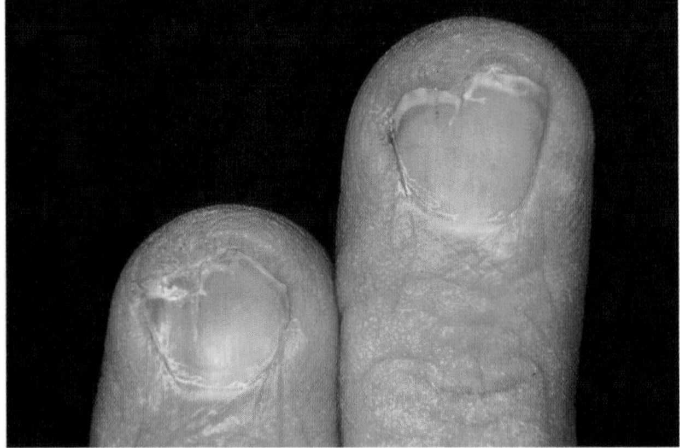

Fig. 6.72. Acanthosis nigricans (courtesy of H. Baker, London).

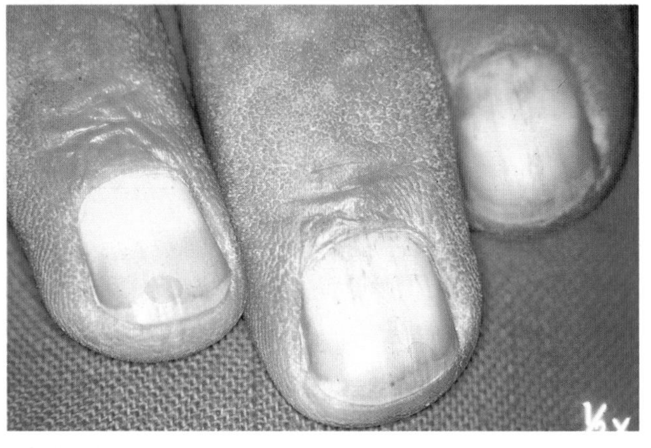

Fig. 6.73. Leuconychia in malignant acanthosis nigricans (courtesy of A. Puissant, Paris).

Reference

Hickman J.W. (1977) Onycholysis associated with carcinoma of the lung. *J. Am. Med. Assoc.* **238**, 1246.

Acanthosis nigricans

Nail ridging and brittleness can be associated with palmar hyperkeratosis in some patients with malignant acanthosis nigricans (Von Fischer, 1949; Ebling *et al.*, 1979); patchy (Ive, 1963) or complete leuconychia and nail thickening have also been reported (Azizi, 1980) (Figs 6.72 & 6.73). Hypertrophic pulmonary osteoarthropathy and bullous pemphigoid can occasionally be associated with acanthosis nigricans (Ive, 1963). Warty excrescences were present around the free margin of a thumbnail in a patient of Baker and Barth (1983).

References

Azizi E., Trau H., Schewach-Millet M., Rosenberg V., Schneebaum S. & Michalevicz R. (1980) Generalized malignant acanthosis nigricans. *Arch. Dermatol.* **116**, 381.

Baker H. & Barth J.H. (1983) Acanthosis nigricans. *Br. J. Dermatol.* **109** (Suppl.), 101–103.

Ebling F.J.G., Marks R. & Rook A. (1979) Disorders of keratinization. In: *Textbook of Dermatology*, eds Rook A., Wilkinson D.S., Ebling F.J.G., Champion R.H. & Burton J.L., pp. 1393–1468. Blackwell Scientific Publications, Oxford.

Ive F.A. (1963) Metastatic carcinoma of cervix with acanthosis nigricans, bullous pemphigoid and hypertrophic pulmonary osteoarthropathy. *Proc. Roy. Soc. Med.* **56**, 910.

Von Fischer F. (1949) Acanthosis nigricans. *Dermatologica* **98**, 319–320.

Digital ischaemia

Raynaud's phenomenon and digital necrosis can be early signs of an occult neoplasm (Hawley *et al.*, 1967; Vayssairat *et al.*, 1978). Onset of symptoms is not related to cold exposure. Pain and paraesthesia of fingers may precede development of digital ischaemia. Splinter haemorrhages were also observed in three patients (Palmer, 1974).

Gastrointestinal, genital and blood malignancies have been associated with digital ischaemia. Removal of neoplasms is usually followed by improvement of ischaemic signs (Barriere, 1984; Garioch *et al.*, 1991). The mechanism of digital ischaemia associated with malignancy is probably multifactorial. Metastatic involvement of the sympathetic ganglion, hypergammaglobulinaemia, production of cryoglobulins, hypercoagulable states, production of catecholamine or other neurohumoral factors have been implicated (Albin *et al.*, 1986).

References

Albin G., Lapeyre A.C., Click R.L. & Callahan M.J. (1986) Paraneoplastic digital thrombosis: a case report. *Angiology* **37**, 203–206.

Barriere H. (1984) Syndromes cutanés para-néoplasiques. *Ann. Med. Intern.* **135**, 662–668.

Garioch J.J., Todd P., Soukop M. & Thomson J. (1991) T-cell lymphoma presenting with severe digital ischaemia. *Clin. Exp. Dermatol.* **16**, 202–203.

Hawley P.R., Johnston A.W. & Rankin J.T. (1967) Association between digital ischemia and malignant disease. *Br. Med. J.* **ii**, 208.

Palmer H.M. (1974) Digital vascular disease and malignant disease. *Br. J. Dermatol.* **91**, 476.

Vayssairat M., Fiessinger J.N., Bordet F. & Housset F. (1978) Rapports entre nécroses digitales du membres supérieur et affections malignes. *Nouv. Presse. Med.* **7**, 1279–1282.

Papuloerythroderma

Since the first report (Ofuji *et al.*, 1984), 35 cases of papuloerythroderma have been reported in the Japanese literature (Ofuji, 1990). This is a clinically distinctive entity associated with blood eosinophilia characterized by a pruritic eruption that quickly develops into a papular erythroderma with notable sparing of compressed abdo-

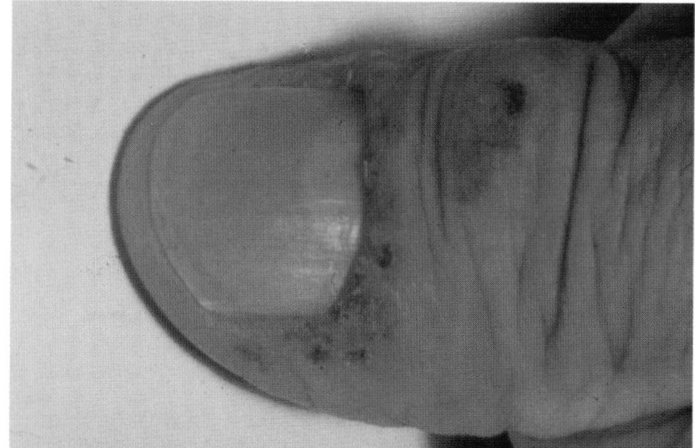

Fig. 6.74. Papuloerythroderma (courtesy of R. Staughton, London).

minal folds (deck chair sign). Splinter haemorrhages in the nails were noted by Grob *et al.* (1989). Thrombosed capillaries in the nail folds were a striking feature in Staughton *et al.*'s case (1987) (Fig. 6.74). Multiple causative factors (lymphoma, gastric and lung cancer, etc.) underlie the pathogenesis of papuloerythroderma (Ofuji, 1990). Langerhans' cells may possibly have a central role in the pathogenesis of this condition (Wakeel *et al.*, 1991).

References

Grob J.J., Collet-Villette A.M., Herchowski N. & Ofuji S. (1989) Papuloerythroderma. Report of a case with T-cell skin lymphoma and discussion of the nature of the disease. *J. Am. Acad. Dermatol.* **20**, 927–931.

Ofuji S. (1990) Papuloerythroderma. *J. Am. Acad. Dermatol.* **22**, 697.

Ofuji S., Furukawa F., Miyachi Y. *et al.* (1984) Papuloerythroderma. *Dermatologica* **169**, 125–130.

Staughton R., Laugry J., Rowland-Payne C. *et al.* (1987) Papuloerythroderma: the first European case. In: *Clinical Dermatology*, eds Wilkinson D.S., Mascaro J.M. & Orfanos C.E., pp. 181–182. The CDM Case Collection, Berlin. Stuttgard, Schattawer.

Wakeel R.A., Keefe M. & Chapman R.S. (1991) Papuloerythroderma. *Arch. Dermatol.* **127**, 96–98.

Breast carcinoma

Longitudinal hyperpigmented nail banding unrelated to chemotherapy occurred in a 49-year-old woman with breast carcinoma (Krutchik *et al.*, 1978). Leuconychia striata of all fingernails has been reported in a 67-year-old woman with breast cancer (Hortobagyi, 1983).

References

Hortobagyi G.N. (1983) Leukonychia striata associated with breast carcinoma. *J. Surg. Oncol.* **23**, 60–61.

Krutchik A.N., Tashima C.K., Buzdar A.U. & Blumenschein G.R. (1978) Longitudinal nail banding associated with breast carcinoma unrelated to chemotherapy. *Arch. Intern. Med.* **138**, 1302–1303.

Intestinal leiomyosarcoma

Facial and nail hyperpigmentation occurred in a 47-year-old man affected by intestinal leiomyosarcoma. Skin and nail pigmentation faded dramatically 3 months after surgery (Suda *et al.*, 1985).

Reference

Suda M., Ishii H., Kashiwazaki K. & Tsuchiya M. (1985) Hyperpigmentation of skin and nails in a patient with intestinal leiomyosarcoma *Dig. Dis. Sci.* **30**, 1108–1111.

Multicentric reticulohistiocytosis (see p. 219)

A large number of malignancies have been reported in association with multicentric reticulohistiocytosis.

Nasopharyngeal carcinoma

Thirty-two of 1300 patients affected by nasopharyngeal carcinoma developed a paraneoplastic syndrome. Hypertrophic osteoarthropathy was observed in 17 patients, while 13 patients exhibited finger clubbing. One patient had dermatomyositis and one patient had myelaemia. Pulmonary metastases were present in 15 of the 17 patients with hypertrophic osteoarthropathy and in all of the 13 patients with finger clubbing. Most of the patients with a paraneoplastic syndrome were young and had undifferentiated nasopharyngeal carcinoma with lung metastases (Maalej *et al.*, 1985).

Reference

Maalej M., Ladgham A., Ennouri A., Ben Attia A., Cammoun M. & Ellouze R. (1985) Le syndrome paranéoplasique du cancer du nasopharynx. *Presse Med.* **14**, 471–474.

Castelman tumour

There is a remarkable association between Castelman tumours and skin diseases. A 45-year-old patient with a retroperitoneal Castelman tumour developed a severe lichen planus involving the skin, mouth, nails and pemphigus vulgaris of the oral cavity. Both dermatoses regressed after surgical removal of the tumour (Plewig *et al.*, 1990). POEMS syndrome has also been associated with Castelman's disease (Thajeb *et al.*, 1989).

References

Plewig G., Jansen T., Jungblut R.M. & Roher H.D. (1990) Castelman-Tumour, lichen ruber und pemphigus vulgaris:

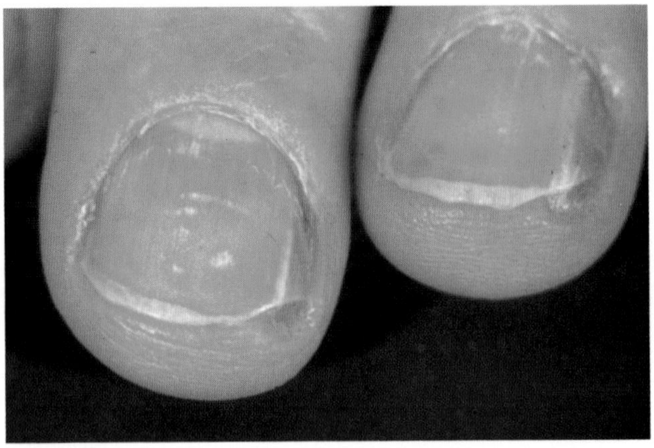

Fig. 6.75. Cowden's disease (courtesy of R. Happle, Münster, Germany).

paraneoplastische association immunologischer erkrankungen? *Hautarzt* **41**, 662–670.

Thajeb P., Chee C.Y., Lo S.F. & Lee N. (1989) The POEMS syndrome among Chinese: association with Castelman's disease and some immunological abnormalities. *Acta Neurol. Scand.* **80**, 492–500.

Cowden's disease (Fig. 6.75)

A linear nail dystrophy with changes resembling an evergreen tree that extends distally from the cuticle to the edge of the nail plate has been described in a patient with Cowden's disease, an autosomal dominant genodermatosis (Lazar, 1986). Siegel (1974) reported a patient with Cowden's disease who presented a solitary subungual fibrotic nodule on the great toe of the right foot and a similar lesion starting under a fingernail. Linear subungual hyperkeratosis resembling longitudinal leuconykia may involve several fingers (Happle, 1989).

References

Lazar A.P. (1986) Cowden's disease (multiple hamartoma and neoplasia syndrome) treated with isotretinoin. *J. Am. Acad. Dermatol.* **14**, 142–143.

Happle R. (1989) Genodermatosen an Handen und Fusser. In: *Handsymposium Dermatologische Erkrankungen der Hande und Fusse* , eds Altmeyer P., Schultz-Ehrenburg U. & Luther H., pp. 109–111. Springer-Verlag, Berlin.

Siegel J. (1974) Tuberous sclerosis (forme fruste) vs. Cowden syndrome. *Arch. Dermatol.* **110**, 476–477.

Metastases (see Chapter 11)

Metastases to the nail unit can cause diffuse inflammation of periungual tissues resembling acute paronychia. Involvement of the phalangeal bones is common (Baran & Tosti, 1994). The metastatic malignancy is usually a visceral carcinoma, most commonly seen in the lung, breast and gastrointestinal tract.

Reference

Baran R. & Tosti A. (1994) Metastatic bronchogenic carcinoma to the terminal phalanx with review of 116 non-melanoma metastatic tumors to the distal digit. *J. Am. Acad. Dermatol.* (in press).

Leukaemias (Fig. 6.76)

Splinter haemorrhages as well as subungual and periungual haematomas can occur in patients with leukaemia. Pallor of the nail bed due to anaemia can also be observed. A nail dystrophy is a common symptom in longstanding erythroderma independent of its aetiology and may therefore be observed as a non-specific lesion in about 25% of patients with chronic lymphocytic leukaemia. Non-tender swelling of the proximal nail fold mimicking chronic paronychia has been reported in a patient affected by chronic lymphocytic leukaemia. All fingers except the thumbs were affected. Fingernails were mildly dystrophic with brownish discoloration. Histopathological findings of leukaemia cutis were present in the skin biopsy. Lesions drammatically resolved after irradiation (High *et al.*, 1985).

Clubbing and distal digital periosteal bone destruction due to leukaemic infiltration of the distal phalanges have also been reported (Hirschfeld, 1925). A patient presented spatulate fingers due to marginal and dorsal leukaemic infiltration and subungual deposits that caused bulbous tips and splintered nails. Onychogryphosis of toenails was also present (Calvert & Smith, 1955). A patient developed subungual tumours involving several fingers and the left toenail early in the course of chronic lymphocytic leukaemia. The affected nails showed an increased curvature as well as an elevation of the nail plates (Simon

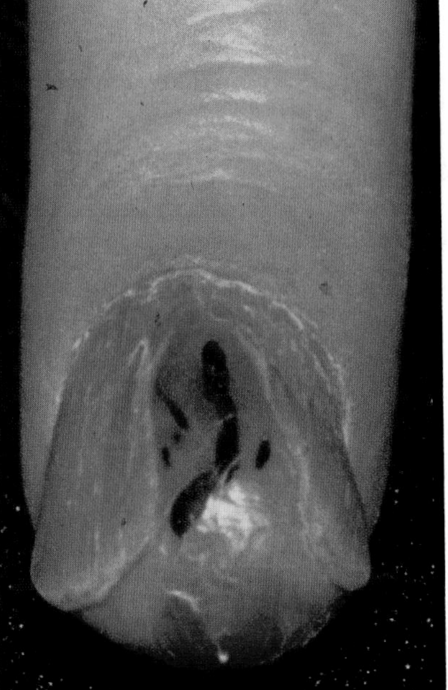

Fig. 6.76. Leukaemic infiltrate in the nail apparatus (courtesy of W.P.D. Su, USA).

et al., 1990). Histopathology showed a massive leukaemic infiltrate in the reticular dermis and subcutaneous tissue sparing a grenz zone in the papillary dermis of the nail bed. The epidermis was normal.

Leukaemic infiltration in the distal phalanx of the thumb resulting in a chronic whitlow with bone involvement has been reported in a patient affected by acute monomyelocytic leukaemia (Chang *et al.*, 1975). A syndrome resembling pachydermoperiostosis has also been described in this condition (Mackenzie, 1986).

Perniotic lesions on fingers, toes, nose and ears have been seen in three elderly men during the pre-leukaemic phase of monocytic leukaemia (Marks *et al.*, 1969). Norwegian scabies was the presenting symptom of adult T-cell leukaemia in two members of a Japanese family (Egawa *et al.*, 1992).

References

Beek C.H. (1948) Skin manifestation associated with lymphatic-leukaemia. *Dermatologica* **96**, 350–356.

Calvert R.J. & Smith E. (1955) Metastatic acropachy in lymphatic leukemia. *Blood* **10**, 545–549.

Chang Y.D., Whitaker L.A. & La Rossa D. (1975) Acute monomyelocytic leukemia presenting as a felon. *Plast. Reconstr. Surg.* 623–624.

Egawa K., Johmo M., Hayashibara T. & Ono T. (1992) Familial occurrence of crusted (Norwegian) scabies with adult T-cell leukaemia. *Br. J. Dermatol.* **127**, 57–59.

High D.A., Luscombe H.A. & Kauh Y.C. (1985) Leukemia cutis masquerading as chronic paronychia. *Int. J. Dermatol.* **24**, 595–597.

Hirschfeld H. (1925) Leukamic und verewandte zustände. In: *Handbuch der Krankheiten der Blutbildenen Organe* Vol. I, ed. Schittenhelm A., p. 258. Springer, Berlin.

Mackenzie C.R. (1986) Pachydermoperiostosis: a paraneoplastic syndrome. *New York State J. Med.* 153–154.

Marks R., Lim C.C. & Borrie P.F. (1969) A perniotic syndrome with monocytosis and neutropenia: a possible association with a preleukaemic state. *Br. J. Dermatol.* **81**, 327–332.

Simon C.A., Su W.P.D. & Li C.Y. (1990) Subungual leukemia cutis. *Int. J. Dermatol.* **29**, 636–639.

Plasmocytoma

Multiple large tumours involving the digits of the hands represented the initial symptom of multiple myeloma in a patient (Pobanz *et al.*, 1955). Nail changes can be observed in patients with systemic amyloidosis secondary to plasmocytoma (see p. 203).

Clinical symptoms of hyalinosis cutis et mucosae occurred in a 66-year-old patient affected by plasmacytoma with monoclonal IgG light chain gammopathy. A severe onychodystrophy characterized by onychoschisis and onycholysis was also present (Von der Helm *et al.*, 1989). Digital ischaemia due to cryoglobulins can occur in patients with Waldenström's macroglobulinaemia or multiple myeloma. Finger clubbing and Terry's nails have been described in patients with POEMS syndrome associated with plasmocytoma (see p. 207).

References

Pobanz D.M., Condon J.V. & Baker L.A. (1955) Plasma-cell myelomatosis. *Arch. Intern. Med.* **96**, 828–832.

Von der Helm D., Ring J., Schmoeckel C. & Braun-Falco O. (1989) Erworbene hyalinosis cutis et mucosae bei Plasmozytom mit monoklonaler IgG-lambda-Gammopathie. *Hautarzt* **40**, 153–157.

Lymphoma

Cutaneous B-cell lymphomas rarely affect the nails. A 70-year-old patient affected by chronic lymphocytic leukaemia developed nail lesions that clinically resembled onychomycosis associated with slowly growing pink tumours in the toenails. A nail biopsy established the diagnosis of non-Hodgkin's, B-cell type centrocytic/centroblastic malignant lymphoma. Treatment with chlorambucil and prednisolone produced striking effects (Moller Pedersen *et al.*, 1992).

The nail abnormalities observed in patients with cutaneous T-cell lymphoma may be non-specific or may be a direct consequence of the localization of the neoplastic cells in the nail constituents.

Onychodystrophy has been reported to occur in 32% of patients affected by Sézary syndrome (Wieselthier & Koh, 1990). The nail changes may be indistinguishable from the onychodystrophy of other erythrodermal affections such as pityriasis rubra pilaris, psoriasis or actinic reticuloid (Toonstra *et al.*, 1985; Sonnex *et al.*, 1986). Nail bed hyperkeratosis (Tomsick, 1982) along with nail plate thickening and discoloration are the most common clinical features. Ridging, roughness and shedding of the nail plate can also occur. A nail biopsy can reveal lymphomatous infiltration of the nail apparatus (Dalziel *et al.*, 1989; Tosti *et al.*, 1990; Zaias, 1990) (Figs 6.77 & 6.78).

In mycosis fungoides of the digits, nail changes are not uncommon (Figs 6.79–6.81) and have been reported even in childhood (Wilson *et al.*, 1991). The nail changes occasionally improve with chemotherapy. Gangrene of the right finger due to cutaneous T-cell lymphoma has been described by Lund *et al.* (1990). Combination chemotherapy produced a complete remission of digital ischaemia in a patient (Garioch *et al.*, 1991).

An elephantiasis-like tumescence of the third left finger associated with multiple nodular lesions on several other fingers and dystrophic nail changes were the unusual manifestations of mycosis fungoides in a 56-year-old patient (Voigtlander *et al.*, 1988). Yellow nail syndrome has been reported in a 72-year-old patient suffering from mycosis fungoides (Stosiek *et al.*, 1993).

Fig. 6.77. T-cell lymphoma of nail apparatus.

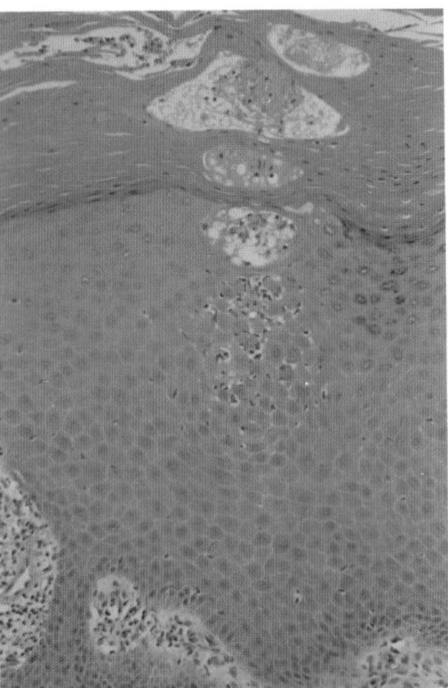
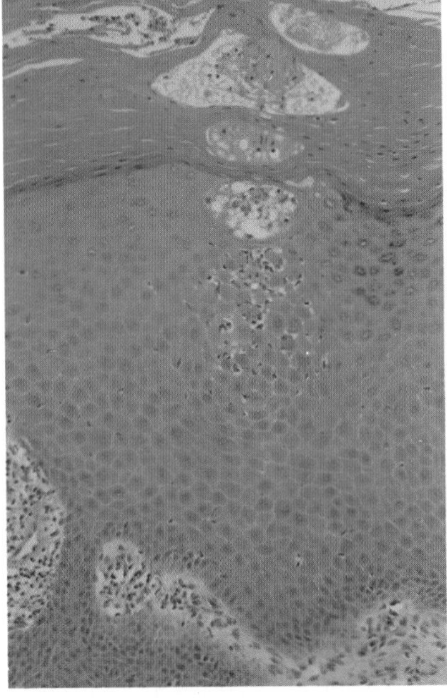

Fig. 6.78. Same case as Fig. 6.77 showing nail dermal infiltrate and epidermotropism.

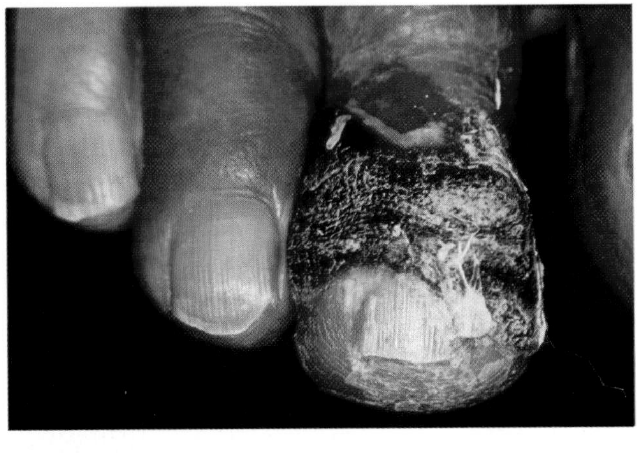

Fig. 6.79. Mycosis fungoides – tumour of the nail apparatus.

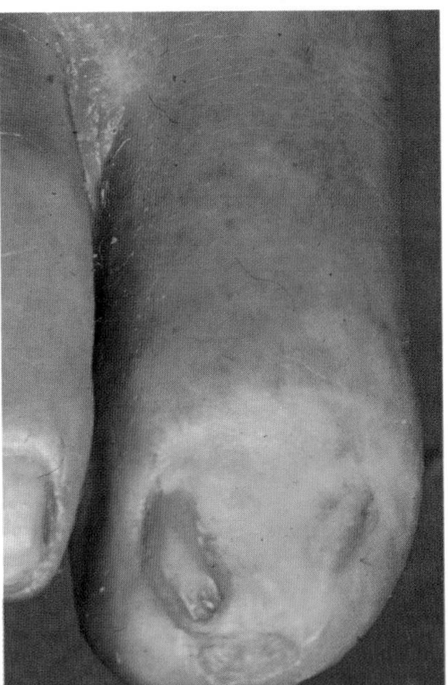

Fig. 6.80. Mycosis fungoides.

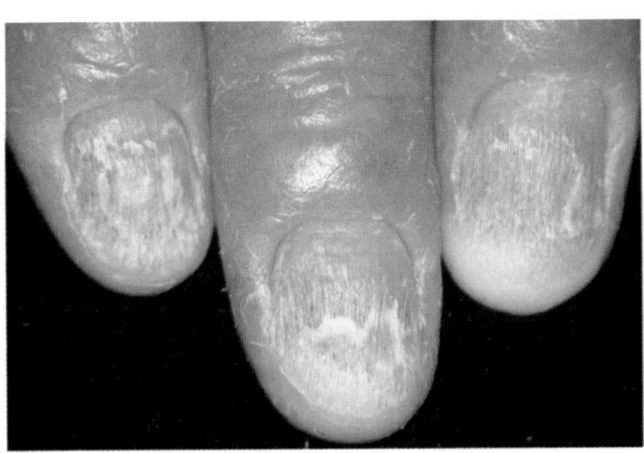

Fig. 6.81. Mycosis fungoides after electron beam therapy.

References

Dalziel K.L., Telfer N.R. & Dawber R.P.R. (1989) Nail dystrophy in cutaneous T-cell lymphoma. *Br. J. Dermatol.* **120**, 571–574.

Garioch J.J., Todd P., Soukop M. & Thomson J. (1991) T-cell lymphoma presenting with severe digital ischaemia. *Clin. Exp. Dermatol.* **16**, 202–203.

Lund K.A., Parker C.M., Norins A.L. & Tejada E. (1990) Vesicular cutaneous T cell lymphoma presenting with gangrene. *J. Am. Acad. Dermatol.* **23**, 1169–1170.

Moller Pedersen L., Nordin H., Nielsen H. & Lisse I (1992) Non Hodgkin malignant lymphoma in the nails in the course of a chronic lymphocytic leukemia. *Acta Dermatol. Venereol.* **72**, 277–278.

Sonnex T.S., Dawber R.P.R., Zachary C.B., Millard P.R., Path M.R.C. & Griffiths A.D. (1986) The nails in adult type 1 pityriasis rubra pilaris. *J. Am. Acad. Dermatol.* **15**, 956–960.

Stosiek N., Peters K.P., Hiller D. *et al.* (1993) Yellow nail syndrome in a patient with mycosis fungoides. *J. Am. Acad. Dermatol.* **28**, 792–794.

Tomsick R.S. (1982) Hyperkeratosis in mycosis fungoides. *Cutis* **29**, 621–623.
Toonstra J., Van Weelden H., Gmelin Meyling F.H.J., Van der Putte S.C.J., Schiere S.I.M. & Baart de la Faille H. (1985) Actinic reticuloid simulating Sézary syndrome. Report of two cases. *Arch. Dermatol. Res.* **277**, 159–166.
Tosti A., Fanti P.A. & Varotti C. (1990) Massive lymphomatous nail involvement in Sézary syndrome. *Dermatologica* **181**, 162–164.
Voigtlander V., Hartmann A.A., Adam W. & Friedrich W. (1988) Mycosis fongoide. Etiologie inattendue d'un eczéma chronique des mains avec gigantisme digital. *Ann. Dermatol. Venereol.* **115**, 1212–1214.
Wieselthier J.S. & Koh H.K. (1990) Sézary syndrome: diagnosis, prognosis, and critical review of treatment options. *J. Am. Acad. Dermatol.* **22**, 381–401.
Wilson K.G., Cotter F.E., Lowe D.G. *et al.* (1991) Mycosis fungoides in childhood: An unusual presentation. *J. Am. Acad. Dermatol.* **25**, 370–372.
Zaias N. (1990) *The Nail in Health and Disease*, 2nd edn, p. 227. Appleton & Lange, Norwalk, CN.

HTLV-1 positive cutaneous T-cell lymphoma

A 34-year-old German woman noticed painless swelling and blackish discoloration which had developed within 2 weeks on several finger- and toenails. The nails were blackish red, thickened and leathery. An unusual haemorrhagic, epidermotrophic lymphocytic infiltrate with T-cell pattern and numerous large Pautrier's abscesses, transepithelial elimination and infiltration of the subungual keratin and nail plate was seen histologically. The nail changes resolved completely within 4 months and did not recur although she later developed opportunistic infections and eventually died. HTLV-1 was confirmed serologically whereas HIV-1 and HIV-2 were negative (Wolter *et al.*, 1991).

Hodgkin's disease

In a review of 50 patients with Hodgkin's disease, four patients (three males and one female) showed transverse leuconychia. All four patients had from one to three transverse white lines; one patient had dark brown discoloration of the distal part of the affected nail. All changes were more marked in the finger than in the toenails. In these patients the nail changes reflected a poor prognosis, death occurring within 4 months of the development of leuconychia. No relationship between nail anomalies and chemotherapy or radiotherapy was evident (Shahani & Blackburn, 1973).

References

Shahani R.T. & Blackburn E.K. (1973) Nail anomalies in Hodgkin's disease. *Br. J. Dermatol.* **89**, 457–458.
Wolter M., Schleussner-Samuel P. & Marsh W. (1991) HTLV-1 Infektion: unguales T-Zell-Lymphon als Primarmanifestation. *Hautarzt* **42**, 50–52.

Systemic drugs

Drug-induced photoonycholysis (Figs 6.82–6.85)

Numerous drugs have occasionally been incriminated as causing photoonycholysis. These include trypaflavine, acriflavine hydrochloride, chloramphenicol, chlorpromazine, thiazides, clorazepate dipotassium, systemically administered 5-fluorouracil, oral contraceptives, benoxaprofen, thorazine, practolol, captopril, quinine sulphate and quinolones (flumequine, nalidixic acid, pefloxacine, ofloxacine) (Baran, 1986; Baran & Brun, 1986).

Drug-induced photoonycholysis, however, most commonly occurs with the use of tetracycline or psoralens, both with natural sunlight (Zala *et al.*, 1977) and with ar-

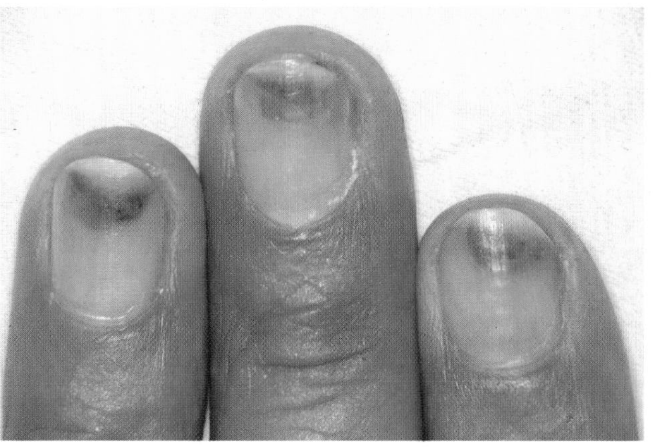

Fig. 6.82. Photoonycholysis, type I.

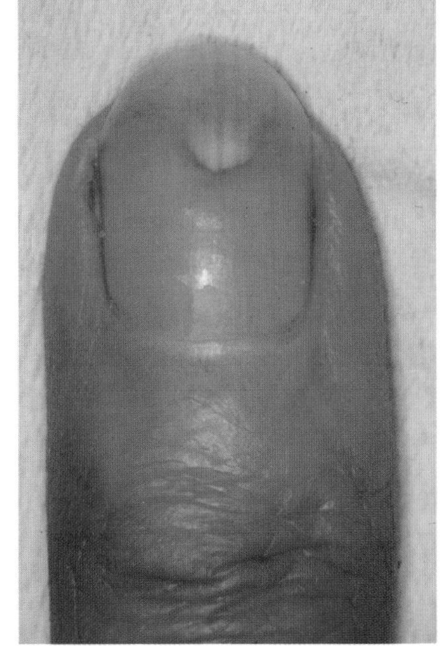

Fig. 6.83. Photoonycholysis, type II.

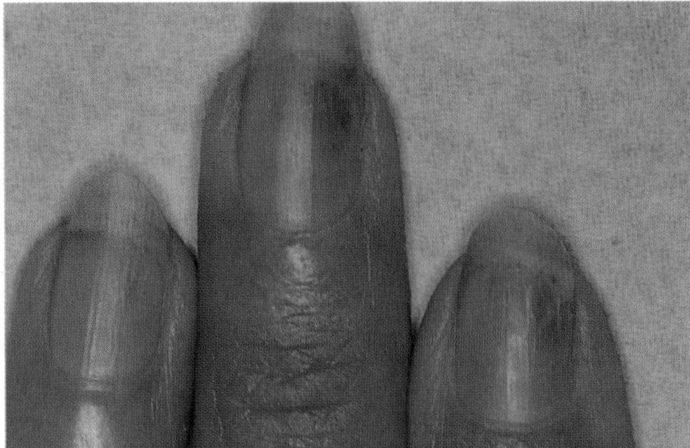

Fig. 6.84. Photoonycholysis, type III.

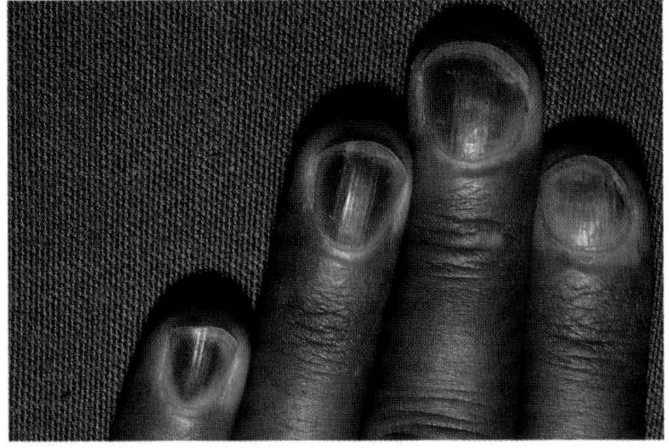

Fig. 6.85. Photoonycholysis, type III.

tificial light sources in psoralen and ultraviolet A (PUVA) treatment (Ortonne & Baran, 1978; Mackie, 1979; Morgan *et al.*, 1992). Development of photoonycholysis is not related to the cumulative UV dose (Segal, 1963; Baran & Barthélémy, 1990).

Three different clinical varieties of drug-induced photoonycholysis have been described. In all three varieties the lateral margins of the nails are never involved by the process and thumbs are only rarely affected (Baran, 1986; Baran & Juhlin, 1987). In the first variety (Fig. 6.82), the detachment is half-moon-shaped, variably pigmented and presents a well-demarcated proximal convex border. This is the most frequent clinical variety of drug-induced photoonycholysis and usually involves several digits. In the second variety (Fig. 6.83), which usually involves only one nail, the proximal border of the detachment presents a well-defined, distally opened circular notch that is surrounded by a proximal brownish margin. In the third variety (Fig. 6.84), which usually affects several digits, the detachment is localized in the central part of the pink nail bed showing initially a round yellow stain which turns into a reddish colour after several days (photohaemorrhages; Fig. 6.85). It may be seen initially as part of Segal's triad: photosensitivity followed by discoloration of the nails and onycholysis (Segal, 1963). Photoonycholysis due to tetracycline derivatives or psoralens can be painful (Mackie, 1979), and pain may occasionally precede onycholysis (Zala *et al.*, 1977). The development of photoonycholysis can be preceded or followed by a sunburn reaction on sun-exposed areas (Segal, 1963). Painful bullae under the nails have been reported with tetracycline hydrochloride after 1 month of intensive sun bathing (Ibsen & Andersen, 1983).

Photoonycholysis can occur early in treatment as well as after prolonged therapy. Interruption of the drug does not prevent the onset of onycholysis, which may be delayed, even by 1 month. Long-term persistence of the drug in the skin has been suggested to explain such delayed onset of photoonycholysis in some patients (Baran & Barthélémy, 1990).

Attempts to induce photoonycholysis experimentally have been unsuccessful, and onycholysis does not necessarily recur with readministration of the drug. Psoralen-induced photoonycholysis is not an indication for discontinuing treatment since the nail changes spontaneously resolve even if the therapy is not stopped (Mackie, 1979). A single layer of opaque adhesive strapping or the liberal application of coloured nail varnish has been shown to prevent development of nail changes. The mechanism of drug-induced photoonycholysis remains undetermined (Baran & Juhlin, 1987). Concentration of UV irradiation by the nail plate has been proposed. The possible role of melanin in the prevention of photoonycholysis is suggested by the observation that black or Mongoloid individuals are not apparently affected.

Since skin lipids can reduce UV transmission, the absence of sebaceous glands in the subungual area may also be important. UV irradiation between 310 and 313 nm has been suggested to have a major role in inducing the reaction. The observation that 3–20% of irradiation with wavelength 313–500 nm can penetrate normal nails but not psoriatic nails possibly explains the poor effect of psoralens in nail psoriasis.

The origin of pigmentation observed in most cases of photoonycholysis is poorly understood. Haemosiderin deposits due to blood extravasation and keratin dust have been implicated.

References

Baran R. (1986) Les onycholyses. *Ann. Dermatol. Venereol.* **113**, 159–170.

Baran R. & Barthélémy H. (1990) Photo-onycholyse induite par le 5-MOP (Psoraderm) et application de la méthode d'imputation des effects medicamenteux. *Ann. Dermatol. Venereol.* **117**, 367–369.

Baran R. & Brun P. (1986) Photo-onycholysis induced by the fluoroquinolones pefloxacine and ofloxacine. *Dermatologica* **176**, 185–188.

Baran R. & Juhlin L. (1987) Drug induced photo-onycholysis Three subtypes identified in a study of 15 cases. *J. Am. Acad. Dermatol.* **17**, 1012–1016.

Ibsen H.H. & Andersen B.L. (1983) Photo-onycholysis due to tetracycline-hydrochloride. *Acta Derm. Venereol.* **63**, 555–557.

Mackie R.M. (1979) Onycholysis occurring during PUVA therapy. *Clin. Exp. Dermatol.* **4**, 111–113.

Morgan J.M., Wellen R. & Adams S.J. (1992) Onycholysis in a case of atopic eczema treated with PUVA photochemotherapy. *Clin. Exp. Dermatol.* **17**, 65–66.

Ortonne J.P. & Baran R. (1978) Photo-onycholyse induite par la photochimiothérapie orale. *Ann. Dermatol. Venereol.* **105**, 887–888.

Segal B.M. (1963) Photosensivity, nail discoloration, and photo-onycholysis: side effects of tetracycline therapy. *Arch. Int. Med.* **112**, 165–167.

Zala L., Omar A. & Krebs A. (1977) Photo-onycholysis induced by 8-methoxypsoralen. *Dermatologica* **154**, 203–215.

Nail changes associated with drug-induced erythroderma

Beau's lines and onychomadesis are commonly observed in drug-induced erythroderma. A distinctive nail abnormality, which has been referred to as 'shoreline nails', has been described in three patients. All fingernails and toenails presented a transverse line of discontinuity in the nail plate that was preceded by a transverse band of leuconychia. This indicates that the drug reaction initially caused a defective keratinization of the nail matrix which was followed by a total matrix arrest. Thickened toenails showed less dramatic changes. Readministration of the drug caused the appearance of multiple bands in one patient (Shelley & Shelley, 1985).

Reference

Shelley W.B. & Shelley ED (1985) Shoreline nails: sign of drug-induced erythroderma. *Cutis* 220–224.

Nail changes associated with exposure to systemic medications in early pregnancy

Occurrence of malformations depends on the time of fetal exposure and dose of teratogen. Nails are infrequently affected except in complete expression of each syndrome. Hydantoin, trimethadione, carbamazepine (see p. 239), alcohol (see p. 196) and warfarin (see p. 251) are all reported to cause hypoplastic nails. Valproic acid has been associated with hyperconvex nails (see p. 239).

Drugs acting on the central nervous system

Anticonvulsant drugs

Hypoplasia of the fingernails and terminal phalanges of the fingers and sometimes the toes can occur in children whose mothers had been treated with trimethadione (Kosem & Lightner, 1978) or diphenylhydantoin during the first months of pregnancy (Hanson & Smith, 1975; Runne & Orfanos, 1981). Nail hyperpigmentation may also be seen (Johnson & Goldsmith, 1981). Phenytoin may cause an acute lichen planus-like eruption with nail involvement (Haneke, unpubl.). Fingernail and toenail hypoplasia has been described in the newborn of a 29-year-old epileptic woman who had been treated with carbamazepine during gestation. Regression of nail hypoplasia was observed during the first months of life (Niesen & Froscher, 1985).

Reversible onychomadesis with subsequent development of bluish-black discoloration of the nails has been reported in a 31-year-old Indian man treated with carbamazepine for a generalized partial seizure disorder. A band of longitudinal melanonychia was also present in three fingernails (Mishra *et al.*, 1989).

Digital abnormalities with long, thin, partly overlapping fingers and toes, and hyperconvex nails have been reported in infants of women with epilepsy who were receiving valproic acid monotherapy (Jager-Roman *et al.*, 1986).

References

Hanson J.W. & Smith D.W. (1975) The fetal hydantoin syndrome. *J. Pediatr.* **87**, 285–290.

Jager-Roman E., Deichl A., Jakob S. *et al.* (1986) Fetal growth, major malformations, and minor anomalies in infants born to women receiving valproic acid. *J. Pediatr.* **108**, 997–1004.

Johnson R.B. & Goldsmith L.A. (1981) Dilantin digital defects. *J. Am. Acad. Dermatol.* **5**, 191–196.

Kosem R.C. & Lightner E.S. (1978) Phenotypic malformations in association with maternal trimethadione therapy. *J. Pediatr.* **92**, 240.

Mishra D., Singh G. & Pandey S.S. (1989) Possible carbamazepine-induced reversible onychomadesis. *Int. J. Dermatol.* **28**, 460–461.

Niesen M. & Froscher W. (1985) Finger and toenail hypoplasia after carbamazepine monotherapy in late pregnancy. *Neuropediatrics* **16**, 167–168.

Runne U. & Orfanos C.E. (1981) The human nail. *Curr. Prob. Dermatol.* **9**, 102–149.

Benzodiazepines

Photoonycholysis and subungual haemorrhages occurred in a 36-year-old woman treated with clorazepate dipotassium 10 mg/day for several weeks (Torras *et al.*, 1989).

Reference

Torras H., Mascaro J.M. & Mascaro J.M. (1989) Photo-onycholysis caused by clorazepate dipotassium. *J. Am. Acad. Dermatol.* **21**, 1304–1305.

Tricyclic antidepressant

Leuconychia has been reported in patients treated with trazodone hydrochloride (Longstreth & Hershman, 1985; Gupta *et al.*, 1987).

References

Gupta M.A., Gupta A.K. & Ellis C.N. (1987) Antidepressant drugs in dermatology. *Arch. Dermatol.* **123**, 647–652.

Longstreth G.F. & Hershman J. (1985) Trazodone-induced hepatotoxicity and leukonychia. *J. Am. Acad. Dermatol.* **13**, 149–150.

Phenothiazines

High doses of chlorpromazine and related substituted phenothiazines taken for prolonged periods produce pigmentation on exposed areas of skin, ranging from tan or slate blue to a deep blue–black or purple colour. In severe cases the nail beds are also involved. The pigmentation is cumulative and increases in intensity in the summer months, fading only slightly in the winter. The mechanism is thought to be due to increased melanin deposition. Rarely, photoonycholysis may be caused by phenothiazines.

Reference

Satanove A. (1965) Pigmentation due to phenothiazines in high and prolonged dosage. *J. Am. Med. Assoc.* **191**, 263–268.

Lithium carbonate

Lithium therapy may induce a rich golden colour in the nail plate distally, the proximal part remaining pink (Hooper, 1971). Nail growth alteration occurs on reducing the dose of lithium. Transverse brown–black pigmented bands of the fingernails followed by latent onychomadesis have also been reported (Don & Silverman, 1988). Psoriasis is often aggravated or precipitated by lithium treatment. Rudolph (1991) has observed a case of psoriatic trachyonychia of the fingernails as the sole manifestation of lithium ingestion (Fig. 6.86).

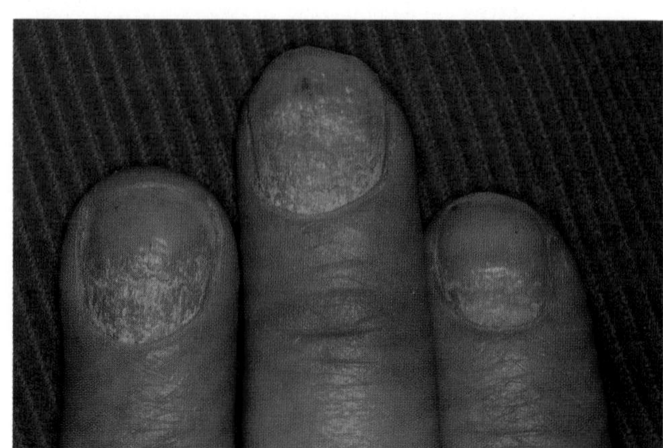

Fig. 6.86. Lithium-induced nail dystrophy (courtesy of R.I. Rudolph, USA).

References

Don P.C. & Silverman R.A. (1988) Nail dystrophy induced by lithium carbonate. *Cutis* **84**, 19–21.

Hooper J.F. (1971) Lithium carbonate and toenails. *Am. J. Psychiatr.* **138**, 1519.

Rudolph R.I. (1991) Lithium induced psoriasis of the fingernails *J. Am. Acad. Dermatol* **26**, 135–136.

Buspirone

Nail thinning can be a consequence of buspirone treatment (Daniel & Scher, 1990).

Reference

Daniel C.R. & Scher R.K. (1990) Nail changes secondary to systemic drugs or ingestants. In: *Nails: Therapy, Diagnosis, Surgery*, eds Scher R.K. & Daniel C.R., pp. 192–201. W.B. Saunders, Philadelphia.

L-Dopa

Accelerated nail growth and hardness of the nail has been described in patients treated with L-dopa for Parkinson's disease (Miller, 1973).

Reference

Miller E. (1973) Levodopa and nail growth. *New Engl. J. Med.* **208**, 916.

Cocaine

A patient developed livedo reticularis, acrocyanosis, generalized myalgia and proximal muscle weakness after inhalation of cocaine in a base pipe. Periungual erythema, microinfarctions and diffuse swelling of the fingers were prominent features (Zamora-Quezada *et al.*, 1988).

Reference

Zamoda-Quezada J.C., Dineman H., Stadecker M.J. & Kelly J.J. (1988) Muscle and skin infarction after free-basing cocaine (crack). *Ann. Intern. Med.* **108**, 564–566.

Retinoids (Figs 6.87–6.92)

Synthetic retinoids have evident effects on nail keratinization. Most of the side effects induced by retinoids on

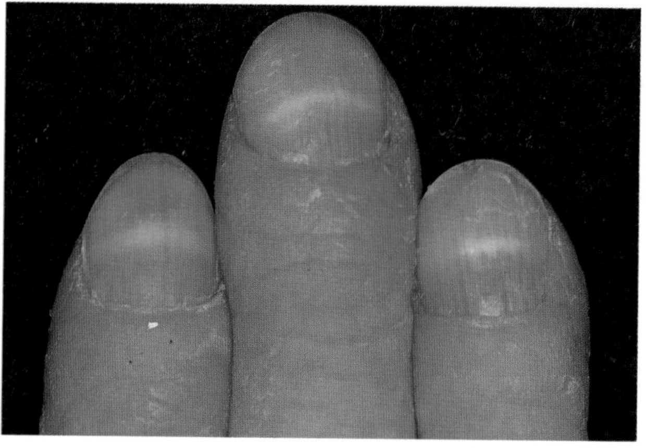

Fig. 6.87. Transverse leuconychia.

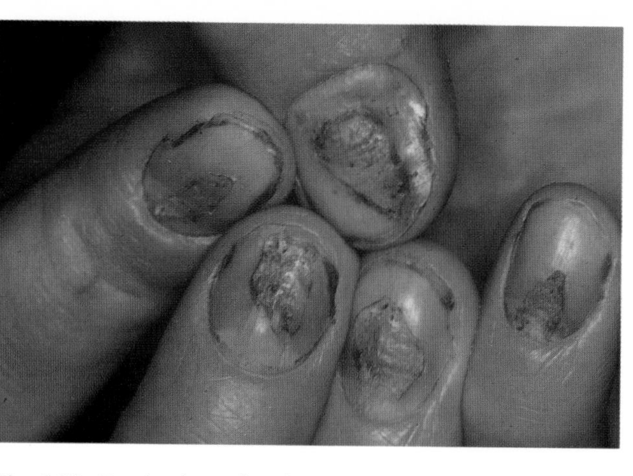

Fig. 6.88. Proximal onychoschizia.

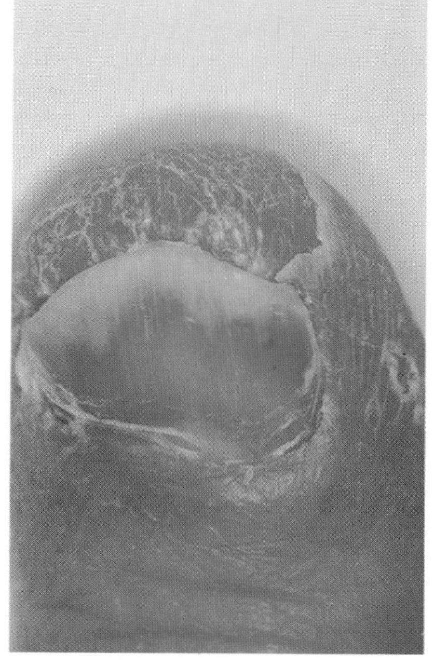

Fig. 6.89. Fingertip peeling and onycholysis.

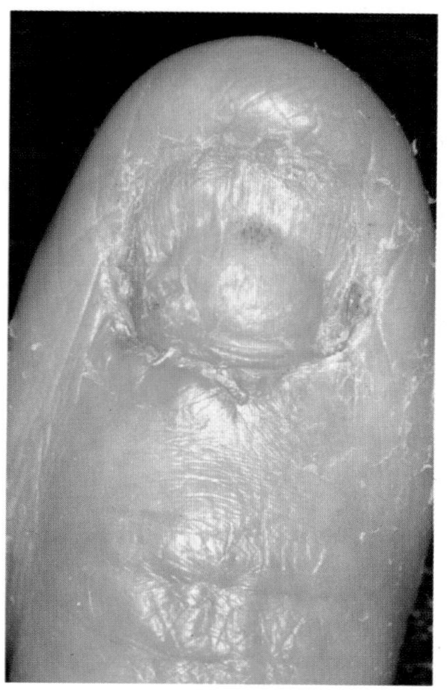

Fig. 6.90. Nail shedding.

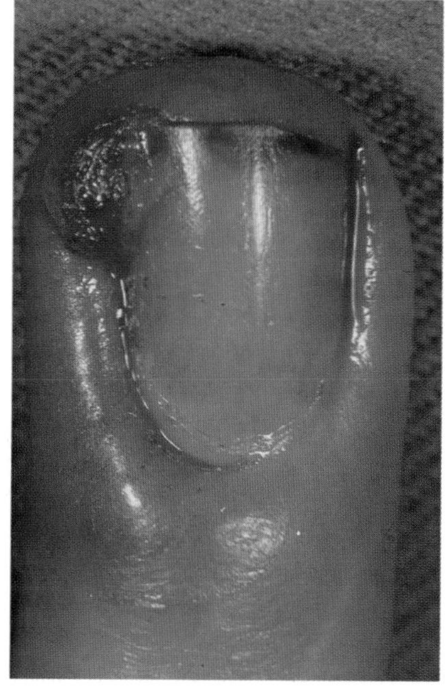

Fig. 6.91. Paronychia associated with pyogenic granuloma (courtesy of H. Zaun, Homburg, Germany).

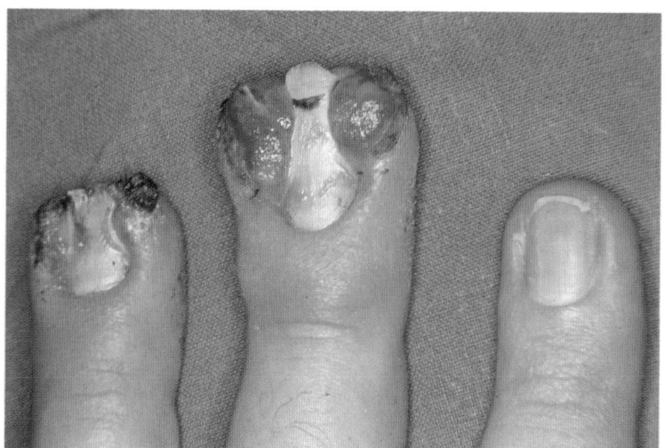

Fig. 6.92. Pyogenic granuloma (courtesy of J. Delescluses, Brussels).

Figs 6.87–6.92. Nail changes due to etretinate.

the nail apparatus can be explained as part of the general desquamative process. The delay in the appearance of nail complications ranges from 2 weeks to 18 months after the commencement of therapy. Their occurrence is unpredictable, but the changes are far more frequent in psoriatic patients than in other subjects. Sometimes the nail changes are transient even when medication is continued (Baran, 1982, 1986, 1990). Linear nail growth may be normal or more frequently decreased (Baran, 1982). Accelerated fingernail growth has however been documented in patients with psoriasis (Galosi *et al.*, 1985).

Nail thinning, splitting, softening and fragility are commonly seen during etretinate treatment (Ellis & Voorhees, 1987). A nail biopsy obtained from a patient who developed softening, thinning and depression of the proximal nail plate showed inadequate keratinization of the nail plate in the absence of inflammatory changes (Lindskov, 1982).

Although thinning of the nails can be regarded as a positive result in patients with thick psoriatic nails, some patients complain of increased sensitivity to external pressure and inability to use the nails in a functional way (Ellis & Voorhees, 1987). Beau's lines, latent or complete onychomadesis, proximal onychoschizia (Fig. 6.88) and transverse leuconychia (Fig. 6.87) are possible consequences of nail matrix damage (Baran *et al.*, 1983; Ferguson *et al.*, 1983; Garioch & Simpson, 1989).

Progressive onychoatrophy may lead to nail loss (Baran, 1986) (Fig. 6.90). Onycholysis (Fig. 6.89) is an uncommon complication of etretinate therapy (Orfanos *et al.*, 1978; Baran, 1982). Elkonyxis has also been reported (Cannata & Gambetti, 1990). A 35-year-old female treated with etretinate 0.25 mg/kg/day developed distal hemitorsion of the nail plates of several fingernails. This unusual side effect of etretinate has been referred to as 'curly nails' (Griffiths, 1990). A case of median nail dystrophy associated with isotretinoin therapy is unique (Bottomley & Cunliffe, 1993).

Chronic paronychia originating from periungual psoriasis foci frequently occurs in patients with psoriasis treated with etretinate, and has been related to retention of scales on the undersurface of the proximal nail fold (Baran, 1986). Pyogenic granuloma-like lesions of the nail folds (Figs 6.91 & 6.92) may be associated with chronic paronychia or may occur separately (Hodak *et al.*, 1984). Increased skin fragility along with nail plate brittleness resulting in fine spicules that break through the lateral nail grooves are possibly responsible for this peculiar side effect (Baran, 1990). Pyogenic granuloma-like lesions can also occur during isotretinoin treatment (Blumental, 1984; De Raeve *et al.*, 1986). Ingrowing nails can occasionally be observed.

References

Baran R. (1982) Action thérapeutique et complications du rétinoide aromatique sur l'appareil unguéal. *Ann. Dermatol. Venereol.* **109**, 367–371.

Baran R. (1986) Etretinate and the nails (study of 130 cases) possible mechanisms of some side-effects. *Clin. Exp. Dermatol.* **11**, 148–152.

Baran R. (1990) Retinoids and the nails. *J. Dermatol. Treat.* **1**, 151–154.

Baran R., Brun P. & Juhlin L. (1983) Leuconychie transversale induite par étrétinate. *Ann. Dermatol. Venereol.* **110**, 657.

Blumental G. (1984) Paronychia and pyogenic granuloma-like lesions with isotretinoin. *J. Am. Acad. Dermatol.* **4**, 677–678.

Bottomley W.W. & Cunliffe W.J. (1993) Median nail dystrophy associated with isotretinoin therapy. *Br. J. Dermatol.* **127**, 447–448.

Cannata G. & Gambetti M. (1990) Elkonyxis: une complication méconnue de l'étrétinate. *Nouv. Dermatol.* **9**, 251.

De Raeve L., Willemsen M., De Coninck A. & Roseeuw D. (1986) Paronychie et formation de tissu granuleux au cours d'un traitement par isotrétinoine. *Dermatologica* **172**, 278–280.

Ellis C.N. & Voorhees J.J. (1987) Etretinate therapy. *J. Am. Acad. Dermatol.* **16**, 267–291.

Ferguson M.M., Simpson N.B. & Hammersley N. (1983) Severe nail dystrophy associated with retinoid therapy. *Lancet* **ii**, 974.

Galosi A., Plewig G. & Braun-Falco O. (1985) The effect of aromatic retinoid RO 10-9359 (Etretinate) on fingernail growth. *Arch. Dermatol. Res.* **277**, 138–140.

Garioch J. & Simpson N.B. (1989) Etretinate and severe nail plate dystrophies. *Clin. Exp. Dermatol.* **14**, 261–262.

Griffiths W.A.D. (1990) 'Curly nails' – an unusual side-effect of etretinate. *J. Dermatol. Treat.* **1**, 265–266.

Hodak E., David M. & Feuerman E.J. (1984) Excess granulation tissue during etretinate therapy. *J. Am. Acad. Dermatol.* **11**, 1166–1167.

Lindskov R. (1982) Soft nails after treatment with aromatic retinoids. *Arch. Dermatol.* **118**, 535–536.

Orfanos C.E., Landes E. & Bloch P.H. (1978) Traitement du psoriasis pustuleux par un nouveau rétinoide aromatique (RO 10-9359). *Ann. Dermatol. Venereol.* **105**, 807–811.

Psoralens

Photoonycholysis can develop in patients submitted to PUVA therapy or treated with sunlight and orally administered psoralens (see Figs 6.82–6.85). It is often painful and has been reported after administration of both 8-methoxypsoralen (Zala *et al.*, 1977; Mackie 1979; Balato *et al.*, 1984) and 5-methoxypsoralen (Baran & Barthélémy, 1990). Fingernails are more commonly affected. Both splinter haemorrhages and subungual haematoma frequently occur and can possibly result in secondary onycholysis (Zala *et al.*, 1977; Balato *et al.*, 1984). The nail biopsy of a patient who developed photoonycholysis after 8-methoxypsoralen treatment showed multinucleate cells in the nail epithelium and multinucleate fibroblasts in the dermis of the nail bed (Zala *et al.*, 1977). Beau's lines have been occasionally associated with photoonycholysis

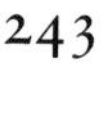

(Rau *et al.*, 1978; Mackie, 1979). Longitudinal melanonychia can also be seen in the fingernails of patients treated with 8-methoxypsoralen or 5-methoxypsoralen and ultraviolet irradiation (Naik & Singh, 1979; Weiss & Sayegh-Carreno, 1989). Pigmentation of the proximal portion of fingernail plates has been reported by Hann *et al.* (1989).

References

Balato N., Giordano C., Montesano M. & Lembo G. (1984) 8-Methoxypsoralen-induced photo-onycholysis. *Photodermatology* **1**, 202–203.

Baran R. & Barthélémy H. (1990) Photo-onycholyse induite par le 5-MOP (Psoraderm) et application de la méthode d'imputation des effets medicamenteux. *Ann. Dermatol. Venereol.* **117**, 367–369.

Briffa D.V. & Warin A.P. (1977) Photo-onycholysis caused by photochemotherapy. *Br. Med. J.* **2**, 1150.

Hann S.K., Hwang S.Y. & Park Y.K. (1989) Melanonychia induced by systemic photochemotherapy. *Photodermatology* **6**, 98–99.

Mackie R.M. (1979) Onycholysis occurring during PUVA therapy. *Clin. Exp. Dermatol.* **4**, 111–113.

Naik R.P.C. & Singh G. (1979) Nail pigmentation due to oral 8-methoxypsoralen. *Br. J. Dermatol.* **100**, 229–230.

Rau R.C., Flowers F.P. & Barrett J.L. (1978) Photo-onycholysis secondary to psoralen use. *Arch. Dermatol.* **114**, 448.

Weiss E. & Sayegh-Carreno R. (1989) PUVA-induced pigmented nails. *Int. J. Dermatol.* **28**, 188–189.

Zala L., Omar A. & Krebs A. (1977) Photo-onycholysis induced by 8-methoxypsoralen. *Dermatologica* **154**, 203–215.

Antimicrobial agents

Tetracyclines

A yellow fluorescence of the lunulae under Wood's lamp examination can be seen in patients taking tetracycline hydrochloride in dosages of 1 g or more daily. It can be useful for monitoring the patient compliance to the drug. A reversible yellow pigmentation of the lunulae occurred in a 26-year-old man treated with tetracycline hydrochloride for acne. The yellow lunulae fluoresced yellow on Wood's lamp examination (Hendricks, 1980). Yellow discoloration of the entire nail plate has also been reported during tetracycline treatment. Reddish nail fluorescence may follow demethylchlortetracycline therapy (Zaun, 1980).

Photoonycholysis is a possible side effect of treatment with tetracyclines (see p. 237). Among the tetracycline group, demetylchlortetracycline is the most common cause followed by doxycycline (Orentreich *et al.*, 1961; Cavens, 1981; Jeanmougin *et al.*, 1982). Minocycline has been occasionally incriminated whereas oxytetracycline, tetracycline chloridrate and tetracycline hydrochloride rarely induce this side effect. Beau's lines and subungual haemorrhages can occur in association with photoonycholysis (Harris, 1950; Domonkos, 1973). A patient who

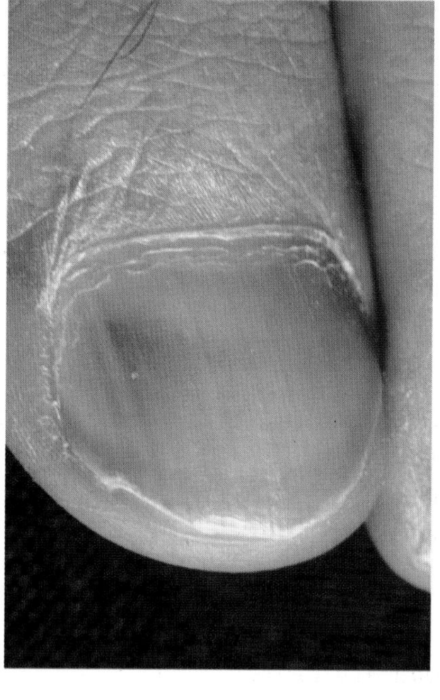

Fig. 6.93. Minocycline-induced nail pigmentation.

developed Raynaud's phenomenon of the left middle finger and photoonycholysis of the left hand after treatment with demethylchlortetracycline has been reported (Carter, 1966). Onycholysis that is not sun-related can also occur in patients on tetracycline (Daniel & Scher, 1984).

Minocycline can occasionally cause abnormal pigmentation of the skin, thyroid, nails (Fig. 6.93), bone, sclera, conjunctive as well as permanent discoloration of the teeth (Poliak *et al.*, 1985). Nail pigmentation during minocycline treatment is rare and is accompained by cutaneous pigmentation. A blue-grey or slate grey discoloration of the proximal portion of the nail bed as well as longitudinal brown pigmented bands or diffuse darkening and hyperpigmentation of the nail plate have been reported (Angeloni *et al.*, 1987). Pigmentation of the proximal nail folds can also occur (Mooney & Bennet, 1988).

An iron chelate of minocycline has been suggested as the cause of the nail pigmentation. Elemental analysis of nail clippings from a minocycline-treated patient showed the presence of a large amount of iron in pigmented areas of the nail but not in the adjacent normal nail. The possibility that nail polish is the source of iron in the pigmented nails is supported by the observation that minocycline-induced nail pigmentation occurs almost exclusively in women (Gordon *et al.*, 1985).

References

Angeloni V.L., Salasche S.J. & Ortiz R. (1987) Nail, skin and scleral pigmentation induced by minocycline. *Cutis* **40**, 229–233.

Carter W.I. (1966) Disorders of the nails. *Br. Med. J.* **2**, 1198–1199.
Cavens T.R. (1981) Onycholysis of the thumbs probably due to a phototoxic reaction from doxycycline. *Cutis* **27**, 53–54.
Daniel C.R. & Scher R.K. (1984) Nail changes secondary to systemic drugs or ingestants. *J. Am. Acad. Dermatol.* **10**, 250–258.
Domonkos A.N. (1973) Phototoxic onycholysis. *Arch. Dermatol.* **108**, 733.
Gordon G., Sparano B.M. & Iatropoulos M.J. (1985) Hyperpigmentation of the skin associated with minocycline therapy. *Arch. Dermatol.* **121**, 618–623.
Harris H.J. (1950) Aureomycin and chloramphenicol in brucellosis. *J. Am. Med. Assoc.* **142**, 161–165.
Hendricks A.A. (1980) Yellow lunulae with fluorescence after tetracycline therapy. *Arch. Dermatol.* **116**, 438–440.
Jeanmougin M., Morel P. & Civatte J. (1982) Photoonycholyse induite par la doxycycline. *Ann. Dermatol. Venereol.* **109**, 165–166.
Mooney E. & Bennett R.G. (1988) Periungual hyperpigmentation mimicking Hutchinson's sign associated with minocycline administration. *J. Dermatol. Surg. Oncol.* **14**, 1011–1013.
Orentreich N., Harber L.C. & Tromovitch T.A. (1961) Photosensitivity and photo-onycholysis due to demethylchlortetracycline. *Arch. Dermatol.* **83**, 730–737.
Poliak S.C., Di Giovanna J.J., Gross E.G., Gantt G. & Peck G.L. (1985) Minocycline-associated tooth discoloration in young adults. *J. Am. Med. Assoc.* **254**, 2930–2932.
Zaun H. (1980) *Krankhafte Veranderungen des Nagels* ed., Perim, p. 40. Erlangen.

Cephalosporin

A periungual inflammatory reaction resembling acute paronychia has been described in two fingers of a patient taking cephalexine (Fig. 6.94). The reaction resolved without residual pigmentation but recurred after readministration of the drug (Baran & Perrin, 1991). Shedding of the nails resulted from the administration of large doses of cephaloridine and cloxacillin in patients on maintenance haemodialysis (Eastwood *et al.*, 1969).

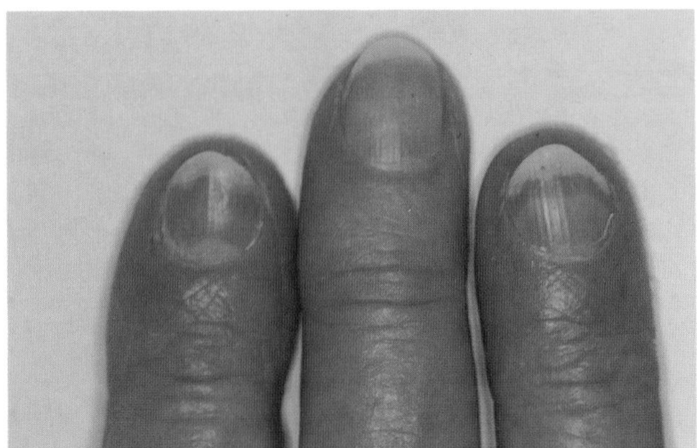

Fig. 6.94. Acute paronychia due to cephalexine involving the second and fourth fingers.

References

Baran R. & Perrin C. (1991) Fixed drug eruption presenting as an acute paronychia. *Br. J. Dermatol.* **125**, 592–595.
Eastwood J.B., Curtis J.R., Smith E.K.M. & De Wardener H.E. (1969) Shedding of nails apparently induced by the administration of large amounts of cephaloridine and cloxacillin in two anephric patients. *Br. J. Dermatol.* **81**, 750–752.

Chloramphenicol

Onycholysis and photoonycholysis are rare complications of chloramphenicol treatment (Runne & Orfanos, 1981).

Reference

Runne U. & Orfanos C.E. (1981) The human nail. *Curr. Prob. Dermatol.* **9**, 102–149.

Clofazimine

Two patients developed brown discoloration of the nail plate, subungual hyperkeratosis and onycholysis during treatment with clofazimine at high doses for lepromatous leprosy (Dixit *et al.*, 1989). Clofazimine crystals were demonstrated in the nail plate and in the nail bed. The nail changes regressed when the drug dosages were reduced. Reversible melanonychia has also been reported in a 55-year-old man treated with 300 mg/day of clofazimine for 6 months (Tosti *et al.*, 1992).

References

Dixit V.B., Chaudhary S.D. & Jain V.K. (1989) Clofazimine induced nail changes. *Ind. J. Lepr.* **61**, 476–478.
Tosti A., Piraccini B.M., Guerra L. & Bardazzi F. (1992) *Reversible Melanonychia Due to Clofazimine.* 18th World Congress of Dermatology, Book of Abstracts, 13A.

Quinolones

Photoonycholysis has been reported after treatment with flumequine, pefloxacine and ofloxacine (Revuz & Pouget, 1983; Baran & Brun, 1986). Subungual haemorrhages were associated with photoonycholysis in one patient (Baran & Brun, 1986).

References

Baran R. & Brun P. (1986) Photoonycholysis induced by the fluoroquinolones pefloxacine and ofloxacine. *Dermatologica* **176**, 185–188.
Revuz J. & Pouget F. (1983) Photo-onycholyse à l'apurone. *Ann. Dermatol. Venereol.* **110**, 765.

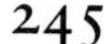

Sulphonamides

Onychomadesis, Beau's lines, paronychia, partial leuconychia and reduction of the nail growth may occur in patients who develop a photosensitivity reaction during sulphonamide treatment (Baran & Témime, 1973).

Reference

Baran R. & Témime P. (1973) Les onychodystrophies toxi-medicamenteuses et les onycholyses. *Conc. Med.* **95**, 1007–1023.

Dapsone

Beau's lines occurred in a 35-year-old female with borderline lepromatous leprosy who developed dapsone hypersensivity with erythroderma (Patki & Mehta, 1989). A severe but temporary hair loss and the appearance of transverse grooves followed the dapsone syndrome (high temperature, morbilliform rash, lymphadenopathy and hepatitis) (Kromann *et al.*, 1982).

References

Patki A.K. & Mehta J.M. (1989) Dapsone-induced erythroderma with Beau's lines. *Lepr. Rev.* **60**, 274–277.

Kromann N.P., Vilhelmsen R. & Stahl D. (1982) The dapsone syndrome. *Arch. Dermatol.* **118**, 531–532.

Emetine

White nails have been described in patients treated with emetine (Daniel & Scher, 1984).

Reference

Daniel C.R. & Scher R.K. (1984) Nail changes secondary to systemic drugs or ingestants. *J. Am. Acad. Dermatol.* **10**, 250–258.

Azidothymidine (AZT, zidovudine)

Various patterns of nail pigmentation have been described in patients receiving azydothymidine. Black or heavily pigmented patients more commonly develop nail hyperpigmentation, which has been estimated to occur in about 12–67% of patients using the drug (Groark *et al.*, 1990; Don *et al.*, 1990; Tosti *et al.*, 1990). Bluish to brown diffuse nail discoloration (Fig. 6.95) as well as transverse or longitudinal banding have been described (Furth & Kazakis, 1987; Panwalker, 1987; Azon-Masoliver *et al.*, 1988).

A faint blue pigmentation of the lunulae has also been reported (Greenberg & Berger, 1990). Fingernails seem to be more commonly affected than toenails. Nail pigmentation usually develops within 8 weeks but could occur after 1 year of therapy. It appears to be reversible when the use of AZT is discontinued or the dosage is reduced significantly.

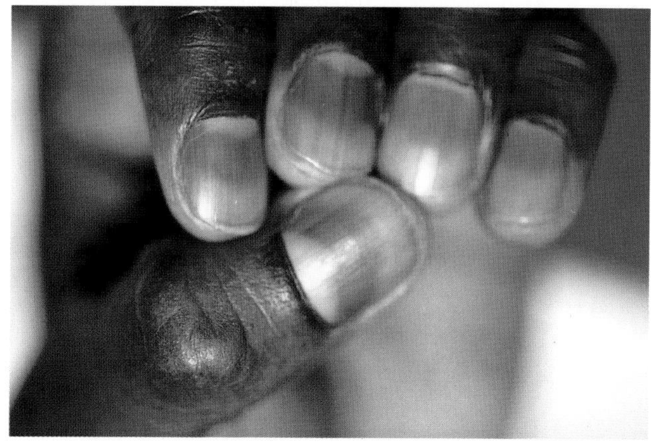

Fig. 6.95. AZT (azidothymidine, zidovudine)-induced nail pigmentation.

Histological studies have shown that AZT-induced nail pigmentation is due to melanin deposition (Grau-Massanes *et al.*, 1990; Tosti *et al.*, 1990). Nail matrix toxicity induced by the drug may result in matrix melanocyte stimulation (Fisher & McPoland, 1989; Groark *et al.*, 1990).

Slow nail growth has also been reported (Fisher & McPoland, 1989).

References

Azon-Masoliver A., Mallolas J., Gatell J. & Castel T. (1988) Zidovudine-induced nail pigmentation. *Arch. Dermatol.* **124**, 1570–1571.

Don P.C., Fusco F., Fried P. *et al.* (1990) Nail dyschromia associated with zidovudine. *Ann. Intern. Med.* **112**, 145–146.

Fisher C.A. & McPoland P.R. (1989) Azidothymidine-induced nail pigmentation. *Cutis* **43**, 552–554.

Furth P.A. & Kazakis A.M. (1987) Nail pigmentation changes associated with azidothymidine (zidovudine). *Ann. Intern. Med.* **107**, 350–351.

Grau-Massanes M., Millan F., Febrer M.I. *et al.* (1990) Pigmented nail bands and mucocutaneous pigmentation in HIV-positive patients treated with zidovudine. *J. Am. Acad. Dermatol.* **22**, 687–688.

Greenberg R.G. & Berger T.G. (1990) Nail and mucocutaneous hyperpigmentation with azidothymidine therapy. *J. Am. Acad. Dermatol.* **22**, 327–330.

Groark S.P., Hood A.F. & Nelson K. (1990) Nail pigmentation associated with zidovudine. *J. Am. Acad. Dermatol.* **21**, 1032–1033.

Panwalker A.P. (1987) Nail pigmentation in the acquired immunodeficiency syndrome (AIDS). *Ann. Intern. Med.* **107**, 943–944.

Tosti A., Gaddoni G., Fanti P.A., D'Antuono A. & Albertini F. (1990) Longitudinal melanonychia induced by 3′-azidodeoxythymidine. *Dermatologica* **180**, 217–220.

Anti-inflammatory agents

Acetanilid

Acetanilid can produce purple discoloration of the nails (Positano *et al.*, 1989).

Reference

Positano R.G., DeLauro T.M. & Berkowitz B.J. (1989) Nail changes secondary to environmental influences. *Clin. Pod. Med. Surg.* **6**, 417–429.

Aspirin

Purpura of the nail bed can be seen in patients taking aspirin.

Benoxaprofen

Benoxaprofen is a non-steroidal anti-inflammatory agent that has been withdrawn from the market because of its serious side effects. Photoonycholysis was a common side effect of benoxaprofen treatment (McCormack *et al.*, 1982). Benoxaprofen-induced photosensitivity and onycholysis are possibly related to the ability of the drug to stimulate spontaneous oxidative metabolism and degranulation of human leucocytes (Anderson & Anderson, 1982). Onycholysis was seen in toes, without photo-onycholysis (Fenton, 1982). Accelerated nail growth has been reported in patients treated with benoxaprofen (Fenton *et al.*, 1982; Fenton & Wilkinson, 1983). Koilonychia has also been described.

References

Anderson R. & Anderson I.F. (1982) The possible value of retinoic acid in the treatment of benoxaprofen-induced photosensitivity and onycholysis. *Afr. Med. J.* **26**, 985.

Fenton D.A. (1982) Side effects of benoxaprofen. *Br. Med. J.* **284**, 1631.

Fenton D.A. & Wilkinson J.D. (1983) Milia, increased nail growth and hypertrichosis following treatment with benoxaprofen. *J. R. Soc. Med.* **76**, 525–527.

Fenton D.A., English J.S. & Wilkinson J.D. (1982) Reversal of male-pattern baldness, hypertrichosis, and accelerated hair and nail growth in patients receiving benoxaprofen. *Br. Med. J.* **284**, 1228–1229.

McCormack L.S., Elgart M.L. & Turner M.L. (1982) Benoxaprofen-induced photo-onycholysis. *J. Am. Acad. Dermatol.* **7**, 678–680.

Ibuprofen

Longitudinal melanonychia has been reported by Daniel and Scher (1990).

Reference

Daniel C.R. & Scher R.K. (1990) Nail changes secondary to systemic drugs or Ingestant In: *Nails: Therapy, Diagnosis, Surgery*, eds Scher R.K. & Daniel C.R., pp. 192–201. W.B. Saunders, Philadelphia.

Cardiovascular drugs

β-blockers

β-blockers have been implicated in the cause of psoriasiform skin eruptions and the exacerbation of preexisting psoriasis (Gold *et al.*, 1988). Histopathology in a case with mucous membrane, scrotal and nail involvement showed a mixed psoriasiform and lichenoid reaction. There was a mild acanthosis of matrix and nail bed epithelium, a spongiosis with mononuclear exocytosis, a hypergranulosis and hyperorthokeratosis. Some polymorphonuclear leucocytes were found just beneath the keratosis. A band-like mainly lymphocytic infiltrate was found in the subepidermal connective tissue. Although some basal cells were swollen, hydrotic degeneration of the basal layer was not a pronounced feature (Haneke, unpubl.). Psoriasis-like nail changes have been reported during treatment with the β-blocker agent practolol. Reversible pincer nails occurred in a 48-year-old woman treated with practolol. Painful narrowing of the nail bed and excessive transverse overcurvature were associated with subungual hyperkeratosis, onycholysis and brownish discoloration of the nail plate (Tegner, 1976).

Pitting, thickening and discoloration of the nail plate have been described during propanolol treatment. Periungual tiny pustules can also occur (Jensen *et al.*, 1976). Beau's lines and alopecia have been reported during metoprolol treatment (Graeber & Lapkin, 1981).

Cold extremities and Raynaud's phenomenon are possible side effects of β-blocker treatment of hypertension. Pterygium inversum unguis can also occur. Peripheral ischaemia leading to digital gangrene is a rare complication of β-blocker treatment, which almost exclusively occurs in patients with hypertension. Although both cardioselective (atenolol, metoprolol acebutolol) and non-selective (propanolol, timolol, oxyprenol) β-blockers can cause digital necrosis, propanolol is more commonly responsible (Stringer & Bentley, 1986; Dompmartin *et al.*, 1988). Reversion of symptoms does not always follow withdrawal of the drug and digit or limb amputation has been the final outcome in several patients. The occurrence of acral skin necrosis is related to the twofold effect of β-blockers on peripheral circulation. In fact, the reflex vasoconstriction (mediated by β-adrenoreceptors), which occurs in response to the reduction in cardiac output, cannot be compensated by vasodilation because of the β-receptor blockage. Elderly and hypertensive patients who have an acquired deficiency of β-receptors are more sensitive to the ischaemic effects of β-blockers.

A patient with phaeochromocytoma developed acral skin necrosis along with splinter haemorrhages and periungual telangiectasias after taking atenolol. Her skin biopsy showed epidermal and sweat-gland necrosis (Naeyaert *et al.*, 1987). Reversible symmetrical brown discoloration of fingernails and toenails has been reported in a 56-year-old woman affected by glaucoma who was treated with timolol maleate 0.5% eyedrops (Feiler-Ofry *et al.*, 1981).

References

Dompmartin A., Le Maitre M., Letessier D. & Leroy D. (1988) Nécroses digitales sous beta-bloquants. *Ann. Dermatol. Venereol.* **115**, 593–596.

Feiler-Ofry V., Godel V. & Lazar M. (1981) Nail pigmentation following timolol maleate therapy. *Ophthalmologica* **182**, 153–156.

Gold M.H., Holy A.K. & Roenigk H.H. Jr (1988) Beta-blocking drugs and psoriasis: A review of cutaneous side-effects and retrospective analysis of their effects on psoriasis. *J. Am. Acad. Dermatol.* **19**, 837–841.

Graeber C.W. & Lapkin R.A. (1981) Metoprolol and alopecia. *Cutis* **28**, 633–634.

Jensen H.A.E., Mikkelson H.I., Wadskov S. & Sondergaard J. (1976) Cutaneous reactions to propanolol (Inderal). *Acta Med. Scand.* **199**, 363–367.

Naeyaert J.M., Deram E., Santosa S. & Rubens R. (1987) Sweat-gland necrosis after beta-adrenergic antagonist treatment in a patient with pheochromocytoma. *Br. J. Dermatol.* **117**, 371–376.

Stringer M.D. & Bentley P.G. (1986) Peripheral gangrene associated with β-blockade. *Br. J. Surg.* 73, 1008.

Tegner E. (1976) Reversible overcurvature of the nails after treatment with practolol. *Acta Derm. Venereol. (Stock.)* **56**, 493–495.

Captopril

Reversible onycholysis has been reported in patients treated with captopril (Brueggemeyer & Ramirez, 1984). A lichenoid skin eruption associated with hair loss, ageusia and nail dystrophy (Fig. 6.96) occurred in a patient with renal insufficiency treated with captopril (Smit *et al.*, 1983).

References

Brueggemeyer C. & Ramirez G. (1984) Onycholysis associated with captopril. *Lancet* **i**, 1352–1353.

Smit A.J., Hoorntje S.J. & Donker A.J.M. (1983) Zinc deficiency during captopril treatment. *Nephron* **34**, 196–197.

Clonidine

Raynaud's syndrome is a possible side effect of clonidine treatment (Delanoe & Puissant, 1974).

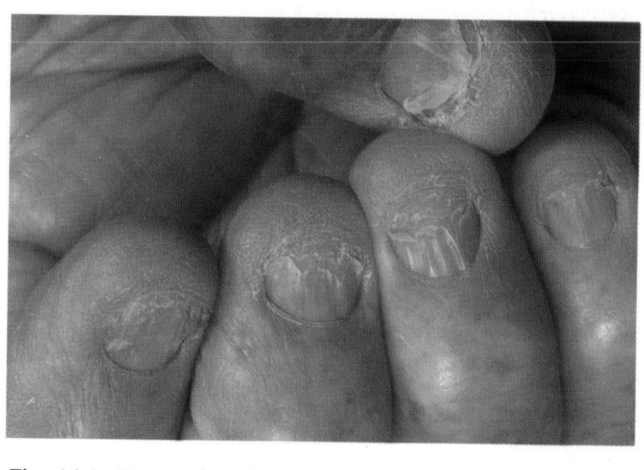

Fig. 6.96. Captopril nail atrophy (lichen planus-like).

Reference

Delanoe J. & Puissant A. (1974) Les principaux medicaments responsable des toxidermies. *Rev. Med.* **19**, 1199–1212.

Calcium channel blockers

A 'nail dystrophy' has been reported in association with nifedipine, verapamil or diltiazem treatment (Stern & Khalsa, 1989).

Reference

Stern R. & Khalsa J.H. (1989) Cutaneous adverse reactions associated with calcium channel blockers. *Arch. Intern. Med.* **149**, 829–832.

Quinidine

Horizontal blue-grey discoloration of the nail bed has been described in the fingernails and toenails of an 83-year-old man receiving quinidine (Mahler *et al.*, 1986). This antiarhythmic agent is the D-isomer of quinine and presents structural similarities with synthetic antimalarials (see p. 251).

Reference

Mahler R., Sissons W. & Watters K. (1986) Pigmentation induced by quinidine therapy. *Arch. Dermatol.* **122**, 1062–1064.

Amrinone

Nail discoloration has been observed during amrinone therapy (Wilsmhurst & Webb-Peploe, 1983).

Reference

Wilsmhurst P.T. & Webb-Peploe M.M. (1983) Side effects of amrinone therapy. *Br. Heart J.* **49**, 447–451.

Purgatives

A bluish discoloration of the lunulae can be observed in patients treated with phenolphthalein (Campbell, 1931). Paronychia-like changes and nail plate ridging have also been described (Wise & Sulzberger, 1933). Differential diagnosis includes azure lunulae due to argyria or to Wilson's disease. Reversible finger clubbing has been reported in purgative abuse (see p. 210).

References

Campbell G.G. (1931) Peculiar pigmentation following the use of a purgative containing phenolphthalein. *Br. J. Dermatol.* **43**, 186–187.

Wise F. & Sulzberger M.B. (1933) Drug eruptions. *Arch. Dermatol. Syphil.* **27**, 549–567.

Intoxicants

Toxic oil syndrome

In 1981 a multisystem disease occurred in Spain, after ingestion of denatured rapeseed oil. Raynaud's phenomenon and scleroderma-like changes were commonly observed during the chronic phase of the disease (Noriega *et al.*, 1982; Alonso-Ruiz *et al.*, 1984).

References

Alonso-Ruiz A., Zea-Mendoza A.C., Gonzàles-Lanza M. & Go'mez-Catalàn E. (1984) Digital tuft alterations in toxic oil syndrome. *Lancet* **ii**, 520–521.

Noriega A.R., Go'mez-Reino J., Lopéz-Encuentra A. *et al.* (1982) Toxic epidemic syndrome, Spain 1981. *Lancet* **ii**, 697–702.

Polychlorinated biphenyl intoxication

Nail pigmentation has been reported in PCB-exposed workers. Nail deformities occurred in 68% of patients with polychlorinated biphenyl poisoning due to consumption of rice-bran cooking oil contaminated by large amounts of polychlorinated biphenyls and congeners. Flattened nails were noted in one-fourth of Urabe and Asahi's patients (1984), ingrowing nails and lamellar dystrophy were also particularly common. Dark brown pigmentation was frequently seen on the finger- and toenails (Wong *et al.*, 1982). Nail deformities were also frequently observed in children born from a few months to several years after maternal PCB poisoning. Specific nail deformities included koilonychia, transverse grooves, ridging, thinning, longitudinal splitting, onychauxis and transverse overcurvature. Hyperpigmentation of the nail plate and bed was also observed. Toenails were affected more than fingernails (Taylor, 1988; Gladen *et al.*, 1990).

References

Gladen B.C., Taylor J.S., Wu Y.C., Ragan N.B., Rogan W.J. & Hsu C.C. (1990) Dermatological findings in children exposed transplacentally to heat-degraded polychlorinated biphenyls in Taiwan. *Br. J. Dermatol.* **122**, 799–808.

Taylor J.S. (1988) Congenital Yucheng – dermatological findings. *Proc. Am. Dermatol. Assoc. St Moritz*, p. 30.

Urabe H. & Asahi M. (1984) Past and current dermatological status of Yusho patients. *Am. J. Indust. Med.* **5**, 5–12.

Wong C.K., Chen C.J., Cheng P.C. & Chen P.H. (1982) Mucocutaneous manifestations of polychlorinated biphenyls (PCB) poisoning: a study of 122 cases in Taiwan. *Br. J. Dermatol.* **107**, 317–323.

Carbon monoxide

A cherry red discoloration of the nail bed is a symptom of carbon monoxide intoxication (Baran, 1981).

Reference

Baran R. (1981) Modifications of colour: chromonychias or dyschromias. In: *The Nail*, ed. Pierre M., pp. 30–38. Churchill Livingstone, Edinburgh.

Selenium

Nail loss has been described in selenium intoxication (MMWR, 1984).

Reference

Morbidity and Mortality Weekly Report (1984) Selenium intoxication. *J. Am. Med. Assoc.* **251**, 1938.

Vinyl chloride

Clubbing-like nail changes in the fingers have been observed in vinyl chloride disease (Runne & Orfanos, 1981). Scleroderma-like changes and acroosteolysis can also occur.

Reference

Runne U. & Orfanos C.E. (1981) The human nail. *Curr. Prob. Dermatol.* **9**, 102–149.

Heavy metal intoxications

Arsenic

Colorimetry polarography, atomic absorption and neutron activation analysis can be used to detect arsenic in body tissues, hairs and nails. Nail samples containing more than 3 ppm of arsenic are diagnostic for arsenic intoxication (Massey *et al.*, 1984).

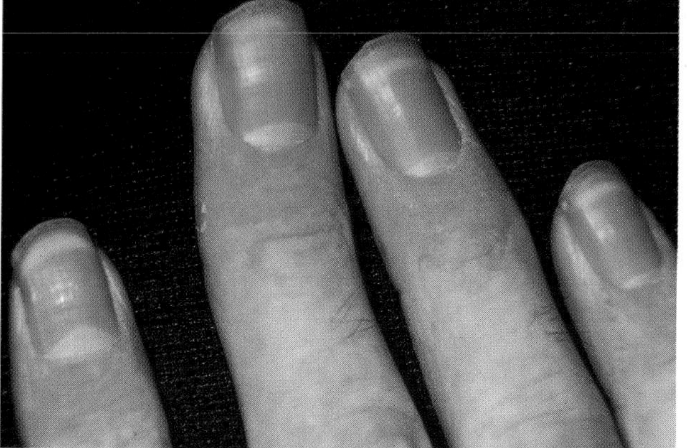

Fig. 6.97. Arsenic poisoning – transverse white band (Mees' lines) (courtesy of J. Mascaro, Barcelona).

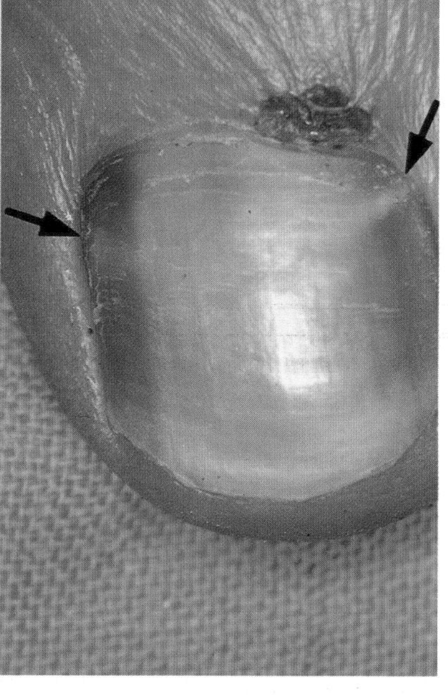

Fig. 6.98. Arsenic poisoning – periungual and subungual keratoses.

Mees' lines are a typical symptom of arsenic poisoning. They appear as transverse white bands (Thomas, 1964) (Fig. 6.97) that move distally with nail growth (true leuconychia). A single broad band is usually seen (Welter *et al.*, 1982), but multiple lines are occasionally observed (Aldrich, 1904).

Beau's lines, onychomadesis, longitudinal brown hyperpigmented bands as well as diffuse blackish-brown discoloration of the nail plate and keratosis have also been described in arsenic intoxication (De Nicola *et al.*, 1974) (Fig. 6.98).

An endemic peripheral vascular disorder resembling Buerger's disease has been described in a limited area of southern Taiwan. The disorder, which has been referred to as 'black foot disease', results in gangrene in the extremities. It has been associated with drinking of artesian well water containing both arsenic and chemically unknown fluorescent substances. A similarity between fluorescent substances and ergot alkaloids has been suggested (Yu *et al.*, 1984).

References

Aldrich C.J. (1904) Leuconychia striata arsenicalis transversus with report of 3 cases. *Am. J. Med. Sci.* **127**, 702–709.

De Nicola P., Morsiani M. & Zavagli G. (1974) *Nail Diseases in Internal Medicine*. Charles C. Thomas, Springfield, IL.

Massey W., Wold D. & Heyman A. (1984) Arsenic: homicidal intoxication. *South. Med. J.* 77, 848–851.

Thomas H.M. (1964) Transverse bands in fingernails. *Bull. Johns Hopkins Hosp.* **115**, 238–244.

Welter A., Michaux M. & Blondeel A. (1982) Lignes de Mees dans un cas d'intoxication aigue à l'arsenic. *Dermatologica* **165**, 482–483.

Yu H.S., Sheu H.M., Ko S.S., Chiang L.C., Chien C.H., Lin S.M., Tserng B.R. & Chen C.S. (1984) Studies on blackfoot disease and chronic arsenism in Southern Taiwan. *J. Dermatol.* **11**, 361–370.

Silver

A bluish-black pigmentation of the skin of sun-exposed areas including the periungual regions is a cardinal feature of argyria. A slate-blue discoloration of the proximal nail beds is typical, the pigmentation being more evident in the lunulae (Figs 6.99 & 6.100). The toes are not usually involved. The pigmentation is permanent (Plewig *et al.*, 1977; Tanner & Gross, 1990).

Differential diagnosis includes azure lunulae observed in patients with Wilson's disease and bluish discoloration occurring after systemic administration of phenolphthalein. Deposition of silver granules in the dermal tissue can be detected both in light-exposed and non-exposed areas of patients with argyria. The reduction of colourless silver salts to black metallic silver under the influence of light has been suggested to explain the pathogenesis of skin and nail pigmentation in argyria (Shelley *et al.*, 1987).

References

Plewig G., Lincke H. & Wolff H.H. (1977) Silver-blue nails. *Acta Derm. Venereol. (Stock.)* **57**, 413–419.

Shelley W.B., Shelley E.D. & Burmeister V. (1987) Argyria: the intradermal 'photograph', a manifestation of passive photosensivity. *J. Am. Acad. Dermatol.* **16**, 211–217.

Tanner L.S. & Gross D.J. (1990) Generalized argyria. *Cutis* **45**, 237–239.

Mercury

Acrodynia is a rare disorder that principally occurs in infancy and is due to chronic exposure to mercury. Excruciating pain in the hands and feet together with inter-

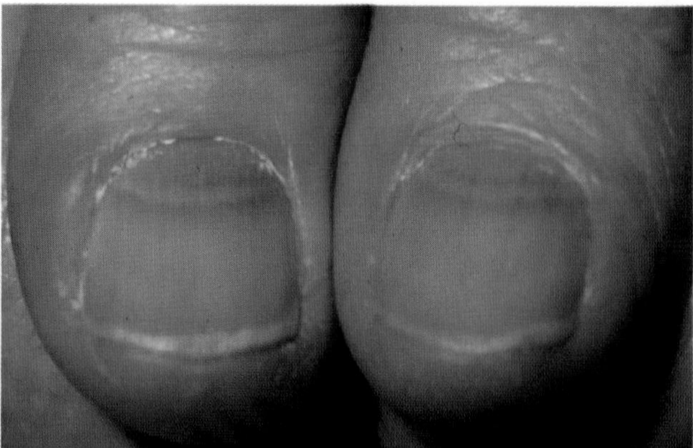

Fig. 6.99.

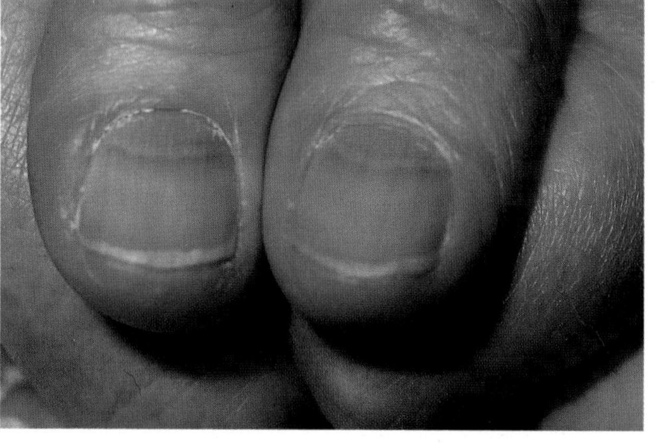

Fig. 6.100.

Figs 6.99 & 6.100. Argyria (silver), showing slate blue, mainly lunular, pigmentation.

mittent pink discoloration of the tips of the fingers, toes and nose is an early manifestation of the disease (Dinehart *et al.*, 1988). Ridging, fragility and dark discoloration of the nail plates is frequently observed. Alopecia and nail loss have been reported in severe cases. Gangrene of the extremities may develop (Boissière, 1971).

Oral treatment with DMPS (sodium dimercaptopropane sulphonate) has been successfully used in a child with acrodynia (Bockers *et al.*, 1984).

A greyish-brown discoloration of the nails can occur after chronic exposure to topical preparations containing mercury (Butterworth & Strean, 1963). Hair loss and a brown pigmentation of the distal portion of the fingernails occurred in a patient with chronic mercury poisoning caused by the use of mercury-containing cosmetic bleaches. The mercury content of the patient's nails was extremely high (Wustner & Orfanos, 1975). A similar case has been also reported by Böckers *et al.* (1985).

References

Bockers M., Schonberger W. & Neumann P. (1984) Klinik und Therapie der Akrodynie infolge inhalative Quecksilberintoxikation. *Int. Cong. Eur. Soc. Ped. Dermatol.*, Munster Dia-Klinik, pp. 24–25.

Bockers M., Wagner R. & Oster O. (1985) Nageldyscromie als leitsymptom einer chronischen Quecksilberintoxication Durch ein Kosmetisches Bleichmittel. *Z. Autkz.* **60**, 821–829.

Boissière H. (1971) Les gangrènes cutanées du nourrisson. *Conc. Med.* **24**, 3138–3154.

Butterworth T. & Strean L.P. (1963) Mercurial pigmentation of nails. *Arch. Dermatol.* **88**, 55–57.

Dinehart S.M., Dillard R., Raimer S.S., Diven S., Cobos R. & Pupo R. (1988) Cutaneous manifestations of acrodynia (Pink disease). *Arch. Dermatol.* **124**, 107–109.

Wustner H. & Orfanos C.E. (1975) Nagelverfarbung und haaranusfall. *Dtsch. Med. Wschr.* **100**, 1694–1697.

Gold

Gold levels in skin, hair and nails do not appear to correlate with gold toxicity (Gottlieb *et al.*, 1974). Yellow to dark brown nail plate pigmentation can occur after parenteral gold therapy (Fam & Paton, 1984). Nail thinning, softening, fragility, onycholysis and onychomadesis can also be seen (Voigt & Holzegel, 1977). Slow nail growth has been reported by Sertoli (1956).

References

Fam A.G. & Paton T.W. (1984) Nail pigmentation after parenteral gold therapy for rheumatoid arthritis: 'gold nails'. *Arth. Rheum.* **27**, 119–120.

Gottlieb N.L., Smith P.M., Penneys N.S. & Smith E.M. (1974) Gold concentrations in hair, nail and skin during chrysotherapy. *Arth. Rheum.* **17**, 56–62.

Sertoli P. (1956) Fisiopatologia del complesso ungueale. *Ed. Min. Med.* 250.

Voigt K. & Holzegel K. (1977) Bleibende Nagelveranderungen nach goldtherapie. *Hautarzt* **28**, 121–123.

Lead

Onychomadesis, leuconychia and onychalgia have been reported in lead poisoning (Pardo Castello & Pardo, 1960; Daniel & Scher, 1990). Diffuse hyperpigmentation of fingernails and toenails occurred in a 55-day-old boy after the use of an astringent powder with a high lead content (Wenynan & Mingyu, 1989). Partial leuconychia and nail bed hyperkeratosis have also been described (Sertoli, 1956; Baran, 1981).

References

Baran R. (1981) Modifications of colour: chromonychias or dyschromias. In: *The Nail*, ed. Pierre M., pp. 30–38. Churchill Livingstone, Edinburgh.

Daniel C.R. & Scher R.K. (1990) Nail changes secondary to

systemic drugs or Ingestants. In: *Nails: Therapy, Diagnosis, Surgery*, eds Scher R.K. & Daniel C.R., pp. 192–201. W.B. Saunders, Philadelphia.

Pardo Castello V. & Pardo O. (1960) *Diseases of the Nails*, 3rd edn., p. 244. Charles C. Thomas, Springfield, IL.

Sertoli P. (1956) Fisiopatologia del complesso ungueale. *Ed. Min. Med.* p. 250.

Wenyuan Z. & Mingyu X. (1989) Hyperpigmentation of the nail from lead deposition. *Int. J. Dermatol.* **28**, 273–275.

Thallium

Diffuse or partial brownish discoloration of the nails has been described in thallium poisoning. Onychorrhexis and Mees' lines can be observed in acute intoxication (De Nicola *et al.*, 1974; Baran, 1981). Dry scaling of the distal parts of the extremities can also occur (Heyl & Barlow, 1989).

References

Baran R. (1981) Modifications of colour: chromonychias or dyschromias. In: *The Nail*, ed. Pierre M., pp. 30–38. Churchill Livingstone, Edinburgh.

De Nicola P., Morsiani M. & Zavagli G. (1974) *Nail Diseases in Internal Medicine*, pp. 47 & 84. Charles C. Thomas, Springfield, IL.

Heyl T. & Barlow R.J. (1989) Thallium poisoning: a dermatological perspective. *Br. J. Dermatol.* **121**, 787–792.

Aniline

A purplish-blue discoloration of the nail bed due to cyanosis has been reported in aniline poisoning (Baran, 1981). Softening of the nail plate can also occur (Sertoli, 1956).

References

Baran R. (1981) Modifications of colour: chromonychias or dyschromias. In: *The Nail*, ed. Pierre M., pp. 30–38. Churchill Livingstone Edinburgh.

Sertoli P. (1956) Fisiopatologia del complesso ungueale. *Ed. Min. Med.* 250.

Chromium salts

Dichromates produce a yellow ocre colour of the nails (Baran, 1981) (see chromonychia, Chapter 7).

Reference

Baran R. (1981) Modifications of colour: chromonychias or dyschromias. In: *The Nail*, ed. Pierre M., pp. 30–38. Churchill Livingstone, Edinburgh.

Anticoagulants

Nail growth can be reduced during heparin treatment (Ludwig, 1965). Transverse red banding, separated from the lunula by a pink area, and subungual haematoma are also recognized signs of anticoagulation. A purple discoloration of the toenails can be seen after a few weeks of treatment with warfarin (Feder & Auerbach, 1961; Lebsack & Weilbert, 1982). Hypoplasia of the fingernails and terminal phalanges, associated with stippled epiphyses, can occur in children whose mothers have been treated with warfarin during the first trimester of pregnancy (Pettiform *et al.*, 1975). Ross (1963) noted intermittent diffuse, orange-coloured staining of the finger nails in patients submitted to long-term treatment with phenindione.

References

Feder W. & Auerbach R. (1961) 'Purple toes'; an uncommon sequela of oral coumarin drug therapy. *Ann. Intern. Med.* **55**, 911–917.

Lebsack C.S. & Weilbert R.T. (1982) Purple toes syndrome. *Postgrad. Med.* **71**, 81.

Ludwig E. (1965) Nebenwirkungen der heparinoide auf haare und nagel. In: *Webenwirkungen und Bluntingen bei Antikoagulation und Fibrinolytika*, eds Zukschwerd L. & Thies H.A. Schattauer-Verlag, Stuttgard.

Pettiform J.M. *et al.* (1975) Congenital malformation with the administration of oral anticoagulants during pregnancy. *J. Pediatr.* **86**, 459–462.

Ross J.B. (1963) Side effects of phenindione. *Br. Med. J.* **1**, 866.

Antimalarial agents

Since chloroquine is stored in the fingernails over a long period of time, determination of chloroquine in nail clippings can be useful in assessing drug intake dating back at least 1 year (Ofori-Adjei & Ericsson, 1985).

Development of pigmentary changes, which is most commonly observed in Caucasians, is a characteristic side effect of antimalarial usage (Tuffanelli *et al.*, 1963). A bluish-black or bluish-brown pigmentation of the nail beds can be seen following prolonged treatment with amodiaquine, mepacrine (quinacrine) and chloroquine (Baden & Zaias, 1987; Dodd & Sarkany, 1988). Diffuse nail bed pigmentation (Figs 6.101 & 6.102) as well as transverse hyperpigmented bands can occur. The nature of the pigment is still undetermined but both melanin and haemosiderin deposits appear to be present (Tuffanelli *et al.*, 1963). The presence of a complex containing the antimalarial has also been suggested.

Nail pigmentation usually takes several months to decrease in intensity after cessation of therapy and it may not disappear completely. An increased incidence of retinopathy has been noted in patients with cutaneous hyperpigmentation (Tuffanelli *et al.*, 1963).

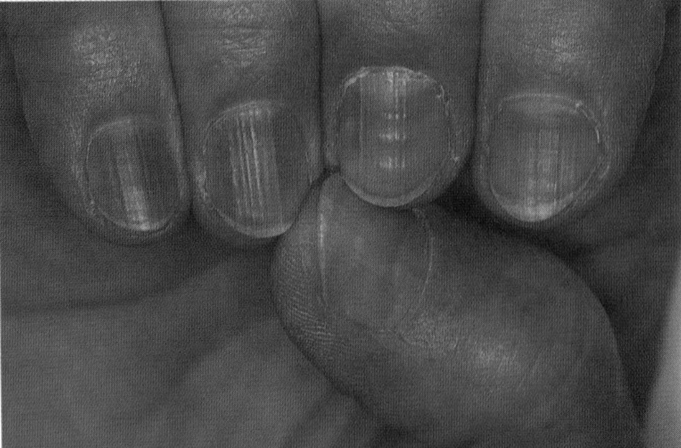

Fig. 6.101.

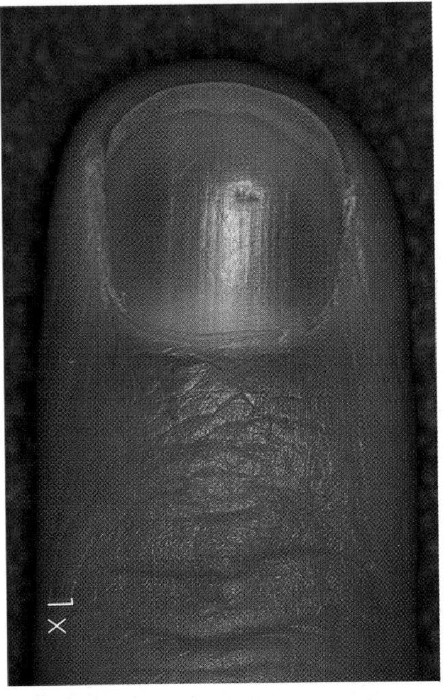

Fig. 6.102.

Figs 6.101 & 6.102. Antimalarial diffuse nail pigmentation (courtesy of J.L. Verret, Angers, France).

A nail discoloration varying from white, diffuse yellow or lemon-green to blue-green or grey has been described in patients taking mepacrine. Both blue and yellow discoloration of the nail bed may be seen together (Baran & Témime, 1973). A purplish-blue transverse pigmentation of the nail bed has been described during chloroquine treatment (Baran & Témime, 1973). A characteristic green-yellow or whitish fluorescence of the nails under the Wood's light is also commonly observed during mepacrine treatment (Kierland *et al.*, 1946). Nail pitting, ridging and shedding can occur in association with mepacrine treatment (Baran & Témime, 1973).

Photoonycholysis associated with a lichenoid eruption has been described in a 66-year-old man receiving quinine sulphate (Tan *et al.*, 1989).

References

Baran R. & Témime P. (1973) Les onychodystrophies toxi-medicamenteuses et les onycholyses. *Conc. Med.* **95**, 1007–1023.

Baden H. & Zaias N. (1987) Nails. In: *Dermatology in General Medicine*, eds Fitzpatrick T.B., Eisen A.Z., Wolff K., Freedberg I.M. & Austen K.F., pp. 651–666. McGraw Hill, New York.

Dodd H.J. & Sarkany I. (1988) Chronic discoid lupus erythematosus with mepacrine pigmentation bands in the nails. *Br. J. Dermatol.* **119**, (Suppl.), 33, 74–75.

Kierland R.R., Sheard C., Mason H.L. & Lobitz W.C. (1946) Fluorescence of nails from quinacrine hydrochloride. *J. Am. Med. Assoc.* **131**, 809–810.

Ofori-Adjei D. & Ericsson O. (1985) Chloroquine in nail clippings. *Lancet* **ii**, 331.

Tan S.V., Berth-Jones J. & Burns D.A. (1989) Lichen planus and photo-onycholysis induced by quinine. *Clin. Exp. Dermatol.* **14**, 335.

Tuffanelli D., Abraham R.K. & Dubois E.I. (1963) Pigmentation from antimalarial therapy. *Arch. Dermatol.* **88**, 113–120.

Hormones

Oral contraceptive pill

Some postmenopausal women on the oral contraceptive pill report an increased growth rate of nails and reduced splitting and 'chipping' (Knight, 1974). Photoonycholysis may occur in patients with porphyria who take the oral contraceptive pill thus revealing an underlying occult porphyria cutanea tarda or variegata (Byrne *et al.*, 1976). Nail shedding has also been reported following oral contraceptive treatment.

References

Byrne J.P.H., Boss J.M. & Dawber R.P.R. (1976) Contraceptive-pill-induced porphyria cutanea tarda presenting with onycholysis of the fingernails. *Postgrad. Med. J.* **52**, 535–538.

Knight J.F. (1974) Side benefits of the pill. *Med. J. Aust.* **November**, 680.

Androgens

Half-and-half nail-like changes have been described in a breast cancer patient after androgen therapy (Nixon *et al.*, 1981).

Reference

Nixon D.W., Pirrozi D., York R.M. *et al.* (1981) Dermatologic changes after systemic cancer therapy. *Cutis* **27**, 181.

Parathyroid extracts

Onychomadesis has been reported with parathyroid extract medication (Perrot *et al.*, 1973).

Reference

Perrot H., Tourniaire J. & Fournier M. (1973) Onychopathie induite par la parathormone. *Bull. Soc. Fr. Dermatol. Syphil.* **80**, 313.

Cortisone

Topical steroids can produce distal phalangeal atrophy. The so-called 'disappearing digit' may result from the frequent application of potent local steroids even without occlusion (Wolf *et al.*, 1990). There may be atrophic tapering of the fingertip after just 1 month of treatment (Deffer & Goette, 1987). This gives the finger a sharpened pencil appearence. Striking atrophy of the terminal phalanges of the fingers was noted in both hands in a case reported by Requena *et al.* (1990) showing a sharp limitation at the level of the proximal interphalangeal joints. The affected areas were characterized by severe thinning, erythema and scaling. The nails exhibited diffuse yellow discoloration and subungual hyperkeratosis whereas the nails of both thumbs were lost. After discontinuing the use of topical high-potency fluorinated corticosteroids with occlusion, it took 2 years to recover a relatively normal appearance of the hands with slight persistence of some degree of acroatrophy.

Intralesional steroids might be used in the treatment of psoriasis and lichen planus. Side effects include hypopigmentation (Bedi, 1977) and intramatricial haemorrhages, which may be unsightly when they appear on the nail plate. Permanent damage to the matrix may result from injections given either too frequently or in too concentrated dosages.

Dermojet steroid injection

J. Mascaro (personal communication) observed a psoriatic patient who was treated with steroids by dermojet; this produced multiple implantation epidermoid cysts which necessitated the amputation of some of the distal phalanges.

Systemic steroids

A white caucasoid woman developed a single band of transverse leuconychia in all fingernails and toenails after cortisone administration (Thomas, 1964). Transverse melanonychia due to prednisone has been described by Thomsen (personal communication).

References

Bedi T.R. (1977) Intradermal triamcinolone treatment of psoriatic onychodystrophy. *Dermatologica* **155**, 24–27.

Deffer T.A. & Goette K. (1987) Distal phalangeal atrophy secondary to topical steroid therapy. *Arch. Dermatol.* **123**, 571–572.

Requena L., Zamora E. & Martin L. (1990) Acroatrophy secondary to long-standing applications of topical steroids. *Arch. Dermatol.* **126**, 1013–1014.

Thomas H.M. (1964) Transverse bands in fingernails. *Bull. Johns Hopkins Hosp.* **115**, 238–244.

Thomsen K. (1992) *Nail Changes after Chemotherapy*. 18th World Congress of Dermatology, New York.

Wolf R., Tur E. & Brenner S. (1990) Corticosteroid induced 'disappearing digit'. *J. Am. Acad. Dermatol.* **23**, 755–756.

Adrenocorticotrophic hormone (ACTH), melanocyte-stimulating hormone (MSH)

Transverse hyperpigmented bands have been described in patients taking ACTH or MSH (Thomas, 1964).

Reference

Thomas H.M. (1964) Transverse bands in fingernails. *Bull. Johns Hopkins Hosp.* **115**, 238–244.

Cancer chemotherapeutic agents (Table 6.6; Figs 6.103–6.106)

Patients receiving cancer chemotherapeutic agents frequently exhibit nail abnormalities (Malacarne & Zavagli, 1977; Dunagin, 1982; Delaunay, 1989). Nail pigmentation (Figs 6.103 & 6.104) is the most frequent change. This has been reported following treatment with numerous antineoplastic agents including cyclophosphamide, doxorubicin, bleomycin sulphate, methotrexate, nitrogen mustard, nitrosurea, dacarbazine, 5-fuorouracil, daunorubicin hydrochloride, melphalan hydrochloride, etoposide, tegafur and hydroxyurea. The pigmentation, which is more common and intense in heavily pigmented than in fair-skinned individuals, usually appears 3–8 weeks after the initiation of chemotherapy. It is more commonly observed with combination chemotherapy than with the use of a single drug (Nixon, 1976). The pigmentation of either the nail plate or the nail bed may occur as horizontal or longitudinal bands or as a diffuse darkening. The same chemotherapeutic agent can cause different patterns of nail pigmentation and simultaneous presence of any type on the same nails is possible. Pigmentation may affect hands or feet or both and may involve one or more digits. Hyperpigmentation of the skin, especially over the finger joints, is commonly associated with nail pigmentation. Patients submitted to intermittent therapy can develop transverse pigmented bands that correspond

Fig. 6.103. Cancer chemotherapy – pigmentation and transverse leuconychia.

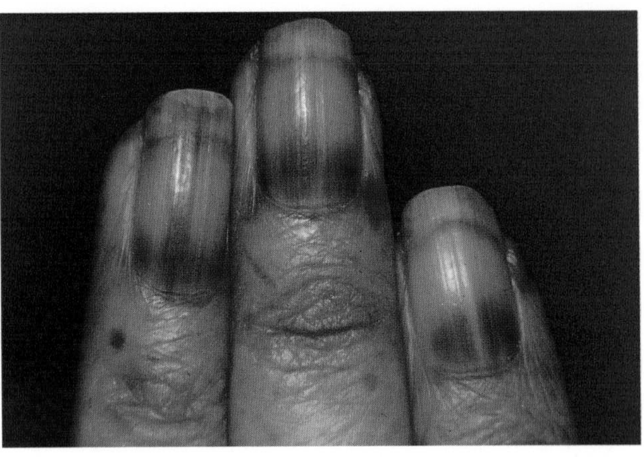
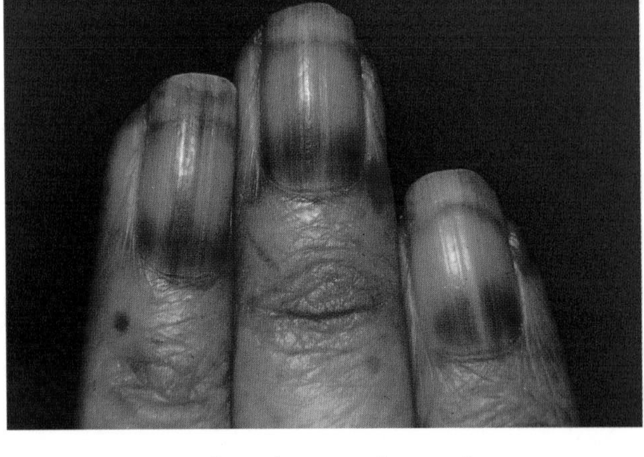
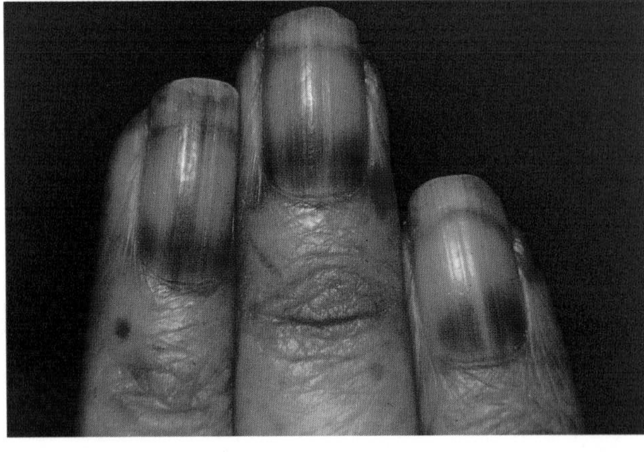

Fig. 6.104. Cancer chemotherapy – pigmentation.

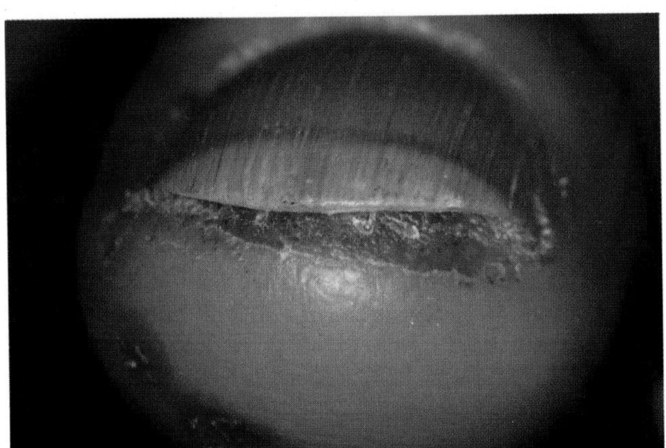

Fig. 6.105. Cancer chemotherapy – onycholysis and inflammation (courtesy E. Groishaus, Strasbourg, France).

Fig. 6.106. Cancer chemotherapy – paronychial inflammation.

to the time of drug administration and are separated by bands of normal colour (Jeanmougin *et al.*, 1982). The pigmentation disappears 6–8 weeks after discontinuation of treatment.

The mechanism of hyperpigmentation produced by chemotherapeutic agents remains obscure. Stimulation of melanocyte activity in the nail matrix and epidermis probably accounts for most of the pigmentary changes. It seems independent of both MSH and ACTH activity (Arakawa *et al.*, 1978) as well as ultraviolet light. A possible genetic predisposition has been suggested by the occurrence of the pigmentation in some consanguineous patients and by the high incidence seen in patients from Sardinia (Sulis & Floris, 1980).

Beau's lines, true transverse leuconychia (Fig. 6.103) and onychomadesis reflect transitory inhibition of the nail matrix. They occur most frequently after short and intensive chemotherapy, especially combined chemotherapy (Jeanmougin *et al.*, 1982; Kochupillai *et al.*, 1983; Tucker & Church, 1984; Singh & Kaur, 1986; Shetty, 1988; Bader-Meunier *et al.*, 1990; Hogan *et al.*, 1991; Requena, 1991). Transverse white bands limited to left fingernails have been reported after isolated cytostatic perfusion of the left arm (Zaun & Omloz, 1992). Intralesional bleomycin treatment of periungual warts can result in onychomadesis and permanent onychodystrophy (Baran, 1985; Gonzales *et al.*, 1986). Apparent leuconychia is an other side effect of cancer chemotherapy. Both transverse white bands of the nail bed, resembling Muehrcke's lines, and half-and-half nails have been occasionally reported (Schwartz & Vickerman, 1979; Nixon *et al.*, 1981; James & Odom, 1983; Bianchi *et al.*, 1992; Unamino *et al.*, 1992). Apparent leuconychia may be explained by haematological involvement.

Onycholysis (Fig. 6.105) and paronychia (Fig. 6.106) are uncommonly observed. They may be painful (Katz & Hansen, 1979; Cunningham *et al.*, 1985; Van Belle *et al.*, 1989). High-dose methotrexate and leucovorin calcium regimen can cause an acute severe bullous dermatitis associated with onycholysis, which can be serious enough to require a modification in the treatment programme (Chang, 1987). Acute paronychia in toenails has also been

Table 6.6. Cancer chemotherapeutic agents – nail changes

Drug	Colour change	Pattern: Diffuse	Pattern: Longitudinal	Pattern: Horizontal	Site: Nail plate	Site: Nail bed	Site: Lunulae	Remarks
Adriamycin (Doxorubicin)	Bluish, grey, brown, black	+	+	+	+	+		Hyperpigmentation of mouth, palms, soles and dorsum of the hands, painful desquamating erythema of palms and soles, onycholysis (Pratt & Shanks, 1974; Prietsman & James, 1975; Morris *et al.*, 1977; Levine & Greenwald, 1978; Runne *et al.*, 1980; Sulis & Floris, 1980; Daniel & Scher, 1984; Lokich & Moore, 1984; Curran, 1990)
Azathioprine	Pink	+					+	Reduced nail growth (Dawber, 1970; Koranda *et al.*, 1974)
Bleomycin (systemic or intralesional)	Brown		+	+	+	+		Brittleness, Beau's lines, onycholysis, onychomadesis, thickening of the nail bed, dark cuticles, Raynaud's phenomenon, acropachy, gangrene, sclerodermatous changes (Halnan *et al.*, 1972; Ohnuma *et al.*, 1972; Shetty, 1977; Norton, 1980; Nixon *et al.*, 1981; Snauwaert & Degreef, 1984; Baran, 1985; Gonzales *et al.*, 1986; Veraldi *et al.*, 1987; Epstein, 1991)
5-Bromodeoxyuridine and radiation	Yellow, brown, white			+				Beau's lines, onychomadesis (McCuaig *et al.*, 1989)
Busulphan	Brown		+			+		Skin pigmentation in 5–10% of the patients (Levantine & Almeyda, 1974; Malacarne, 1978; Baran, 1981)
Cyclophosphamide	Brown, black	+	+	+	+	+		Reduced nail growth, pigmentation of palms, soles, dorsum of hands and teeth (Harrison & Wood, 1972; Markenson *et al.*, 1975; Shah *et al.*, 1978; Sulis & Floris, 1980). Erythema of the onychodermal band and proximal nail folds due to cyclophosphamide and/or vincristine (Kowal-Vern, 1993)
Cytosine arabinoside								Painful desquamating erythema of palms and soles (Horwitz & Dreizen, 1990)
Daunorubicin	Brown, black			+	+			Reduced nail growth (De Marinis *et al.*, 1978)
Dacarbazine (DTIC)	Brown			+		+		(Nixon *et al.*, 1981)
Etoposide	Brown					+		(Wong *et al.*, 1984)

continued on p. 256

reported with high-dose methotrexate and leucovorin calcium therapy (Wantzin & Thomsen, 1983).

Onycholysis can occur following the topical use of 5-fluorouracil with occlusive dressing for warts located around the nails. It may be associated with tenderness, swelling, maceration and oozing of the proximal nail fold (Goldman *et al.*, 1963).

Raynaud's phenomenon and sclerodermatous changes

Table 6.6. *Continued*

Drug	Colour change	Pattern			Site			Remarks
		Diffuse	Longitudinal	Horizontal	Nail plate	Nail bed	Lunulae	
5-Fluorouracil (systemic or topical)	Blue, brown, half-and-half nails	+	+	+	+	+		Nail brittleness and cracking, pigmentation of dorsum of the hands and skin overlying the veins used for infusion, Beau's lines, paronychia, onycholysis, half-and-half nail-like changes, onychomadesis, painful desquamating erythema of palms and soles, superficial blue hue can be scraped off (Falkson & Schulz, 1962; Goldman *et al.*, 1963; Hrushesky, 1976; Levine & Greenwald, 1978; Katz & Hansen, 1979; Nixon *et al.*, 1981; Baran & Laugier, 1985; Guillame *et al.*, 1988)
Hydroxyurea	Melanic, slate, brown		+	+	+	+	+	Brittle atrophic nails, onychoschizia, pigmentation of flexural pressure areas, onycholysis, acral erythema, dermatomyositis-like eruption (Barety *et al.*, 1975; Kennedy *et al.*, 1975; Richard *et al.*, 1989; Vomvouras *et al.*, 1991; Kelsey, 1992)
Ifosfamide	Brown		+					(Teresi *et al.*, 1993)
Melphalan	Brown		+		+			Beau's lines (Malacarne & Zavagli, 1977; Malacarne, 1978)
Methotrexate	Brown			+		+		Horizontal hyperpigmented bands of the hair, acute paronychia, onychomadesis, reduced nail growth (Dawber, 1970; Wantzin & Thomsen, 1983; Wheeland *et al.*, 1983)
Mercaptopurine								Onychomadesis, periungual erythema, painful desquamating erythema of palms and soles (Daniel & Scher, 1984; Cox & Robertson, 1986)
Mitotane (O, *p*-DDD)								Painful desquamating erythema of palms and soles, onychomadesis (Levine & Greenwald, 1978)
Mitoxantrone	Blue	+						Nail softening and splitting, painful onycholysis, nail bed haemorrhages (Speechly-Dick & Owen, 1988; Scheithauer *et al.*, 1989)
Nitrogen mustard	Brown			+				(Nixon *et al.*, 1981)
Nitrosurea	Brown			+				(Nixon *et al.*, 1981)
Razoxane								Beau's lines (Tucker & Church, 1984)
Tegafur	Brown, black		+		+			Spotted hyperpigmentation of lips, palms, soles and glans penis (Llistosella *et al.*, 1991)

are possible consequences of systemic bleomycin therapy (Snauwaert & Degreef, 1984). They can also occur after intralesional bleomycin administration treatment of periungual warts (Bovenmyer, 1985; Epstein, 1985, 1991; Smith *et al.*, 1985). In a retrospective study of 60 patients, Vogelzang *et al.* (1981) found an incidence of 37%. Fingertip gangrene can occur in severe cases. These side effects usually occur from 3 months to 2 years after bleomycin injections and are irreversible. The possibility that bleomycin causes alterations in the dermal matrix has been postulated to explain these particular side effects. The observation that the drug is capable of stimulating the synthesis of collagen and glucosaminoglycans both *in vivo* and *in vitro* further supports this hypothesis (Snauwaert & Degreef, 1984).

Painful desquamating erythema of the palms, soles and periungual regions of the hands is a common complication of continuous infusion of cytosine arabinoside, adriamycin or 5-fluorouracil (Lokich & Moore, 1984; Guillaume *et al.*, 1988; Horwitz & Dreizen, 1990). It has also been occasionally reported with other cytotoxic agents (Cox & Robertson, 1986). In chemotherapy-induced acral erythema, tingling on the palms and soles usually precedes the development of painful, symmetric, well-defined swelling and erythema, often more pronounced over the pads of the distal phalanges. After several days the indurated erythematous plaques become dusky and develop areas of pallor that subsequently blister and desquamate. The desquamation is frequently more obvious than the original erythema. Periungual areas and nails can also be affected (Baack & Burgdorf, 1991).

Splinter haemorrhages and subungual haematoma can occur as a consequence of thrombocytopaenia. Shortening or complete disappearance of the lunulae have also been described. Delayed onychomadesis of all the fingernails and some toenails occurred in a series of 25 patients affected by malignant astrocytomas treated with continuous intracarotid 5-bromodeoxyuridine radiosensitization and radiotherapy for 8.5 weeks. Nail shedding was preceded by the formation of a depressed horizontal white band with slight discoloration superimposed. Completely normal nail regrowth occurred within 6 months. All patients also experienced ipsilateral facial dermatitis, epilation of eyebrows and eyelashes, ocular irritation and scalp alopecia (McCuaig *et al.*, 1989).

References

Adrean R.M., Hood A.F. & Skarin A.T. (1980) Mucocutaneous reactions to antineoplastic agents. *Cancer* **80**, 143.

Arakawa S., Takamatsu T., Imashuku S. & Kusumoki T. (1978) Plasma ACTH and melanocyte-stimulating hormone in nail pigmentation. *Arch. Dis. Child.* **53**, 249–258.

Baack B.R. & Burgdorf W.H.C. (1991) Chemotherapy-induced acral erythema. *J. Am. Acad. Dermatol.* **24**, 457–461.

Bader-Meunier B., Garel D., Dommergues J.P. & Venencie P.Y. (1990) Leuconychies transversales et chimiothérapie antileucémique. *Ann. Pédiatr. (Paris)* **37**, 337–338.

Baran R. (1981) Modifications of colour: chromonychias or dyschromias. In: *The Nail*, ed. Pierre M. pp. 30–38. Churchill Livingstone, Edinburgh.

Baran R. (1985) Onychodystrophie induite par injection intralésionnelle de bléomycine pour verrue périunguéale. *Ann. Dermatol. Venereol.* **112**, 463–464.

Baran R. & Laugier P. (1985) Melanonychia induced by topical 5-fluorouracil. *Br. J. Dermatol.* **112**, 621–625.

Barety M., Audoly P. & Migozzi B. (1975) Pigmentation unguéale et cutanée au cours d'un traitement par hydroxyurée. *Bull. Soc. Fr. Derm. Syph.* **82**, 208.

Bianchi L., Iraci S., Tomassoli M., Carrazzo A.M. & Nini G. (1992) Coexistence of apparent transverse leuconychia (Muehrcke's lines-type) and longitudinal melanonychia after F.A.C. chemotherapy. *Dermatology.* **185**, 216–217.

Bovenmyer D.A. (1985) Persistent Raynaud's phenomenon following intralesional bleomycin treatment of finger warts. *J. Am. Acad. Dermatol.* **13**, 470–471.

Chang J.C. (1987) Acute bullous dermatosis and onycholysis due to high-dose methotrexate and leucovorin calcium. *Arch. Dermatol.* **123**, 990–992.

Cox G.J. & Robertson D.B. (1986) Toxic erythema of palms and soles associated with high-dose mercaptopurine chemotherapy. *Arch. Dermatol.* **122**, 1413–1414.

Cunningham D., Gilchrist N.L., Forrest G.J. & Soukop M. (1985) Onycholysis associated with cytotoxic drugs. *Br. Med. J.* **290**, 675–676.

Curran C.F. (1990) Onycholysis in Doxorubicin-treated patients. *Arch. Dermatol.* **126**, 1244.

Daniel C.R. & Scher R.K. (1984) Nail changes secondary to systemic drugs or ingestants. *J. Am. Acad. Dermatol.* **10**, 250–258.

Dawber R.P.R. (1970) The effect of methotrexate, corticosteroids and azathioprine on fingernail growth in psoriasis. *Br. J. Dermatol.* **83**, 680–683.

Delaunay M. (1989) Effects cutanés indésirables de la chimiothérapie antitumorale. *Ann. Dermatol. Venereol.* **116**, 347–361.

De Marinis M., Hendricks A. & Stoltzner G. (1978) Nail pigmentation with daunorubicin therapy. *Ann. Intern. Med.* **89**, 516–517.

Dunagin W.G. (1982) Clinical toxicity of chemotherapeutic agents: dermatologic toxicity. *Semin. Oncol.* **9**, 14–22.

Epstein E. (1985) Persisting Raynaud's phenomenon following intralesional bleomycin treatment of finger warts. *J. Am. Acad. Dermatol.* **13**, 468–469.

Epstein E. (1991) Intralesional bleomycin and Raynaud's phenomenon. *J. Am. Acad. Dermatol.* **24**, 785–786.

Falkson G. & Schulz E.J. (1962) Skin changes in patients treated with 5-fluorouracil. *Br. J. Dermatol.* **74**, 229–236.

Goldman L., Blaney D.J. & Cohen W. (1963) Onychodystrophy after topical 5 fluorouracil. *Arch. Dermatol.* **88**, 529–530.

Gonzales F.U., Del Carmen Cristobal Gil M., Martinez A.A., Rodriguez P.G., DePaz F.S. & Garcia-Perez A. (1986) Cutaneous toxicity of intralesional bleomycin administration in the treatment of periungual warts. *Arch. Dermatol.* **122**, 974–975.

Guillaume J.C., Carp E., Rougier P. *et al.* (1988) Effets secondaires cutanéomuqueux des perfusions continues de 5 fluorouracile: 12 observations. *Ann. Dermatol. Venereol.* **115**, 1167–1169.

Halnan K.E., Bleehen N.M., Brewin T.B. *et al.* (1972) Early clinical experience with bleomycin in the United Kingdom in series of 105 patients. *Br. Med. J.* **2**, 635–638.

Harrison B.N. & Wood C.B.S. (1972) Cyclophosphamide and pigmentation. *Br. Med. J.* **1**, 352.

Hogan P.A., Krafchik B.R. & Boxall L. (1991) Transverse striate leuconychia associated with cancer chemotherapy. *Pediatr. Dermatol.* **8**, 67–68.

Horwitz L.J. & Dreizen S. (1990) Acral erythemas induced by chemotherapy and graft-versus-host diseases in adults with hematogenous malignancies. *Cutis* **46**, 397–404.

Hrushesky W.J. (1976) Serpentine supravenous 5 fluorouracil hyperpigmentation. *Cancer Treat. Rep.* **60**, 639.

James W.D. & Odom R.B. (1983) Chemotherapy-induced transverse white lines in the fingernails. *Arch. Dermatol.* **119**, 334–335.

Jeanmougin M., Civatte J., Bonvalet D. & Martinet C. (1982) Chromonychies et chimiothérapie anti-cancéreuse. *Ann. Dermatol. Venereol.* **109**, 169–172.

Katz M.E. & Hansen T.W. (1979) Nail plate-nail bed separation. *Arch. Dermatol.* **115**, 860–861.

Kennedy B.J., Smith L.R. & Goltz R.W. (1975) Skin changes secondary to hydroxyurea therapy. *Arch. Dermatol.* **111**, 183–187.

Kelsey P.R. (1992) Multiple longitudinal pigmented bands during hydroxyurea therapy. *Clin. Lab. Haematol.* **14**, 337–338.

Kochupillai V., Prabhu M. & Bhide N.K. (1983) Cancer chemotherapy and nail loss (onychomadesis). *Acta Haematol.* **70**, 137.

Koranda F.C., Dehemel E.M., Kahn G. *et al.* (1974) Cutaneous complications in immunosuppressed renal homograft recipients. *J. Am. Med. Assoc.* **229**, 419.

Kowal-Vern A. & Eng A. (1993) Unusual erythema of the proximal nail fold and onychodermal band. *Cutis* **52**, 43–49.

Levantine A. & Almeyda J. (1974) Cutaneous reactions to cytostatic agents. *Br. J. Dermatol.* **90**, 239–242.

Levine N. & Greenwald E.S. (1978) Mucocutaneous side effects of cancer chemotherapy. *Cancer Treat. Rev.* **5**, 67–84.

Llistosella E., Codina A., Alvarez R., Pujol R.M. & De Moragas J.M. (1991) Tegafur-induced acral hyperpigmentation. *Cutis* **48**, 205–207.

Lokich J.J. & Moore C. (1984) Chemotherapy-associated palmar-plantar erythrodysesthesia syndrome. *Ann. Intern. Med.* **101**, 798–800.

Malacarne P. (1978) Chemioterapia antineoplastica e melanonichia striata. *G. Ital. Dermatol. Venereol.* **113**, 223–226.

Malacarne P. & Zavagli G. (1977) Melphalan-induced melanonychia striata. *Arch. Dermatol. Res.* **258**, 81–83.

Markenson A.L., Chandra M. & Miller D.R. (1975) Hyperpigmentation after cancer chemotherapy. *Lancet* **ii**, 1128.

McCuaig C.C., Ellis C.N., Greenberg H.S., Hegarty T.J. & Page M.A. (1989) Mucocutaneous complications of intraarterial 5-bromodeoxyuridine and radiation. *J. Am. Acad. Dermatol.* **21**, 1235–1240.

Morris D., Aisner J. & Wiernik P.H. (1977) Horizontal pigmented banding of the nails in association with adriamycin chemotherapy. *Cancer Treat. Rep.* **61**, 499–501.

Nixon D.W. (1976) Alterations in nail pigment with cancer chemotherapy. *Arch. Intern. Med.* **136**, 1117–1118.

Nixon D.W., Pirrozi D., York R.M. *et al.* (1981) Dermatologic changes after systemic cancer therapy. *Cutis* **27**, 181.

Norton L.A. (1980) Nail disorders. *J. Am. Acad. Dermatol.* **22**, 451–467.

Ohnuma T., Selawry O.S., Holland J.F. *et al.* (1972) Clinical study with bleomycin: tolerance to twice weekly dosage. *Cancer* **30**, 914–922.

Pratt C.B. & Shanks E.C. (1974) Hyperpigmentation of nails from doxorubicin. *J. Am. Med. Assoc.* **228**, 460.

Priestman T.J. & James K.W. (1975) Adriamycin and longitudinal pigmented banding of fingernails. *Lancet* **i**, 1337–1338.

Requena L. (1991) Chemotherapy-induced transverse ridging of the nails. *Cutis* **48**, 129–130.

Richard M., Truchetet F., Friedel J., Leclech C. & Heid E. (1989) Skin lesions simulating chronic dermatomyositis during long-term hydroxyurea therapy. *J. Am. Acad. Dermatol.* **21**, 797–799.

Runne U., Pleiff B. & Mitrenga D. (1980) Braunes nagelbett und onycholyse durch adriamycin; schwellung, pigmentierung und hyperkeratosen durch bleomycin. *Z. Hautkr.* **55**, 1590–1593.

Scheithauer W., Ludwig H., Kotz R. & Depisch D. (1989) Mitoxantrone-induced discoloration of the nails. *Exp. J. Cancer Clin. Oncol.* **25**, 763–765.

Schwartz R.A. & Vickerman C.E. (1979) Muehrcke's lines of the fingernails. *Arch. Intern. Med.* **139**, 242.

Shah P.C., Rao K.R.P. & Patel A.S. (1978) Cyclophosphamide induced nail pigmentation. *Br. J. Dermatol.* **98**, 675–680.

Shetty M.R. (1977) Case of pigmented banding of the nail caused by bleomycin. *Cancer Treat. Rep.* **61**, 501.

Shetty M.R. (1988) White lines in the fingernails induced by combination chemotherapy. *Br. Med. J.* **297**, 1635.

Singh M. & Kaur S. (1986) Chemotherapy-induced multiple Beau's lines. *Int. J. Dermatol.* **25**, 590–591.

Smith E.A., Harper F.E. & LeRoy E.C. (1985) Raynaud's phenomenon of a single digit following local intradermal bleomycin sulphate injection. *Arth. Rheum.* **28**, 459–461.

Snauwaert J. & Degreef H. (1984) Bleomycin-induced Raynaud's phenomenon and acral sclerosis. *Dermatologica* **169**, 172–174.

Speechly Dick M.E. & Owen E.R.T.C. (1988) Mitoxantrone-induced onycholysis. *Lancet* **i**, 113.

Sulis E. & Floris C. (1980) Nail pigmentation following cancer chemotherapy. A new genetic entity? *Eur. J. Cancer* **16**, 1317–1319.

Teresi M.E., Murry D.J. & Coznelius A.S. (1993) Ifosamide-induced hyperpigmentation. *Cancer* **71**, 2873–2875.

Tucker W.F.G. & Church R.E. (1984) Beau's lines after razoxane therapy for psoriasis. *Arch. Dermatol.* **120**, 1140.

Unamino P., Fernàndez-Lopez E. & Santos C. (1992). Leuconychia due to cytostatic agents. *Clin. Exp. Dermatol.* **17**, 273–274.

Van Belle S.J.P., Dehou M.F., De Bock V. & Volckaert A. (1989) Nail toxicity due to the combination adriamycin–mitoxantrone. *Cancer Chemother. Pharmacol.* **24**, 69–70.

Veraldi S., Renzi D., Schianchi R., Sala F. & Marin D. (1987) Iperpigmentazione ungueale come unico segno di tossicità da bleomicina. *G. Ital. Dermatol. Venereol.* **122**, 443–445.

Vogelzang J.N., Bosl G.J., Johnson K. & Kennedy B.J. (1981) Raynaud's phenomenon: a common toxicity after combination chemotherapy for testicular cancer. *Ann. Intern. Med.* **95**, 288–292.

Vomvouras S., Pakula A.S. & Shaw J.M. (1991) Multiple pigmented nail bands during hydroxyurea therapy: an uncommon finding. *J. Am. Acad. Dermatol.* **24**, 1016–1017.

Wantzin G.L. & Thomsen K. (1983) Acute paronychia after high-dose methotrexate therapy. *Arch. Dermatol.* **119**, 623–624.

Wheeland R.G., Burgdorf W.H.C. & Humphrey G.B. (1983) The flag sign of chemotherapy. *Cancer* **51**, 1356–1358.

Wong L.C., Choo Y.C. & Ma H.K. (1984) Oral etoposide in

gestational trophoblastic disease. *Cancer Treat. Rep.* **68**, 775–777.

Zaun H. & Omloz G. (1992) Einseitige leukopathia unguis toxica und diffusez haarasfall nach zytostatischer extremitaten perfusion. *Hautarzt* **43**, 215–216.

Radiation

Melanonychia striata has been reported after UVB and UVA phototherapy (Beltrani & Scher, 1991). Onychomadesis, Beau's lines and nail hyperpigmentation can be consequences of X-ray therapy (Shelley *et al.*, 1964; Runne & Orfanos, 1981). Nail ridging has been reported in six patients who developed late chronic radiation changes after electron beam therapy (Price, 1978).

References

Beltrani V.P. & Scher R.K. (1991) Evaluation and management of melanonychia striata in a patient receiving phototherapy. *Arch. Dermatol.* **127**, 319–320.

Price N.M. (1978) Radiation dermatitis following electron beam therapy. *Arch. Dermatol.* **114**, 63–66.

Runne U. & Orfanos C.E. (1981) The human nail. *Curr. Prob. Dermatol.* **9**, 102–149.

Shelley W.B., Rawnsley H.M. & Pillsbury D.M. (1964) Post-irradiation melanonychia. *Arch. Dermatol.* **90**, 174–176.

Pulse oximetry

Digital skin necrosis can be a complication of pulse oximetry monitoring of critically ill or anaesthetized patients. Lesions are caused by pressure necrosis and occur at the site of application of the probe sentor (Stogner *et al.*, 1991; Pettersen *et al.*, 1992). Inaccuracy of the oxygen saturation determinations can be due to excessively long nails (Tweedie, 1989).

References

Pettersen B., Konsgaard V. & Aune H. (1992) Skin injury in an infant with pulse oximetry. *Br. J. Anaesth.* **69**, 204–205.

Stogner S.W., Owens M.W. & Baethge B.A. (1991) Cutaneous necrosis and pulse oximetry. *Cutis* **48**, 235–237.

Tweedie I.E. (1989) Pulse oximeters and long fingernails. *Anesthesia* **44**, 268.

Miscellaneous drugs

Antihistamines

Exacerbation of psoriasis, liver dysfunction and thrombocytopenia have been associated with mebhydrolin treatment (McKenna & McMillan, 1993).

Reference

McKenna K.E. & McMillan J.C. (1993) Exacerbation of psoriasis, liver dysfunction and thrombocytopenia associated with mebhydrolin. *Clin. Exp. Dermatol.* **18**, 131–132.

Carotene

Long-term treatment with carotene can produce yellow discoloration of the nails.

Cyclosporin

Two patients experienced Raynaud's phenomenon 2 days after treatment with cyclosporin 10 mg/kg/day was started. The therapy was interrupted in one patient who developed Raynaud's phenomenon again after reintroduction of the drug at a dose of 5 mg/kg/day (Deray *et al.*, 1986). Increase of linear nail growth has been noticed by R. Baran (personal observation).

Reference

Deray G., Lehoang P., Achour L., Hornych A., Landault C. & Caraillon A. (1986) Cyclosporin and Raynaud's phenomenon. *Lancet* **ii**, 1092–1093.

Dimercaptosuccinic acid (DMSA)

A 16-year-old boy developed longitudinal nail striations after DMSA administration for mercury poisoning therapy (Thomas *et al.*, 1987).

Reference

Thomas G., Fournier L., Garnier R. & Dally S. (1987) Nail dystrophy and dimercaptosuccinic acid. *J. Toxicol. Clin. Exp.* **7**, 285–287.

Diuretics

Thiazide diuretics have been reported to produce onycholysis (Krull, 1981).

Reference

Krull E. (1981) Fingernail abnormalities as indicators of systemic disease. *Topics Dermatol.*, **March** 1981.

Ergotamine

Peripheral gangrene leading to limb amputation is a well-known complication of ergotamine overdosage (Cranley *et al.*, 1963). It can also occur after administration of standard dosages of the drug to patients presenting contraindications to its use. These include peripheral vascular disease, hypertension, coronary disease, pregnancy, thyrotoxicosis, sepsis, hepatic and renal disease as well as anaemia, and treatment with macrolides (Cameron & French, 1960).

References

Cameron E.A. & French E.B. (1960) St. Anthony's fire rekindled: gangrene due to therapeutic dose of ergotamine. *Br. Med. J.* **2**, 28–30.

Cranley J.J., Krause R.J., Strasser E.S. & Hafner C.D. (1963) Impending gangrene of four extremities secondary to ergotism. *New Engl. J. Med.* **269**, 727–729.

Fluorine

Prolonged fluorine ingestion produces changes in the skin and its appendages including teeth, nails and hair. Various nail dystrophies occur including brittleness, longitudinal striations (onychorrhexis), Beau's lines as well as pitting, punctate and transverse leuconychia producing 'mottled' nails of both fingers and toes (Spira, 1943, 1946).

References

Spira L. (1943) Mottled nails as an early sign of fluorosis. *J. Hyg. Camb.* **43**, 69–71.

Spira L. (1946) Disturbance of pigmentation in fluorosis. *Acta Med. Scand.* **126**(1) , 65–84.

Gelatin, biotin, cystine and methionine

These drugs have been claimed to accelerate nail growth (Runne & Orfanos, 1981).

Reference

Runne U. & Orfanos C.E. (1981) The human nail. *Curr. Prob. Dermatol.* **9**, 102–149.

Hydroquinone

A reversible brown or orange-brown pigmentation of the nails can be a consequence of topical hydroquinone treatment for melasma or actinic lentigines of the hands with a relationship to light exposure (Mann & Harman, 1983) (see Chapters 2 and 7).

Reference

Mann R.J. & Harman R.R.M. (1983) Nail staining due to hydroquinone skin-lightening creams. *Br. J. Dermatol.* **108**, 363–365.

Ketoconazole

Splinter haemorrhages and longitudinal pigmented bands have been described in patients taking ketoconazole (Positano *et al.*, 1989).

Reference

Positano R.G., DeLauro T.M. & Berkowitz B.J. (1989) Nail changes secondary to environmental influences. *Clin. Pod. Med. Surg.* **6**, 417–429.

Peloprenoic acid

Nail fragility was observed in psoriatics treated with peloprenoic acid derivatives (Ohkido, personal communication).

Penicillamine

Longitudinal ridging, onychoschizia, elkonyxis and Beau's lines have been reported during penicillamine treatment. Absence of the lunulae and leuconychia can also be seen (Thivolet *et al.*, 1968; Levy *et al.*, 1983; Bjellerup, 1989). Nail changes are reversible with cessation of treatment. Yellow nail syndrome has been described in patients taking penicillamine (Lubach & Marghescu, 1979; Ilchyshyn & Vickers, 1983).

References

Bjellerup M. (1989) Nail-changes induced by penicillamine. *Acta Derm. Venereol. (Stock.)* **69**, 339–341.

Ilchyshyn A. & Vickers C.F.H. (1983) Yellow nail syndrome associated with penicillamine therapy. *Acta Derm. Venereol. (Stock.)* **63**, 554–555.

Levy R.S., Fisher M. & Alter J.N. (1983) Penicillamine: review and cutaneous manifestations. *J. Am. Acad. Dermatol.* **8**, 548.

Lubach D. & Marghescu S. (1979) Yellow-nail-syndrome durch d-Penizillamin. *Hautarzt* **30**, 547–549.

Thivolet J., Perrot H. & François R. (1968) Glossite, stomatite et onychopathie provoquées par la pénicillamine. *Bull. Soc. Fr. Dermatol. Syphil.* **75**, 61–63.

Phenylephrine

Purpura of the nail bed has been reported with phenylephrine treatment (Baran & Témime, 1973).

Reference

Baran R. & Témime P. (1973) Les onychodystrophies toxi-medicamenteuses et les onycholyses *Conc. Med.* **95**, 1007–1023.

Salbutamol

Periungual and palmoplantar erythema has been described in pregnant women treated with salbutamol (Lacour *et al.*, 1987).

Reference

Lacour J.P., Reygagne P., Grimaldi M., Gillet J. & Ortonne J.P. (1987) Erythème pseudo-lupique des extrémités au cours de grossesses pathologiques traitées par salbutamol. *Press Med.* 32, 1599.

L-Tryptophan

Eosinophilic myalgia syndrome has been linked to L-tryptophan ingestion. Eosinophilic fasciitis (Gordon *et al.*, 1991) as well as a reversible scleroderma-like illness (Connolly *et al.*, 1990) have been reported after ingestion of L-tryptophan for the treatment of insomnia (Connolly *et al.*, 1990).

References

Connolly S.M., Quimby S.R., Griffing W.L. & Winkelmann R.K. (1990) L-tryptophan: a possible explanation of the eosinophilia-myalgia-syndrome. *J. Am. Acad. Dermatol.* **23**, 451–457.

Gordon M.L., Lebwohl M.G., Phelps R.G., Cohen S.R. & Fleischmayer R. (1991) Eosinophilic fasciitis associated with tryptophan ingestion. *Arch. Dermatol.* **127**, 217–220.

Vitamin A

Nail dystrophy and brittle nails have been described with vitamin A treatment (Positano *et al.*, 1989).

Reference

Positano R.G., DeLauro T.M. & Berkowitz B.J. (1989) Nail changes secondary to environmental influences. *Clin Pod. Med. Surg.* **6**, 417–429.

Chapter 7
Occupational Abnormalities and Contact Dermatitis

R.J.G. RYCROFT & R. BARAN

Definition
Diagnosis
Reaction patterns
Occupational nail hazards
- Physical hazards
  - Cold
  - Burns
  - Ionizing radiation
  - Microwave radiation
  - Plants and woods
  - Bulbs
  - Glass fibre, splinters of hair
  - Victualler's thumbnail
  - Friction and pressure
  - Vibrating power tools
- Chemical sensitizers
  - Rhus dermatitis
  - Tulip fingers
  - Alstroemeria
  - Hydrangea
  - Turpentine
  - Thiourea
  - Codeine
  - 1-Methylquinoxalinium-*p*-toluene sulphonate
  - Acrylics
  - Cyanoacrylate
  - Epoxy resin
  - PTBP resin
  - Nonoxynol-6
  - Hydroxylamine
  - 'Caine' local anaesthetics and propanidid
  - Mydriatic agents
  - Dicyandiamide derivatives
  - Escavenitis (seaworm) and bryozoans
  - Plate makers
  - Onion dermatitis
  - Cement
- Chemical irritants
  - Alkalis
  - Hydrofluoric acid
  - Oxalic acid
  - Formaldehyde
  - Diquat, paraquat,
  - Dinitroorthocresol
  - Dinobuton
  - Aminoethyl ethanolamine
- Bacterial infections
- Viral infections
- Fungal infections
- Systemic conditions
- Principal signs associated with occupational origin
  - Gradual nail plate destruction
  - Brittle and atrophic nails
  - Paronychia
  - Alteration in colour
  - Koilonychia
  - Clubbing, pseudoclubbing
  - Onycholysis
  - Distal bone anomaly

Non-occupational nail hazards
- Physical hazards
  - Synthetic nail covers
- Chemical sensitizers
  - Nail base coat
  - Nail varnish
- Chemical irritants
  - Nail hardeners
  - Enzyme detergent
  - Thioglycolates
- Discoloration of the nail plate

Nail protection at work

Definition

Occupational nail disorders represent those abnormalities of the nail apparatus produced or aggravated by the working environment. The predisposing factors are those for occupational disorders elsewhere, that is:

1 inexperienced workers;
2 inadequate personal hygiene;
3 excess use of irritants;
4 temperature and humidity;
5 inadequate protection.

Accurate diagnosis depends on

1 appearance of nail condition;
2 location of the lesion;
3 patient's history.

Diagnosis of occupational nail disorders

The fingernails are used as 'tools' in many occupations (Ronchese, 1953, 1955, 1969) and the way they look is of importance in all occupations where personal contact occurs. Nail disorders can therefore be more disabling at work than might at first appear. Most are confined to the hands.

The subject of the first part of this chapter is the wide

range of nail disorders that are primarily caused by the working environment. Some of these look very like certain endogenous (constitutional) nail disorders. This makes their diagnosis more difficult. Nail changes in dermatoses such as psoriasis, tinea and lichen planus may be misinterpreted as being caused by work. Conditions such as psoriasis of the nails may be exacerbated by occupational trauma (Baran & Levy, 1992), or this may even precipitate an underlying tendency to the disease (isomorphic phenomenon); in patients with rheumatoid arthritis, lichen planus and secondary syphilis an identical phenomenon may occur (Fisher & Baran, 1992).

In assessing a nail condition suspected of being occupational:

1 visualize what the hands do;
2 look for functional distribution;
3 look for occupational stigmata of the nails;
4 examination of the whole skin surface should never be omitted. The correct diagnosis may be evident at a site distant from the nails.

There are some laboratory tests, such as mycological and bacteriological examinations, which are essential diagnostic aids. A punch biopsy of the nail can sometimes assist. An X-ray of the terminal phalanx is occasionally relevant, e.g. exostosis of occupational origin.

Clinical reaction patterns

Clinical reaction patterns include:

1 changes in the texture and contour of the nail plate, onychauxis, worn-down nail plate (usure des ongles), brittle nails, koilonychia, clubbing and pseudoclubbing;
2 changes in the surface of the nail plates resulting from direct trauma, matrix involvement or paronychia, with sometimes onychomadesis leading to nail shedding;
3 changes in colour by nail plate staining or subungual alteration.
4 distal bony phalanx anomalies.

Occupational nail hazards

Physical hazards

Prolonged exposure to *cold* may result in injury to the nail matrix, leading to derangement of the nail plate ranging from Beau's lines to complete shedding. Cold injury, particularly to peripheral parts, is common amongst such groups as armies on active service – adequate protective measures now make this rarer than in the past; conditions such as trench foot (Fairbairn *et al.*, 1972), acute perniosis (chilblains) and frostbite (Washburn, 1962) may damage the nail apparatus. Seasonal koilonychia in Ladakh, in north-west India, is due to exposure to cold wet mud while repairing walls and irrigation canals (Dolma *et al.*, 1990). Frostbite, the freezing of tissues in response to cold air, metals or liquids, may cause tissue loss due to vasospasm with thrombus formation and extracellular ice crystal formation; venous pressure increases, capillary perfusion decreases and intravascular 'sludging' is evident. Depending on the acuteness of the cold injury to the nail apparatus, changes such as chilblains, Raynaud's phenomenon or disease, and early acrosclerosis may be seen, including necrosis or gangrene of skin or deeper tissues.

Numbness of the tip of the right index finger and thumb has been noted as a side effect of cryotherapy in the treating physician. It would seem that even brief contact with the nitrogen-cooled nozzle of a cryosurgical unit is sufficient to induce superficial neural damage in the fingertips, provided that exposure occurs repeatedly (Heidenheim & Jemec, 1991). It should be noted that the nail apparatus possesses a good anastomotic blood supply and large numbers of glomus bodies which help to protect against all but the worst of cold injuries.

Burns, when mild, cause onycholysis. When severe, disfiguring scars and fissured nails may result (Chapter 10).

Ionizing radiation may cause loss of nails (Gallaghar *et al.*, 1955), with late changes of chronic radiodermatitis (Messite *et al.*, 1957) and subsequent Bowen's disease or squamous cell carcinomas (Dulanto & Camacho, 1979), up to 30 years after exposure. The earliest signs are brittleness and longitudinal ridging (Fig. 7.1). Later the nail plates become dull and slightly opaque with a brownish hue. The thumb is never involved in X-ray dermatitis. The skin at the same stage shows atrophy, telangiectasia and keratoses. A verrucous lesion appearing on the hyponychium (Fig. 7.2) or adjacent nail bed may herald the development of malignant change (Fig. 7.3). Minute black spots, known as 'coal spots', appear beneath the nail plate and slowly spread over large areas of nail, often in longitudinal bands. A chronic relapsing paronychia commonly occurs. Occupational radiodermatitis from

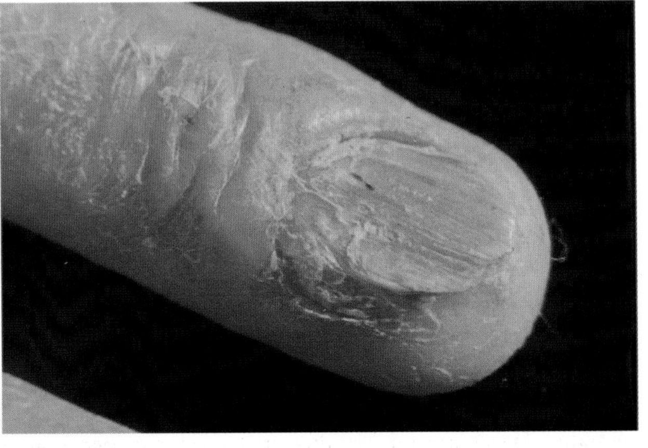

Fig. 7.1. X-irradiation nail changes – brittleness and longitudinal ridging.

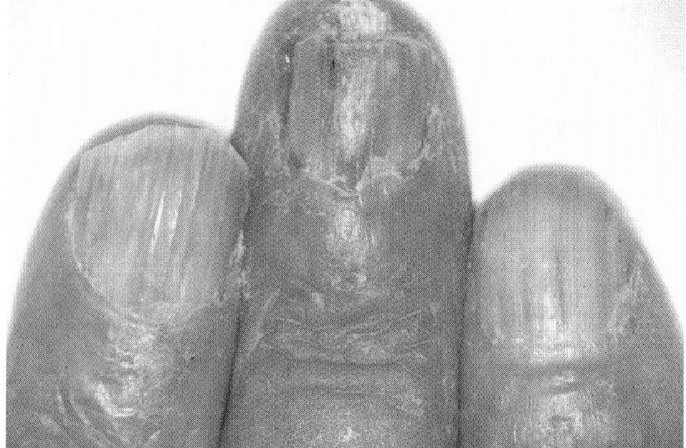

Fig. 7.2. X-irradiation nail damage – distal subungual warty lesion of the third finger.

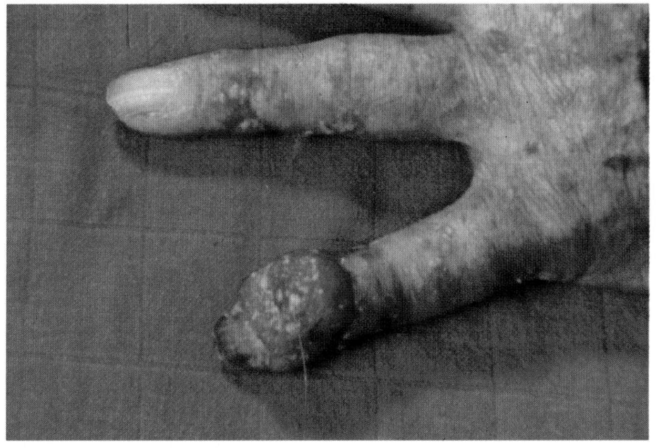

Fig. 7.3. X-irradiation squamous carcinoma.

^{192}Ir exposure was reported in three Spanish industrial radiologists (Condé-Salazar *et al.*, 1986). After a brief episode of acute radiodermatitis, which may elude diagnosis, an asymptomatic period of many months may precede the typical picture of chronic radiodermatitis.

Microwave radiation can cause transverse ridging, onycholysis and other plate dystrophies. Brodkin and Bleiberg (1973) reported nail damage in restaurant workers exposed to a faulty microwave oven. They emphasized that the nail matrix may be damaged by microwave-induced thermal injury without the sensation of heat being felt by the oven user.

Exposure to certain *plants and woods* may cause nail trauma. Thorns, thistles and sharp-edged leaves may injure the nails, especially cactus thorns in desert areas. Secondary infection is a likely complication.

Hyacinth and narcissus bulbs possess raphide cells containing bundles of needle-shaped crystals of calcium oxalate. These crystals readily penetrate the periungual skin causing erythema and oedema with pain and itching (Hjorth & Wilkinson, 1968).

Glass fibre, above approximately 5 mm in diameter, mechanically irritates the periungual tissue. Paronychia may result from the penetration of glass spicules beneath the proximal nail fold. It may also cause onycholysis with darkening of the nail plate (Rogaïlin *et al.*, 1975). Introduction of *splinters of hair* beneath the nail may produce onycholysis (Stubbart, 1956), and even subungual trichogranuloma (Hogan, 1988). Chronic paronychia, which is sometimes seen in hairdressers, usually deserves surgical management (Baran & Bureau, 1981).

Victualler's thumb nail, a condition of subungual osmotrauma, is the consequence of small foreign bodies of dehydrated food becoming embedded below the nails (Head, 1984).

Friction and pressure gradually wear down the nail (Fig. 7.4) and are characteristic of particular occupations (occupational stigmata). Pottery workers and workers who repeatedly lift heavy bags (Fig. 7.5) (Schubert *et al.*, 1977) are examples. Onycholysis, koilonychia, longitudinal splitting and occasional splinter haemorrhages

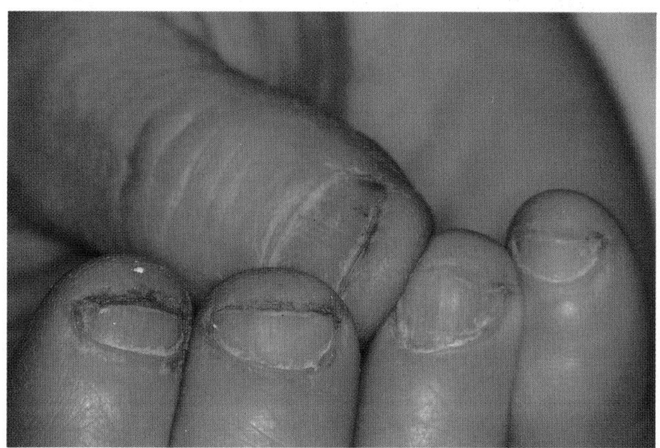

Fig. 7.4. Worn-down nails due to occupational friction and pressure.

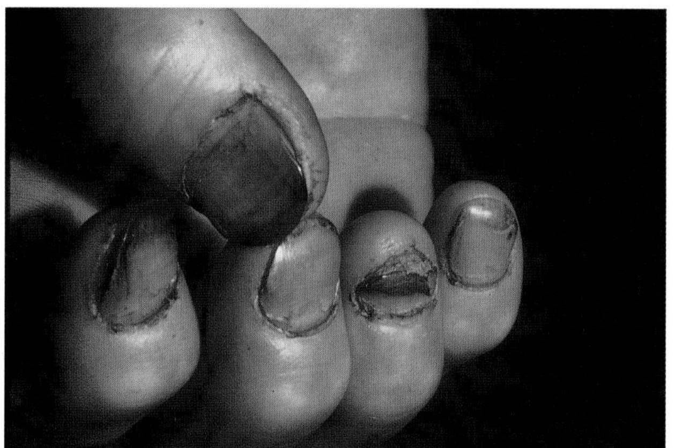

Fig. 7.5. Nail dystrophy due to lifting heavy plastic bags.

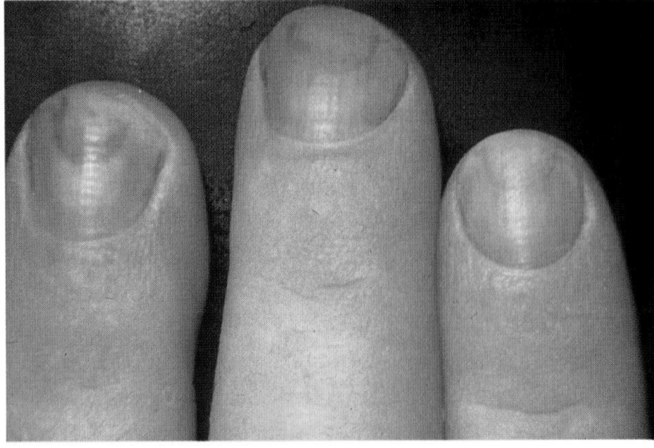

Fig. 7.6. 'Rectangular' onycholysis – slaughterhouse workers' dystrophy (courtesy of T. Menne, Denmark).

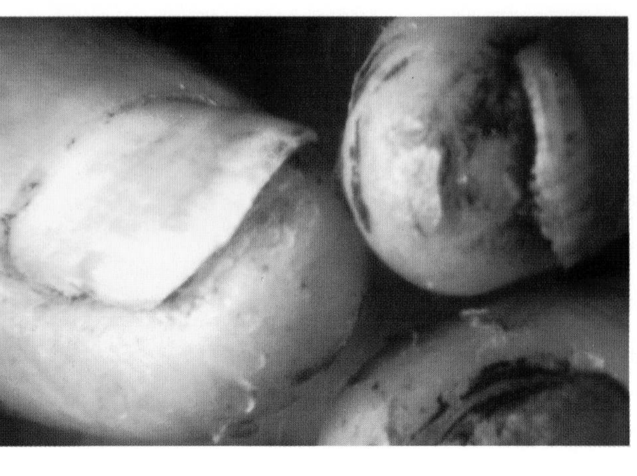

Fig. 7.7. 'Tulip fingers' dystrophy (courtesy of the late N. Hjorth, Denmark).

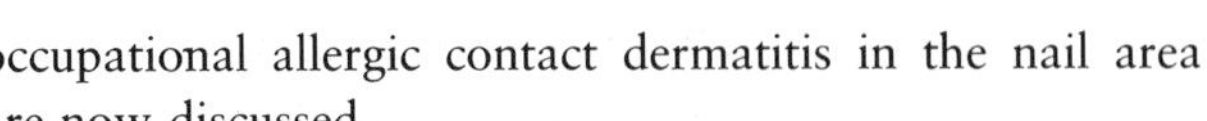

may also be seen. Subungual haemorrhages have been reported in three inexperienced male dishwashers using heavy rubber gloves while working in the United States (Long, 1958), and are frequent in sportsmen's toes (Gibbs, 1973; Baran, 1978) and in the toes of dancers, where there may be associated subungual exostosis (Sebastian, 1977). Slaughterhouse workers, manually skinning cattle, develop a rectangular onycholysis of the central nail plate and, in one case necrosis of the nail bed was reported (Menné *et al.*, 1985) (Fig. 7.6).

Transverse leuconychia has been described in Japan from the mechanical pressure of keypunching (Honda *et al.*, 1976).

Vibrating power tools, such as pneumatic drills and chainsaws, cause nail thickening, brittleness and splitting of the free edges. Yellow-white longitudinal bands may extend distally from the lunula, sometimes becoming confluent. Distally the nails become darkly tinged and may turn black. The nail plate may develop ridging and eventually be shed entirely (Kulcsár, 1966). The same stimulus causes Raynaud's phenomenon in the skin (vibration white finger), especially when vibrating power tools are operated in cold climates (Taylor, 1982; Yu *et al.*, 1988), or in carpal tunnel syndrome (Boyle *et al.*, 1988; Veccherini-Blineau & Guiheneuc, 1988). The hand that holds and guides the tool is often more severely affected. Raynaud's phenomenon has also been seen in typists, violinist and pianists. Ekenvall (1987) has usefully reviewed the clinical assessment of patients between attacks.

Chemical sensitizers

While it is debatable whether contact sensitization ever occurs through the nail plate, rather than via periungual skin, the nail plate can certainly be altered by subsequent allergic contact dermatitis. Sensitizers causing occupational allergic contact dermatitis in the nail area are now discussed.

Rhus dermatitis (from poison ivy, oak and sumac) may result in onycholysis and a yellowish discoloration of the nail plate (Fulghum, 1972).

'Tulip fingers' (Fig. 7.7) is a painful dry fissured hyperkeratotic eczema caused by contact with tulip bulbs. It starts beneath the free margin of the nails and extends to the fingertips and periungual regions. Suppurative granulating erosions may be seen on the fingertips in long-standing cases. At times the face, hands, forearms and genitals may also become involved. The highest concentration of the allergen, α-methylene-γ-butyrolactone, is to be found in the outermost cell layers of the inner bulb scales (Klaschka *et al.*, 1964; Hjorth & Wilkinson, 1968; Verspyck Mijnssen, 1969; Hausen, 1982; Gette & Marks, 1990).

Alstroemeria dermatitis can result in onycholysis, in addition to dermatitis of the thumbs and index fingers (Rycroft & Calnan, 1981; Marks, 1988).

Hydrangea dermatitis may present with a clinical picture including chronic paronychia and associated nail dystrophy (Bruynzeel, 1986).

The wooden *orange stick* traditionally used for applying cuticle remover has been responsible for a persistent eczema of the right hand in a manicurist (Brun, 1978).

Turpentine, the oleoresin from pine trees, is now a much less common sensitizer that it used to be, owing to its gradual replacement as a solvent by less expensive substitutes. In craft workers, it can still occasionally cause an eczema of the peringual tissues and fingers with subungual hyperkeratosis.

Thiourea contained in silver polish may produce contact and photocontact allergy with vesicular eruption of the fingertips and invasion under the fingernails (Dooms-Goossens *et al.*, 1988).

Codeine sensitization in pharmaceutical workers has

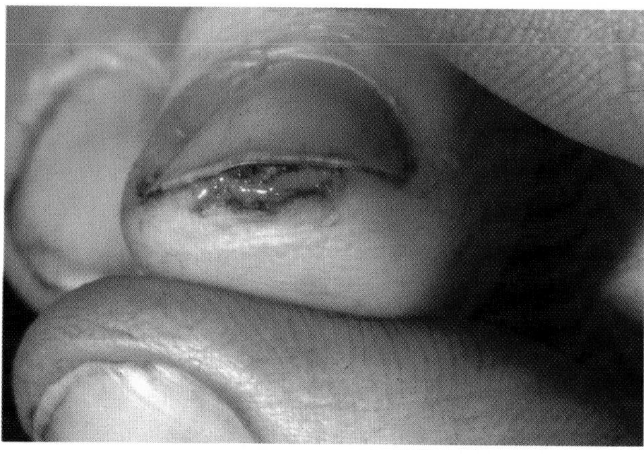

Fig. 7.8. Codeine sensitization – pharmaceutical industry workers (courtesy of C. Romaguera, Spain).

been associated with subungual hyperkeratosis, onycholysis and nail atrophy, as well as dermatitis of the hands, arms and face (Romaguera & Grimalt, 1983) (Fig. 7.8).

1-Methylquinoxalinium-p-toluene sulphonate sensitization, from a conditioner applied to offset lithography plates to render the image receptive to ink, causes dermatitis of the fingertips and periungual areas, particularly of the index, middle and ring fingers of the right hand (English *et al.*, 1986).

Repeated contact with *acrylic* materials, especially the sensitizing liquid monomers, has long been known to be responsible for contact dermatitis in dentists, dental technicians (Farli *et al.*, 1990) and orthopaedic surgeons (Rycroft, 1977). People have also been affected due to the practice of wearing sculptured artificial nails (Fisher *et al.*, 1957). Manicurists who apply these artificial nails to clients may become sensitized. The thumb and index (Condé-Salazar *et al.*, 1986) or middle (Canizares, 1956) fingers of the left hand are constantly exposed as the manicurist holds the client's finger during building-up of the sculptured nails. Even exposure to the vapour from open bottles may subsequently elicit dermatitis in highly sensitized persons. Sculptured nails are marketed as a kit containing an artificial nail called the template, a liquid monomer and a powdered polymer (Chapter 8). By mixing the monomer and polymer together polymerization is effected because of the presence of an organic peroxide catalyst and an accelerator. The material can be moulded onto the client's natural nail and hardening occurs at room temperature or in a photobonding box (Fisher, 1990). First the natural nail is roughened with a burr, then it is painted with the acrylic compound to produce, on hardening, an artificial nail, which is gradually enlarged and elongated by repeated applications. The prosthesis can be filed and manicured to the desired shape and as the nail plate grows out further infillings of acrylic can be made to maintain the natural contour.

After 2–4 months of application, patients may begin to show an allergic contact dermatitis, usually of the dorsal aspects of some of the fingers and paronychial tissue, the face and the eyelids. Symptoms include pain and persistent paraesthesia, but permanent paraesthesia may occur without allergic reaction (Baran & Schibli, 1990). Paronychial inflammation may be quite severe. Nail discoloration may occur and the nail bed itself usually becomes dry and thickened. Onycholysis of the natural nail occurs with thinning and splitting (Goodwin, 1976). This disfiguration of the nail plate can last for many months.

On patch testing the patients react strongly to the liquid acrylic monomer but not to the polymer, except for an anecdotal report of Lane and Kost (1956). Until recently methyl methacrylate was used, but in 1976 the Food and Drug Administration in the United States banned its use. Since then ethyl and butyl methacrylates have been used instead. These also sensitize (Marks *et al.*, 1979).

A laboratory technician working in the manufacture of disposable contact lenses developed neurologic and gastrointestinal symptoms after working with UV-curable acrylic monomers. The only skin symptom was transient onycholysis of the fingernails (Andersen, 1986).

Dental personnel are exposed to many sensitizing compounds such as coconut diethanolamide from handwashing liquids, *N*-ethyl-4-toluene sulfonamide, a resin carrier in dental materials for isolating cavities underneath restorations, and 4-tolyldiethanolamine, an accelerator for inducing polymerization of dental acrylic resins at room temperature. They may be responsible for finger dermatitis and paronychia (Kaneva *et al.*, 1993a,b).

Industrial sealants which polymerize rapidly under anaerobic conditions in the presence of the metals in steel and brass contain sensitizing *dimethacrylates*. These products have immensely useful applications in the locking of screws firmly into position. Allergic contact dermatitis from such sealants affects principally the pulps of the fingers (Cronin, 1980a) and can extend as scaly eczema under the free margin of the nails (Condé-Salazar *et al.*, 1986). Onycholysis developed in one patient described by Mathias and Maibach (1984).

Printing workers sensitized to *photopolymerizable acrylic resin* may show eczematous lesions on the fingers and around the nail plate, extending to the distal subungual area (Calas *et al.*, 1977).

Ethyl-cyanocrylate-containing glue used in nail wrapping, in which linen or silk is glued to the abraded nail and filed down, can cause a periungual contact dermatitis in manicurists and/or clients (Shelley & Shelley, 1988) with spread to the eyelids and patchily over the backs of the hands (Belsito, 1981), and simulating small-plaque parapsoriasis (Shelley & Shelley, 1984).

Epoxy resin dermatitis (Castelain *et al.*, 1992) especially involves the right first two fingertips, producing erosion

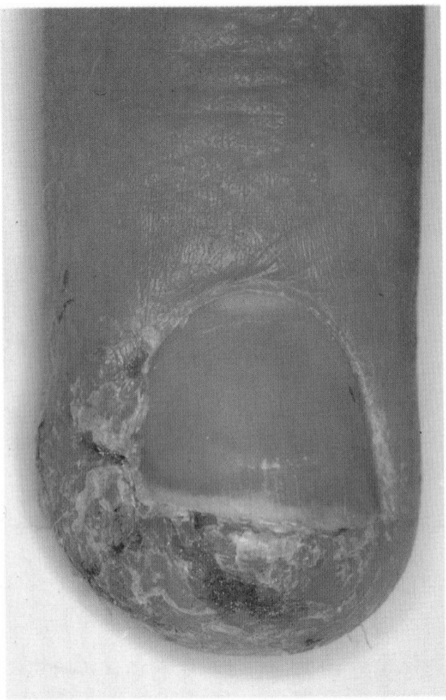

Fig. 7.9. Epoxyresin 'dermatitis'.

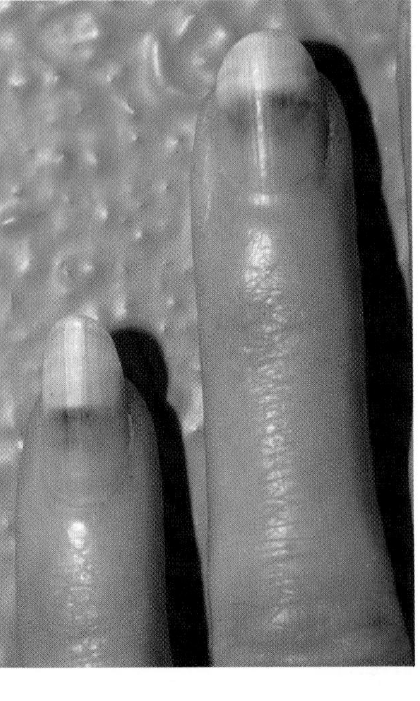
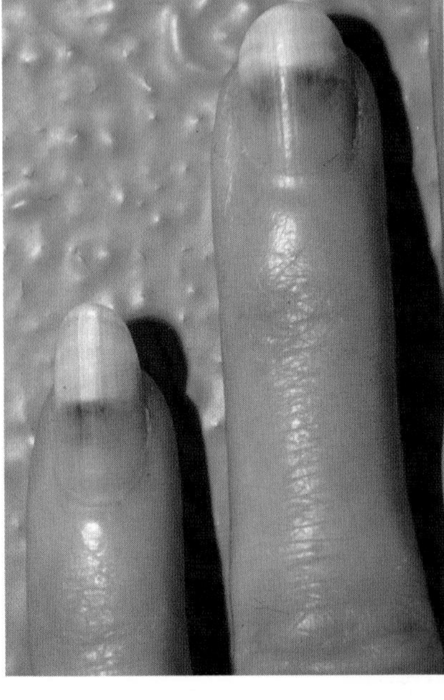

Fig. 7.11. Nail dystrophy with subungual haemorrhage due to formaldehyde.

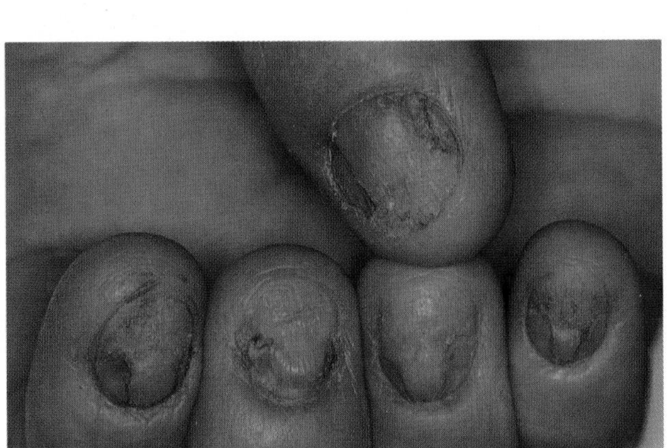

Fig. 7.10. Dystrophy due to PTBP resin.

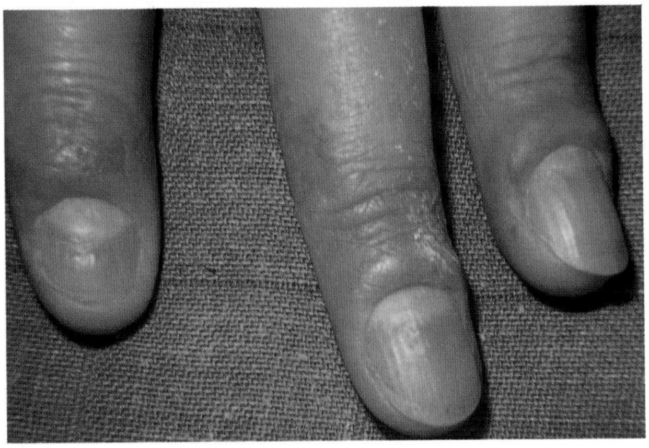

Fig. 7.12. Propanidid paronychia, usually seen in anaesthetists (courtesy of P.Y. Castelain, France).

and crusting or necrotic appearing lesions (Fowler, 1990); the resin oligomer may collect under the free edge of the nail and polymerise slowly as it dries (Fig. 7.9).

Allergic contact dermatitis from *nonoxynol-6*, a non-ionic emulsifier in an industrial waterless hand cleanser, was associated with a transverse dystrophy of the fingernails (Nethercott & Lawrence, 1984).

During the summer of 1979, women in Britain using adhesive to attach a brand of plastic artificial nails began to present with onycholysis, subungual hyperkeratosis, atrophy of the nail plate, and dermatitis of the periungual skin (Rycroft *et al.*, 1980). This was traced to contact sensitization by *p-tertiary butylphenol (PTBP) formaldehyde resin* in a particular batch of the adhesive (Fig. 7.10). Patients using these nails tended to have occupations in which they were in the public eye.

Formaldehyde (Fig. 7.11) itself sensitizes many occuptional groups including hospital staff; eczema of the fingers with nail dystrophy may result (Cronin, 1980b).

Hydroxylamine, which is both a sensitizer and an irritant, may produce onycholysis and/or paronychia (Pellerat & Chabeau, 1976; Goh, 1990; Baran, 1991). It has been widely used in colour photograph processing, the chemical industry (oximes synthesis), the pharmaceutical industry (bactericide, fungicide, antialgal) and in the manufacture of rubber and plastic compounds, cosmetics and soap.

'Caine' local anaesthetics, especially amethocaine and procaine, cause an allergic contact dermatitis in dental personnel, particularly on the pulps of the first three digits, either due to contact with the topical preparation or the liquid to be injected. *Propanidid* can give a similar pattern

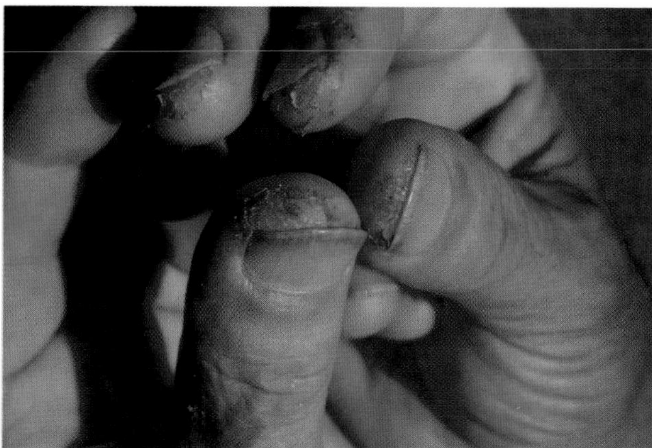

Fig. 7.13. Fisherman's dystrophy due to Escavenitis (caused by sea worm coelomic fluid) (courtesy of P. Angelini, Bari, Italy).

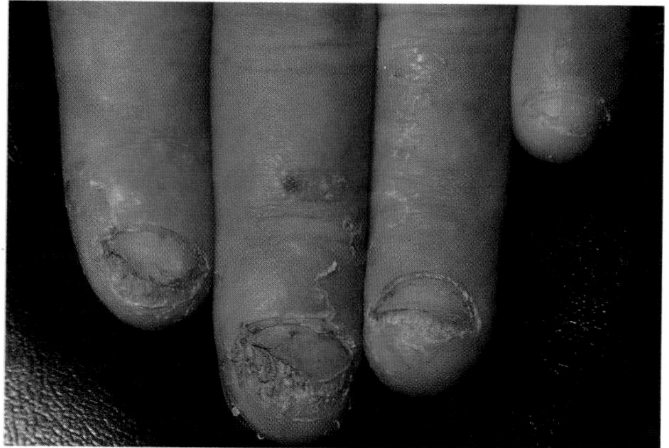

Fig. 7.14. Severe dermatitis and nail dystrophy due to bryozoans (courtesy of C. Audebert, le Havre, France).

with paronychia, sometimes of both hands, in anaesthetists (Castelain & Piriou, 1980) (Fig. 7.12).

Contact sensitivity to a cycloplegic *mydriatric agent* and to its pharmacologic components tropicamide and phenylephrine hydrochloride was reported on the finger of a nurse. Her work included the instillation of eyedrops into patients undergoing routine fundoscopic examination. The lesions showed well-demarcated brownish erythema with scaling on the second and third fingers of the left hand, which are used for opening the eyes of patients and are subjected routinely to contact with leaking mydriatic drops (Okamato & Kawai, 1991).

Among hairdressers in continental Europe many cases of allergic contact dermatitis due to *dicyandiamide derivatives* have been reported (Lépine & Fachot, 1971). This chemical was used in wave-setting lotions to restore split ends and thinning hair. The dermatitis began on the sides of the second, third and fourth fingers of the left hand and the webs between them. Onycholysis developed later, associated with a brownish discoloration of the

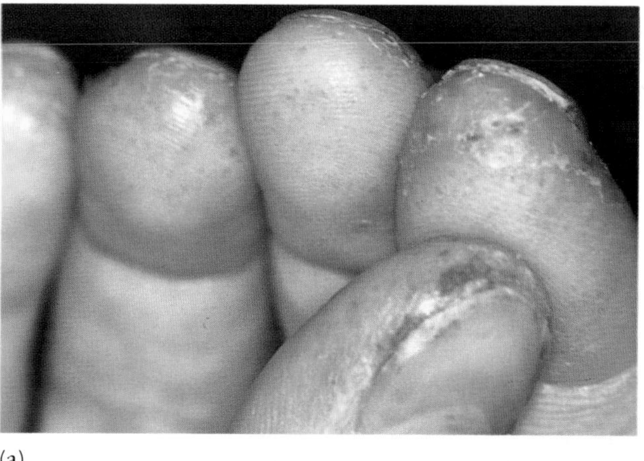

(a)

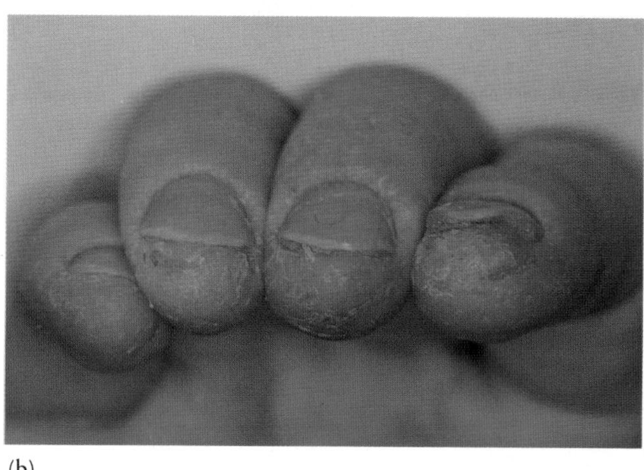

(b)

Fig. 7.15. (a & b) Nail changes due to contact with onions.

distal part of the nail bed. The company manufacturing the product has since replaced the sensitizing chemical, a formaldehyde releaser, with a different substance.

Escavenitis (Montel & Gouyer, 1957): the coelomic fluid of a sea-worm (*Nesreis diversicolor*), used as bait, can cause an exudative onychopathy with onycholysis of the first three fingers of the right hand in fishermen (Fig. 7.13). *Bryozoans* ('moss animals'), invertebrate animals resembling seaweeds, cause contact and photocontact dermatitis with nail involvement, the signs including pitting, paronychia, extensive distal nail dystrophy and subungual hyperkeratosis (Audebert & Lamoureux, 1978) (Fig. 7.14). Plate makers and those with *food* allergy, such as to onions, may develop finger pulp dermatitis and onycholysis (Fig. 7.15).

Cement dermatitis may be allergic, due to the dichromate content, or may result from alkaline irritation and burns. Dermatitis of the dorsum of the proximal nail fold and koilonychia are frequent. The latter is usually accompanied by disto-lateral subungual hyperkeratosis lifting the lateral edges of the nail (Fig. 7.16). Painful fissures in the same area are common (Calnan, 1960).

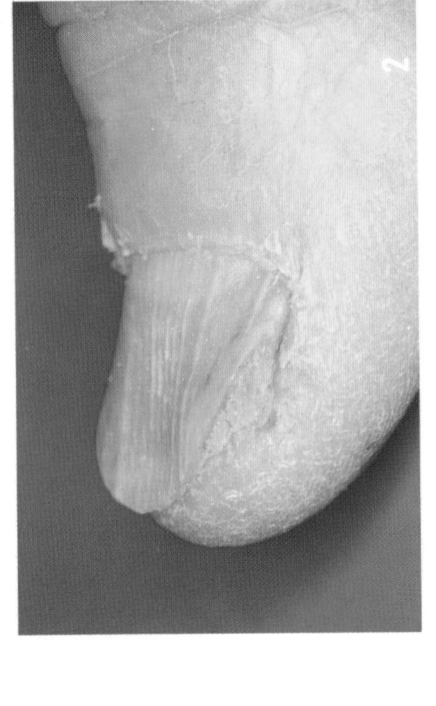

Fig. 7.16. Cement dermatitis nail signs with lateral subungual hyperkeratosis.

Chemical irritants

The nails can be softened and gradually destroyed by prolonged immersion in water containing high concentration of *alkalis*, *alkaline chlorine-containing compounds* (Coskey, 1974) or powerful *detergents* (Fig. 7.17(a) & (b)). Irritant reactions appear around and under the nails when the hands come into contact with concentrated

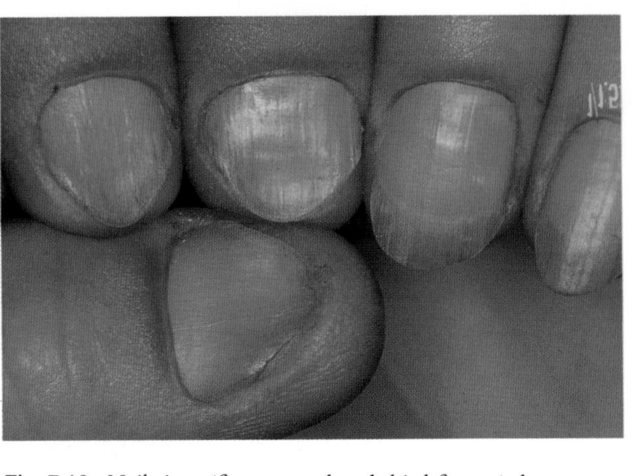

Fig. 7.18. Nail signs (first, second and third fingers) due to oven cleaning foam.

enzyme powder. Bleeding ulcerations under the nails may be seen (Göthe *et al.*, 1972).

Organic solvents (Fig. 7.18) and *motor oils* also soften the nail plate. Mineral oil may cause onycholysis and subungual hyperkeratosis (Fig. 7.19(a) & (b)). *Gold potassium cyanide* is responsible for a purplish-brown discoloration and onycholysis of the nails among electroplaters and electronics workers (Budden & Wilkinson, 1978).

Hydrofluoric acid especially damages the subungual tissues (Fig. 7.20(a) & (b)), which are a common portal of entry for this highly destructive chemical. The acid readily diffuses through minute holes in rubber gloves. Frequently the burn is unrecognized until up to 24 h later when excruciating pain begins: specific treatment with a topical 2% calcium gluconate preparation is indicated

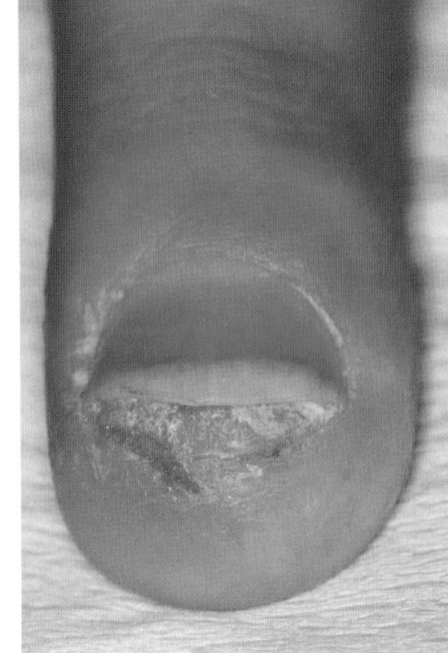

(a)

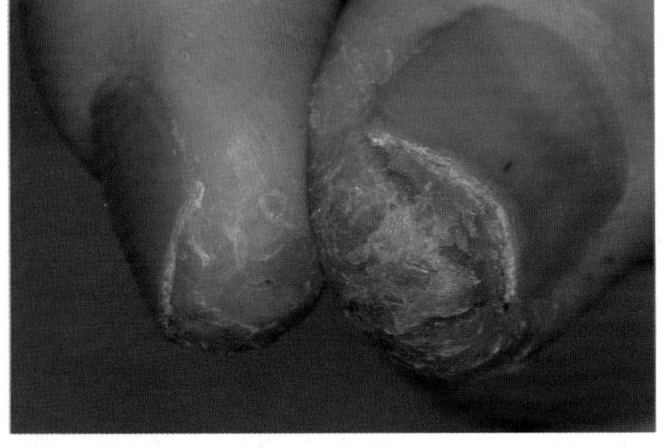

(b)

Fig. 7.17. (a & b) Subungual and fingertip inflammatory eruption due to powerful detergents.

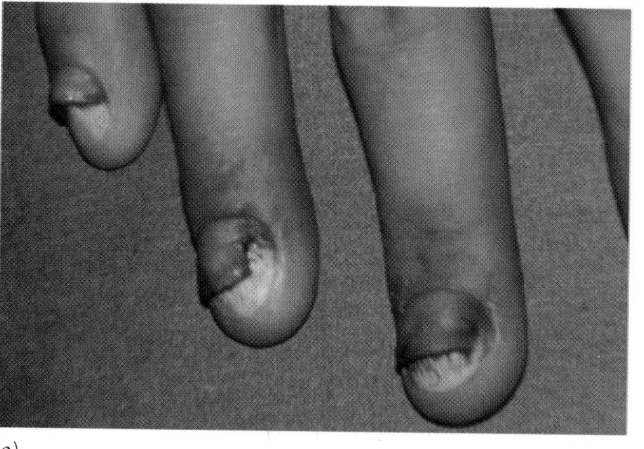
(a)

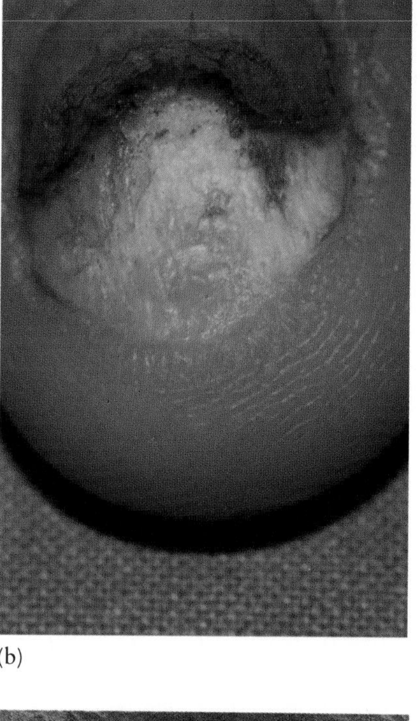
(b)

Fig. 7.19. (a & b) Onycholysis and subungual thickening due to mineral oils.

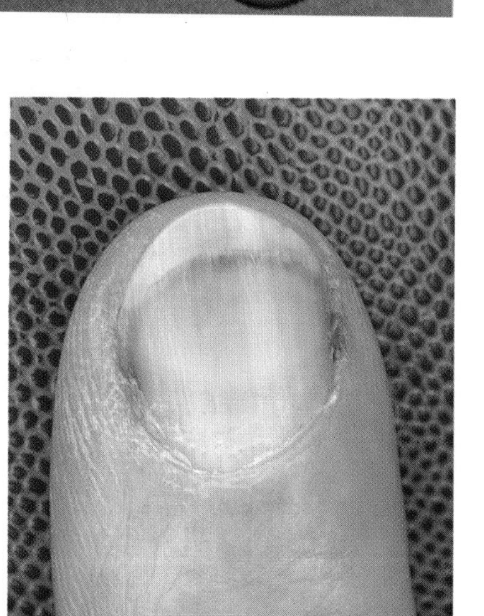
(a)

(b)

Fig. 7.20. (a & b) Terminal, subungual hyperkeratosis and onycholysis due to hydrofluoric acid.

(MacKinnon, 1986; Julie *et al.*, 1988). Hydrofluoric acid is widely used in the semiconductor industry and can be a component of rust-removing agents (Shewmake & Anderson, 1979; Baran, 1980; Pedersen, 1980). It is used, considerably diluted, to remove rust stains from fabrics prior to laundering and dry cleaning. It is also used in the manufacture of plastics, germicides, dyes, tanning solutions, solvents and fire-proofing materials; the glazing of pottery; photography; chemical digestion; metal electropolishing; graphite processing; cleaning brick, stone, iron and steel; and in the brewing of beer to control fermentation and to cleanse rubber pipes.

Oxalic acid, which is used in bleaching animal and vegetable materials, can cause redness and swelling of the fingertips together with a bluish discoloration and brittleness of the nails (Schwartz *et al.*, 1957a).

Prolonged occupational contact with *formaldehyde* solutions can cause softening and brown discoloration of the nail plate (Schwartz *et al.*, 1957b). Formalin (37–50% solution of formaldehyde in water) is widely used in-

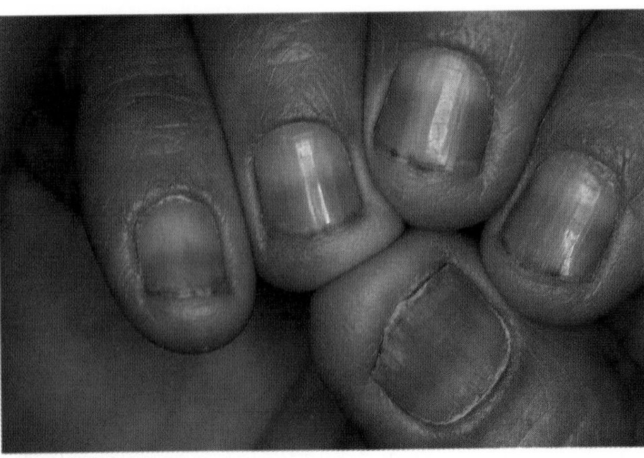

Fig. 7.21. Nail discoloration and onycholysis due to 5% dinitroorthocresol.

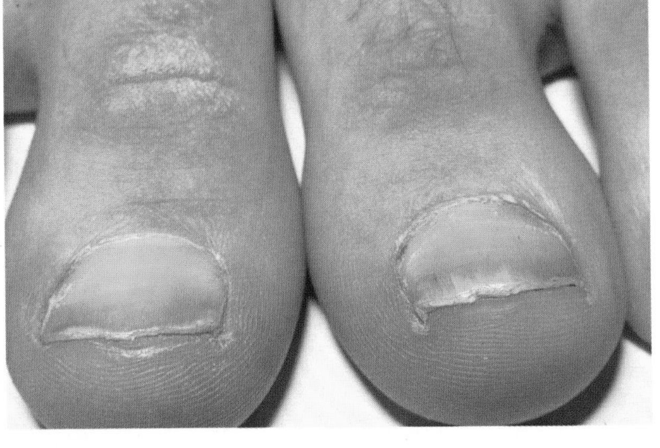

Fig. 7.22. Yellow nails in a Dinobuton handler (Wahlberg, Sweden, 1974).

dustrially. It can be used as a preservative, a tanning agent and an increaser of the water resistance of paper.

The weed killers *diquat* and *paraquat* can also soften and discolour the nail plate, leading to nail loss (Botella *et al.*, 1985). This can happen either from contact with the chemicals in concentrated form (Samman & Johnston, 1969) or following gross contamination with diluted solutions (Hearn & Keir, 1971). Similar changes have been described in a man using 5% *dinitroorthocresol*, without further recommended dilution, for spraying fruit trees (Baran, 1974) (Fig. 7.21). *Dinobuton* handlers may present with yellow nails and hair (Wahlberg, 1974) (Fig. 7.22).

Aminoethylethanolamine-containing soldering flux in the electronics industry can cause usually irritant, sometimes allergic, contact dermatitis (Goh, 1985), beginning periungually, with onycholysis, and spreading down the fingers and patchily onto the backs of the hands.

The application of a solution containing arsenic, copper acetate and hydrochloric acid, used to give a patina to belt

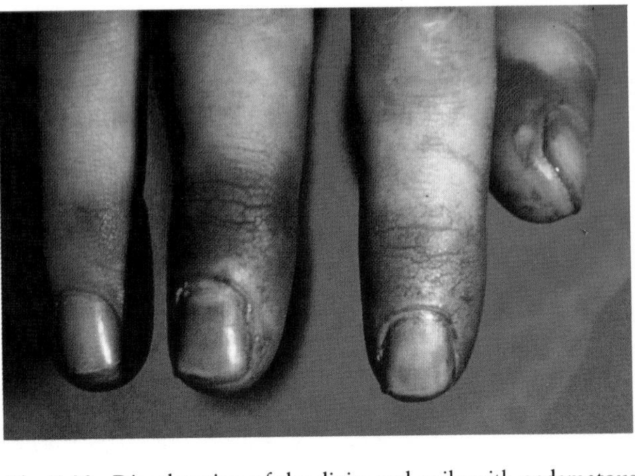

Fig. 7.23. Discoloration of the digits and nails with oedematous changes – due to solution used to give patina to belt buckles (courtesy of X. Balguerie, France).

buckles, produced after 3 days a marked throbbing pain in the distal phalanx of all the fingers of the right hand. A green-blue colour appeared in the nails, in the surrounding tissues and in the pulp, together with oedema of the affected region (Fig. 7.23). Onycholysis, slight subungual hyperkeratosis and acropulpitis were still evident after 6 months.

Bacterial infections

Even trivial abrasions and lacerations of the periungual skin may lead to more serious conditions such as cellulitis, erysipelas and septicaemia. The usual microorganisms are coagulase-positive staphylococci and various streptococci. *Pseudomonas* infection results in the cosmetically distressing green nail syndrome. Health care personnel with green nails may be a source of nosocomial infections (Greenberg, 1975). Interestingly, certain genera of bacteria, e.g. *Serratia*, Acinetobacter and *Pseudomonas*, were recovered only from nurses with artificial nails (Senay, 1991).

Paronychial infections are common and usually caused by a mixture of pathogenic organisms. Kitchen employees, agricultural workers and pianists are particulary liable to develop this condition. Acute paronychia is frequently seen in meat handlers (Barnham & Kerby, 1984). Streptoccal paronychia has been reported in a chicken factory (Barnham *et al.*, 1980).

Inoculation of the spores of *Clostridium tetani*, which are widespread in soil, through the periungual tissues may lead to a full-blown tetanus infection.

Erysipeloid is a bacterial infection of the hand usually seen in meat and fish handlers. The paronychial areas are occasionally involved (Fig. 7.24). Zahaff (1987) has described a case of leishmaniasis mimicking erysipeloid.

The prosector's paronychia is a primary inoculation infection with *Mycobacterium tuberculosis* (Fig. 7.25).

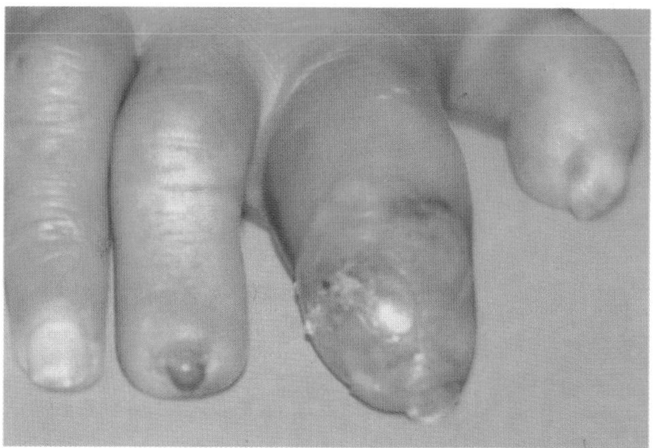

Fig. 7.24. Leshmaniasis mimicking erysipeloid, usually seen in meat or fish handlers (courtesy of A. Zahaff, Tunisia).

The prosector's wart (tuberculosis verrucosa cutis, verrucosa necrogenica) signifies a reinoculation cutaneous tuberculosis (Fig. 7.26) more often than a primary inoculation infection. The usual source of infection is an autopsy on a tuberculotic cadaver, and it may occasionally be seen in pathologists, morgue attendants and other hospital personnel (Jetton & Coker, 1969; O'Donnell *et al.*, 1971; Goette *et al.*, 1978; Hooker *et al.*, 1979; Hoyt, 1981). Penetrating trauma is necessary for the initiation of the infection because the tubercle bacillus cannot traverse the normal skin barrier. Such primary inoculation tuberculosis is associated with a negative tuberculin test prior to infection, compared with reinoculation cutaneous tuberculosis; the differential diagnosis includes chancriform conditions of deep fungal or bacterial origin.

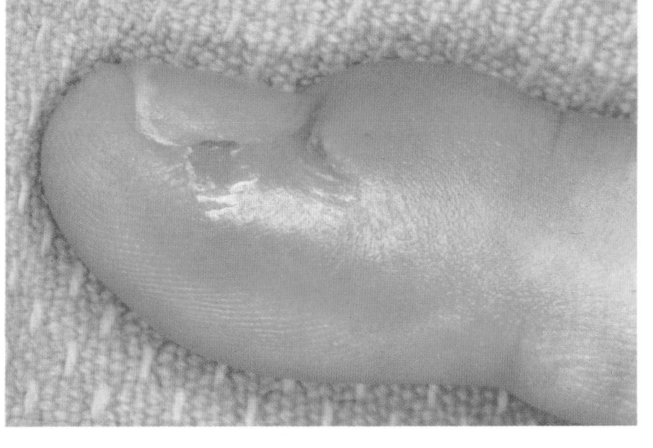

Fig. 7.25. TB infection – primary (prosector's paronychia) (courtesy of D. Goette, USA).

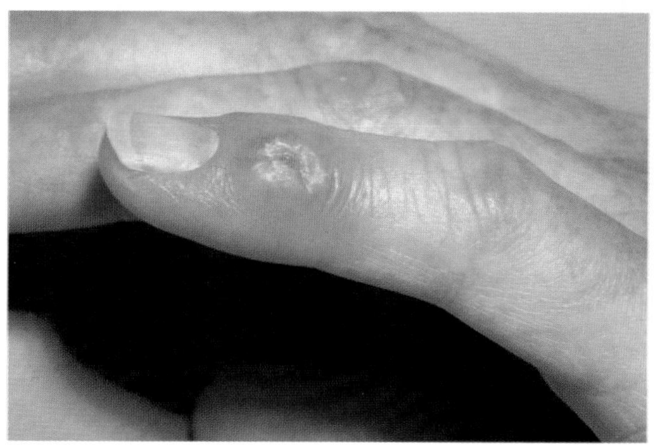

Fig. 7.27. *Mycobacterium marinum* infection (swimming pool granuloma) (courtesy of D. Sigal, France).

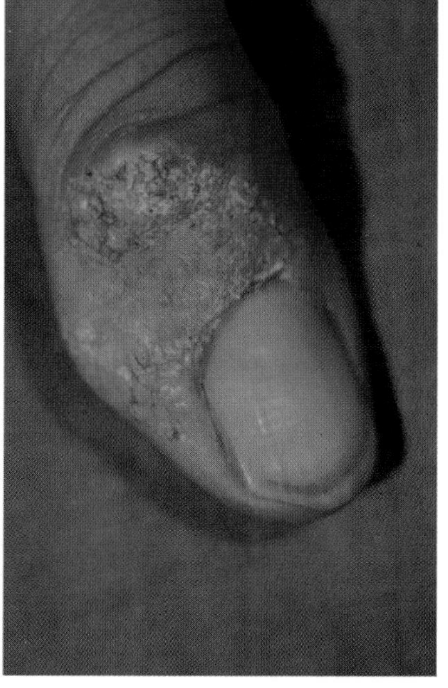

Fig. 7.26. Verrucous TB – reinoculation type (prosecutor's wart).

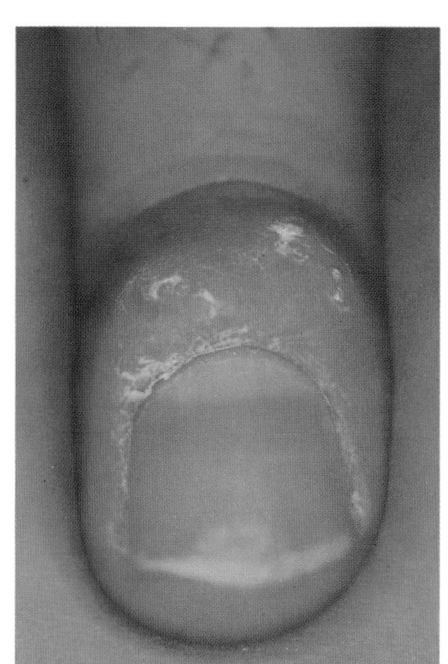

Fig. 7.28. *Mycobacterium marinum* infection (swimming pool granuloma) (courtesy of S. Salasche, USA).

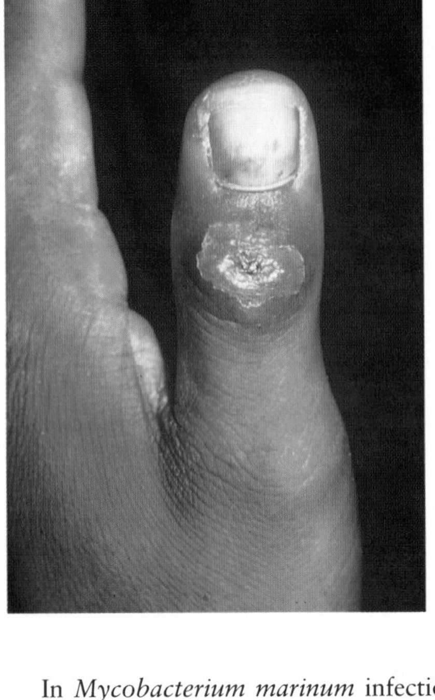

Fig. 7.29. Tularaemia – inoculation lesion (courtesy of R. Arenas, Mexico DF).

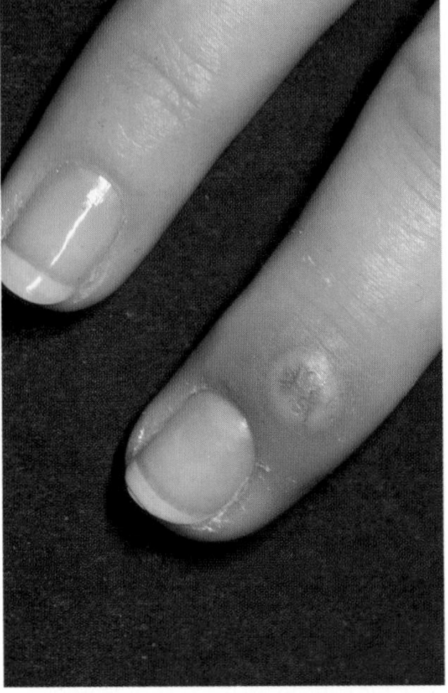
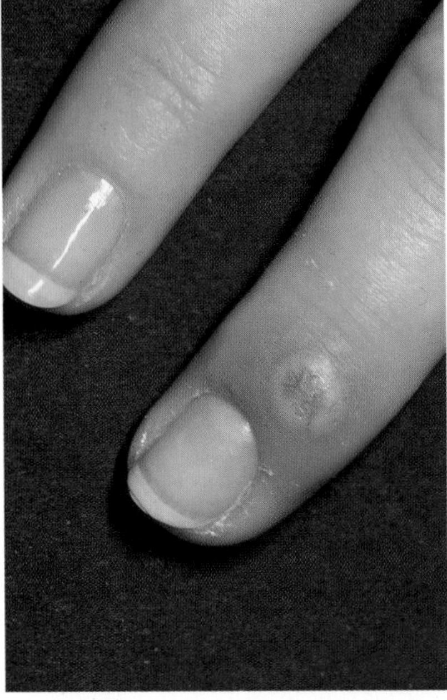

Fig. 7.30. Orf virus infection (courtesy of J. Gill, Canada).

In *Mycobacterium marinum* infection (swimming pool granuloma) (Figs 7.27 & 7.28), a slightly tender papule develops at the proximal nail fold which becomes pustular and drains; the latter ceases within a week but the papule persists gradually increasing in size. The dorsal surface of the distal phalanx of the finger appears erythematous and verrucous (Horn, 1981). The differential diagnosis includes atypical mycobacterial infection, sporotrichosis, and tuberculosis verrucosa cutis. Frequently, swimming pool granuloma is a self-limited infection which may last for several months. Small lesions may be satisfactorily excised (Pettit, 1982). However, if the infectious material is not completely eradicated, relapse can be expected. Tetracyline in doses ranging from 1 to 2 g/day (or minocycline, 100 mg b.i.d.) should be considered the treatment of choice in swimming pool granuloma.

Tularaemia results from infection with the coccobacillus, *Pasterurella tularensis*. Infection around the nail may be transmitted to man by direct contact with infected wildlife (rabbits are the principal reservoirs of tularaemia in nature). However most infections are due to contact with animal carcasses (Lewis, 1982). Ulceroglandular tularaemia, the most common form, consists of a primary papule which becomes ulcerated, suppurative and granulomatous at the site of inoculation, with regional lymphadenitis (bubonic tularaemia) (Fig. 7.29). Over half the patients with any cutaneous ulcers present with multiple lesions including shallow erosions into subungual tissues (Young *et al.*, 1969). Streptomycin is generally the drug of choice, but chloramphenicol, gentamicin and tetracycline are also used in the treatment of tularaemia.

Primary syphilis may be acquired occupationally, e.g. by doctors.

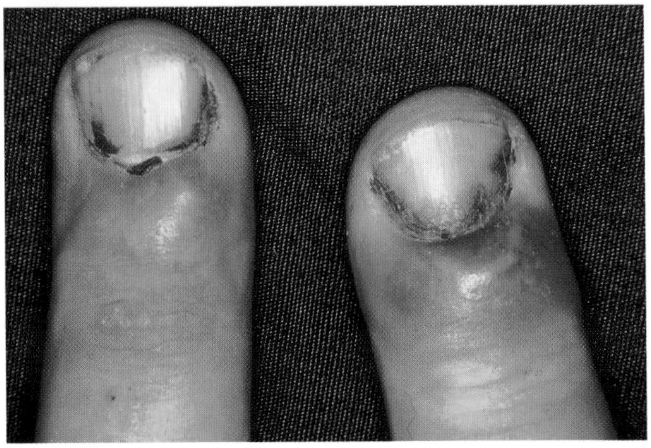

Fig. 7.31. Milker's nodules (paravaccinia infection) (courtesy of R.K. Scher, New York, USA).

Viral infections

The orf virus infects sheep, goats and even reindeer in and around the mouth and can be transmitted to man. The lesion in the human is most commonly on the dorsum of the right index finger. It can take on a target-like appearance (Fig. 7.30). Spontaneous healing occurs within 4–6 weeks, leaving a small scar (Arnaud *et al.*, 1986). Examination of an aspirate by electron microscopy confirms the diagnosis. The lesion resolves spontaneously within 6 weeks (Gill *et al.*, 1990).

Milker's nodules is a clinically similar viral infection (Fig. 7.31) caused by a paravaccinia virus, and afflicts mostly agricultural workers and veterinarians. Viral cultures permit differentiation from orf. This condition passes through the same clinical sequence as orf, in appearance and timing, and heals spontaneously in 21–70 days without scarring (Marriot, 1982). In 'farmyard pox', Shelley and Shelley (1983) recommend a less conservative attitude, suggesting its complete removal by epidermal subsection using a Gillette 'super blue' blade.

Orf and milker's nodule infection have distinctive histopathologic features, and viral changes may frequently be found (Groves *et al.*, 1991).

Herpes simplex infection is an occupational hazard of dentists (Rames *et al.*, 1984), nurses (Kanaar, 1967), surgeons and anaesthetists (Rosato *et al.*, 1970) and pathologists (Haedicke *et al.*, 1989). The eruption may resemble pyogenic paronychia to some extent, but the presence of several closely grouped vesicles on an erythematous base should suggest the diagnosis (Louis & Silva, 1979). Two or more fingers may be involved at the same time.

Viral warts are more common in butchers (Jablonska *et al.*, 1987; Aloi *et al.*, 1988), poultry handlers (Moragon *et al.*, 1987) and fish handlers (Rüdlinger *et al.*, 1984), in whom many of the lesions are periungual or subungual.

Fungal infections

Fungal infection of the nails and periungual region are common occupational problems, particularly candidiasis. Those with occupations requiring the hands to be wet or exposed to detergents for prolonged periods, such as dishwashers in restaurants, are prone to candidal paronychia and onycholysis. Candidal infections are also often seen in poultry and fish handlers.

Dermatophytic toenail infections are known to occur with increased prevalence in coal miners and others who work in hot humid environments and share washing facilities. Infection with *Trichophyton rubrum* often involves both feet and only one hand, a curious and unexplained phenomenon. Either the dominant or the other hand may be involved (Gellin, 1972). A useful diagnostic feature of fungal nail involvement is the sparing of one or more nails, as opposed to psoriatic nail involvement where all the nails tend to be affected.

Alkiewicz and Sowinski (1967) noted two cases of *Trichophyton* infection of the fingernails, a cashier and a teacher; their occupations required moistening of the tips of the fingers continually with a wet sponge. Fungal infections of the toenails have been reported in 6.5–27% of miners (Götz & Hantschke, 1965; Tappeiner & Male, 1966) often associated to *Hendersonula toruloidea* and *Scytalidium hyalinum* (Gugnani & Oyeka, 1989).

Primary cutaneous blastomycosis can be an occupational hazard to pathologists (Larson *et al.*, 1983). A reddish-purple furuncle of the distal part of the finger presents 2 weeks after accidental inoculation into a deep cut in the same area (Fig. 7.32).

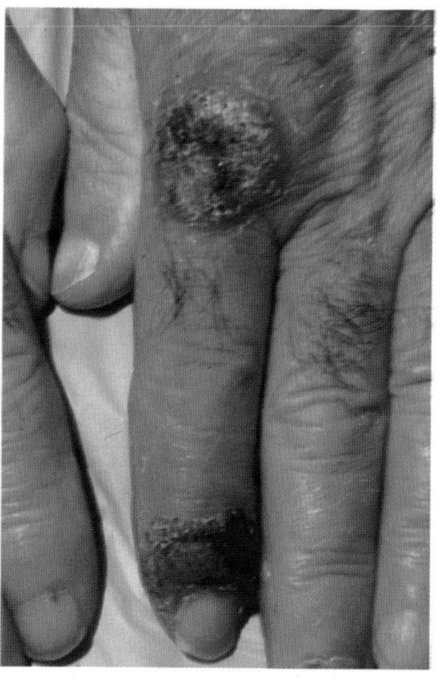

Fig. 7.32. Blastomycosis – primary lesion in a pathologist (courtesy of D. Sweeny, USA).

Systemic conditions

Besides chemical percutaneous absorption, which may be responsible for methaemoglobinaemia, systemic conditions, such as neurologic and gastrointestinal symptoms related to patch tests with UV curable acrylic monomers (Andersen, 1986) and even death (Ford *et al.*, 1978), may be due to chemical absorption by the inhalational route. Pneumoconiotic lung diseases can produce clubbing after exposure to asbestos (Petry, 1966), talc, beryllium, silica (Kern, 1990), cobalt and tungsten (Desoille *et al.*, 1962).

Systemic sclerosis may develop after occupational exposure to excessive levels of vinyl chloride monomer (with pseudoclubbing) (Fig. 7.33), epoxy resin vapour, trichlorethylene and trichlorethane and silica (Rustin *et al.*, 1989). Sclerodactyly with nail fold capillary changes, Raynaud's phenomenon and acroosteolysis (Fig. 7.34) are characteristic (Bachurzewska & Borucka, 1986; Flindt-Hansen & Isager, 1987). Lupus erythematosus-like erythema and periungual telangiectasia have been reported among coffee plantation workers (Narahari *et al.*, 1990). Davies *et al.* (1990) reported on cutaneous haemangioendothelioma developed on a toenail bed of a patient who had worked with polyvinyl chloride.

Principal signs associated with occupational origin

Tables 7.1–7.6 demonstrate the principal signs found in occupational nail disorders.

When dealing with occupational nail dyschromia, examination of the abnormal nails should follow the directions indicated in the chapter on chromonychia.

1 When the discoloration is due to nail plate–nail bed

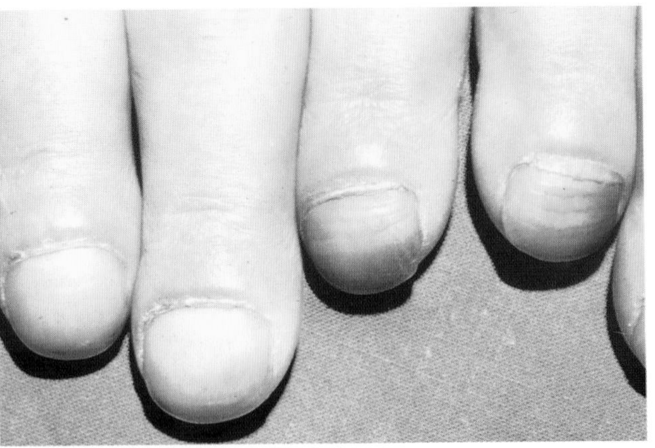

Fig. 7.33. 'Pseudoclubbing' due to occupational acroosteolysis.

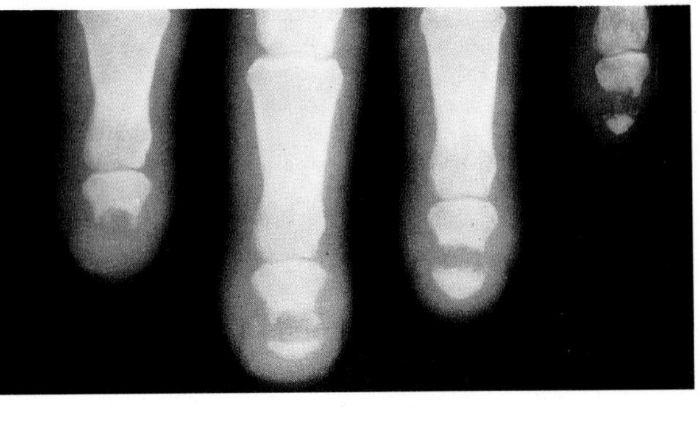

Fig. 7.34. Occupational acroosteolysis – X-ray changes in terminal phalanges.

Table 7.1. Gradual destruction of the nail plate (Ronchese 1962a,b, 1969)

Butchers
Cement workers (Fig. 7.35)
File-makers
Optical glass handlers
Packers
Rope workers
Silk weavers (Ronchese, 1955)
Shoemakers
Shoe-shiners
Workers handling small instruments
Workers required to lift repeatedly heavy plastic bags frequently (Schubert *et al.*, 1977)

Table 7.2. Brittle and atrophic nails

Bean shellers and potato peelers (paronychia)
Chemists and laboratory workers (paronychia)
Dentists (onycholysis, subungual hyperkeratosis, dermatitis)
Engravers (paronychia)
Etchers (paronychia)
Glaziers (paronychia)
Hat cleaners (paronychia)
Nurses
Painters (paronychia)
Photographers (paronychia, discoloration)
Physicians
Plasterers (corroded nails)
Porcelain workers (serrated nails)
Radio workers (paronychia and nail loss)
Radium workers (radium dermatitis)
Shoemakers (onycholysis and paronychia)
Wet work (paronychia)
Wood workers (paronychia and stains)
Workers exposed to microwave radiation (onycholysis)

Table 7.3. Paronychia

Automotive workers (sulphuric acid exposure from batteries)
Bakers and pastry cooks
Barbers and hairdresser (onycholysis)
Bartenders
Bean shellers
Book binders (paste)
Bricklayers (limes, cement, mortar)
Builders and carpenters (including glass fibre)
Button makers
Cement workers
Chemists and laboratory workers
Cooks
Cosmetic workers
Dyers (aniline dyes, producing stains and necrosis)
Engravers (brittle nail)
Etchers, glass etchers (brittle nail)
Fishermen
Fishmongers
Florist and gardeners (onycholysis) (hyacinth, narcissus bulbs, tulip fingers)
Glaziers (brittle nail)
Ground keepers
Janitorial and domestic workers
Mechanics
Milkers (onycholysis from bristle)
Oil-rig workers
Painters
Photographic developers (brittle nail, discoloration)
Pianists
Physicians, dentists' nurses
Potato peelers
Radio workers (methanol, causing pigmentation and nail loss)
Salt plant workers (ulcers)
Shoe workers (brittle nails)
Tanners (whitlow)
Textile workers (threads of fabric)
Violinists (nail dystrophy)
Wood workers (brittle nails, stains)
Wool workers (wool thread)

Table 7.4. Alterations in colour of nail plate

Sign	Workers affected
Leuconychia	Arsenic workers Butchers (Fig. 7.36) Keypunchers (Honda *et al.*, 1976) Salt plant workers and contact with salted intestines (Ferreira Marques, 1939; Frenk & Leu, 1966) Weedkillers (paraquat) (transverse leuconychia) (Botella *et al.*, 1985) Workers manufacturing thallium rodenticides Fly tyer's finger apparent leuconychia (MacAulay, 1990)
Black	Electric bulb cleaners (hydrochloric acid) Gunsmiths Vintners (red wine)
Blue	Anodisers (aluminium) Local argyria (Bergfeld & McMahon, 1987; Sarsfield *et al.*, 1992) Auto mechanics (oxalic acid in radiators) Cyanosis from methaemoglobinaemia or sulphhaemoglobinaemia Dye makers Electroplaters Gold platers Metal cleaners, metal patina solution (Fig. 7.23) Ink makers Paint removers Photographers Rust remouvers Silver workers (Bleehen *et al.*, 1981) presenting generalized argyria. Textile workers
Brown	Cigar makers Cobblers Coffee bean workers Cooks and bakers (burnt sugar) Hairdressers (Fig. 7.37) Photographers Roadway pavers Shoe-shiners Walnut pickers (pecans; Fig. 7.38) Woodworkers (varnish) Woodworkers (ebony, mahogany) (Harris & Rosen, 1989)
Green (usually caused by *Pseudomonas* infection)	Bartenders Dish-washers Electricians Fruit handlers Laundry workers Metallurgists Restaurant workers Sugar factory workers

continued

Table 7.4. *Continued*

Sign	Workers affected
Yellow	Epoxy system handlers: metaphenylenediamine and 4,4′-methylenedianiline (Cohen, 1985) Flower handlers Pesticide workers: diquat (Samman & Johnston, 1969; Clark & Hurst, 1970), paraquat (Samman & Johnston, 1969; Hearn & Keir, 1971; Dobbelaere & Bouffioux, 1974), dinitro-orthocresol (Baran, 1974), dinobuton (Wahlberg, 1974) Workers handling chromium salts Workers handling dyestuffs: dinitrosalicylic acid (Fregert & Trulson, 1980), dinitrobenzene, dinitrotoluene, and trinitrotoluene

Table 7.5. Koilonychia. After a while, nail changes may become irreversible (Pedersen, 1982)

Automotive workers (Dawber, 1974)
Chimney sweeps
Coil winders (Smith *et al.*, 1980)
Glass workers
Hairdressers (thioglycolates)
Mushroom growers
Organic chemists (organic solvents) (Ancona-Alayón, 1975)
Rickshaw pullers (feet) (Bentley-Phillips & Bayles, 1971)
Slaughterhouse workers (Meyer-Hamme & Quadripur, 1983)

Table 7.6. Onycholysis. Occupational onycholysis is most frequently due to chemical irritants or sensitizers as described in the text. In addition, there are infective causes, which tend to be limited to medical personnel (*Herpes*) (Louis & Silva, 1979) and occupations with entail prolonged soaking of the hands (*Candida* and *Pseudomonas*); there are also traumatic causes

Traumatic onycholysis caused by repeated minor injuries (Ronchese, 1962a; Forck & Kästner, 1967; Somov *et al.*, 1976; Menné *et al.*, 1985)	Cropping Milking Nut cracking Poultry plucking Separating meat from bone Scraping Shell casing Destalking mushrooms
Caused by introduction of foreign bodies	Bristles Glass fibre (Rogaïlin *et al.*, 1975) Hair (Stubbart, 1956, Hogan, 1988) (Fig. 7.40) Metal Thorns

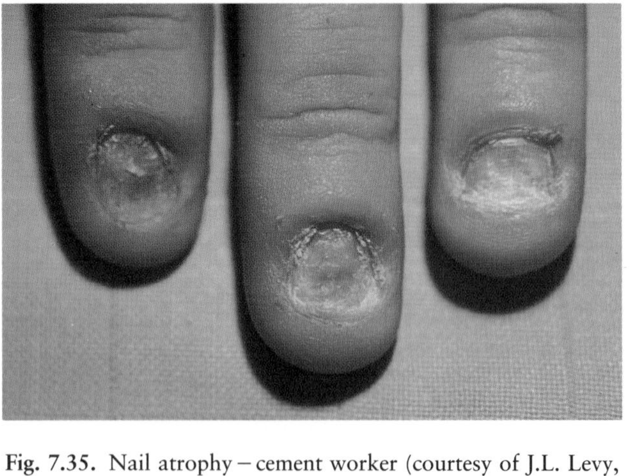

Fig. 7.35. Nail atrophy – cement worker (courtesy of J.L. Levy, Marseilles, France).

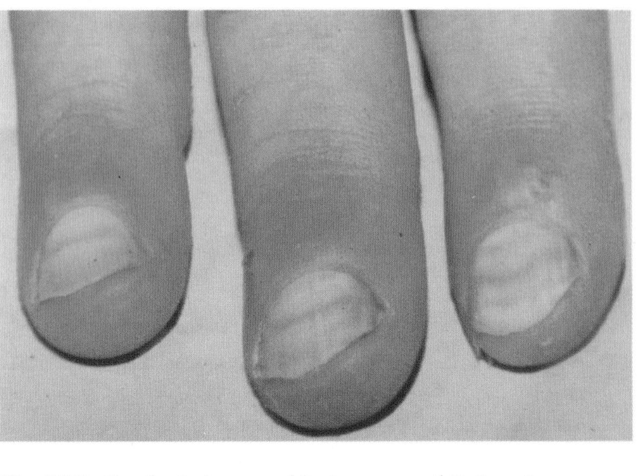

Fig. 7.36. Butcher's leuconychia (courtesy of F. Leu, Lausanne, Switzerland).

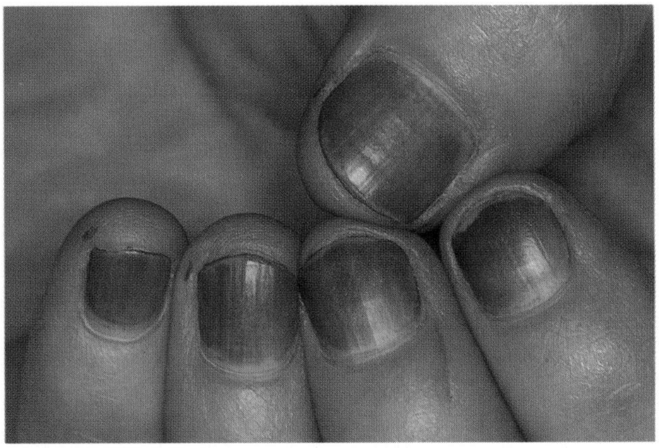

Fig. 7.37. Brown discoloration of nails due to dye (in a hairdresser).

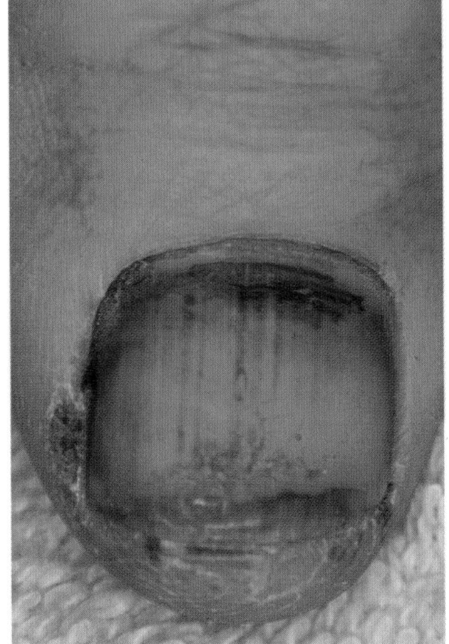

Fig. 7.38. Colour changes (walnut picker) (courtesy of S. Salasche, USA).

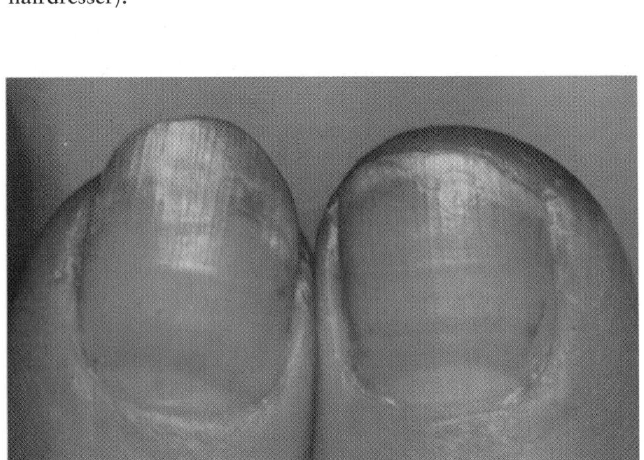

Fig. 7.39. Yellow staining in a handler of epoxy resin system chemicals (courtesy of S.R. Cohen, USA).

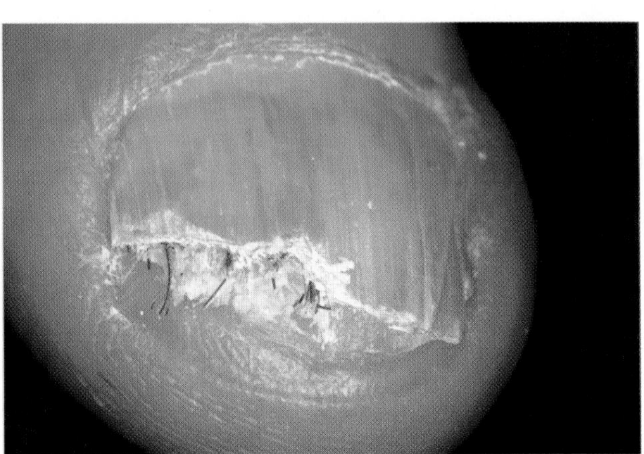

Fig. 7.40. Onycholysis and subungual thickening associated with subungual hairs in a hairdresser.

separation, the history of the condition will help to find its cause. Onycholysis is most frequently due to chemicals and often due to prolonged soaking of the hands. It may also be traumatic or infective.

2 When the discoloration is restricted to the nail plate, fingertip pressure producing blanching does not alter the pigmentation, nor does the pen-torch placed against the pulp. The discoloration may follow the shape of the proximal nail fold, which is the signature of an exogenous cause. History of the condition may confirm the traumatic origin of a haematoma. But the possibility of malignant melanoma following trauma to a nail as a coincidental or causal event should be kept in mind.

3 When pigmentation is due to systemic absorption of a chemical through the skin or lungs, it involves all the digits.

(a) Disappearance of the pigmentation on the nail bed blanching test means that the pigment originates from the blood vessels. In such a case, methaemoglobinaemia, for example, that manifests as bluish discoloration of the terminal digits, should be looked for in an otherwise asymptomatic worker, i.e. following exposure to aromatic nitro and amino compounds that penetrate all glove materials. The colour disappears within 16 h of leaving work, in contrast to sulfhaemoglobinaemia, presenting with the same distal discoloration as an early warning sign of intoxication (Pinkus *et al.*, 1963), but disappearing only with the normal life span of the red blood cells, i.e. 4 months (Kern, 1990).

(b) If the pigmentation is not altered on the nail blanching test, it may be obliterated by the pen-torch pressed against the pulp. This means that the pigment is deposited in the nail bed, as observed in the blue nails of silver refinery workers (Bleehen *et al.*, 1981).

4 When systemic absorption of a chemical is oral, the discoloration is more likely to correspond to the shape of the lunula. Transverse leuconychia known as Mees' lines is likely to occur in occupational arsenic and thallium poisoning, for example.

Non-occupational nail hazards

There are few direct hazards to the nails that are not occupational, and these largely consist of cosmetic applications to the nails. Nail preparations rarely damage the nails themselves. When they do, their effect is usually quickly perceived and the product either radically altered or withdrawn from the market.

The principles of diagnosis of these rare non-occupational but exogenous nail disorders are the same as those for occupational nail disorders outlined in a previous section of this chapter. Besides the cosmetic hazards that are specified in this second part of the chapter, there are several conditions described in the first part that can sometimes also arise non-occupationally from leisure pursuits, e.g. 'do-it-yourself' activities, or housework. These are not repeated here. Allergic contact dermatitis from acrylic sculptured nails has been included earlier because of its occurrence in manicurists as well as in their clients. Permanent loss of fingernails due to allergic reaction to an acrylic nail preparation seems unique (Fisher, 1989). The use of cyanoacrylate glue nail preparations may produce allergic reaction of the nail plate and paronychial area, which may be prolonged with resultant marked dystrophy of the nails (Shelley & Shelley, 1988) and even partial loss that may eventually prove permanent (Fisher, 1987).

Physical hazards

Synthetic nail covers were once introduced as an alternative to nail varnish. They caused flaking, roughness and ridging of the nail plate, onycholysis, recession of the cuticle and even the lunula, and mild paronychia (Calnan, 1958; Calnan & Sarkany, 1958). This was thought to be caused by a combination of occlusion and the cumulative trauma of repeatedly pulling them off (Samman, 1961).

Chemical sensitizers

Nail base coats are applied before nail varnish to help prevent it from chipping off. In the past there was a base coat formulation that sensitized its users because of its content of phenol formaldehyde resin (Sulzberger *et al.*, 1948; Rein & Rogin, 1950). This caused only minimal skin changes but striking nail changes. These included discoloration of the nail plate, progressing from yellow to almost black, subungual hyperkeratosis and haemorrhage, and onycholysis. Later Reisch (1959) reported discoloration and onycholysis from a base coat not containing formaldehyde resin. Patch tests with all its ingredients were negative and occlusion rather than sensitization was blamed.

Nail varnish itself can cause allergic contact dermatitis, which is usually due to sensitization to its content of arylsulphonamide formaldehyde resin. It is rare, however, for the periungual skin or fingers to be affected and excessively rare for the nails themselves to show any changes. Scaly fissured proximal nail folds can very occasionally be seen in sensitized women, particularly perhaps if nail varnish is wiped onto the skin during removal (Cronin, 1980c). The three principal sites of nail varnish dermatitis arise by direct contact between the nails and the skin and are the eyelids, the lower half of the face and the sides of the neck and upper chest (Calnan & Sarkany, 1958). Away from the eyelids the dermatitis has a characteristically patchy distribution. A case of contact

Table 7.7. General guidance on glove materials*

Material	Protective against	Additional notes
Natural rubber	Soaps and detergents, water-soluble irritants, dilute acids and alkalis	Not good for organic solvents, strong acids and alkalis, many other organic compounds
Butyl rubber	Aldehydes, most amines, amides, ketones, formaldehyde resins, epoxy resins, most acrylates, isocyanates	
Chloroprene	Soaps and detergents, dilute acids and alkalis, certain amines and esters, most alcohols, vegetable oils	Not good for aldehydes, ketones, nitro- and halogenated compounds
Fluorocarbon	Organic solvents, particularly halogenated and aromatic hydrocarbons	Cost 30–40 times as much as natural rubber
Nitrile rubber	Organic acids, certain alcohols, amines, ethers, peroxides, inorganic alkalis, vegetable oils	Also protect against organophosphorus compounds to some extent
Styrene-butadiene rubber		Hypoallergenic surgical gloves only
Polyethylene	Mainly for food handlers and medical personnel	Chemical resistance dependent on seams
Polyvinyl alcohol	Several organic solvents, most esters	Not resistant to water or aqueous solutions
Polyvinyl chloride	Soaps and detergents oils, metalworking fluids dilute acids and alkalis, vegetable oils	Not good for most organic solvents

* Actual protection depends on glove thickness, manufacturing quality, chemical concentration, duration of contact, environmental temperature and humidity, etc.

dermatitis from hypoallergenic nail varnish has been reported (Shaw, 1989), a polyester resin being identified as the sensitizer.

Nickel may cause onycholysis, acting as a local sensitizer (B. Magnusson, personal communication, 1972).

Nail damage resulting in onycholysis and subungual hyperkeratosis has been reported as secondary to a hairspray (Daniel & Scher, 1991).

Chemical irritants

Nail hardeners are marketed to help prevent lamellar splitting of the free edge of the nail plate. They usually contain *formaldehyde* and this can cause, especially when over-used, a leuconychia of the distal half of the nail plate and onycholysis (Mitchell, 1981) with mild subungual hyperkeratosis and paronychia (March, 1966; Cronin, 1980d). Painful thickening of the hyponychium (pterygium inversum unguis) has been reported from application of a nail hardener to the ventral as well as the dorsal nail surfaces (Daly & Johnson, 1986). The formaldehyde usually acts as an irritant rather than as a sensitizer. A nail hardener containing both formaldehyde and toluenesulphonamide formaldehyde resin caused an outbreak of contact dermatitis of the face and neck in The Netherlands, due to allergy to the resin (de Wit *et al.*, 1988). One case also had fissures on the fingertips, but there was no nail damage.

Enzyme detergent can cause acute onychia and onycholysis (Hodgson & Mayon-White, 1971); symptoms appeared after 2 weeks of using an enzyme detergent for approximately an hour each day without gloves. Patch tests with 1 and 2% aqueous solutions of the detergent were negative.

Thioglycolates in depilatories (chemical hair removers) are a further domestic cause of acute chemical onycholysis, several fingernails being involved at the same time (Baran, 1980).

Discoloration of the nail plate (see Chapters 2 and 8)

Perhaps the most familiar instance of simple discoloration of the nail plate are the yellow-brown nails of heavy cigarette smokers. The vegetable hair dye, henna, will stain nails red-brown (Wilkinson, 1973).

Certain nail varnishes have had nail plate discoloration as an unwanted side effect. Calnan (1967) reported some that produced a non-removable yellow-orange discoloration. One particularly striking example was traced to the presence of the pigment Transparent Yellow Lake 16901. Benzophenone-2, a UV filter contained in a nail laquer, induced a light-dependent discoloration of the fingernails in two female patients (Schauder, 1990). Some topical dermatological therapies, such as potassium permanganate and ammoniated mercury ointment (Butterworth & Strean, 1963), can stain the nails brown. Discoloration from the combined effect of nail varnish and dermatological treatment was reported by Loveman and Fliegelman (1955). They were consulted by several patients because of yellow-orange discoloration of the nails; all had been using lotions containing either resorcinol or resorcinol monoacetate, but only nails previously lacquered were affected. The contribution of nail varnish was narrowed down to its content of nitrocellulose.

An anecdotal case report concerned acquired pachyonychia of the 20 digits due to presence of lead in a scalp lotion (Esteves *et al.*, 1983). Its withdrawal was followed by a remarkable improvement.

Nail protection at work

Gloves are the best form of protection, but only if they are considered safe to wear and if they are made of material appropriate to the agent against which protection is required. Neither natural rubber nor polyvinyl chloride (PVC) gloves, for example, are good protection against organic solvents. Further general guidance is given in Table 7.7. Expert detailed advice is now available on computer (Mellströme, 1985; Forsberg & Keith, 1989). The novel 4H glove could minimize the risks of working with hazardous chemicals (Tobler & Freiburghaus, 1992).

References

Alkiewicz J. & Sowinski W. (1967) Die Trichophytie der Fingernägel als berufliches Problem. *Mycosen* **10**, 463.

Aloi F.G., Molinero A., Passera A. *et al.* (1988) Viral warts in Butchers. Clinical and statistical study. *G. Ital. Dermatol. Venereol.* **123**, 341–344.

Ancona-Alayón A. (1975) Occupational koilonychia from organic solvents. *Contact Derm.* **1**, 367–369.

Andersen K.E. (1986) Systemic symptoms related to patch test with UV curable acrylic monomers. *Contact Derm.* **14**, 180.

Arnaud J.P., Bernard P., Souyri N. *et al.* (1986). Human orf disease localized in the hand. A study of eight cases. *Ann. Chir. Main.* **5**, 129–132.

Audebert C. & Lamoureux P. (1978) Eczema professionnel du marin pêcheur par contact de bryozoaires en baie de Seine. *Ann. Dermatol. Venereol.* **105**, 187–192.

Bachurzewska B. & Borucka I. (1986) Gefässläsionen bei Einsenbahnnarbeiterinnen die mit Epoxidharzen in Berührung kommen. *Dermatosen* **34**, 77–79.

Baran R. (1974) Nail damage caused by weed killers and insecticides. *Arch. Dermatol.* **110**, 467.

Baran R. (1978) Pigmentations of the nails (chromonychia). *J. Dermatol. Surg. Oncol.* **4**, 250–254.

Baran R. (1980) Acute onycholysis from rust-removing agents. *Arch. Dermatol.* **116**, 382–383.

Baran R. (1991) Onycholysis from hydroxylamine. *Contact Derm.* **24**, 158.

Baran R. & Bureau H. (1981) Surgical treatment of recalcitrant chronic paronychias of the fingers. *J. Dermatol. Surg. Oncol.* **7**, 106–107.

Baran R. & Levy J.L. (1992) Onychopathies et travail. *Rev. Med. Travail* **19**, 47–49.

Baran R. & Schibli H. (1990) Permanent paresthesia to sculptured nails. A distressing problem. *Dermatol. Clin.* **8**, 139–141.

Barnham M. & Kerby J. (1984) A profile of skin sepsis in meat handlers. *J. Infect.* **9**, 43–50.

Barnham M. Kerby J. & Skillin J. (1980) An outbreak of streptococcal infection in a chicken factory. *J. Hyg. Camb.* **84**, 71–75.

Belsito D.V. (1981) Contact dermatitis to ethyl-cyanoacrylate-containing glue. *Contact Derm.* **17**, 234–236.

Bentley-Phillips B. & Bayles M.A.H. (1971) Occupational koilonychia of the toe nails. *Br. J. Dermatol.* **85**, 140–144.

Bergfeld W.F. & McMahon J.T. (1987) Cutaneous metalloid hyperpigmentation. In: *Advances in Dermatology*, eds Callen J.P., Dahl M.V., Golitz L.E. & Stegman S.J., Vol. 1, pp. 123–124. Year Book, Chicago.

Bord A. & Castelain P.Y. (1966) Les dermatoses professionnelles dans l'industrie aéronautique. *Bull. Soc. Fr. Dermatol. Syphil.* **73**, 396–401.

Botella R., Sastre A. & Castells A. (1985) Contact dermatitis to paraquat. *Contact Derm.* **13**, 123–124.

Boyle J.C., Smith N.J. & Burke F.D. (1988) Vibration white finger. *Hand Surg.* **13B**, 171–175.

Brodkin R.H. & Bleiberg J. (1973) Cutaneous microwave injury. A report of two cases. *Acta Derm. Venereol. (Stock.)* **53**, 50–52.

Brun R. (1978) Contact dermatitis to orange-wood in a manucurist. *Contact Derm.* **4**, 315.

Bruynzeel D.P. (1986) Allergic contact dermatitis to hydrangea. *Contact Derm.* **14**, 128.

Budden M.G. & Wilkinson D.S. (1978) Skin and nail lesions from gold potassium cyanide. *Contact Derm.* **4**, 172–173.

Butterworth T. & Strean L.P. (1963) Mercurial pigmentation of nails. *Arch Dermatol.* **88**, 55–57.

Calas E., Castelain P.Y., Raulot Lapointe H. *et al.* (1977) Allergic contact dermatitis to a photopolymerizable resin used in printing. *Contact Derm.* **3**, 186–194.

Calnan C.D. (1958) Onychia from synthetic nail coverage. *Trans. St Johns Hosp. Dermatol. Soc.* **41**, 66–68.

Calnan C.D. (1960) Cement dermatitis. *J. Occupat. Med.* **2**, 15.

Calnan C.D. (1967) Reactions to artificial colouring materials. *J. Soc. Cos. Chem.* **18**, 215–223.

Calnan C.D. & Sarkany I. (1958) Studies in contact dermatitis; III Nail varnish. *Trans. St Johns Hosp. Dermatol. Soc.* **40**, 1–11.

Canizares O. (1956) Contact dermatitis due to the acrylic materials used in artificial nails. *Arch. Dermatol.* **74**, 141–143.

Castelain P.Y., Com J. & Castelain M. (1992) Occupational

dermatitis in the aircraft industry: 35 years of progress. *Contact Derm.* **27**, 311–316.

Castelain P.-Y. & Piriou A. (1980) Contact dermatitis due to propanidid in an anesthetist. *Contact Derm.* **6**, 360.

Clark D.G. & Hurst E.W. (1970) The toxicity of diquat. *Br. J. Indust. Med.* **27**, 51–55.

Cohen S.R. (1985) Yellow staining caused by 4,4'-methylenedianiline exposure. *Arch. Dermatol.* **121**, 1022–1027.

Condé-Salazar L., Guimaraens D. & Romero L.V. (1986) Occupational allergic contact dermatitis from anaerobic acrylic sealants. *Contact Derm.* **18**, 129–132.

Coskey R.J. (1974) Onycholysis from sodium hypochlorite. *Arch. Dermatol.* **109**, 96.

Cronin E. (1980a) *Contact Dermatitis*, p. 586. Churchill Livingstone, Edinburgh.

Cronin E. (1980b) *Contact Dermatitis*, p. 792. Churchill Livingstone, Edinburgh.

Cronin E. (1980c) *Contact Dermatitis*, p. 153. Churchill Livingstone, Edinburgh.

Cronin E. (1980d) *Contact Dermatitis*, p. 158. Churchill Livingstone, Edinburgh.

Daly B.M. & Johnson M. (1986) Pterygium inversum unguis due to nail fortifier. *Contact Derm.* **15**, 256–257.

Daniel C.R. & Scher R.K. (1991) Nail damage secondary to a hair spray. *Cutis* **47**, 165–166.

Davies M.F.P., Curtis M. & Howat J.M.T. (1990) Cutaneous hemangioendothelioma: possible link with chronic exposure to vinyl chloride. *Br. J. Indust. Med.* **47**, 65–67.

Dawber R. (1974) Occupational koilonychia. *Br. J. Dermatol.* **91** (Suppl. 10), 11.

Desoille H., Brouet G., Assouly M. *et al.* (1962) Fibrose pulmonaire diffuse chez un sujet exposé aux poussières de cobalt et de carbure de tungstène. *Arch. Mal. Prof.* **23**, 570–578.

de Wit F.S., de Groot A.C., Weyland J.W. *et al.* (1988) An outbreak of contact dermatitis from toluenesulfonamide formaldehyde resin in a nail hardener. *Contact Derm.* **18**, 280–283.

Dobbelaere F. & Bouffioux J. (1974) Leuconychie en bandes due au paraquat. *Arch. Belges Dermatol.* **30**, 283–384.

Dolma T, Norboo T, Yayha M. *et al.* (1990) Seasonal koilonychia in Ladakh. *Contact Derm.* **22**, 78–80.

Dooms-Goossens A., Dubusschère K., Morren M. *et al.* (1988) Silver polish: another source of contact dermatitis reactions to thiourea. *Contact Derm.* **19**, 133–135.

Dulanto (De) F. & Camacho F. (1979) Radiodermatitis. *Acta Derm. Sif.* **70**, 67–94.

Ekenvall L. (1987) Clinical assessment of suspected damage from hand-held vibrating tools. *Scand. J. Work Environ. Health* **13**, 271–274.

English J.S.C., White I.R. & Rycroft R.J.G. (1986) Sensitization by 1-methylquinoxalinium-*p*-toluene sulfonate. *Contact Derm.* **14**, 261–262.

Esteves J., Amaro J.A. Nogueira M.R. *et al.* (1983) Paquionyquia adquirida (Pelochumbo?). *Trab. Soc. Port. Derm. Ven.* **41**, 129–134.

Fairbairn J.F., Juergeas J.L. & Spittell J.A. (1972) *Peripheral Vascular Disease*, 4th edn, p. 428. W.B. Saunders, Philadelphia.

Farli M., Gasperini M., Francalanli S. *et al.* (1990) Occupational contact dermatitis in 2 dental technicians. *Contact Derm.* **22**, 282–287.

Ferreira Marques J. (1939) Une forme particulière de leuconychia, la leuconychie en large bande longitudinale (stigmate professionnel). *Ann. Dermatol.* **10**, 688–691.

Fisher A.A. (1987) Allergic reactions to cyanoacrylate 'Crazy glue' nail preperations. *Cutis* **40**, 475–476.

Fisher A.A. (1989) Permanent loss of fingernails due to allergic reaction to an acrylic nail preparation: a sixteen-year follow-up study. *Cutis* **43**, 404–406.

Fisher A.A. (1990) Adverse nail reactions and paresthesia from photobonded acrylate sculptured nails. *Cutis* **45**, 293–294.

Fisher A.A. & Baran R. (1992) Occupational nail disorders with a reference to Koebner's phenomenon. *Am. J. Contact Derm.* **3**, 16–23.

Fisher A.A., Franks A. & Glick H. (1957) Allergic sensitization of the skin and nails to acrylic plastic nails. *J. Allergy* **28**, 84–88.

Flindt-Hansen H. & Isager H. (1987) Scleroderma after occupational exposure to trichlorethylene and trichlorethane. *Acta Derm. Venereol.* **67**, 263–264.

Fowler J.F. (1990) Patch test clinic. *Am. J. Contact Derm.* **1**, 210–211.

Forck G. & Kästner H. (1967) Charakteristische onycholysis traumatica bei Fleissbandarbeiter in Geflügelschlachterei. *Hautarzt* **18**, 85–87.

Ford R., Shkor J., Akman W.V. *et al.* (1978) Deaths from asphyxia among fisherman. *MMWR* **27**, 309–315.

Forsberg K. & Keith L.H. (1989) *Chemical Protective Clothing Performance Index Book*. Wiley, New York.

Fregert S. & Trulson L. (1980) Yellow stained skin from dinitrosalicylic acid. *Contact Derm.* **6**, 362.

Frenk E. & Leu F. (1966) Leukonychie durch beruflichen Kontakt mit gesalzenen Därmen. *Hautarzt* **17**, 233–235.

Fulghum D.D. (1972) Allergic contact onycholysis due to poison ivy oleoresin. *Contact Derm. Newsletter* **11**, 266.

Gallaghar R.G., Zavon M. & Doyle H.N. (1955) Radioactive contamination in a radium therapy clinic. *Pub. Health Rep.* **70**, 617–624.

Gellin G.A. (1972) *Occupational Diseases*, p. 78. American Medical Association, Chicago.

Gette M.T. & Marks J.E. (1990) Tulip fingers. *Arch. Dermatol.* **126**, 203–205.

Gibbs R.C. (1973) Tennis toe. *Arch. Dermatol.* **107**, 918.

Gill M.J., Arlette J., Buchan K.A. *et al.* (1990). Human orf. *Arch. Dermatol.* **126**, 356–358.

Goette D.K., Jacobson K.W. & Doty R.D. (1978) Primary inoculation tuberculosis of the skin. Prosecutor's paronychia. *Arch. Dermatol.* **114**, 567.

Goh C.L. (1985) Occupational dermatitis from soldering flux among workers in the electronic industry. *Contact Derm.* **13**, 85–90.

Goh C.L. (1990) Allergic contact dermatitis and onycholysis from hydroxylamine sulphate in colour developer. *Contact Derm.* **22**, 109.

Goodwin P. (1976) Onycholysis due to acrylic nail applications. *Clin. Exp. Dermatol.* **1**, 191.

Göthe C.J., Nilzen A., Holmgren A. *et al.* (1972) Medical problems in the detergent industry caused by proteolytic enzymes from bacillus subtiles. *Acta Allerg.* **27**, 63.

Götz H. & Hantschke D. (1965) Einblicke in die Epidemiologie der Dermatomykosen im Kohlenbergbau. *Hautarzt* **16**, 543.

Greenberg J.H. (1975) Green fingenails: a possible pathway of nosocomial pseudomonas infection. *Milit. Med.* **145**, 356.

Groves R.W., Wilson-Jones E. & MacDonald D.M. (1991) Human orf and milkers' nodules: a clinicopathologic study. *J. Am. Acad. Dermatol.* **25**, 706–711.

Gugnani H.C. & Oyeka C.A. (1989) Foot infections due to *Hendersonula toruloidea* and *Scytalidium hyalinum* in coal miners. *J. Med. Vet. Mycol.* **27**, 169–179.

Haedicke G.J., Crossman J.A.I. & Fisher A.E. (1989) Herpetic whitlow of the digits. *J. Hand Surg.* **14B**, 443–446.

Harris A.O. & Rosen T. (1989) Nail discoloration due to mahogany. *Cutis* **43**, 55–56.

Hausen B.M. (1982) Airborne contact dermatitis caused by tulip bulbs. *J. Am. Acad. Dermatol.* 7, 500–503.

Head S. (1984) Victualler's thumb nail – a condition of subungual osmotrauma. *J. R. Coll. Gen. Pract.* **34**, 118.

Hearn C.E.D. & Keir W. (1971) Nail damage in spray operators exposed to paraquat. *Br. J. Indust. Med.* **28**, 399.

Heidenheim M. & Jemec G.B.E. (1991) Side effects of cryotherapy. *J. Am. Acad. Dermatol.* **24**, 653.

Hjorth N. & Wilkinson D.S. (1968) Contact dermititis IV: Tulip fingers, hyacinth itch and lily rash. *Br. J. Dermatol.* **80**, 696.

Hodgson G. & Mayon-White R.T. (1971) Acute onychia and onycholysis due to an enzyme detergent. *Br. Med. J.* **3**, 352.

Hogan D.J. (1988) Subungual trichogranuloma in a hairdresser. *Cutis* **42**, 105–106.

Honda M., Hattori S., Koyama L. *et al.* (1976) Leukonychia striae. *Arch. Dermatol.* **112**, 1147.

Hooker R.P., Eberts T.J. & Strickland J.A. (1979) Primary inoculation tuberculosis. *J. Hand Surg.* **4**, 270.

Horn M.S. (1981) Mycobacterium marinum infection. *J. Assoc. Milit Dermatol.* 7(**2**), 25.

Hoyt E.M. (1981) Primary inoculation tuberculosis. Report of a case. *J. Am. Med. Assoc.* **245**, 1556.

Jablonska S., Obalek S., Favre M. *et al.* (1987) The morphology of butcher's warts as related to papilloma-virus types. *Arch. Dermatol. Res.* **279**, 566–572.

Jetton R.L. & Coker W.L. (1969) Tuberculosis verrucosa cutis (prosecutor's wart) *Arch. Dermatol.* **100**, 380.

Julie R., Barbier F., Lambert J. *et al.* (1988) Brûlures par acide fluorhydrique. A propos d'une série de 32 cas. *Sem. Hop. Paris* **64**, 31–39.

Kanaar P. (1967) Primary herpes simplex infection of fingers in nurses. *Dermatologica* **134**, 346.

Kanerva L., Jolanki R. & Estlander T. (1993a) Dentist's occupational allergic contact dermatitis caused by coconut diethanolamide, *N*-ethyl-4-toluene sulfonamide and 4-tolylethanolanine. *Acta Derm. Venereol.* 73, 126–129.

Kanerva L., Estlander T., Jolanki R. *et al.* (1993b) Occupational contact dermatitis caused by exposure to acrylates during work with dental protheses. *Contact Derm.* **28**, 268–275.

Kern D.G. (1990) Occupational disease. In: *Nails: Therapy, Diagnosis, Surgery*, eds Scher R. & Daniel C., pp. 224–243. W.B. Saunders, Philadelphia.

Klaschka F., Grimm W. & Biersdorff H.U. (1964) Tulpen-Kontaktekzem als. *Berufsdermatosem* **15**, 317.

Kulcsár S. (1966) Deformity of the finger nails caused by vibrations. A case report. *Berufsdermatosen* **14**, 244.

Lane C.W. & Kost L.B. (1956) Sensitivity to artificial nails. *Arch. Dermatol.* **74**, 671–672.

Larson D.M., Eckman M.R., Albert R.L. *et al.* (1983). Primary cutaneous (inoculation) blastomycosis: An occupational hazard to pathologists. *Am. J. Clin. Pathol.* **79**, 253–255.

Lépine M.J. & Fachot M.L. (1971) Dermite allergique des mains des coiffeurs par un nouveau produit capillaire: l'Inéral. *Bull. Soc. Fr. Dermatol. Syphil.* **78**, 250.

Lewis J.E. (1982) Suppurative inflammatory eruption occurring in septicemic tularemia. *Cutis* **30**, 92.

Long P.I. (1958) Subungual hermorrhage in pan washer. *J. Am. Med. Assoc.* **168**, 1226.

Louis D.S. & Silva J. Jr. (1979) Herpetic whitlow: herpetic infections of the digits. *J. Hand Surg.* **4**, 90.

Loveman A.B. & Fliegelman M.T. (1955) Discoloration of the nails. Concomitant use of nail lacquer with resorcinol or resorcinol monoacetate (Eurosol) as cause. *Arch. Dermatol.* **72**, 153.

MacAulay J.C. (1990) Fly tiers finger. *Can. J. Dermatol.* **2**, 67.

MacKinnon M.A. (1986) Treatment of hydrofluoric acid burns. *J. Occup Med.* **22**, 804.

March C.H. (1966) Allergic contact dermatitis to a new formula to strengthen nails. *Arch. Dermatol.* **93**, 720.

Marks J.G. (1988) Allergic contact dermatitis to alstroemeria. *Arch. Dermatol.* **124**, 914–916.

Marks J.G., Bishop M.E. & Willis W.F. (1979) Allergic contact dermatitis to sculptured nails. *Arch. Dermatol.* **115**, 100.

Marriot W. (1982) Some viral disease: Orf and milker's nodule: tropical dermatology syllabus. XVI Congressus Internationalis Dermatologiae, Tokyo.

Mathias C.G. & Maibach H.I. (1984) Allergic contact dermatitis from anaerobic acrylic sealants. *Arch. Dermatol.* **120**, 1202–1205.

Mellströme G. (1985) Protective effect of gloves – compiled in a date base. *Contact Derm.* **13**, 162–165.

Menné T., Roed-Petersen J. & Hjorth N. (1985) Pressure onycholysis in slaughterhouse workers. *Acta Derm. Venereol.* **65** (suppl. 120), 88–89.

Messite J., Troisi F.M. & Kleinfeld M. (1957) Radiological hazards due to X-radiation in veterinarians. *Arch. Indust. Health* **16**, 48–51.

Meyer-Hamme S. & Quadripur S.A. (1983) Berufsbedingte Koilonychie. *Hautarzt* **34**, 577–579.

Mitchell J.C. (1981) Non-inflammatory onycholysis from formaldehyde-containing nail hardener. *Contact Derm.* 7, 173.

Montel M.L. & Gouyer E. (1957) L'Escavenite. *Bull. Soc. Fr. Dermatol. Syphil.* **64**, 672.

Moragon M., Ibañez M.D., San Juan L. *et al.* (1987) L'incidence des verrues vulgaires chez les travailleurs d'abattoirs industriels de volaille de la province de Valence. *Arch. Mal. Prof.* **48**, 41–43.

Narahari S.R., Skinivas C.R. & Kelkar S.K. (1990) L.E.-like erythema and periungual telangiectasia among coffee plantations workers. *Contact Derm.* **22**, 296–297.

Nethercott J.R. & Lawrence M.J. (1984) Allergic contact dermatitis due to nonylphenol ethoxylate. *Contact Derm.* **10**, 235–239.

O'Donnell T.F., Jurgenson P.F. & Weyerich N.F. (1971) An occupational hazard, tuberculous paronychia. *Arch. Surg.* **103**, 757.

Okamoto H. & Kawai S. (1991) Allergic contact sensitivity to mydriatic agents on a nurse's fingers. *Cutis* **47**, 357–358.

Pedersen N.B. (1980) Edema of fingers from hydrogen fluoride containing aluminium blancher. *Contact Derm.* **6**, 41.

Pedersen N.B. (1982) Persistent occupational koilonychia. *Contact Derm.* **8**, 134.

Pellerat M. & Chabeau G. (1976) Hydroxylamine et dermatoses professionnelles. *Soc. Fr. Dermatol. Syphil.* **83**, 238–239.

Petry H. (1966) Uhrglasnägel und Trommelschlegelfinger bei Asbestose. *Int. Arch. Geweberpath. Geweberghyg.* **22**, 55–59.

Pettit J.H.S. (1982) Skin tuberculosis and mycobacterial ulcers. Tropical dermatology Syllabus. XVI Congressus Internationalis Dermatologicae, Tokyo.

Pinkus J., Djaldetti M., Joshua H. *et al.* (1963) Sulfhemoglobinemia and acute hemolytic anemia with Heinz bodies following contact with a fungicide – zinc ethylene bisdithiocarbamate in a subject with glucose-6-phosphate dehydrogenase deficiency and hypocatalasemia. *Blood* **21**, 484–494.

Rames S., Folkmar T. & Roed-Petersen B. (1984) Herpes simplex as a possible occupational disease in dentists of the county of Aarhus, Denmark. *Acta Derm. Venereol.* **64**, 163–165.

Rein C.R. & Rogin J.R. (1950) Allergic eczematous reactions of the nail bed due to 'under coats'. *Arch. Dermatol.* **61**, 971.

Reisch M. (1959) Nail changes due to new base coat. *Arch. Dermatol.* **80**, 230.

Rogaïlin V.I., Selisski G.D. & Zakharov G.A. (1975) Clinical characteristics of skin disease in production of glass fibre. *Sovietsk Med.* **9**, 154.

Romaguera C. & Grimalt F. (1983) Dermatitis de contacto profesional por codeina. *Bol. Inform. G.E.I.D.C.* **5**, 21–23.

Ronchese F. (1953) Occupational nail marks, true and false. *Ind. J. Med. Surg.* **22**, 45–48.

Ronchese F. (1955) Peculiar silk weavers' nails. A new type of artefacts. *Arch. Dermatol.* **71**, 525–526.

Ronchese F. (1962a) Nail defect and occupational trauma. *Arch. Derm.* **85**, 404.

Ronchese F. (1962b) *Nails: Injuries and Disease in Traumatic Medicine and Surgery for the Attorney*, Vol. 6, pp. 626–639. Butterworth, Washington.

Ronchese F. (1969) Occupational nails. *Cutis* **5**, 164–165.

Rosato F.E., Rosato E.F. & Plotkin S.A. (1970) Herpetic paronychia, an occupational hazard of medical personnel. *New Engl. J. Med.* **282**, 804–805.

Rüdlinger R., Bunney M.H., Grab R. *et al.* (1984) Warts in fish handlers. *Br. J. Dermatol.* **120**, 375–381.

Rustin M.H.A., Bull H.A., Ziegler V. *et al.* (1989) Silica exposure and silica-associated systemic sclerosis. *Br. J. Dermatol.* **121** (Suppl. 34), 29–30.

Rycroft R.J.G. (1977) Contact dermatitis from acrylic compounds. *Br. J. Dermatol.* **96**, 685–687.

Rycroft R.J.G. & Calnan C.D. (1981) Alstroemeria dermatitis. *Contact Derm.* **7**, 284.

Rycroft R.J.G., Wilkinson J.D., Holmes R. *et al.* (1980) Contact sensitization to *p*-tertiary butylphenol (PTBP) resin in plastic nail adhesive. *Contact Derm.* **5**, 441–445.

Samman P.D. (1961) Onychia due to synthetic nail coverings. Experimental studies. *Trans. St Johns Hosp. Dermatol. Soc.* **46**, 68–73.

Samman P.D. & Johnston E.N.M. (1969) Nail damage associated with handling of paraquat and diquat. *Br. Med. J.* **1**, 818–819.

Sarsfield P., White J.E. & Theaker J.M. (1992) Silverworker's finger: an unusual occupational hazard mimicking a melanocytic lesion. *Histopathology* **20**, 73–75.

Schauder S. (1990) Adverse reactions to sunscreening agents in 58 patients. *Z. Hautkr.* **66**, 294–318.

Schubert B. Minard J.J., Baran R. *et al.* (1977) Onychopathie des champignonnistes. *Ann. Dermatol. Venereol. (Paris)* **104**, 627–630.

Schwartz L., Tulipan L. & Birmingham D.J. (1957a) *Occupational Disease of the Skin*, 3rd edn, pp. 242, 760. Henry Kimpton, London.

Schwartz L., Tulipan L. & Birmingham D.J. (1957b) *Occupational Diseases of the Skin*, 3rd edn, pp. 759–760. Henry Kimpton, London.

Sebastian G. (1977) Subungual Exostose der Grosszche, Berufsstigma bei Tänzern. *Derm. Monatsschr.* **163**, 998–1000.

Senay H. (1991) Acrylic nails and transmission of infection. *Can. J. Infect. Control* **6**, 52.

Shelley W.B. & Shelley E.D. (1983) Surgical treatment of farmyard pox. *Cutis* **31**, 191–192.

Shelley D.E. & Shelley W.B. (1984) Chronic dermatitis simulating small-plaque parapsoriasis due to cyanoacrylate adhesive used in fingernails. *J. Am. Med. Assoc.* **252**, 2455–2456.

Shelley D.E. & Shelley W.B. (1988) Nail dystrophy and periungual dermatitis due to cyanoacrylate glue sensitivity. *J. Am. Acad. Dermatol.* **19**, 574–575.

Shewmake S.W. & Anderson B.G. (1979) Hydrofluoric acid burns. *Arch. Dermatol.* **115**, 593–596.

Smith S.J., Yoder F.W. & Knox D.W. (1980) Occupational koilonychia. *Arch. Dermatol.* **116**, 861.

Somov B.A., Lipets M.E., Ivanov V.V. *et al.* (1976) Occupational onycholysis. *Vestn. Derm. Venereol.* **2**, 51–55.

Stubbart F.J. (1956) Onycholysis of the fingernails of beauticians due to imbedded hair. *Arch. Dermatol.* **74**, 430.

Sulzberger M.B., Rein C.R., Fanburg S.J. *et al.* (1948) Allergic eczematous reactions of the nail bed. Persistent subungual an ungual changes based on contact with 'undercoats' containing artificial resins and rubbers. *J. Indust. Dermatol.* **11**, 67–72.

Tappeiner J. & Male O. (1966) Nagelveränderungen durch Schimmelpilze. *Derm. Int.* **5**, 145.

Taylor W. (1982) Vibration white finger in the workplace. *J. Soc. Occup. Med.* **32**, 159–166.

Tobler M. & Freidburghaus A.U. (1992) A glove with exceptional protective features minimizes the risks of working with hazardous chemicals. *Contact Derm.* **26**, 299–303.

Veccherini-Blineau M.F. & Guiheneuc P. (1988) Syndrome digital des vibrations et syndrome du canal carpien: deux entités électrophysiologiques différentes? *Neurophysiol. Clin.* **18**, 541–548.

Verspyck Mijnssen G.A.W. (1969) Pathogenesis and causative agent of 'tulip finger'. *Br. J. Dermatol.* **81**, 737–745.

Wahlberg J.E. (1974) Yellow staining of hair and nails and contact sensitivity to dinobuton. *Contact Derm. Newsletter* **16**, 481.

Washburn B. (1962) Frostbite: What is it? How to prevent it. Emergency treatment. *New Engl. J. Med.* **266**, 974–989.

Wilkinson J.B. (1973) *Harry's Cosmeticology*, 6th edn, pp. 439–440. Leonard Hill Books, Aylesbury.

Young L.S., Bicknell D.S., Archer B.G. *et al.* (1969) Tularemia epidemic: Vermont 1968. Forty-seven cases linked to contact with muskrats. *New Engl. J. Med.* **280**, 1253.

Yu Hsin-Su, Yao Tsing-Hua, Tseng Ho-Ming *et al.* (1988) Vibration syndrome with special reference to the effects of temperature on vibration-induced white finger. *J. Dermatol.* **15**, 466–72.

Zahaff A., Sevestre H., Fraitag S. *et al.* (1987) Leishmaniox curanéé dans le sud-ouest tunisien. *Nouv. Dermatol.* **6**, 551–555.

Chapter 8
Cosmetics: The Care and Adornment of the Nail

E. BRAUER & R. BARAN

The art of nail care
- Manicure routine
- Special products and procedures
  - Mending kits
  - Hardeners
  - Wrappings
  - Sculptured nails
  - Artificial nails
  - Press-on nail colour

Nail care and adornment in medical practice
- Benefits
- Adverse effects (see also Chapter 7)
  - Paronychia
  - Ridging
  - Discoloration
  - Granulation
  - Onycholysis
  - Contact dermatitis
  - Risk of adverse reactions

This chapter is directed towards showing the importance of the care and adornment of the normal nail, free from disease or obvious genetic defect, though variations in physical characteristics such as colour, nail plate thickness, contour, flexibility and surface smoothness are considered. The human nail, chemically similar to horn and hoof, is not essential for the survival of *Homo sapiens*, but has many important functions that are crucial for the efficient use of the hands and feet (Chapter 1). The nail is a prime source for the transmission of organisms, both macro- and microscopic, toxins, irritants and allergens. Maintaining nail cleanliness is essential to many aspects of health and 'confidence'.

The nail is also aesthetically a site of critical importance (Figs 8.1 & 8.2). For many, cleanliness does not achieve aesthetic satisfaction. A multitude of products, implements and procedures are now on sale to fulfil the quest of those seeking nails with enhanced attractiveness (Figs 8.3 & 8.4). While the cosmetic industry encourages and caters for the trappings of nail care and adornment, the motivation is probably innate; nail beautification was an established practice in societies long past (Barnett & Scher, 1992); the long fingernail, often accentuated by gold and jewelled fingertip extenders, was indicative of high rank and station in society.

The principle is the same today, only style and intensity has changed. The appearance of the nail remains the major distinguishing feature of the hands of the labourer, male or female. Basic nail grooming is a universal practice; nail adornment is not limited to, only more obvious in, the female. Attractive fingertips, in conjunction with many other grooming characteristics, contribute towards improvement in confidence and self-image. The physician, when debating whether to treat a dystrophy or not, is advised to recognize this means of achieving a psychological 'lift' in the patient. The great benefit achieved makes the small risk of adverse reaction insignificant (Arnold *et al.*, 1973; Adams & Maibach, 1985). A thorough discussion of the principles of good hygiene and cosmetic usage follows, including descriptions of products and implements (Figs 8.4–8.7) (Brauer, 1969).

The purist might easily discuss nail care as requiring only soap, water, and perhaps a brush. The same can be said for the maintenance of any hard surface, even a kitchen floor. One easily recognizes that abrasives, solvents, waxes, stains, varnishes, paints and floor coverings (which do not exhaust the catalogue of items in daily use) not only create a clean, sanitary deck, but an attractive one as well. The nail, whose exposure to environmental insult is greater, is a vital surface that reproduces itself, imperfections included, every few months. With its delicate biological system it cannot be expected to be served by fewer agents if cleanliness, beauty and personal taste are to be satisfied. Table 8.1 lists, with a brief description, the major items in general use for nail care.

The art of nail care

The method by which each of the items in Table 8.1 is used and the sequence for performing the professional manicure in a beauty salon follows. An individual at home will usually shorten or omit completely selected steps because of the limits of time and dexterity. The physician, familiarizing himself or herself with the procedure, will gain insight into the use and abuse which occasionally may lead to ungual and periungual problems.

An attractive fingernail is oval in shape, but there are three other basic nail shapes: round, rectangular and pointed. Length creates the impression of thin, tapered

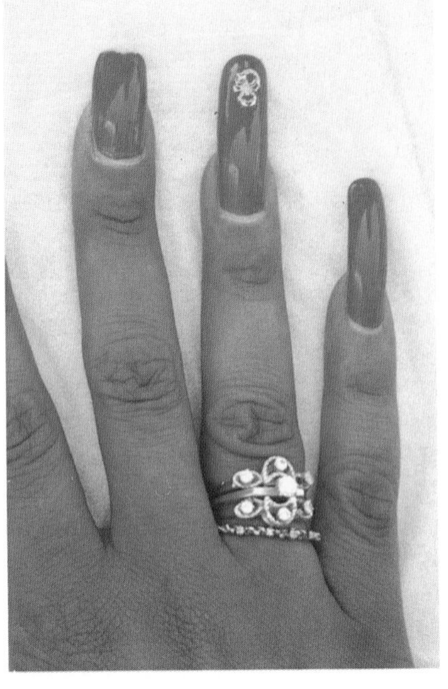

Fig. 8.1. Long artificial painted nails; cf. Fig. 8.2.

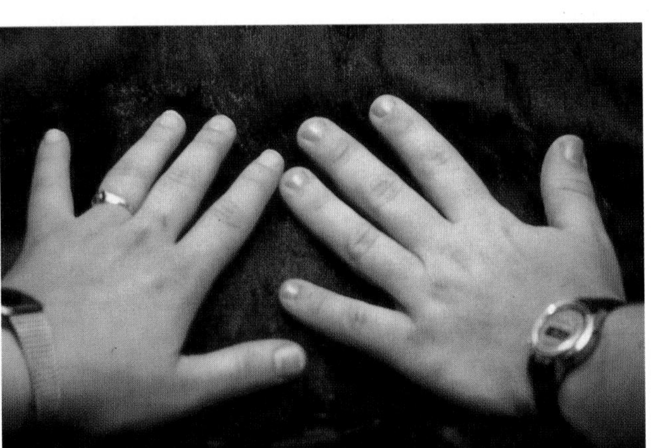

Fig. 8.2. Short 'stubby' nails; cf. Fig. 8.1 – less attractive.

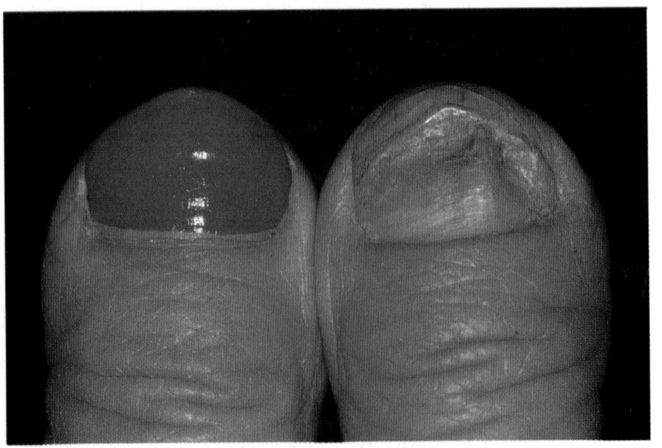

Fig. 8.3. Varnish adds little in cosmetic improvement to a broad, short fingernail.

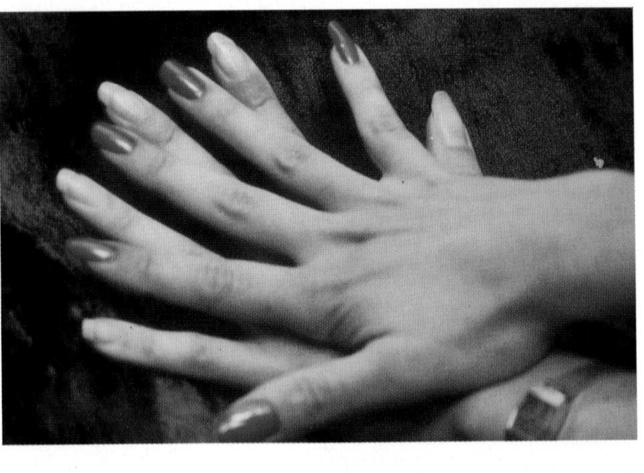

Fig. 8.4. Showing the aesthetic difference between long red nails and uncoloured ones, same individual.

and graceful fingers. Exessive length interferes with the efficiency of the hand's performance (Fig. 8.8).

Manicure routine (Fig. 8.9)

1 Old nail enamel or buffer waxes and oils are thoroughly removed with a cotton ball saturated with nail enamel remover.

2 The nails are shaped with a file or emery board in preference to clipping. The latter tends to cause a shearing action on the nail plate, promoting fissures and fracturing.

3 The tissues of the fingertip are then softened by soaking them in a bath of warm, soapy water for several minutes; the cuticular edge is next gently and bluntly retracted from the nail plate. The best and safest way to achieve this is by covering the nail with a soft fabric. The operator then grasps the subject's fingertip between her thumb (placed on the dorsal surface) and index finger. The operator then pushes the thumb in a proximal direction exerting gentle pressure on the cuticular rim that surrounds the nail. The stretch created on the fibrous band gradually causes it to thin while more of the proximal nail is exposed, creating an oval shape. This desired appearance will only be achieved after a number of treatments of this type over several weeks. The novice may try to accomplish this rapidly by pressure with a 'cuticle-pusher'; this may damage the softened nail matrix/bed following which a horizontally ridged defect may occur.

4 As necessary, cuticle remover is then applied to the exposed new nail growth. After several minutes it is rinsed off thoroughly with water. Any remnants of cuticle adhering to the plate can be gently rubbed away with an orange stick or similar implement to create a smooth, even surface.

5 Any ragged edges are then trimmed from the cuticle. No attempt is made to eliminate this rather fibrous band

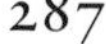

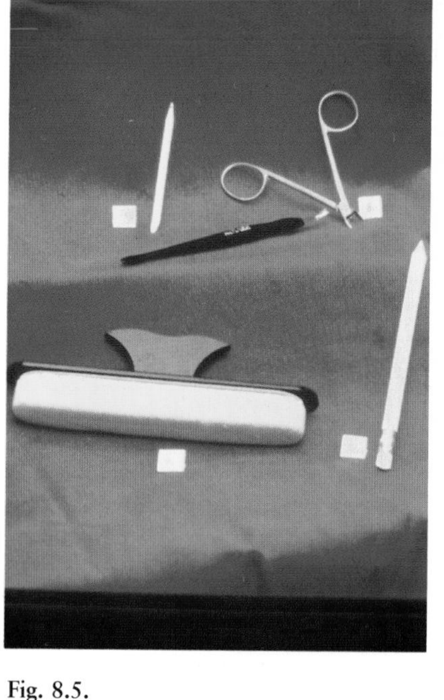

Fig. 8.5.

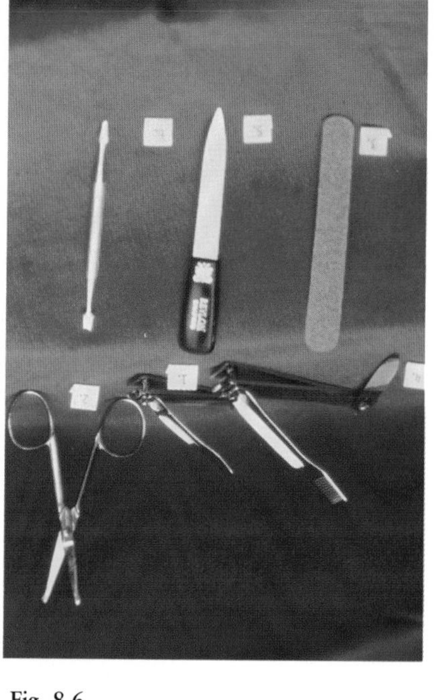

Fig. 8.6.

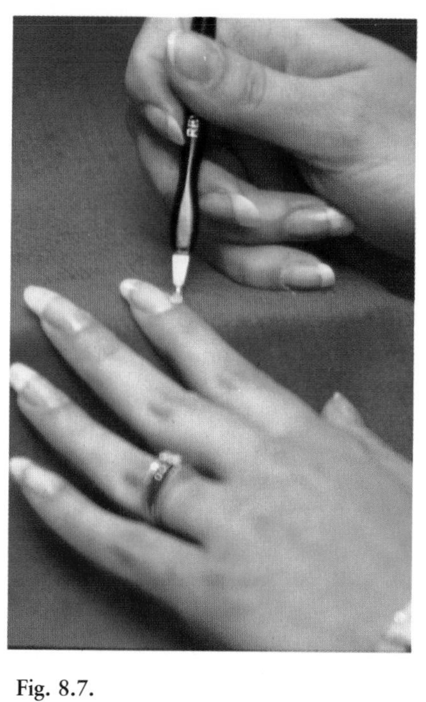

Fig. 8.7.

Figs 8.5–8.7. 'Tools of the trade' for nail apparatus manicure (see Table 8.1).

Table 8.1. Items for nail care (Figs 8.5–8.7)

Item	Description	Item	Description
Orange stick	A reed-like wooden or flexible pencil-shaped plastic implement that is used as the cuticle pusher above. It is less likely to cause injury to the nail fold. It was originally fabricated from orange wood	Clippers	Slightly curved, jaw-like blades operated by a spring mechanism for severing the free edge of the nail plate. Available in many sizes
Cuticle trimmer	Tiny, clipper-jawed scissors for cutting frayed cuticle. Recently, a curette-like V-shaped blade, mouted in a plastic handle has been introduced to efficiently shave down this tissue	Scissors	Slightly curved blades for cutting soft, thin, flexible nail plates. Note: blunted ends of blades to minimize injury to soft tissue
Nail buffer	Chamois or similar fabric, usually padded and mounted on a convenient holding device for polishing the nail plate. It is used in conjunction with mild pumice-type abrasive creams or waxes to produce a high lustre to the nail surface	Emery board	A flat, disposable, 'paper-board' wand, coated with powdered emery to shape as well as file down length, or smoothen sharp, rough portions of the free edge of the nail
Nail whitener	This is a pencil-like device with a white clay (kaolin) core that is used to deposit colour on the under surface of the free edge of the nail	Nail file	A rough, scored, flat steel wand used as the emery board but with less delicacy and poor efficiency
Wet sanitizer	Receptacle large enough to hold the disinfectant solution in which items to be sanitized are immersed	Metal particle file	Fine metallic particles are electroplated on a metal wand; performs indefinitely with the delicacy, speed and efficiency of the emery board
Toileteries and cosmetics		Acrylic nippers	They are designed specifically to chip back the acrylic at the base of the nail in preparation for a fill
Nail enamel solvents	Solvents of acetone and/or ethyl acetate or similar compounds that quickly soften and solubilize nail enamel, oils and waxes for quick and easy cleansing	Cobalt steel fibreglass shear	
		Cuticle pusher	A polished, metallic probe with various shaped ends for separating the cuticle edge from the nail plate and loosening cuticle remnants. The probe has rounded edges to minimize injury to soft tissue

continued on p. 288

Table 8.1. *Continued*

Item	Description
	cuticular ridge. Their purpose is to 'digest' the remnants of cuticle that adhere to the nail plate as it grows outward. The lotion is left in place for approximately 10 min and then washed off. These products are not meant to remove the fibrous cuticular ridge
Base coats, top coats, and nail enamel	These three products have similar basic formulas. They consist of a film former, such as nitrocellulose, a thermoplastic resin for gloss and adhesion (e.g. toluensulfonamide/formaldehyde*) and a plasticizer (e.g. dibutyl phthalate) for flexibility; these are incorporated in an acetate and ketone solvent. (A nail enamel differs only in containing pigments and suspending agents to achieve colour.) The quantities of the basic ingredients vary with desired product performance. For example, with a base coat good adhesion or bonding to the nail plate and the superimposed nail enamel is accentuated at the price of gloss; with a top coat, which is applied over the nail enamel, the gloss factor is dominant
Film drying accelerant	Mineral oil is sprayed or brushed over freshly applied enamel to give fast protection from minor environmental insults while the enamel sets
Sanitation	It can include physical agents (ultraviolet rays, moist and dry heat) or chemicals (alcohol, quaternary compounds, etc.). We prefer the use of the dry heat temperature for 10 s in the electric glass bead sterilizer that reaches 475°F

* New analytic technology reveals that this resin may contain a trace of formaldehyde (Nater *et al.*, 1985).
Pedicures demands a special set of implements due to the size and thickness of toenails. A typical toenail cutter works with a squeeze grip action.

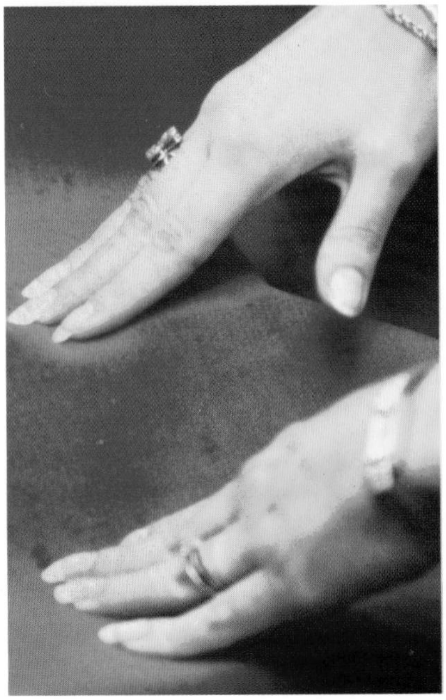

Fig. 8.8. 'Lever' effect of long nails, may lead to onycholysis. Excessively long nails may interfere with the subtle functions of the hands.

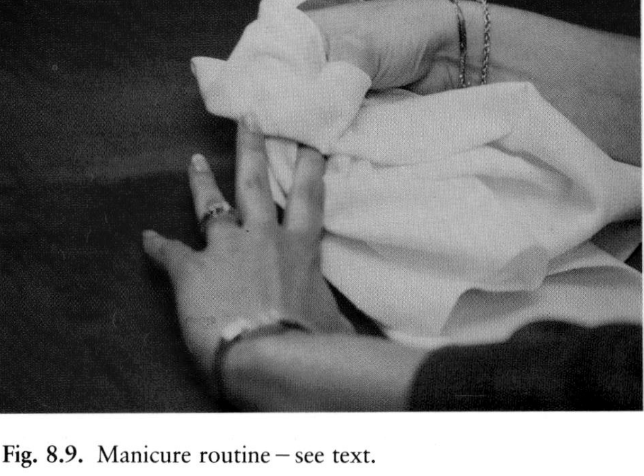

Fig. 8.9. Manicure routine – see text.

which creates a thin, attractive, framed edge to the proximal nail.

6 The nail plate should be cleansed again with nail enamel remover. It may now be polished with the application of wax and suitably buffed or coated with nail enamel.

7 Nail enamel provides gloss and colour in a broad spectrum of shades. Two or three coats are necessary for an even, attractive finish with five polish options: full coverage, free edge, hair line tip, slim line or free wall, halfmoon unpolished. A nail base coat applied before nail enamel will increase bonding of the enamel to the plate and reduce the tendency for some shades of nail enamel to stain the nail plate (see 'Discoloration of nails' below). The application of a top coat product to the dried enamel will increase gloss and enhance wear characteristics.

These details mainly relate to fingernails. Toenails require similar care for cleanliness. However, toenail plates should be clipped and filed to achieve an almost square or slightly oval free edge carried just beyond the toe, in order not to interfere with the pressure of footwear, and to prevent the nail from ingrowing. Adornment is usually less vigorous, especially when self-administered, due to difficulty in accessibility. It is easier to groom toenails if a firm, pencil-thick roll of cotton wool is placed between the digits.

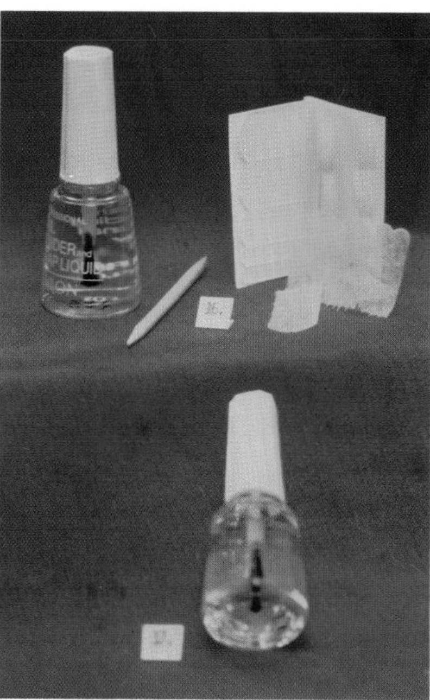

Fig. 8.10. Nail mending kit – see text.

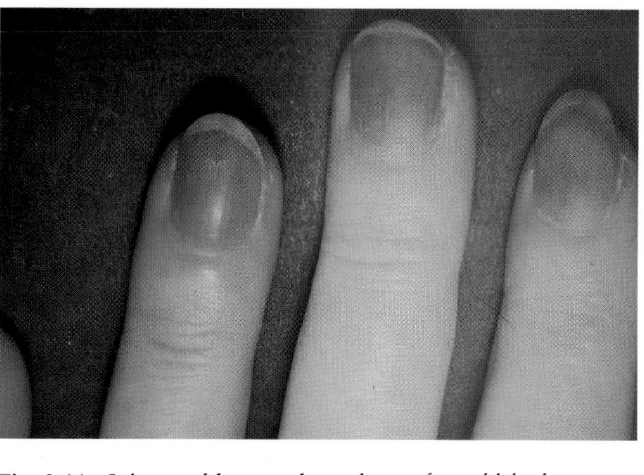

Fig. 8.11. Subungual haemorrhage due to formaldehyde.

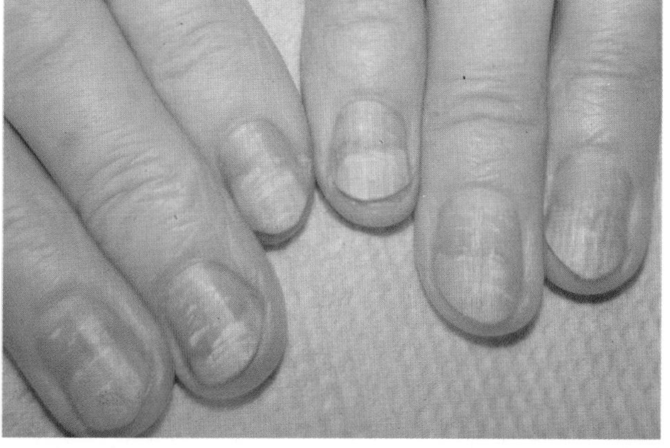

Fig. 8.12. Onycholysis.

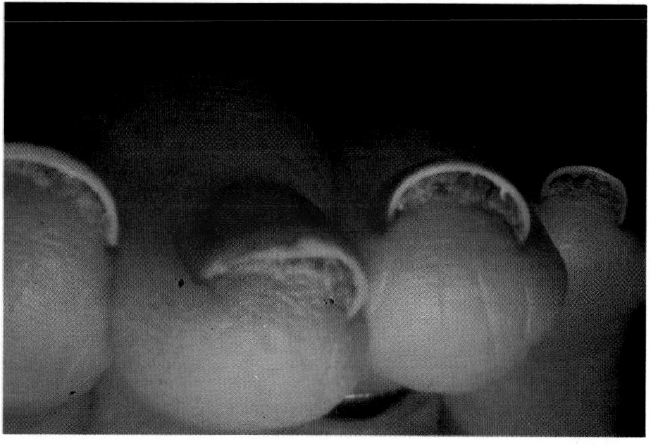

Fig. 8.13. Subungual hyperkeratosis.

Figs 8.11–8.13. Reactions to nail hardeners (courtesy of P. Lazar, Chicago).

Special products and procedures

Nail mending kits (Fig. 8.10)

Cultivating nails of pleasing, matched length demands an investment in time, care and devotion. The reward is aesthetic satisfaction and considerable pride; damage to such a 'prized' possession is of significant concern. Fracture to the free edge can be splinted by the application of mending papers that are saturated with clear, thickened basic nail enamel substance. When dry, conventional nail enamel may be applied with reasonably good cosmetic effect so that the damaged plate can be protected until normal growth permits filing to the length and shape desired. Quick, efficient nail mending kits are available that consist of transparent plastic film strips which are applied to the nail fracture with a cyanoacrylate glue. Even a totally severed nail plate tip can be mended by this method. Since application is made to a non-viable portion of the nail, the possibility of an allergic reaction is minimized. However, this substance requires much care and skill in its use. It dries rapidly and firmly: fingers, and even eyelids, have been bound together by this substance, requiring medical attention for resolution.

Nail hardeners (Figs 8.11–8.13)

Fragile, or very flexible nail plates pose difficulties to those desiring long, tapered nails. Regular application of 5–10% aqueous formalin will successfully 'harden' nails. However, local irritation, allergic dermatitis, pain, onycholysis, subungual hyperkeratosis and even subungual haemorrhage have been reported (Lazar, 1966). For approximately 20 years the United States Food and Drug Administration (FDA) has restricted the marketing of such commercial products. Formaldehyde is also prohibited in Japan. In the European community, products containing formaldehyde must state this clearly on the label. They may be dispensed on prescription. Because of the ability of nail enamel films to protect, splint and modestly fortify the nail plate itself, products with minor modifications in quality and quantity of the resin are now offered as 'hardeners'. These contain no formaldehyde other than a trace which may result from the chemical reaction used to create the basic resin. The FDA permits a formaldehyde concentration of 0.2% or less which is far too low to have any hardening benefit. Formaldehyde is merely the chemical moiety upon which the resin is formed.

Nail wrapping

This procedure is performed in salons; each operator has her own technique and product mix. Essentially, the free edge of each nail is splinted with layers of a fibrous substance, such as cotton wool, paper, silk, linen, plastic film or fibre glass and affixed with cyanoacrylate glue. After drying, the edge is fashioned to suit, and the nail is coated with enamel. Fibre glass has become very popular. Most fibre glass systems consist of three basic elements: resin or adhesive, fibre glass mesh, and an activator or catalyst which speeds up the resin (cyanoacrylate) polymerization.

Depending on skill and quality of workmanship, the procedure may require as long as 2 h to perform. The reinforced, durable, free edge resists wear and tear and allows the nail to grow quite long. Fresh nail enamel is applied after several days and the entire procedure repeated every 2 weeks. The previous wrappings are easily removed with nail enamel remover. This is a costly, time-consuming procedure, but which gives much satisfaction. Care must be taken to keep the edge of the nail coated with nail enamel to prevent snagging as it wears.

Sculptured nails (Figs 8.14–8.17)

This procedure is only performed in salons. A plastic 'nail' is actually constructed upon the natural nail or nail sub-

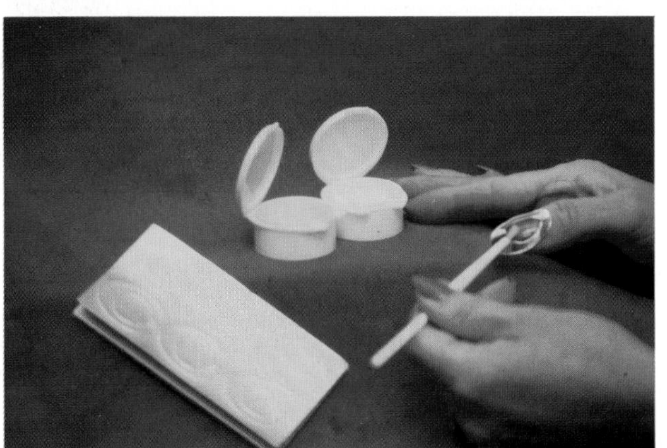

Fig. 8.14.

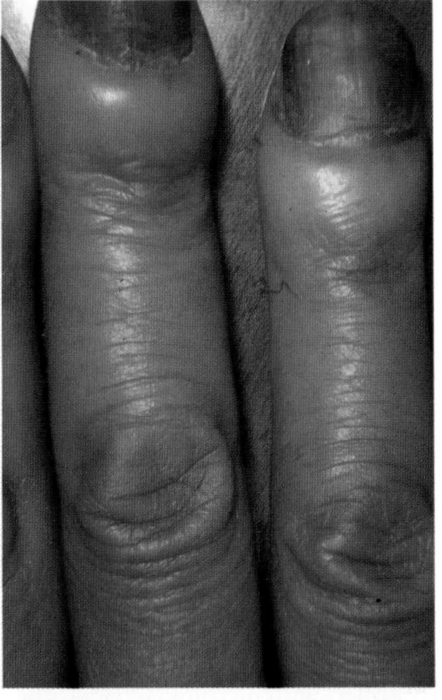
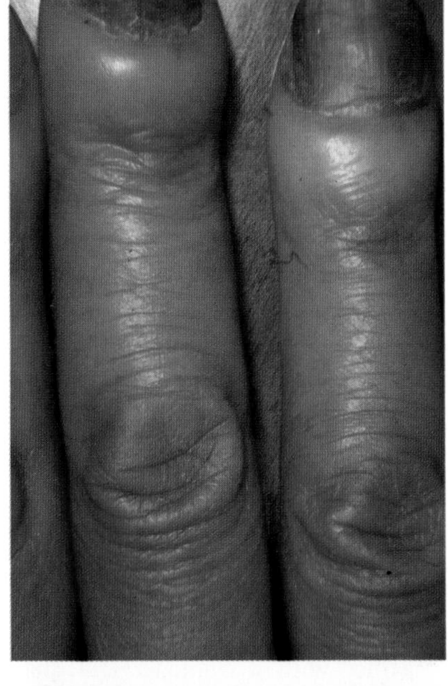

Fig. 8.15. Paronychia (courtesy of A. Fisher, New York, USA).

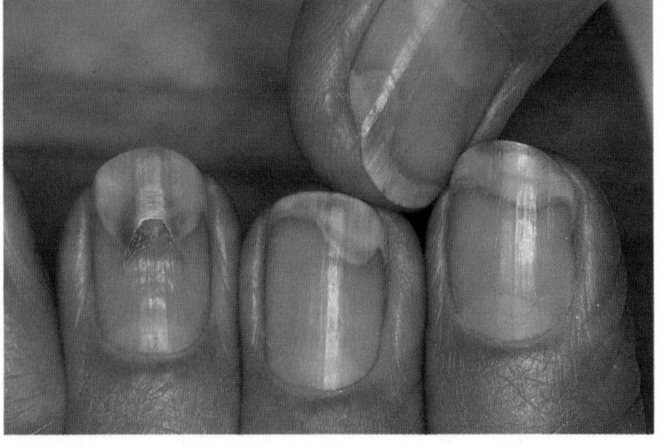

Fig. 8.16.

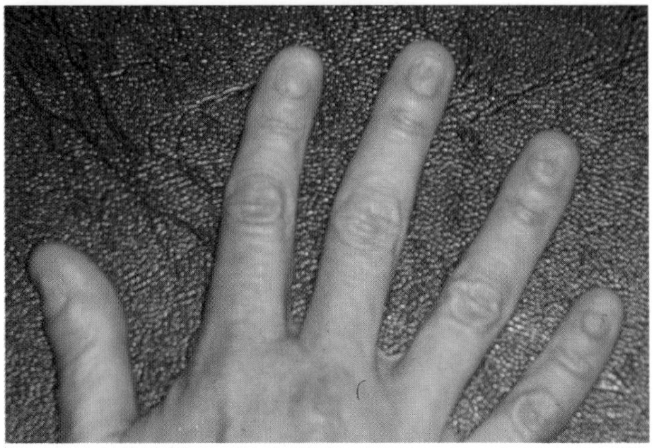

Fig. 8.17. Permanent anonychia.

Figs 8.14–8.17. Nail sculptering, side-effects and complications (see text).

stance of each fingertip. A metallized paperboard template is placed upon the natural nail surface to frame the 'nail' to be. A fresh acrylic mixture of ethyl methacrylate (or related moieties) monomer and polyethyl polymer is moulded within the template so that a plastic 'nail' of desired thickness and length is created (Fig. 8.1). When hardened, the template is removed. The prosthesis is then filed to shape and the surface polished. Nail enamel is then applied. It is cosmetically elegant and exceedingly durable. Depending on the skill and quality of the workmanship, several hours are required to complete a very costly procedure which must be redone every few weeks to fill in the surface defect apparent at the lunula as the new growth becomes obvious. The bonding created is essentially permanent, defying usual chemical solvents. One specific solvent, acetonitrile, will liberate inorganic cyanide when metabolized. Paediatric cyanide deaths following ingestion have been reported. Removal, if necessary, can be a painful surgical event. Allergic contact-type inflammation of ungual and periungual areas, infection, foreign body reactions, haemorrhage, and severe pain have been reported; secondary nail dystrophy is not unusual. Fisher (1980, 1989) described a single case of persistent paraesthesia and anonychia from the procedure. Baran and Schibli (1990) reported a case of permanent paraesthesia without anonychia or sensitization to the acrylic monomer. Many individuals, however, happily tolerate the method regularly over many years.

There are different types of acrylic, giving the technician more choice in treating clients (hard acrylic, acrylic with high UV absorbency and a clearer acrylic). The new odourless products contain hydroxy ethyl methacrylate. They require proper ventilation, as do traditional products.

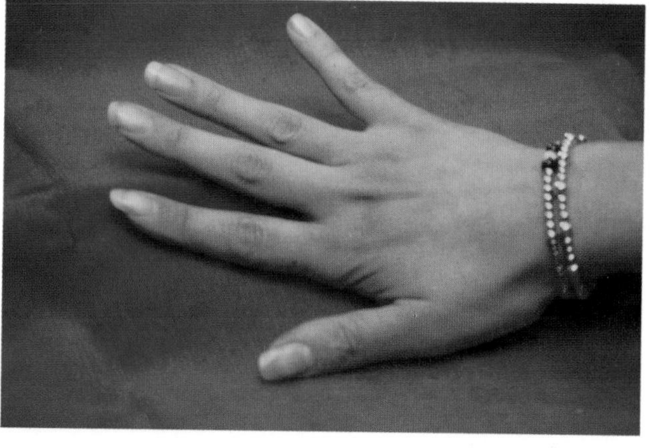

Fig. 8.18.

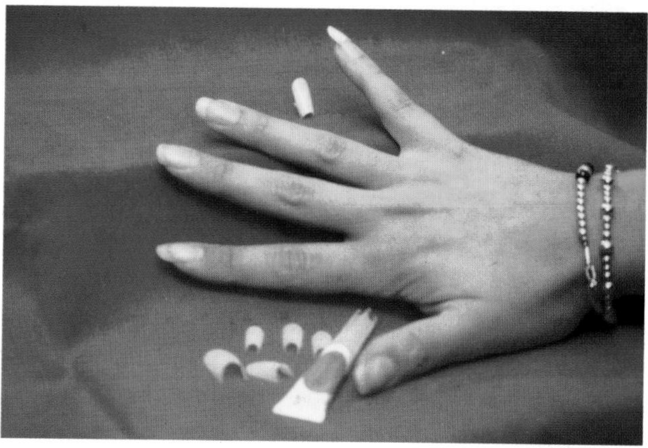

Fig. 8.19.

Figs 8.18 & 8.19. Preformed artificial nails.

Premixed acrylic gels

These products contain UV initiator to activate the polymerization process. The UV gel system typically contains a blend of monomers, i.e. polyurethane oligomers, acrylates, methacrylates, epoxyacrylate and diacrylates.

Coloured gels may be recommanded to clients who do not change polish colour often.

To improve adhesion between the natural nail and the artificial nail, a substance called 'primer' may be needed. There are two types of primer: acid primer (acrylic acids) and non-acid primer or non-etching primer (without methacrylic acid).

Primer should be used when recommended by the manufacturer. Any formula which uses only ethyl, methyl (outlawed in the US) or isobutyl methacrylate has a low affinity for the natural nail. In contrast, cyanoacrylates form extremely strong bonds and require no primers.

Preformed artificial nails (Figs 8.18 & 8.19)

Preformed, plastic prosthetic full nails, or just nail tips, are cut to fit a finger or the free edge of the nail and cemented in place with various type glues. The cosmetic effect is good (Figs 8.18 & 8.19) but short-lived unless the new ethyl cyanoacrylate adhesive is used – with its accompanying hazard as mentioned previously (Fisher, 1987; Shelley & Shelley, 1988). Significant improvement has been made in adhesives for cosmetic use. The setting time has been slowed down, while removal with ordinary nail enamel removers is now possible.

'Press-on' nail colour

Self-adherent, various sized, nail-shaped, coloured plastic films are affixed to the nail plate to duplicate a nail enamel effect (Fig. 8.20). Although the cosmetic benefit is achieved quite quickly and easily, the wear is poor and its use not popular (Calnan, 1958).

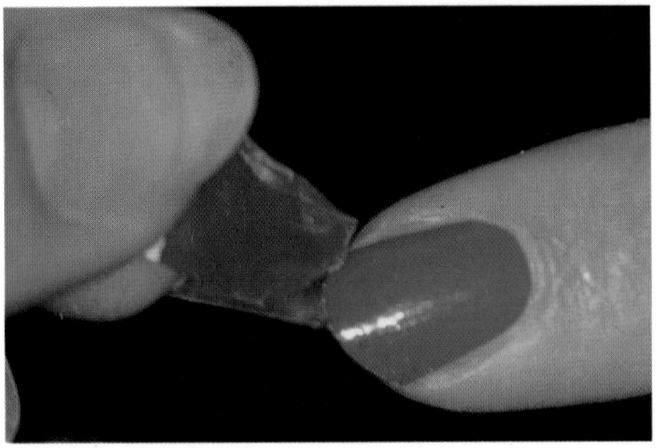

Fig. 8.20. Self-adherent plastic nails, press-on type.

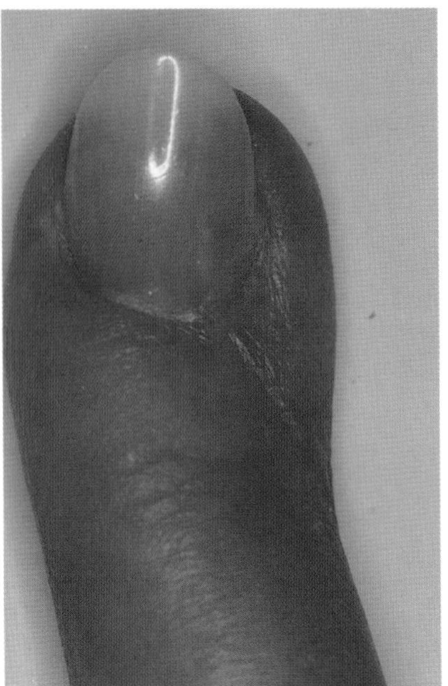

Fig. 8.22. After nail prosthesis applied (see Fig. 8.21).

Nail care and adornment in medical practice

Benefits

General

A clean, well-groomed nail is important to one's health and self-esteem. Nail adornment is a common practice among fashion-conscious individuals in order to project attractiveness and social status. It is a mistake for the physician to view a patient's complaint of unattractive nails as too trivial for medical consideration. Many of the products and procedures previously described will help overcome cosmetic defects.

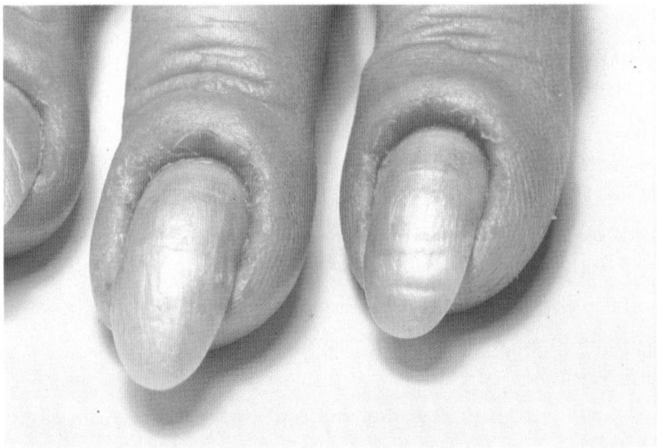

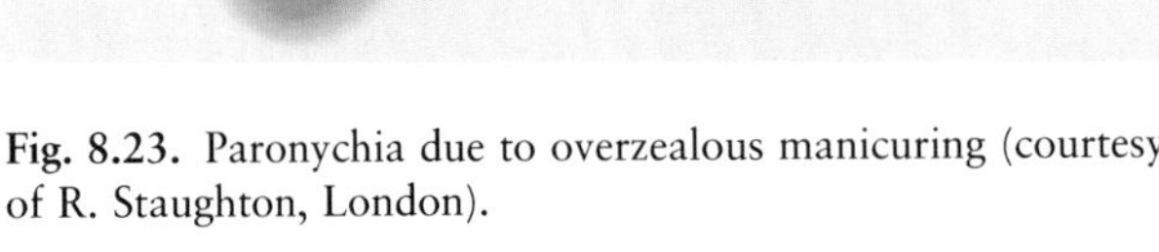

Fig. 8.23. Paronychia due to overzealous manicuring (courtesy of R. Staughton, London).

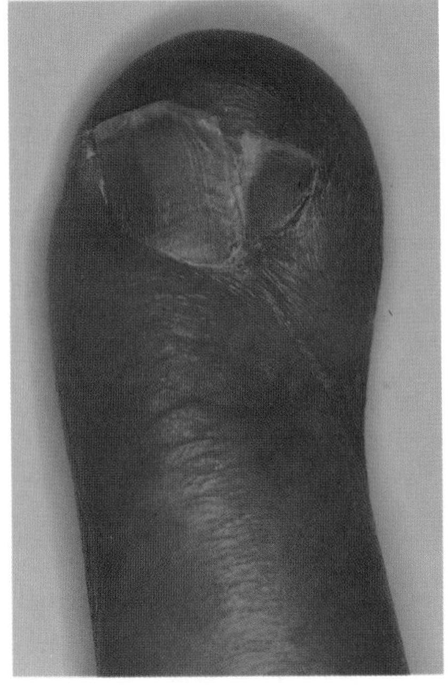

Fig. 8.21. Dystrophic nail.

Specific

A regimen of nail care, particularly with added colour, may discourage the habit of nail biting and cuticle picking and 'tearing'.

Dystrophic, atrophic, absent, or diseased nails, particulary where only few are involved, can be improved cosmetically with one of the procedures previously described (Figs 8.21 & 8.22). Due to the severity of adverse reactions with the 'permanently' adhering sculptured nail, caution should be exercised in its recommendation.

Adverse effects (see also Chapter 7)

Paronychia (Fig. 8.23)

This occasionaly appears when poor manicuring skill causes skin penetration by sharp and pointed implements.

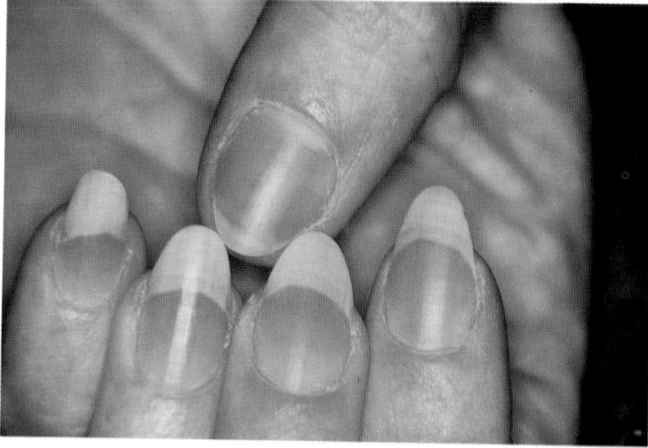

Fig. 8.24. Discoloration of the nails due to nail enamels.

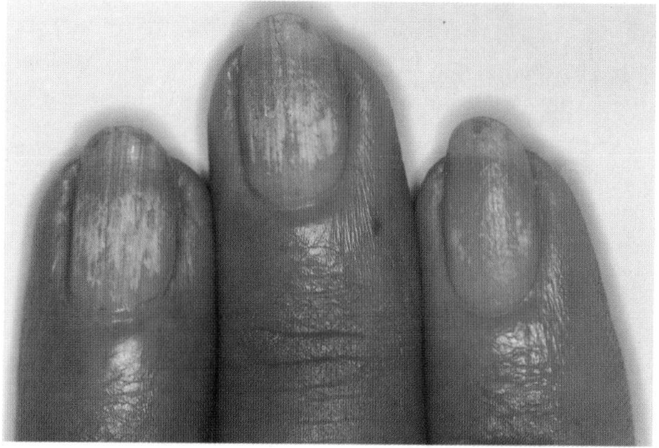

Fig. 8.25. 'Granulation' of the nail plate due to multiple layers of enamel.

Ridging

Transverse ridging of nail plates, as well as transverse leuconychia, may result from excessive manipulation with implements in the vicinity of the lunula, particularly in association with the use of cuticle removers.

Discoloration of the nail (Fig. 8.24)

Deeper shades of red and brown nail enamel may cause mild staining of nail keratin (Calnan, 1967). This phenomenon occurs in only a few users and is without satisfactory explanation. It is asymptomatic and self-limiting as new nail growth appears. It poses a cosmetic problem only if the user decides not to continue with a coloured nail enamel. The staining is significantly, or completely, avoided by the application of a base coat prior to the use of the offending nail enamel.

Benzophenone-2, a UV filter contained in a nail laquer, induced a light-dependent discoloration of the fingernails in two female patients (Schauder, 1990).

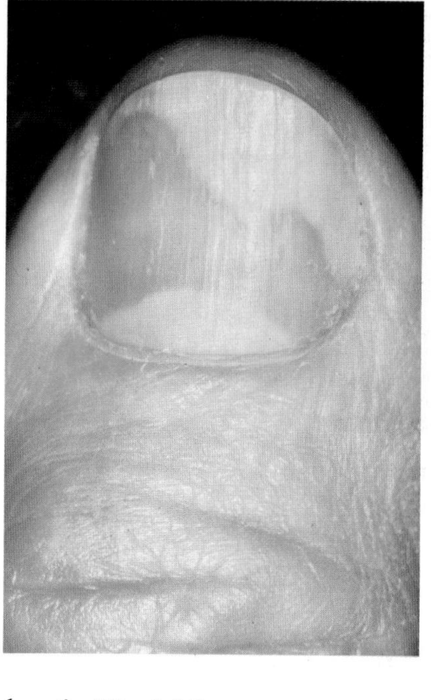

Fig. 8.26. Onycholysis due to nail cosmetic procedures – patch testing is required to find the cause, but here the nail plate–bed separation was due to overzealous cleaning with an orange stick (sculptured onycholysis).

Granulation of nail keratin (Fig. 8.25)

Granulation is occasionally observed in individuals who apply fresh coats of enamel on top of old, worn enamel, for several weeks in succession. It results in superficial friability (Baran, 1985). It may be avoided by following a 5–7-day nail care schedule as described previously.

Onycholysis (Fig. 8.26)

Impervious coatings, such as cemented, preformed artificial nails, sculptured nails, or similar films may cause spontaneous, uncomplicated separation of the natural plate from its bed due to the interference with normal vapour exchange.

Nail enamels and related products reduce, but do not eliminate the vapour exchange from nail bed to the environment. Although nail enamels have been mentioned in association with onycholysis, considering the extensive worldwide use, the cause-and-effect relationship must be most unusual.

Significant attention to nail care often yields longer nails. Onycholysis of the distal portion of the fingertip may be caused by the increased kinetic force (lever action) created by the length of nail beyond the fingertip (Fig. 8.8).

Contact dermatitis (allergic) (Figs 8.27 & 8.28) (Kechijian, 1991; Norton, 1991; Liden *et al*., 1993; Tosti *et al*., 1993)

Conventional nail care and nail enamel products are rarely associated with local (fingertips) allergic, eczematous-type, contact reactions. A patchy eruption on distant sites, such

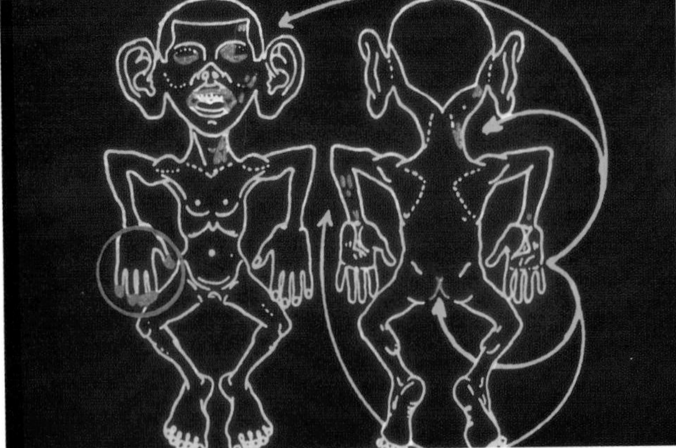

Fig. 8.27. Sites of origin and transfer of allergens (courtesy of C. Bonu, Italy).

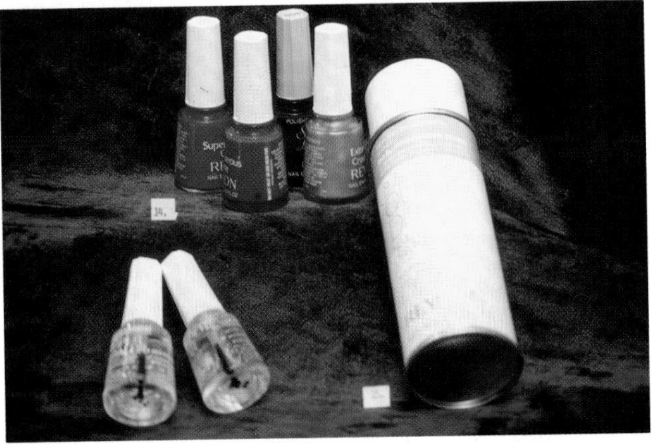

Fig. 8.28. Some of the agents causing type IV hypersensitivity.

as eyelids, neck, deltoid areas, and even the genitals, may appear due to contact with fingers. Besides ectopic dermatitis, allergic airborne contact dermatitis should be suspected when the lesions involving face, neck and ears are symmetrical. The allergen in nail enamels is usually the thermoplastic resin. Diagnostic skin patch testing with nail enamel should be performed without occlusive covering, or with dry enamel films to avoid false-positive reactions from solvent.

The recommendation to a patient to use a product labelled 'hypoallergenic' is naive, as is it used in the cosmetic industry purely for promotion. Dermatologically, it is without any merit. It serves only to mislead the practitioner and confuse the patient. There are as many patients that react to products labelled 'hypoallergenic' as to any other. All reputable manufacturers are committed to market products with as low a sensitizing potential as possible. A patient with an allergic sensitivity to substance R can benefit only if the product is free of substance R. If substance W is substituted for it, the product can hardly be hypoallergenic to another patient with an allergic sensitivity to substance W. Frequently, so-called hypoallergenic products are identical in ingredient content to products not so labelled. The physician may wish to subject a particular patient to an extensive, time-consuming battery of skin patch tests to identify the offending substance and then seek a product free of it. However, initially, the patient is pragmatically better served by being asked to change the type of the product (e.g. from cream to lotion or powder form), or the brand name or manufacturer.

In the case of nail enamel resins, there are several different types used in manufacture, so switching brands to present a different resin is a reasonable approach. In countries that require ingredient disclosure on the label, product differences may be readily identified; allergen identification by means of detailed skin patch test work-up may be worthwhile. When the practice proves successful, the new product, though tolerated, still cannot be called hypoallergenic. The patient may eventually become allergically sensitive to another substance in the new product.

Haemorrhage, paronychia and foreign body reactions have been associated with unusual contact-type reactions (see 'sculptured nails', above).

Overall risk of adverse reactions

Precise figures are not available for the number of adverse reactions related to the use of cosmetics in general, and certainly none for nail care products in particular. However, by reviewing data collected from several sources, a reasonable estimate can made.

Industry

Several years ago the cosmetic industry of the Unites States agreed to participate in a voluntary programme for reporting product experience to the FDA. Although not all companies cooperate in this voluntary programme, a sufficient number of the major manufacturers, accounting for the vast majority of total sales, do. For all types of cosmetic products there are only approximately two instances of adverse reaction per million units sold. Analysis of the data from these industry reports reveals that for all the many nail care products marketed, there are approximately 45 instances of unclassified experiences per million units sold. Not included in this figure is the small class designated as nail extenders – the sculptured nail product – which alone accounted for 125 reactions per million units.

FDA

The FDA tabulates complaints it receives directly from consumers. This number is relatively small, 400–600 per year. Most consumers, probably because of the trivial nature of this self-limiting complaint, do not write to regulatory agencies. However, the information has some value for identifying classes of products which users believe have been responsible for poor performance or personal injury. A recent FDA report establishes that less than 5% of the products identified are associated with nail care. Again, the sculptured nail category alone accounted for one-fifth of this figure.

NEISS

A third source of information is the National Electronics Injury Surveillance System (NEISS). A network of approximately 120 hospital emergency rooms provide accident data to the US Consumer Product Safety Commission (CPSC) which is extrapolated as a 'statistically valid' report for the contiguous United States. For a recent year there were 698 non-ingestion cosmetic-related 'injuries' of which approximately 10% could be classified as associated with nail care products.

North American Contact Dermatitis Group

In a 64-month interval between 1977 and 1983, 12 dermatologists representing various geographic areas of the United States studied 713 patients with cosmetic dermatitis. Of this number, 55 (8%) had adverse reactions to the entire category of nail preparation.

Summary

No matter how one reviews and analyses the figures from all above sources, the incidence of untoward reactions related to the use of cosmetics by the general population is very small (approximately 2 per million units sold). Nail care products as a subgroup probably account for under 10% of cosmetic reactions. The rare injury of any significance is caused by the cyanoacrylate resins where the monomer and polymer are mixed on the fingertip to create the sculptured nail. These are products of low volume use which are not marketed, presently, by any of the large, well-known cosmetic manufacturers.

Typical of cosmetics, nail care products are fashion oriented. Short-lived fads have not been considered in this discussion since they would lack pertinence. Likewise, this chapter is not meant to be an historic review of past irrelevant literature. For example, nail care products with ingredient compositions that are no longer available commercially have been omitted. Regrettably, current dermatologic literature continues to cite nail enamel base coats as singularly responsible for adverse reactions, when the product formula in question has not been marketed for 40 years.

There are many products, implements and devices for maintaining clean, well-groomed nails to satisfy individual needs. These benefits are obtained with small risk. The physician can and should be well versed in nail care and adornment to aid patients in achieving an improved, positive self-image.

References

Adams R.M. & Maibach H.I. (1985) A five year study of cosmetic reactions. *J. Am. Acad. Dermatol.* **13**, 1062–1069.

Arnold H.L., Rees R.B. & Izumi A.K. (1973) Report: American Academy of Dermatology, 1972. *Cutis* **11**, 365–398.

Balsam M.S. & Sagarin E. (eds) (1972–74) *Cosmetics: Science and Technology*, 2nd edn (3 vols). Wiley-Interscience, New York.

Baran R. (1982) Pathology induced by the application of cosmetics to the nail. In: *Principles of Cosmetics for the Dermatologist*, eds Frost P. & Horwitz S., p. 181. Mosby, St Louis.

Baran R. (1985) Cosmetics and the fingernails – old and new facts. Soc. Cosm. Sci., Symposium on Recent Advances in Skin Biology in Relation to Cosmetics, Paper 14.

Baran R. & Schibli H. (1990) Permanent paresthesia to sculptured nail. A distressing problem. *Dermatol. Clin.* **8**, 139–141.

Barnett J.M. & Scher R.K. (1992) Nail cosmetics. *Int. J. Dermatol.* **31**, 675–681.

Brauer E.W. (1969) *Your Skin and Hair: A Basic Guide to Care and Beauty*. Macmillan, New York.

Brauer E.W. (1980) Letters to the editor. *Cutis* **26(6)**.

Calnan C.D. (1958) Onychia from synthetic nail coverage. *Trans. St Johns Hosp. Dermatol. Soc.* **41**, 66–68.

Calnan C.D. (1967) Reactions to artificial colouring materials. *J. Soc. Cosm. Chem.* **18**, 215–223.

Caravati E.M. & Litovitz T.L. (1988) Pediatric cyanide intoxication and death from an acetonitrile-containing cosmetic. *J. Am. Med. Assoc.* **260**, 3470–3473.

Fisher A.A. (1973) *Contact Dermatitis*, 2nd edn. Lea & Febiger, Philadelphia.

Fisher A.A. (1980) Permanent loss of finger nails from sensitization and reaction to acrylic in a preparation designed to make artificial nails. *J. Dermatol. Surg. Oncol.* **6**, 70–71.

Fisher A.A (1987) Allergic reactions to cyanoacrylate 'Krazy glue' nail preparations. *Cutis* **40**, 475–476.

Fisher A.A. (1989) Permanent loss of finger nails due to allergic reaction to an acrylic nail preparation. A sixteen-year follow-up study. *Cutis* **43**, 404–406.

Fisher A.A. & Baran R. (1991) Adverse reactions to acrylate sculptured nails with particular reference to prolonged paresthesia. *Am. J. Contact Derm.* **2**, 38–42.

Gibbs R.C. & Leider M. (1979) Foot notes–a comprehensive, annotated, and partially illustrated table of conditions in, under, and around toe and finger nails. *J. Dermatol. Surg. Oncol.* **5**, 467–473.

Kechijian P. (1991) Nail polish removers: are they harmful? In: *Seminars in Dermatology*, ed. Baran R., pp. 26–28. W.B. Saunders, Philadelphia.

Lazar P. (1966) Reactions to nail hardeners. *Arch. Dermatol.* **94**, 446–448.

Linden C., Berg M., Faärm G. *et al.* (1993) Nail varnish allergy with far-reaching consequences. *Br. J. Dermatol.* **123**, 57–62.

Marks J.G., Bishop M.E. & Willis W.F. (1979) Allergic contact dermatitis to sculptured nails. *Arch. Dermatol.* **115** 100.

Mitchell J.C. (1981) Non-inflammatory onycholysis from formaldehyde-containing nail hardener. *Contact Derm.* 7, 173.

Nater J.P., de Groot A.C. & Miem D.H. (1985) Unwanted effects of cosmetics and drugs used. In: *Dermatology*, 2nd edn, pp. 337–342. Excerpta Medica, Amsterdam.

North American Contact Dermatitis Group (1982) *Prospective Study of Cosmetics Reactions*, 1977–1980. Vol. 6, pp. 909–917.

Norton L.A. (1991) Common and uncommon reactions to formaldehyde-containing nail hardeners. In: *Seminars in Dermatology*, ed. Baran R., pp. 29–33. W.B. Saunders, Philadelphia.

Orentreich N. & Schmucker S. (1971) *Nails – Care and Treatment.* American Medical Association, Committee on Cutaneous Health and Cosmetics.

Schauder S. (1990) Adverse reactions to sunscreening agents in 58 patients. *Z. Hautkz.* **66**, 294–318.

Shelley E.D. & Shelley W.D. (1988) Nail dystrophy and periungual dermatitis due to acrylate glue sensitivity. *J. Am. Acad. Dermatol.* **19**, 574–575.

Tosti A., Guerra L., Vincenzi C. *et al.* (1993) Contact sensitization caused by toluene sulfonamide-formaldehyde resin in women who use nail cosmetics. *Am. J. Contact Derm.* **4**, 150–153.

Chapter 9
Hereditary and Congenital Nail Disorders

L. JUHLIN & R. BARAN

Embryology
Anonychia
Hereditary ectodermal dysplasias
Disease loci and chromosomal anomalies
Predominent skeletal anomalies
Hyperplastic thick nails
Clubbing, acropachy
Broad nails and pseudoclubbing
Koilonychia
Overcurvature of the nails
Ectopic nails (onychoheterotopia)
Congenital malformations due to drugs or infections
Nail discoloration and secondary nail changes
Epidermolysis bullosa
Miscellaneous dystrophies

Introduction

Many of the defects of the nails are accompanied by developmental changes in other organs, such as skin, teeth, brain and bones. The many abnormalities of the nails described here are often of minor importance when making a diagnosis. Of greater interest are apparently isolated nail defects, since they may help in the diagnosis of hidden syndromes or more generalized disease. In categorizing these disorders we have placed the nail in the 'centre' but we have also grouped disorders according to the most obvious symptoms. Such a practical division aims to aid the physician observing nail changes as a help to diagnosis.

In view of the large number of unique and rare syndromes with nail involvement, we have resolved much of this chapter into comprehensive tables stressing the nail apparatus changes and major associated abnormalities.

Nail embryology (see Chapter 1)

The human nail apparatus begins to develop during the ninth week of intrauterine life; nail plate growth is evident by 14 weeks and may be complete by 20 weeks (see Chapter 1). Nail defects occurring during this period are called embryopathies and those appearing later are the fetopathies. The embryopathies are often hereditary whereas the fetopathies as a rule are caused by vascular or mechanical factors. Some hereditary defects do not become apparent until later in life, mainly because they are due to increased susceptibility to infections or secondary damage. Telfer *et al.* (1988) classified the congenital and hereditary nail dystrophies according to whether the defects occurred in the nail matrix, the nail field or the nail bed. A defect in the nail matrix is the most common cause of abnormal nails. The matrix can have an abnormal position, size or quality. The nail field is the area in which the entire nail unit (nail matrix and nail bed) develops. Proliferation of the nail bed will produce a thickened nail which, as in pachyonychia congenita, is not evident until early childhood.

Reference

Telfer N.R., Barth J.H. & Dawber R.P.R. (1988) Congenital and hereditary nail dystrophies – an embryological approach to classification. *Clin. Exp. Dermatol.* 13, 160–163.

Anonychia

Total absence of all nails from birth is rare. Often there are rudimentary nails on some fingers or toes; therefore there is frequently only a quantitative difference between anonychia and hyponychia and they often occur together (Timerman *et al.*, 1969). The first two cases with anonychia were described in 1842 by the physician to the King of Saxony, Dr F.A. Amman; Cockayne (1933) reviewed some of the earlier cases.

Isolated anonychia (Fig. 9.1) without other symptoms can be inherited as a dominant, recessive or sporadic abnormality (see Salamon, 1966; Mahloudji & Amidi 1971; Hopsu-Havu & Jansen, 1973). Cockayne (1933) and Strandskov (1939) described families with absent thumbnails from birth. If an X-ray is undertaken an underlying bone abnormality is generally found (Baran & Juhlin 1986). There will be no nail if the distal phalanx is lacking; when the latter is hypoplastic the nails may be absent, dystrophic or normal. Often anonychia is combined with other symptoms (Nevin *et al.*, 1982) (Fig. 9.2) such as broad, small hands, due to various skeletal anomalies such as loss of phalanges or isolated fingers and toes (ectrodactyly), syndactyly (Figs 9.3 & 9.4) or polydactyly

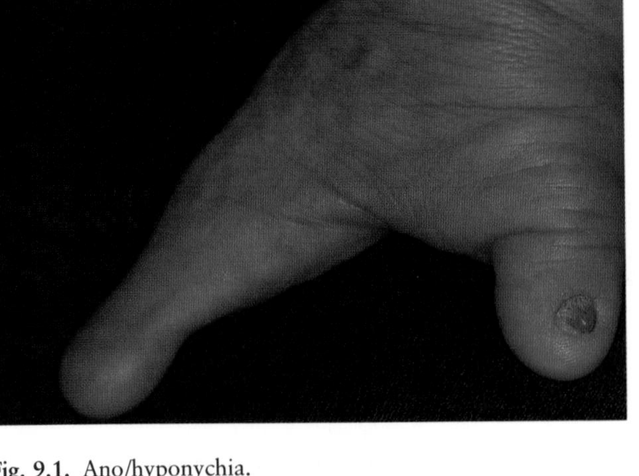

Fig. 9.1. Ano/hyponychia.

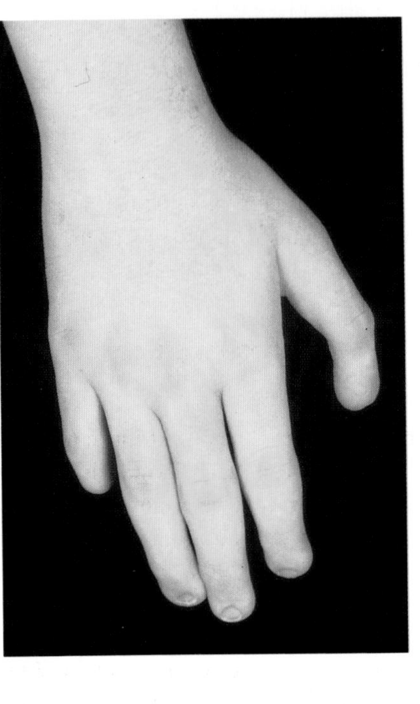

Fig. 9.2. Anonychia in DOOR syndrome (Prof. Nevin, Belfast).

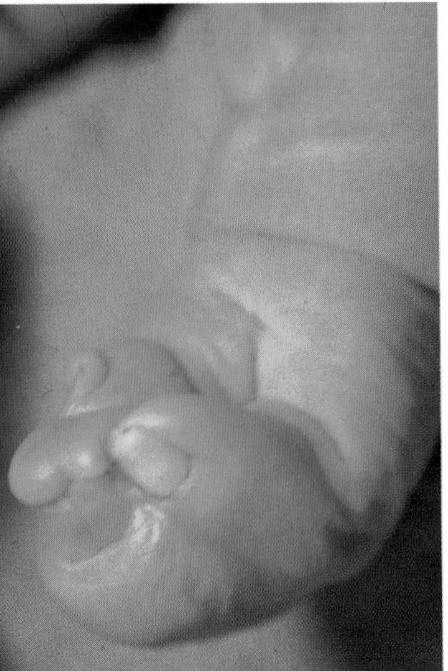

Fig. 9.3. Syndactyly.

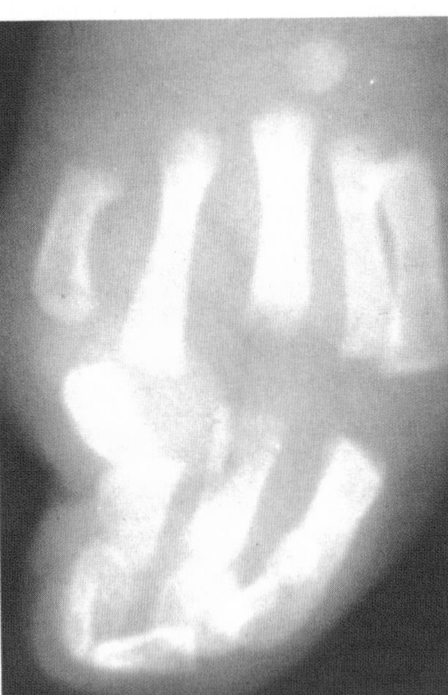

Fig. 9.4. Syndactyly – X-ray changes in digits of patient in Fig. 9.3.

(Salamon, 1966; Lawrence, 1969; Rahbari *et al.*, 1975; Kurgan *et al.*, 1976. Goldschlag-Cooks *et al.*, 1985; Kumar & Levick, 1986). In the brachydactyly variant called apical dystrophy of MacArthur and McCullough (1932) or banana fingers, the four ulnar digits barely project beyond the thumb and the fingers look amputated and have no nails (Fig. 9.5). Absence of nails on the ring fingers and rudimentary nails on other fingers with brachydactyly in six generations was reported by Schott (1978).

Anonychia with other symptoms

Anonychia can occur with retarded development of teeth (Baisch, 1931). Freire-Maia and Pinheiro (1979) described recessive total anonychia with a dominant dental anomaly and aplasia or hypoplasia of upper lateral incisors, spaced teeth and lack of some molars. Loss of toenails and brachydactyly with dental changes was reported by Tennstedt *et al.* (1985). Congenital absence of three toenails with linear skin atrophy, scaring alopecia and scar-like lesions of the tongue was reported by Sequerios and Sack (1985). Absence or hypoplasia of nails on thumbs and halluces can together with gingival fibromatosis, be diagnostic features for Zimmerman–Laband syndrome (Chodriker *et al.*, 1986). Anonychia can be combined with deafness, onychoosteodystrophy (DOO) and mental retardation (Fig. 9.2) (DOOR syndrome) (Table 9.3). These patients have an inborn metabolic error with an increase of 2-

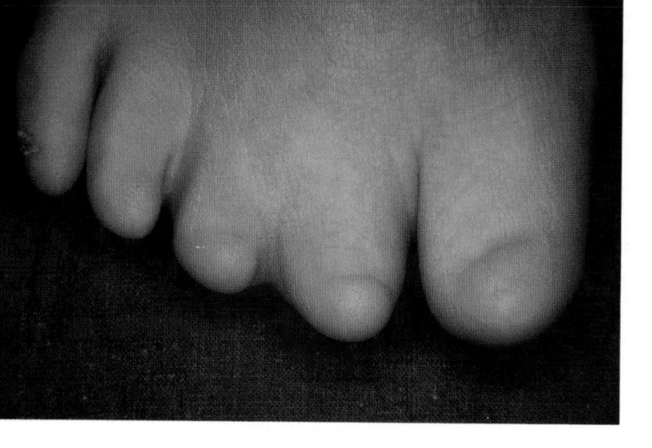

Fig. 9.5. Anonychia – pseudo-amputee appearance.

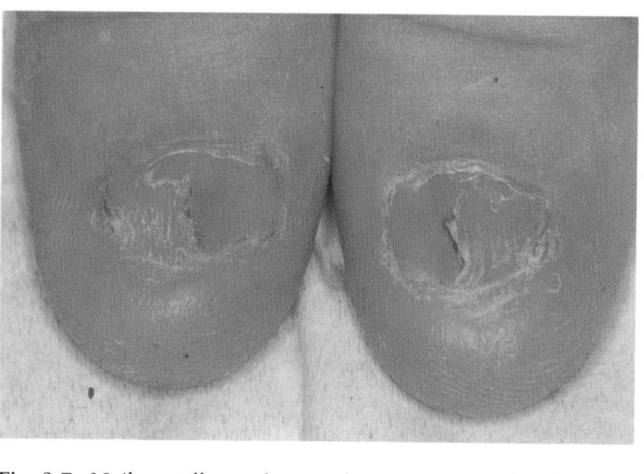

Fig. 9.7. Nail–patella syndrome – hypoplastic thumbnails.

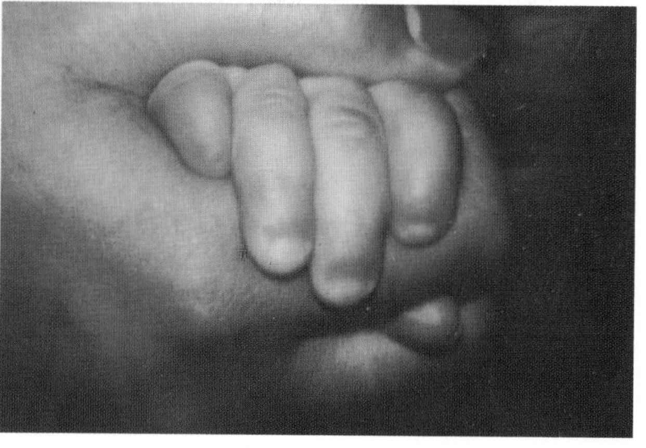

Fig. 9.6. Coffin–Siris syndrome (courtesy of Professor Schinzel, Zurich, Switzerland).

oxyglutarate in plasma and urine (Patton *et al.*, 1987). Pfeiffer (1982) reported the otoonychoperoneal syndrome with absence of nails on thumbs, index fingers and big toes with dysplastic ears and hypoplasia of the fibula.

Anonychia is described in the rare glossopalatine ankylosis syndrome in which the mouth is abnormal, the tongue being attached to the temporo-mandibular joint (Gorlin *et al.*, 1976). A family with dominant anonychia with bizarre flexural pigmentation and hair abnormalities was reported by Verbov (1975). Anonychia has also been described in the dyscephalic-mandibulo-oculofacial syndrome of Hallerman–Streiff–Francois (Guérineau & Plassart, 1965) and craniofrontal nasal dysplasia (Table 9.6). Familial absence of the fifth fingernails (Fig. 9.6) in combination with mental retardation, coarse facies with full lips and scalp hypotrichosis were first described by Coffin and Siris (1970). Carey and Hall (1978) and Haspeslagh *et al.* (1984) have reviewed the literature and described new cases. This disorder belongs to the group of epidermal dysplasias which often have other abnormalities as described in Table 9.2. In Klein's syndrome the nails are missing on the fifth toe. The patients also have pterygium and fissures on the first toe with syndactyly (Klein, 1962). In congenital onychodysplasia of the index finger (COIF) or Iso and Kikuchi syndrome the nail on the index finger can be missing (see p. 314 and Table 9.6). Lack of thumbnails can occur in the nail patella syndrome.

Nail–patella syndrome or hereditary osteoonychodysplasia (HOOD)

This was described by Chatelain (1820) and Little (1897) (cited in Raman & Haslock, 1983). Early diagnosis of this syndrome can be made by examining the nails which give clues to the possibility of other organs being involved.

Nails (Fig. 9.7)

The nail changes are most pronounced on the ulnar side of the thumbs and decrease towards the fifth finger. The toenails are rarely affected. The nails, especially on the thumbs, might be absent or short, narrow, spoon-shaped, soft and/or fragile. The lunula can be triangular or V-shaped (Fig. 9.8), which is almost pathogonomic for the condition (Norton & Mescon, 1968; Daniel *et al.*, 1980).

Bones

The patella is aplastic or luxated in 90% of patients (Fig. 9.10). Pain in the knee or gait problems after exercise often bring the patient to the doctor. The changes can result in early osteoarthritis. The radius head is small which can cause limitation in elbow motion or subluxation of radius. Bilateral posterior iliac horns are pathognomic (Fig. 9.10). Other bone changes can be seen such as scapular hypoplasia, scoliosis, genu valgum and hypoplastic lateral humerus epicondyle.

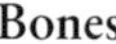

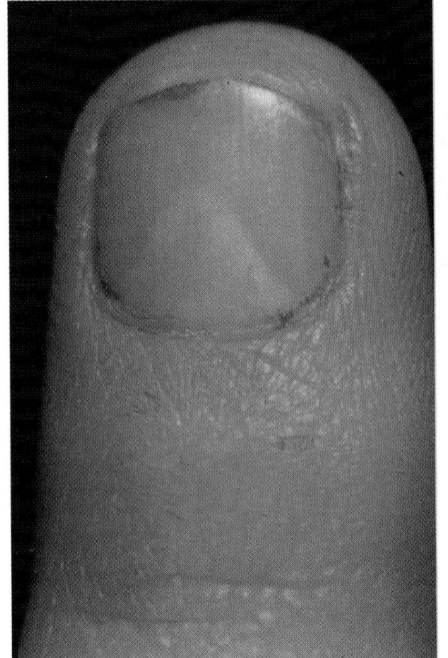

Fig. 9.8. Nail–patella syndrome – triangular, pointed lunula.

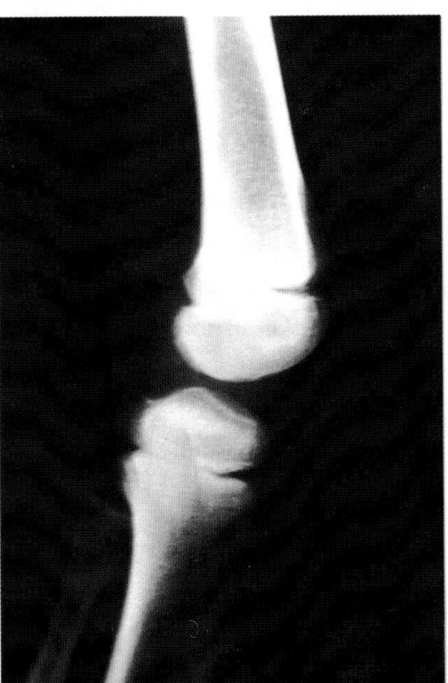

Fig. 9.9. Nail–patella syndrome – X-ray to show aplastic patellae.

Kidney

Renal involvement is seen in 42% of the cases with various degree of dysfunction (Carbonara & Albert, 1964; Croock *et al.*, 1987). It has recently been described as the only manifestation of the syndrome (Dombros & Katz, 1982; Salcedo, 1984; Gubler *et al.*, 1990). The presence of collagen-like fibrils in the glomerular basement membrane as revealed by electron microscopy is diagnostic (Morita *et al.*, 1973). The renal symptoms are usually first discovered in adults as asymptomatic proteinuria. The end

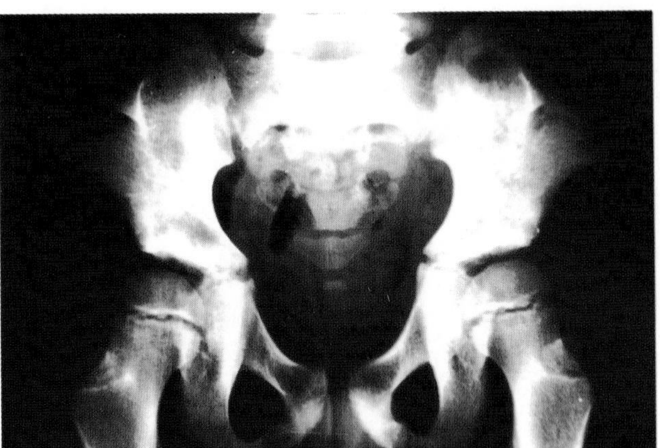

Fig. 9.10. Nail–patella syndrome – X-ray showing bilateral posterior iliac horns.

result can be a nephrotic-like picture which can result in renal failure.

Eye

Heterochromia of the iris with hyperpigmentation of the papillary margin are also helpful diagnostic signs. Microcornea and glaucoma have also been reported.

Other signs

Webs on fingers in the popliteal area can occur.

Genetics

The syndrome is autosomal dominant and the gene located on the long arm of the ninth chromosome (Westerveld *et al.*, 1976). The locus is linked to that of the ABO group (Renwick & Lawler, 1955).

References

Baisch A. (1931) Anonychia congenita, kombiniert mit Polydactylie und verzögertem abnormen Zahndurchbruch. *Dtsch. Z. Chir.* **232**, 450.

Baran R. & Juhlin L. (1986) Bone dependent nail formation. *Br. J. Dermatol.* **114**, 371.

Carbonara P. & Albert M. (1964) Hereditary osteo-onychodysplasia (HOOD). *Am. J. Med. Sci.* **248**, 139.

Carey J.C. & Hall B.D. (1978) The Coffin–Siris syndrome. Five new cases including two siblings. *Am. J. Dis. Child.* **132**, 667.

Chodriker B.N., Chudley A.E., Toffler M.A. & Reed M.H. (1986) Brief clinical report: Zimmerman–Laband syndrome and profound mental retardation. *Am. J. Med. Genet.* **25**, 543.

Cockayne E.A. (1933) Abnormalities of the nails. In: *Inherited Abnormalities of Skin and its Appendages*, Ch. IX, p. 265, Oxford University Press, London.

Coffin G.S. & Siris E. (1970) Mental retardation with absent fifth fingernail and terminal phalanx. *Am. J. Dis. Child.* **119**, 433.

Croock A.D., Kahaleh M.B. & Powers J.M. (1987) Vasculitis and renal disease in nail–patella syndrome: case report and literature review: *Ann. Rheum. Dis.* **46**, 562.

Daniel C.R., Osment L.S. & Noojin R.O. (1980) Triangular lunulae. *Arch. Dermatol.* **116**, 448.

Dombros N. & Katz A. (1982) Nail patella-like renal lesions in the absence of skeletal abnormalities. *Am. J. Kidney Dis.* **1**, 237.

Freire-Maia N. & Pinheiro M. (1979) Recessive anonychia totalis and dominant aplasia (or hypoplasia) of upper lateral incisors in the same kindred. *J. Med. Genet.* **16**, 45.

Goldschlag-Cooks R., Hertz M., Katznelson M. & Goodman R.M. (1985) A new nail dysplasia syndrome with onychonychia and absence and/or hypoplasia of distal phalanges. *Clin. Genet.* **27**, 85.

Gorlin R.J., Pindborg J.J. & Cohen M.M. (1976) *Syndromes of the Head and Neck*, 2nd edn. McGraw Hill, New York.

Gubler M.C., Dommersures J.P., Furioli J. *et al.* (1990) Syndrome de 'nail-patella' sans atteinte extrarenale. Une nouvelle nephropathie hereditaire glomerulaire. *Ann. Pediatr. (Paris)* **37**, 78.

Guerinéau P. & Plassart H. (1965) Syndrome dyscéphalique de Francois a propos d'un nourrison de race maure. *Arch. Fr. Pediart.* **22**, 882.

Haspeslagh M., Fryns J.P. & van den Berghe H. (1984) The Coffin–Siris syndrome: report of a family and further delineation *Clin. Genet.* **26**, 374.

Hopsu-Havu V.K. & Jansen C.T. (1973) Anonychia congenita. *Arch. Dermatol.* **107**, 752.

Klein D. (1962) Cheilo-palatoschizis avec fistules de la levre inférieure associé a une syndactylie, une onychodysplasie particuliere, un pterygion poplité unilatéeral et des pieds varus équins. *J. Genet. Hum.* **11**, 65.

Kumar D. & Levick R.K. (1986) Autosomal dominant onychodystrophy and anonychia with type B brachydactyly and ectrodactyly. *Clin. Genet.* **30**, 219.

Kurgan A., Hirsch M. & Williams F.J. (1976) Aplasia of toe phalanges and nails. *Isr. J. Med. Sci.* **12**, 570.

Lawrence R. (1969) Absence of phalanges and toe nails. *Med. Radiogr. Photogr.* **45**, 46.

MacArthur J.W. & McCullough F. (1932) Apical dystrophy, an inherited defect of hands and feet. *Hum. Biol.* **4**, 179.

Mahloudji M. & Amidi M. (1971) Simple anonychia. Further evidence for autosomal recessive inheritance. *J. Med. Genet.* **8**, 478.

Morita T., Laughlin O., Kawano K. & Kimmelstiel P. (1973) Nail-patella syndrome. *Arch. Intern. Med.* **131**, 271.

Nevin N.C., Thomas P.S., Calvert J. & Reid M. (1982) Deafness, onycho-osteodystrophy, mental retardation (DOOR) syndrome. *Am. J. Med. Genet.* **13**, 325.

Norton L.A. & Mescon H. (1968) Nail–patella–elbow syndrome. *Arch. Dermatol.* **98**, 372.

Patton M.A., Krywawych S., Winter R.M., Brenton D.P. & Baraitser M. (1987) DOOR syndrome (deafness, onycho-osteo-dystrophy and mental retardation). Elevated plasma and urinary 2-oxyglutamate in three unrelated patients. *Am. J. Med. Genet.* **26**, 207.

Pfeiffer R.A. (1982) The oto-onycho-peroneal syndrome. A probably new genetic entity. *Eur. J. Paediat.* **138**, 217.

Rahbari H., Heath L. & Chapel T. (1975) Anonychia with ectrodactyly. *Arch. Dermatol.* **111**, 1482.

Raman D. & Haslock I. (1983) The nail-patella syndrome – A report of two cases and a literature review. *Br. J. Rheumatol.* **22**, 41.

Renwick J.H. & Lawler S.D. (1955) Genetical linkage between the ABO and nail–patella loci. *Ann. Hum. Genet.* **19**, 312.

Salamon T. (1966) Erbkrankheiten der Nägel. In: *Handbuch der Haut und Geschlechtkrankheiten Erganzungswerk*, Vol. 7, p. 409. Springer, Berlin.

Salcedo J.R. (1984) An autosomal recessive disorder with glomerular basement membrane abnormalities similar to those seen in the nail patella syndrome: Report of a kindred. *Am. J. Med. Genet.* **19**, 579.

Schott G.D. (1978) Hereditary brachydactyly with nail dysplasia. *J. Med. Genet.* **15**, 119.

Sequeiros J. & Sack G.H. Jr (1984) Linear skin atrophy, scaring alopecia. *Am. J. Med. Genet.* **17**, 579.

Strandskov H.H. (1939) Inheritance of absence of thumb nails. *J. Hered.* **30**, 53.

Tennstedt D., Lachapelle J.-M. & Baran R. (1985) Brachydactylie avec anonychia. *Ann. Dermatol. Venereol.* **112**, 901.

Timerman I., Museteanu C. & Simionescu N.N. (1969) Dominant anonychia onychodystrophy. *J. Med. Genet.* **6**, 105.

Verbov J. (1975) Anonychia with bizarre flexural pigmentation – An autosomal dominant dermatosis. *Br. J. Dermatol.* **92**, 469.

Westerveld A., Jongsma A.P.M., Meera Khan P., Van Someren H. & Bootsma D. (1976) Assignment of the AK$_1$:Np:ABO linkage group to human chromosome 9. *Proc. Natl. Acad. Sci.* 73, 895–899.

Hereditary ectodermal dysplasias

The term hereditary ectodermal dysplasia (HED) was introduced by Weech (1929). It is used to cover a heterogenous group of primary epidermal disorders where at least one of the following signs occur: hypotrichosis, hypodontia, onychodysplasia and anhidrosis, plus at least one sign affecting other structures of epidermal origin as classified by Freire-Maia (1977) and Freire-Maia and Pinheiro (1988). Solomon and Keuer (1980) prefer to exclude diseases which are progressive. The list of HED now includes over 60 different conditions. Whether there is a reduction in sweating in certain areas has in many cases not been fully tested, which makes this part of the classification weak (Berg *et al.*, 1990). We therefore prefer to list skin changes instead of hidrotic changes. Additional ectodermal tissues which can be involved are ears, lens of eyes, anterior pituitary gland, central nervous system and adrenal medulla. Other embryologic germ layers may also be involved, but when they dominate and when epidermal changes are secondary they are not considered as HED.

Tables 9.1, 9.2 and 9.3 list the combinations and features where the nails are involved (Figs 9.11–9.13). Since thickening of the soles and palms is an easily recognized sign, those with keratoderma palmoplantare have been grouped together (Table 9.1). The nail changes in other ectodermal dysplasias with changes of teeth and hair or skin are listed in Table 9.2 and those where the teeth are

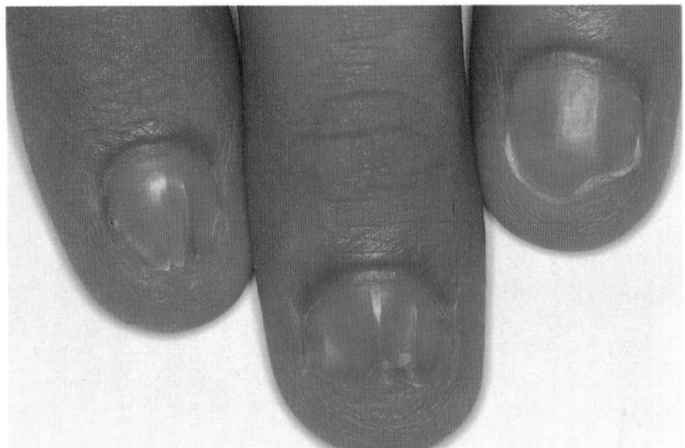

Fig. 9.11. Hidrotic ectodermal dysplasia – small 'nail fields'.

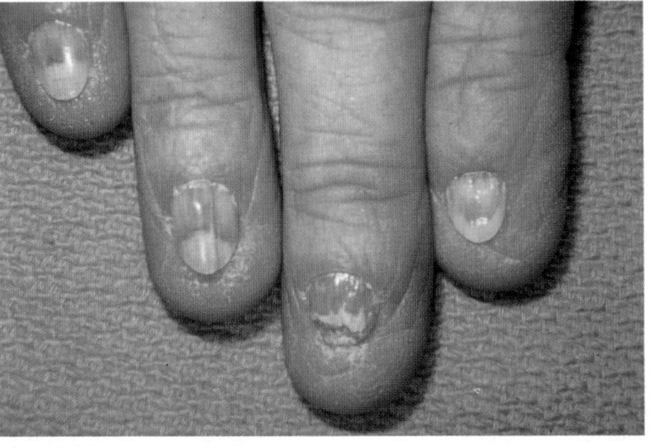

Fig. 9.12. Hidrotic ectodermal dysplasia – small 'nail fields' with short, overcurved nails (courtesy of L. Norton, USA).

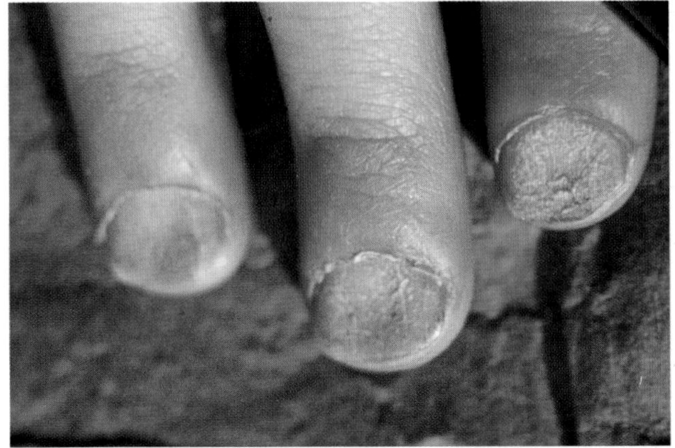

Fig. 9.13. Hidrotic ectodermal dysplasia – thin nails with koilonychia.

normal in Table 9.3. Four important conditions will here be further described.

Anhidrotic and hypohidrotic ectodermal dysplasia (Fig. 9.14)

One type is the X-linked Christ–Siemens–Touraine syndrome (Reed *et al.*, 1970; Norval *et al.*, 1988; Sybert, 1989) and one autosomal recessive (Passarge & Fried, 1977). The prominent features are the typical facies suggestive of congenital syphilis often with a depressed nasal bridge (saddle back nose), large and conspicuous nostrils, high cheek bones and a narrow lower face. The eyebrows are scanty and the eyes slant upwards. The lips can be thick and the buccal commisures have radiating furrows. Sebaceous gland hyperplasia and telangiectases are often seen on the cheeks. The hair of scalp and body is thin and sparse. There is hypodontia, reduced sweating and decreased function of lacrimal ducts. The nails can be normal, fragile, dystrophic or absent at birth (Fig. 9.14). A combination with hypothyroidism and ciliary dyskinesia was described by Pabst and Groth (1981). Other syndromes are described where cleft lip and palate (Rapp–Hodgkin syndrome, AEC syndrome), ectrodactyly (EEC syndrome) or genitourinary anomalies are combined with anhidrotic dysplasia (Freire-Maia & Pinheiro, 1984; Schwayder *et al.*, 1986; Schroeder & Sybert, 1987; Rollnick & Hao, 1988). Pike and Baraitser (1986), Morris *et al.* (1987) and Pinheiro *et al.* (1989) called this condition another syndrome (alopecia nail dystrophy, ophthalmic complications, thyroid dysfunction, hypohidrosis, ephelides and enteropathy, and respiratory tract infections).

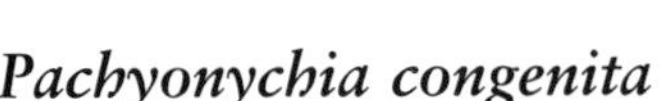

Pachyonychia congenita

This is a hereditary ectodermal dysplasia with thickening of the nails and subungeal hyperkeratosis appearing within the first 6 months of life but late onset has also been reported (Paller *et al.*, 1991; Iraci *et al.*, 1993) (Figs 9.15–9.17). There is also abnormal keratinization of skin and mucosa membranes.

The nail changes with keratosis of palms and soles were described in 1897 by Colcott-Fox. In 1904 Müller reported the condition, as did Garrick–Wilson in 1905. The following year Jadassohn and Lewandowski described the full syndrome in two siblings. Today pachonychia congenita is classified into four types with increasing clinical symptoms.

Type I is most common (Feinstein *et al.*, 1988). The yellow-brown nails show subungual hyperkeratosis and become progressively thicker. The patients also have palmoplantar hyperkeratosis, follicular hyperkeratosis of the body and oral leukokeratoses.

Table 9.1. Hereditary ectodermal dysplasia (ED) with keratoderma palmoplantare and nail changes. Inheritances are indicated as follows: AD, autosomal dominant; AR, autosomal recessive; XL, sex-linked transmission; ASD, autosomal semi-dominant

Condition	Inheritance	Nails	Hair	Skin with hyperkeratosis palmoplantaris+	Teeth	Ear	Eye	Other findings
Dermatopathia pigmentosa reticularis (Rycroft *et al.*, 1977)		Longitudinal ridging and lamellar splitting	Sparse over vertex	Hyperpigmented macules and hypopigmentation. Slight hyperkeratosis of soles and feet	Normal	—	—	—
Dyskeratosis congenita, Zinsser–Engman–Cole syndrome (Connor & Teague, 1981; Kalb *et al.*, 1986) p. 312	XL	Short, atrophic after late childhood, most prominent on fingers where they often are lost	Nornal or scarring alopecia	Mainly palmar hyperkeratosis. Hyperhidrosis of palms and soles. Reticulated hyperpigmentation of neck, face and chest	Sometimes malformed	Deafness	Blepharitis with loss of cilia. Leucoplakia on conjunctive. Lacrimal duct obstruction	Acrocyanosis. Aplastic anaemia. Pancytopaenia. Oral lesions and leukoplakia. Immunological abnormalities. Testicular atrophy. Avascular necrosis of femor
Scoggins' type (1971)	AD	Short, atrophic after late childhood, most prominent on fingers where they often are lost	Nornal or scarring alopecia	Mainly palmar hyperkeratosis. Hyperhidrosis of palms and soles. Reticulated hyperpigmentation of neck, face and chest	Sometimes malformed	Deafness	Blepharitis with loss of cilia. Leukoplakia on conjunctive. Lacrimal duct obstruction	Acrocyanosis. Aplastic anaemia. Pancytopaenia. Oral lesions and leukoplakia. Immunological abnormalities. Testicular atrophy. Avascular necrosis of femor
ED-AOHD syndrome (Freire-Maia *et al.*, 1977)	AD	Onychodysplasia: thick, dark and deformed toenails	*Alopecia* or fair thin hair	*Hypohidrosis. Hyperkeratosis* of knees and elbows. Dermatoglyphics abnormal	Normal	Neural *deafness*	Photophobia hyperopia	Palpebral slanting EEG abnormal, retarded bone age. Unusual face, prominent nose
Ectrodactyly – clefting (EEC) syndrome. (Cockayne, 1936; Ogur & Yüksel, 1988; Rollnick & Hoo, 1988)	AD	Deformed, thin, brittle, striated: pitted and terminated irregular (Fig. 9.8)	Wiry, hypopigmented	Fair, hypopigmented, scaly skin with comedo-naevus (Leibowitz & Jenkins, 1984)	Dysplasia. Partial anodentia. Caries		Blue sclera. Photophobia. Absence of lacrimal puncta. Tearing. Blepharitis. Meibom's glands deficient. Corneal scarring. Blindness	Cleft lip + palate. Short stature. Ectrodactyly + syndactyly. Claw-shaped hands. Genital and urinary tract abnormalities. Growth hormone deficiency (Knudtzon & Aarskog, 1987)
Focal dermal hypoplasia. Goltz & Gorlin syndrome (Goltz *et al.*, 1970; Malfait *et al.*, 1989; Mallory & Moore, 1989; Pujol *et al.*, 1992)	XL	Thin, spoon-shaped. Can be absent in 50%. No lunula	Sparse in focal areas of scalp and pubis	Focal thin skin with herniation of fat. Linear hypo- and hyperpigmentation. Papillomas	Normal	—	Multiple severe anomalies	Small stature. Asymmetric face. Cranial, spinal and bone anomalies. Cleft lip and palate. Multiple lip papillomas of mucous membranes. Urinary abnormality
Hidrotic ED, (Clouston, 1929; Wilkey & Stevenson, 1945; Freire-Maia & Pinhero, 1984; Haneke, 1987; Ando *et al.*, 1988)	AD	Dystrophic nails. Grow slowly. Change more marked with age. Onycholysis, pits ridges. Often small and conical. Paronychia. Hyperkeratotic nailbed looks like thickened nails (Figs 9.11–9.13)	In 50% sparse, short and thin. Eyebrows and eyelashes often absent	Normal sweat. Hyperpigmentation especially over joints. Clubbing of fingers	Normal but occasionally hypodontia and natal teeth	—	Occasionally strabism and cataracts	—

continued on p. 304

Table 9.1. *Continued*

Condition	Inheritance	Nails	Hair	Skin with hyperkeratosis palmoplantaris+	Teeth	Ear	Eye	Other findings
Hyperpigmentaton, hypotrichosis and dystrophy of nails (Sparrow *et al.*, 1976)	AD	Distal thickening, subungual hyperkeratosis, onycholysis	Normal	Symmetrical hyperpigmentation most marked on neck and in axillae. Hypohydrosis. Hypoplastic dermatoglyphic pattern. Punctate keratosis on palms and soles	Normal	—	—	—
Hyper- and hypopigmentation with dystrophic nails (Moon-Adams & Slatkin, 1955)	—	Thin, brittle with longitudinal furrows	Normal	Symmetrical pigmentation and hyperkeratosis of non-exposed skin with areas of hypopigmentation	Normal	—	—	Probably same as dermopathia pigmentosa recularis (see above)
Hyperpigmentation, palmoplantar keratosis and childhood blistering (Boss *et al.*, 1981)	AD	Terminal onycholysis, 'peaked' lunula	Normal	Speckled hyperpigmentation. Blistering tendency of hands and feet in infancy. Punctate keratosis of palms and soles	Normal	—	—	—
Hypoplastic – enamel-onycholysis – hypohidrosis syndrome (Witkop *et al.*, 1975)	AD	Onycholysis	Normal	Hypohidrosis. Seborrhoeic dermatitis of scalp	Hypoplastic hypocalcified enamel	—	—	—
Lacrimo-auriculo-dento-digital syndrome (Hollister *et al.*, 1973)	AD	Ectopic nails. Large thumbnail	Normal	Normal	Enamel poor. Peg-shaped incisors. Darkening of teeth	Hearing loss. Cup shaped ears	Aplasia of lacrimal punctata. Eye infections	Digital malformations. Kidney anomalies can occur
Nail, tooth, ear syndrome (Robinson *et al.*, 1962)	AD	Hypoplastic and dysplastic with furrows and cracks	Normal	Chloride increased in sweat	Anodontia	Sensory deafness	—	Syndactyly. Polydactyly may occur
Oculo-*dentodigital* (ODD or ODOD) syndrome (O'Rourk & Bravos, 1969; Traboulsi *et al.*, 1986)	AD or AR	Dysplastic; fusion of nails and phalanges between fourth and fifth fingers	Hypotrichosis	Normal	Microdontia. Hypodontia. Conical incisive. Enamel hypoplasia		Microphthalmia. Ectropia. Nystagmus. Iris atrophy	Small alae nasi. Anteversion of nostrils. Microstomia, micrognathia. Polydactyly, syndactyly, hypophalangy
Oculo-*tricho-dysplasia* (OTD) syndrome (Cecatto de Lima *et al.*, 1988)	AR	Fragile, brittle	Hypohidrosis	Normal	Small, widely spaced	—	—	Retinitis pigmentosa
Odonto-thichomelic hypohidrotic ED (Cat *et al.*, 1972)	AR	Hypoplastic nails and no nail on some fingers	Hypotrichosis	Thin, dry, shiny	Hypodontia	Auricles abnormal	—	Protruding lips, enlarged nose hypoplastic nipples and areola. Tetramelic reductions Oligophreny. Metabolic defects. ECG anormalities. Retarded growth
Keratosis, ichthyosis and deafness (KID syndrome) (Senter *et al.*, 1978; Skinner *et al.*, 1981; Langer *et al.*, 1990; McGrae, 1990).	AR	Thick white nails most marked on fingers	Hypotrichosis. Eyebrows and eyelashes absent	Erythrokeratoderma On knees and palms pitted type of hyperkeratosis. Plaques on central portion of face. Hypohidrosis	Normal or abnormal	Neuro-sensory deafness	Vascularization of cornea; keratitis	Tight heel cords may occur. Fungal infections common

continued

Table 9.1. *Continued*

Condition	Inheritance	Nails	Hair	Skin with hyperkeratosis palmoplantaris+	Teeth	Ear	Eye	Other findings
Keratoderma palmoplantare (Thost-Unna)	AD	Thick	Normal	Hyperhidrosis of palms and soles	Normal	—	—	A mutilating type described (Gamborg–Nielsen, 1983)
Keratoderma palmoplantare progressiva (type Meleda) (Salamon, 1982; Protonotarius *et al.*, 1986)	AR	Onychogryphosis koilonychia, short subungual hyperkeratosis; proximal part of nail pink, distal pale	Normal	Hyperhidrosis of palms and soles. Erythema of face and sacral region. Keratosis of elbows and knees	Normal	—	—	Cardiomegaly. Mental retardation may occur
Keratoderma palmoplantare and alopecia (Stevanovic, 1959)	SD	Dystrophic nail plate. Proximal parts hyperkeratotic and brittle	Scanty hair. Eyebrows and eyelashes absent	Otherwise normal	Normal	—	—	—
Keratoderma palmoplantare (Raphael *et al.*, 1968; Gorlin *et al.*, 1976)	—	Sub- and periungual hyperkeratosis	Normal	Changes marked on friction areas. Appear at age 5 on fingers. Later on toes	Normal	—	—	Gingival hyperplasia
Keratoderma palmoplantare with periodontosis (Papillon & Lefevre, 1924; Gorlin *et al.*, 1964; Haneke, 1979; Nazzaro *et al.*, 1988)	AR	Punctate depressions. Occasionally spoon-shaped or thick	Normal or sparse after 25 years	Hyperhidrosis of palms and soles. Erythema of face and sacral region. Hyperkeratosis of elbows, knees and Achilles area. Pyogenic infections	Periodontosis. Premature loss of teeth. Bleeding of gingiva	Deafness (Thorel, 1964)	—	Calcification of the dura common. Acroosteolysis. Pyogenic infections (Bergman & Friedman–Birnbaum, 1988)
Keratoderma palmoplantare with periodontosis and onychogryphosis (Puliyel & Sridharan Iyer, 1986)	AR	Onychogryphosis of thumbs and big toe	Normal	Hyperkeratosis after extending onto dorsum of hands and feet and on extensor area of arms and legs	Periodontosis	—	—	Pes planus. Arachnodactyly, acroosteolysis
Keratoderma palmoplantare type Buschke – Fischer (Shirren & Dinger, 1965)	AD	Subungual hyperkeratosis, onychogryphosis, longitudinal furrows	Normal	Papuloverrucoid palmoplantar lesions after puberty and progressively increasing. Hyperhidrosis of palms and soles may occur as well as hyperkeratosis over knees	Normal	—	—	—
Keratoderma with leuconychia totalis (Crosti *et al.*, 1983)	—	Leuconychia totalis	Coiled with furrows	Follicular hyperkeratosis	Transversal furrows of incisors	Deafness	—	—
Keratoderma palmoplantare with leuconychia and deafness (Schwann, 1963; Bart & Pumphrey, 1967)	AD	Leuconychia on thumbs and big toes. Longitudinal white spots on other nails. Frequently koilonychia	Normal	Hyperkeratotic areas knuckle pads on the dorsal side of the fingers	Normal	Deafness since birth	—	Dupuytren's contracture
Keratoderma palmoplantare mutilans with deafness (Vohwinkel, 1929; Bhatia *et al.*, 1989)	AD	Pseudo-ainhum	Alopecia	Polygonal papules on knees, elbows, backs of hands and feet	Normal	Deafness	—	—
Keratoderma palmoplantare with atrophic fibrosis of the extremities (Huriez *et al.*, 1969) (de Berker & Kavanagh, 1993)	AD	Hypoplastic with fracture of free edge. Sometimes apparent prominent lunulae, leuconychia, koilonychia and complete aplasia.	Retroauricular alopecia	Scleroderma-like atrophy of hands, squamous cell carcinoma	Microdontia	—	—	Increased risk of intestinal cancer

continued on p. 306

Table 9.1. *Continued*

Condition	Inheritance	Nails	Hair	Skin with hyperkeratosis palmoplantaris+	Teeth	Ear	Eye	Other findings
		Transverse and longitudinal ridging increased longitudinal curvature						
Keratoderma palmoplantare and clubbing of nails (Bureau *et al.*, 1959)	—	Thick, with clubbing	Normal	Increased sweating expecially on extremities. Recidivating leg ulcers	Normal	—	—	Tall massive body but small head. Hypertrophy of long bones. Decreased bone density with thin cortex. Distal phalanges enlarged
Keratoderma palmoplantare and neuropathy (Tholmie *et al.*, 1988b)	AD	Dystrophic nails at birth or early childhood with painful longitudinal cracks	Normal	Focal hyperkeratosis on palms and soles	Not mentioned	—	—	Motor and sensory neuropathy
Keratoderma palmoplantare with cystic eyelids, hypodontia and hypotrichosis (Schöpf *et al.*, 1971; Font *et al.*, 1986; Happle & Rampen, 1987; Nordin *et al.*, 1988)	AR	Fragile with longitudinal and oblique furrows	Sparse on vertex	—	Hypodontia	—	Cyst on upper and lower eyelids. Senile cataract	Squamous cell carcinoma on a finger in one patient
Kindler's syndrome (Forman *et al.*, 1989; Hovnanian *et al.*, 1989)	AD, AR or sporadic	Dystrophic	Normal	Poikiloderma gradually appearing with cutaneous atrophy and reticulated pigmentation. Friction blisters in infancy. Hyperkeratosis of palms and soles, often mild	Poor dention can occur	—	—	Photosensitivity in childhood. Gingival fragility. Leukokeratosis. Webbing of digits. Ainhum-like constrictions. Urethral and oesophageal stenoses
Lamellar ichthyosis (ichthyosiformis erythroderma)	AR	Thick-striated subungual hyperkeratosis. Can be normal or absent	Normal	Ichthyosis on erythemic skin. Hyperhidrosis of soles and palms	Normal	—	Ectropion. Corneal dystrophies. Photophobia	Occasionally small stature and mental retardation (see BIDS syndrome)
Olmsted's syndrome (Poulin *et al.*, 1984; Atherton *et al.*, 1990)	AD	Thick, transversal, rigid. Subungual hyperkeratosis	Alopecia or hypohidrosis	Keratotic plaques around body orifices and in groins. Linear keratosis of flexor surfaces, later mutilating contractions of fingers. Anhidrosis. Constricting bands on fingers	Premolar can be lacking	Audio-gram abnormal for higher fre-quencies	—	Leukokeratosis. Hyperlaxity of joints. Atresia of distal phalanges
Pachyonychia congenita (Jadassohn & Lewandowsky, 1906; Thomas *et al.*, 1984)	AD	Yellow or brown at age 3–5 months, followed by thickening of nail bed. Paronychia common. Onycholysis	Normal	Hyperhidrosis palmoplantare. Follicular hyperkeratosis with hyperpigmentation Leukokeratosis of tongue. Steatocystoma multiplex may occur	Natal teeth caries or normal	Deafness	Cataract and corneal dyskeratosis	Short statute. mental retardation. Hoarseness
Pachyonychia congenita with amyloidosis and hyperpigmentation (Buckly & Cassuto,	AD	Thick and discoloured in infancy but improving in adulthood	Normal	Diffuse rippled and macular. Hyperpigmentation of neck, axilla, trunk, thighs and	Normal	Normal	Normal	—

continued

Table 9.1. *Continued*

Condition	Inheritance	Nails	Hair	Skin with hyperkeratosis palmoplantaris+	Teeth	Ear	Eye	Other findings
1962; Tidman *et al.*, 1987)				popliteal fossa. Fading when adult. Amyloid deposits in papillary dermis of hyperpigmented areas				
Pachyonychia congenita (Jackson & Lawler, 1951; Clementi *et al.*, 1986)	AD	Very thick subungual hyperkeratosis at early age	Dry, sometimes alopecia	Palmar and plantar hyperhidrosis. Follicular keratosis	Teeth present at birth	—	—	Epidermoid cysts
Pachyonychia congenita with leuconychia (Haber & Rose, 1986)	AR	Proximal leuconychia with obliteration of lunula after age 12. Mild onycholysis of toes with slight elevation of nailplate	—	Bulla on plantar surface. Punctate keratoderma. Hyperkeratotic papules on dorsa of toes and fingers. Angular cheilitis	Normal	Normal	Normal	—
Trichothiodystrophy IBDS or Tay syndrome (Jorizzo *et al.*, 1982)	AR	Thick, convex curvature subungual hyperkeratosis	Brittle, short, trichoschizis, trichorrhexis nodosa in some	Collodion baby. Ichthyosisform erythroderma	Normal	Normal	Punctate cataracts. Nystagmus	Intellectual impairment common. Decreased fertility. Short stature common Poor motor coordination. Hypogonadism Photosensitivity (PIBIDS)

Table 9.2. Ectodermal dysplasias with nail and teeth changes: hair and skin often involved. Inheritances are indicated as follows: AD, autosomal dominant; AR, autosomal recessive; XR, sex-linked recessive

Condition	Inheritance	Nails	Hair	Skin	Teeth	Ear	Eye	Other findings
AEC syndrome (Hay & Wells, 1976; Schwayder *et al.*, 1986)	AD	Absent or dystrophic	Partial or complete loss	Dry. Partial anhidrosis, often thick palms and soles	Widely spaced	Auricular deformities common	Ankyloblepharon. Lacrimal duct atresia	Cleft lip and palate. Syndactyly, supernumerary nipples
ADULT syndrome (Propping & Zerres, 1983)	AD	Concave Dysplastic	Thin	Excessive freckling	Hypodontia Loss of teeth	—	Obstruction of lacrimal duct	Ectrodactyly
ANOTHER syndrome (see p. 298) (Pike *et al.*, 1986)	AR	Ridged, fragile, brittle	Thin, sparse	Dry. Hypohidrosis	Hypodontia. Conical teeth	Conductive hearing deficit. Otitis media	—	Respiratory tract infection. Infantile hypothyroidism. Absent breast tissue
Anhidrotic ED. Christ–Siemens–Touraine syndrome (Pinheiro *et al.*, 1981; Sybert, 1989) pp. 298, 307–8	XR	Often normal. May be dystrophic	Thin, sparse on scalp and body	Thin, dry shiny. No or decreased sweating. Dermoglyphic changes	Delayed eruption. Hypodontia. Peg shaped, conical	Hearing loss may occur	—	Saddle shaped nose. Small nostrils. Oral dryness causes hoarseness
AREDYLD syndrome (Pinheiro *et al.*, 1983)	?	Transverse and longitudinal	Hypotrichosis	Reduced sweating	Hypodontia Anodontia	—	—	Diabetes and hypomastia
Chondroectodermal dysplasia (Ellis & van Creveld, 1940; Christian *et al.*, 1980)	AR	Dystrophic koilonychia	Sparse, thin, brittle and hypochromic	Normal	Natal teeth in 25%. Hypodontia. Oligodontia Conically crowned	—	—	Broad nose, Short limbs. Polydactyly. Fusion of bones. Respiratory difficulties and heart defects common
Chondroectodermal dysplasia (Curry & Hall, 1979; Shapiro *et al.*, 1984)	AD	As above + nails splitting	Normal	Normal	As above	—	—	As above
Coffin–Siris syndrome (Coffin & Siris, 1970; Carey & Hall, 1978;	AD	Fifth finger and toenails hypoplastic or	Sparse on scalp eyebrows and lashes.	Dermatoglyphic changes	Delayed eruption. Microdontia	—	—	Thick lips. Low nasal bridge. Microcephaly.

continued on p. 308

Table 9.2. *Continued*

Condition	Inheritance	Nails	Hair	Skin	Teeth	Ear	Eye	Other findings
Lucaya *et al.*, 1981; Patel *et al.*, 1987)		absent, other nails sometimes hypoplastic (Fig. 9.3)	Hirsutism of limbs, forehead and back					Psychomotor and growth retardation. Absence or hypoplasia of distal phalanges especially of finger 5 and toe 5. Patellae dysplasia. Respiratory infections
Congenital hypoparathyroidism (Moshkowitz *et al.*, 1969; Braverman, 1981)	—	Distal half brittle. Irregular grooves. Onychorrhexia. Leuconychia	Normal	Normal	Malocclusion caries. Loss of enamel	—	Cataract	Hypoparathyroidism. Epilepsy
Dentooculocutaneous syndrome (Ackerman *et al.*, 1973)	AR	Horizontal ridging with distal onychoschizia	Scanty, no beard	Indurated and hyperpigmented over finger joints	Taurodont, pyramidal or fused molar roots	—	Juvenile glaucoma. Ectropion lower lids	Upper lip lacking. Cupid bow. Philtrum thick and wide. Syndactyly. Clinodactyly
Fried's tooth and nail syndrome (Fried, 1977)	AR	Thin on finger. On toes also small and concave	Fine, short and scanty eyebrows	Hypodontia peg-shaped	—	—	—	Prominent lip and chin. Cleft lip, brachial cyst on the neck
Hay – Wells syndrome; see AEC syndrome								
Hypohidrotic ED (Marshall, 1958; Passarge *et al.*, 1966; Gorlin *et al.*, 1970)	AR	As above or koilonychia AEC?	As above	Mild hypohidrosis	Adontia or normal teeth	Hearing loss may occur	Cataract myopia	As above
Hypohidrotic ED with multiple anomalies (Rapp & Hodgkin, 1968; Schroeder & Sybert, 1987; O'Donnell & James, 1992)	AD	Small, disfigured with distal soft tissue. Subungual keratosis	On scalp sparse, short, slow growing, wiry. Body hair sparse or lacking	Hypohidrosis	Slow development. Hypodontia conically shaped. Caries	—	Aplasia of lacrimal punctate	As above + short stature + cleft lip and palate. Hypospadias. Syndactyly
Odontoonychodysplasia with alopecia (Pinheiro *et al.*, 1985)	AR	Fragile and brittle with a subungual corneal layer	Almost total alopecia. Absent axillary and pubic hair. Abnormal dermatoglyphics	Mild palmoplantar keratosis. One or more café au lait spots	Micro- and hypodentia. Widely spaced teeth with hypoplastic enamel		—	Syndactyly. Irregular arreata mammae
Popliteal pterygium syndrome (Gorlin *et al.*, 1976; Escobar & Weaver, 1978)	AD	Dystrophic longitudinal stria. Brittle. Subungual hyperkeratosis	Hypotrichosis. No eyebrows or eyelashes. Fair and depigmented	Hypohidrosis. Cutaneous folds on limbs	Microdontia. Conical	Hypoplasia or earlobes	Black iris	Hare lip. Supernumary nipples. Right thumb lacking. Alteration of genitalia. Popliteal and perianal pterygia
Salamon syndrome (Salamon *et al.*, 1967)	AR	Dystrophic	Sparse, dry lustreless. Pili torti. Trichorhexis nodosa	Normal	Hypodontia. Microdontia	—	Chronic blepharoconjunctivitis. Punctate keratitis. Atrophia retina. Trichiasis palpebra	Piriform nose. Slight osteoporosis of arms and legs
Tooth and nail syndrome (Witkop *et al.*, 1975; Kinch *et al.*, 1983)	AD	Small and spoon-shaped. Slow growth in children. Longitudinal ridging	Fine and brittle	Dry. Wrinkles in face	Hypodontia. Cone shaped. Widely spaced	Big ears	—	Everted lips
Variant of above (Ellis & Dawber, 1980)	AD	As above. Nail fold thick	Fine and brittle	Reduced palmar sweat duct potency	As above	Big ears	—	Mental retardation
Tricho-donto-osseous (TDO) syndrome. Enamel hypoplasia and curly hair (Robinson *et al.*, 1966; Lichtenstein *et al.*, 1972)	AD	Flat, thick, malformed, striated. Break off easily	Thick with short curls. Dry and rough	Normal	Small pitted, widely spaced. Caries. Hypoplastic enamel	—	—	Sclerosteosis especially of the skull

continued

Table 9.2. *Continued*

Condition	Inheritance	Nails	Hair	Skin	Teeth	Ear	Eye	Other findings
Tricho-odonto-onycho dermal (TOOD) syndrome (Pinheiro *et al.*, 1981, 1983, 1985, 1990)	AR	Dystrophic nails, some absent	Hypotrichosis	Dry, atrophic, poikiloderma like spots. Palmar keratosis	Delayed eruption. Hypodontia. Enamel hypoplasia. Abnormal shape. Supernumerary teeth	—	—	Microstomia. Thin lips. Hypoplastic nose. Eyelids hyperpigmented. Absent nipple. Phalangeal changes
Tricho-rhino-phalangeal syndrome I (TRP I) (Giedion, 1967; Parizel *et al.*, 1987)	AD and AR	Thin, short with stria. Flattened thumbnail. Koilonychia	Sparse, blond fine and slow growing. Eyebrows laterally sparse	Normal	Supernumerary, peg-shaped	—	—	Prominent lip and chin. Pear-shaped nose. Short fingers. Brachial cyst on the neck. Cleft lip seen. High arched palate
Tricho-rhino-phalangeal syndrome II (TRP II) (Langer *et al.*, 1984; Sánchez *et al.*, 1985; Bühler *et al.*, 1987)	AR	Thin, short with stria. Flattened thumbnail. Koilonychia	Sparse, blond fine and slow growing. Eyebrows laterally sparse	Normal	Supernumerary, peg-shaped	—	—	As above + multiple exostosis
Triphalangy of thumbs and toes (Qazi & Smithwick, 1970)	AR	Hypoplastic	Normal	Dermatoglyphic abnormalities	Widely spaced. Poorly formed	—	—	Three phalanges in both thumbs and big toes. Hypoplasia of distal phalanges
Xeroderma, talipes and enamel defect (XTE) syndrome (Moynahan, 1970)	AD	Small malformed	Dry, slow growing. No lower lashes	Hypohidrosis	Yellow enamel	—	Photophobic	Clubfoot. Oligophrenia

Table 9.3. Ectodermal dysplasia with hair and/or skin changes but without dental changes. Inheritances are indicated as follows: AD, autosomal dominant; AR, autosomal recessive; XL, sex-linked transmission; XD, sex-linked dominant

Condition	Inheritance	Nails	Hair	Skin	Teeth	Ear	Eye	Other findings
Aplasia cutis congenita. See focal dermal hypoplasia								
Aplasia cutis with dystrophic nails (Harari *et al.*, 1976)	?	Short thin grey nail plate. Longitudinal stria. Some onychogryphotic	Normal	Aplasia cutis of scalp and/or trunk	Normal	—	—	—
Apical dysplasia of fingers (Dodinval, 1972)	AD	Transverse depressions	Normal	Epidermal dysplastic ridges. Fingerpads hypoplastic with painful chaps	Normal	—	—	—
Atrichia with nail dystrophy (Vogt *et al.*, 1988)	AR	Distal parts dystrophic and brittle	Alopecia. A few pigmented short hairs on scalp. Eyebrows and lashes sparse	Normal	Normal	—	—	Moderate retardation with delayed speaking. Abnormal facies with depressed nasal bridge, hypertelorism and long philtrums
BIDS, IBIDS and PIBIDS syndromes; see trichothiodystrophy (Tables 9.1 and 9.3)								
CHANDS syndrome (curly hair, ankyloblepharon, nail dysplasias) (Baughman, 1971; Toriello *et al.*, 1979)	AR	Small, hypoplastic	Curly	Normal	Normal	—	Ankyloblepharon	Ataxia
Chondrodysplasia punctata (Happle, 1979; O'Brien, 1990)	XD	Flattened and split into layers (Fig. 9.9)	Circumscribed alopecia. Trichorrhexis nodosa. Sparse lashes and eyebrows	Ichthyosis. Athrophoderma. Pseudopelade. Pigmentary changes	Normal	Dysplastic auricles described	Cataract common. Epicanthus. Nystagmus and hazy cornea also described	Flat nose bridge and peculiar shape of face. Malformation of limbs and vertebral column

continued on p. 310

Table 9.3. *Continued*

Condition	Inheritance	Nails	Hair	Skin	Teeth	Ear	Eye	Other findings
DOO syndrome (Feinmesser & Zelig, 1961)	AD	Onychodystrophy since birth. Nails do not grow	Normal or alopecia	Abnormal dermatoglyphics. Spiny hyperkeratosis	Normal	Deafness	—	Osteodystrophy (phalangeal)
DOOR syndrome (Walbaum, 1970; Cantwell, 1975; Qazi & Nangia, 1984; Patton *et al.*, 1987)	AR	Onychodystrophy. since birth. Nails do not grow	Normal or alopecia	Abnormal dermatoglyphics. Spiny hyperkeratosis	Normal	Deafness	—	Osteodystrophy. Mental retardation seizures. Increase of 2-oxyglutarate
ED with onychogryphosis (Freire-Maia *et al.*, 1975)	—	Severe onychogryphosis	Eyebrows lacking, scarce eyelashes	Dry. Hypohidrosis. Follicular hyperkeratosis, hyper- and hypochromic spots	Normal	—	Nuclear cataract	Psychomotor and growth retardation. Frontal bossing. Depressed bridge of the nose
ED with abnormal papillar ridging (Basan, 1965)	AD	Transverse over-curvature, irregular, atrophic with central fissures and ridging	Normal	Papillar ridging lacking. Abnormal furrows of hands	Normal	—	—	—
Focal dermal hypoplasia. Goltz & Gorlin syndrome (Goltz *et al.*, 1970; Hall & Terezhalmy, 1983; Sybert, 1985; Moore & Mallory, 1989)	XL	Thin, spoon-shaped. Can be absent in 50%	Sparse in focal areas of scalp and pubis	Focal thin skin with herniation of fat. Papilloma, telangiectasis. Linear hypo- and hyperpigmentation. Keratotic lesions in palms and soles in 11%. Epidermolysis bullosa (Jones *et al.*, 1992)	Normal or enamel defects	—	Multiple severe anomalies	Small stature. Asymmetric face. Cranial, spinal and bone anomalies. Cleft lip and palate. Striated pattern of long bones (Larrègue & Duterque, 1975)
Hair-nail dysplasia (Pinheiro & Freire-Maia, 1992)	AD	Short, fragile, spoon-shaped	Thin and fragile, slow growing, sparse	—	—	—	—	—
Hypohidrotic ectodermal dysplasia with hypothyroidism (Pabst *et al.*, 1981; Pike *et al.*, 1986)	AR?	Ridged dystrophic shrivelled appearance	No or scanty hair on scalp. Eyelashes long	Speckled brown pigmentation. Dry skin. Hypohidrosis. Dermographism	Normal	—	Cicatricial conjunctivities in one patient	Hypothyroidism susceptible to respiratory infections
Ichthyosis follicularis with alopecia (Rothe *et al.*, 1990)	AD	Onychodystrophy and paronychia	Total alopecia	Follicular hyperkeratosis. Hyperkeratosis of extensive aspect of hands, knees and elbows. Perineal plaques	Normal	Hearing defect	Photophobia	Angular cheilitis
Ichthyosis follicularis-alopecia-photophobia IFAP syndrome (Martino *et al.*, 1992)	XR?	Dystrophic hyperconvex	Atrichia	Erythematous follicular ichthyosis hypohidrosis	Normal or enamel dysplasia	Large ears	Myopia. Corneal dystrophy	Vertebral defects. Short stature. Megacolon. Renal anomalies. Brain atrophy
Onychotrichodysplasia with neutropenia (Cantú *et al.*, 1975; Hernandez *et al.*, 1979, Verhage *et al.*, 1987)	AR	Hypoplastic. Onychorrhexis. Koilonychia	Trichorrhexis. Dry, short curly, sparse	Mild keratosis follicularis. Thick, wrinkled palms and soles with pustules	Normal	—	Conjunctivitis. Ectropion	No or mild mental retardation. Neutropenia and repeated infections. Sulphur deficient hairs (Itin & Pittelkow, 1990)
Pili torti and onychodysplasia (Calzavara-Pinton *et al.*, 1991)	AR	Dystrophic of distal part	Scalp, beard, pubic and axillary hair broken at 1–10 mm length. Eyebrows, eyelashes and body hair absent	Normal	Normal	Normal	Normal	Facial dysmorphism with long philthrum
Retinal angiomas with hair and nail defects (Tolmie *et al.*, 1988a)	AR	Dysplastic	Sparse	Normal	Normal	Normal	Strabismus. Retinal angioma	Intracranial calcification

continued

Table 9.3. *Continued*

Condition	Inheritance	Nails	Hair	Skin	Teeth	Ear	Eye	Other findings
Thumb deformity and alopecia (Winter *et al.*, 1988)	AD	—	Alopecia	Hyper- and depigmentation in the groin	Single upper. Incisor in some patients	—	—	Short stature. Mental retardation (Chiba & Miura, 1979). Hypoplastic thumbs
Tricho-oculo-dermal vertebral syndrome (Alves *et al.*, 1981)	AR	Thin and brittle fingernails. Toes wide and short with paronychia	Hypotrichosis Dry and rough	Dry. Fissures. Infections. Hyperkeratotic spots, especially on soles. Scaling. Skin webbing of fingers. Dermoglyphic changes	Normal	—	Bilateral nuclear cataract. Narrow palperal fissures. Entropion	Wide nasal bridge and hypoplasia of nasal alae. Micrognathia. Enlarged interphalanged joints. Genu valga. Kyphoscoliosis. Spina bifida oculta
Trichothiodystrophy (Price *et al.*, 1980). BIDS syndrome (see italic letters). (Jackson *et al.*, 1974). Sabin's syndrome (Itin & Pittelkow, 1990) p. 308	AR	Break easily. Do not grow long	*B*rittle, short, trichoschizis, trichorrhexis nodosa in some	Normal or dry	Normal or carious	Normal	Punctate cataracts	*I*ntellectual, impairment common. *D*ecreased fertility. *S*hort stature common. Poor motor coordination
Trichothiodystrophy with PIBI(D)S syndrome (van Neste *et al.*, 1980, 1988; Rebora & Crovato, 1987)	AR	Hypoplastic or dystrophic with spotted leuconychia and lamellar splitting	*B*rittle, short, trichoschizis, trichorrhexis nodosa in some	Normal at birth. Later xerosis or non-congenital *i*chthyosis vulgaris. Xeroderma pigmentosum	—	Neurosensory loss	Nystagmus, Myopia, Retinal dystrophia can occur	*I*ntellectual impairment. *S*hort stature. Smiling outgoing personality. *P*hotosensitivity
Trichothiodystrophy with transient immunodeficiency (Baden & Katz, 1988)	—	Short with horizontal splitting. Thin and often spoon-shaped	Short, sparse or uneven length	Normal	Normal	Normal	Normal	Transient immunodeficiency in one patient, otherwise healthy
Trichothiodystrophy with neutropenia (see onychotrichodysplastic with neutropenia)								

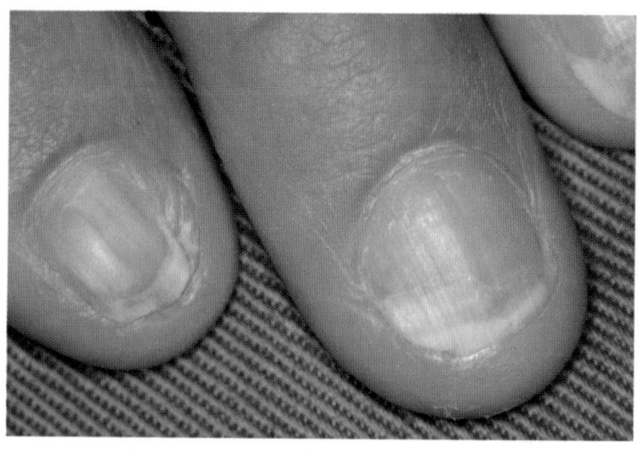

Fig. 9.14. Hypohidrotic ectodermal dysplasia – nail dystrophy.

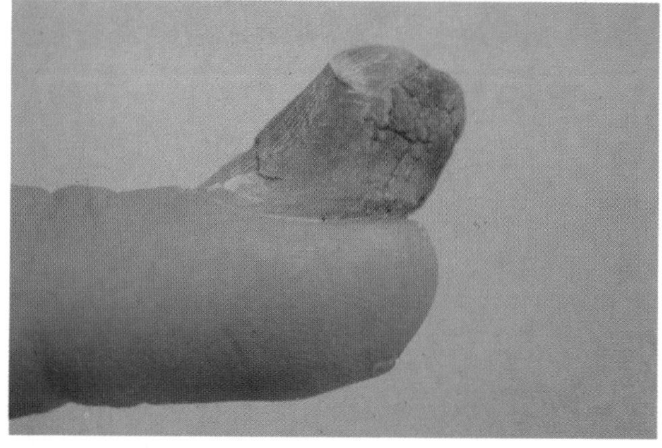

Fig. 9.15. Pachyonychia congenita.

Type II has clinical findings as in type I but also bullae and hyperhidrosis of palms and soles, early dentition and steatocystoma multiplex.

Type III occurs in 12% of the patients and has in addition angular cheilosis, corneal dyskeratosis and cataracts. Type IV (7%) has these features plus laryngeal lesions, hoarseness, mental retardation and hair anomalies.

The differential diagnosis can be epidermolysis bullosa, onychogryphosis, psoriasis and oral thrush but the presence of thick wedge-shaped, pinched-up or claw-like nails with yellowish-brown pigmentation together with other symptoms rarely offers any diagnostic problems.

Treatment with retinoids has been tried with, as a rule, only moderate improvement of skin and nail lesions, but positive results have also been reported (Hoting &

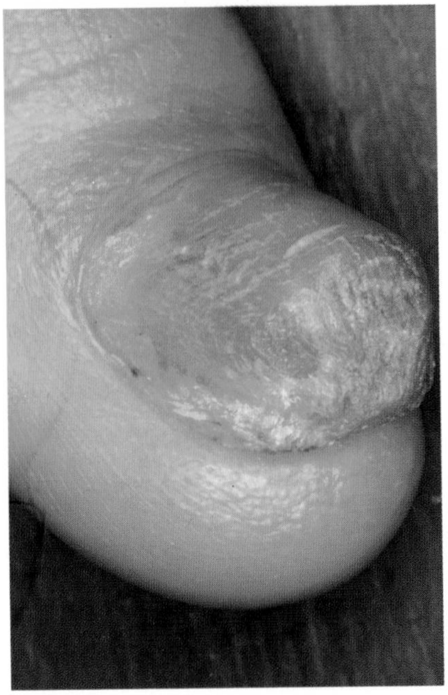

Fig. 9.16. Pachyonychia congenita.

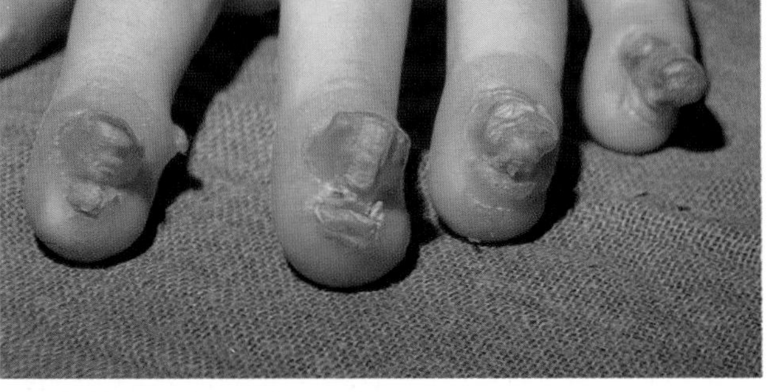

Fig. 9.17. Pachyonychia congenita.

Wassilew, 1985). Distal avulsion with nail bed scarification and matrix destruction is needed to prevent growth of nails. Areas of ulceration should be observed for possible skin malignancy (Su *et al.*, 1990).

Dyskeratosis congenita (Zinser–Engman–Cole syndrome)

Here one finds short and atrophic fingernails appearing after late childhood. The nail changes are progressive and the nails may later be lost (Fig. 9.18). At the same time appear crops of vesicles in the mouth which ulcerate and leave an atrophic mucosa. There is palmar hyperkeratosis and hyperhidrosis and almost always a reticulated hyperpigmentation of the face, neck and chest. The complete syndrome is not apparent until the second or third decade of life (Connor & Teague, 1981; Kalb *et al.*, 1986; Ogden *et al.*, 1988). Continuous lacrimation due to atresia of the

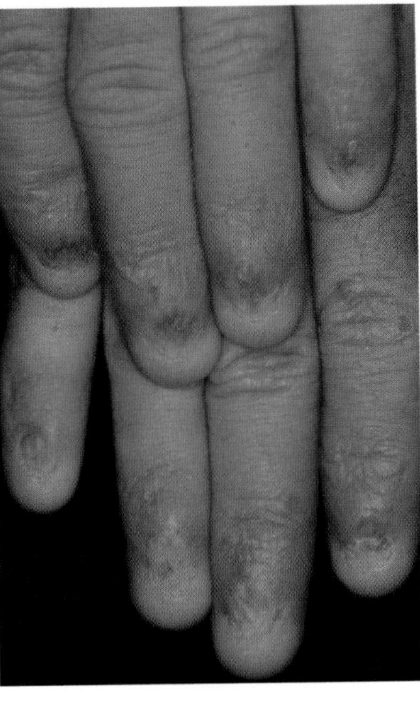

Fig. 9.18. Dyskeratosis congenita.

lacrimal duct and thickened fissured mucosal leukoplakia are common not only in the mouth but also in the oesophagus, anus, urethra and vagina. There is a high risk of developing early malignancy in these lesions and frequent biopsies are often needed. Dental caries and early loss of teeth is seen. The eye manifestations are epiphora, fundus changes, blepharitis and loss of eyelashes. The ear manifestations include transparent tympanic membrane, meatal atresia and malformations of the middle ear. Intracranial calcification and increased fragility of bones have been reported. Abnormal immunology with haematopoietic disorders occur in 50% of patients in the second and third decades and may be the presenting changes. The manifestations include anaemia, bone marrow hypoplasia, thrombocytopenia and pancytopenia (Dodd *et al.*, 1985).

The inheritance is X-linked recessive and the gene has been assigned to Xq28 by linkage of DNA markers (Connor *et al.*, 1986).

Trichothiodystrophy

Several types of this rare disorder with sulphur-deficient brittle hair have been described. In addition the patients frequently have nail dysplasia, splitting and koilonychia (Fig. 9.19) as well as symptoms from skin and other organs such as mental and growth retardation. Trichothiodystrophy was associated with keratodermia in the IBDS or Tay syndrome (Table 9.1). In other types the palms and soles could be thickened and fissured, but keratodermia is not mentioned in the review of 95 cases by Itin and Pittelkow (1990). Minor dental abnormalities such as caries were mentioned in 10% of the cases: we have therefore listed these disorders in Table 9.3. Recently

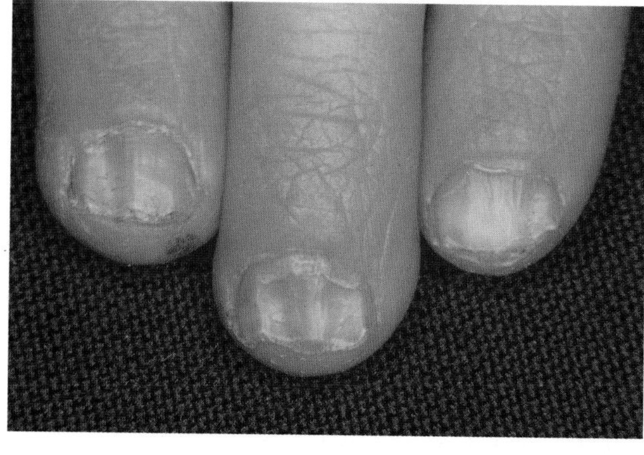

Fig. 9.19. Trichothiodystrophy (thin nails and slight koilonychia).

Itin and Pittelkow (1991) described sulphur-deficient hair in a patient who also had neutropenia. Such a syndrome has earlier been described (but not examined for sulphur) as onychotrichodysplasia with neutropenia (Table 9.3) by Cantu *et al.* (1975), Hernandez *et al.* (1979) and Verhage *et al.* (1987). It is possible therefore that the family of trichothiodystrophies will increase in the future as more cases with hair anomalies are examined for sulphur content.

References

Ackerman J.L., Ackerman A.L. & Ackerman A.B. (1973) A new dental ocular and cutaneous syndrome. *Int. J. Dermatol.* **12**, 285.

Alves A.F.P., dos Santos P.A.B., Castelo-Branco-Neto E. & Freire-Maia N. (1981) Brief clinical report: An autosomal recessive ectodermal dysplasia syndrome of hypotrichosis, onychodysplasia, hyperkeratosis, kyphoscoliosis, cataract, and other manifestations. *Am. J. Med. Genet.* **10**, 213.

Ando Y., Tanaka T., Horiguchi Y., Ikai K. & Tomono H. (1988) Hidrotic ectodermal dysplasia: A clinical and ultrastructural observation. *Dermatologica* **176**, 205.

Atherton D.J., Sutton C. & Jones B.M. (1990) Mutilating palmoplantar keratoderma with periorificial keratotic plaques (Olmsted's syndrome). *Br. J. Dermatol.* **122**, 245.

Baden H.P. & Katz A. (1988) Trichothiodystrophy without retardation: One patient exhibiting transient combined immunodeficiency syndrome. *Pediatr. Dermatol.* **5**, 257.

Bart R.S. & Pumphrey R.E. (1967) Knuckle pads, leukonychia and deafness. A dominantly inherited syndrome. *N. Engl. J. Med.* **276**, 202.

Basan M. (1965) Ektodermale Dysplasie. Fehlendes Papillarmuster Nagelveraenderungen und Vierfingerfurche. *Arch. Klin. Exp. Dermatol.* **222**, 546.

Baughman F.A. Jr (1971) CHANDS: the curly hair-ankyloblepharon–nail dysplasia syndrome. *Birth Defects* **7**, 100.

Berg D., Weingold D.H., Abson K.G. & Olsen E.A. (1990) Sweating in ectodemal dysplasia syndromes. *Arch. Dermatol.* **126**, 1075.

Bergman R. & Friedman-Birnbaum R. (1988) Papillon–Lefevre syndrome: a study of the long-term clinical course of recurrent pyogenic infections and the effects of etretinate treatment. *Br. J. Dermatol.* **119**, 731.

Bhatia K.K., Chaudhary S., Pahwa U.S. & Mehrotra G.C. (1989) Keratoma hereditaria mutilans (Vohwinkel's disease) with congenital alopecia universalis (atrichia congenita). *J. Dermatol.* **16**, 231.

Boss J.M., Matthews C.N.A., Peachey R.D.G. & Summerly R. (1981) Speckled hyperpigmentation, palmo-plantar punctate keratoses and childhood blistering: a clinical triad, with variable associations. A report of two families. *Br. J. Dermatol.* **105**, 579.

Breslau–Siderius E.J., Toonstra J., Baart J.A., Koppeschaar H.P.F., Maassen J.A. & Beemer F.A. (1992) Ectodermal dysplasia, lipoatrophy, diabetes mellitus and amastia: A second case of the AREDYLD syndrome. *Am. J. Med. Genet.* **44**, 374.

Braverman I.M. (1981) In: *Skin Signs of Systemic Disease*, 2nd edn, p. 640. W.B. Saunders, Philadelphia.

Buckly W.R. & Cassuto J. (1962) Pachyonychia congenita. *Arch. Dermatol.* **85**, 397.

Bühler E.M., Bühler U.K., Beutler C. & Fessler R. (1987) A final word on the trichorhino-phalangeal syndromes. *Clin. Genet.* **31**, 273.

Bureau Y., Barrière H. & Thomas M. (1959) Hippocratisme digital congénital avec hyperkératose palmo-plantaire et troubles osseux. *Ann. Dermatol. Venereol.* **86**, 611.

Calzavara-Pinton P., Carlino A., Benetti A. & de Panfilis G. (1991) Pilitorti and onychodysplasia. Report of a previously underscribed hidrotic ectodermal dysplasia. *Dermatologica* **182**, 184.

Cantú J.M., Arias J., Foncerada M. *et al.* (1975) Syndrome of onycho-trichodysplasia with chronic neutropenia in an infant from con-sanguineous parents. *Birth Defects: Original Article Series* **XI**, 2.63.

Cantwell R.J. (1975) Congenital sensori-neural deafness associated with onycho-osteo-dystrophy and mental retardation (DOOR syndrome). *Humangenetik* **26**, 261.

Carey J.C. & Hall B.D. (1978) The Coffin-Siris syndrome. Five new cases including two siblings. *Am. J. Dis. Child.* **132**, 667.

Cat I., Costa O. & Freire-Maia N. (1972) Odontotrichomelic hypohidrotic dysplasia. A clinical reappraisal. *Hum. Hered.* **22**, 91.

Cecatto de Lima L., Pinheiro M. & Freire-Maia N. (1988) Oculotricho-dysplasia (OTD): a new probably autosomal recessive condition. *J. Med. Genet.* **25**, 430.

Chiba A. & Miura T. (1979) A family with hypotrichosis associated with congenital hypoplasia of the thumb. *Japan J. Genet.* **24**, 111.

Christan J.C., Dexter R.N., Palmer C.G. & Muller J. (1980) A family with three recessive traits and homozygosity for a long 9gh + chromosome segment. *Am. J. Med. Genet.* **6**, 301.

Clementi M., Cardin de Stefani E., Dei Rossi C., Avventi V. & Tenconi R. (1986) Pachyonychia congenita Jackson-Lawler type: a distinct malformation syndrome. *Br. J. Dermatol.* **114**, 367.

Clouston H.R. (1929) A hereditary ectodermal dystrophy. *Can. Med. Assoc. J.* **21**, 10.

Cockayne E.A. (1936) Cleft palate-lip, hare lip, dacrocystitis, and cleft hand and foot. *Biometrika* **28**, 60.

Coffin G.S. & Siris E. (1970) Mental retardation with absent fifth fingernail and terminal phalanx. *Am. J. Dis. Child.* **119**, 433.

Colcott-Fox T. (1897) Symmetrical hyperkeratosis of the nail beds of the hands and feet and other areas chiefly on the

palms and soles. *Clin. Soc. Trans. (London)* **30**, 242.
Connor J.M. & Teague R.H. (1981) Dyskeratosis congenita. Report of a large kindred. *Br. J. Dermatol.* **105**, 321.
Connor J.M., Gatherer D., Gray F.C., Pirrit A. & Affara N.A. (1986) Assignment of the gene for dyskeratosis congenita to Xq28. *Hum. Genet.* **72**, 348.
Crosti C., Sala F., Bertani E., Gasparini G. & Menni S. (1983) Leuconychie totale et dysplasie ectodermique. Observation de deux cas. *Ann. Dermatol. Venereol.* **110**, 617.
Curry C.J.R. & Hall B.P. (1979) Polydactyly, conical teeth, nail dysplasia, and short limbs: A new autosomal dominant malformation syndrome. *J. Bone Joint Surg.* **53B**, 101.
de Berker D. & Kavanagh G. (1993) Distinctive nail changes in scleroatrophy of Huriez. *Br. J. Dermatol.* **129** (Suppl. 42) 36.
Dodd H.J., Devereux S. & Sarkany J. (1985) Dyskeratosis congenita with pancytopenia. *Clin. Exp. Dermatol.* **10**, 73.
Dodinval P. (1972) The dysplasia of epidermal ridges revisited. Evidence of an apical dysplasia of the fingers. *Humangenetik* **15**, 20.
Ellis J. & Dawber R.P.R. (1980) Ectodermal dysplasia syndrome: a family study. *Clin. Exp. Dermatol.* **5**, 295.
Ellis R.W.B. & van Creveld S. (1940) A syndrome characterized by ectodermal dysplasia, polydactyly, chondro-dysplasia and congenital morbus cordis: Report of three cases. *Arch. Dis. Child.* **15**, 65.
Escobar V. & Weaver D.D. (1978) The facio-genito-popliteal syndrome. *Birth Defects: Original Article Series* **XIV**, 6B: 185.
Feinmesser M. & Zelig S. (1961) Congenital deafness associated with onychodystrophy. *Arch. Otolaryng.* **74**, 507.
Feinstein A., Friedman J. & Schewach-Millet M.S. (1988) Pachyonychia congenita. *J. Am. Acad. Dermatol.* **19**, 705.
Font R.L., Seabury Stone M., Schanzer M.C. & Lewis R.A. (1986) Apocrine hidrocystomas of the lids, hypodontia, palmar-plantar hyperkeratosis, and onychodystrophy – A new variant of ectodermal dysplasia. *Arch. Ophthalmol.* **104**, 1811.
Forman A.B., Prendiville J.S., Esterly N.B., Herbert A.A. *et al.* (1989) Kindler syndrome: Report of two cases and review of the literature. *Pediatr. Dermatol.* **6**, 91.
Freire-Maia N. (1977) Ectodermal dysplasias revisited. *Acta Genet. Med. (Roma)* **26**, 121.
Freire-Maia N. & Pinheiro M. (1984) *Ectodermal Dysplasias, a Clinical and Genetic Study.* Alan R. Liss, New York.
Freire-Maia N. & Pinheiro M. (1988) Ectodermal dysplasias – some recollections and a classifications. *Birth Defects: Original Article Series* **24**, 3.
Freire-Maia N., Fortes V.A., Pereira L.C., Opitz J.M., Marcallo F.A. & Cavalli I.J. (1975) A syndrome of hypohidrotic ectodermal dysplasia with normal teeth, peculiar facies, pigmentary disturbances, psychomotor and growth retardation, bilateral nuclear cataract, and other signs. *J. Med. Genet.* **12**, 308.
Freire-Maia N., Cat I. & Rapone Gaidzinsky R. (1977) An ectodermal dysplasia syndrome of alopecia, onychodysplasia, hypohidrosis, hyperkeratosis, deafness and other manifestations. *Hum. Hered.* **27**, 127.
Fried K. (1977) Autosomal recessive hydrotic ectodermal dysplasia. *J. Med. Genet.* **14**, 137.
Gamborg Nielsen P. (1983) Mutilating palmo-plantar keratoderma. *Acta Derm. Venereol. (Stockh.)* **63**, 365.
Garrick-Wilson A. (1905) Three cases of hereditary hyperkeratosis of the nail bed. *Br. J. Dermatol.* **17**, 13.
Giedion A. (1967) Cone-shaped epiphyses of the hands and their diagnostic value: The tricho-rhino-phalangeal syndrome. *Ann. Radiol. (Paris)* **10**, 322.
Goltz R.W., Henderson R.R., Hitch J.M. & Ott J.E. (1970) Focal dermal hypoplasia syndrome. *Arch. Dermatol.* **101**, 1.
Gorlin R.J., Sedano H. & Anderson V.E. (1964) The syndrome of palmar-plantar hyperkeratosis and premature periodontal destruction of the teeth. *J. Pediatr.* **65**, 895.
Gorlin R.J., Old T. & Anderson V.A. (1970) Hypohidrotic ectodermal dysplasia in females: A critical analysis and argument for genetic heterogeneity. *Z. Kinderheilk* **108**, 1.
Gorlin R.J., Pindborg J.J. & Cohen M.M. (1976) *Syndromes of the Head and Neck*, 2nd edn. McGraw-Hill, New York.
Haber R.M. & Rose T.H. (1986) Autosomal recessive pachyonychia congenita. *Arch. Dermatol.* **122**, 919.
Hall E.M. & Terezhalmy G.I. (1983) Case report and literature review. *J. Am. Acad. Dermatol.* **9**, 443.
Haneke E. (1979) The Papillon–Lefèvre syndrome: Keratosis palmoplantaris with periodontopathy. *Hum. Genet.* **51**, 1.
Haneke E. (1987) Hidrotic ectodermal dysplasias. In: *Pediatric Dermatology*, eds Happle R. & Grosshans E. Springer-Verlag, Berlin.
Happle R. (1979) X-linked dominant chondrodysplasia punctata. *Humangenetik* **53**, 65.
Happle R. & Rampen F.H.J. (1987) Multiple eyelid hidrocystoma syndrome: a new cancer syndrome? Proc 17 World Congr. Dermatol. (Berlin) Clinical Dermatology p. 290. Eds. Wilkinson D.S., Mascaro J.M., Orfanos C.E. & Schattawer, Stuttgart.
Harari Z., Pasmanik A., Dvoretzky I., Schewach-Millet M. & Fischer B.K. (1976) Aplasia cutis congenita with dystrophic nail changes. *Dermatologica* **153**, 363.
Hay R.J. & Wells R.S. (1976) The syndrome of ankyloblepharon, ectodermal defects and cleft lip and palate: an autosomal dominant condition. *Br. J. Dermatol.* **94**, 277.
Heimer W.L., Brauner G. & James W.D. (1992) Dermatopathia pigmentosa reticularis: A report of a family demonstrating autosomal dominant inheritance. *J. Am. Acad. Dermatol.* **26**, 298.
Hernandez A., Olivares F. & Cantu J.M. (1979) Autosomal recessive onychotrichodysplasia, chronic neutropenia and mild mental retardation. *Clin. Genet.* **15**, 147.
Hollister D.W., Klein S.N., de Jager H.J., Lachman R.S. & Rimoin D.L. (1973) The lacrimo-auriculo-dento-digital syndrome. *J. Pediatr.* **83**, 438.
Hoting E. & Wassilew S.W. (1985) Systemische Retinoidtherapie mit Etretinat bei Pachyonychia congenita. *Hautarzt* **36**, 526.
Hovnanian A., Blanchet-Bardon C. & de Prost Y. (1989) Poikiloderma of Thereas Kindler: Report of a case with Ultrastructural study, and review of the literature. *Pediatr. Dermatol.* **6**, 82.
Huriez C.L., Deminati M., Agache P., Delmas-Marsalet Y. & Mennecier M. (1969) Génodermatose scléro-atrophiante et kéeratodermique des extrémitées. *Ann. Dermatol. Syph. (Paris)* **6**, 135.
Iraci S., Bianchi L. & Gatti S. (1993) Pachynychia congenita syndrome: A case with late definition. *Clin. Exp. Dermatol.* in press.
Itin P.H. & Pittelkow M.R. (1990) Trichothiodystrophy: Review of sulfur-deficient brittle hair syndromes and association with the ectodermal dysplasias. *J. Am. Acad. Dermatol.* **22**, 705.
Itin P.H. & Pittelkow M.R. (1991) Trichothiodystrophy with chronic neutropenia and mild mental retardation. *Arch. Dermatol.* **24**, 356.
Jackson A.D.M. & Lawler S.D. (1951) Pachyonychia congenita: a report of six cases in one family. *Ann. Eugen (Lond.)* **16**, 141.

Jackson C.E., Eiss L. & Watson J.H.L. (1974) 'Brittle' hair with short stature; intellectual impairment and decreased fertility: An autosomal recessive syndrome in an amish kindred. *Pediatrics* **54**, 201.

Jadassohn J. & Lewandowsky F. (1906) Pachyonychia congenita. *Ikonogr. Dermatol.* **1**, 29.

Jones E.M., Hersch J.H. & Yusk J.W. (1992) Aplasia cutis congenita, cleft palate, epidermolysis bullosa, and ectrodactyly. A new syndrome? *Pediatr. Dermatol.* **9**, 293.

Jorizzo J.L., Atherton D.J., Crounse R.G. & Wells R.S. (1982) Ichthyosis, brittle hair, impaired intelligence, decreased fertility and short stature (I.B.D.S. syndrome) *Br. J. Dermatol.* **106**, 705.

Kalb R.E., Grossman M.E. & Hutt C. (1986) Avascular necrosis of bone in dyskeratosis congenita. *Am. J. Med.* **80**, 511.

Knudtzon J. & Aarskog D. (1987) Growth hormone deficiency associated with the ectrodactyly-ectodermal dysplasia-clefting syndrome and isolated absent septum pellucidum. *Pediatrics* **79**, 410.

Langer K., Konrad K. & Wolff K. (1990) Keratitis, ichthyosis and deafness (KID)-syndrome: report of three cases and a review of the literature. *Br. J. Dermatol.* **122**, 689.

Langer L.O., Krassikoff N., Laxova R. *et al.* (1984) The tricho-rhino-phalangeal syndrome with exostoses (or Langer-Gideon syndrome): Four additional patients without mental retardation and review of the literature. *Am. J. Med. Genet.* **19**, 81.

Larregue M. & Duterque M. (1975) Striated osteopathy in focal dermal hypoplasia. *Arch. Dermatol.* **111**, 1365.

Leibowitz M.R. & Jenkins T. (1984) A newly recognized feature of ectrodactyly, ectodermal dysplasia, clefting (EEC) syndrome: comedone naevus. *Dermatologica* **169**, 80.

Levan N.E. (1961) Congenital defect of thumbnails. *Arch. Dermatol.* **83**, 938.

Lichtenstein J., Warson R. & Jorgenson R. (1972) The tricho-dento-osseous (T.D.O.) syndrome. *Am. J. Hum. Genet.* **24**, 569.

Lucaya J., Garcia-Conesa J.A., Bosch-Banyeras J.M. & Pons-Peadejordi G. (1981) The Coffin-Siris syndrome. A report of four cases and review of the literature. *Pediatr. Radiol.* **11**, 35.

Malfait Y., Decroix J., Vandaele R. & Bourlond A. (1989) Un nouveau cas de syndrome de Goltz. *Ann. Dermatol. Venereol.* **116**, 715.

Marshall D. (1958) Ectodermal dysplasia. Report of a kindred with ocular abnormalities and hearing defect. *Am. J. Ophthalmol.* **45**, 143.

Martino F., D'Eufemia P., Pergola M.S. *et al.* (1992) Child with manifestations of dermotrichic syndrome and ichthyosis follicularis-alopecia-photophobia (IFAP) syndrome. *Am. J. Med. Genet.* **44**, 233.

McGrae J.D. (1990) Keratitis, ichthyosis, and deafness (KID) syndrome. *Int. J. Dermatol.* **29**, 89.

Moon-Adams D. & Slatkin M.H. (1955) Familial pigmentation with dystrophy of the nails. *Arch. Dermatol.* **71**, 591.

Moore D.J. & Mallory S.B. (1989) Goltz syndrome. *Pediatr. Dermatol.* **6**, 251.

Morris C.A., Carey J.C. & Demsey S.A. (1987) Another case. *Proc. Greenwood Genet. Center* **6**, 145.

Moshkowitz A., Abrahamov A. & Pisanti S. (1969) Congenital hypoparathyroidism simulating epilepsy, with other symptoms and dental signs of intra-uterine hypocalcemia. *Pediatrics* **44**, 401.

Murdoch-Kinch C.A., Miles A.D. & Poon C.-K. (1993) Hypodontia and nail dysplasia syndrome. *Oral Surg. Oral Med. Oral Pathol.* **75**, 403.

Müller C. (1904) On the causes of congenital onychogryphosis. *München Med. Wochenscr.* **49**, 2180.

Nazarro V., Blanchet-Bardon C., Mimoz C., Revuz J. & Puissant A. (1988) Papillon-Lefèvre syndrome. Ultrastructural study and successful treatment with acitretin. *Arch. Dermatol.* **124**, 533.

Nordin H., Månsson T. & Svensson A. (1988) Familial occurrence of eccrine tumours in a family with ectodermal dysplasia. *Acta Derm. Venereol. (Stockh.)* **68**, 523.

Norval E., van Wyk C.W., Basson N.J. & Coldrey J. (1988) Hypohidrotic ectodermal dysplasia: a genealogic, stereomicroscope, and scanning electron microscope study. *Pediatr. Dermatol.* **5**, 159.

O'Brien T.J. (1990) Chondrodysplasia punctata (Conradi disease). *Int. J. Dermatol.* **29**, 472.

O'Donnell B.P. & James W.D. (1992) Rapp-Hodgkin ectodermal dysplasia. *J. Am. Acad. Dermatol.* **27**, 323.

Ogden G.R., Connor E. & Chishlom D.M. (1988) Dyskeratosis congenita: report of a case and review literature. *Oral Surg. Med. Oral Pathol.* **65**, 586.

Ogur G. & Yüksel M. (1988) Association of syndactyly, ectodermal dysplasia, and cleft lip and palate: report of two sibs from Turkey. *J. Med. Genet.* **25**, 37.

O'Rourk T.R. & Bravos A (1969) An oculo-dento-digital dysplasia. *Birth Defects* 5: 226.

Pabst H.F., Groth O. & McGy E.E. (1981) Hypohidrotic ectodermal dysplasia with hypothyroidism. *J. Pediatr.* **98**, 223.

Paller A.S., Moore J.A. & Scher R.K. (1991) Pachyonychia congenita tarda. *Arch. Dermatol.* **127**, 701.

Papillon P. & Lefevre P. (1924) Deux cas de kéeratodermie plamaire et plantaire symétrique familiale (maladie de Méléeda) chez le frère et la soeur: coexistence dans les 2 cas d'altérations dentaires graves. *Bull. Soc. Fr. Derm. Syph.* **31**, 82.

Parizel P.M., Dumon J., Vossen P., Rigaux A. & De Scheppes A.M. (1987) The trichorhino-phalangeal syndrome revisited. *Eur. J. Radiol.* **7**, 154.

Passarge E. & Fried E. (1977) Autosomal recessive hypohidrotic ectodermal dysplasia with subclinical manifestations in the heterozygote. In: *Birth Defects*, ed. Bersma D. XIII (3C), pp. 95–100. Williams and Wilkins, Baltimore.

Passarge E., Nuzum L.T. & Schubert W.K. (1966) Anhidrotic ectodermal dysplasia as autosomal recessive trait in an inherited kindred. *Humangenetik* **3**, 181.

Patel Z.M., Mulye V.R., Raghavan & Shah S.B. (1987) Translocation in Coffin Sirris syndrome. *Indian Pediatr.* **24**, 435.

Patrizi A., Di Lernia V. & Patrone P. (1992) Palmoplantar keratoderma with sclerodactyly (Huriez syndrome). *J. Am. Acad. Dermatol.* **26**, 855.

Patton M.A., Krywawych S., Winter R.M., Brenton D.P. & Baraitser M. (1987) DOOR syndrome (deafness, onycho-osteodystrophy, and mental retardation): Elevated plasma and urinary 2-oxoglutarate in three unrelated patients. *Am. J. Med. Genet.* **26**, 207.

Pike M.G., Baraitser M., Dinwiddie R. & Atherton D. (1986) A distinctive type of hypohidrotic ectodermal dysplasia featuring hypothyrodism. *J. Pediatr.* **108**, 109.

Pinheiro M., Ideriha M.T., Chautard-Freire-Maia E.A., Freire-Maia N. & Primo-Parmo S.L. (1981) Christ–Siemens–Touraine syndrome. Investigations on two large Brazilian kindreds with a new estimate of the manifestation rate among carriers. *Hum. Genet.* **57**, 428.

Pinheiro M., Freire-Maia N., Chautard-Freire-Maia E.A., Araujo L.M.B. & Libermar B. (1983) A syndrome combining an acrorenal field defect, ectodermal dysplasia, lipoatrophic diabetes and other manifestations. *Am. J. Med. Genet.* **16**, 29–33.

Pinheiro M., Freie-Maia N. & Gollop T.R. (1985) Odonto-onychodysplasia with alopecia: a new pure ectodermal dysplasia with probable autosomal recessive inheritance. *Am. J. Med. Genet.* **20**, 197.

Pinheiro M. & Freire-Maia N. (1992) Hair-nail dysplasia – a new pure autosomal dominant ectodermal dysplasia. *Clin. Genet.* **41**, 296.

Pinheiro M., José Penna F. & Freire-Maia N. (1989) Two other cases of another syndrome? Family report and update. *Clin. Genet.* **35**, 237.

Pinheiro M., Gomes-de-Sá-Filho & Freire-Maia N. (1990) New cases of dermoodontodysplasia? *Am. J. Med. Genet.* **36**, 161.

Poulin Y., Perry H.O. & Muller S.A. (1984) Olmsted syndrome – congenital palmoplantar and periorificial keratoderma. *J. Am. Acad. Dermatol.* **10**, 600.

Price V.H., Odom R.B., Ward W.H. & Jones F.T. (1980) Trichothiodystrophy. *Arch. Dermatol.* **116**, 1375.

Propping P. & Zerres K. (1993) ADULT syndrome: An autosomal-dominant disorder with pigment anomalies, ectrodactyly, nail dysplasia, and hypodontia. *Am. J. Med. Genet.* **45**, 642.

Protonotarios N., Tsatsopoulou A., Patsourakos P. *et al.* (1986) Cardiac abnormalities in familial palmoplantar keratosis. *Br. Heart J.* **56**, 321.

Pujol R.M., Casanova J.M., Pérez M., Matias-Guiu X., Planagumà M. & de Moragas J.M. (1992) Focal dermal hypoplasia (Goltz syndrome). Report of two cases with minor cutaneous and extracutaneous manifestations. *Pediatr. Dermatol.* **9**, 112.

Puliyel J.M. & Sridharan Iyer K.S. (1986) A syndrome of keratosis palmo-plantaris congenita, pes planus, onychogryphosis, periodontosis, arachnodactyly and a peculiar acroosteolysis. *Br. J. Dermatol.* **115**, 243.

Qazi Q.H. & Nangia B.S. (1984) Abnormal distal phalanges and nails; deafness, mental retardation; and seizure disorder: A new familiar syndrome. *J. Pediatr.* **104**, 391.

Qazi Q.H. & Smithwick E.M. (1970) Triphalangy of thumbs and great toes. *Am. J. Dis. Child.* **120**, 255.

Raphael A.L., Baer P.N. & Lee W.B. (1968) Hyperkeratosis of gingival and plantar surfaces. *Periodontics* **6**, 118.

Rapp R.S. & Hodgkin W.E. (1968) Anhidrotic ectodermal dysplasia: autosomal dominant inheritance with palate and lip anomalies. *J. Med. Genet.* **5**, 269.

Rebora A. & Crovato F. (1987) PIBI(D)S syndrome – trichothiodystrophy with xeroderma pigmentosum (group D) mutation. *J. Am. Acad. Dermatol.* **16**, 940.

Reed W.B., Lopez A. & Landing B. (1970) Clinical spectrum of anhidrotic ectodermal dysplasia. *Arch. Dermatol.* **102**, 134.

Robinson G.C., Miller J.R. & Bensimon J.R. (1962) Familial ectodermal dysplasia with sensori-neural deafness and other anomalies. *Pediatrics* **30**, 797.

Robinson G.C., Miller J.R. & Worth HM (1966) Hereditary enamel hypoplasia: Its association with characteristic hair structure. *Pediatrics* **37**, 498.

Rollnick B.R. & Hoo J.J. (1988) Genitourinary anomalies are a competent manifestation in the ectodermal dysplasia, ectrodactyly, cleft lip/palate (EEC) syndrome. *Am. J. Med. Genet.* **29**, 131.

Rothe M.J., Weiss D.S., Dubner B.H., Weitzner J.M., Lucky A.W. & Schachner L. (1990) Ichthyosis follicularis in two girls: An autosomal dominant disorder. *Pediatr. Dermatol.* **7**, 287.

Rycroft R.J., Calnan C.D. & Allenby C.F. (1977) Dermatopathia pigmentosa reticularis. *Clin. Exp. Dermatol.* **2**, 37.

Salamon T. (1982) Nagelveränderungen bei des krankheit von mijet. *Z. Hautkr.* **57**, 1496.

Salamon T., Cubela V., Bogdanovic B., Lazovic O. & Bulatovic N. (1967) Uber ein Geschwisterpaar mit einer eigenartigen ektodermalen Dysplasie. *Arch. Klin. Exp. Dermatol.* **230**, 60.

Sánchez J.M., Laberta J.D., de Negrotti T.C. & Migliorini A.M. (1985) Complex translocation in a boy with trichorhinophalangeal syndrome. *J. Med. Genet.* **22**, 314.

Schapiro S.D., Jorgenson R.J. & Salinas C.F. (1984) Brief clinical report: Curry-Hall syndrome. *Am. J. Med. Genet.* **17**, 579.

Schöpf E., Schultz H. & Passarge E. (1971) Syndrome of cystic eyelids, palmo-plantar keratosis. Hypodontia and hypotrichosis as a possible autosomal recessive trait. *Birth Defects: Original Article Series* **VII**, 8: 219.

Schroeder H.W. & Sybert V.P. (1987) Rapp-Hodgkin ectodermal dysplasia. *J. Pediatr.* **110**, 72.

Schwann J. (1963) Keratosis palmaris et plantaris cum surditate congenita et leuconychia totali ungium. *Dermatologica* **126**, 335.

Schwayder T.A., Lane A.T. & Miller M.E. (1986) Hay-Wells syndrome. *Pediatr. Dermatol.* **3**, 399.

Scoggins R.B., Prescott K.J., Asher G.H., Blaylock W.K. & Bright R.W. (1971) Dyskeratosis congenita with Fanconi-type anemia: Investigations of immunologic and other defects. *Clin. Res.* **19**, 409.

Senter T.P., Jones K.L., Sahati N. & Nyham W.L. (1978) Atypical ichthyosiform erythroderma and congenital meurosensory deafness. A distinct syndrome. *J. Pediatr.* **92**, 68.

Shirren V. & Dinger R. (1965) Untersuchungen bei keratosis palmo-plantaris papulosa. *Arch. Klin. Exp. Dermatol.* **221**, 481.

Skinner B.A., Greist M.C. & Norins A.L. (1981) Keratitis, ichthyosis and deafness (K.I.D.) syndrome. *Arch. Dermatol.* **117**, 285.

Solomon L.M. & Keuer E.J. (1980) The ectodermal dysplasias. Problems of classification and some newer syndromes. *Arch. Dermatol.* **116**, 1295.

Sparrow G.D., Samman P.D. & Wells R.S. (1976) Hyperpigmentation and hypohidrosis. *Clin. Exp. Dermatol.* **1**, 127.

Stevanovic D.V. (1959) Alopecia congenita. *Acta Genet. Med. (Roma)* **9**, 127.

Su W.P.D., Chun S.I., Hammond D.E. & Gordon H. (1990) Pachyonychia congenita: A clinically study of 12 cases and review of the literature. *Pediatr. Dermatol.* **7**, 33.

Sybert V.P. (1985) Aplasia cutis congenita: A report of 12 new families and review of the literature. *Pediatr. Dermatol.* **3**, 1.

Sybert V.P. (1989) Hypohidrotic ectodermal dysplasia: Argument against an autosomal recessive form clinically indistinguishable from X-linked hypohidrotic ectodermal dysplasia (Christ-Siemens-Touraine syndrome). *Pediatr. Dermatol.* **6**, 76.

Thomas D.R., Jorizzo J.L., Brysk M.M., Tschen J.A., Miller J. & Tschen E.H. (1984) Pachyonychia congenita. *Arch. Dermatol.* **120**, 1475.

Thorel F.M. (1964) Un cas de maladie de Méléda, variété Papillin-Lefèvre avec surdité. *Bull. Soc. Franc. Derm. Syph.* **71**, 707.

Tidman M.J., Wells R.S. & MacDonald D.M. (1987) Pachyonychia congenita with cutaneous amyloidosis and hyperpigmentation – a distinct variant. *J. Am. Acad. Dermatol.* **16**, 935.

Tolmie J.L., Browne B.H., McGettrick P.M. & Stephenson J.B.P. (1988a) A familial syndrome with coats' reaction retinal angiomas, hair and nail defects and intracranial calcification. *Eye* **2**, 297.

Tolmie J.L., Wilcox D.E., McWilliam R., Assindi A. & Stephenson J.P.B. (1988b) Palmoplantar keratoderma; nail dystrophy, and hereditary motor and sensory neuropathy: an autosomal dominant trait. *J. Med. Genet.* **25**, 754.

Toriello H.V., Lindstrom J.A., Waterman D.F. & Baugham F.A. (1979) Reevaluation of CHANDS. *J. Med. Genet.* **16**, 316.

Traboulsi E.I., Faris B.M. & Kaloustian V.M. (1986) Persistant hyperplastic primary vitreous and recessive oculodento-osseous dysplasia. *Am. J. Med. Genet.* **24**, 95.

van Neste D., Thomas P. & Desmons F. (1980) Trichoschisis, Photosensibilité. Retard staturopondéral. Nouveau syndrome congénital. *Ann. Dermatol. Vénéréol. (Paris)* **107**, 718.

van Neste D., Miller X. & Bohnert E. (1988) Trichothiodystrophie. *Akt. Dermatol.* **14**, 191.

Verhage J., Habbema L., Vrensen G.F.J., Roord J.J. & Bleeker-Wagemakers E.H. (1987) A patient with onychotrichodysplasia, neutropenia and normal intelligence. *Clin. Genet.* **31**, 374.

Vogt B.R., Traupe H. & Hamm H. (1988) Congenital atrichia with nail dystrophy, abnormal facies, and retarded psychomotor development in two siblings: A new autosomal recessive syndrome? *Pediatr. Dermatol.* **5**, 236.

Vohwinkel K.H. (1929) Keratoma hereditarium mutilans. *Arch. Dermatol.* **158**, 354.

Walbaum R., Fontaine G., Lienhardt J. & Piquet J.J. (1970) Surdite familiale avec osteo-onycho-dysplasie. *J. Genet. Hum.* **18**, 101.

Weech A.A. (1929) Hereditary ectodermal dysplasia (congenital ectodermal defect). A report of two cases. *Am. J. Dis. Child.* **37**, 766.

Wilkey W.D. & Stevenson G.H. (1945) A family with inherited ectodermal dystrophy. *Can. Med. Assoc. J.* **53**, 226.

Winter R.M., MacDermott K.D. & Hill F.J. (1988) Sparse hair, short stature, hypoplastic thumbs, single upper central incisor and abnormal skin pigmentation: a possible 'new' form of ectodermal dysplasia. *Am. J. Med. Genet.* **29**, 209.

Witkop C.J., Brearly L.J. & Gentry W.D. (1975) Hypoplastic enamel, onycholysis and hypohidrosis inherited as an autosomal dominant trait. *Oral Surg.* **39**, 71.

Disease loci and chromosome anomalies

Chromosomal localization has now been established for several genetic traits (Table 9.4). Mapping of important disease loci has increased rapidly during the last years (Harper *et al.*, 1989; Moss, 1991). As the specific genes and their products are discovered for particular disorders, disease names no longer appear in the individual chromosome tables.

Syndromes with chromosome anomalies usually have mental deficiency and dysmorphic changes as the main features together with multiple defects (Jones, 1988; de Grouchy & Turleau, 1982; McKusick, 1992). The nails are often convex or hypoplastic from birth (Table 9.5).

References

Allansson J.E. (1987) Noonan syndrome. *J. Med. Genet.* **24**, 9.

Dubowitz V., Cooke P., Colver D. & Harris F. (1971) Mental retardation, unusual facies and abnormal nails associated with a Group G ring chromosome. *J. Med. Genet.* **8**, 195.

de Grouchy J. & Turleau C. (1982). *Atlas des Maladies Chromosomiques*, 2nd edn. Expansion, Scientifique, Paris.

Harper P.S., Frézal J., Ferguson-Smith M.A. & Schinzel A. (1989) Report of the committee on clinical disorders and chromosomal deletion syndromes. *Cytogenet. Cell Genet.* **51**, 563.

Jones K.L. (1988) *Smith's Recognizable Patterns of Human Malformation*, 4th edn. W.B. Saunders, Philadelphia.

McKusick V.A. (1992) *Mendelian Inheritance in Man*, 10th edn. Johns Hopkins University Press, Baltimore.

Moss C. (1991) Dermatology and the human gene map. *Br. J. Dermatol.* **124**, 3.

Nail change in syndromes with predominant skeletal anomalies

In patients with bradydactyly, syndactyly, zygodactyly and polydactyly the nails are sometimes malformed or absent. When the distal phalanges are involved the nails are often longitudinally convex and/or broad (Figs 9.20 & 9.21). Skeletal changes are also found in syndromes with ectodermal dysplasia (Tables 9.1, 9.2) and with chromosomal anomalies (Table 9.4).

Hypoplastic or atrophic nails with skeletal anomalies

These disorders are listed in Table 9.6. Here we will especially discuss the congenital onychodysplasia of the index fingers (COIF), also termed the Iso and Kikuchi's syndrome (Figs 9.22–9.25). Baran (1980) suggested that it was congenital and characterized by a variety of nail deformities affecting one or both index fingers (Fig. 9.22) and by bone abnormalities, such as a Y-shaped bifurcation of the distal phalanx, visible on lateral X-ray pictures (Fig. 9.25). Such a bone abnormality may occur under both normal and abnormal nails. The defects are mainly seen on the radial side of the index fingers. Kikuchi *et al.* (1981) related this to the smaller calibre of the artery on the radial side. Micronychia is the commonest clinical manifestation. The so-called 'rolled micronychia' is a rare variant. Anonychia, haemionychogryphosis or simple malalignment are also less frequent presentations. A deformed lunula was described by Baran and Stroud (1984). Millman and Strier (1982), in an extensive article, described nine members of one family who suffered from the COIF syndrome; the clinical spectrum was broadened to include autosomal dominant inheritance. Kikushi (1991) described a case where both thumbnails also were involved. He thought that it could be related to an abnormal handgrip in fetal life. Kitayama and Tsukada (1983) prefer the term congenital onychodysplasia since it is not only located on the index finger. They assumed that it is due to ischaemic damage in embryonic life. Miura and Nakamura (1990) suggest that impediments to the membranous ossification centre can lead to a dysplastic crescent-shaped cap with nail anomalies. Another strong

Table 9.4. Chromosomal localization known for genetic traits mentioned in the text. The regions are numbered from the centromera (cen) outwards along the short (p) and long (q) arms to the termini (ter)

Disease	Locus symbol	Map location
Acanthocytosis nigricans	INSR	19p13.3-p13.2
Chondrodysplasia punctata, X-linked recessive	CDPX	Xp22.32
Coprophorphyria	CP	3q23-q25
Dyskeratosis congenita	DKC	Xq27-q28
Epidermolysis bullosa dystrophica (Pasini)	COL 7A1	3p21
Epidermolysis bullosa progresiva (Gedde-Dahl)	EBR3	ULG
Focal dermal hypoplasia	D40F, FODH	Xp22-31
Epidermolysis bullosa simplex (Ogna)	EBS1	8q24
Epidermolysis bullosa, dystrophic recessive	CLG	11q21-q22
Gout, PPRPS overexpression	PRSP2	Xpter-q21
Haemochromatosis	HFE	6p21.3
Hyperuricaemia, gout	PRSPI	Xq21-q27
Hypohidrotic ectodermal dysplasia	HED	Xq13.1
Ichthyosis (X-linked), steroid sulphatase deficiency	STS	Xp22.32
Incontinentia pigmenti	IP1	Xp11.21-cen
	IP2	Xq27-q28
Lesch–Nyhan syndrome	HPRT	Xq26-q27,2
Nail–patella syndrome	NPS1	9q34
Neurofibromatosis 1	NF1	17q11.2
Porphyria cutanea tarda	UROD	1p34
Porphyria variegata	VD	14q
Porphyria, acute, hepatic	ALAD	9q34
Porphyria, acute, intermittent	PBGD	11q23.2-qter
Tricho-rhino-phalangeal syndrome I	TRP I	8q23.3-924.13
Tricho-rhino-phalangeal syndrome II (Langer Gideon)	LGS TRP II	8q24.1-q24.1
Tuberous sclerosis 1	TSC1	9q33-q34
Tuberous sclerosis 2	TSC2	11q23
Wilson disease	WND	13q14.2-q21

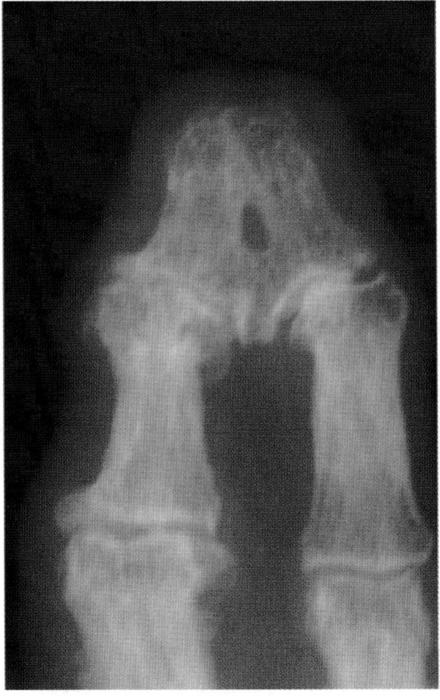

Fig. 9.20. Fused digits and nails.

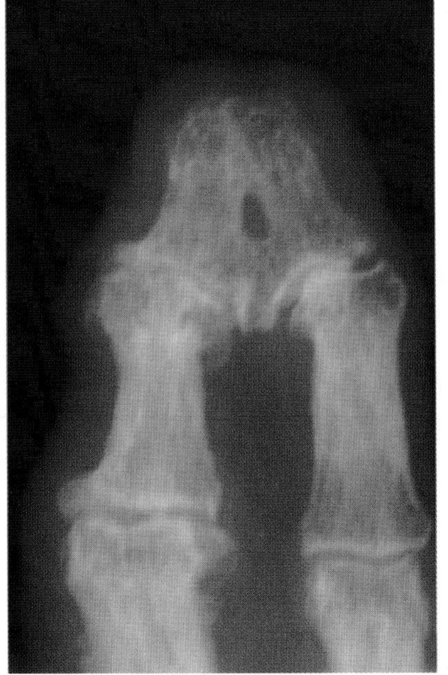

Fig. 9.21. X-ray of digits in Fig. 9.20 – only terminal phalanges are fused.

influence on the cause is that the critical period of intra-uterine life in COIF may be the same time as the critical period of the syndactylyl and Grachy mesophalangy because these anomalies are the most commonly associated anomalies of COIF.

References

Badame A.J. (1989) Progeria. *Arch. Dermatol.* **125**, 540.

Baran R. (1980) Syndrome d'Iso et Kikuchi. *Ann. Dermatol. Venereol.* **107**, 431.

Baran R. & Stroud J.D. (1984) Congenital onychodysplasia of

Table 9.5. Disorders with chromosome anomalies. See de Grouchy and Turleau (1982) and Jones (1988) for references

Diseases	Nails	Other findings
Trisomy 3q partial	Hypoplastic	Finger anomalies
Trisomy 4p	Hypoplastic	Finger anomalies. Facial dysmorphy. Mental and growth deficiency
4p syndrome	Convex, narrow, transvers striae. Lunula lacking	Microcephaly. Mental deficiency. Facial dysmorphy
Trisomy 7q	Convex	Mental deficiency. Dysmorphies of face and skull
Trisomy 8	Hypoplastic. May be absent at birth	Mental deficiency. Facial dysmorphy, bone and joint anomalies. Stiffness
Trisomy 8p	Dysplastic toenails	Mental deficiency. Often dysmorphies of hands and feet
Trisomy 9p	Dysplastic and sometimes claw-shaped toes	Mental defects. Brachycephalia. Big nose and other dysmorphies
9p syndrome	Convex square and wide	Mental defects. Trigonocephaly. Long upper lip
Trisomy 13	Small convex and narrow	Mental retardation. Dysmorphia face and skull. Micropthalmia. Hexadactyly. Haemangioma. Failure to thrive
Trisomy 18	Hypoplastic	Mental deficiency. Dysmorphia. Cutis laxa. Hand and visceral deformities. High neonatal mortality. Failure to thrive
Turner's syndrome 45,X (female), Noonan's syndrome (male) (Allanson, 1987), Bonnevie–Ullrich's syndrome	Convex, narrow, hypoplastic. Sometimes missing (Fig. 9.31, p. 329)	Small stature. Precocious puberty and senility. Webbing of neck and toes. Lymphoedema of hands and feet
Group G-ring chromosome (Dubowitz *et al.*, 1971)	Pachyonychia of toenails	Mental retardation and unusual faces
Trisomy 21 Down's syndrome	Can be large	Mental defects. Dysmorphies and malformations. Retardation of growth. Short fingers. Dry skin. Hypoplastic teeth

the index finger (Iso and Kikuchi syndrome). *Arch. Dermatol.* **120**, 243.

Bass H.N. (1968) Familial absence of middle phalanges with nail dysplasia: a new syndrome. *Pediatrics* **42**, 318.

Beighton P.H. (1970) Familial hypertrichosis cubiti: Hairy elbows syndrome. *J. Med. Genet* **7**, 158.

Bittar E.O., Parra C.A., de Prieto G.L., Briggs E. & Baeza O.O. (1988) Kongenitale ischämische Onychodystrophie (Iso-Kikuchi-Syndrom) und chronischer Lupus erythematodes. *Hautarzt* **39**, 750.

Brunzlow H., Lorck D. & Neumann J. (1987) Beitrag zum Iso-Kikuchi-Syndrom Kongenitale Onychodysplasie. *Radiol. Diagn. (Berl.)* **6**, 773.

Carney R.G. & Carney G. Jr (1970) Incontinentia pigmenti. *Arch. Dermatol.* **102**, 157.

Cartwright J., Nelson M. & Fryns F.P. (1991) Pre- and postnatal growth retardation – severe mental retardation – acral limb deficiences with poorly keratinized nails. *Genet. Couns.* **2**, 147.

Table 9.6. Atrophic or hypoplastic nails with skeletal anomalies. Inheritances are indicated as follows: AD, autosomal dominant; AR, autosomal recessive; XD, sex-linked dominant

Disease	Inheritance	Nails	Other symptoms
Absence of middle phalanges with hypoplastic nails (Bass, 1968; Cuevas-Sosa & Garcia-Segur, 1971)	AD	Hypoplasia of several nails	Brachydactyly. Duplicated phalanges of thumbs. Sometimes syndactyly
Acrogeria. Gottron syndrome (Grüneberg, 1960; DeGroth *et al.*, 1980)	—	Atrophic nails	Senile changes limited to distal extremities
Brachymorphism-onychodysplasia-dysphalingism (BOD) syndrome (Verloes *et al.*, 1993)	AD?	Hypoplasia or absent	Hypoplasia distal phalanges. Facial dysmorphism
Brachydactyly with nail dysplasia (Schott, 1978; Bass, 1968)	AD	Absence of nail of fourth digit. Dysplastic nails on other fingers	Asymmetrical brachydactyly
CHARGE association (Meinecke *et al.*, 1989)	AR	Hypoplastic	Colomboma, heart anomaly, choanal atresia. Retardation. Genital and ear anomalies
COIF syndrome (see below)			
Congenital hemidysplasia with ichthyosiform erythroderma and limb defects. CHILD syndrome (Happle *et al.*, 1980; Christiansen *et al.*, 1984; von Schlenzka *et al.*, 1989)	XD	Dystrophic on affected side	Only in females
Craniofrontonasal dysplasia (Grutzner & Gorlin, 1988; Orlov, 1992)	XD	Longitudinally grooved nails, heminychia or anonychia	Hypertelorism, broad nasal root, syndactyly craniosynostosis
Frontometaphyseal dysplasia (Gorlin & Cohen, 1969)	AD	Short nails	Marked supraorbital bony ridge. Skeletal alteration. Deafness
Fryns syndrome (Fryns, 1987)	AR	Hypoplastic and small	Characteristic facies with broad nasal bridge, cleft palate, distal digital hypoplasia and urogenital anomalies
Hairy elbows syndrome (Beighton, 1970)	AR	Short	Hypertrichosis of elbows. Short stature
Incontinentia pigmenti, Bloch-Sulzberger syndrome (Carney & Carney, 1970; El-Benhawi & George, 1988; Dolan *et al.*, 1992)	XD	Dystrophic. In 7% koilonychia. At 15 years subungual tender tumours which clear spontaneously (Hartman, 1966; Pinol Aguade *et al.*, 1973; Mascaro *et al.*, 1985)	Vesicular, verrucous and pigmented macular lesions. Anomalies of eyes (30–50%), nervous system (30%), teeth (65%), skeleton (13%), alopecia (40%)

continued

Table 9.6. *Continued*

Disease	Inheritance	Nails	Other symptoms
Iso and Kikuchi COIF syndrome, congenital onychodysplasia of the index fingers (Brunzlow *et al.*, 1987; Millman & Strier, 1982; Bittar *et al.*, 1988; Miura & Nakamura, 1990)	AD	Anonychia, micronychia or polyonychia of index finger (Figs 9.4–9.6)	See pp. 314, 317
Lethal syndrome with cloudy cornea, diaphragmatic and distal defects (Fryns *et al.*, 1979; Young *et al.*, 1986)	AR	Small, hypoplastic	Stillborn or dead shortly after birth. Coarse face, small eyes, cleft palate, hypoplasia of lungs; diaphragm and distal bone deformation
Osteo-onycho dysplasia. Nail–patella syndrome (Pye-Smith, 1893; Gibbs *et al.*, 1964) (see p. 295)	AD	Short, narrow, fragile, changes most pronounced on the thumb where the nails might be missing. Sometimes koilonychia. Toes rarely affected. Pterygium. Lunula missing or V-shaped (Fig. 9.2)	Patella absent 92%. Radius head small. Iliac crest exostosis. Eyes and kidney abnormalities as well as other changes occasionally. Linked to ABO blood group. Locus localized on chromosome
Poikiloderma congenita. Rothmund Thomson syndrome (Silver, 1966; Vennos *et al.*, 1992)	AR	Nails small; thin and dystrophic in 25%	Short phalanges. Small stature. Frontal bossing: Photosensitive cataracts. Skin of cheeks red and swollen about the third month of age, then on extensor surface of extremities. Later atrophy, pigmentation and telangiectasia
Pre- and postnatal growth retardation, mental retardation and acral limb deficiences (Cartwright *et al.*, 1991)	—	Small, hyperconvex and poorly keratinized	Facial dysmorphism
Progeria. Hutchinson–Gilford syndrome (De Busk, 1972; Jimbow *et al.*, 1987; Badame, 1989)	AR	Thin, yellow, atrophic	Dwarfism, pseudosenility. Small face giving a hydrocephalic appearance. Bird face. Narrow chest, other bone deformations. Arterosclerosis. Atrophic skin
Rüdiger syndrome (Rüdiger *et al.*, 1970)	AR	Hypoplastic	Somatic retardation, small fingers, ureteral stenosis, cleft palate, coarse facies. Death within first year of life
Weaver syndrome (Fitch, 1980)	?	Thin, deep set nails	Increased weight, height and bifrontal diameter. Hypertonia. Prominent fingerpads

continued on p. 322

Table 9.6. *Continued*

Disease	Inheritance	Nails	Other symptoms
Werner syndrome (Epstein *et al.*, 1966)	AR	Atrophic nails	Short stature, premature greying and baldness. Juvenile cataracts. Hypogonadism, diabetes, calcification of blood vessels, osteoporosis. Atrophic skin. Wasting of musculature
Williams elfin facies syndrome (Jones & Smith, 1975)	—	Short, deep set or brittle	Coarse facies, depressed nasal bridge, hoarse voice, aortic stenosis, growth deficiency and mental retardation

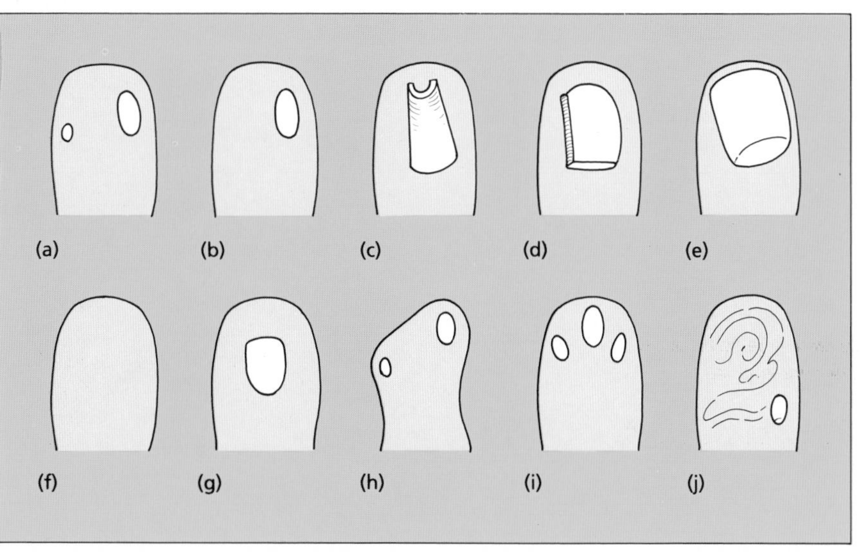

Fig. 9.22. Types of micronychia and other dystrophies seen particularly in congenital onychodystrophy of the index fingers (COIF). (a) Polyonchia in COIF; (b) micronychia in COIF; (c) 'rolled' micronychia in COIF; (d) hemionychogryposis in COIF; (e) malalignment in COIF; (f) anonychia in COIF; (g) usual micronychia; (h) polyonchia in syndactyly; (i) polyonchia in congenital skin disease; (j) onychoheterotopia (Ohya's type). (After Baran, 1980; Kikuchi, 1991; Millman & Strier, 1982.)

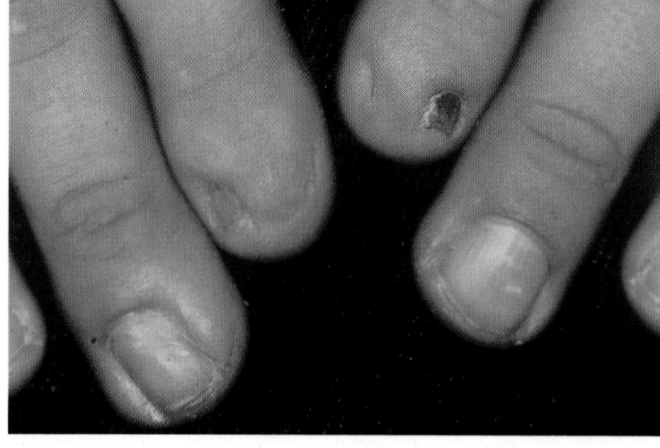

Fig. 9.23. Iso–Kikuchi (COIF) syndrome – see Fig. 9.22; classical involvement of the index fingers.

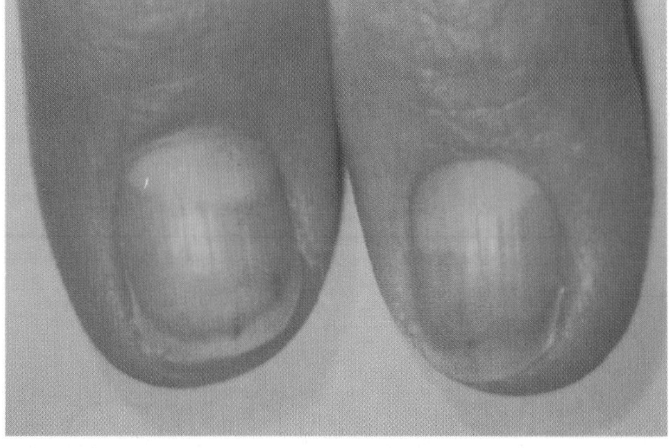

Fig. 9.24. COIF syndrome – asymmetrical lunula.

Christiansen J.V., Petersen H.O. & Søgaard H. (1984) The CHILD-syndrome–Congential hemidysplasia with ichthyosiform erythroderma and limb defects. A case report. *Acta Derm. Venereol. (Stockh.)* **64**, 165.

Cuevas-Sosa A. & Garcia-Segur F. (1971) Brachydactyly with absence of middle phalanges and hypoplastic nails. A new herediatry syndrome. *J. Bone Joint Surg.* **53B**, 101.

De Busk F.L. (1972) The Hutchinson-Gilford progeria syndrome. *J. Pediatr.* **80**, 697.

de Groot W.P., Tafelkruyer J. & Woerdeman M.J. (1980) Fam-

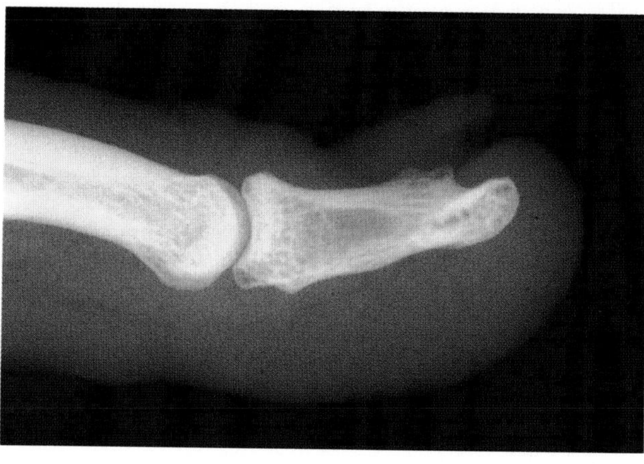

Fig. 9.25. COIF syndrome – X-ray showing Y-shaped bifurcation of the distal phalanx.

ilial acrogeria (Gottron). *Br. J. Dermatol.* **103**, 213.
Dolan O.M., Bingham E.A. & Corbett J.R. (1992) Incontinentia pigmenti. *Br. J. Dermatol.* **127**, Suppl. 40, 54.
El-Benhawi M.O. & George W.M. (1988) Incontinentia pigmenti: A review. *Cutis* **41**, 259.
Epstein C.J., Martin G.M., Schultz A.L. & Motulsky A.G. (1966) Werner's syndrome. Review of its symptomatology, natural history, pathology features, gentics and relationships to natural aging process. *Med. (Baltimore)* **45**, 177.
Fitch N. (1980) The syndromes of Marshall and Weaver. *J. Med. Genet.* **17**, 174.
Fryns J.P. (1987) Fryns syndrome: a variable MCA syndrome with diaphragmatic defects, coarse face, and idstal limb hypoplasia. *J. Med. Genet.* **24**, 271.
Fryns J.P., Moerman F., Goddeeris P., Bossuyt C. & van den Berghe H. (1979) A new lethal syndrome with cloudy corneae, diaphragmatic defects and distal limbs deformities. *Hum. Genet.* **50**, 65.
Gibbs R., Berczellar P.H. & Hyman A.B. (1964) Nail–patella–elbow syndrome. Arch. Dermatol. **89**, 196.
Gorlin R.J. & Cohen M.M. Jr (1969) Frontometaphyseal dysplasia: A new syndrome. *Am. J. Dis. Child.* **118**, 487.
Grüneberg T. (1960) Die Akrogerie (Gottron). *Arch. Klin. Exp. Dermatol.* **210**, 409.
Grutzner E. & Gorlin R.J. (1988) Craniofrontonasal dysplasia: Phenotypic expression in females and males and genetic considerations. *Oral Surg. Oral Med. Oral Pathol.* **65**, 436.
Happle R., Kich H. & Lenz W. (1980) The CHILD-syndrome. Congenital hemidysplasia with ichthyosiform erythroderma and limb defects. *Eur. J. Pediatr.* **134**, 27.
Hartman D.L. (1966) Incontinentia pigmenti associated with subungual tumour. *Arch. Dermatol.* **94**, 632.
Jimbow K., Ohtani S., Ishii M. & Ohyanagi K. (1987) Progeria and hyperplastic scar-like lesions: Immunohistochemical and electron-microscopic characterization. *Clin. Dermatol.* **125**.
Jones K. & Smith D.W. (1975) The Williams elfin facies syndrome. *J. Pediatr.* **86**, 718.
Kikuchi I. (1991) Congenital onychodysplasia of the index fingers: A case involving the thumbnails. *Semin. Dermatol.* **10**, 7.
Kikuchi I., Ishii Y., Idemori M. & Ogata K. (1981) Congenital onychodysplasia of the index fingers. *J. Dermatol.* **8**, 51.
Kitamaya Y. & Tsukada S. (1983) Congenital onychodysplasia: Report of 11 cases. *Arch. Dermatol.* **119**, 8.
Mascaro J.M., Palou J. & Vives P. (1985) Painful subungual keratotic tumors in incontinentia pigmenti. *J. Am. Acad. Dermatol.* **13**, 913.
Meinecke P., Pole A. & Schmiegelow P. (1989) Limb anomalies in the CHARGE association. *J. Med. Genet.* **26**, 202.
Millman A.J. & Strier R.P. (1982) Congenital onychodysplasia of the index fingers. *J. Am. Acad. Dermatol.* **7**, 57.
Miura T. & Nakamura R. (1990) Congenital onychodysplasia of the index fingers. *J. Hand. Surg.* **15A**, 793.
Orlow S.J. (1992) Cutaneous findings in craniofacial malformation syndromes. *Arch. Dermatol.* **128**, 1379.
Pinol Aguade J., Mascaro J.M., Herrero C. & Castel T. (1973) Tumeurs sous-unguéales dyskératosiques douloureuses et spontanément résolutives. Les rapports avec l'Incontinentia Pigmenti. *Ann. Dermatol. Syphil. (Paris)* **100**, 159.
Pye-Smith R.J. (1893) Notes on a family presenting in most of its members certain deformities of the joints of both limbs. *Med. Press.* **34**, 504.
Rüdiger R.A., Haase W. & Passarge E. (1970) Association of ectrodactyly, ectodermal dysplasia and cleft lip-palate. *Am. J. Dis. Child.* **120**, 160.
Schott G.D. (1978) Hereditary brachydactyly with nail dysplasia. *J. Med. Genet.* **15**, 119.
Silver H.K. (1966) Rothmund-Thomson syndrome: an oculocutaneous disorder. *Am. J. Dis. Child.* **111**, 182.
Vennos E.M., Collins M. & James W.D. (1992) Rothmund–Thomson syndrome: Review of the world literature. *J. Am. Acad. Dermatol.* **27**, 750.
Verloes A., Bonneau D., Guidi O. *et al.* (1993) Brachymorphism-onychodysplasia-dysphalangism syndrome. *J. Med. Genet.* **30**, 158.
von Schlenzka K., Gehre M., Neumann H.-J. & Sochor H. (1989) CHILD-Syndrome – kasuistischer Beitreag zur Kenntnis dieser seltenen Genodermatose. *Dermatol. Monatschr.* **175**, 100.
Young I.D., Simpson K. & Winter R.M. (1986) A case of Fryns syndrome. *J. Med. Genet.* **23**, 82.

Hyperonychia, hyperplastic thick nails

Large nails are seen in patients with macrodactylia due to epidermal naevus, gigantism and various connective tissue syndromes (Greenberg *et al.*, 1987). Thick nails are common in patients with various types of keratoderma (Table 9.1) and in ichthyosiform dermatitis (Table 9.2). Schulze (1966), Burg (1975) and Bazex *et al.* (1990) described families with thick and hard nails with partial onycholysis but without other anomalies (Fig. 9.26). Thick nails that split into double layers (matrix doubling syndrome) on fingers and toes was reported by Vigh and Pinter (1973). The patients also showed oculomotor paresis, debility and external ear aplasia. Three cases of nail-bed hyperkeratosis where the base is normal, the surface smooth but the distal part of the nail is raised up from the nail bed by a dark friable horny mass, was described by Garrick Wilson and Cantab (1905). A special form is pachonychia, i.e. thickening of the nail bed with elevation of the nail plate, which occurs in pachonychia congenita (p. 298). Pachonychia on the toes was found in patients having a rare

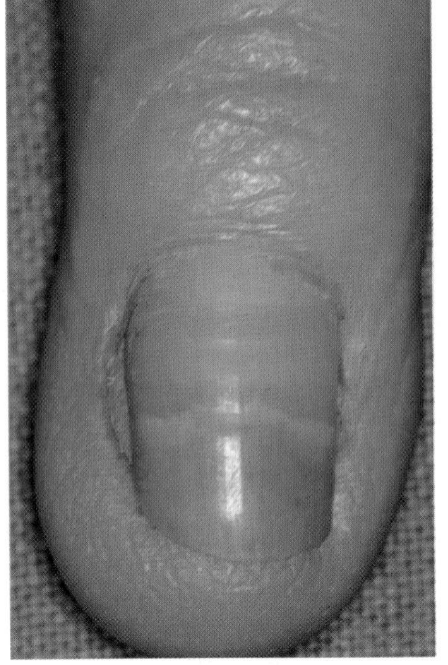

Fig. 9.26. Congenital 'onycholysis'.

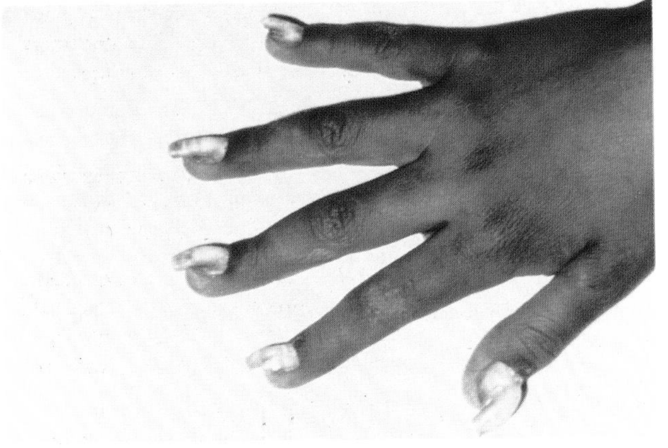

Fig. 9.27. Onychogryphosis.

syndrome with severe mental retardation and unusual facies together with large ears; this is associated with a stable ring group G chromosome (Dubowitz *et al.*, 1971).

Onychogryphosis (Fig. 9.27) can occur with autosomal dominant inheritance, but usually appears first in early childhood (Heller, 1927; Clement, 1928; Orel, 1928; Videbaeck, 1948; Lubach, 1982). It can also be seen with other ectodermal malformations (Tables 9.1 and 9.2).

References

Bazex J., Baran R., Monbrun F., Griforieff-Larrue N. & Marguery M.C. (1990) Hereditary distal onycholysis – a case report. *Clin. Exp. Dermatol.* **15**, 146.

Burg G. (1975) Onycholysis partialis hereditaria cum skleronychia. *Hautarzt* **26**, 386.

Clement L.S. (1928) A claw-fingered family. The inheritance of nail mutation in man. *J. Hered.* **19**, 529.

Dubowitz V., Cooke P., Colver D. & Harris F. (1971) Mental retardation, unusual facies and abnormal nails associated with a group G ring chromosome. *J. Med. Genet.* **8**, 195.

Garrick Wilson A. & Cantab M.B. (1905) Three cases of hereditary hyperkeratosis of the nail bed. *Br. J. Dermatol.* **17**, 13.

Greenberg G.M., Pess G.M. & May J.W. (1987) Macrodactyly and the epidermal nevus syndrome. *J. Hand Surg.* **12**, 730.

Heller J. (1927) Die Krankheiten der Näger. In: Jadassohn J (Hrsg) *Handbuch der Haut und Geschlechtskrankheiten*, Bd VIII/2. Springer, Berlin.

Lubach D. (1982) Erbliche Onychogryposis. *Hautarzt* **33**, 331.

Orel H. (1928) Über eine Familie mit erblicher Onychogryposis. *Arch. Rassenbiol.* **20**, 169.

Schulze H.D. (1966) Hereditary Onycholysis partialis mit Skleronychie. *Derm. W.* **30**, 766.

Videbaeck A. (1948) Hereditary onychogryphosis. *Ann. Eugen (Lond.)* **14**, 139.

Vigh G. & Pinter L. (1973) Nagelmatrix-Verdoppelungssyndrom. *Z. Haut-u. Geschl.-Kr.* **48**, 125.

Clubbing, acropachy, hippocratic nails

Here the nails are thick and curved. Most common are the acquired forms seen in association with pulmonary and other systemic diseases. A hereditary form of clubbing without any other symptoms has been reviewed by Fischer *et al.* (1964). It has a gradual onset from puberty. The cause of the clubbing is unknown and it is usually not evident before early childhood. Clubbing can also be seen as a part of various syndromes which are listen in Table 9.7.

References

Andren L., Dymling J.F., Hogeman K.E. & Wendeberg B. (1962) Oseopetrosis acroosteolytica: a syndrome of osteopetrosis, acro-osteolysis and open sutures of the skull. *Acta Chir. Scand.* **12**, 496.

Bureau Y., Barrière H. & Thomas M. (1959) Hippocratisme digital congénital avec hyperkératose palmo-plantaire et trobules osseux. *Ann. Dermatol. Venerol.* **86**, 611.

Cheney W.D. (1965) Acro-osteolysis. *Am. J. Roentgenol.* **94**, 595.

David T.J. & Burwood R.L. (1972) The nature and inheritance of Kirner's deformity. *J. Med. Genet.* **9**, 430.

Dore D.D., MacEwen G.D. & Boulos M.I. (1987) Cleidocranial dysostosis and syringomyelia: Review of the literature and case report. *Clin. Orthop.* **214**, 229.

Elias A.N., Pinals R.S., Andersson C.H., Gould L.V. & Streeten D.H.P. (1978) Hereditary osteodysplasia with acro-osteolysis (the Hajdu–Cheney syndrome). *Am. J. Med.* **65**, 627.

Fischer D.R., Singer D.H. & Feldman S.M. (1964) Clubbing, a review with emphasis on hereditary acropachy. *Med.* **43**, 459.

Kirner J. (1927) Doppelseitige Verkrümmungen des Kleinfingerendglides als selbständiges Kranheitsbild. *Fortschr. Röntgenstr.* **36**, 804.

Kitano Y., Matsunaga E., Morimoto T., Okada N. & Sano S. (1985) A syndrome with nodular erythema, elongated and thickened fingers, and emaciation. *Arch. Dermatol.* **121**, 1053.

Lacroux R., Delahaya R.P. & Laynaud S. (1965) Dystrophies

Table 9.7. Hereditary forms of clubbed fingernails. Inheritances are indicated as follows: AD, autosomal dominant; AR, autosomal recessive

Disease	Inheritance	Comments
Acroosteolysis with osteoporosis (Cheney, 1965; Elias *et al.*, 1978; Udell *et al.*, 1986)	AD	Broad distal phalanges with two ossicles. Increase of bitemporal diameter of the skull and flattening of the vertex. Osteoporosis of the mandible
Cartilage–hair hypoplasia, (McKusick *et al.*, 1965; Polmat & Pierce, 1986)	AR	Short fingers, especially of terminal phalanges. Short stature and thin sparse hair. Impaired cell function
Cleido-cranial dysostosis (Lacroux *et al.*, 1965; Dore *et al.*, 1987)	AD	Aplasia of clavicles, delayed ossification of fontanelles, typical facies, coxa vara, abnormal terminal phalanges. Multiple associated anomalies. Micronychia. Syringomyelia
Dystelephalangy (Kirner, 1927; David & Burwood, 1972)	AD	Distal phalange of digit V is curved. Sometimes with absence of middle finger
Hereditary clubbing of digits (Fischer *et al.*, 1964)	AD	Gradual onset puberty
Ichthyosiform dermatosis with linear keratotic flexural papules and sclerosing palmoplantar keratodermia (Barrière *et al.*, 1977; Pujol *et al.*, 1989)	AR	Increased curvature of the nail plate and clubbing of nails. Pseudohainum of fingers. Dental abnormalities
Keratoderma palmoplantare and clubbing of nails (Bureau *et al.*, 1959)	?	See Table 9.1. Recidivating leg ulcers. Small head. Bone changes with enlarged distal phalanges
Nodular erythema with digital changes. Nakajo syndrome (Kitano *et al.*, 1985)	AR	Nodular erythema. Long and thick fingers. Joint mobility restricted. Loss of adipose tissue of the upper part of body. Large eyes, nose, lips and ears
Oto-onycho-peroneal syndrome (Pfeiffer, 1982)	AR	Enlarged fingertips, dysmorphic cranofacial features, hypoplasia of fibula, contractures of hip, knee and ankle joints
Pachydermoperiostosis (Pramatarov *et al.*, 1988)	AD	Thickening and furrowing of face and scalp. Clubbing of digits and periosteal new bone, formation starting about puberty
Peutz–Jeghers–Touraine syndrome (Valero & Sherf, 1965)	AD	Pigmented macule and intestinal polyps. See Table 9.8
Pycnodysostosis (Maroteaux & Lamy, 1965; Andren *et al.*, 1962)	AR	Stubby digits simulating clubbing. Short, brittle nails. Dystrophy. Dwarfism, sclerotic bones which easily fracture

unguéales et macrocheilite dans la dysostose cleido-cranienne. *Bull. Soc. Fr. Dermatol. Syphil.* 72, 366.

Maroteaux P. & Lamy M. (1965) The malady of Tolouse-Lautrec. *J. Am. Med. Assoc.* **191**, 715.

McKusick V.A., Elridge R., Hostetler J.A., Egeland J.A. & Ruangwit U. (1965) Dwarfism in the Amish II. Cartilage-hair hypoplasia. *Bull. Johns Hopk. Hosp.* **116**, 285.

Pfeiffer R.A. (1982) The oto-onycho-peroneal syndrome. A probably new genetic entity. *Eur. J. Pediatr.* **138**, 317.

Polmat S.H. & Pierce G.F. (1986) Cartilage hair hypoplasia: immunological aspects and their clinical implications. *Clin. Immun. Immunpathol.* **40**, 87.

Pramatarov K., Daskarev L., Schurliev L. & Tonev S. (1988) Pachydermoperiostose (Touraine-Solente-Golé-syndrome). *Z. Hautkrank.* **63**, 55.

Pujol R.M., Moreno A., Alomar A. & de Moragas J.M. (1989)

Table 9.8. Hereditary forms of broad nails and some also with pseudoclubbing. Inheritances are indicated as follows: AD, autosomal dominant; AR, autosomal recessive; XL, sex-linked transmission; XD, sex-linked dominant; XR, sex-linked recessive

Diseases	Inheritance	Comments
Acrocephalosyndactyly (Apert, 1906; Pfeiffer, 1964; Rasmussen & Frias, 1988).	AD	Craniosynostosis. Syndactyly. Ankylosis and other skeletal deformities
Acrodysostosis (Maroteaux & Malamut, 1968; Robinow *et al.*, 1971)	AD	Fingernails short, broad and oval in shape. Short fingers. Nasal and midface hypoplasia. Mental retardation. Growth failure. Pigmented naevi
Berk–Tabatznik syndrome (1961)	?	Stub thumb, short terminal phalanges of all fingers except digit V. Bilateral optic atrophy, cervical kyphosis
Dwarfism–brachydactyly syndrome (Tonoki *et al.*, 1990)	XL	Nails broad, deformed and hypoplastic. Mental retardation. Multiple anomalies
Greig cephalopolysyndactyly syndrome (Kunze & Kaufmann, 1985)	AD	Hexdactyly, syndactyly craniofacial abnormalities. Nails small; broad and dystrophic
Larsen's syndrome (Larsen *et al.*, 1950; Marques 1980; Tsang *et al.*, 1986)	AR or AD	Stub thumbs, cylindrical fingers, flattened peculiar facies, widespread eyes. Multiple dislocations, short metacarpals
Mandibuloacral dysplasia (Zina *et al.*, 1981; Tenconi *et al.*, 1986)	AR	Club-shaped terminal phalanges. Mandibular hypoplasia, delayed cranial closure. Dysplastic clavicles. Atrophy of skin over hands and feet. Alopecia
Macrodactyly (Barsky, 1967)	AD	One or two fingers markedly enlarged
Nanocephalic dwarfism (Seckel, 1960; Butler *et al.*, 1987)	AR	Low birth weight with adult head circumference. Mental retardation. Beak-like protrusion of nose. Multiple osseous anomalies. Clubbing of fingers
Nasodigitoacoustic syndrome (Keipert *et al.*, 1973; Gorlin *et al.*, 1976)	AR	Facial abnormalities. Broad distal phalanges. Deafness
Otopalatodigital syndrome (Taybi, 1962; Pazzaglia & Beluffi, 1986)	XR or AR	Broad, short nails of thumbs and big toes. Mental retardation. Prominent occiput. Hypoplasia of facial bones. Cloven palate. Conductive deafness.
Pleonosteosis (Léri, 1921)	?	Short stature. Spade-like hand with thick palmar pads. Massive knobby thumbs. Short flexed fingers. Limited joint motion with contractures
Pseudohypoparathyroidism, hereditary osteodystrophy (Gorlin *et al.*, 1976; Fitch, 1982)	XD or AR	Short stature. Round face. Depressed nasal bridge. Short metacarpals. Mental retardation. Cataracts in 25%. Enamel hypoplasia. Calcification of skin

continued

Table 9.8. *Continued*

Diseases	Inheritance	Comments
Puretic syndrome fibramatosis systemic hyalinosis (Puretic *et al.*, 1962; McKusick, 1992)	AR	Subcutaneous tumours causing deformities of face and skull. Osteolysis of peripheral phalanges. Stunted growth. Contracture of joints. Multiple subcutaneous nodes, atrophic sclerodermic skin. Gingival fibromatosis
Rubinstein–Taybi syndrome (Rubinstein & Taybi, 1963; Berry 1987)	AR	Broad thumb and great toes. High palate, short stature, mental retardation; peculiar facies, keloid formation
Spiegler tumours and racquet nails (Tsambaos *et al.*, 1979; Greither & Rehrmann, 1980)	?	Brachydactyly. Turban tumors
Stub thumb with racquet nail (Zaun *et al.*, 1987)	AD	No other defects

Congenital ichthyosiform dermatosis with linear keratotis flexural papules and sclerosing palmoplantar keratoderma. *Arch. Dermatol.* **125**, 103.

Udell J., Schumacher H.R. Jr, Kaplan F. & Fallon M.D. (1986) Idiopathic familial acroosteolysis: histomorphometric study of bone and literature review of the Hajdu–Cheney syndrome. *Arth. Rheum.* **29**, 1032.

Valero A. & Sherf K. (1965) Pigmented nails in Peutz-Jeghers syndrome. *Am. J. Gastroentereol.* **43**, 56.

Broad nails and pseudoclubbing

When the terminal phalanx is short or dysmorphic, the nail is sometimes curved which is termed pseudoclubbing. In other cases the nail appears only broad and short. Stub thumb (brachydactyly type D, 'murderer's thumb') is a rather common genetic disorder without any other defects. The overlying nail is often called 'racquet nail'–see Chapter 2. It is also seen in connection with the various syndromes listed in Table 9.8.

References

Apert E. (1906) De l'acrocéphalosyndactylie. *Bull. Soc. Med. (Paris)* **23**, 1310.

Barrière H., Litoux P., Bureau B. *et al.* (1977) Kératose liqénoide striée: Forme congenitale. *Ann. Dermatol. Venereol.* **104**, 767.

Barsky A.J. (1967) Macrodactyly. *J. Bone Joint Surg.* **49A**, 1255.

Berk M.E. & Tabatznik B. (1961) Cervical kyphosis form posterior hemivertebrae with brachyphalangy and congenital optic artrophy. *J. Bone Joint Surg.* **43B**, 77.

Berry A.C. (1987) Rubinstein-Taybi syndrome. *J. Med. Genet.* **24**, 562.

Butler M.G., Hall B.D., Maclean R.N. & Lozzio C.B. (1987) Do some patients with Seckel syndrome have haematological problems and/or chromosome breakage? *Am. J. Med. Genet.* **27**, 645.

Fitch N. (1982) Albright's hereditary osteodystrophy: A review. *Am. J. Med. Genet.* **11**, 11.

Gorlin R.J., Pindborg J.J. & Cohen M.M. (1976) *Syndromes of the Head and Neck*, 2nd edn. McGraw & Hill, New York.

Greither A. & Rehrmann A. (1980) Spiegler-Karzinome mit assoziierten Symptomen. Ein neues Syndrom? *Dermatologica* **160**, 361.

Keipert J.A., Fitzgerald M.G. & Danks D.M. (1973) A new syndrome of broad terminal phalanges and facial abnormalities. *Aust. Paediatr. J.* **9**, 10.

Kunze J. & Kaufmann H.J. (1985) Greig cephalopolysyndactyly syndrome. Report of a sporadic case. *Helv. Paediatr. Acta* **40**, 489.

Larsen L.J., Schottstaedt E.R. & Bost F.C. (1950) Multiple congenital dislocations associated with characteristic facial abnormality. *J. Pediatr.* **37**, 574.

Léri A. (1921) Une maladie congénitale et héréditarire: La pléonostéose familiale. *Bull. Soc. Med. (Paris)* **45**, 1228.

Maroteaux P. & Malamut G. (1968) L'acrodysostose. *Presse Med.* **76**, 2189.

Marques M.N.T. (1980) Larsen's syndrome: Clinical and genetic aspects. *J. Genet. Hum.* **28**, 83.

McKusick V.A. (1992) *Mendelian Inheritance in Man*, 10th edn. Johns Hopkins Univ. Press, Baltimore.

Pazzaglia U.E. & Beluffi G. (1986) Oto-Palato-Digital syndrome in four generations of a large family. *Clin. Genet.* **30**, 338.

Pfeiffer R.A. (1964) Dominant erbliche Akrocephalosyndaktylie. *Z. Kinderheilk* **90**, 300.

Puretic S., Puretic B., Fiser-Herman M. & Adamcic M. (1962) A unique form of mesenchumal dysplasia. *Br. J. Dermatol.* **74**, 8.

Rasmussen S.A. & Frias J.L. (1988) Mild expression of the Pfeiffer syndrome. *Clin. Genet.* **33**, 5.

Robinow M., Pfeiffer R.A., Gorlin R.J. *et al.* (1971) Acrodysostosis: a syndrome of peripheral dysostosis, nasal hypoplasia, and mental retardation. *Am. J. Dis. Child.* **121**, 195.

Rubenstein J.H. & Taybi H. (1963) Broad thumbs and toes and facial abnormalities. *Am. J. Dis. Child.* **105**, 588.

Seckel H.P.G. (1960) *Bird-Headed Dwarfs: Studies in Devel-*

opmental *Anthropology including Human Proportion*. C. Thomas, Springfield, IL.
Taybi H. (1962) Generalized skeletal dysplasia with multiple anomalies. A note on Pyle's disease. *Am. J. Roentgenol.* **88**, 450.
Tenconi R., Miotti F., Miotti A., Audino G. *et al.* (1986) Another Italian family with mandibuloacral dysplasia: why does it seem more frequent in Italy? *Am. J. Med. Genet.* **24**, 357.
Tonoki H., Kishino T. & Niikawa N. (1990) A new syndrome of dwarfism, brachydactyly, nail dysplasia, and mental retardation in sibs. *Am. J. Med. Genet.* **36**, 89.
Tsambaos D., Greither A. & Orfanos C.E. (1979) Multiple malignant Spiegler tumors with brachydactyly and racket-nails. *J. Cutan. Pathol.* **6**, 31.
Tsang M.C.K., Ling J.Y.K., King N.M. & Chow S.K. (1986) Oral and craniofacial morphology of a patient with Larsen syndrome. *J. Craniofac. Genet. Dev. Biol.* **6**, 357.
Zaun H., Payeur M. & Stenger D. (1987) Brachyonychie unterschiedlichen Typs bei Mutter und Tochter. *Hautarzt* **38**, 104.
Zina A.M., Cravario A. & Bundino S. (1981) Familial mandibuloacral dysplasia. *Br. J. Dermatol.* **105**, 719.

Koilonychia – spoon nails

In koilonychia the contour is concave instead of convex. Acquired forms are often associated with anaemia, thyroid dysfunction or trauma. Familial koilonychia without other defects is rare, but the cases reported suggest autosomal dominant transmission (Bumpers & Bishop, 1980; Almagor & Haim, 1981; Crosby & Petersen, 1989). Koilonychia with dominantly inherited leuconychia was described by de Graciansky and Boule (1961) and Baran and Achten (1969), and with leuconychia, keratoderma palmoplantare, knuckle pads and deafness by Bart and Pumphrey (1967). Koilonychia is also seen with keratoderma palmoplantare progressiva (type Meleda; Table 9.1); some other ectodermal dysplasias (Tables 9.2 & 9.3); monilethrix (Walzer, 1930; Lewis 1942); onychogryphosis (Curtis & Netherton, 1939); the nail–patella syndrome (p. 295); incontinentia pigmenti (Table 9.6); trichoepithelioma multiplex (Cramers, 1981); and in a syndrome with abnormally long eyelashes (Zaun *et al.*, 1984). In trichomegaly koilonychia has otherwise not been reported (Gray, 1944).

References

Almagor G. & Haim S. (1981) Familial koilonychia. *Dermatologica* **162**, 400.
Baran R. & Achten G. (1969) Les associations congénitales de koilonychie et de leuconychie totale. *Arch. Belg. Dermatol.* **25**, 13.
Bart R.S. & Pumphrey R.E. (1967) Knuckle pads, leukonychia and deafness. A dominantly inherited syndrome. *N. Engl. J. Med.* **276**, 202.
Bumpers R.D. & Bishop M.E. (1980) Familial koilonychia. *Arch. Dermatol.* **116**, 845.
Cramers M. (1981) Trichoepithelioma multiplex and dystrophia unguis congenita. A new syndrome? *Acta Derm. Venereol. (Stockh.)* **61**, 364.
Crosby D.L. & Petersen M.J. (1989) Familial koilonychia. *Cutis* **44**, 209.
Curtis G.H. & Netherton F.W. (1939) Congenital koilonychia and onychogryphosis. *Arch. Dermatol.* **40**, 839.
de Graciansky P. & Boule S. (1961) Association de koilonychie et de leuconychie transmises en dominance. *Bull. Soc. Fr. Dermatol. Syphil.* **68**, 15.
Gray H. (1944) Trichomegaly or movie lashes. *Stanford Med. Bull.* **2**, 157.
Lewis G.M. (1942) Monilethrix, koilonychia. *Arch. Dermatol.* **45**, 209.
Walzer A. (1930) Monilethrix and koilonychia. *Arch. Dermatol.* **21**, 1054.
Zaun H., Stenger D., Zabransky S. & Zankl M. (1984) Das Syndrom der langen Wimpern ('Trichomegaliesyndrom', Oliver-McFarlane). *Hautarzt* **35**, 162.

Curved nail of the fourth toe

Plantarly curved nail deformity of the fourth toe with hypoplasia of the bone and soft tissue of the distal phalange was described by Iwasawa *et al.* (1990).

Reference

Iwasawa M., Hirose T. & Matsao K. (1991) Congential curved nail of the fourth toe. *Plast. Rec. Surg.* **87**, 553.

Overcurvature of the nails

This is an excessive transverse curvature of one or more nails giving the effect of an ingrowing toenail, often causing considerable discomfort (Chapman, 1973; Samman, 1978). In hidrotic ectrodermal dysplasia (Table 9.1) the nails are conical with distal ingrowing and increased convexity. They often fail to reach the end of the digit, appear small and may have onycholysis and/or spontaneous shedding. Circumferential nails (Table 9.12) also have an excessive curvature (Chauda & Crosby, 1993).

References

Chapman. R.S. (1973) Overcurvature of the nails. An inherited disorder. *Br. J. Dermatol.* **89**, 317.
Chavda D.V. & Crosby L.A. (1993) Circumferential toenail. *Foot & Ankle* **14**, 111.
Samman P.D. (1978) Great toe nail dystrophy. *Clin. Exp. Dermatol.* **3**, 81.

Ectopic nails, onychoheterotopia

(Figs 9.28–9.30)

After trauma to the nail matrix a portion of it can produce a nail outside the nail fold. A normal looking congenital ectopic nail on the palmar aspect of the thumb was described by Ohya (1931; cited in Kikuchi *et al.*, 1978).

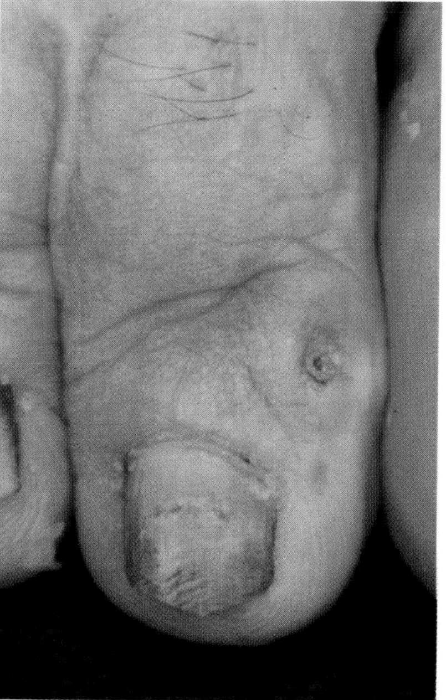

Fig. 9.28. Ectopic nail (courtesy of K. Aoki, Japan).

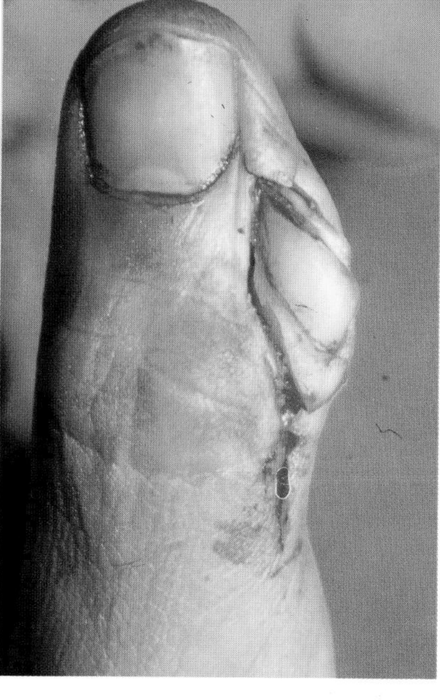

Fig. 9.29. Ectopic nail – in the process of removal.

Kalisman and Kleinert (1983) reported a boy with circumferential nail growth over all sides of the small finger. A similar case was associated with Pierre Robin syndrome (Roger *et al.*, 1986). A fingernail and dorsal skin on the palmar surface with a normal nail on the dorsal surface was reported by Keret and Ger (1987). Two patients with congenital ectopic palmar nails of the little finger were associated with absent flexion in the finger (Rider, 1992). In other reported cases the nails have been abnormally shaped (Kikuchi *et al.*, 1978, 1984; Miura, 1978; Aoki & Suzuki, 1984; Yamasaki *et al.*, 1984; Markinson *et al.*, 1988). They all appeared on the palmar (Fig. 9.30) or dorsal side 1 cm from the normal nail. Kinoshita *et al.*

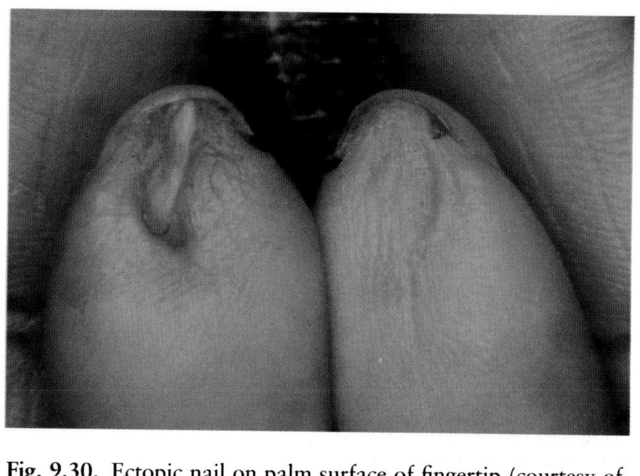

Fig. 9.30. Ectopic nail on palm surface of fingertip (courtesy of Lindsay, USA).

(1993) reported a clam-like deformity of the little finger expressing the unusual appearance of the nail wrapping around the fingertip. Ectopic nails should be differentiated from rudimentary polydactyly (Baden *et al.*, 1976), from COIF (Millman & Strier, 1982) and from the nail matrix doubling syndrome of Vigh and Printer (1973), with thick nails, oculomotor paresis, debility and aplasia of the external ear.

References

Aoki K. & Suzuki H. (1984) The morphology and hardness of the nail in 2 cases of congenital onychoheterotopia. *Br. J. Dermatol.* **110**, 717–723.

Baden H.P., Alper J.C. & Lee L.D. (1976) Rudimentary polydactyly presenting as a claw. *Arch. Dermatol.* **112**, 1006.

Kalisman M. & Kleinert H.E. (1983) A circumferential fingernail–fingernail on the palmar aspect on the finger. *J. Hand Surg.* **8**, 58.

Keret D. & Ger E. (1987) Double fingernails on the small fingers. *J. Hand Surg.* **12A**, 608.

Kikuchi I., Ono T. & Ogata K. (1978) Ectopic nail. *Plast. Reconstr. Surg.* **61**, 781.

Kikuchi I., Ogata K. & Idemori M. (1984) Vertically growing ectopic nail. Nature's experiment on nail growth direction. *J. Am. Acad. Dermatol.* **10**, 114.

Kinoshita Y., Kojima T. & Ushida M. (1993) Clam nail deformity of the little finger. *Plast. Reconstr. Surg.* **91**, 158.

Markinson B., Brenner A.R. & McGrath M. (1988) Congenital ectopic nail. A case study. *J. Am. Podiatr. Med. Assoc.* **78**, 318.

Millman A.J. & Strier R.P. (1982) Congenital onychodysplasia of the index fingers. *J. Am. Acad. Dermatol.* **7**, 57.

Miura T. (1978) Two families with congenital nail anomalies: Nail formation in ectopic areas. *J. Hand Surg.* **3**, 348.

Rider M.A. (1992) Congenital palmar nail syndrome. *J. Hand Surg.* **17B**, 371.

Roger H., Souteyrand P., Collin J.P., Vanneuville G. & Teinturier (1986) Onychohétérotopie avec polyonychie associée a un syndrome de Pierre Robin: A propos d'une nouvelle observation. *Ann. Dermatol. Venereol.* **113**, 235.

Vigh G. & Pinter L. (1973) Nagelmatrix-Verdoppelungssyndrom. *Z. Haut. Geschl.-Krankh.* **48**, 125.

Yamasaki R., Yamasaki M., Kokoroishi T. & Jidoi J. (1984) Ectopic nail associated with bone deformity. *J. Dermatol.* **11**, 295.

Congenital malformations caused by drugs or infections

Hydantoin (phenytoin) taken during pregnancy is known to cause malformations, including hypoplasia of nail and fingers, a broad short nose, ocular hypertelorism, ptosis, strabismus and ear and mouth abnormalities. Cleft lip, ventricular septum defects and psychomotor retardation can also occur (Silverman *et al.*, 1988). Trimethadione, paramethadione and valproic acid can produce similar multiple defects (Gorlin *et al.*, 1976; Rosen & Lightner, 1978; Jäger-Roman *et al.*, 1986). After valproic acid the nails were long and hyperconvex. After carbamazepine only hypoplastic nail changes were reported which normalized after some months (Niesen & Fröscher, 1985). After phenobarbitone hypoplasia of nails and phalanges was observed (Thakker *et al.*, 1991). Hyperpigmentation of several fingernails after hydantoin has also been described (Johnson & Goldsmith 1981; Verdeguer *et al.*, 1988). It can be distal with detachment of the nail plate, diffuse or occur as dark longitudinal streaks.

Anticoagulant therapy with warfarin during the first trimester of pregnancy may give hypoplasia of nasal bones and the terminal phalanges together with stippled epiphyses: the fingernails are small and malformed. The syndrome has many features in common with the dominant type of chondrodysplasia punctata (Pettifor & Benson, 1975). Malformations in infants of chronically alcoholic women are common and include growth deficiency, bone, eye and cardiac anomalies as well as hirsutism and nail hypoplasia (Crain *et al.*, 1983). Taylor *et al.* (1988) reported koilonychia, transverse growth, hyperpigmentation and thinning of nails in children born after maternal poisoning with polychlorinated biphenyls (PCB) in rice oil.

Congenital cutaneous candidiasis is uncommon and can involve only the nails (Arbegast *et al.*, 1990). In congenital acquired immune deficiency syndrome (AIDS) the nails appear yellow (Chernosky & Finley, 1985; Daniel, 1986).

References

Arbegast K.D., Lamberty L.F., Koh J.K. *et al.* (1990) Congenital candidiasis limited to the nail plates. *Pediatr. Dermatol.* **7**, 310.

Chernosky M.E. & Finley V.K. (1985) Yellow nail syndrome in patients with acquired immunodeficiency disease. *J. Am. Acad. Dermatol.* **13**, 731.

Crain L.S., Fitsmaurice N.E. & Mondry C. (1983) Nail dysplasia and fetal alcohol syndrome. *Am. J. Dis. Child.* **137**, 1069.

Daniel C.R. III (1986) Yellow nail syndrome and acquired immunodeficiency disease. *J. Am. Acad. Dermatol.* 14:844.

Gorlin R.J., Pindborg J.J. & Cohen M.M. (1976) *Syndromes of the Head and Neck*, 2nd edn. McGraw Hill, New York.

Jäger-Roman E., Deichl A., Jakob S. *et al.* (1986) Fetal growth, major malformations, and minor anomalies in infants born to women receiving valproic acid. *J. Paediatr.* **108**, 997.

Johnson R.B. & Goldsmith L.A. (1981) Dilantin digital effects. *J. Am. Acad. Dermatol.* **5**, 191.

Niesen M. & Fröscher W. (1985) Finger- and toenail hypoplasia after carbamazepine monotherapy in late pregnancy. *Neuropediatrics* **16**, 167–168.

Pettifor J.M. & Benson R. (1975) Congenital malformations associated with the administration of oral anticoagulants during pregnancy. *J. Pediatr.* **86**, 459.

Rosen R.C. & Lightner E.S. (1978) Phenotypic malformations in association with maternal trimethadione therapy. *J. Pediatr.* **92**, 240.

Silverman A.K., Fairley J. & Wong R.C. (1988) Cutaneous and immunologic reactions to phenytoin. *J. Am. Acad. Dermatol.* **18**, 721.

Thakker J.C., Kothari S.S., Deshmu K.L. *et al.* (1991) Hypoplasia of nails and phalanges: A teratogenic manifestation of phenobarbitone. *Indian Pediatr.* **28**, 73.

Verdeguer J.M., Ramon D., Moragon M. *et al.* (1988) Onychopathy in a patient with fetal hydantoin syndrome. *Pediatr. Dermatol.* **5**, 56.

Taylor J.S., Rogan W.J. & Cwi J. (1988) Congenital Yucheng-dermatological findings. *Proc. Am. Dermatol. Assoc.* 30.

Nail discoloration

Discoloration of nails is common. Abnormal colour due to external factors staining the nail have been reviewed by Daniel (1985) and the influence of drugs and systemic disorders have recently been discussed (Daniel, 1990). Leuconychias and their classification have been reviewed by Grossman and Scher (1990). The conditions with congenital and/or hereditary discoloration are listed in Table 9.9 according to colour changes. Several of them are combined with other abnormalities and are therefore also mentioned elsewhere.

References

Albright S.D. & Wheeler C.I. (1964) Leukonychia. Total and partial leukonychia in a single family with a review of the literature. *Arch. Dermatol.* **90**, 392.

Baran R. & Achten G. (1969) Les associations congénitales de koilonychie et de leuconychie totale. *Arch. Belg. Dermatol.* **25**, 13.

Bart R.S. & Pumphrey R.E. (1967) Knuckle pads, leukonychia and deafness. A dominantly inherited syndrome. *N. Engl. J. Med.* **176**, 202.

Bart B.J., Gorlin R.J., Anderson E.V. & Lynch F.W. (1966) Congenital localized absence of skin and associated abnormalities resembling epidermolysis bullosa. *Arch. Dermatol.* **93**, 296.

Bearn A. & McKusick V.A. (1958) Azure lunulae an unusual change in the fingernails in two patients with hepatolenticular degeneration (Wilson's disease). *J. Am. Med. Assoc.* **166**, 903.

Buskshell L.L. & Gorlin R.J. (1975) Leukonychia totalis, mul-

Table 9.9. Conditions with congenital and/or hereditary discoloration of nails listed according to colour changes. Inheritances are indicated as follows: AD, autosomal dominant; AR, autosomal recessive

Disease	Colour of nail	Inheritance	Comments and references
Keratitis, ichthyosis and deafness	White, thick	AR	See Table 9.1, KID syndrome
Keratoderma palmoplantare with atrophic fibrosis of extremities	White	AD	(Huriez *et al.*, 1969)
Leopard syndrome	White with koilonychia	AD	Lentigines, electrocardiographic changes, ocular hypertelorism, pulmonary stenosis, abnormalities of genitalia, retarded growth, deafness (Selmanowitz *et al.*, 1971; Voron *et al.*, 1976)
Leuconychia totalis	Milky or porcelain	AD	(Albright & Wheeler, 1964; Kates *et al.*, 1986)
Leuconychia subtotalis	Milky or porcelain	AD	Pink area (2–4 mm), distal to white area (Juhlin, 1963).
Leuconychia striatus	Milky or porcelain	AD	Longitudinal or transverse band (Sibley, 1922; Higashi, 1971; Mahler *et al.*, 1987)
L. striatus + eruptive milia	Milky or porcelain		(Schimpf & Pons, 1974)
Leuconychia + koilonychia	Milky or porcelain	AD	(de Graciansky & Boule, 1961; Baran & Achten, 1969)
Leuconychia + koilonychia + deafness + knuckle pads + keratoderma palmoplantare	Milky or porcelain	AD	(Bart & Pumphrey, 1967; Crosti *et al.*, 1983)
Leuconychia + multiple sebaceous cysts + renal calculi, FLOTCH syndrome)	Milky or porcelain	AD	(Bushkell & Gorlin, 1975; Friedel *et al.*, 1986)
Leuconychia + onychorhexis + hypoparathyroidism + dental changes + cataract	Milky or porcelain	AR	(Moshkowitz *et al.*, 1969)
Leuconychia duodenal ulcer and gallstones	Milky or porcelain	?	(Ingegno & Yatto, 1982)
Leuconychia + pili torti	White		(Giustina *et al.*, 1985)
Acrokeratosis verruciformis (Hopf's disease)	White in early years. Brown with ridging and subungual hyperkeratosis in later life	AD	Verrucuos or lichenoid papules on the dorsa of hands and fingers. Palms and soles may be involved as translucent punctae (Niedelman & McKusick, 1962; Herndon & Wilson, 1966; Schueller, 1972)
Haemochromatosis	White, grey or brownish	AD	Koilonychia in 50%. Periungual area brown (Chevrant-Breton *et al.*, 1977; Kalk, 1957)

continued on p. 332

Table 9.9. *Continued*

Disease	Colour of nail	Inheritance	Comments and references
Familial amyloidosis with polyneuropathy	Yellow	—	More marked on distal toenails (Hendricks, 1980)
Incontinentia pigmenti	Slightly yellow	AD	See Table 9.6
Macular amyloidosis with familial nail dystrophy	Yellow-brown	AD	Resolution of nail changes during third or fourth decade (Shaw *et al.*, 1983)
Aplasia cutis with dystrophic nails	Grey-yellow, brown periungual skin	AD	(Bart *et al.*, 1966)
Pachyonychia congenita	Yellow or brown	AD	See Table 9.7
Progeria	Yellow, atrophic	AR	See Table 9.7
Yellow nail syndrome congenital	Yellow	—	Family history of lymphoedema (Marks & Ellis, 1970)
Acrodermatitis enteropathica	Brownish		(Kamatani *et al.*, 1978)
Acanthosis nigricans	Grey-brown	AD	(Magid *et al.*, 1987)
Aplasia cutis with dystrophic nails	Grey-yellow, brown periungual skin	AD	(Bart *et al.*, 1966)
Darier's disease	Brown, red or white	AD	Usually as longitudinal white and red streaks. Subungeal, V-shaped keratoses (Ronchese, 1965; Zaias & Ackerman, 1973)
Congenital phenytoin effect	Brown, red and white	—	—
Congenital pigmented naevi of the nails	Brown, sometimes as longitudinal band	AD	(Caron, 1962; Coskey, 1983)
Epidermal naevus	Dark	?	—
Hereditary ectodermal dysplasia syndromes	Dark, brown		See Table 9.1
Congenital porphyria (Günther's)	Brown	AR	Possible mutilation of hands and feet. Koilonychia
Porphyria cutanea tarda	Yellow brown. Pigmentation in bands Photoonycholysis	AR	Usually distal. Absence of lunula, early koilonychia (Puissant *et al.*, 1971)
Erythropoetic protoporphyria	Grey-blue-brown, opaque. Can be red in Wood's light. Photoonycholysis (white). Absence of lunula	AR	(Redeker & Berke, 1962; Thivolet *et al.*, 1968; Marsden & Dawber, 1977)
Ochronosis	Grey blue	AR	Appears in adults (Teller & Winkler, 1973) With alkaptonuria (Christensen & Manthrope, 1983)

continued

Table 9.9. *Continued*

Disease	Colour of nail	Inheritance	Comments and references
Angioma	Bluish-red nail bed	—	—
Coat's syndrome	Bluish-red nail bed with telangiectasia	AR	Telangiectasis of face conjunctiva, retina. Deafness, muscles weakness. Mental retardation (Small, 1968)
Congenital heart disease	Red-bluish lunula	AD	Clubbing
Hepatolenticular degeneration, Wilson's disease	Azure lunula	AR	(Bearn & MacKusick, 1958)
Hereditary acrolabial teleangiectasia	Blue lunula and nail bed	AD	Blue lips and nipples, telangiectasia of chest, elbows and dorsal of hands. Varicosities of lower legs (Millns & Dicken, 1979)
Hereditary haemorrhagic teleangiectasia (Rendu–Olser–Weber syndrome)	Blue fine blood vessels (Fig. 9.11)	AD	Telangiectasia of face conjunctiva, fingers, mucosa of nasopharynx, gastrointestinal tract and bladder (Gorlin & Sedano, 1978; Graft, 1983)
Klippel–Trénaunay syndrome	Bluish	AD	Large haemangioma with hypertrophy of bones and soft tissue
Nigraemia. Hemoglobin M disease	Blue cyanotic	AD	Cyanosis of face. No clubbing. Brown haemoglobin M band on electrophoresis (Shibata *et al.*, 1967)
Pernicious anaemia	Blue	AD or AR	Hair changes (Carmel, 1985; Noppakun & Swasdikul, 1986)
Peutz–Jeghers–Touraine syndrome	Black	AD	Longitudinal bands; unusual clubbing (Valero & Sherf, 1965)

tiple sebacous cysts, renal calculi. *Arch. Dermatol.* **111**, 899.

Carmel R. (1985) Hair and fingernail changes in acquired and congenital pernicious anema. *Arch. Intern. Med.* **145**, 484.

Caron G.A. (1962) Familial congenital pigmented naevi of the nails. *Lancet* **i**, 508.

Chevrant-Breton J., Simon M., Bourel M. & Ferrand B. (1977) Cutaneous manifestations of idiopathic hemochromatosis. *Arch. Dermatol.* **113**, 161.

Christensen K. & Manthrope R. (1983) Alkaptonuria and ochronosis: a survey and 5 cases. *Human Hered.* **33**, 140.

Coskey R. (1983) Congenital subugual naevus. *J. Am. Acad. Dermatol.* **9**, 747.

Crosti C., Sala F., Bertani E., Gasparini G. & Menni S. (1983) Leuconychie totale et dysplasie ectodermique. Observation de deux cas. *Ann. Dermatol. Venereol.* **110**, 617.

Daniel C.R. III (1985) Nail pigmentation abnormalities. *Dermatol. Clin.* **3**, 431.

Daniel C.R. III (1990) Pigmentation abnormaties. In: *Nails: Therapy, Diagnosis, Surgery*, p. 153. eds Scher & Daniel, W.B. Saunders, Philadelphia.

de Graciansky P. & Boule S. (1961) Association de koilonychie et de leuconychie transmises en dominance. *Bull. Soc. Fr. Dermatol. Syphil.* **68**, 15.

Friedel J., Heid E. & Grosshans (1986) Le Syndrome 'Flotch'. Survenue Familiale d'une LeucOnychie totale, de kystes Trichilemmaux et d'une dystrophie Ciliaire à Hérédité autosomique dominante. *Ann. Dermatol. Venereol.* **113**, 549.

Giustina T.A., Woo T.X., Campbell J.P. & Ellis C.N. (1985) Association of pili torti and leukonychia. *Cutis* **35**, 533.

Gorlin R.J. & Sedano H.O. (1978) Hereditary hemorrhagic telangiectasia. The Rendu–Weber–Osler syndrome. *J. Dermatol. Surg. Oncol.* **4**, 864.

Graft G.E. (1983) A review of hereditary hemorrhagic teleangiectasia. *J. Am. Osteopathol. Assoc.* **82**, 412.

Grossman M. & Scher R.K. (1990) Leukonychia. Review and classification. *Int. J. Dermatol.* **29**, 535.

Hendricks A.A. (1980) Yellow lunulae with fluorescence after tetracycline therapy. *Arch. Dermatol.* **116**, 438.

Herndon J.H. & Wilson J.D. (1966) Acrokeratosis verruciformis (Hopf) and Darier's disease. *Arch. Dermatol.* **93**, 305.

Higashi N. (1971) Leukonychia striata longitudinalis. *Arch. Dermatol.* **104**, 142.

Huriez C., Deminati M., Agache P., Delmas-Marsalet Y. & Mennecier M. (1969) Génodermatose scléro-atrophiante et kératodermique des extrémités. *Ann. Dermatol. Syphil. (Paris)* **96**, 135.

Ingegno A.D. & Yatto R.P. (1982) Hereditary white nails (leuconychia totalis), duodenal ulcer and gallstones: genetic implications. *NY State J. Med.* **82**, 1797.

Juhlin L. (1963) Hereditary leuconychia. *Acta Derm. Venereol. (Stockh.)* **43**, 136.

Kalk H.O. (1957) Über Hautzeichen bei Leberkrankheiten. *Dtsch. Med. Wochenschr.* **38**, 1637.

Kamatani M., Rai A., Hen H. *et al.* (1978) Yellow nail syndrome associated with mental retardation in two siblings. *Br. J. Dermatol.* **99**, 329.

Kates S.L., Harris G.D. & Nagle D.J. (1986) Leukonychia totalis. *J. Hand Surg. (Br.)* **11B**, 465.

Magid M., Esterly N.B., Prendiville J. & Fujisaki C. (1987) The yellow nail syndrome in an 8-year-old girl. *Pediatr. Dermatol.* **4**, 90.

Mahler R.H., Gerstein W. & Watters K. (1987) Congenital leukonychia striata. *Cutis* **39**, 453.

Marks R. & Ellis J.P. (1970) Yellow nails. A report of six cases. *Arch. Dermatol.* **102**, 619.

Marsden R.A. & Dawber R.P.R. (1977) Erythropoeitic protoporphyria with onycholysis. *Proc. Roy. Soc. Med.* **70**, 252.

Millns J.L. & Dicken C.H. (1979) Hereditary acrolabial telangiectasia. *Arch. Dermatol.* **115**, 474.

Moshkowitz A., Abrahamov A. & Pisanti S. (1969) Congenital hypoparathyroidism simulating epilepsy, with other symptoms and dental signs of intra-uterine hypocalcemia. *Pediatrics* **44**, 401.

Niedelman M.L. & McKusick V. (1962) Acrokeratosis verruciformis (Hopf). *Arch. Dermatol.* **86**, 779.

Noppakun N. & Swasdikul D. (1986) Reversible hyperpigmentation of skin and nails with white hair due to vitamin B_{12} deficiency. *Arch. Dermatol.* **122**, 896.

Puissant A., David V., Lachiver D. & Aitken G. (1971) Formes cliniques atypiques de la porphyrie cutanée tardive. *Boll. Ist Derm. San Gallicano* **7**, 19.

Redeker A. & Berke M. (1962) Erythropoietic protoporphyria with eczema solare. *Arch. Dermatol.* **86**, 569.

Reilly P.J. & Nostrant T.T. (1984) Clinical manifestations of hereditary hemorrhagic teleangiectasia. *Am. J. Gastroenterol.* **79**, 363.

Ronchese F. (1965) The nail in Darier's disease. *Arch. Dermatol.* **91**, 617.

Schimpf A. & Pons F. (1974) Multiple eruptive Millien und striäre leukonychia. *Z. Hautkrankh.* **49**, 207.

Schueller W.A. (1972) Acrokeratosis verruciformis of Hopf. *Arch. Dermatol.* **106**, 81.

Selmanowitz V.J., Orentreich N. & Felsenstein J.M. (1971) Lentiginous profusa syndrome (multiple lentigines syndrome). *Arch. Dermatol.* **104**, 393.

Shaw M., Jurecka W., Black M.M. & Kurwa A. (1983) Macular amyloidosis associated with familial nail dystrophy. *Clin. Exp. Dermatol.* **8**, 363.

Shibata S., Miyagi T., Iuchi I., Ohba Y. & Yamamoto K. (1967) Hemoglobin M's of the Japanese. *Bull. Yamaguchi Med. Sch.* **14**, 141.

Sibley K. (1922) Leukonychia striata. *Br. J. Dermatol. Syphil.* **34**, 238.

Small R.G. (1968) Coat's disease and muscular dystrophy. *Trans. Am. Acad. Ophthalmol.* **72**, 225.

Teller H. & Winkler K. (1973) Zur Klinik und Histopathologie der endogenen Ochronose. *Hautarzt* **12**, 537.

Thivolet J., Freycon J., Perrot H., Gauibaud P. & Beyvin A.J. (1968) Protoporphyrie érythropoietique. *Bull. Soc. Fr. Dermatol. Syphil.* **75**, 829.

Valero A. & Sherf K. (1965) Pigmented nails in Peutz-Jeghers syndrome. *Am. J. Gastroenterol.* **43**, 56.

Voron D.A., Hatfield H.H. & Kalkhoff R.K. (1976) Multiple lentigines syndrome. Case report and review of literature. *Am. J. Med.* **60**, 446.

Zaias N. & Ackerman B. (1973) The nail in Darier–White disease. *Arch. Dermatol.* **107**, 193.

Epidermolysis bullosa (Figs 9.32–9.42)

The various forms of epidermolysis bullosa and their nail changes which might help in diagnosis are listed in Table 9.10. We have used a slight modification of the classification recommended by a consensus group on epidermolysis bullosa (Fine *et al.*, 1991). A comprehensive review of epidermolysis bullosa has recently been published (Priestley *et al.*, 1990). Epidermolysis bullosa with congenital skin defects described as a new syndrome by Bart *et al.* (1966) has been excluded since it is regarded as damage caused *in utero* which can occur in most types of epidermolysis bullosa (Wojnarowska *et al.*, 1983; Bedane *et al.*, 1990).

References

Altomare G.F., Polenghi M., Pigatto P.D. *et al.* (1990) Dystrophic epidermolysis bullosa inversa: A case report. *Dermatologica* **181**, 145.

Bart B.J., Gorlin R.J., Anderson E.V. & Lynch F.W. (1966) Congenital localized absence of skin and associated abnormalities resembling epidermolysis bullosa. *Arch. Dermatol.* **93**, 296.

Bedane C., Barbeau C., Ronayette D. *et al.* (1990) Dystrophic epidermolysis bullosa with congenital skin defect: A variant of Bart's syndrome? In: *Epidemolysis Bullosa*, eds Priestley *et al.*, p. 87. DEBRA, Crowthorne, Berkshire.

Bruckner-Tuderman L., Vogel A., Rüegger S., Odermatt B., Tönz O. & Schnyder U.W. (1989) Epidermolysis bullosa simplex with mottled pigmentation. *J. Am. Acad. Dermatol.* **21**, 425.

Buchbinder L.H., Lucky A.W., Ballard E. *et al.* (1986) Severe infantile epidermolysis bullosa simplex: Dowling–Meara type. *Arch. Dermatol.* **122**, 190.

Fine J.-D., Johnson L. & Wright T. (1989) Epidermolysis bullosa simplex superficialis: a new variant of epidermolysis bullosa characterized by subcorneal skin cleavage mimicking peeling skin syndrome. *Arch. Dermatol.* **125**, 633.

Fine J.-D., Bauer E.A., Briggaman R.A. *et al.* (1991) Revised clinical and laboratory criteria for subtypes of inherited epidermolysis bullosa. *J. Am. Acad. Dermatol.* **24**, 119.

Fischer T. & Gedde-Dahl T. Jr (1979) Epidermolysis bullosa simplex and mottled pigmentation: a new dominant syndrome. *Clin. Genet.* **15**, 228.

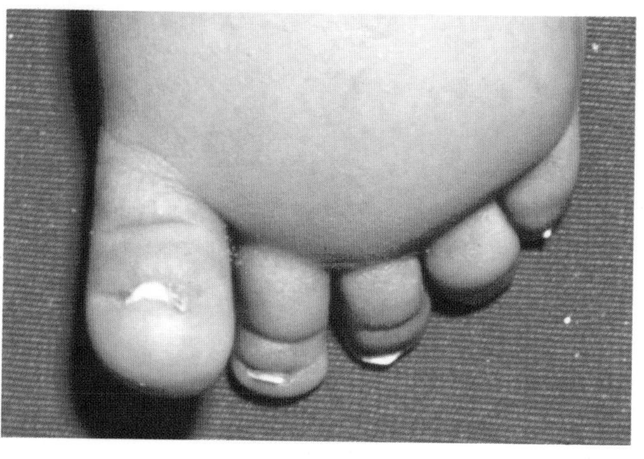

Fig. 9.31. Turner's syndrome (see Table 9.5). Narrow hypoplastic nails associated with limb lymphoedema (courtesy of L. Tamayo, Mexico DF).

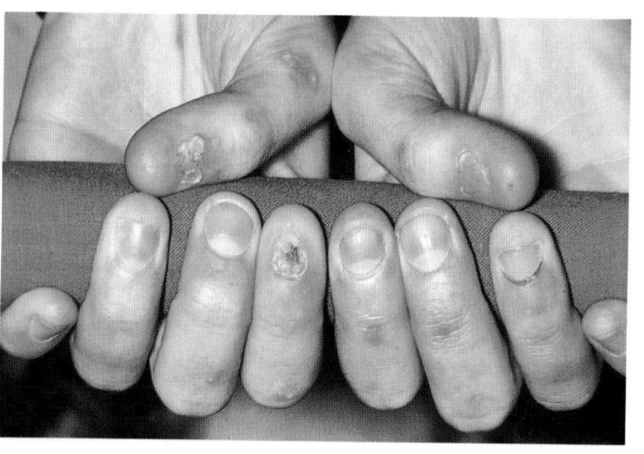

Fig. 9.32. Recessive epidermolysis bullosa dystrophica (Hallopeau–Siemens). Twenty-four-year-old female – some nails normal, some dystrophic, some absent.

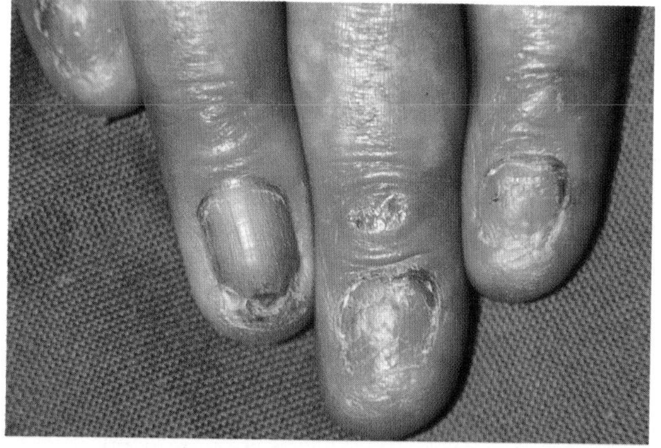

Fig. 9.33. Recessive epidermolysis bullosa dystraphica (Hallopeau–Siemens). Forty-two-year old male – severe nail dystrophy; mutilating epidermolysis bullosa with widespread blistering.

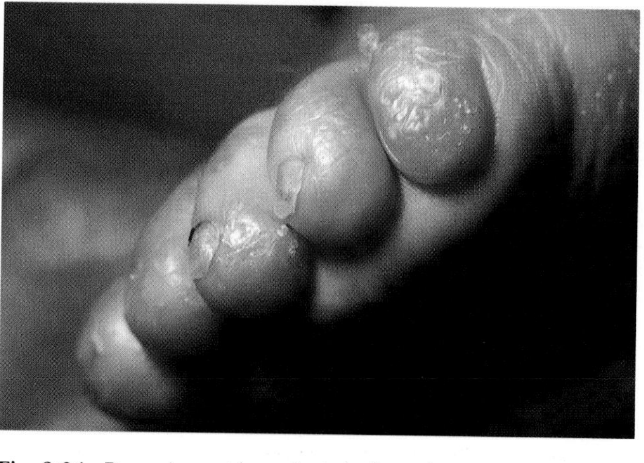

Fig. 9.34. Recessive epidermolysis bullosa dystrophica – nails of 11-month-old female.

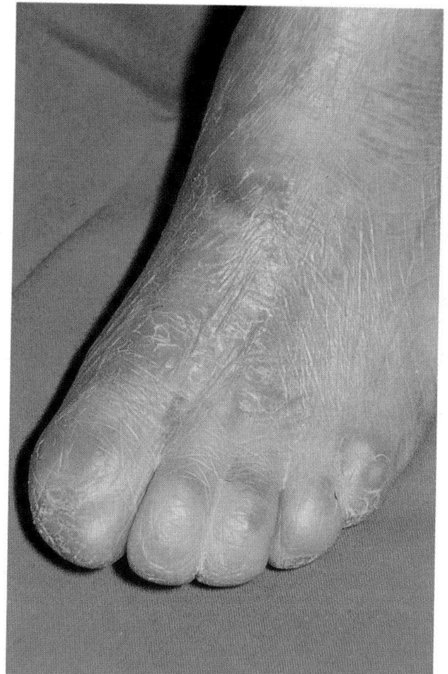

Fig. 9.35. Recessive epidermolysis bullosa dystrophica – 11-month-old male; complete loss of nails.

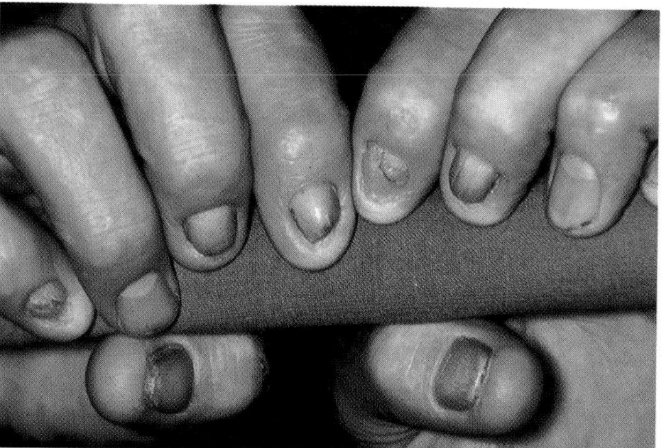

Fig. 9.36. Dominant epidermolysis bullosa dystrophica (Cockayne–Touraine) – 36-year-old male with nail dystrophy and blisters limited to hands and feet.

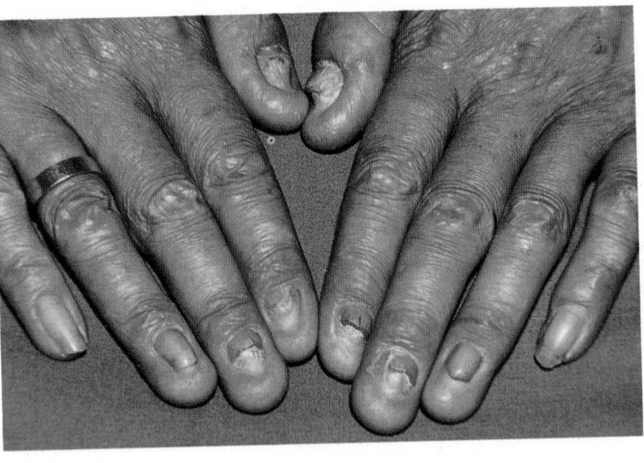

Fig. 9.37. Dominant epidermolysis bullosa dystrophica, albulopapuloid (Pasini) – 41-year-old male with thickened, short and brittle nails.

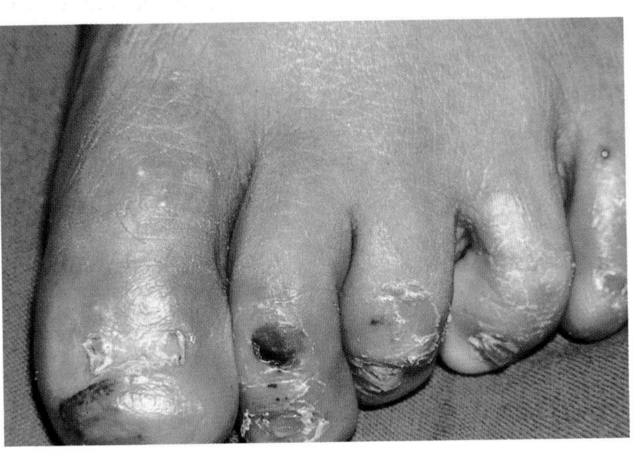

Fig. 9.38. Dominant epidermolysis bullosa dystrophica, albulopapuloid (Pasini) – 5-year-old daughter of patient in Fig. 9.37; toe blisters and nail dystrophy.

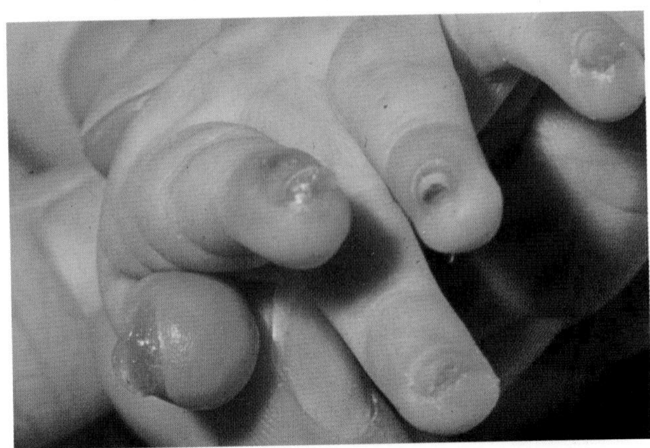

Fig. 9.39. Epidermolysis bullosa atrophicans gravis, generalized (Herlitz) – 4-week-old male with heaped-up nails and subungual granulation tissue (Voigtländer *et al*., 1979).

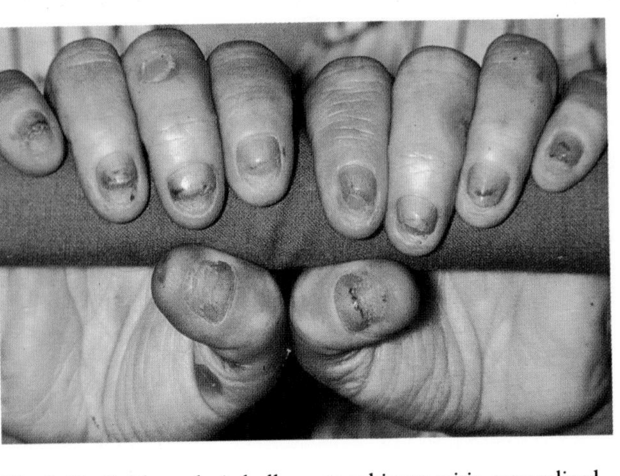

Fig. 9.40. Epidermolysis bullosa atrophicans mitis, generalized (Hashimoto *et al.*) – 42-year-old female with thickened, raised nails with early onychogryphosis.

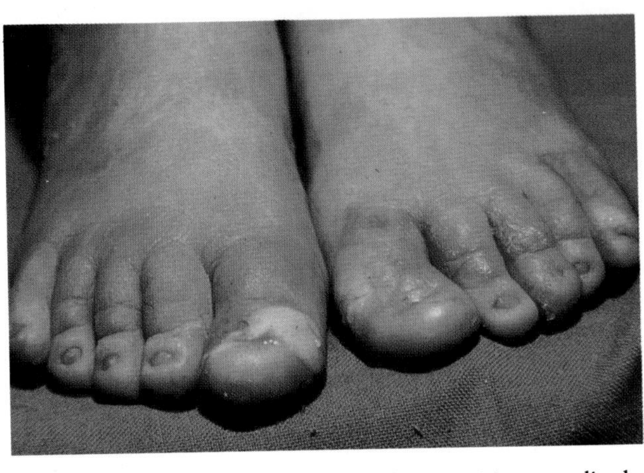

Fig. 9.41. Epidermolysis bullosa atrophicans mitis, generalized (Hashimoto *et al.*) – 5-year-old male with severe toenail dystrophy and generalized blistering.

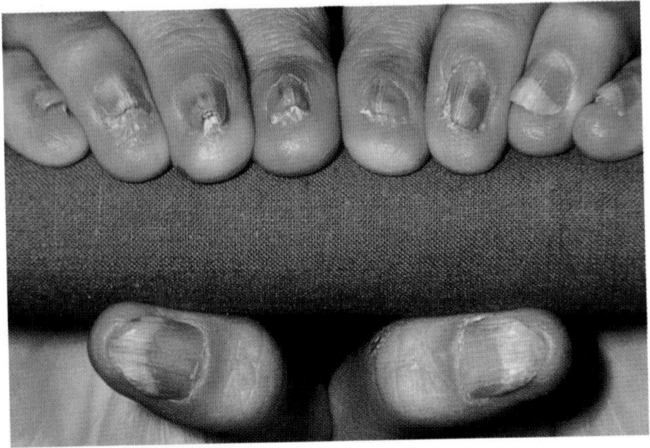

Fig. 9.42. Epidermolysis bullosa atrophicans, localized (Schnyder & Anton-Lamprect) – 27-year-old female with raised, dome-shaped, partly onychogryphotic nails.

Table 9.10. Nails in patients with epidermis bullosa. Table modified after Fine *et al.* (1991). Inheritance: AD, autosomal dominant; AR, autosomal recessive; XR, sex-linked recessive

Type of disease	Nails	Inheritance	Comments
INTRAEPIDERMAL			
EB simplex localized			
Hands and feet (Weber Cokayne type)	Normal. Rarely dystrophic	AD	Mainly palmoplantar with callus
With anodontia (Kallin's syndrome) (Gamborg Nielsen & Sjölund, 1985)	Thick or curved	AR	Alopecia, blisters mainly on hands and feet. No teeth
EB simplex, generalized			
Koebner type	Usually normal	AD	—
Herpetiformis (Dowling – Meara Buchbinder *et al.*, 1986)	Loss of nails with regeneration. End result dystrophic or normal nails	AD	Herpetiform groups of bloody blister since birth. Keratodermia
EBS with mottled pigmentation (Fischer & Gedde-Dahl, 1979; Bruckner–Tuderman *et al.*, 1989). Can overlap with Dowling–Meara	Peculiar curving Partially dystrophic	AD	Pigmentation neck, abdomen. Variant with punctate keratoderma (Medenica-Mojsilovic *et al.*, 1986)
Ogna variant	Onychogryphosis of big toe in adulthood	AD	Haemorrhagic blisters
Superficialis (Fine *et al.*, 1989)	Often dystrophic	AD	Subcorneal blisters
With neuromuscular disease (Salih *et al.*, 1985; Niemi *et al.*, 1988)	Can be dystrophic	AR	Scarring alopecia. Mysthenica gravis
Mendes da Costa variant	Normal	XR	Alopecia
JUNCTIONAL			
Junctional localized			
Inversa (Altomare, 1990)	Dystrophic or absent sometimes heaped up. Easily shed	AR	Teeth dystrophic
Acral (minimus)	Nails often absent	AR	Enemal hypoplasia
Progressive type (Gedde-Dahl, 1981)	Nails hypoplastic. Do not regrow at old age	AR	Childhood onset or blisters on hand and feet. Progressive atrophy of papillary ridges and lingual papilla
Junctional generalized			
Gravis (Herlitz)	Absent, hypoplastic or partly normal. Sometimes heaped up. Easily shed	AR	Pitted enamel hypoplasia. Anaemia. Growth retardation
Mitis	Absent, hypoplastic or partly normal. Sometimes heaped up. Easily shed	AR	Enamel hypoplasia
Cicatricial (Haber *et al.*, 1985)	Normal	AR	Alopecia. Enamel hypoplasia

continued on p. 338

Table 9.10. *Continued*

Type of disease	Nails	Inheritance	Comments
DERMAL			
Dystrophic localized			
Inversa (Gedde-Dahl, 1971)	Thick nails on toes	AR	Lesions of neck, groin, axilla
Acral (minimus)	Dystrophia on toes	AD	Improves in childhood
Pretibial (Lichtenwald *et al.*, 1990)	Short, thick, dystrophic or normal	AD	—
Centripetal	Dystrophic or absent	AR	Acral blisters with centripetal spread
Dystrophic generalized			
Albupapuloides (Pasini var.) (Ramelet & Boillat, 1985)	Thick, short split or absent	AD	Blisters mainly acral. Papules with white stria and spots on trunk
Hyperplastic (Cockayne–Touraine var.)	Dystrophic or absent nails. Onychogryphosis can occur	AD	Blisters on hands, feet, elbows, knees and malleoles. Oesophagus involved in some cases
Transient bullous dermolysis of newborn	Normal	AD AR?	Lesions disappear within first year of life. Hypopigmentation on healed areas seen
Gravis (Hallopeau–Siemens var.) (Schurig *et al.*, 1987)	Short, split or absent	AR	Scaring alopecia and oral lesions. Oesophagus stenosis. Pseudodactyly
Mitis	Dystrophic on absent nails	AR	—

Gamborg Nielsen P. & Sjölund E. (1985) Epidermolysis bullosa simplex localisata associated with anodontia, hair and nail disorders: a new syndrome. *Acta Derm. Venereol. (Stockh.)* **65**, 526.

Gedde-Dahl T. Jr (1971) *Epidermolysis Bullosa. A Clinical, Genetic and Epidemiologic Study*, p. 1. The Johns Hopkins Press, Baltimore.

Gedde-Dahl T. Jr (1981) Sixteen types of epidermolysis bullosa. *Acta Derm. Venereol. (Stockh.)* Suppl. 95, 74.

Haber R., Hanna W., Ramsay C.A. *et al.* (1985) Cicatricial junctional epidermolysis bullosa. *J. Am. Acad. Dermatol.* **12**, 836.

Lichtenwald D.J., Hanna W., Sauder D.N., Jakubovic H.R. & Rosenthal D. (1990) Pretibial epidermolysis bullosa: Report of a case. *J. Am. Acad. Dermatol.* **22**, 346.

Medenica-Mojsilovic L., Fenske N.A. & Espinoza C.G. (1986) Epidermolysis bullosa herpetiformis with mottled pigmentation and an unusual punctate keratoderma. *Arch. Dermatol.* **122**, 900.

Niemi K.-M., Sommer H., Kero M. *et al.* (1988) Epidermolysis bullosa simplex associated with muscular dystrophy with recessive inheritance. *Arch. Dermatol.* **124**, 551.

Priestley G.C., Tidman M.J., Weiss J.B. & Eady R.A.J. (1990) *Epidermolysis Bullosa: A Comprehensive Review of Classification, Management and Laboratory Studies.* DEBRA, Crowthorne, Berkshire.

Ramelet A.A. & Boillat C. (1985) Epidermolyse bulleuse dystrophique albupapuloide autosomique recessive. *Dermatologica* **171**, 397.

Salih M.A.M., Lake B.D., El Hag M.A. *et al.* (1985) Lethal epidermolytic epidermolysis bullosa: a new autosomal recessive type of epidermolysis bullosa. *Br. J. Dermatol.* **113**, 135.

Schurig B., Krieg T., Landthaler M. & Braun-Falco O. (1987) Epidermolysis bullosa hereditaria dystrophica (Hallopeau–Siemens). *Hautarzt* **38**, 619.

Wojnarowska F.T., Eady R.A.J. & Wells R.S. (1983) Dystrophic epidermolysis bullosa presenting with congenital absence of skin: report of four cases. *Br. J. Dermatol.* **108**, 477.

Secondary nail changes and some miscellaneous nail conditions

Various hereditary disorders with secondary nail changes appear in Table 9.11. In Table 9.12 we have listed disorders with non-classified nail involvement.

Table 9.11. Hereditary disorders with secondary nail changes. Inheritances are indicated as follows: AD, autosomal dominant; AR, autosomal recessive; XD, sex-linked dominant

Disease	Inheritance	Nails	Comments
Acanthosis nigricans (benign hereditary) (Tasjian & Jarrat, 1984)	AD	Thick, friable, dull, grey or normal	Pigmented, thick skin neck, axilla of inguinal region
Acrodermatitis enteropathica	AR	Periungual eczema, candida infections. Multiple Beau's lines	Alopecia, typical acral skin lesion, enteropathia
Aminogenic alopecia deficiency (Shelley & Rawnsley, 1965)	AR	Brittle	Argininosuccinic aciduria. Loss of hair
Citrullinaemia (Bonafe *et al.*, 1984)	AR	Clubbed. Red transverse band distally	Trichorrhexis. Cutaneous atrophy. Hyperammoniaemia
Congenital loss of pain (Thomson *et al.*, 1980)	AR	Brittle	Argininosuccinic synthetase deficiency
Diabetes	AR	*Candida* infection. Thick finger and toenails	—
Gingival fibromatosis, Zimmerman–Laband syndrome (Laband *et al.*, 1964; Chodirker *et al.*, 1986)	AD	Small or absent nails of thumb and big toe	Gingival fibroma. Big nose and ears. Hepatosplenomegaly. Distal phalanges short. Sometimes hypertrichosis mental retardation or ocular changes
Hyper-IgE syndrome (Davies *et al.*, 1966; Koch *et al.*, 1992)	AR	Hyperkeratotic or atrophic nails due to candida infections. Mild clubbing	Defect in polymorphonuclear neutrophil function. Red scaly skin lesions. Cold staphylococcal abscess High IgE levels. Craniosynostosis (Hoger *et al.*, 1985)
Hyperuricaemia (Gospos, 1976)	AD	Thick, split, dystrophic	—
Lesh-Nyhan syndrome (Gharbi *et al.*, 1989)	XL	Destroyed	Self-mutilation
Lichen planus hereditaria (Copeman *et al.*, 1978; Mahood, 1983; Valsechi *et al.*, 1990)	—	Destroyed	—
Lymphoedema with yellow nails (Wells, 1966) and mental retardation (Kamatani *et al.*, 1978)	AD	Thick yellow nails	Congenital lymphoedema with adult onset and respiratory tract infection
Multiple cartilaginous exostosis–Diaphyseal aclasis (Krooth *et al.*, 1961: Soloman, 1964; Hazen & Smith, 1990)	AD	Non-tender nodules of proximal part of nail fold with elevation and splitting of nail	Retardation of growth of long bones and sarcomatous degeneration reported

continued on p. 340

Table 9.11. *Continued*

Disease	Inheritance	Nails	Comments
Neurofibromatosis (Recklinghausen) (Chao, 1959; Ricchardi & Eichner, 1986)	AD	One or more hypertrophic fingers or toes with dislocation of nails	Multiple neurofibromas, cutaneous pigmentation, central nervous involvement
Porokeratosis Mibelli	AD	Thick, ridged or fissured	—
Psoriasis. Pityriasis rubra pilaris	AD	One or more hypertrophic	—
Tuberous sclerosis, epiloia, (Bourneville–Pringle)	AD	Koenen's tumours. Subungual fibroma dislocating nails	Epilepsy, mental retardation. Angiofibroma of face and oral mucosa, intracranial calcification
Zimmerman–Laband syndrome (see gingival fibromatosis above)			

Table 9.12. Various hereditary, familial or congenital disorders with nail involvement. Inheritance: AD, autosomal dominant; AR, autosomal recessive; XL, sex-linked transmission; XD, sex-linked dominant; XR, sex-linked recessive

Disease	Nails	Inheritance	Comments
Acrorenal ocular syndrome (Halal *et al.*, 1984)	Thumbnail hypoplasia	AD	Renal and ocolar anomalies. Ptosis
Ainhum, amniotic constriction band (Feingold, 1984).	Dysplastic	—	Swelling, brachydactylia or amputations *in utero*
Circumferential, curved fingernail. Congenital claw-like fingers and toes (Egawa, 1977; Kalisman & Kleinert, 1983; Allieu *et al.*, 1985; Iwasawa *et al.*, 1991)	Nails cover both dorsal and lateral or all sides of one or more fingers	AR	One case combined with Pierre – Robin syndrome
Congenital ingrown toenails (Hendricks, 1979) resulting in malalignment of the big toe nail (Baran *et al.*, 1979; Baran & Bureau, 1982; 1983; Barth *et al.*, 1986)	Thick with transverse ridging onycholysis, shedding. Panonychia common. Fibrous tumours of nailfold (Hammerton & Shrank, 1988)	?	Early surgical operation advised. Seen in monozygotic twins
Congenital subungual pterygium (Odom *et al.*, 1974; Christophers, 1975; Dugois *et al.*, 1975; Chams-Davatchi, 1980; Runne & Orfanos, 1981; Nogita *et al.*, 1991)	Aberrant hyponychium. Painful fractures of nails may occur	?	Mainly females
Dysplasia of the fifth toenail (Hundeiker, 1969)	After age 2 on the fifth toe longitudinal furrows and distal onycholysis with splitting of nails	AD?	—

continued

Table 9.12. *Continued*

Disease	Nails	Inheritance	Comments
Epidermodysplasia verruciformis-like dermatoses with nail changes (Salamon *et al.*, 1987)	Thick with longitudinal furrows. White, yellow pigmentation. Subungual hyperkeratoses	XD	Symmetric flat warts. Hyper- and hypopigmented spots
Familial twenty-nail dystrophy (Knöll *et al.*, 1989, Commens, 1990)	Longitudinal ridging, rough, loss of lustre	AD	Trachonychia can also be acquired
Great toenail dystrophy (Samman, 1978)	Affected nails, dystrophic and brownish	—	(See congenital malalignment of big toe nail)
Hypocalcified enamel and dystrophic nails (Takeda *et al.*, 1989)	Dysplastic, striated on finger and toes	XR	Hypoplastic enamel on permanent teeth. Patients otherwise normal
Inherited toenail dystrophy (Dawson, 1979, 1982)	Said to be identical to Samman's dystrophy	AD	Spontaneous resolution can occur
Laryngoonycho-cutaneous syndrome (Shabbir *et al.*, 1986; Ainsworth *et al.*, 1992)	Dystrophic nails sometimes thick	AR	Hoarseness in early life. Ulcerative pyogenic granuloma-like lesions mainly around mouth and nose. Teeth showed notching and crenations
Leprechaunism (Roth *et al.*, 1981; Cantani *et al.*, 1987)	Hyperconvex	—	Wrinkled loose skin. Decreased subcutaneous fat. Thick lips. Acanthosis nigricans. Hypotrichosis. Hyperinsulinaemia
Macular amyloidosis with familial nail dystrophy (Shaw *et al.*, 1983)	See Table 9.8	—	—
Pili torti (Beare) syndrome (Beare, 1952)	Onychodysplasia	AD	Appears after puberty. See also pili torti, p. 306
Rud syndrome (Wallach *et al.*, 1987)	Increased lunula on hands. Micronychia on toes	AR or XL	Congenital ichthyosis, epilepsy, mental retardation, retinitis pigmentosa
Soft nail disease (Prandi & Caccialanza, 1977)	Atrophic short soft nail. Absence of lunula		A single case
Trichoepithelioma multiplex and dystrophic nails (Cramers, 1981)	Thumb nails most affected. Koilonychia of index finger	AD?	Only dystrophic nails in some
Trichomegaly syndrome (Zaun *et al.*, 1984)	Koilonychia	AD	Abnormally long eyelashes. Sparse scalp hair, eye disorders and mental retardation can occur (Goldstein & Hutt, 1972)

References

Ainsworth J.R., Shabbir G., Spencer A.F. & Cockburn F. (1992) Multisystem disorder of Punjabi children exhibiting spontaneous dermal and submucosal granulation tissue formation: LOGIC syndrome. *Clin. Dysmorphol.* **1**, 3.

Allieu Y., Benichou M., Teissier J. & Baldet P. (1985) L'ongle annulaire, une malformation congénitale exceptionnelle de la main. *Ann. Chir. Plast. Esthét.* **30**, 217.

Baran R. & Bureau H. (1982) Malalignment of the big toenail as a cause of ingrowing toenail in infancy. Pathology and treatment. *Br. J. Dermatol.* **107**, 33.

Baran R. & Bureau H. (1983) Congenital malalignment of the big toe-nail as a cause of ingrowing toe-nail in infancy. Pathology and treatment (a study of thirty cases). *Clin. Exp. Dermatol.* **8**, 619.

Baran R., Bureau H. & Sayag J. (1979) Congenital malalignment of the big toenail. *Clin. Exp. Dermatol.* **4**, 359.

Barth J.H., Dawber R.P.R., Ashton R.E. & Baran R. (1986) Congenital malalignment of great toenails in 2 sets of monocygotic twins. *Arch. Dermatol.* **122**, 379.

Beare J.M. (1952) Congenital defect showing features of pili torti. *Br. J. Dermatol.* **64**, 566.

Björnberg A. (1961) Adenoma sebaceum. Review, case reports and discussion of eugenic aspects. *Acta Derm. Vernereol. (Stockh.)* **41**, 213.

Bonafe J.L., Pieraggi M.T., Abravanel M., Benque A. & Abravanel G. (1984) Skin, hair and nail changes in a case of citrullinemia with late manifestation. *Dermatologica* **168**, 213.

Cantani A., Ziruolo M.G. & Tacconi M.L. (1987) Un syndrome polydysmorphique rare: Le Lepréchaunisme. *Ann. Genet.* **30**, 221.

Chams-Davatchi C. (1980) Pterygium inversum ungueal. *Ann. Dermatol. Venereol.* **107**, 83.

Chao D.H.-C. (1959) Congenital neurocutaneous syndromes in childhood. *J. Pediatr.* **55**, 189.

Chodirker B.N., Chudley A.E., Toffler M.A. & Reed M.H. (1986) Brief clinical report: Zimmerman-Laband syndrome and profound mental retardation. *Am. J. Med. Genet.* **25**, 543.

Christophers E. (1975) Familiäre subunguale pterygion. *Hautarzt* **26**, 543.

Commens C.A. (1990) Twenty nail dystrophy in identical twins. *Pediatr. Dermatol.* **5**, 117.

Copeman P.W.M., Tan R.S.-H., Timlin D. & Samman P.D. (1978) Familial lichen planus. Another disease or a distinct people? *Br. J. Dermatol.* **98**, 573.

Cramers M. (1981) Trichoepithelioma multiplex and dystrophia unguis congenita. A new syndrome? *Acta Derm. Venereol. (Stockh.)* **61**, 364.

Davis S.D., Schaller J. & Wedgwood R.J. (1966) Job's syndrome. Recurrent 'cold' staphylococcal abscesses. *Lancet* **i**, 1013.

Dawson T.A.J. (1979) An inherited nail dystrophy principally affecting the great toenails. *Clin. Exp. Dermatol.* **4**, 309.

Dawson T.A.J. (1982) An inherited nail dystrophy principally affecting the great toenails: further observations. *Clin. Exp. Dermatol.* **7**, 455.

Dugois P., Amblard P., Martel C. & Reymond J.L. (1975) Pterygium inversum unguis familial. *Bull. Soc. Fr. Dermatol. Syphil.* **82**, 283.

Egawa T. (1977) Congenital claw-like fingers and toes. Case report of two siblings. *Plast. Reconstr. Surg.* **59**, 569.

Feingold M. (1984) Amniotic constriction bands (Streeter dysplasia, ring constrictions). *Am. J. Dis. Child.* **138**, 199.

Gharbi M.-R., Fazaa B., Ferchiou A., Mokhtar I. & Lahmar M.L. (1989) Le syndrome de Lesch et Nyhan. *Rev. Eur. Dermatol. MST* **2**, 87.

Goldstein J.H. & Hutt A.E. (1972) Trichomegaly, cataract, and hereditary spherocytosis in two siblings. *Am. J. Oththalmol.* **73**, 333.

Gospos C. (1976) Gicht. Subacute periarticuläre knotige Hautgicht der Endphalangen mit Nageldystrophie. *Z. Haut.* **51**, 29.

Halal F., Homsy M. & Perreault G. (1984) Actro-renal-ocular syndrome: Autosomal dominant thumb hypoplasia, renal ectopia, and eye defect. *Am. J. Med. Genet.* **17**, 753.

Hammerton M.D. & Shrank A.B. (1988) Congenital hypertrophy of the lateral nail folds of the hallux. *Pediatr. Dermatol.* **5**, 243.

Hazen P.G. & Smith D.E. (1990) Hereditary multiple exostoses: Report of a case presenting with proximal nail fold and nail swelling. *J. Am. Acad. Dermatol.* **22**, 132.

Hendricks W.M. (1979) Congenital ingrown toenails. *Cutis* **24**, 393.

Hoger P.H., Boltshauser E. & Hitzig W.H. (1985) Craniosynostosis in hyper IgE syndrome. *Eur. J. Pediatr.* **144**, 414.

Hundeiker M. (1969) Herditäre Nageldysplasie der 5. Zehe. *Hautarzt* **20**, 282.

Iwasawa M., Hirose T. & Matsuo K. (1991) Congenital curved nail of the fourth toe. *Plast. Reconstr. Surg.* **87**, 553.

Kalisman M. & Kleinert H.E. (1983) A circumferential fingernail. Fingernail on the palmar aspect of the finger. *J. Hand Surg.* **8**, 58.

Kamatani M., Rai A., Hen H. *et al.* (1978) Yellow nail syndrome associated with mental retardation in two siblings. *Br. J. Dermatol.* **99**, 329.

Knöll R., Ulrich R. & Schäfer R. (1989) Autosomal-dominant verebte 20-Nägel-Dystrophie. *Arch. Dermatol.* **15**, 213.

Koch P., Wettstein A., Knauber J. & Zaun H. (1992) A new case of Zimmermann–Laband syndrome with atypical retinitis pigmentosa. *Acta Derm. Venereol. (Stockh.)* **72**, 376.

Krooth R.S., Macklin M.T. & Hilbish T.F. (1961) Diaphysial aclasis (multiple exostosis) on Guam. *Am. J. Human Genet.* **13**, 340.

Laband P.F., Habib G. & Humphreys G.S. (1964) Hereditary gingival fibromatosis. Report of anaffected family with associated splenomegaly and skeletal and soft-tissue abnormalities. *Oral Surg.* **17**, 339.

Mahood J.M. (1983) Familial lichen planus. *Arch. Dermatol.* **119**, 292.

Nogita T., Yamashita H., Kawashima M. & Hidano A. (1991) Pterygium inversum unguis. *J. Am. Acad. Dermatol.* **24**, 787.

Odom R.B., Stein K.M. & Maibach H. (1974) Congenital, painful, abberant hyponychium. *Arch. Dermatol.* **110**, 89.

Prandi G. & Caccialanza M. (1977) An unusual congenital nail dystrophy ('soft nail disease'). *Clin. Exp. Dermatol.* **2**, 265.

Riccardi V.M. & Eichner J.E. (1986) *Neurofibromatosis: Phenotype, Natural History and Pathogenesis.* Johns Hopkins University Press, Baltimore.

Roth S.I., Schedewie H.K., Herzberg V.K., Olefsky J., Elders M.J., & Rubinstein A. (1981) Cutaneous manifestations of leprechaunism. *Arch. Dermatol.* **117**, 531.

Runne U. & Orfanos C.E. (1981) The human nail. *Curr. Prob. Dermatol. (Basel)* **9**, 102.

Salamon T., Halepovic E., Berberovic L. *et al.* (1987) Epidermodysplasia verruciformis-ähnliche Genodermatose mit Veränderungen der Nägel. *Hautarzt* **38**, 525.

Samman P.D. (1978) Great toe nail dystrophy. *Clin. Exp. Dermatol.* **3**, 81.

Shabbir G., Hassan M. & Kazmi A. (1986) Laryngo-onychocutaneous syndrome. A study of 22 cases. *Biomed.* **2**, 15.

Shaw M., Jurecka W., Black M.M. & Kurwa A. (1983) Macular amyloidosis associated with familial nail dystrophy. *Clin. Exp. Dermatol.* **8**, 363.

Shelley W. & Rawnsley H.M. (1965) Aminogenic alopecia: Hair loss associated with argininosuccinic aciduria. *Lancet* **ii**, 1327.

Solomon L. (1964) Herediatry multiple exostosis. *Am. J. Human Genet.* **16**, 351.

Takeda Y., Itagaki M. & Ishibashi K. (1989) Hypoplastic-hypocalcified enamel of teeth and dysplastic nails: an undescribed ectodermal dysplasia syndrome. *Int. J. Oral Maxillofac. Surg.* **18**, 73.

Tasjian D. & Jarrattt M. (1984) Familial acanthosis nigricans. *Arch. Dermaol.* **120**, 1351.

Thomson C.C., Park R.I. & Prescot G.H. (1980) Oral manifestations of the congenital insensitivity to pain syndrome. *Oral Surg.* **50**, 220.

Valsecchi R., Bontempelli M., di Landro A., Barcella A. & Lainelli T. (1990) Familial lichen planus. *Acta Derm. Venereol. (Stockh.)* **70**, 272.

Voigtländer V., Schnyder U.W. & Anton-Lamprect I. (1979) In: *Dermatologie in Praxis und Klinik*, Band III, p. 2245. Georg Thieme Verlag, Stuttgart.

Wallach D., Foldes C., Cattan E. & Dulac O. (1987) Syndrome de Rud. *Ann. Dermatol. Venereol.* **144**, 1462.

Wells G.C. (1966) Yellow nail syndrome with familial primary hypoplasia of lymphatics, manifest late in life. *Proc. Roy. Soc. Med.* **59**, 447.

Zaun H., Stenger D., Zabransky S. & Zankl M. (1984) Das Syndrom der langen Wimpern ('Trichomegaliesyndrom', Oliver-McFarlane). *Hautarzt* **35**, 162.

Chapter 10
Nail Surgery and Traumatic Abnormalities

E. HANEKE & R. BARAN
(with the participation of G.J. BRAUNER)

History and examination
Materials and instruments
Anaesthesia and dressing
Postoperative care
Biopsy
Dorsal exposure of the distal finger
Microscopically controlled surgery
Non-scalpel techniques
- Cryosurgery
- Electroradiosurgery
- Carbon dioxide laser (G. Brauner)
- Nail avulsion

Trauma
- Acute injuries
  - Haemorrhages
  - Splinter type
  - Haematomas
  - Lacerating wounds
  - Crush fractures
  - Denudation of terminal phalanx
  - Foreign bodies
  - Fingertip amputations
- Delayed post-traumatic deformities
  - Onycholysis
  - Split nail deformity
  - Hook nails
  - Malaligned nail due to matrix damage
- Nail prosthesis
- Repeated minor trauma
  - Self-inflicted injury
  - Subungual haemorrhage
  - Frictional melanonychia
  - Traumatic onycholysis
  - Hyperkeratotic reaction
  - Subungual exostosis
  - Onychogryphosis
  - Hallux valgus

Miscellaneous nail disorders
- Nail narrowing
- Congenital and hereditary disorders
- Ingrowing toenails

Complications of nail surgery
Infection
- Acute paronychia
- Chronic paroncyhia
- Subungual infection
- Lectitis purulenta et granulomatosa
- Management of diabetics and others at risk from infection

Burns
Chemical burns
The painful nail

The surgery of the nail and its associated structures has generated considerable interest during the last decade; a deformed nail has always been an unpleasant cosmetic stigma but, until recently, the possibilities for surgical correction were limited. The application by the dermatologist of the techniques of plastic surgery and the more refined skills of the specialized hand surgeon have brought fresh optimism to the field. The objectives of surgery are:

1 to facilitate diagnosis, which may entail biopsy;
2 to alleviate pain;
3 to treat infection, which may or may not be directly associated;
4 to correct or prevent anatomical, traumatic, congenital, infection-induced, parasitic or iatrogenic deformities;
5 to remove local tumours;
6 to ensure the best cosmetic result.

These objectives are often closely interrelated and must be viewed as a therapeutic whole.

History and patient examination

General examination of the patient should be carried out to exclude such potential contraindications to surgery as peripheral vascular disease, diabetes and blood dyscrasias, collagen disease, peripheral neurologic disease, prosthetic cardiac valves, elderly and incapacited patients in poor general health, and immunocompromised patients. The concomitant administration of drugs should be noted: these may affect anaesthesia, e.g. monoaminoxidase inhibitors, β-blockers or phenothiazines; prolong bleeding, e.g. aspirin or anticoagulants; delay healing, e.g. systemic or topical steroids; or have toxic effects on nail, e.g. retinoids. Additionally there may be a history of allergy to lidocaine or carbocaine, or preservatives such as parabens; local anaesthetics may be contraindicated in patients with cardiac disease such as heart block. Acknowledge of previous anti-tetanus immunization is important since tetanus toxoid is advisible when handling the toenail area or in traumatic lesions that come into contact with soil. The affected digit should be inspected with regard to the quality and colour of the surrounding skin and compared to the unaffected contralateral digit. The presence of signs of

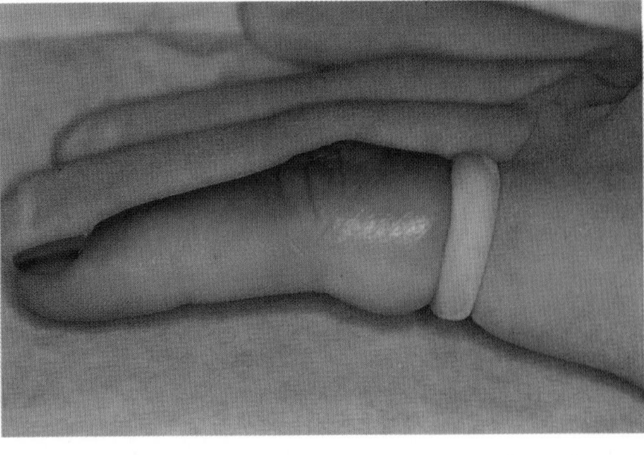

Fig. 10.1. Simple method for aseptic technique using the 'rolled-up' rubber glove finger method.

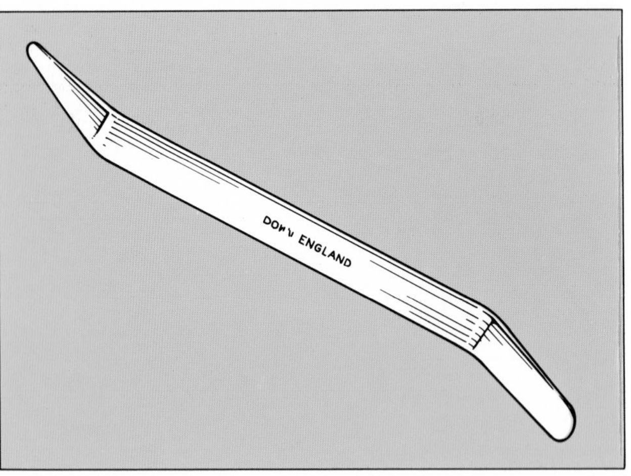

Fig. 10.2. McKay nail elevator, for finger- or toenail.

infection, particularly in association with pyrexia, may delay surgery until appropriate systemic antibiotic therapy has had effect or at least may modify the site or type of anaesthesia.

Xeroradiography, echography, and magnetic resonance imaging (MRI) enable the phalanx and soft tissues to be carefully evaluated.

Preoperative measures

The hand is prepared for fingernail surgery using a surgical scrub with povidone-iodine or alternative disinfectant soap. A sterile surgical glove with the tip of the appropriate finger removed provides an aseptic covering of the patient's hand (Fig. 10.1). The foot should first be soaked in an appropriate antiseptic solution before surgery is performed on the toenails. If cutting the nail plate is needed it is wise to soak the digit for about 10 min in water to soften it, thus facilitating nail section. The foot is draped in the usual aseptic manner with sterile towels which are secured with towel clamps.

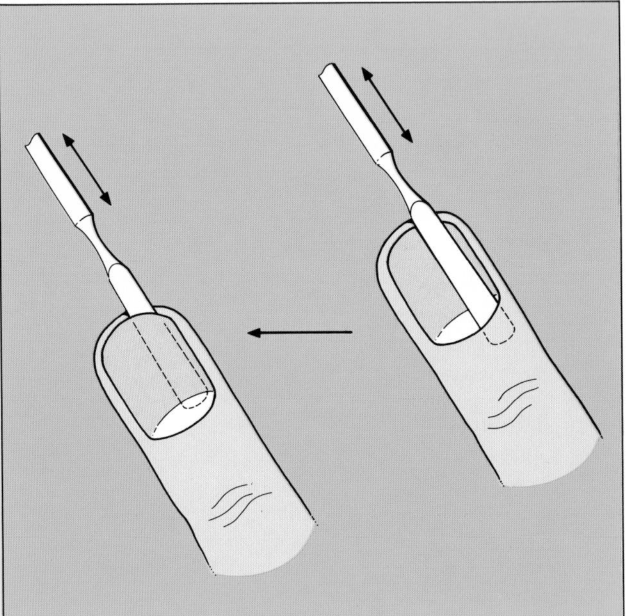

Fig. 10.3. Nail avulsion with a dental spatula (after M. Albom).

Instruments for nail surgery (Figs 10.2–10.6)

The instruments used in nail surgery are the same as those normally used in cutaneous surgery; in addition the following are required: (a) nail elevators (dental spatula or Freer septum elevator); (b) single or double pronged skin hooks (flexible retractors); (c) double action nail clippers (bone rongeur); (d) nail splitting scissors; (e) English nail splitter (the lower blade is unique, with its smooth under-surface that glides atraumatically along the nail bed, while the anvil-like upper surface slides under the nail (Fig. 10.6) the regular scissor's upper blade then cuts through the nail plate; (f) pointed scissors (Gradle scissors); (g) curved iris scissors; (h) small-nosed mosquito haemostats; (i) No. 11 and 15 scalpel blades; (j) the chisel-like No. 81 blade of the Beaver system is useful as a nail splitter for thickened or friable nails (Salasche & Peters, 1985); (k) disposable punches (2, 3, 3.5, 4, 5 and 6 mm); (l) tourniquet (Penrose drains); (m) Luer–Lok syringe; and (n) 30-gauge needle. The sutures most commonly used are monofil non-absorbable polypropylene (e.g. Prolene) or 6-0 colourless absorbable threads (e.g. PDS).

The use of a magnifier lens (×3 or ×5) or a microscope may be valuable or even mandatory for detailed close-up or microsurgery and for subtle microrepair.

Anaesthesia

Anaesthesia is a key factor in this type of surgery, which for economical, psychological and social reasons must enable the patient to remain ambulatory.

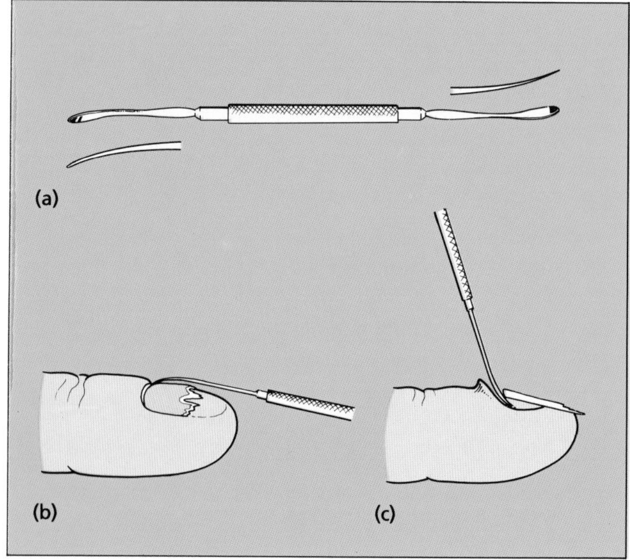

Fig. 10.4. Cordero's method of nail plate avulsion. (a) Freer septum elevator. (b) The instrument shown is a pushed under the proximal nail fold to the far edge of the nail plate and in process of freeing it from side to side. (c) The instrument is shown slipped along the natural plane of cleavage between nail plate and bed, thus freeing it entirely.

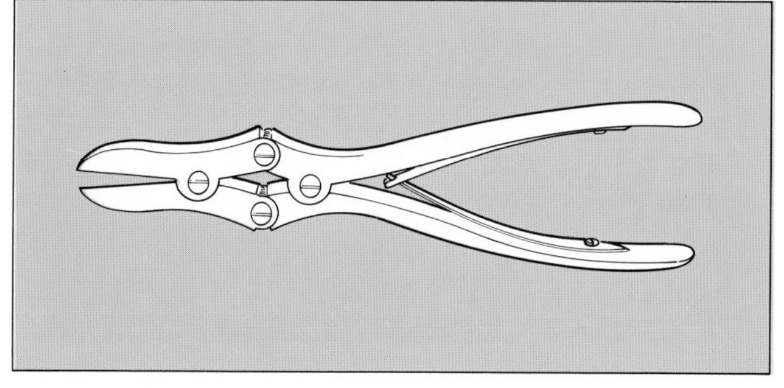

Fig. 10.5. Double action nail clippers (bone rongeur).

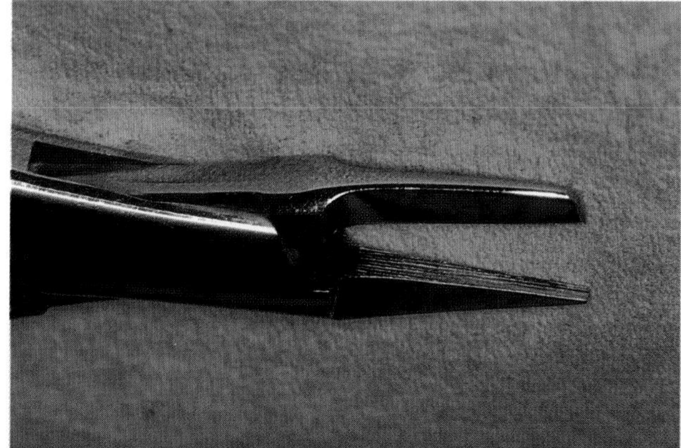

Fig. 10.6. The English nail splitter.

The four properties of anaesthetics that one must consider in selecting the most appropriate agent are: (1) time of onset of anaesthesia; (2) duration of anaesthesia; (3) potency of action of the agent; and (4) the risk of allergic and toxic reactions.

Since all local anaesthetic agents are potentially toxic, the physician should be familiar with the agent selected and be prepared for any untoward side effects. Emergency resuscitation measures must be available, including provisions for the maintenance of an adequate airway, oxygen administration, and the control of convulsions. Although emergencies related to minor surgery occur very rarely, the ready availability of certain resuscitation equipment and procedures is essential. Lidocaine is widely used. A buffered local anaesthesia solution produces significantly less pain (McKay *et al.*, 1987; Pontasch & Brodell, 1988) and can be accomplished by adding 1 ml of sodium bicarbonate to a 10 ml vial of lidocaine. The simple procedure of warming to 37°C reduces the pain associated with subcutaneous injection of lidocaine (Davidson & Boom, 1992). The incidence of allergy to lidocaine is very small. Carbocaine, which is said not to be a vasodilator, has been advocated. Bupivacaine has a long duration of action and is more potent than lidocaine. Its slow onset of action may be overcome by mixing it with equal part of 2% lidocaine solution (Auletta & Grekin, 1991). Adrenaline should not be used.

Local anaesthesia may be induced by several alternative methods.

Peripheral nerve block

'Wing' block local distal digital anaesthesia
(Salasche & Peters, 1985) (Fig. 10.7)

Using a 30-gauge needle, the injection is started 2–3 mm proximal to the junction of the proximal and lateral nail fold. It is continued distally and downward to deaden the lateral digital nerve and its branches. The injection is then carried across the proximal nail fold, to involve the transverse nerve, and finally to the other side of the digit: the lateral and proximal nail folds will be seen to distend and blanch; the anaesthetic solution partially acts as a tourniquet. For distal nail bed operations, a supplementary injection at the tip of the digit is often necessary. Unilateral 'wing' block is used for isolated surgery of the nail border. This method of anaesthesia takes effect almost immediately.

Central local distal digital anaesthesia (Zaias, 1990)
(Fig. 10.8)

In the digits and small toes of children, a single injection of the anaesthetic into the proximal nail fold area further delivers the anaesthetic into the dermis of the lunula. The

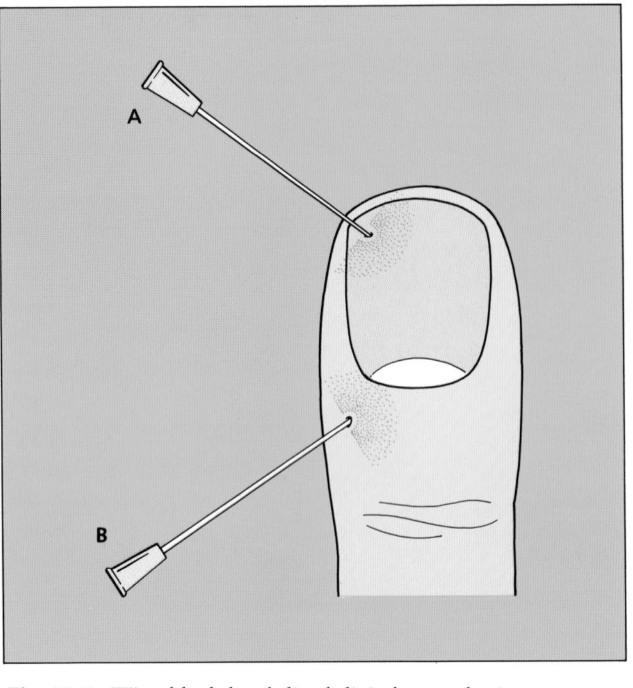

Fig. 10.7. Wing block local distal digital anaesthesia.

anaesthetic will cover all the matrix and nail bed region. We have also obtained good, but inconsistent, results in adults, even for anaesthesia of the great toe.

Local distal digital anaesthesia is contraindicated if there is infection in the terminal phalangeal region.

Digital nerve block (base block) (Figs 10.9(a) & (b))

The needle is inserted at the base of the finger, into the dorsolateral aspect of both sides of it, opposite and just proximal to the volar or plantar flexion crease at the base of the proximal phalanx. The needle is directed tangentially to the sides of the phalanx as far as the lateral side of the flexor tendon. One to 2 ml of the local anaesthesia solution are injected either side plus a small amount across the dorsal aspect. A volume greater than 5 ml may interfere with the circulation.

This technique is slightly modified for anaesthesia of the big toe. The digital nerves of the big toe lie on the plantar side of the coronal plane of the distal phalanx (Fig. 10.10). Anaesthesia is produced by injecting the great toe at its fibular side, injecting downward to the plantar aspect of the great toe. The needle is then retracted, but not withdrawn completely from the dorsal surface of the toe, being redirected horizontally, dorsiflexing the toe so that the needle passes under the extensor hallucis longus tendon. The dorsum of the toe is infiltrated toward its tibial side. The final injection is on the plantar side of the great toe at its fibular side, directing the needle diagonally upward, until an anaesthetic wheal has been created around the base of the toe (Ross, 1969).

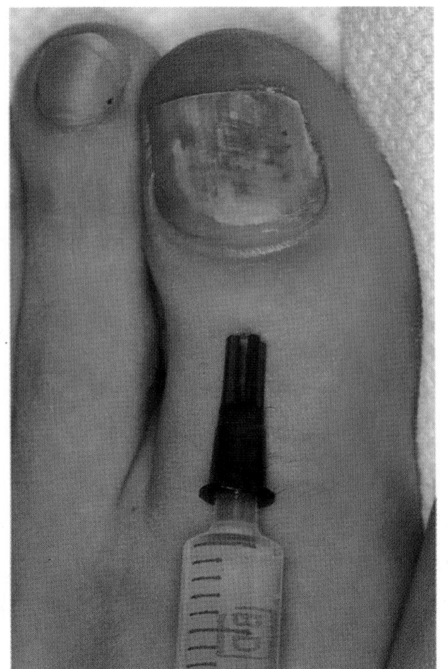

Fig. 10.8. Central local distal digital anaesthesia.

Metacarpal block (Kleinert, 1959) (Fig. 10.11)

A wheal is raised on the dorsum of the hand 2–3 cm proximal to the web. A 30-gauge needle is placed 2–3 cm proximal to the dorsal web and 2 ml of the local anaesthetic agent is infiltrated at the level of the digital nerve which is volar to the deep transverse intermetacarpal ligament. The needle is reinserted on the opposite side of the metacarpal to block the other digital nerve. A small subcutaneous wheal is raised on the dorsum of the hand to block the dorsal sensory branches.

It takes 10–15 min for anaesthesia to develop in digital nerve blocks. Metacarpal blocks and webspace blocks are of use for anaesthetizing the lateral aspect of adjacent digits.

Digital nerve block performed in the web or in the metacarpal area is safer than when performed more distally, because with the latter, the hydrostatic pressure of the injected agent creates a tourniquet effect. In addition, digital block anaesthesia may contribute to the extension of pre-existing infection and carries a risk of spreading it higher up the limb. Therefore most hand surgeons favour general anaesthesia or regional block (if only the distal phalanx is involved).

Transthecal digital block (Chiu, 1990)

The flexor tendon sheath may be used as an avenue for introducing anaesthetic to the core of the digit. Through centrifugal anaesthetic diffusion all four digital nerves are anaesthetized rapidly. This technique involves palmar percutaneous injection of 2 ml of lidocaine into the potential space of the flexor tendon sheath at the level of the

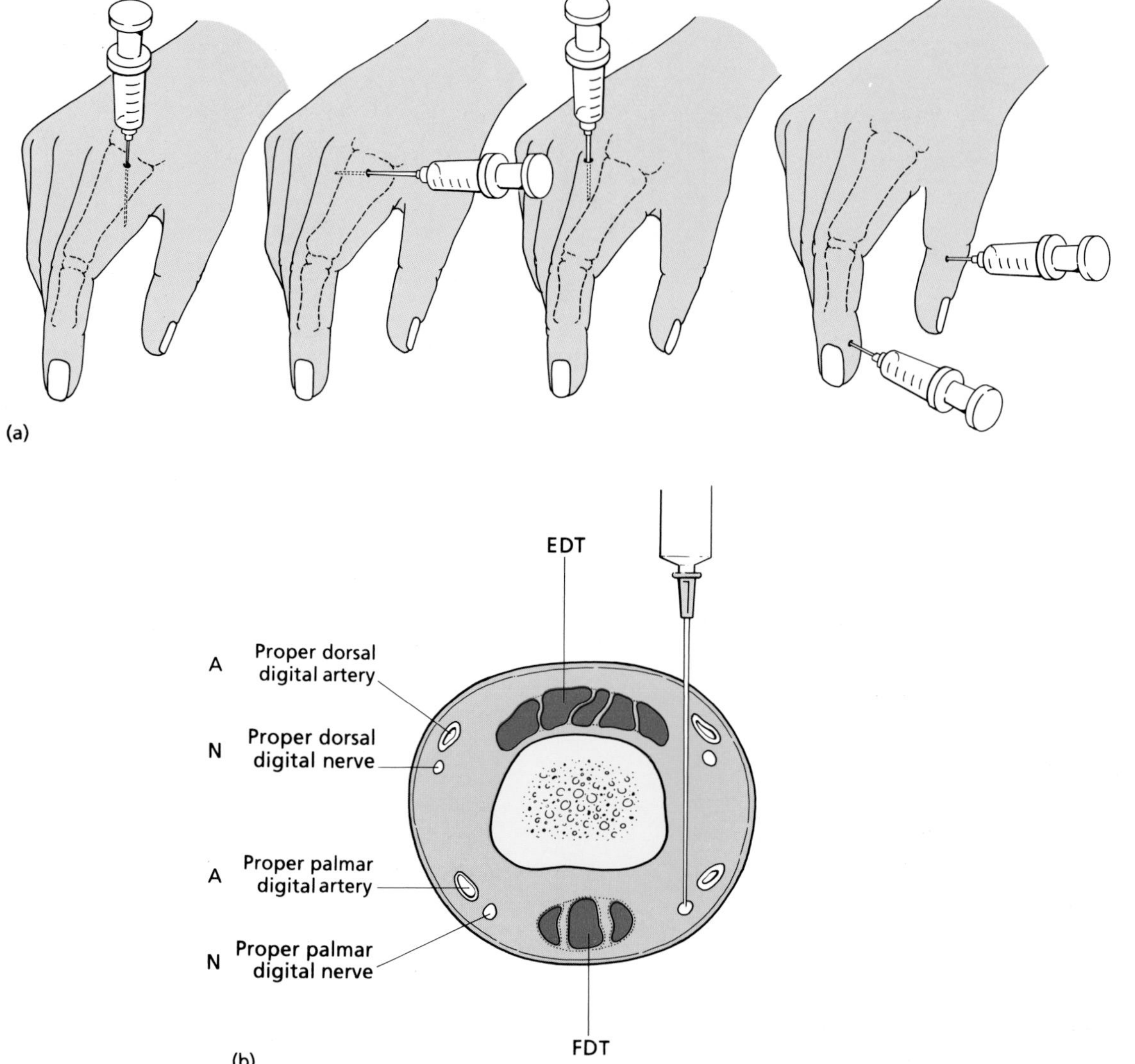

Fig. 10.9. (a) Diagram to show the various digital sites suggested for adequate anaesthesia of the nail apparatus (see text) (after Petres & Hundeiker). (b) Digital cross section showing the various structures present in relation to the nerves to be injected (N); A, artery; EDT, extensor digitorum tendon; FDT, flexor digitorum tendon.

palmar flexion crease with a 3 ml syringe and a No. 25–27 gauge hypodermic needle.

Regional anaesthesia (Kleinert, 1959; Abadir, 1975; Hutton *et al*., 1991)

Regional anaesthesia is indicated for extensive surgery.

Wrist block (Fig. 10.12) is the anaesthesia of choice when treating several fingertips or when there is infection or vascular impairment in the affected digits. This procedure involves truncal infiltration of the median and ulnar nerves.

Median nerve block at wrist

Locate the palmaris longus tendon and flexor carpi radialis by asking the subject to flex the hand against resistance. At the distal crease of the wrist between those two tendons raise a small skin wheel with a 2 cm needle; advance the needle about 8–12 mm. Great care is needed to avoid transfixing the nerve. Advance the needle slowly to contact the nerve if paraesthesia is desired – when this occurs withdraw the needle 1–2 mm. Then inject 5–8 ml of suitable anaesthetic to insure success of the block.

Ulnar nerve block

At the proximal crease of the wrist, immediately medial to the ulna, advance a 2 cm needle diagonally pointing posteriorly and proximally until the medial surface of the ulna is contacted by the advancing needle. Withdraw the needle a few mm then readvance in a slightly more medial direction until the tip of the needle is felt 'tenting' the skin of the dorsal surface of the arm by the operator's other

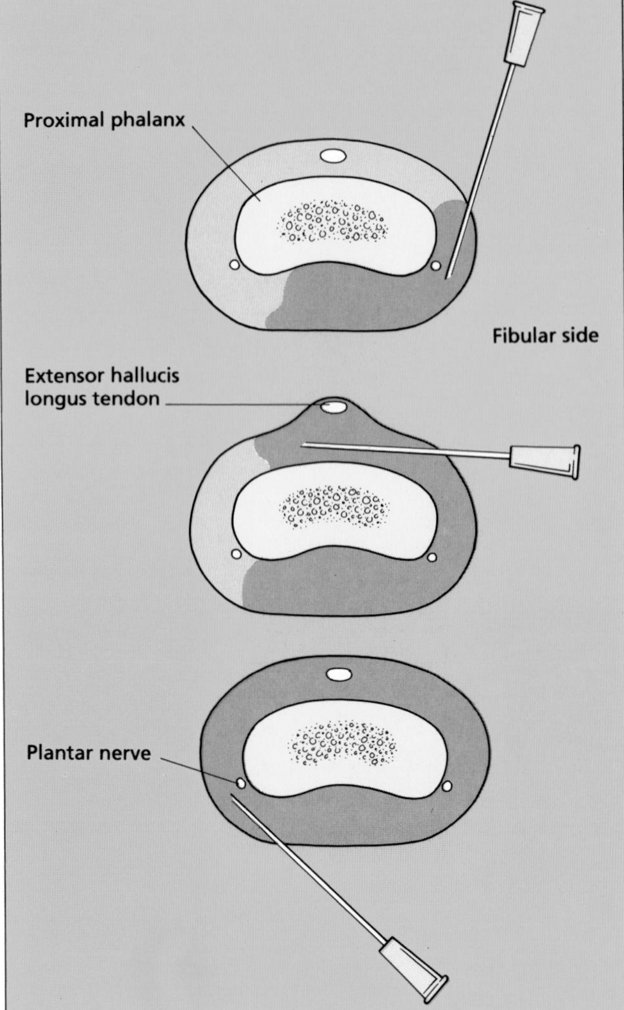

Fig. 10.10. Great toe digital nerves on the planter side of the coronal plane of the phalanx – sites of anaesthesia.

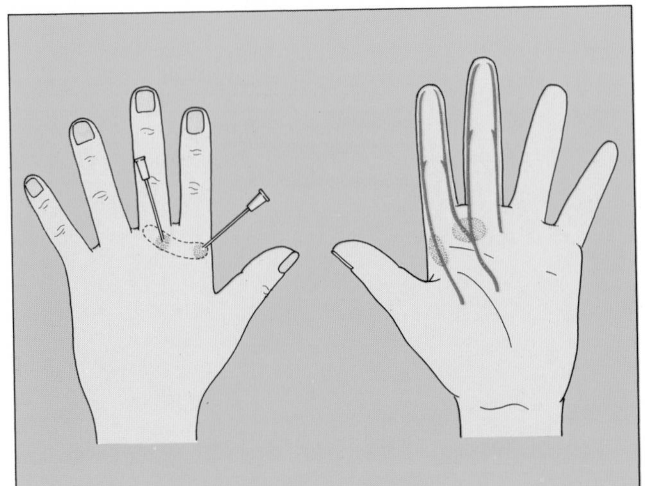

Fig. 10.11. Metacarpal block – useful for the anaesthesia of adjacent digits.

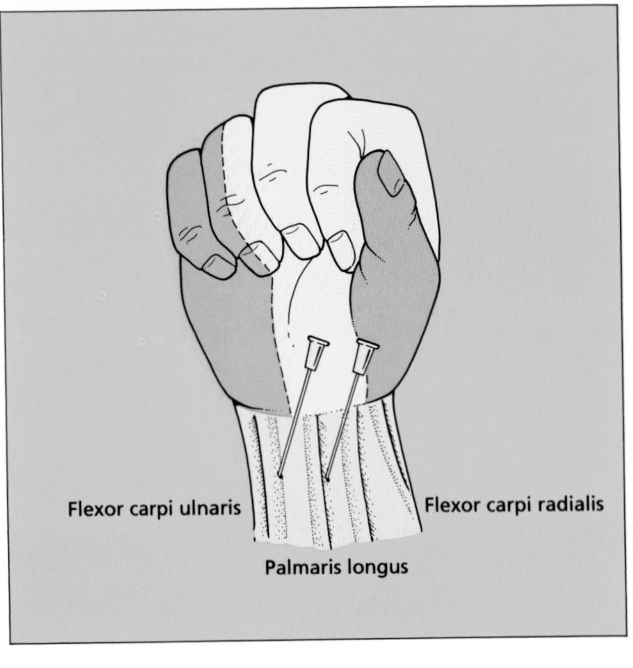

Fig. 10.12. Regional nerve block at the wrist.

hand. Then a spirate, to insure absence of blood; next inject 8–10 ml of any suitable local anaesthetic while at the same time withdrawing the needle. The injection site has to traverse the course of the ulnar nerve and its branches. The success rate is almost 100% with this block (Abadir, 1975).

Radial nerve block

In order to inject the radial nerve, the sharp edge of the curve of the lower end of the radius is used as a guide. The anaesthetic is placed subcutaneously in the deep layer of fat, starting at the edge of the radius 8 cm above the wrist, where the nerve emerges under the brachoradialis tendon and where it may be felt with the finger.

Anaesthesia becomes complete within 5–15 min.

Nerve blocks for the toes (Fig. 10.13)

Digital block is usually adequate for procedures involving the distal part of the toes. However, in selected cases (nail avulsion of several digits, for example), nerve block involving the posterior tibial, deep peroneal, sural or saphenous nerve, or a combination of these should be considered, as indicated by the specific surgical site (Cohen & Roenigk, 1991).

Brachial plexus anaesthesia

This is not usually considered appropriate for nail surgery.

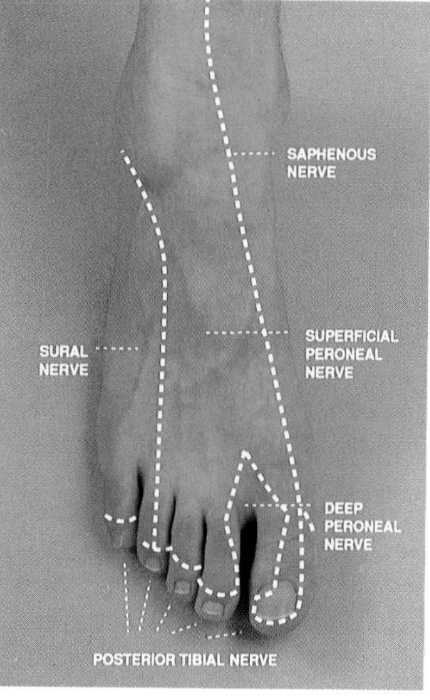

Fig. 10.13. Nerve supply to the foot.

Intravenous regional analgesia

Using lidocaine or bupivacaine, is now less popular. The operative field is exsanguinated either by elevating the limb, or by application of an Esmarch band. It is then excluded from the general circulation by the use of an arterial tourniquet inflated to 30 mmHg above systolic blood pressure. In 20 min, this results in excellent analgesia which lasts for up to 2 h. Pain may be quite severe when the anaesthic wears off. The tourniquet may be removed after 1 h. The analgesia generally persists for a short time, but it is inadequate for haemostasis and satisfactory cutaneous suturing to be carried out. This mode of anaesthesia, which requires a minimum of preoperative tests, may be ideal for ambulatory surgery; but it is not without hazard, expecially with bupivacaine.

Irrespective of the technique used, the following points are relevant.

1 Xylocaine 1 or 2% should be given without adrenaline, since the ischaemia lasts too long and may result in gangrene.

2 Depending on the site of the injection, it takes 3–5 min for anaesthesia to develop.

3 To complement anaesthesia and to provide a bloodless field (as required in phenol matricectomy), Salasche and Peters (1985) recommend an 'exsanguinating' tourniquet (Fig. 10.14). A wide Penrose drain is wound tightly in loops that overlap in a distal to proximal fashion, leaving an exposed loose end distally. This milks the blood from the digit. The loose end is then grasped and unwound, again working distal to proximal until the nail apparatus is exposed; the final proximal loop is secured with a

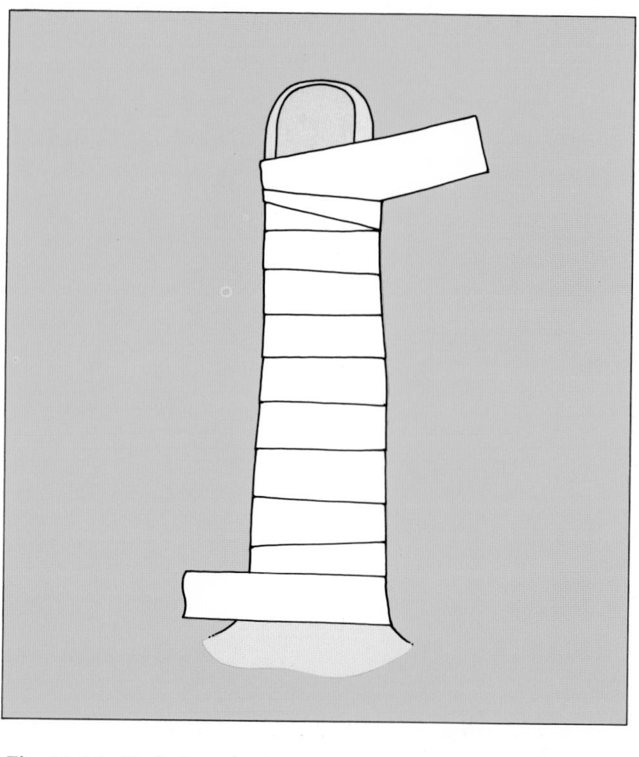

Fig. 10.14. Technique for bloodless field using a Penrose drain wrapped tightly in loops around the digit.

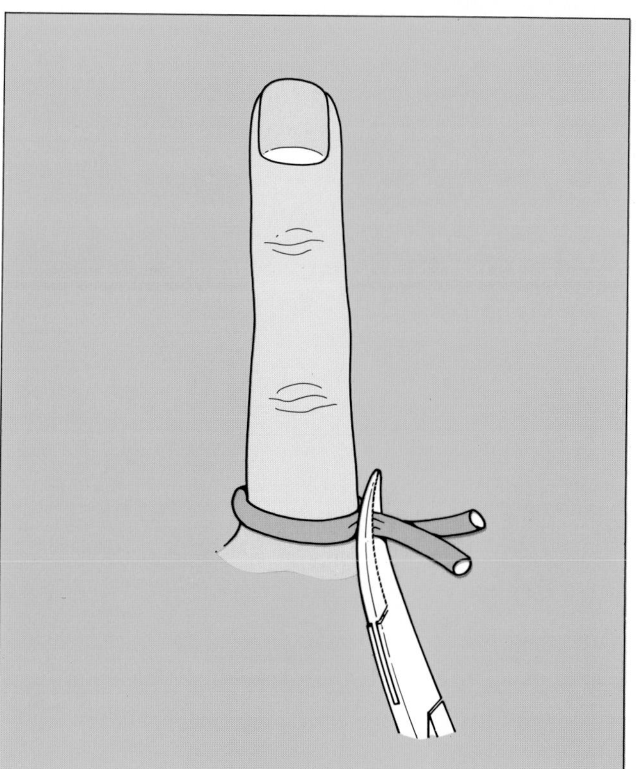

Fig. 10.15. See Fig. 10.14 – the final proximal loop secured with a haemostat.

haemostat to function as a tourniquet (Fig. 10.15). Tourniquets are not a problem if they are wide and applied for less than 15 min. There is an easy and quick alternative to the previous technique; this consists of cutting across the rubber of the tip of finger to be operated on and in rolling the glove down that finger (Fig. 10.1) (Haneke, 1988; Dastgeer, 1990).

General anaesthesia

General anaesthesia may be indicated in children, or for psychological or medical reasons in adults.

References

Abadir A. (1975) Use of local anaesthetics in dermatology. *J. Dermatol. Surg.* **1**, 68–72.

Auletta M.J. & Grekin R.C. (1991) *Local Anesthesia for Dermatologic Surgery*. Churchill Livingstone, New York.

Chiu D.T.W. (1990) Transthecal digital block: Flexor tendon sheath used for anesthetic infusion. *J. Hand Surg.* **15A**, 471–473.

Cohen S.J. & Roenigk R.K. (1991) Nerve blocks for cutaneous surgery on the foot. *J. Dermatol. Surg. Oncol.* **17**, 527–534.

Dastgeer G.M. (1990) Sterile surgical gloving of patients for emergent and ambulatory operations upon the finger. *Surg. Gynecol. Obst.* **170**, 546–548.

Davidson J.A. & Boom S.J. (1992) Warming lignocaine to reduce pain associated with injection. *Br. Med. J.* **305**, 617–618.

Haneke E. (1988) Exzisions-und Biopsieverfahren. *Z. Hautkr.* **63** (Suppl.), 17–19.

Hutton K.P., Podolsky A., Roenigk R.K. *et al.* (1991) Regional anaesthesia of the hand for dermatologic surgery. *J. Dermatol. Surg. Oncol.* **17**, 881–888.

Kleinert H.E. (1959) Fingertip injuries and their management. *Am. Surg.* **25**, 41–45.

McKay *et al.* (1987) Nail elevator. *Lancet* **i**, 864.

Pontasch M.J. & Brodell R.T. (1988) Significant pain reduction with buffered anesthetics (letter). *J. Dermatol. Surg. Oncol.* **14**, 672.

Ross W.R. (1969) Treatment of the ingrown toenail and a new anaesthetic method. *Surg. Clin. North Am.* **49**, 1499–1504.

Salasche S.J. & Peters V.J. (1985) Tips on nail surgery. *Cutis* **35**, 428–438.

Zaias N. (1990) *The Nail in Health and Disease*, 2nd edn. Appleton & Lange, Norwalk, CN.

Post-operative care

Bleeding may be severe, particularly after releasing the tourniquet. It can usually be controlled by the use of Monsel's solution, 35% aluminum chloride or oxycel.

After surgery, the nail area is covered with Telfa or a greasy gauze impregnated with antibiotic ointment or povidone.

The dressing should be bulky. This will enable post-operative bleeding to be absorbed and will provide a cushion against local trauma. The dressing should be sealed with paper tape anchored in a longitudinal manner on the dorsal, ventral and lateral aspects. This method does not impede the blood supply. Several layers of X-span tubing or surgitube complete the bulky dressing (Salasche & Peters, 1985). An aluminium or thermoplastic fingerguard can be placed for protection and splinting of the distal phalanx.

The involved extremity should be elevated during the first 48 h. For toenail surgery the patient should be warned in advance to bring an open-toed shoe, slipper or sandal. The patient has to be kept recumbant. Depending on the type of operation the first dressing should be removed after 24–48 h: any surgical operation of a non-sterile nail area, e.g. ingrowing toenail with oozing granulation tissue, or a nail biopsy on a mycotic nail with subungual hyperkeratosis associated with considerable bleeding, should prompt a change of dressing after 24 h. After removal of the outer layers of the dressing, the extremity is put into lukewarm water containing an antiseptic, e.g. povidone iodine, until the inner layers of the dressing float off. This ensures an entirely painless procedure. If there are any signs of infection, antiseptic soaks should be commenced once to three times daily (Haneke, 1991). If the operation wound does not show any sign of inflammation, the second dressing may be left for 5–7 days.

When the dressing is removed, antiseptic soaks should be commenced for 15 min, three times daily. Pain may be significant and should be treated. Post-operative infection is uncommon following procedures performed with proper surgical technique and appropriate wound care by the patient. When infection is present, the organism should be cultured and treated immediately with systemic antibiotics and soaks.

References

Haneke E. (1991) Operationen am Nagelorgan – Planung, Durchführung, Fehlermöglichkeiten und ihre Vermeidung. *Z. Hautkr.* **66** (Suppl. 3), 132–133.

Salasche S.J. & Peters V.J. (1985) Tips on nail surgery. *Cutis* **35**, 428–438.

Biopsy of the nail area (Figs 10.16–10.20) (Tables 10.1 & 10.2)

Biopsy of the nail area is mostly as simple as at any other site and may be a very useful procedure (André & Achten, 1987; Kechijian, 1987; Rich, 1992).

Why and when? (Baran & Sayag, 1976)

1 To demonstrate pathogenicity of fungal organisms in diseased nails (Chapter 4) (Achten, 1972; Scher & Ackerman, 1980a; Haneke, 1985a; Rich, 1992).

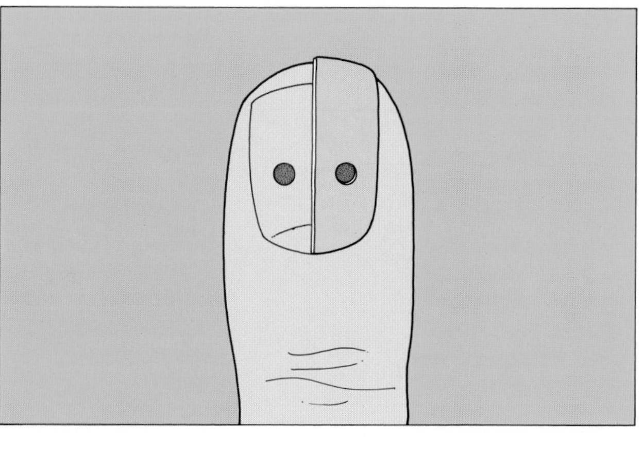

Fig. 10.16. Biopsy of the nail bed: right half showing one punch technique without nail plate avulsion; left half, biopsy after partial nail avulsion.

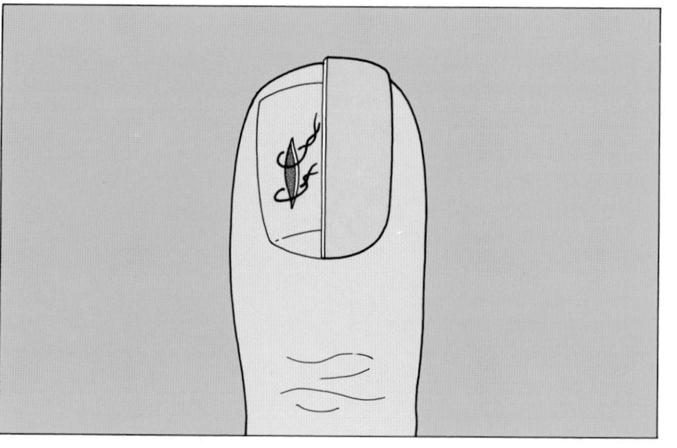

Fig. 10.17. Biopsy of the nail bed; longitudinal ellipse removed after partial nail plate avulsion.

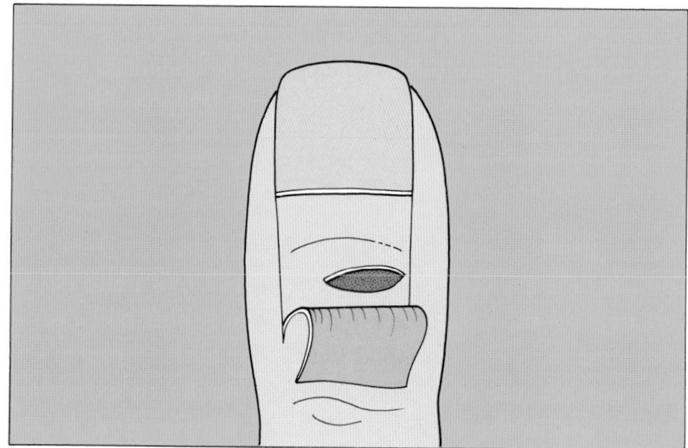

Fig. 10.18. Crescent or fusiform matrix biopsy: only the proximal part of the nail plate is cut to permit biopsy.

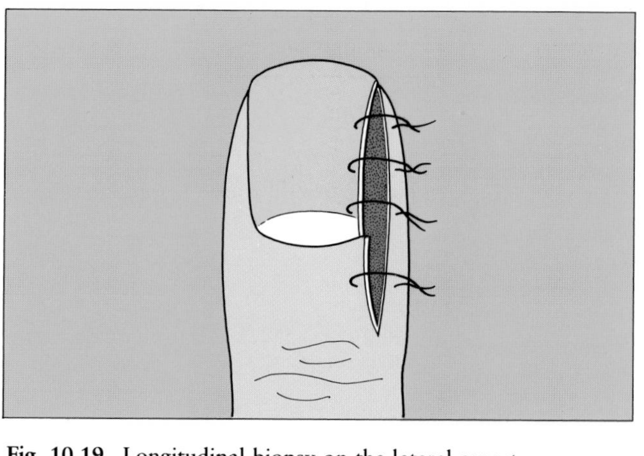

Fig. 10.19. Longitudinal biopsy on the lateral aspect.

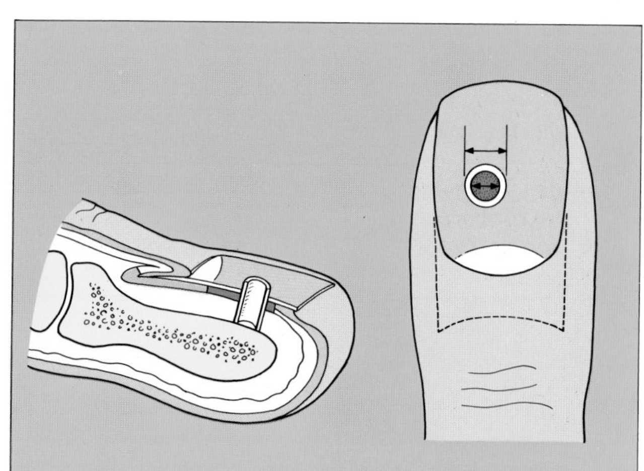

Fig. 10.20. Diagram showing nail bed biopsy using the double punch technique.

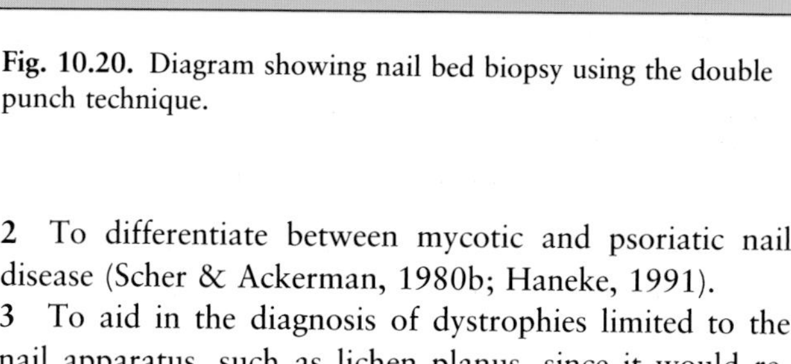

2 To differentiate between mycotic and psoriatic nail disease (Scher & Ackerman, 1980b; Haneke, 1991).
3 To aid in the diagnosis of dystrophies limited to the nail apparatus, such as lichen planus, since it would require special treatment to avoid further nail destruction (Zaias, 1967; Haneke, 1982; Hanno *et al.*, 1986).
4 To establish early diagnosis of malignant subungual and periungual neoplasia or to facilitate the diagnosis of certain benign tumours.

Nail biopsy is not recommended in immunocompromised subjects, diabetes mellitus or peripheral vascular disease.

How and where? (Figs 10.16–10.20)

1 Using scissors or a bone rongeur, it is easy to take specimens that include a piece of the distal plate and the underlying hyponychium. This technique may be adequate

Table 10.1. Nail biopsies (from Gonzalez-Serva, 1990 with permission from the author and publisher)

According to site
Matrix
Bed
Combined (proximal fold–matrix–hyponychium)
Paronychium
Plate

According to field preparation
Without avulsion of plate (translaminar)
With prior avulsion of plate (open)

According to sampling method
Punch
Incisional
Shave (trimming)
(a) Soft tissues
(b) Nail plate

According to orientation
Transverse
Longitudinal

According to comprehensiveness
Local (one component of nail unit)
En-bloc (several components of nail unit), or a large sample of a single component

for the diagnosis of some mycotic nail infections (Achten, 1972).

2 A 3-mm punch biopsy can be restricted to the nail plate. This can be used when there is a possibility that the suspected mycotic pathology is not confined to the distal portion. Soaking in warm water for 10 min immediately prior to punching the nail may be helpful.

3 Except for this purpose, it may also be useful to thin the nail by electric grinding before biopsying the nail bed. This facilitates translaminar punch biopsy. When the punch reaches the periosteum, it is withdrawn and fine (Graddle) scissors are used to release the specimen. Biopsy specimens from the nail matrix or bed are delicate and can be damaged or destroyed by either crushing the tissue with forceps or shredding it while attempting to separate it from its attachment to the bone below. This can be avoided by securely 'skewering' the specimen with a 30-gauge needle after the specimen has been punched or excised down to bone. The distal end of the needle is then bent with a haemostat to prevent the specimen from slipping off (Salasche & Peters, 1985). Pressure on the nail plate also forces the tissue cylinder up so that it can be cut at its base. Only direct pressure or oxycel is used for haemostasis (Stone *et al.*, 1978). Biopsy sites usually heal satisfactorily. Siegle and Swanson (1982) have developed a two-punch technique for the nail bed (Fig. 10.20). The first and larger punch (6 mm) creates a circular defect in the nail plate, and the second smaller 3–4-mm punch biopsies the nail bed through the nail plate defect created by the first larger punch. The 6-mm nail disc is then put back in its original place. The authors prefer this method because it overcomes the difficulty of extracting tissue within the confines of a 3–4-mm window in the nail plate, i.e. the fibrous nail bed, firmly attached both to the periosteum and the surrounding nail bed connective tissue (Kechijian, 1987). In some cases a small area of onycholysis may occur.

4 A 3-mm punch biopsy performed into the matrix will not produce a noticeable or permanent deformity (Higashi, 1970).

Table 10.2. Clinicopathological limitations of nail biopsies (from Gonzalez-Serva, 1990, with permission from the author and publisher)

Regarding inflammatory diseases
1 Clinical and histological signs of dystrophy (plate abnormality) are shared by several diseases, both inflammatory and otherwise
2 Superimposition of common reactional patterns unrelated to primary etiology
(a) metaplastic epidermalization (reversing of specialized nail epithelia to 'genetic' epidermoid squamous epithelium)
(b) lichen simplex chronicus onychalis (post-traumatic orthokeratotic hyperplasia of nail epithelia)
3 Different histologic appearances than homologous cutaneous dermatosis
4 Primary trauma may mimic specific inflammation
5 Microorganisms are difficult to detect or assess as primary agents (i.e. they may represent colonizers)

Regarding solid tumors
1 Non-specific appearance at clinical examination
2 Different behaviour than cutaneous homologue (e.g. keratoacanthoma)
3 Frequent history of trauma obscures neoplastic nature
4 Associated chronic infection
5 Late diagnosis
(a) lack of radiologic studies
(b) reticence to biopsy early in course
(c) insufficient tissue sample
(d) difficult discrimination between some neoplasms and reactive changes

Regarding pigmented lesions
1 Difficult discrimination between pigments. Haemosiderin and melanin may look alike
2 Biopsy may reveal pigment but not its source. The matrix should be assessed because melanocytic lesions, particularily malignant melanoma, primarily reside there.
3 Not all deposition of melanin is neoplastic. Ephelis-like hyperplasia is the most common cause
4 Not all melanocytic neoplasms are malignant. Dysplastic naevi probably exists in the nail field
5 Criteria for diagnosis of melanoma may be of difficult application. 'Acral lentiginous' melanoma traditionally is considered difficult to diagnose

Longitudinal nail bed biopsy (Fig. 10.19)

Sometimes the size of the tissue to be removed necessitates a longitudinal elliptical wedge resection. This is carried out down to bone, the nail plate being fully avulsed, or its longitudinal half partially removed. The wedge biopsy should be long and narrow, parallel with the longitudinal ridges of the nail bed. After the wedge of tissue has been removed, the edges of the ellipse are undermined to facilitate primary closure. Relaxing incisions may be useful at the lateral margins of the nail bed to facilitate primary closure with 6-0 colourless PDS. The indications for this procedure include diagnosis of skin disease, tumours, or unknown lesions.

Transverse matrix biopsy (Fig. 10.18)

Crescent or fusiform matrix biopsy

It is important when performing nail matrix biopsies to maintain the distal curved configuration of the lunula. Two small oblique incisions are made on each side of the proximal nail fold; the fold is then retracted in order to expose the matrix area. The proximal third of the plate is dissected and removed, enabling the distal two-thirds of the plate to be retained for the protection of the distal nail bed. The lesion is identified and either part, or all of the lesion is removed by a crescent-shaped wedge of tissue with the convex portion of the crescent paralleling the anterior border of the lunula. The incision is carried down deep to the bone (Fosnaugh, 1982). Fusiform biopsy is preferable, as a crescent-shaped biopsy often provides specimens of inadequate width. Using a fine hook, the matrix is then undermined to allow primary suture. Closure is accomplished with interrupted 6-0 PDS sutures. As long as the proximal part of the matrix is not disturbed, a transverse biopsy will merely thin the nail plate and will not leave the fissure which may result from a central longitudinal biopsy.

Nail matrix–nail bed biopsy at one time

Lateral longitudinal biopsy

The best speciments for histopathological examination are obtained by a lateral longitudinal nail biopsy that includes the proximal nail fold, matrix, nail bed and hyponychium. It can be done on either side. This method gives as much information as the median longitudinal nail biopsy, but avoids the split-like nail deformity which often results from the latter technique. Beginning in the lateral nail groove, the incisions reach to the bone, parallel for the most part to the lateral margin of the nail plate, including a 3–4-mm nail segment. This ensures that a full thickness

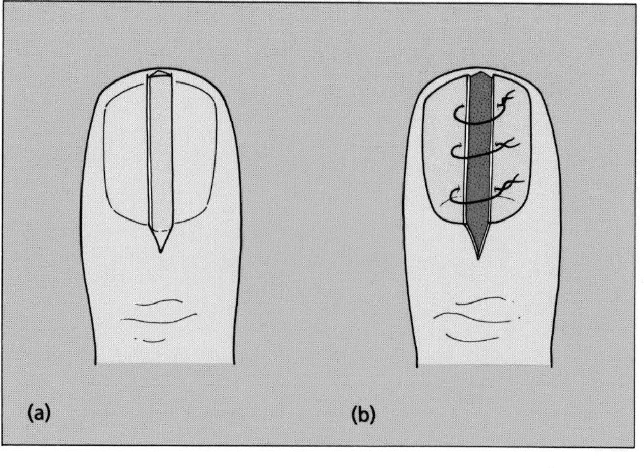

Fig. 10.21. Nail matrix–nail bed biopsy. (a) The nail plate on either side of the area to be biopsied is removed. (b) Excision of a rectangular block down to bone.

fragment of the nail bed and the matrix with its lateral horn is obtained. The most proximal incisions reach the distal crease over the distal interphalangeal joint and the terminal end; they must include the hyponychium. Slightly curved iris scissors or a surgical blade are useful for releasing the tissue from the bone. Starting at the tip of the digit one proceeds proximally while maintaining contact with the bony phalanx. Sutures are placed on the proximal nail fold and the hyponychium. The lateral nail fold is sutured to the nail plate using back-stitches to provide the reconstruction of the lateral nail fold (Haneke, 1985b, 1988) (Fig. 10.25(c)). The method of latteral longitudinal biopsy associated with removal of the homologous lateral nail fold (Bennett, 1976) is not suitable.

In certain cases, it may be necessary to determine the extent of probable malignancy (Siegle & Swanson, 1982). If the nail plate is to be part of the biopsy specimen, then only the plate on each side of the area to be biopsied should be avulsed (Scher, 1980) (Fig. 10.21), but it is quite possible to remove a rectangular block 3-mm wide down to the bone without avulsing the nail plate on either side of it. This will include the hyponychium, nail bed, nail matrix and proximal nail fold. The surrounding tissues are then undermined and closed, again taking care to ensure good lunular approximation.

Biopsy of proximal nail fold

Occasionally the proximal nail fold needs to be biopsied. Depending on the reason, there are three techniques for biopsying this area. When the indications are the same as for routine skin biopsy, a 2-mm punch is advanced down to the nail plate (Stone *et al.*, 1978); the plug can then be lifted free. When a punch biopsy is taken, the distal margin of the proximal nail fold should be preserved. For

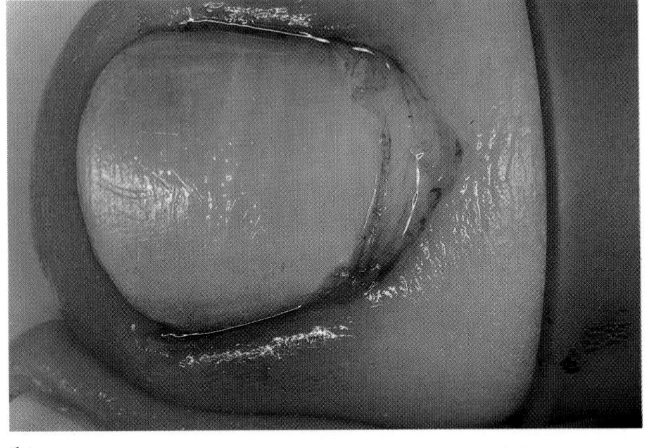

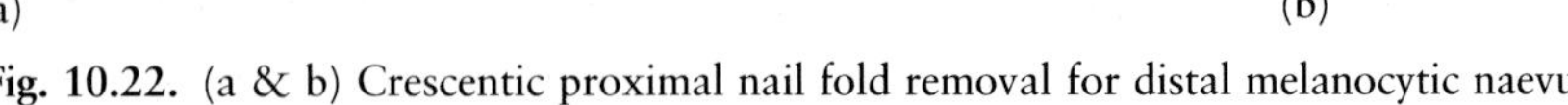

(a) (b)

Fig. 10.22. (a & b) Crescentic proximal nail fold removal for distal melanocytic naevus.

surface biopsy the razor blade technique is ideal (Shelley, 1975). Prior to use, each blade is manually broken into two halves by longitudinal bending. The half blade, which is held securely with the fingers and thumb, is kept perfectly flat or bent to the exact arc which conforms to the depth of tissue one wishes to remove.

Haemostasis is obtained by a sliding gauze pressure and the application of Monsel's solution (or aluminium chloride) to the resultant dry, non-bleeding field. When more tissue is required, for example in collagen diseases, a crescent-shaped tissue excision, 2–3-mm wide, of the edge of the proximal nail fold is performed. This amount of tissue allows histology, immunohistology and electron microscopy examinations to be carried out (Schnitzler *et al.*, 1976, 1980). Healing is rapid – by secondary intention. Usually no scarring is visible after 4 weeks, and no nail dystrophy develops.

The methods of treatment of some tumours of the proximal nail fold are derived from the previous techniques. They may be used according to the type and the location of the tumours in this area.

1 Tumours such as myxoid pseudocysts (Salasche, 1984) and fibrokeratomas (Baran, 1986) for example, may be successfully treated by removing a crescent-shaped piece of proximal nail fold when they are located at its most distal portion. This crescent should not exceed 4–5 mm at its greatest width, to prevent the appearance of a rough nail (Figs 10.22(a) & (b)).

2 Small lesions in the median part of the proximal nail fold may be excised as a wedge. Two lateral incisions are made in the proximal nail fold which is separated from the underlying nail allowing suture of the excisional wound. The narrow secondary defects readily heal by secondary intention (Haneke & Baran, 1991) (Fig. 10.23(a)).

3 A small lesion in the lateral part of the proximal nail fold may be excised as a wedge also. Only one lateral incision is made at the opposite region of the proximal nail fold. To obtain a better healing of the secondary defect which is less narrow than in the previous procedure, the operation may be supplemented by a relaxing crescent-shaped incision in the proximal nail fold (Fig. 10.23(b)).

4 A dorsal flap can be raised from the proximal nail fold using two dorso-lateral incisions and a horizontal one, proximal to the cuticle. This gives complete exposure of subcutaneous tumour, or myxoid pseudocyst.

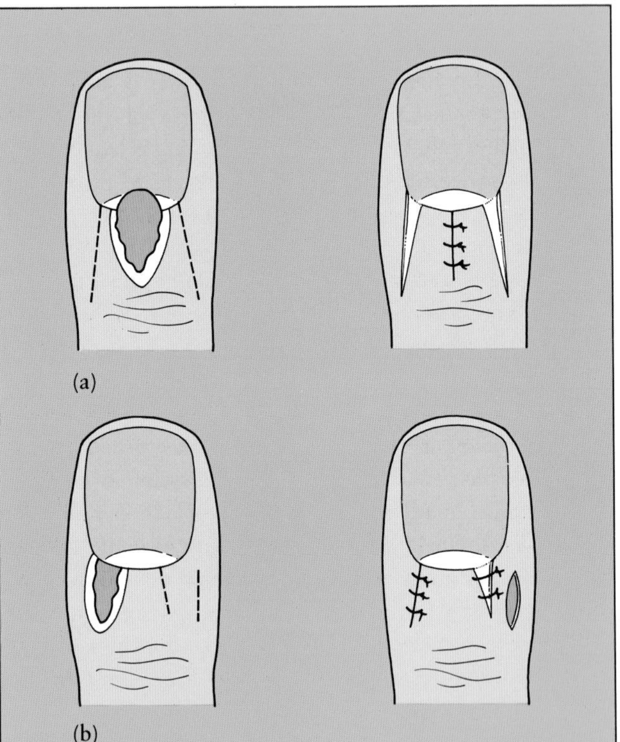

Fig. 10.23. Method for removal of small lesions from the proximal nail fold.

Longitudinal melanonychia and its biopsy

(Baran & Haneke, 1984; Baran & Kechijian, 1989)

Longitudinal melanonychia (LM) is characterized by a brown or black longitudinal streak within the nail plate. LM results from increased melanin deposition in the nail plate. The presence of blood or chromogens, however, may simulate this disorder. LM invariably poses a diagnostic challenge. The causes of LM are numerous and often impossible to differentiate from one another by history and clinical inspection alone. The diagnosis of subungual melanoma must always be included in the differential diagnosis of LM. If the cause of LM is not apparent, it should be established by biopsy. The dangers of an error of judgment in carrying out this diagnostic procedure are two-fold (Sanderson & MacKie, 1979):

1 the proper treatment of a malignant lesion may be delayed and so allow the disease to disseminate;

2 the treatment, correct for a malignant melanoma, may lead to severe, totally unnecessary, cosmetic disability if employed for a benign tumour.

For these reasons, isolated pigmented streaks, involving any portion of the nail apparatus, necessitate biopsy, especially when the thumb or the great toe are involved. The only possible exceptions are in Black and Oriental patients, in whom it could represent a normal finding, in children when the band remains stable and in Laugier–Hunziker–Baran's syndrome (Baran, 1979; Haneke, 1991).

No single biopsy method meets the need of all patients with LM. The following considerations will be helpful in selecting the procedure that is most appropriate.

1 Post-operative dystrophy is less likely to occur with distal matrix biopsies than with biopsies of proximal matrix. However, it is important to exactly locate the origin of pigment production so that the most appropriate surgical procedure can be selected.

2 Complete excision of LM is accomplished more easily and with less cosmetic deformity when the band is located in the lateral third of the nail plate.

3 Thin bands of LM are more amenable to complete excision than wide bands.

4 The features outlined later (e.g. presence or absence of Hutchinson's sign, thumb or great toe involvement, patient age, race, lesion history and clinical features) provide information that is helpful in establishing the likelihood of subungual melanoma. In instances where the likelihood of subungual melanoma is high, biopsy should be pursued with less regard for cosmetic appearance and with greater concern for complete removal.

5 The appearance and functional integrity of the nail are less crucial in the toes than in the fingers.

6 LM in the finger of a person whose occupation depends on the functional and cosmetic integrity of the hand often presents a formidable challenge.

7 Because LM is more likely to represent subungual melanoma in older patients, biopsy should be performed as liberally as thought fit. Fortunately, post-operative appearance and functional nail integrity are less often a critical concern in elderly patients.

8 In general, post-operative appearance is of greater concern in women than in men.

Biopsy methods

Various surgical approaches are available for nail biopsies in LM. The procedure that is ultimately selected will depend on (i) the likelihood of subungual melanoma; (ii)

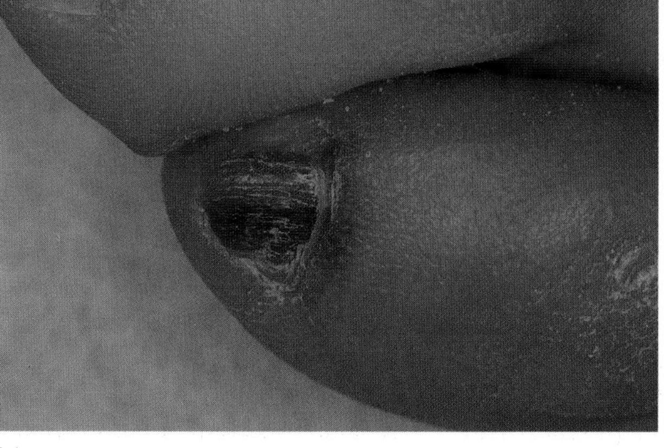

(a)

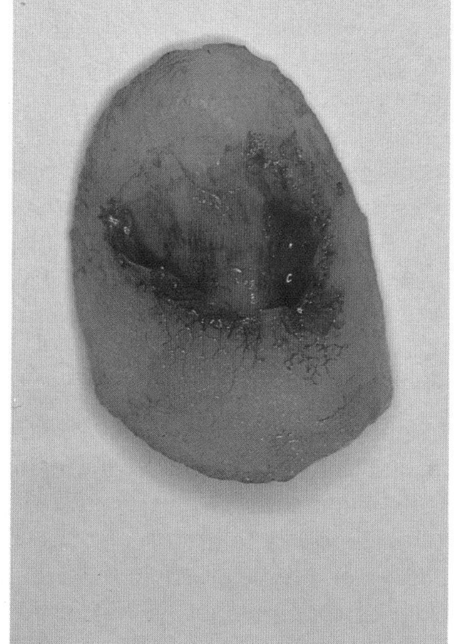

(b)

Fig. 10.24. Periungual (a) and subungual (b) pigmentation – malignant melanoma.

the need to select a procedure that will minimize the risk of post-operative dystrophy; (iii) the location (medial or lateral) of the band within the nail plate; (iv) band width; and (v) matrix origin (proximal or distal) of LM. The patient must be fully advised of the risk of permanent post-operative dystrophy.

Periungual pigmentation present (Figs 10.24(a) & (b))

When LM is accompanied by periungual pigmentation, the likelihood of subungual melanoma is high. X-ray studies should be obtained and the patient examined for lymphadenopathy. If the risk of malignancy (according to the criteria outlined later) is great, if there is no history of previous nail surgery, no history of ingestion of photosensitizing medications, and no evidence for a syndrome associated with hyperpigmentation, and if there is unequivocal evidence that the pigment is located within (and not beneath) the proximal and/or lateral nail folds, all affected portions of the nail apparatus (proximal and lateral nail folds, nail plate, nail bed, hyponychium, and skin) are removed en-bloc down to bone; cosmetic considerations are of secondary importance. To ensure complete biopsy and excision, 1 mm of normal tissue is included in the excision. The advantage of this method lies in completeness of excision. The pathologist is able to study the lesion in its entirety, render a precise diagnosis, and draw salient conclusions regarding prognosis. The conspicuous disadvantage of this approach is the potential for significant post-operative deformity.

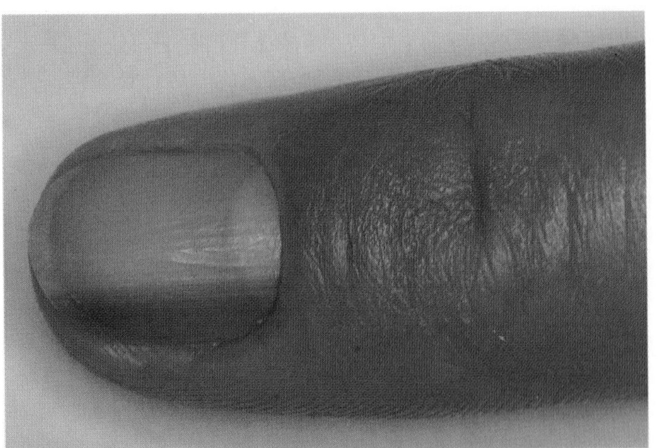

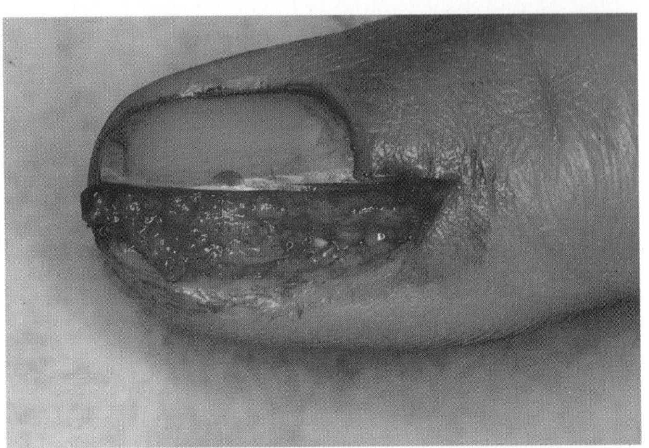

Lateral third of the nail plate involved (Fig. 10.25)

Lateral longitudinal biopsy, is the preferred method when LM involves the lateral third of the nail plate. Advantages of this technique include the following: (i) all affected tissue including the matrix, proximal nail fold, cuticle, upper portion of the lateral nail fold adjacent to the proximal nail fold, nail bed, and nail plate, are completely removed; (ii) the pathologist is able to examine the lesion in its entirety; (iii) pigment recurrence or persistence is unlikely; and (iv) post-operatively, the patient is left with a good cosmetic result with just a narrowed nail.

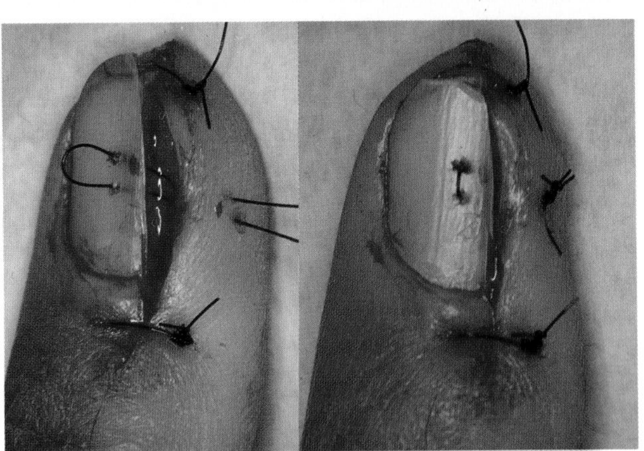

Fig. 10.25. Lateral longitudinal biopsy for lateral nail pigmentation.

Midportion of the nail plate involved

When LM lies within the midportion of the nail plate, the potential for post-operative dystrophy may be great and the selection of the optimal biopsy method is difficult.

It is necessary to identify the origin (proximal or distal matrix) of pigmentation in LM. Pigment histologically localized within the dorsal half of the nail plate indicates a proximal matrix origin; pigment localized within the ventral nail plate indicates a distal matrix origin (Figs 10.26–10.28).

The level of pigment within the nail plate is defined microsopically with Fontana–Masson staining of clippings obtained from the free edge of the nail. When a distal matrix origin seems likely, the cuticle can be retracted proximally to confirm the distal origin of LM without incision and reflection of the proximal nail fold.

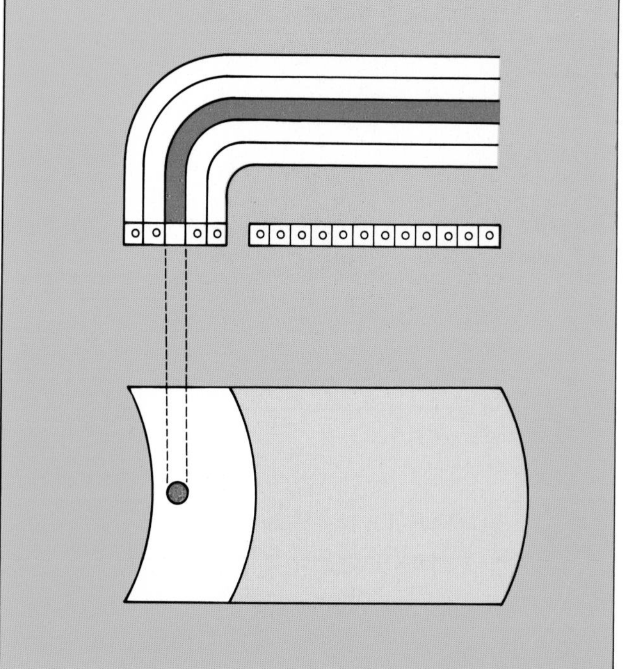

Fig. 10.26. Diagram to show the site of matrix pigment pathology in relation to the depth of nail plate pigmentation (after Higashi, 1970).

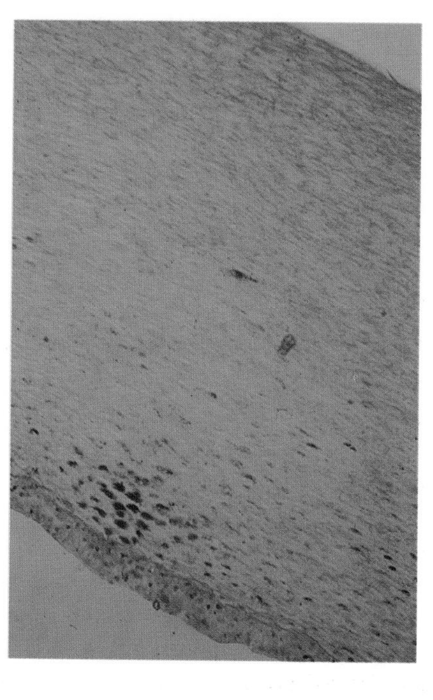

Fig. 10.28. Nail pigmentation localized within the 'ventral' nail plate.

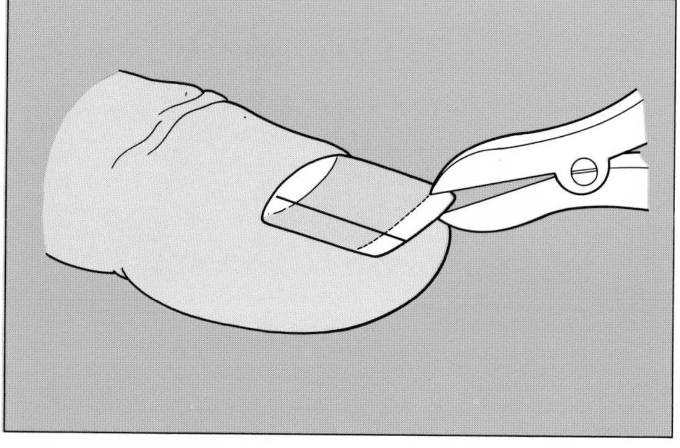

Fig. 10.27. Nail clipping of the free edge to define the depth of pigment with the nail.

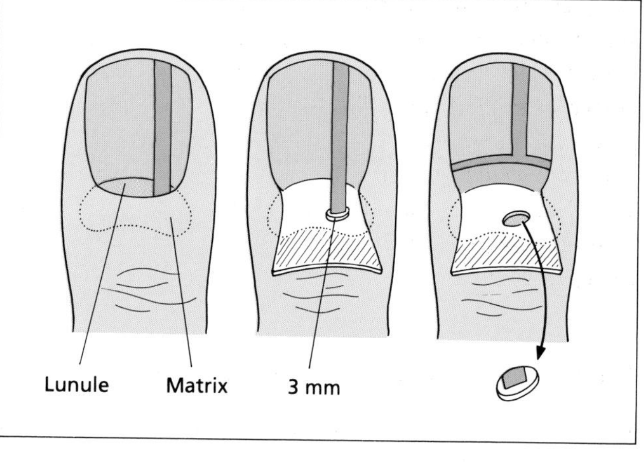

Fig. 10.29. Sites of biopsy for lesions less than 3 mm width; taken through intact nail plate.

Thin band, less than 3 mm in width (Higashi, 1970; Kopf *et al.*, 1984)

When the band is thin, and originates in the distal two-thirds of the matrix it is less likely to be subungual melanoma (e.g. in a young patient with index nail involvement); a 3-mm punch excision is indicated. Punch excision is performed through the nail plate with direct visualization of the band at its origin (Figs 10.29–10.31).

The origin of the band is exposed by reflecting the proximal nail fold with relaxing incisions, if necessary. With a 3-mm punch, a circumferential incision is made around the origin of the band; the cylinder of involved tissue is not removed at this time. The next step consists of removal of the proximal (surrounding) third of the nail plate, leaving in place the cylinder of tissue containing the origin of LM. In the absence of the nail plate, the surgeon is able to inspect the surrounding nail matrix and bed with a head magnifier lens to determine whether pigment extends distally or laterally from the punch incision. The cylinder of tissue containing the origin of LM is then removed. Because the surrounding nail plate has been previously detached, the cylinder of tissue is completely accessible and excised with relative ease. The detached nail plate and cylinder of LM are submitted to the pathologist for sectioning through the band. With assistance from the surgeon, the pathologist is able to orient the speci-

(a)

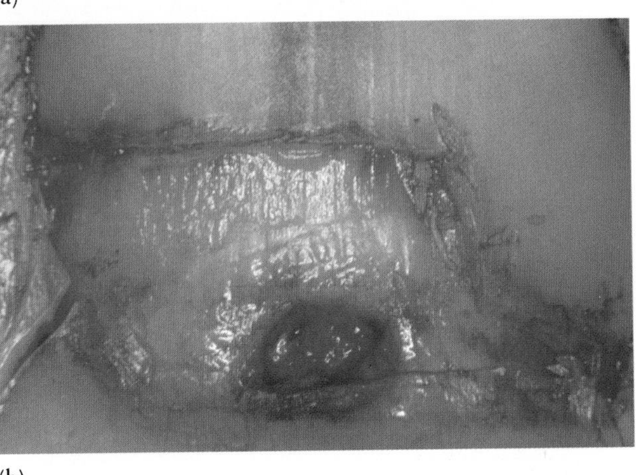
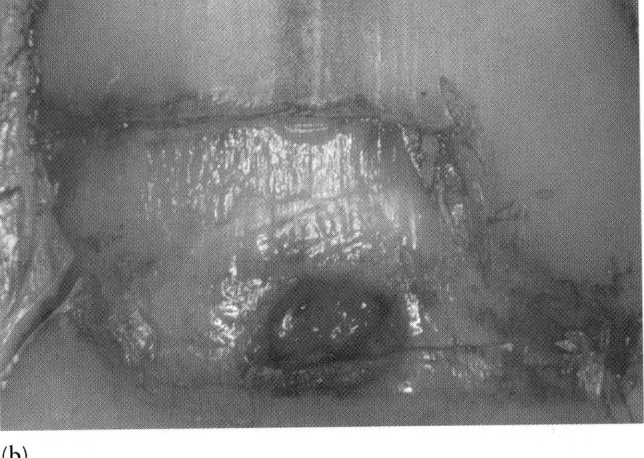

(b)

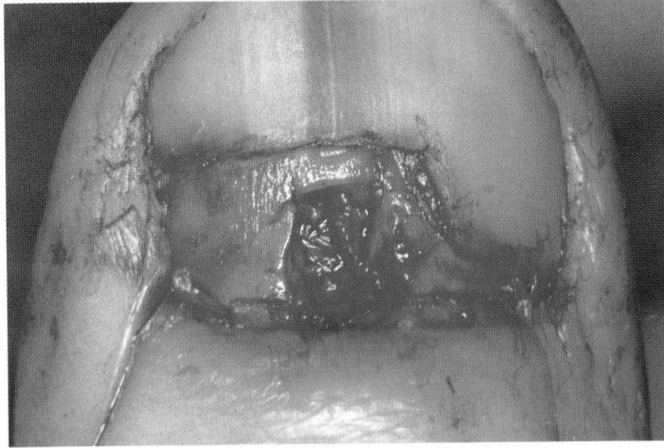

(c)

Fig. 10.30. Punch biopsy through the matrix at the proximal end of a narrow LM band. (a) After biopsy, pigment is still seen in front of the biopsy site, (b) enlargement of the nail window to check the extent of the pigmentation, (c) removal of the latter.

mens properly to ensure optimal sectioning and microscopic interpretation.

Alternatively, a punch biopsy of the LM origin with en-bloc removal of the nail plate and matrix can be performed *without* first removing the surrounding nail plate. Another method is to perform a biopsy on the involved matrix *after* removing the overlying *involved* nail plate.

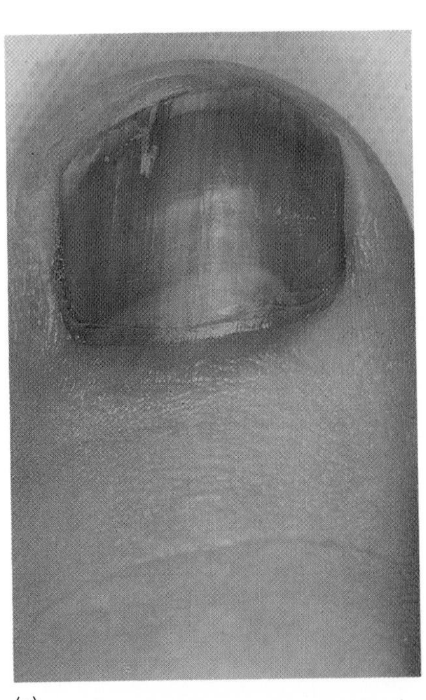
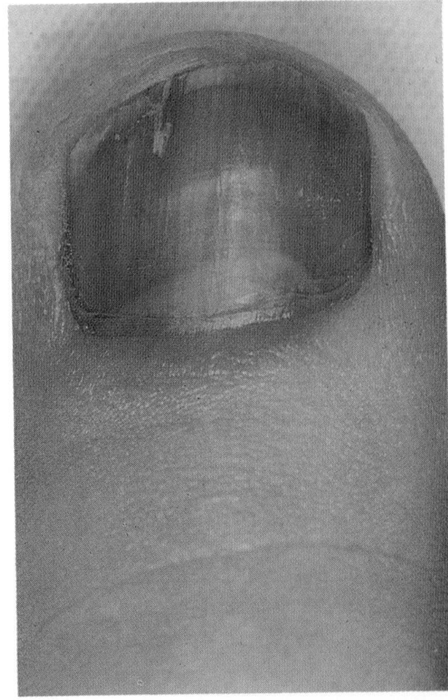

(a)

(b)

(c)

Fig. 10.31. (a) Pigmentation of the whole nail with distal origin in the matrix, (b) proximal nail removal prior to biopsy, (c) transverse biopsy of the matrix.

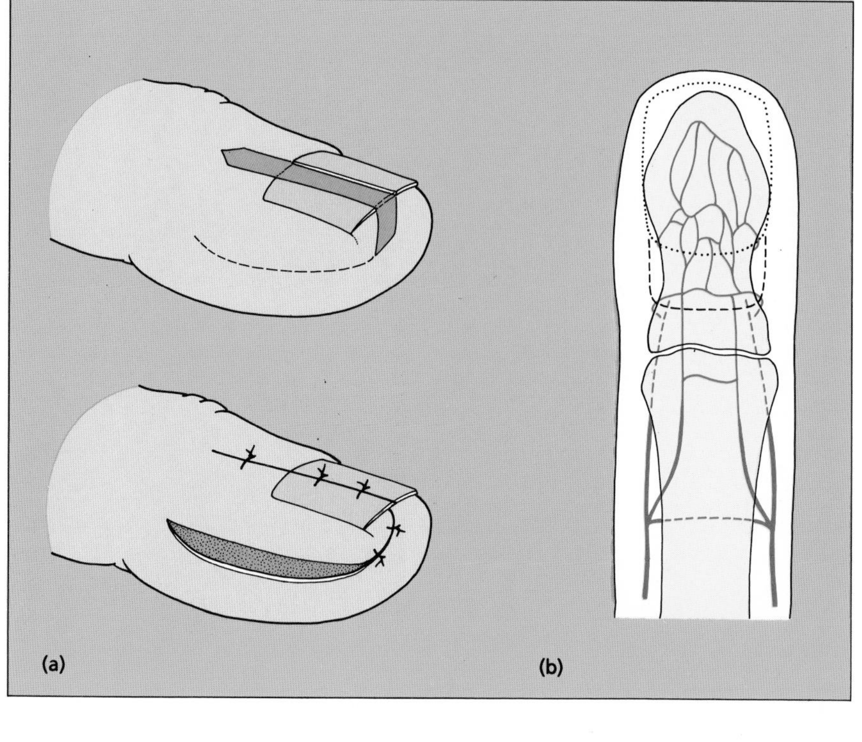

Fig. 10.32. Proximal third of the matrix is involved. Removal of the band using the releasing flap method of Schernberg and Amiel (1985); the flap is revascularized by branches of the medial phalangeal artery (b).

The stage method is preferable for the following reasons.

1 If punch excision is conducted without initially removing the surrounding nail plate, the biopsy cylinder may be difficult to separate from the surrounding tissues. In addition, removal of the proximal third of the nail plate before matrix excision permits direct intraoperative visualization of the underlying nail matrix or bed to verify that the band origin is enclosed within the cylinder of tissue.

2 If involved nail plate is removed before biopsy, the origin of LM (in the underlying matrix) may be 'lost' when the nail is torn off.

3 Punch excision through the affected nail plate and underlying involved matrix ensures that the lesion will be removed en-bloc, usually with the nail plate attached to the underlying matrix.

4 When the origin of LM is completely excised, the likelihood of post-operative pigment recurrence is negligible, and the pathologist is afforded the opportunity to examine the lesion intact and in its entirety. The risk of post-operative dystrophy is minimal because only 3 mm of distal matrix is removed.

Biopsies of bands less than 3 mm in width that originate *in the proximal one-third* of the matrix can also be performed with a 3-mm punch. The proximal nail fold must be reflected completely to ensure full exposure of the band. An attempt may be made to close the (proximal matrix) defect with 6-0 absorbable suture. Because the matrix is fragile and liable to tear easily, it is sufficient to achieve partial approximation rather than to attempt complete closure of the matrix biopsy margins. The risk of post-operative dystrophy is high.

Bands 3–6 mm in width

For bands between 3 and 6 mm wide that involve the *distal two-thirds of the matrix, transverse elliptical excision is necessary* (Fig. 10.31). Although the potential for post-operative dystrophy is significant, an effort should be made, depending on the clinical circumstances, to excise completely the origin of the band, not only to prevent post-operative recurrence of LM, but also to ensure that representative tissue is submitted for study. Because the proximal matrix remains intact, a thinned nail plate will regenerate post-operatively.

When 3–6-mm-wide bands involve the *proximal third of the matrix, the releasing flap method of Schernberg and Amiel* (1985) *is indicated* (Fig. 10.32). This technique enables removal of the proximal portion of the matrix with acceptable post-operative changes in the nail apparatus; the nail plate is diminished in width but is otherwise normal except for slight dystrophy, such as a longitudinal ridge. In this method, the pigmented band is completely excised in a rectangular monoblock comprising involved nail plate, bed, matrix, and proximal nail fold delineated laterally by a curved incision running from the distal end of the monoblock incision to the proximal edge of the matrix. Inferiorly, the nail bed and matrix are separated from the underlying bony phalanx to provide complete mobility. The flap is rotated into position (abutting the incised medial portion of the nail plate, bed, matrix and

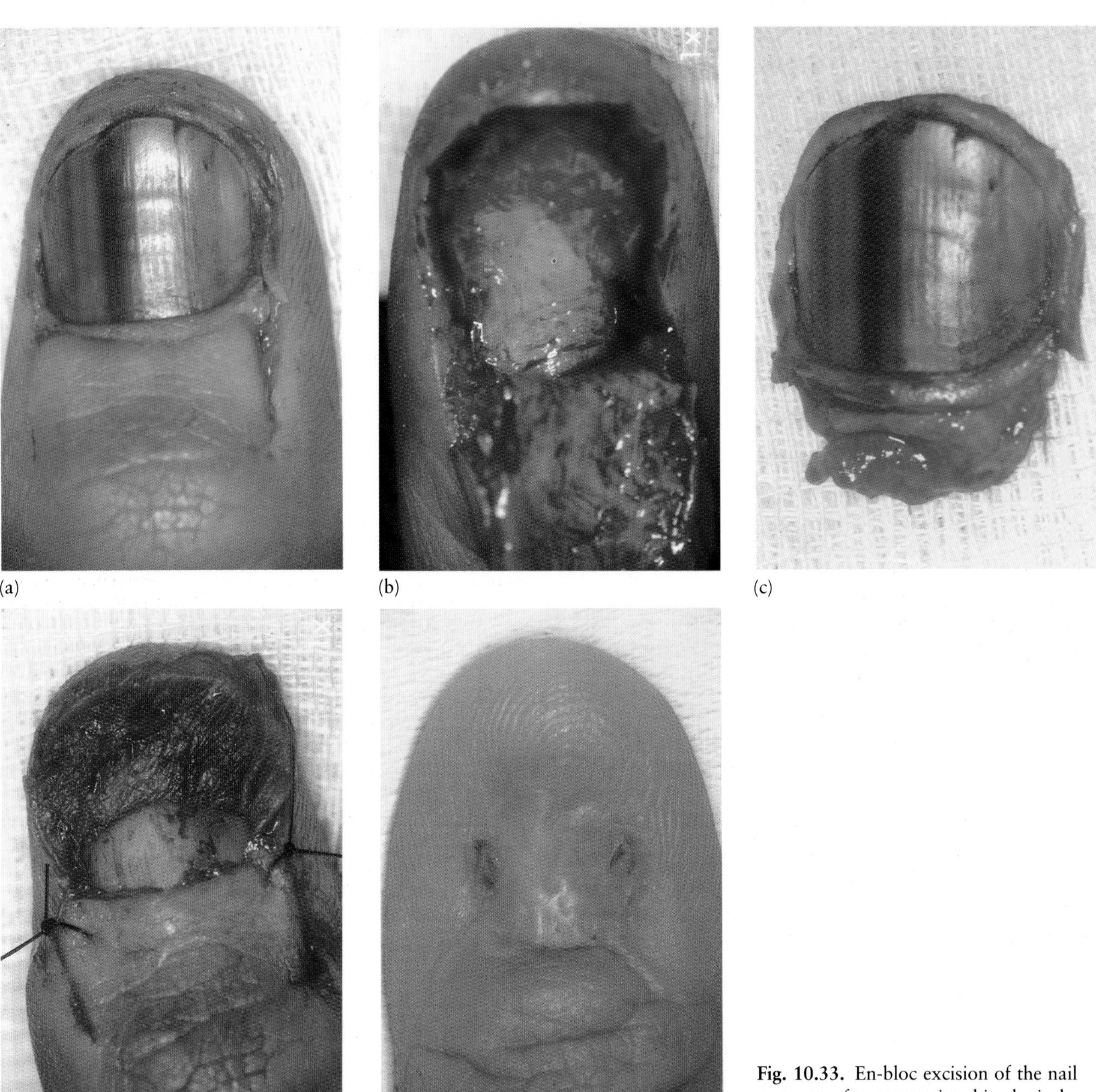

(a) (b) (c) (d) (e)

Fig. 10.33. En-bloc excision of the nail apparatus for appropriate histological examination in a case with very 'broad band' longitudinal melanonychia.

proximal nail fold) and closed with 5-0 nylon sutures. The defect in the lateral nail fold is allowed to heal by secondary intention.

Bands wider than 6 mm (Figs 10.33(a)–(e))

If the band is wider than 6 mm or if the full thickness of the nail is pigmented, a large elliptical portion of the matrix would necessarily be involved. Under these circumstances, the underlying disease process is unlikely to be benign. Depending on the clinical condition, partial longitudinal biopsy, transverse elliptic excision or punch biopsies from selected areas of the matrix can be performed or the entire portion of the involved nail apparatus can be excised enbloc.

Treatment after nail biopsy

After biopsy, whatever the technique employed, the nail area will require careful antiseptic treatment. A simple dressing with an antibiotic ointment, is applied for 3–5 days. The dressing should be thick in order to prevent the pain which might be produced by inadvertant minor trauma. Maintaining the hand or foot elevated for 1–2 days post-operatively will diminish pain during this period. Analgesics are not usually necessary. The first change of the dressing may be painful especially when clotted blood causes the gauze to adhere. Soaking the finger in an antiseptic solution, e.g. 3% hydrogen peroxide, or a mixture of diluted hydrogen peroxide with an antiseptic will make this easier.

'Pulsating' pain after the second post-operative day, mainly at night, may be due to wound infection and the dressing should be changed. If infection is present, the sutures should be removed and the wound drained. Increasing pain after 3–5 days may be an indication of incipient reflex sympathetic dystrophy (Ingram *et al.*, 1987; Haneke, 1992).

Handling biopsy specimens

Nail biopsy specimens are difficult to process. This problem starts with the surgical procedure: artefacts may be produced by tearing and dislocation of the nail plate from the nail bed or by squeezing the tissue.

The portion of the biopsy to be examined should have a straight plane section in order to facilitate tissue orientation in the paraffin block. It is obviously important to ensure that tissue of paramount pathological interest is included in the histological section. The longitudinal (lateral) biopsy (Zaias, 1967; Baran & Sayag, 1976) gives information of the effect of disease on all parts of the nail apparatus. Nail biopsies are difficult to cut. The nail plate is very hard and may be torn from the epithelium. This difficulty can partly be overcome by floating the paraffin block, cut surface down, for 1 h in 1% aqueous polysorbate 40 at 4°C after trimming to expose the surface at the level of the desired section (Lewin *et al.*, 1973).

Entirely flat sections are infrequently obtained. Haematoxylin and eosin (H&E) staining is not always sufficient. Periodic acid Schiff (PAS) and/or Grocott's stain are recommended if onychomycosis is suspected. Intraepithelial polymorphonuclear leucocytes are more easily identified after PAS staining. Physicochemical alterations in the nail keratin are demonstrated with Giemsa's stain, by the abrupt change from red to blue. Masson–Goldner's trichrome stain is particularly valuable in demonstrating keratinization processes.

References

Achten G. (1972) Histologie unguéale. *Boll. Ist. Derm. San Gallicano* **8**, 3.

André J. & Achten G. (1987) Techniques de la biopsie de l'ongle. *Ann. Dermatol. Venereol.* **114**, 889–892.

Baran R. (1979) Longitudinal melanotic streaks as a clue to Laugier–Hunziker syndrome. *Arch. Dermatol.* **115**, 1448–1449.

Baran R. (1986) Removal of the proximal nail fold. Why, when, how? *J. Dermatol. Surg. Oncol.* **12**, 234–236.

Baran R. & Barrière H. (1986) Longitudinal melanonychia with spreading pigmentation in Laugier–Hunziker syndrome: a report of 2 cases. *Br. J. Dermatol.* **115**, 707–710.

Baran R. & Haneke E. (1984) Diagnostik und Therapie der streifenförmigen Nagelpigmentierung. *Hautarzt* **35**, 359–365.

Baran R. & Kechijian P. (1989) Longitudinal melanonychia (melanonychia striata). Diagnosis and management. *J. Am. Acad. Dermatol.* **21**, 1165–1175.

Baran R. & Sayag J. (1976) Nail biopsy. Why, when, where, how? *J. Dermatol. Surg. Oncol.* **2**, 322–324.

Bennett R.G. (1976) Technique of biopsy of nails. *J. Dermatol. Surg. Oncol.* **2**, 325.

Fosnaugh R.F. (1982) Surgery of the nail. In: *Skin Surgery*, 5th edn, eds Epstein E. & Epstein E. Jr, p. 981. C.C. Thomas, Springfield, IL.

Gonzalez-Serva A. (1990) The problem-oriented ungual biopsy. *Pathol. Rev.* **2**, No. 1.

Haneke E. (1984) Segmentale Matrixverschmälerung zur Behandlung des eingewachsenen Zehennagels. *Dtsch. Med. Wschr.* **109**, 1451–1453.

Haneke E. (1985a) Nail biopsies in onychomycosis. *Mykosen* **28**, 473–480.

Haneke E. (1985b) Bahandlung einiger Nagelfehlbildungen. In: *Fehtbidungen, Nävi, Melanome*, eds Wolff H.H. & Schmeller W., pp 71–77. Spinger-Verlag Berlin.

Haneke E. (1988) Exzisions-und Biopsieverfahren. *Z. Hautkr.* **63** (Suppl.), 17–19.

Haneke E. (1991) Laugier–Hunziker–Baran–Syndrom. *Hautarzt* **42**, 512–515.

Haneke E. (1992) Sympathische Reflexdystrophie (Sudeck-Dystro-phie) nach Nagelbiopsie. *Zbl. Haut. Geschl. Kr.* **160**, 263.

Haneke E. & Baran R. (1991) Nails: Surgical aspects. In: *Aesthetic Dermatology*, eds Parish L.C. & Lask G.P., pp. 236–247. McGraw Hill, New York.

Hanno R., Mathes B.M. & Krull E.A. (1986) Longitudinal nail biopsy in evaluation of acquired nail dystrophies. *J. Am. Acad. Dermatol.* **14**, 803–809.

Higashi N. (1970) On the effects of the matrix and nail bed biopsy on the regeneration of the nail plate. *Hifu* 12, 78–80 (in Japanese).

Ingram G.J., Scher R.K. & Lally E.V. (1987) Reflex sympathetic dystrophy following nail biopsy. *J. Am. Acad. Dermatol.* **16**, 253–256.

Kechijian P. (1987) Nail biopsy vignettes. *Cutis* **40**, 331–335.

Kopf A., Albom M. & Ackerman A.B. (1984) Biopsy technique for longitudinal streaks of pigmentation in nails. *Am. J. Dermatopathol.* **6** (Suppl. 1), 309–312.

Lewin K., DeWitt S. & Lawson R. (1973) Softening techniques for nail biopsies. *Arch. Dermatol.* **107**, 223–224.

Rich P. (1992) Nail biopsy: indications and methods. *J. Dermatol. Oncol.* **18**, 673–682.

Salasche S.J. (1984) Myxoid cysts of the proximal nail fold: a surgical approach. *J. Dermatol. Surg. Oncol.* **10**, 35–39.

Salasche S.J. & Peters V.J. (1985) Tips on nail surgery. *Cutis* **35**, 428–438.

Sanderson K.V. & MacKie R.M. (1979) Tumours of the skin. In: *Textbook of Dermatology*, eds Rook A., Wilkinson D.S. & Ebling F.J.G., p. 2129. Blackwell Scientific Publications. Oxford.

Scher R.K. (1980) Longitudinal resection of nails for purposes of biopsy and treatment. *J. Dermatol. Surg. Oncol.* **6**, 805.

Scher R.K. & Ackerman A.B. (1980a) Subtle clues to diagnosis from biopsies of nails. The value of nail biopsy for demonstrating fungi not demonstrable by microbiologic techniques. *Am. J. Dermatopathol.* **2**, 55.

Scher R.K. & Ackerman A.B. (1980b) Subtle clues to diagnosis from biopsies of nails. Histologic differential diagnosis of onychomycosis and psoriasis of the nail unit from cornified cells of the nail bed alone. *Am. J. Dermatopathol.* **2**, 255.

Schernberg F. & Amiel M. (1985) Etude anatomo-clinique d'un lambeau unguéal complet. *Ann. Chir. Plast. Esthet.* **30**, 217–231.

Schnitzler L., Baran R., Civatte J. *et al.* (1976) Biopsy of the proximal nail fold in collagen diseases. *J. Dermatol. Surg. Oncol.* **2**, 313–315.

Schnitzler L., Civatte J., Baran R. *et al.* (1980) Le repli sus-unguéal normal. *Ann. Dermatol. Venereol.* **107**, 771–774.

Shelley W.B. (1975) The razor blade in dermatologic practice. *Cutis* **16**, 843.

Siegle R.J. & Swanson N.A. (1982) Nail surgery: a review. *J. Dermatol. Surg. Oncol.* **8**, 659–666.

Stone O.J., Barr R.J. & Herten R.J. (1978) Biopsy of the nail area. *Cutis* **21**, 257–260.

Zaias N. (1967) The longitudinal nail biopsy. *J. Invest. Dermatol.* **49**, 406–408.

Dorsal exposure of the distal finger (Fig. 10.34)

The ideal incision to expose the distal interphalangeal (DIP) joint is a dorsal S-shaped incision beginning proximally on the ulnar side of the middle phalanx in the midlateral line. At the midpoint of the axis of the DIP joint, the incision turns transversely across the joint in the midjoint skin crease to the midaxis of the radial side. It is extended distally in the midlateral line region as needed. The corners should be gently rounded to avoid tip necrosis.

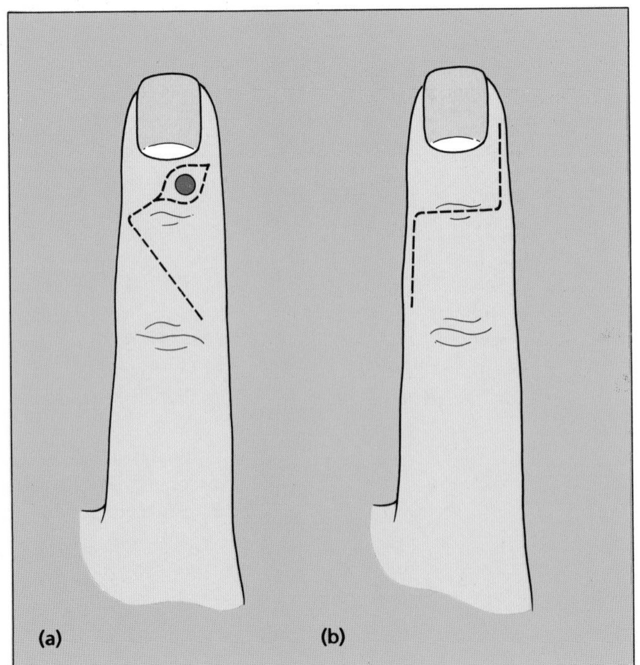

Fig. 10.34. Incisions for the dorsal exposure of distal finger lesions.

An acceptable alternative to this incision is to use only the horizontal limb of the S-shaped incision.

A midline longitudinal incision, if extended onto the base of the nail may result in nail plate damage and nail deformity (Adamson & Fleury, 1988).

Reference

Adamson J.E. & Fleury A.F. (1988) Incisions in the hand and wrist. In: *Operative Hand Surgery*, ed. Green D.P., pp. 1789–1791. Churchill Livingstone, New York.

Microscopically controlled surgery

(Mikhail, 1991; Goldminz & Bennett, 1992)

Mohs' chemosurgery originally involved serial excisions of chemically fixed tissue and immediate thorough histological study of each specimen until completely negative sections were obtained. This method is now usually performed without 'intravital' fixation (fresh tissue technique). Proper orientation of the surgical specimen and the correct histographic reidentification in the histological sections are the crucial points. This is greatly improved by drawing a map of the lesion to be excised and mapping tumour-bearing areas, especially those showing residual involvement.

This technique leads to complete removal of the malignant tumour without sacrificing large amounts of normal tissue. The resulting defect may then be repaired with a free graft or a pedicle flap, depending on the size and location of the defect.

References

Mikhail G.R. (1991) *Mohs Micrographic Surgery.* W.B. Saunders, Philadelphia.

Goldminz D. & Bennett R.G. (1992) Mohs micrographic surgery of the nail unit. *J. Dermatol. Surg. Oncol.* **18**, 721–726.

Non-scalpel techniques

Cryosurgery in the nail region

The fingertips and nail apparatus are well endowed with sensory nerve endings. Therefore, unless adequate pre-treatment analgesia is given, cryosurgery to this area may be relatively painful or resisted by the patient; certainly without such care, repeat treatments for conditions such as warts may be impossible. It should be pointed out that after the initial freeze and thaw, with all but the shortest freeze times, despite the prominent 'burn appearance', pain is considerably less than other methods which cause inflammation, unless the periosteum is frozen. Short freeze times may only induce erythema and blister formation which may be haemorrhagic. Freezing does not damage connective tissue in normal therapeutic doses (Shepherd & Dawber, 1984; Dawber, 1992; Dawber *et al.*, 1992) and for this reason it has recently been suggested as perhaps better than surgery for periungual tumours such as myxoid cysts (Dawber *et al.*, 1983), particularly those which have discharged and may be difficult to dissect surgically.

Cryosurgery has long been used by dermatologists for periungual warts, again because like spontaneous healing, correctly used, scarring should not occur after freezing (Dawber *et al.*, 1992).

References

Dawber R.P.R. (1992) Cryotherapy. In: *Textbook of Dermatology*, eds Champion R.H., Burton J.L. & Ebling F.J.G., 5th edn, pp. 909–910. Blackwell Scientific Publications, Oxford.

Dawber R.P.R., Sonnex T., Leonard J. & Ralfs I. (1983) Myxoid cysts of the finger: treatment by liquid nitrogen spray cryosusgery. *Clin. Exp. Dermatol.* 8, 153.

Dawber R.P.R., Colver G.B. & Jackson A. (1992) *Cutaneous Cryosurgery*. Martin Dunitz, London.

Shepherd J. & Dawber R.P.R. (1984) Wound healing and scarring after cryosurgery. *Cryobiology* **21**, 157–160.

Electroradiosurgery

Electrosurgery has varied in popularity but it is now back in vogue because of the appearance of radiosurgery and the new flexible electrodes on the market with a flattened triangular tip, for treating ingrowing toenail. The insulated matricectomy electrode is specially coated for the protection of the upper tissue while destroying underlying cells. Destruction of the lateral horn of the matrix is thus possible without injuring the ventral aspect of the proximal nail fold using the uncoated side down on the matrix (Fig. 10.35).

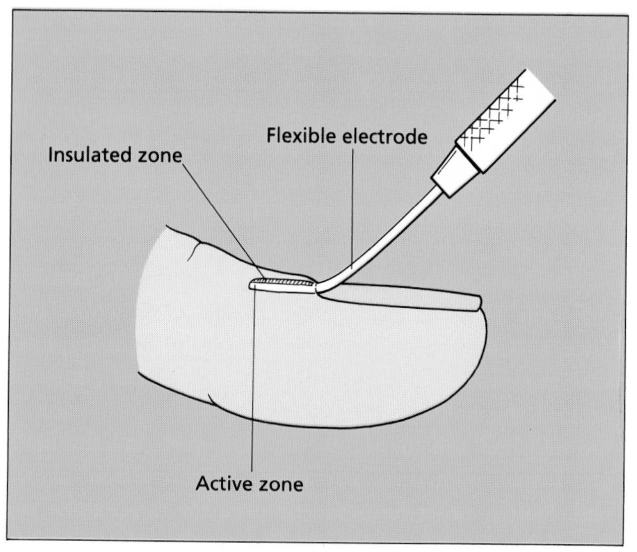

Fig. 10.35. Matricectomy electrode.

Using an English nail splitter the offending lateral border is separated from the nail and the nail segment is removed with forceps. The current selector is then turned to 'partially rectified current' and the electrode is applied for a period of 3 s to the matrix area; the power is then shut off, the electrode removed and after an interval of 10 s the procedure is repeated (twice when treating a great toe). A 0.125 ml dose of dexamethasone phosphate is instilled into the wound. A layer of antibiotic ointment is applied, followed by a sterile compressive dressing (Hettinger *et al.*, 1991). Complete matricectomy is also possible using the same technique after total nail avulsion.

Radiosurgery is used by some to treat warts. When they are subungual they first require partial avulsion of the distal or lateral half of the nail plate, depending on their location. Radiocoagulation is done superficially, followed by careful curettage of the area because of the fragile nature of the tissue in the nail bed. Simply applying pressure with a dressing made of a double thickness of sterile gauze results in adequate haemostasis. If bleeding is persistent, slight pressure with a Q-tip soaked in 35% aluminium chloride is usually sufficient.

Pyogenic granuloma can be excised with a cutting loop electrode, providing a specimen for the histologist whilst coagulating the base (Pollack, 1991).

References

Hettinger D.F., Valinsky M.S., Nucci G. *et al.* (1991) Nail matrixectomies using radio wave technique. *JAPMA* **81**, 317–321.

Pollack S.V. (1991) *Electrosurgery of the Skin*. Churchill Livingstone, New York.

The CO_2 laser in nail surgery (Gary Brauner)

LASER is an acronym for Light Amplification by the Stimulated Emission of Radiation. The CO_2 laser is that laser most utilized for surgery of and around the nail. It produces an intense monochromatic ray of 10 600 nanometers wavelength, absorbed well in water. When it is absorbed by water-bearing tissue it causes the tissue to heat rapidly and vaporize or carbonize. The handpiece of the carbone dioxide laser has a focusing lens which can focus a spot to 0.1–0.2 mm when held at one focal length. Although the CO_2 laser is frequently used in a focused manner where one has a power density of perhaps 50.000 W/cm^2 and haemostatic incisional surgery can be perfomed, it is generally used in and around the nail in a defocused manner, several focal lengths above the surface of the skin so that one has a spot size of 1 mm or more and a power density of hundreds to thousands of W/cm^2.

With such a defocused spot, one can haemostatically vaporize away skin cells and 'peel' the skin with extraordinary ability to visualize the tissue.

Why should one use the laser for diseases of the nail? The major virtue of the CO_2 laser is increased visualization. Because the laser produces a haemostatic wound, one can focus the spot size down to tenths of a millimetre. One can trace abnormal tissue far better than with the smallest curette. Furthermore, because of the haemostasis, one can avoid sacrificing normal surrounding tissue in the attempt to eradicate pathology. Originally, the CO_2 laser was utilized with colposcopic magnification. Magnification will also produce more accurate and better results so that the use of magnifying loupes is a necessary adjunct for laser surgery (Pyrcz & Carlson, 1990). Such loupes should also be used with cold steel surgery alone to produce better results.

Although haemostasis is a critical part of visualization and the CO_2 laser is a very good instrument for providing it, a simple tourniquet provided by an elastic band or Penrose drain is often necessary in CO_2 laser surgery (Borovoy *et al.*, 1983; Kaplan *et al.*, 1985; Rothermel *et al.*, 1987; Wright, 1989). One might therefore argue that adequate haemostasis might be obtainable with such tourniquets in cold steel surgery as well. One certainly does not need to purchase an expensive CO_2 laser to provide post-operative haemostasis when it can be provided with simple application of aluminium chloride or ferric subsulphate solution.

Lastly, one can use the laser to burn through the nail plate or to vaporize it. Simple mechanical avulsion may be faster, but is more traumatizing.

Surprisingly despite extensive and vigorous promotion of laser surgery by podiatrists, there is a paucity of literature concerning the real usefulness of the CO_2 laser for ungual and periungual surgery (Bennett, 1989).

Table 10.3 indicates uses of the CO_2 laser. Subungual haematomas can be treated without the need for local anaesthesia by rapidly penetrating through nail plate with a focused beam. One can use the laser as an incisional instrument to excise squamous cell carcinoma in the Mohs' technique or small tumours such as periungual fibromas or pyogenic granulomas. Excisional surgery generally is done at 15–20 W with a focused spot of approximately 1 mm in size and the beam applied in a continuous fashion. A defocused beam will vaporize myxoid cysts around the nail fold.

The main use of the CO_2 laser is for subungual and periungual warts (Fig. 10.36(a)–(c)). The CO_2 laser allows one to carbonize nail plate in pursuit of the subungual or periungual wart although intra-operative clipping is usually faster. The laser here is operated in a defocused mode with 1–2 mm spot size at 5–10 W output in either intermittent 0.05 s bursts or continuous mode (Apfelberg *et al.*, 1984a,b; Street & Roenigk, 1990). As with electrodesiccation, the infected epidermis tends to boil and bubble and usually separates easily from the underlying dermis. The residual charred area then is snipped at the periphery with iris scissors and the roof is avulsed. The typical fish white appearance of residual wart tissue is easy to demonstrate against the pinker background and evident dermal papillae, particularly when a tourniquet is also used. One can easily vaporize these remnants but they must be traced well down into the lateral sulci for periungual warts and under the nail plate and onto the nail bed for subungual warts. Caution must be used when appoaching the nail matrix lest it be vaporized and produce subsequent nail dystrophy. Healing usually occurs in 3–4 weeks (Apfelberg *et al.*, 1984b).

There are times when the nail growth is so distorted that only total ablation of the affected area would produce a cosmetically acceptable result. Onychogryphosis was the first instance in which a laser was employed around the nail (Kaplan *et al.*, 1976). Vaporization of the nail bed and matrix to the area overlying the interphalangeal joint was perfomed after avulsion of the nail. Similar procedures can be used for onychauxis and have also been used by podiatrists for chronic tinea pedis though appropriate oral medication may be a more

Table 10.3. Use of CO_2 laser for nail diseases

Nail bed
Subungual haematoma
Nail bed or nail fold tumefactions
Periungual fibroma
Pyogenic granuloma
Mohs' surgery
Myxoid cyst
Nail plate dystrophy
Matricectomy total
Onychogryphosis
Onychauxis
Single or double plicature
Matricectomy partial
Single plicature
Nail bed ablation
Pachyonychia congenita
Hyponychial ablation
Partial or double plicature
Nail fold dystrophy
Lateral fold ablation
Hypertrophic lateral nail fold
Matricectomy, partial
Tinea
'Waffling' technique
Nail bed ablation
Matricectomy, total

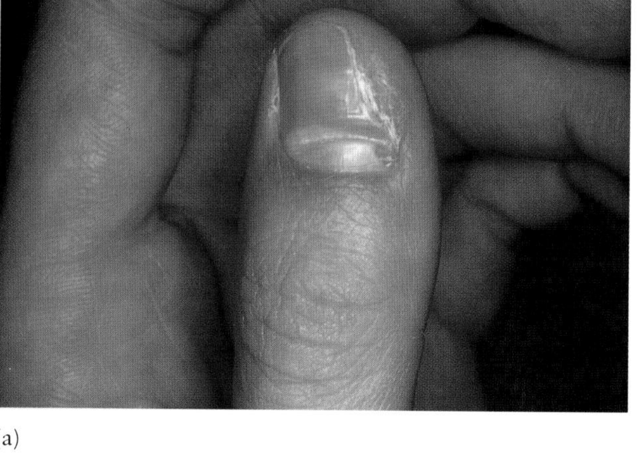
(a)

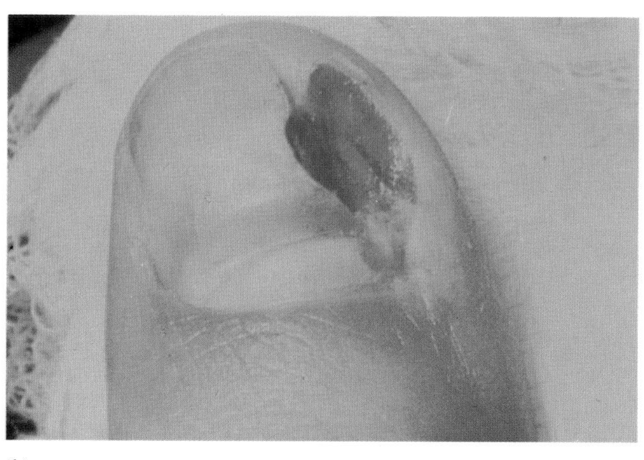
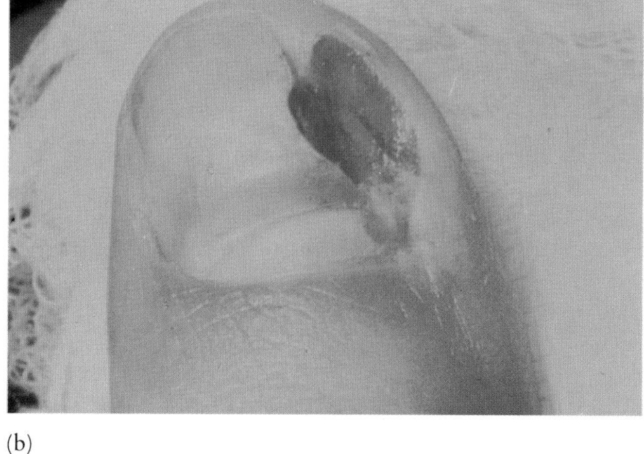
(b)

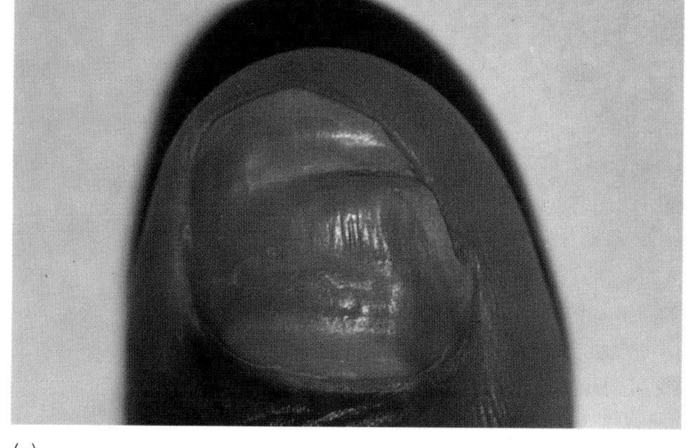
(c)

Fig. 10.36. Periungual and subungual wart treated by CO_2 laser (a) before, (b) immediately after and (c) after healing.

reasonable appoach for the latter patients. The technique involves operating the laser at 2–6 W with an irradiance of approximately 60–160 W/cm^2 (Kaplan *et al.*, 1985; Leshin and Whitaker, 1988) with vaporization of the nail matrix after reflection of the proximal nail fold. The vaporization should include both that portion of the nail matrix extending onto the reflection of the nail fold as well as the lunula, and the vaporization must extend to the lateral horns of the nail unit (Siegle & Swanson, 1982; Leshin & Whitaker, 1988) in order to avoid regrowth of the nail spicules. Although Leshin and Whitaker (1988) found no recurrence after laser surgery, Kaplan *et al.* (1985) had to utilize subsequently 10% sodium hydroxide, which can be used alone to produce a matricectomy. Rothermel and Apfelberg (1987) performed laser, then curettage and relasering (curettage may also be utilized alone successfully). Wright (1989) noted, with a technique involving lasering proximally, medially, and laterally, curetting and relasering, that there was a nail plate recurrence rate of 50% for total matricectomy in 58 nails and 48% for partial matricectomy whereas his own recurrence rate was only 20% for total matricectomy with more traditional surgical techniques; he concluded that the laser was inferior to traditional surgical podiatric techniques. Siegle and Swanson (1982) cited published recurrence rates of 0–5% for phenol or cold steel matricectomies.

Nail bed ablation may be useful palliatively for treatment of nail dystrophies in which the nail bed plays a significant contributing role, such as in pachyonychia congenita (Figs 10.37(a)–(c)). Although Thomsen *et al.* (1982) suggest that surgical ablation of the nail fold, not the nail bed, is appropriate in pachyonychia congenita as a totally destructive method, our patients seem to have had a demonstrably better palliative result by treatment of the nail bed alone rather than the nail fold alone with CO_2 laser surgery.

Partial matricectomy may be useful for nail plate dystrophies in which one has only a partial plicatured nail (partial pincer nail syndrome). The patient must be forewarned about the narrower resultant nail. In this instance, it is easiest to simply either carbonize the offending portion of the nail, or to incise longitudinally the entire nail plate and avulse the offending portion of the nail plate and then destroy the responsible nail matrix, again remembering to laser into the lateral horn of the nail fold after reflecting the fold.

It is not necessary in a partial platonychia to destroy the offending portion of the nail plate and its matrix, if

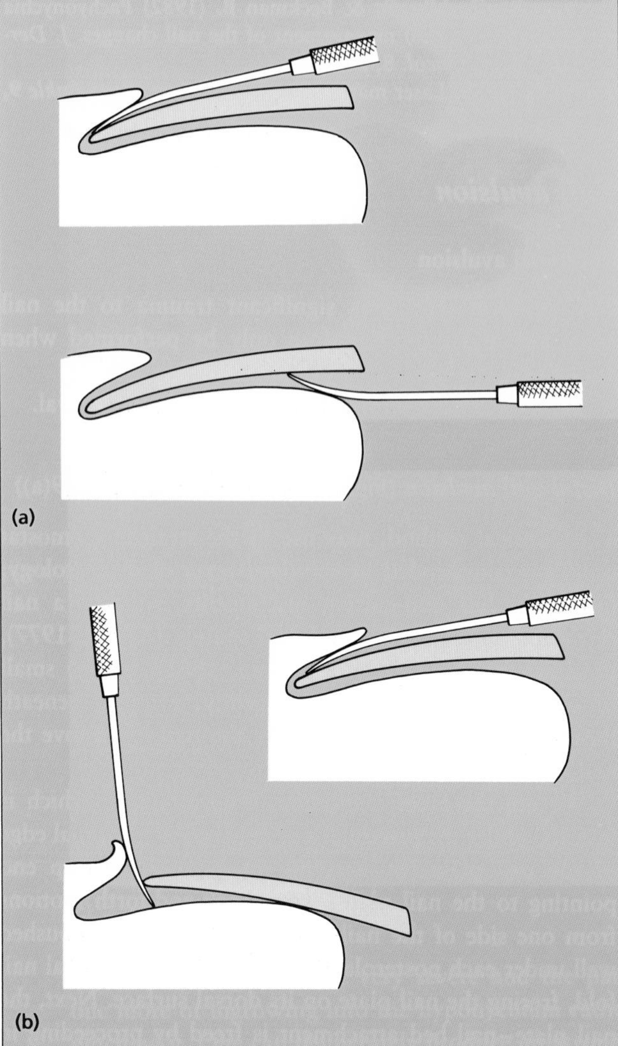

Fig. 10.39. (a) Nail avulsion. (b) Cordero's method of nail avulsion using Freer septum elevator.

techniques, commencing by separating the undersurface of the proximal nail fold from the nail plate, and in the use of a longitudinal back-and-forth motion. During the second stage of surgical avulsion by the proximal to distal technique, the nail elevator is inserted below the proximal edge of the nail plate. It is important to free the postero-lateral angle of the nail plate as the attachment is firm at this site. During the third stage, the lifted proximal part of the nail plate is placed on the proximal nail fold, after which the instrument can be slipped easily along the natural plane of cleavage between nail and bed, allowing the nail plate to be pulled distally. This proximal approach appears to be more valuable when the distal part of the nail has a great deal of subungual hyperkeratosis such as in distal subungual onychomycosis, onychogryphosis, pachyonychia congenita, etc., or when there is no obvious distal fold left.

This technique is feasible because the nail plate, although firmly adherent to the nail bed, has a very loose attachment to the matrix. This explains the histological finding that the epithelium of the nail bed is lining the avulsed nail plate whereas on the part which covers the matrix, there is little or no matrix epithelium attached to it. Incidental to removing the nail plate, it is imperative that the nail grooves be cleared of subungual debris. This is best achieved by wiping the nail bed and grooves with gauze wrapped around the end of a 'mosquito-haemostat'. If any remnants adhere, these can be removed with a curette.

After removal of the nail, Zaias (1990) recommends gently pushing back the proximal nail fold to ensure an 'open' proximal nail groove and to prevent 'pus' pockets in this groove.

Some signs preclude simple nail avulsion: with malformed nails due to matrix disease, large defects of the nail bed or ingrowing toenails, simply extracting the nail is not curative. Indeed, repeated nail avulsion may cause thickening and overcurvature of the nail plate (Runne, 1983). Therefore, it is important to stress that nail avulsion is not a therapy *per se* but enables exposure prior to treatment of the subungual structures.

Keratinization of the nail bed following nail avulsion may be avoided by replacing the original nail with a donor 'nail bank transplant'; this will adapt, adhere and function as an autologous nail in an adequate manner. Preservation of the matrix, the proximal nail fold and the proximal groove is also essential to normal nail regrowth. Whichever method is used, the original nail plate, a 'nail bank transplant' or an artificial nail are necessary for the regeneration of a satisfactory nail.

Partial nail avulsion

Partial nail avulsion may be more suitable than total avulsion in a variety of circumstances. Removing the lateral or

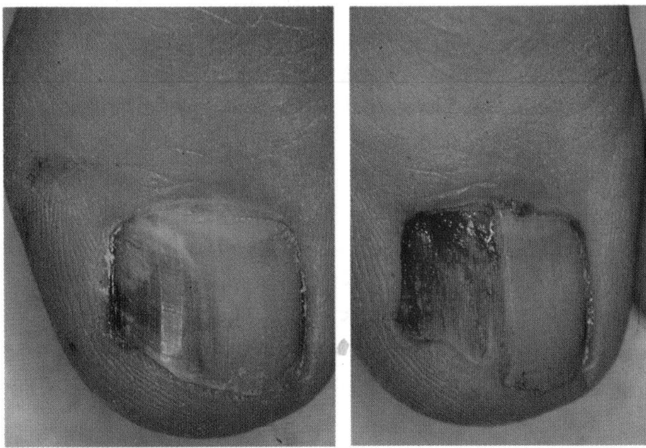

Fig. 10.40. Partial nail avulsion; onycholysis prior to oral and topical therapy.

(a)

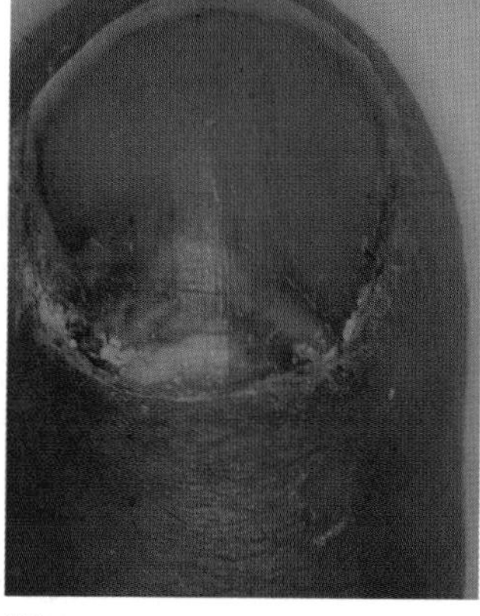
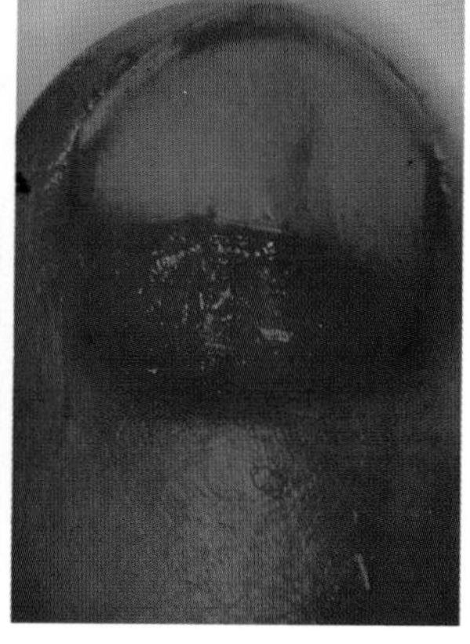

(b)

Fig. 10.41. Proximal subungual onychomycosis – removal of affected proximal nail prior to oral and topical therapy.

medial segment of the nail plate should be encouraged in some onychomycoses of big toes as enough normal nail is left to counteract the upward forces exerted on the distal soft tissue when walking. This will prevent the appearance of a distal nail 'wall'. The involved portion of the nail is separated from the proximal nail fold and the nail bed, then it is incised from the hyponychium to the proximal nail fold with a nail splitter and the freed nail segment is then avulsed (Fig. 10.40). In distal subungual onychomycoses with hyperkeratosis, elevation of the nail plate from the nail bed permits the easy removal of the affected portion of the nail with a double action bone rongeur. In such a case the distal edge of the cut portion of the nail plate has only a short distance to grow to reach the distal nail bed, which prevents the slow development of a distal nail wall.

In proximal subungual onychomycosis, removal of the diseased portion of the nail plate is not difficult: the non-adherent lunula region is cut transversely with a nail splitter, by inserting the instrument beneath the lateral edge of the nail plate. The distal portion of the nail that is left in place decreases discomfort (Fig. 10.41(a)&(b)). Bacterial infection of the nail area and dermatological conditions may benefit from the same techniques. They are also useful when performing some types of nail biopsy.

References

Albom M.J. (1977) Avulsion of a nail plate. *J. Dermatol. Surg. Oncol.* 3, 34–35.

Baran R. (1981) More on avulsion of nail plate *J. Dermatol. Surg. Oncol.* 7, 854.

Cordero C.F.A. (1965) Ablacion ungueal: su uso en la onycomicosis. *Derm. Int.* **14**, 21.

Linares J.L. (1967) Ablacion ungueal. Evaluation terapeutica de la tecnica creada para el Dr FA Cordero. *Dermatol. Rev. Mex.* **11**, 161–172.

McKay I. (1973) Nail elevator. *Lancet* **i**, 864.

Runne U. (1983) Operative Eingriffe an Nagelorgan: Indikationen und Kontraindikationen. *Z. Hautkr.* **58**, 324–332.

Zaias N. (1990) *The Nail in Health and Disease*, 2nd edn. Appleton & Lange, Norwalk, CN.

Trauma

Acute injuries

Trauma may be recent or longstanding; and the lesions may be simple or complex, involving several components of the nail apparatus. Retention of a stable, smooth, functional nail requires preservation of the ungual 'cul-de-sac' plus an adequate matrix and nail bed. The former is repaired in separate layers so as to delineate the ventral proximal nail fold from its dorsum. Loss of the distal nail bed may sometimes be acceptable and usually does not introduce significant functional impairment (Rosenthal, 1983).

The normal functional anatomy of the tip and perionychium depends on the level of the fingertip injuries (Fig. 10.42):

1 distal to the bony phalanx;
2 distal to the lunula (between the distal end of the lunula and the end of the phalanx);
3 proximal to the distal end of the lunula.

The plane of injury (indicator plane) suggests the feasible alternative for pedicle reconstruction. The level of nail bed injury determines the requirements for nail bed management. Nail stability requires at least 5 mm of healthy nail bed distal to the lunula for nail adherence (Rosenthal, 1983).

Recent trauma may produce:

1 partial or total haematomas;
2 lacerating wounds;
3 fractures of the terminal phalanx;
4 denudation of the terminal phalanx.

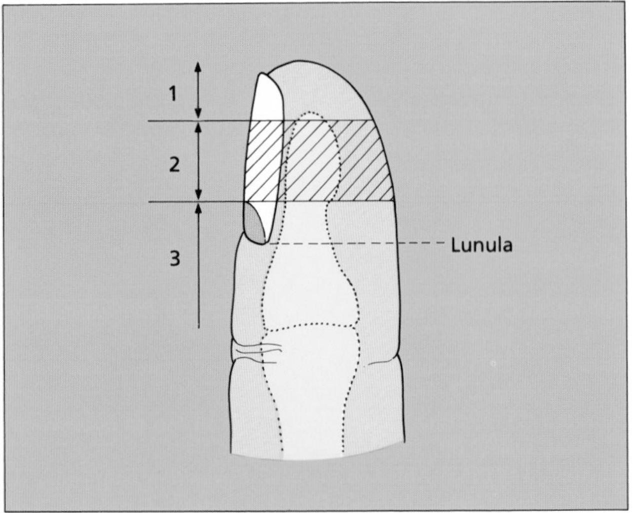

Fig. 10.42. Levels of nail injury. Nail stability requires approx. 5 mm of undamaged nail bed distal to the lunula.

According to Van Beek *et al.* (1990) acute injuries of fingernails can be classified as follows.

1 Type I injury: the small haematoma is associated with a small break in the nail bed. Appropriate decompression would be fenestration of the nail plate over the haematoma.

2 Type II injury: a large haematoma has formed from a significant injury to the nail bed. The nail plate must be removed to permit appropriate examination of the nail bed injury whether in the nail bed or in the matrix.

3 Type III injury: a fracture of the distal phalanx has occurred, and the nail matrix has been injured. This injury often manifests by having the nail plate pulled out of the cul-de-sac and located on top of the proximal nail fold.

4 Type IV injury: this injury is usually associated with severe crush injury. The nail matrix has numerous lacerations creating small islands or flaps of matrix needing surgical repair with loupes and fine suture.

5 Type V injury: amputation of portions or all of the nail matrix is best treated by retrieving the amputed tissue and replacing it as a graft. Often the nail bed may be attached to the nail plate. If the amputated tissue is not available for replacement, treatment requires grafts of nail bed.

Haematomas

1 Splinter haemorrhage (Fig. 10.43), see Chapter 6.

2 Small haemorrhages originating in the nail bed (Fig. 10.44) remain subungual as growth progresses distally (Stone & Mullins, 1963) and will stain the deeper layers of the nail. Trauma to the matrix produces small pockets of dried blood which will be found entrapped in the nail plate. The more proximal the haemorrhage in the matrix, the higher the pocket of dry blood will be in the nail. All haemorrhages beyond the lunula remain subungual. Sometimes patches of leuconychia are seen above the haematoma.

Small haematomas included in the nail plate are not degraded to haemosiderin. The Prussian blue test will be negative in these cases, while the benzidine test (Haemostix) with scrapings boiled in a small test tube will give a positive result. Moderate trauma to the nail area, or blood dyscrasias, affecting extensive numbers of dermal ridges will determine whether the haemorrhages are punctate, or result in large ecchymoses.

3 Subungual haematoma: acute subungual haematomas are usually obvious, occurring shortly after painful trauma involving finger of toenails. The blood which accumulates beneath the nail plate increases pain which may be severe. Depending on the site and intensity of the injury, the haematoma will be visible immediately or grow out from under the proximal nail fold within a few weeks.

The size of the haematoma will determine the technique used for drainage. The objectives of treatment are to prevent both unnecessary delay in the regrowth of the nail plate, and secondary dystrophy which might result from pressure on the matrix due to accumulated blood under the nail.

It is essential to surgically scrub the finger to prevent contamination of the subungual area and the subsequent risk of infection (Zook, 1988).

In partial haematoma of the proximal nail area, drainage of the haematoma with a fine-point scalpel blade or by drilling a hole large enough through the plate will give prompt relief from pain (Figs 10.45(a)–(c)). Hot paper clip cautery is however a useful alternative to trephining the plate. This allows blood to be evacuated; the nail

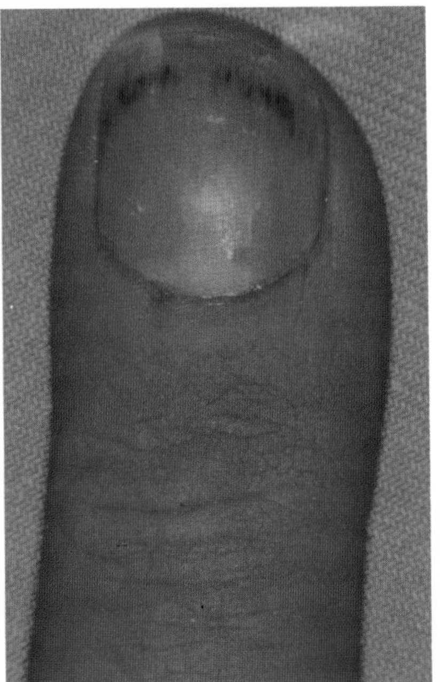

Fig. 10.43. Distal subungual splinter haemorrhages.

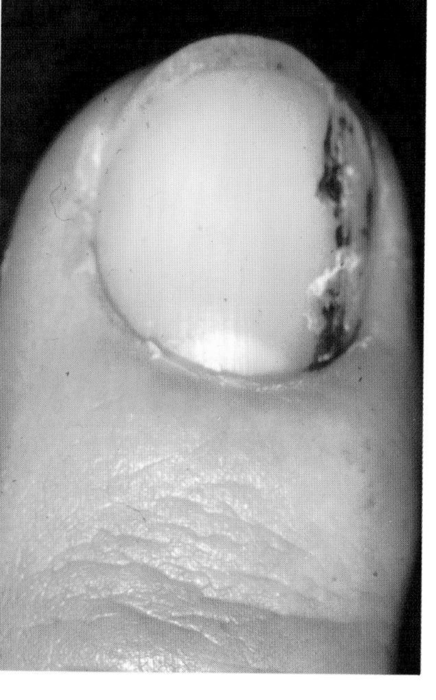

Fig. 10.44. Lateral longitudinal subungual haemorrhage.

is then pressed against the bed by a moderately tight bandage causing the nail plate to adhere. Soaked dressing is advised. This gives good results, unless the haematoma reforms when a clot seals the hole which had not been large enough. The nail will usually slough after some time as the new one regenerates beneath it. If this procedure is not immediately practicable, the pain can be relieved by elevating the hand as high as possible and maintaining this position for approximately 30 min (Rodboard, 1968).

Occasionally subungual haematoma persists under the nail and does not migrate. A reddish-blue colour, an irregular shape, and an absence of colour in the nail plate substance tend to differentiate non-migrating subungual haematoma from naevi or other causes of nail pigmentation (Douglas & Krull, 1981). It is advisable to remove the part overlying the subungual haematoma and identify and remove the old dried blood in order to establish the diagnosis and to eliminate other pathology such as melanoma.

A haematoma involving more than 25% of the visible nail (Figs 10.46(a)–(e)) is the warning sign of severe nail bed injury and possible underlying phalangeal fracture. An X-ray is therefore mandatory. Contusions cause interstitial and subungual haematoma that are painful because of tension developed in limited spaces. The pulp may remain tender for up to 2 months.

The nail is removed, washed and the fibrous soft tissue scraped from it, the haematoma evacuated, and the wound repaired, if necessary with precise suturing of the nail bed, using 6-0 PDS (Fig. 10.46(b)). The subungual tissues are fairly friable and relatively large 'bites' of nail bed tissue should be taken so that the suture material does not pull through when it is tied. Trimming the edges to create a straight edge would remove too much nail bed to allow closure without tension (Zook, 1990). The cleaned nail plate is narrowed and replaced by suturing to the lateral nail folds. A hole is drilled or burned in the replaced nail to allow for adequate drainage (Fig. 10.46(c)). The stitches are removed after 10 days, and usually the nail remains firmly attached (Recht, 1976) (Fig. 10.46(d)).

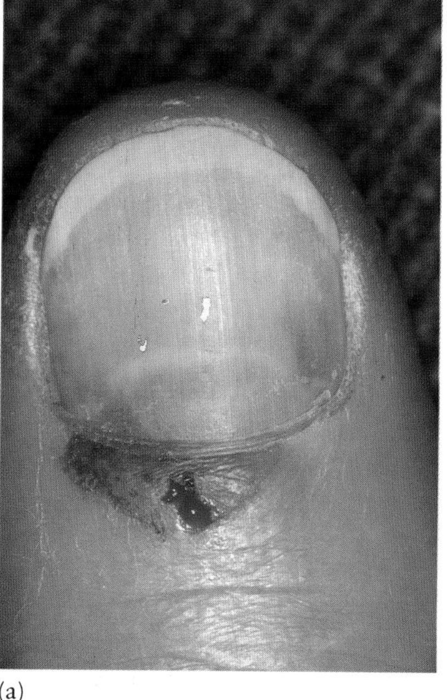

(a)

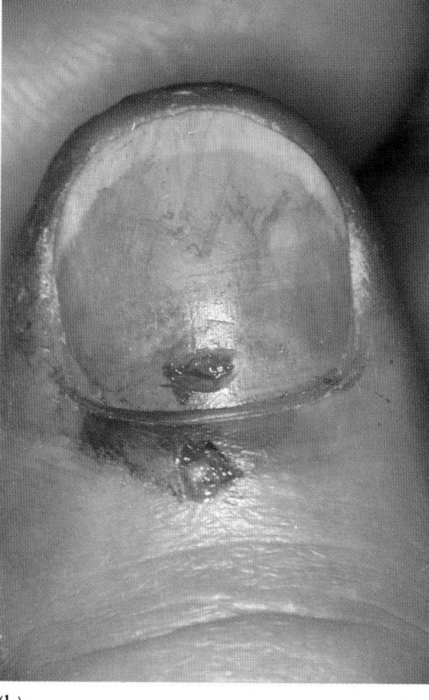

(b)

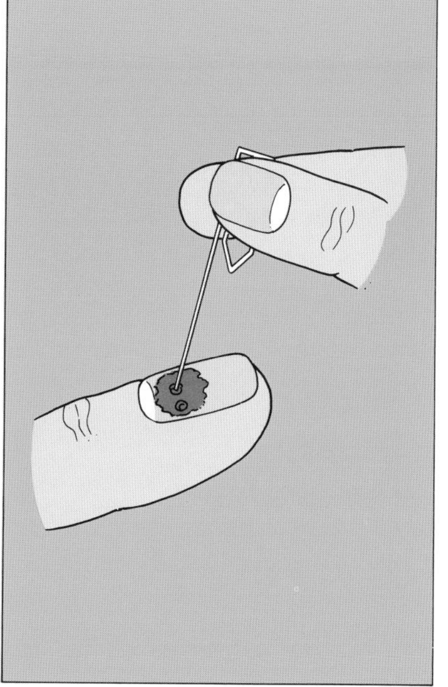

(c)

Fig. 10.45. Proximal subungual haemorrhage (a) with pressure and pain relieved by producing a hole in the nail plate (b & c).

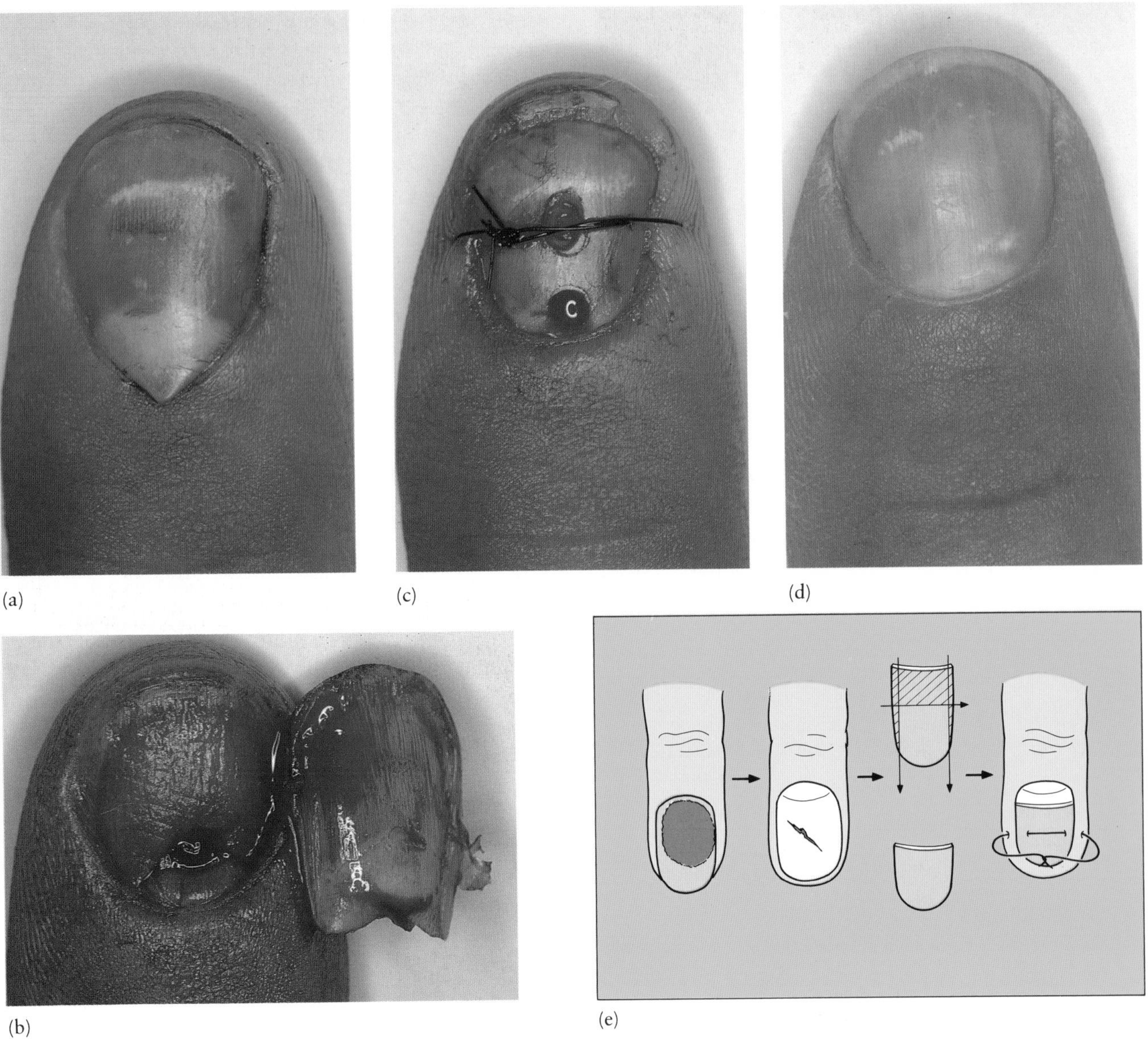

Fig. 10.46. Clinical and diagrammatic changes – severe subungual changes; treatment methods shown. The nail is removed, the wound repaired. The nail plate is then narrowed and replaced by suturing to the lateral nail folds; (d) good healing 6 months after treatment.

Lacerating wounds

These may be simple, complex or avulsive.

Simple incised wounds and lacerations

Avulsion of the nail plate from beneath the proximal nail fold with retained adherence to the nail bed distally is a pathognomonic sign of nail bed laceration. After a round hole has been drilled through avulsed nail at a point not over the repair site to allow drainage from the subungual area, the nail is inserted into the proximal nail groove. Zook (1988) holds it in place with a 5-0 monofilament nylon suture placed through the fingertip and the distal free border of the nail.

1 If the cut is superficial, a simple dressing with adhesive plaster is sufficient (Fig. 10.47(a)).

2 If the cut is deep, in all probability involving the nail bed, the distal portion of the incised nail plate is removed, and the remaining proximal portion of the nail plate is shortened (Fig. 10.47(b)). The edges of the lacerations are undermined 1 mm on each side of the laceration. This will allow slight eversion of the edges for more accurate nail bed approximation (Zook, 1990) using 6-0 PDS sutures. The distal portion of the nail plate (carefully trimmed) is replaced in order to cover the traumatic incision and sutured in position to the lateral nail folds. An alternative to this technique is complete removal of the nail: a round hold is drilled or burned through the nail at a point not over the repair site to allow drainage from the subungual

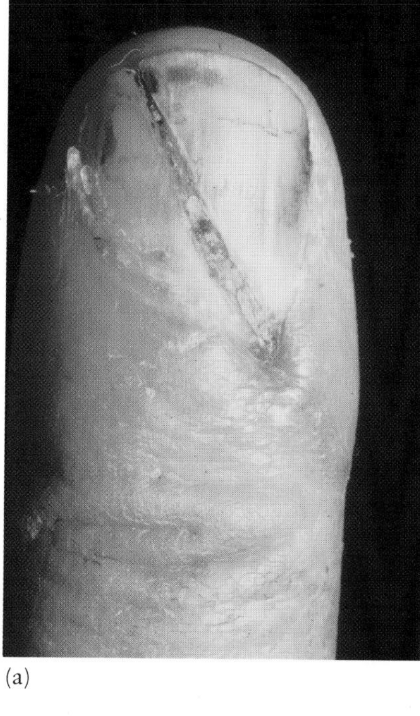

(a)

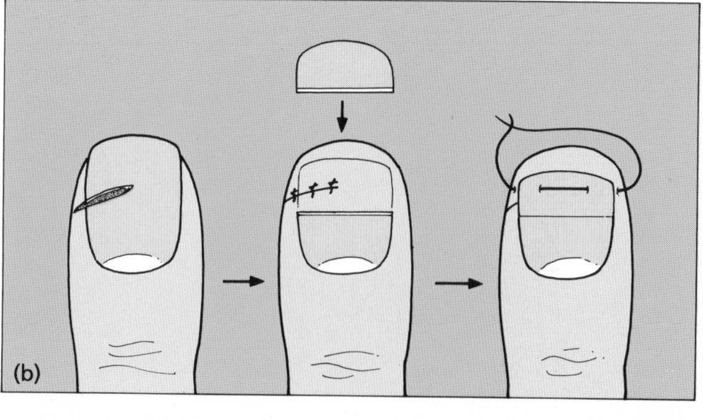

Fig. 10.47. (a) Superficial laceration – good spontaneous healing should occur. (b) Diagram to show technique of repair if laceration is deep (courtesy of P. Maksène, Toulon, France).

area after the nail has been reinserted into the proximal nail groove. The nail is held in place, according to Zook's method described above.

3 If the subungual tissue has been torn in the cul-de-sac and stripped from the proximal nail groove, a horizontal mattress suture through the proximal nail fold is used to replace the nail bed. The nail is then returned to the nail groove to mould the wound edges (Zook, 1988).

4 If the nail has been torn away, it should be trimmed, then replaced, and fixed in the same manner as for 2 (above).

5 If the nail plate is irrevocably damaged or lost, the nail bed should be covered with a nail homograft from a 'nail bank transplant', e.g. nails removed from amputated fingers, stored in mercury antiseptic. Prosthetic nails, silastic sheets, or disposable syringe (Fig. 10.48) cut to the nail shape, are used as temporary nail replacements. The sutures used to hold it in the nail grooves are removed in 2 weeks and the replacement device soon separates from the healed nail groove.

Complex lacerations

These may involve the nail bed, the proximal nail fold and the matrix.

Suturing the different planes will avoid secondary nail dystrophy. The proximal groove should be carefully reconstructed. This requires two incisions in the proximal nail fold made at 90° angles in its lateral curved portions. This will allow retraction, exposing the point of detachment of the nail matrix. The proximal nail fold may be retracted with small skin hooks or sutured to the proximal skin for exposure (Shepard, 1990). The undersurface of the proximal nail fold should be isolated by a non-adherent gauze packing to prevent secondary pterygium.

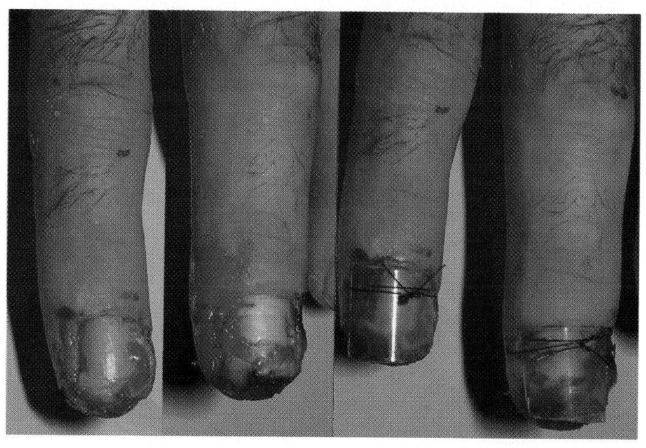

Fig. 10.48. Traumatic nail dystrophy protected by a strip taken from a disposable syringe (courtesy of P. Maksène, Toulon, France).

Avulsive lacerations

Avulsion of the nail bed. All retrievable fragments of nail bed should be replaced as free grafts (Fig. 10.49(a)&(b)). Nail bed avulsion frequently leaves the fragment of nail bed attached to the undersurface of the avulsed nail. It is therefore advisable to replace the nail as accurately as possible onto the avulsion site and to tape it with sterile strips to hold it in place (Zook, 1990).

Since the nail is formed by the nail matrix and moves distally, and the nail bed epithelium desquamates into the anterior limiting furrow, laceration of the nail bed alone, and nail bed defects up to the size of 4 mm in diameter can be left untreated when the avulsed portion of the nail bed is lost (Ogo, 1987). The available alternatives are:

1 healing of a wound larger than 4 mm in diameter by secondary intention. This will be unsightly;

2 split dermal graft would result in adherence in all but the distal portion of the nail plate (Kleinert *et al.*, 1967);

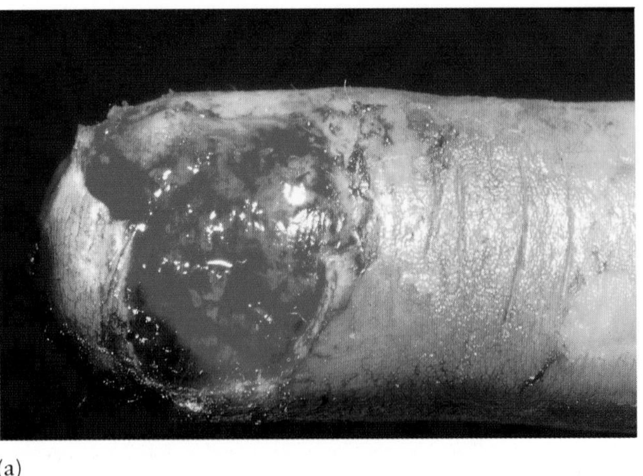

(a)

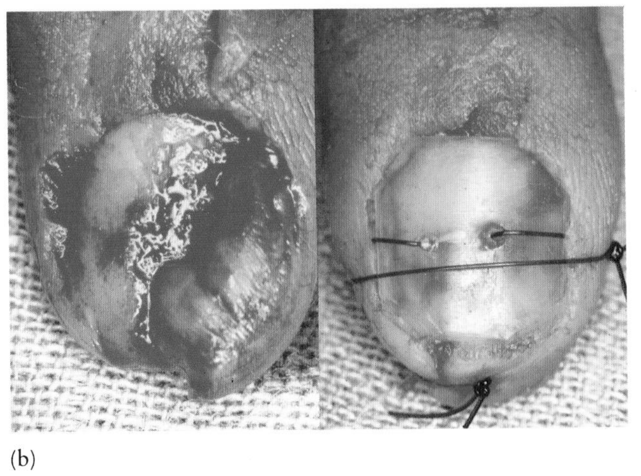

(b)

Fig. 10.49. Traumatic nail avulsion – recovered nail plate sutured back in place (b) (courtesy of P. Maksène, Toulon, France).

3 full thickness toenail bed grafting results in a defect of the donor area;
4 split thickness nail grafts (Fig. 10.50(a) & (b)) (Shepard, 1983, 1990) taken from the lateral third of the great toenail, or from the third toenail, and, when feasible from the adjacent nail bed of the injured finger demonstrate excellent results. Under block anaesthesia a split-thickness nail bed graft of the toenail is removed with a surgical blade used with a back-and-forth sawing technique to tangentially remove a small fragment of nail bed. The blade edge should be visible at all times through the graft being removed, as it is better for the graft to be too thin than too thick. The graft should be 1–2 mm larger than the defect and carefully sutured to existing nail bed segments using 7-0 chromic sutures. Interestingly, the nail bed is one of the few areas in which normal cortical bone, as well as decorticated bone (Matsuba & Spear, 1988), will accept a soft tissue graft.
5 Sometimes patients who present with deformed, functionally intrusive fingernails may be pleased with the results following ablation of the remaining perionychium and application of a full-thickness graft from the non-hair-bearing skin of the groin. The graft is shaped to resemble the nail; it acquires slight pigmentation, and is infinitely better than the nail that had been removed (Rosenthal, 1983).

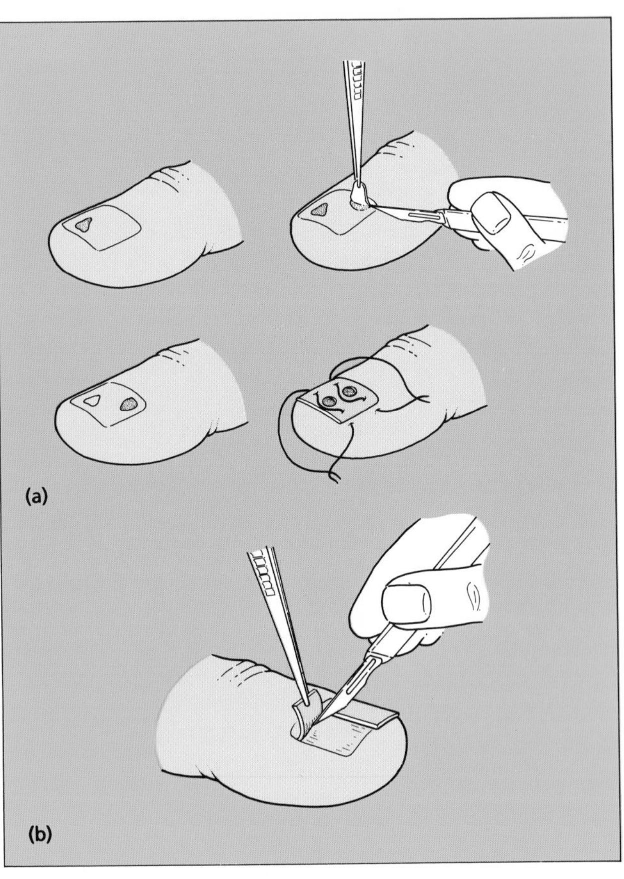

Fig. 10.50. Split thickness skin grafts taken from same digit (a) and toenail bed (b) (after Shepherd, 1983; 1990).

Avulsion of the proximal nail fold. According to Zook (1990) there is no totally satisfactory and uniformly predictable method for recreating a satisfactory nail fold. Imaginative procedures for recreating the fold however have been devised.
1 Recreation of the semilunar proximal nail fold with a single staged transposition flap (Hayes, 1974) modified with a thin split-skin graft to the undersurface of the flap may be successful (Rosenthal, 1983).
2 A nail plasty utilizing a free composite graft from helical rim of the ear has been proposed (Rose, 1980).
3 A subcutaneous pedicle flap can be used to reconstruct the avulsed proximal nail fold and to cover the nail bed and the skin defects on the dorsum of the fingers with tendon, bone and joint exposure (Atasoy, 1982).

4 Restoration of the proximal nail fold lost due to lacerations and thermal or chemical burns may also be performed by using two long, narrow V-shaped flaps from the lateral aspects of the terminal phalanx. They have to be cut in retrograde direction and have therefore to be delayed before being raised and transposed. The small secondary defects rapidly heel by secondary intention virtually without visible scarring (Barfod, 1972; Haneke, 1991).

5 The authors favour, when feasible, excising the jagged tissue in order to recreate the distal curve of the dorsal nail fold. This operation, inspired by the surgical treatment of recalcitrant chronic paronychia (Baran & Bureau, 1981), produces a near perfect restoration of the proximal nail fold (Baran, 1986) (Fig. 10.51(a)&(b)).

Severe avulsive lacerations. These may involve the nail bed, the bone and the finger pulp. Good results may be obtained if the wound is allowed to heal by secondary intention. If healing is not achieved within 6 weeks, a thin split-skin graft can be applied to the wound. The cross-finger technique, using a pedicle flap from the palm can be effective because so much versatility can be incorporated into the design of the repair (Hart & Kleinert, 1993). Frequently however, it gives rise to stiffness, especially when the patient is an elderly manual worker. It may be preferable to graft skin taken from under the shoulder blade, the forearm, or the external surface of the opposite arm.

If the matrix has been severely damaged and the nail avulsed, a free nail graft may be necessary. It is advisable that the patient should be made aware of the high failure rate. McCash (1956) has proposed three alternatives.

1 In the *partial nail graft*, the central portion of the great toenail, including nail plate, nail bed and matrix is used.

2 The *complete nail graft* is taken from one of the lesser toes and consists of nail plate, nail bed and matrix without bone or surrounding skin.

3 In the *composite nail graft* (Fig. 10.52) taken from one of the lesser toes, the graft consists of the complete nail, nail bed and matrix with their vascularization the nail folds and a thin shaving of the upper surface of the terminal phalanx. This alternative is probably the most promising, due to the achievements of microvascular surgery (Morrison, 1990; Foucher *et al.*, 1991).

Crush fractures

Fractures of the distal phalanx

Approximately 50% of nail bed injuries have an accompanying fracture (Zook, 1988). If the fracture involves the phalangal tuft, treatment is easy, even if there are several spurs of bone. Fractures of the shaft are a more serious matter.

Tuft fracture

In most cases, this is due to a blow from a hammer, or slamming a car door on the finger; distal subungual haematoma is common and the pulp is generally well preserved. Numerous small spurs coming away from the tuft almost inevitably produce pseudarthrosis, and painful instability. The spurs should be removed and the cutaneous wound carefully sutured.

Shaft fracture

Three main types occur.

1 Damage to the pulp is limited and the transverse fracture of the bone is clearly discernible. The nail should be removed and replaced, once the bone ends have been carefully reapproximated, with an elastic dressing surrounding the pulp and the nail. The fractured diaphysis can be 'skewered' onto an axial spigot anchored to the

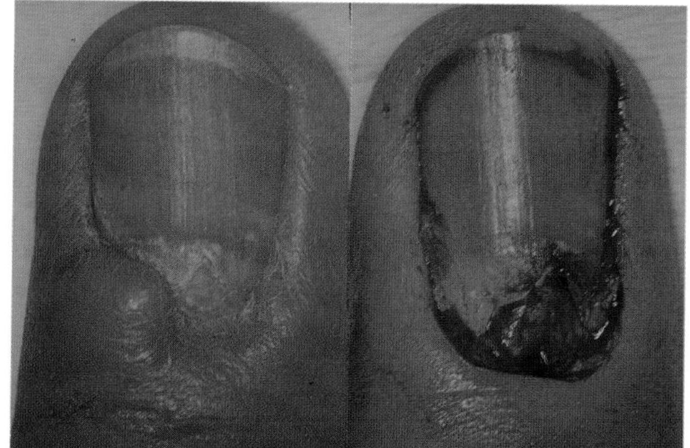
(a)

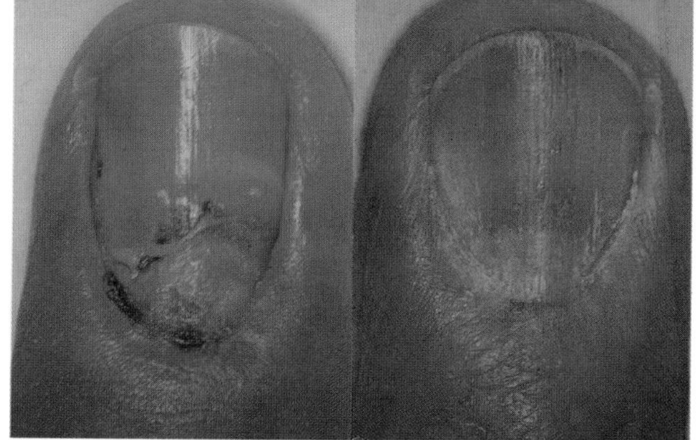
(b)

Fig. 10.51. Procedure to excise jagged proximal nail fold tissue to give a better cosmetic result.

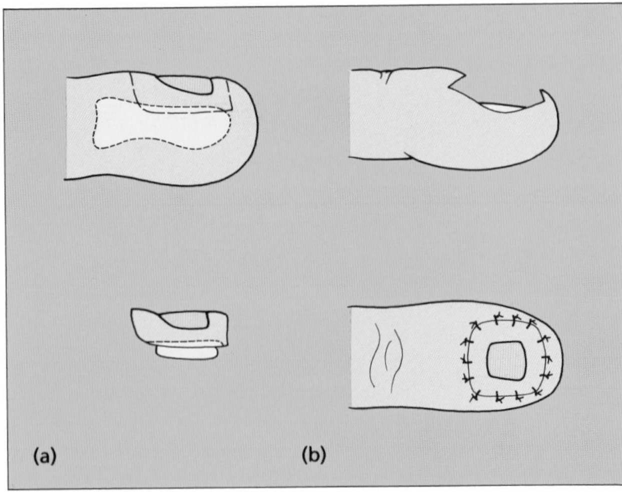

Fig. 10.52. Composite nail graft (McCash, 1956).

middle phalanx and left for 3–4 weeks buried under the skin. This largely eliminates the risk of infection.

2 Damage to the pulp is extensive and the bone is broken into two or more fragments. There are two alternatives: (i) the removal of spurs will shorten the phalanx: this will, however, enable the fracture to reunite; (ii) to opt for plastic surgery, in order to preserve the maximum finger length: in most cases, this allows the affected soft tip to be treated by directed healing. Grafts, even of the great toe pulp, and flaps, often leave scars which may be painful, or anaesthetic; either defect may hamper movement.

3 Open fractures of the joint area will necessitate proper reduction.

Denudation of the terminal phalanx (Fig. 10.53)

The upper surface and tip of the distal phalanx are torn away above the exposed pulp. The operation consists of two successive stages.

1 Any necrotic tissue is excised and the pulp and nail bed replaced using simple skin sutures.

2 The trimmed nail is then carefully reapproximated.

But if the sectioned, transungual extremity has not been preserved, the bias section of the digital extremity should be repaired with advancement flaps. The plane of the injury dictates which flap has application (Rosenthal, 1983). The palmar branches of the proper digital arteries and their anastomoses are the basis of the volar palmar Atasoy V-Y flap (Atasoy *et al.*, 1970). Base of flap is dissected and separated from phalangeal bone. The flap is then advanced and sutured in position. The lateral advancement triangular island flap (Fig. 10.54(a) & (b)) is a routine technique starting at the base of the finger based on only one of the two proper digital arteries while the lateral Kutler V-Y advancement (Fig. 10.55) based on the two neurovascular pedicles is limited to the size of tissue

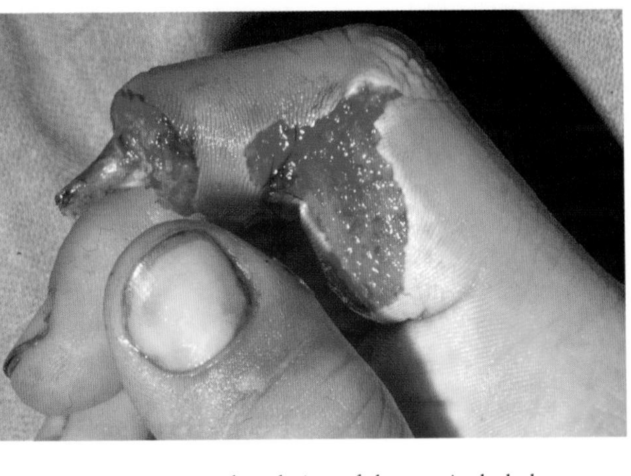

Fig. 10.53. Traumatic denudation of the terminal phalanx (courtesy of P. Maksène, Toulon, France).

that the flaps may contain. These will 'upholster' the extremity and preserve the entire usable length, more or less avoiding the production of a crooked finger. In case of circular denudation of the terminal bony phalanx, utilization of tubular pedicle grafts has been suggested to preserve the entire, usable length of the finger. Multiple surgical steps are required in order to remodel the digit and to re-establish an adequate nerve supply to the area. It is better to attempt some sort of cosmetic, 'tidying-up' operation.

Some suitable cases have been able to benefit from microsurgical techniques, if the artery is large enough. The 'return' supply can usually be established by using a vein on the dorsum of the finger. If this is not available, then the judicious application of leeches will ensure venous decongestion for the first few days.

These cases are not exceptional and, provided the foregoing factors are borne in mind, all or part of the terminal phalanx can be preserved, be it for functional, psychological or cosmetic reasons.

Foreign bodies

Due to its distal position and its role in gripping, the nail and the subungual tissue are very much at risk of penetration by foreign bodies. These can be vegetable (thorns, splinter), animal (urchin, oyster shell), metal, plastic or glass.

Patient seen early

Usually the foreign body cannot be seen. Pain, though severe when the accident occurred, is at this time moderate, but touching the nail increases the pain. The foreign body must be removed immediatly under local anaesthesia with total or partial avulsion of the nail plate. A wet antiseptic dressing must be applied for 2 or 3 days.

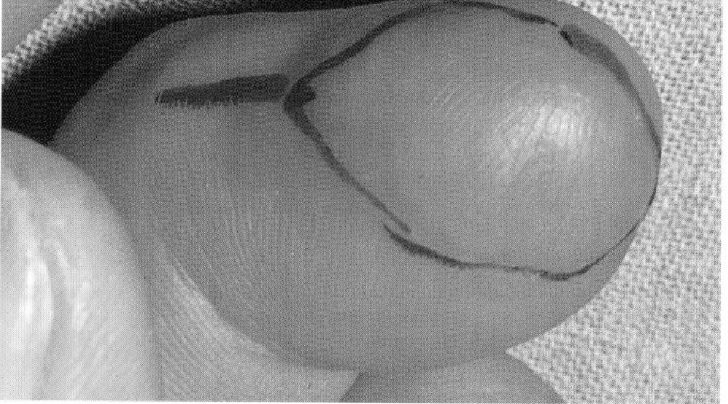
(a)

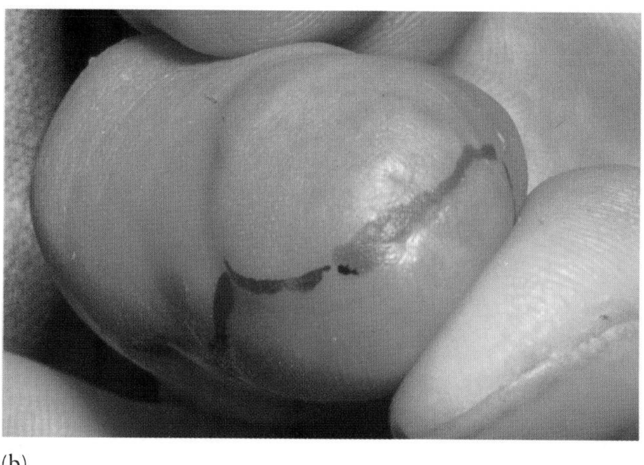
(b)

Fig. 10.54. Lateral advancement triangular island flap (LATI) (courtesy of P. Maksène, Toulon, France).

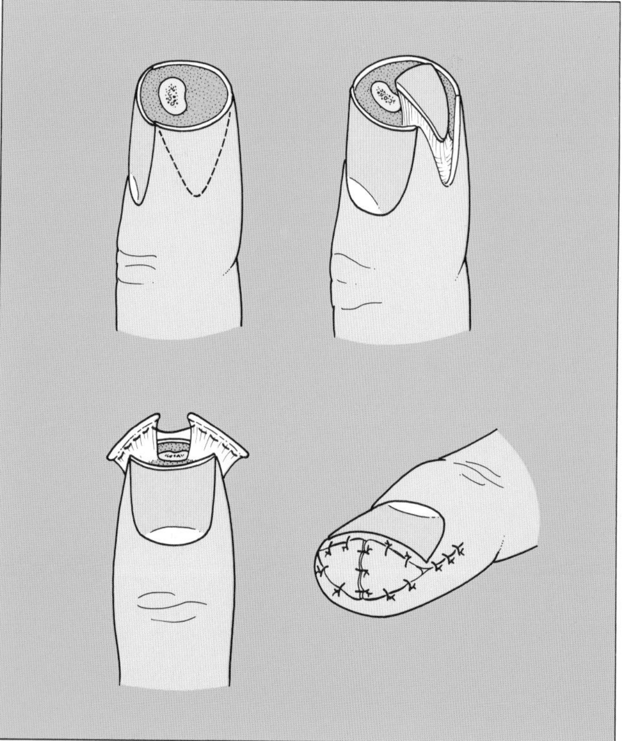

Fig. 10.55. Kutler V-Y advancement flap based on the neurovascular pedicles.

Patient seen later on

Subungual panaritium is the usual reason for the consultation. Diagnosis is easy because of the yellow colour of the nail bed and the pulsating pain, especially during the night. Removal of the nail plate and wide drainage of the cavity should be performed if windowing of the nail is not sufficient (Andrus, 1980). Antibiotics must be avoided and antiseptic dressing applied on the wound. Pain relief is immediately obtained followed by complete recovery within a few days.

Two clinical types deserve special mention.

1 Thorns, of variable origin, may induce non-specific inflammatory responses (Fig. 10.56(a)–(c)), a suppurative dermatitis with eventual expulsion of the foreign material, or a granuloma with central caseation. In a case of a cactus thorn in the nail bed, a mild inflammatory cell infiltrate with some histiocytes, a few giant cells and neutrophils was observed. The foreign body could be identified as a cactus thorn due to its unique structure: on cross section, it is circular, made up of hexagonal cells with a round central canal and lined by a single layer of flat cells; under polarized light, it is strongly birefringent (Hornstein & Haneke, 1980).

Often the initial injury involving the nail matrix has not been noticed and the patient is examined later on, during the second or third month. There is a sensible, but not really painful, oedema of the whole finger, and its mobility is reduced. This is called 'inoculation synovitis'. Surgical treatment is compulsory, consisting of the removal of the foreigh body as well as the oedematous synovial tissue. The colour of the latter is greyish and some clear but turbid fluid comes out of it. There is no bacterial infection. Recovery is obtained with a few days.

A thorn in a subungual position may mimic longitudinal melanonychia (Goldfarb, unpubl.) (Fig. 10.57(a) & (b)).

2 Sea urchin granuloma: this condition resembles a panaritium. A 35-year-old man with sea urchin granulomas on his left foot, including the proximal nail fold and matrix of the fourth toe, was seen. The toe was swollen, reddish blue and tender. The granuloma of the proximal nail fold and matrix had caused a broad split in the nail (Fig. 10.58). Histopathology showed thickening of the proximal fold with loss of the cuticle. There was granulomatous inflammation with lymphocytes, histiocytes and large foreign body-type giant cells, some of which had a large vacuole. Remnants of the sea urchin

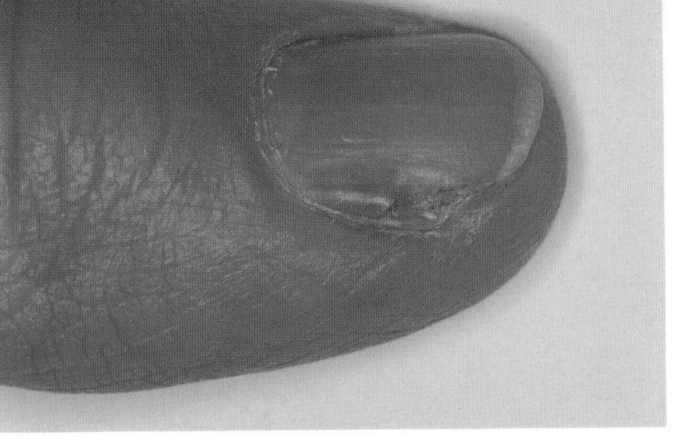

(a)

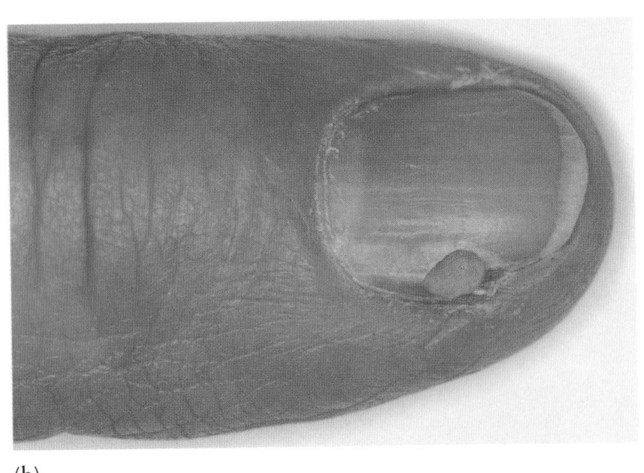

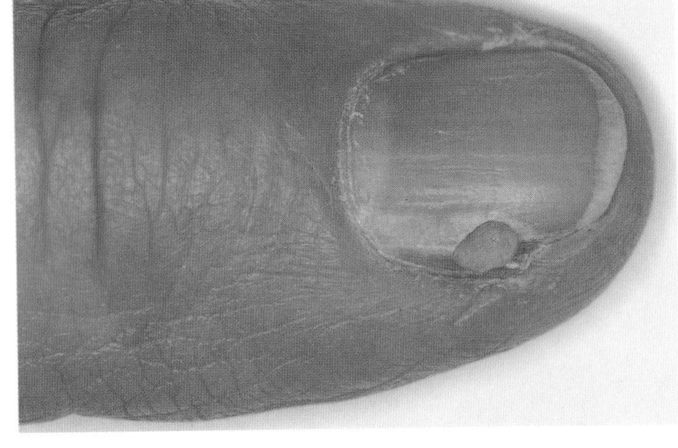

(b)

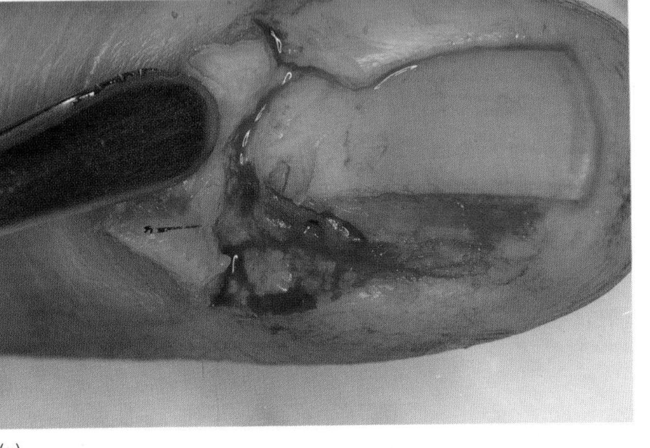

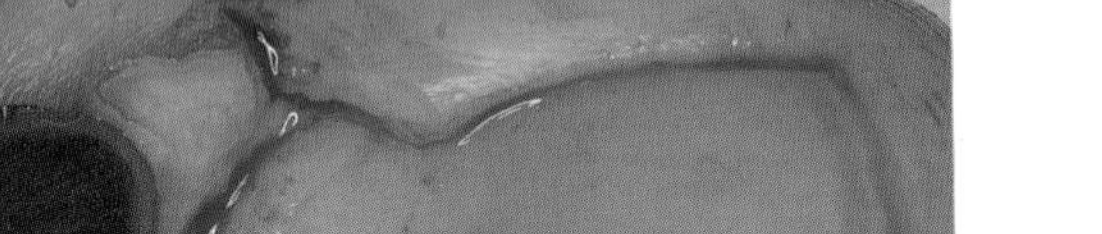

(c)

Fig. 10.56. (a–c) Subungual thorn and its removal.

spicules could not be seen (Haneke & Tosti, 1994). Intralesional long-acting steroids are necessary; complete recovery occurs within 2–3 weeks.

Fingertip amputations

Distal amputation limited to the soft tissues should be left to heal by secondary intention (Fig. 10.59(a) & (b)). Complete section at the level of the matrix jeopardizes the future of the nail apparatus. However in a few cases, notably children (especially where there are transungual lesions), the damaged matrix can be repositioned, become revascularized and act as a real graft. This is well worth attempting in view of the good results in successful cases. The younger the individual the greater the 'take' (Zook, 1990).

Wounds caused by amputation of the bone, or by partial amputation involving the bone and soft tissues, in

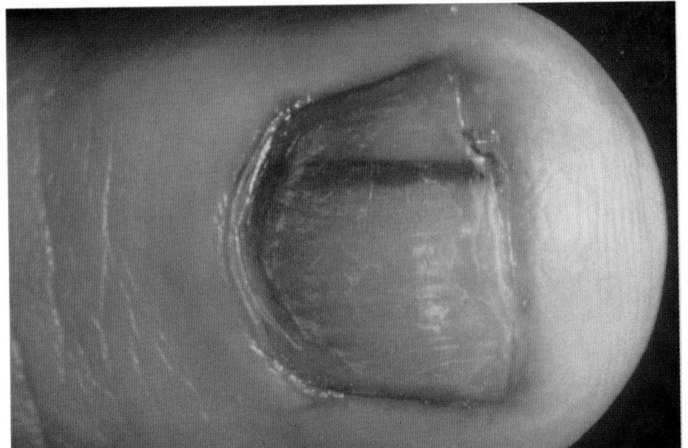

(a)

(b)

Fig. 10.57. Subungual thorn mimicking longitudinal melanonychia (courtesy of N. Goldfarb, USA).

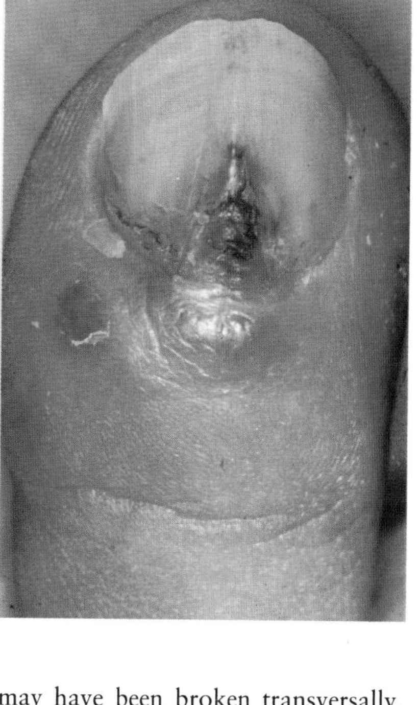

Fig. 10.58. Sea urchin granuloma.

which the phalanx may have been broken transversally, should be allowed to heal by secondary intention or be repaired by advancement flaps (Fig. 10.61(a)–(c)). There are many techniques available. If there is a bias section of the digital extremity it may be repaired with two Kutler flaps. Microsurgery is a gratifying method (Fig. 10.60(a) & (b)).

For amputations at the base of the nail, the matrix should be resected and the diaphysis shortened to facilitate closure without tension.

Delayed post-traumatic deformities

These may be:

1 absence of nail plate – nail bed adhesion (onycholysis);
2 split nail deformity;
3 pterygium;
4 various nail dystrophies;
5 hooked nail;
6 malaligned nail.

Post-traumatic onycholysis (absence of nail plate–nail bed adhesion) (Figs 10.62 & 10.63)

A functionally stable nail requires at least 5 mm of healthy nail bed distal to the lunula for nail adherence but also an even nail bed. If the nail grows normally, but fails to adhere to all or part of the nail bed, treatment consists of removing the nail, scraping the epidermis of the nail bed, and covering it immediately with a 'nail bank transplant' or the original nail, if the latter is adequate. In fact, a more satisfactory result can be obtained with resection of the scar which may cause the nail to loosen, and its replacement by a split-thickness nail bed graft from either an adjacent area of the nail bed or from a toenail bed (Shepard, 1990).

Split nail deformity (Figs 10.64 & 10.65)

1 If the split is very asymmetrical, the best method is to use the technique recommended for lateral longitudinal nail biopsy.

2 If the split is located in the mid-portion of the nail, angular incisions at 90° are made at the radial and ulnar corners of the proximal nail fold and continued proximally to the distal (dorsal) transverse skin crease over the terminal interphalangeal joint. The nail fold is elevated to expose the matrix. Prior to nail avulsion a mark must be made on the proximal nail fold in line with the split deformity and the nail is removed. The deforming scar is excised from its most proximal portion in the matrix to its distal end and the incision is extended to include full thickness tissue down to bone (Johnson, 1971). The entire elliptical defect is undermined to allow for adequate closure. Sometimes relaxing incisions are made at the most

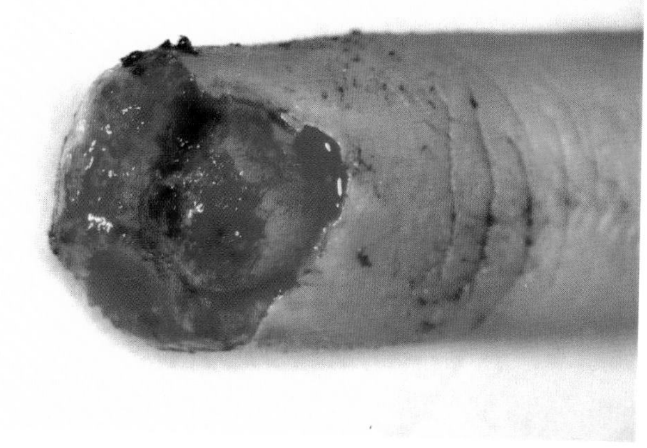

(a)

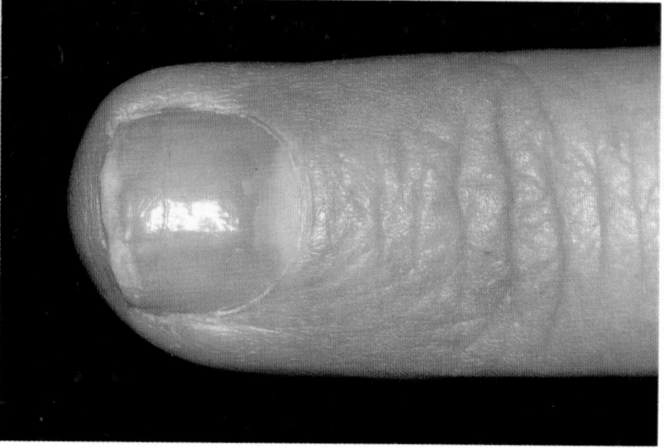

(b)

Fig. 10.59. (a & b) Quite severe distal traumatic soft tissue injuries will heal spontaneously with good results.

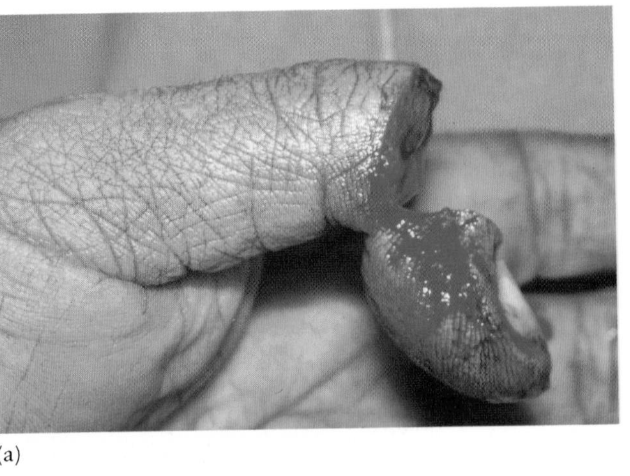
(a)

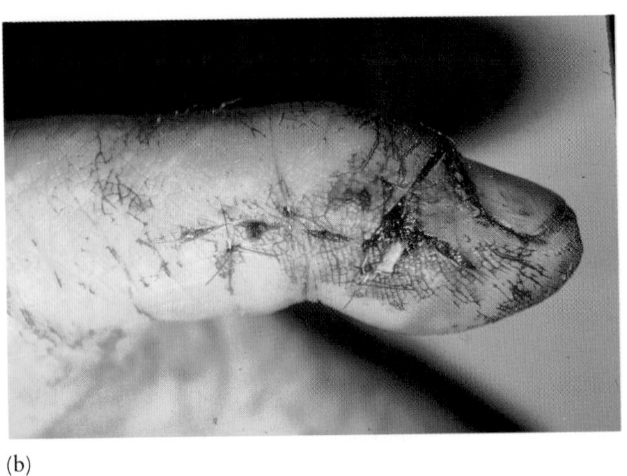
(b)

Fig. 10.60. Severe distal traumatic digital injury (a) and its satisfactory repair after microsurgery (b) (courtesy of P. Maksène, Toulon, France).

(a)

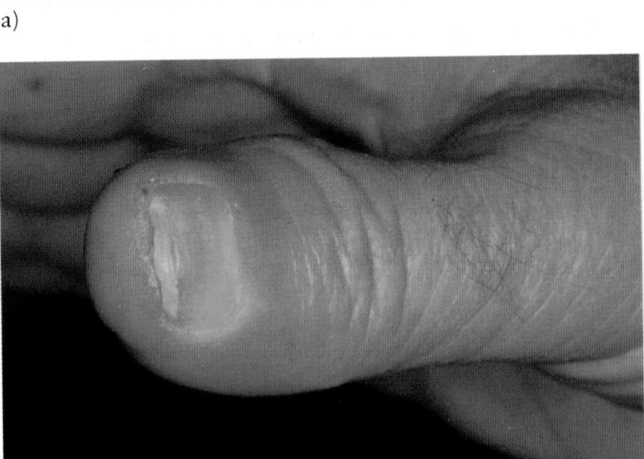
(c)

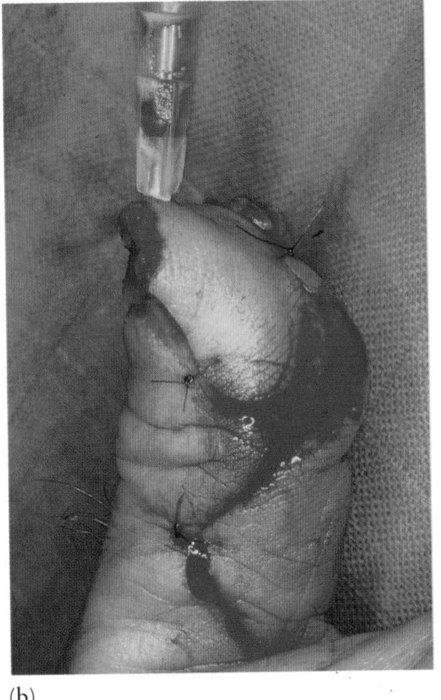
(b)

Fig. 10.61. (a–c) Severe distal traumatic injury repaired by an advancement flap (courtesy of R. Zalta and H. Bureau, Marseilles, France).

medial and lateral margins of the nail bed, which permits easier mobilization, and allows the central margins to be approximated with interrupted sutures of 6-0 monofilament resorbable sutures.

Another modification is to remove only a strip of nail plate corresponding to the split. After excision of the scar, the matrix and nail bed are sutured using fine atraumatic suture material. To prevent cutting of these stitches, 3-0 sutures are placed through the nail plate. When these threads are knotted firmly, matrix and nail bed are further approximated, relaxing the 6-0 sutures, but this may induce a step formation in matrix and nail bed (Haneke & Baran, 1991). The proximal nail fold is replaced in its normal position and the two angular incisions then closed

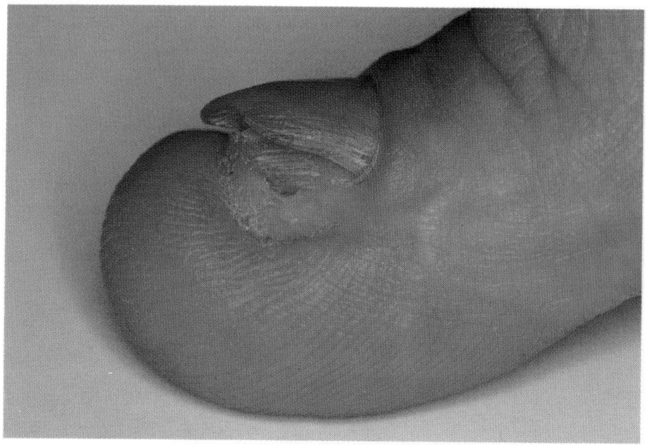

Fig. 10.62. Post-traumatic onycholysis.

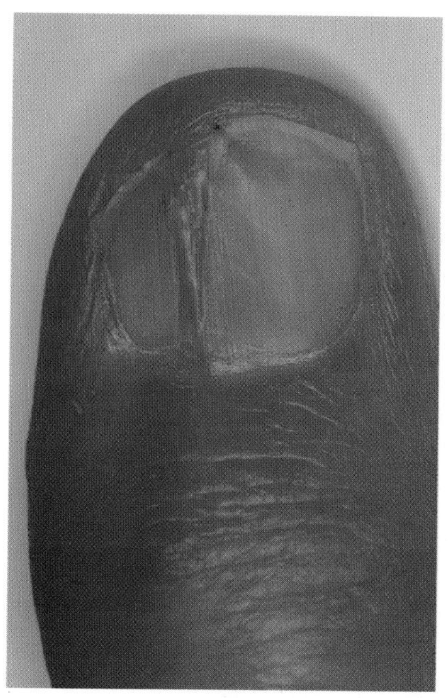

Fig. 10.64. Split nail deformity.

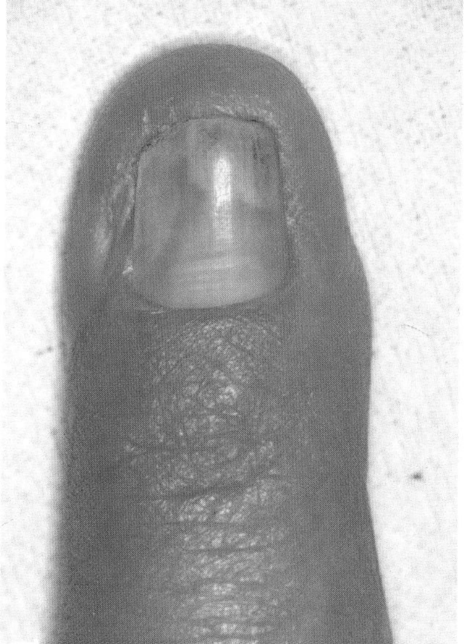

Fig. 10.63. Post-traumatic onycholysis.

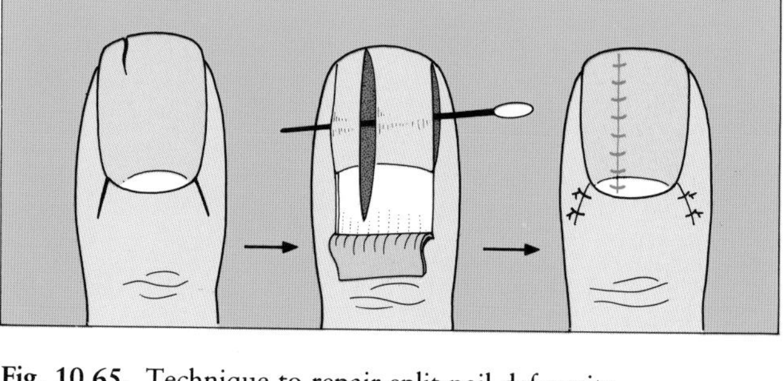

Fig. 10.65. Technique to repair split nail deformity.

with steri-strips. The nail plate, replaced under the proximal nail fold to separate it from the matrix, is sutured to the fingertip. The new nail which regenerates is slightly narrower than the contralateral normal nail. The results of this technique are not always good and improvement may be only marginal (Hoffman, 1973).

The split deformity, when mainly due to nail bed scarring, has successfully been repaired using a split-thickness nail bed graft (Shepard, 1990).

An alternative approach is the formation of a nail bed–matrix flap with an L-shaped incision of the lateral aspect of the nail wall.

In 'non traumatic' split deformity, surgery may also be required (Fig. 10.66(a)–(c)). In distal fissuring of the nail, removal of the distal two-thirds of the nail plate is essential. This may be therapeutic in itself or permit visualization and evaluation of a subungual lesion. It is then possible to undertake the appropriate surgical measures, such as a 3–4-mm punch biopsy in the nail bed, longitudinal elliptical excision or curettage.

Seckel's technique (1986) may be useful. The nail over and around the split nail deformity is elevated with a Freer elevator from the underlying nail bed and excised to create a window through which the defect can be repaired. A 0.02 mm silicone rubber sheet splint is cut to fit under the portion of nail that has been elevated including the nail proximal to the site of repair. The distal end of the splint is sutured to the distal end of the nail on each side of the defect. As the nail grows, the splint advances over the site of repair providing smooth transition for the proximal advancing nail. As the silicone rubber splint is advanced, the nail adheres normally to the site of repair and surrounding nail bed. Sutures are removed after the repair site has been covered by new nail growth, usually at 6 weeks. When the sutures are removed, the splint falls off painlessly.

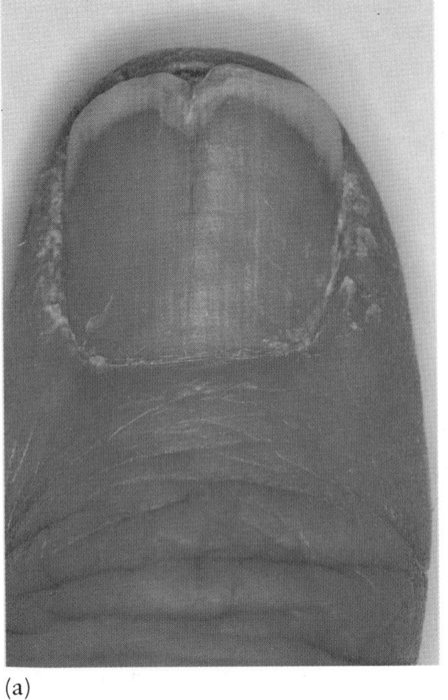

(a)

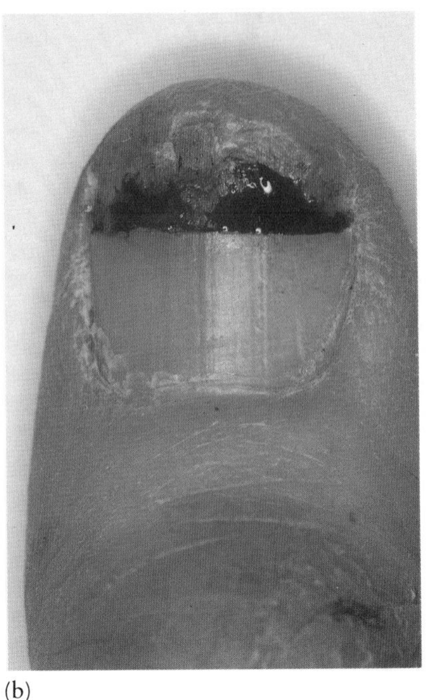

(b)

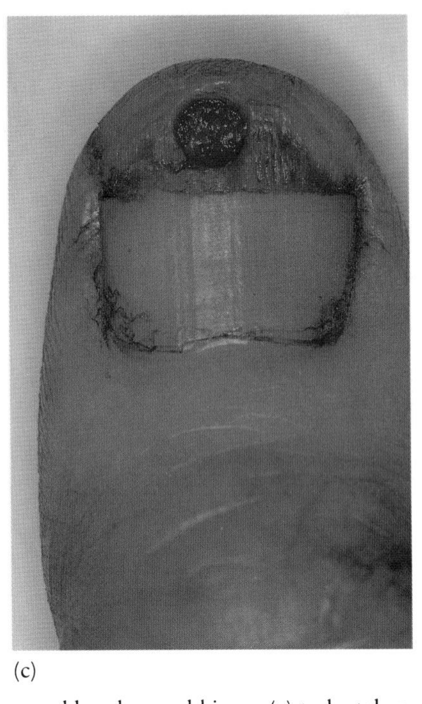

(c)

Fig. 10.66. Distal nail splitting – removal of part of the nail. This may itself be therapeutic or enable subungual biopsy (c) to be taken.

Pterygium (Fig. 10.67(a) & (b))

If the affected area is soaked daily in warm water until it is soft, separation of the pterygium from the nail with an orange wood stick may be successful. If it is not, the proximal nail fold may be elevated surgically from the dorsum of the nail plate and held separated with a strip of silastic or non-adherent gauze. The undersurface of the nail fold epithelializes, releasing the adherence. If it is unsuccessful, a more radical approach is to separate the roof of the 'cul-de-sac' from the nail, and to place a small segment of split-thickness skin graft on the undersurface of the proximal nail fold after freeing it from the nail plate (Zook, 1988).

In the case of total obliteration of the 'cul-de-sac', often encountered as a sequel to burns, Barfod (1972) suggests that the proximal nail fold should be restored by two lateral digital flaps.

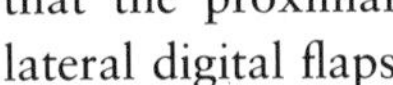

Ventral pterygium

Ventral pterygium is treated by removing the distal 5 mm of nail from the nail bed and hyponychial area. A strip of nail bed and hyponychium 3–4 mm wide is resected and replaced by a split-thickness skin graft. This causes non-adherence in the hyponychial area and usually provides relief from pain (Zook, 1988).

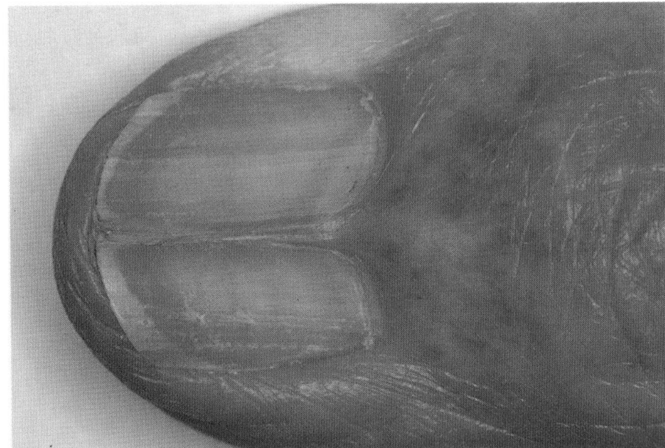

(a)

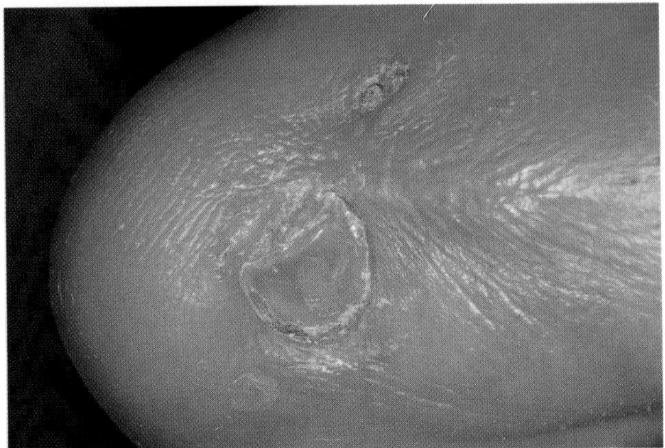

(b)

Fig. 10.67. Dorsal pterygium of the nail – (a) early, (b) late.

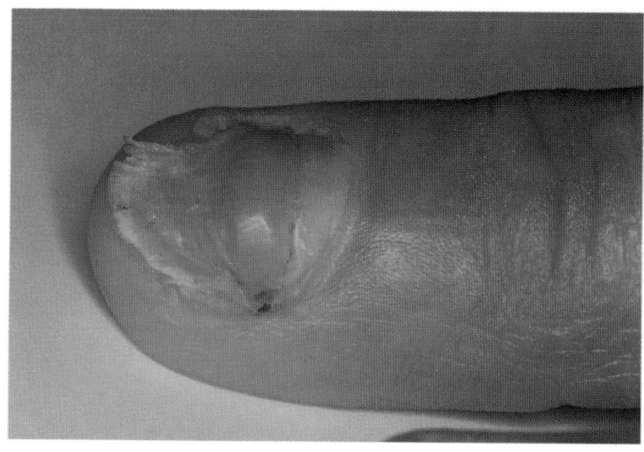

Fig. 10.68. Transient post-traumatic nail thickening.

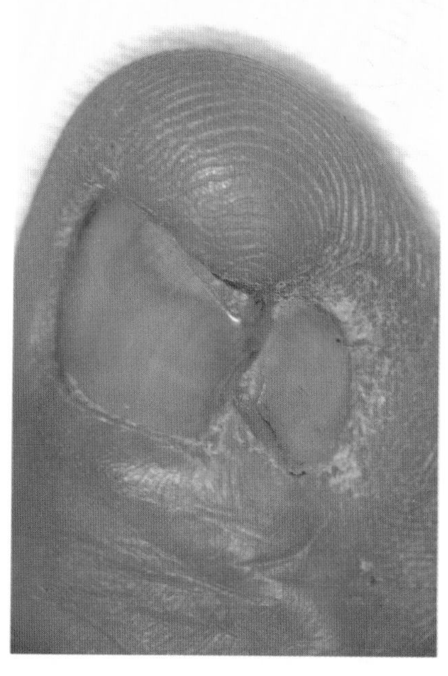

Fig. 10.69. Permanent post-traumatic deformity.

Traumatic nail dystrophies

Transient nail plate thickening is not uncommon (Fig. 10.68). Dystrophic nails may present with varying degrees of severity (Fig. 10.69). Deformities in the form of deep, longitudinal grooves and canals may be left untreated. In exceptional cases it may be necessary to remove the nail plate (Figs 10.70(a) & (b) & 10.71), excise the scar in the matrix and/or nail and approximate the edges of normal tissue with 6-0 PDS sutures. The nail plate should be replaced and sutured in position. However, this procedure may produce a split nail deformity. Some cases require the nail bed to be scraped, even rendered and then covered by a 'nail bank transplant'. This enables the newly formed nail to regenerate normally. Sometimes, deformities arising from defects in the nail bed can be treated by split-thickness nail bed grafts (Yong & Teoh, 1992).

In more advanced cases, only a few dysmorphic nail fragments persist, growing from dystrophic remnants of the matrix. Complete removal of the matrix and the nail bed is effective. The patient may also have continued problems with the keratinized material that grows from the nail bed. This should be excised and a split thickness graft applied; or the nail bed may be cauterized with liquefied phenol.

Dermal inclusion cysts of the bone result from epithelial elements of the nail bed being displaced into a fracture. Over time the cyst enlarges, causing deformity of the distal phalanx and nail (Zook, 1986).

If neuromas form in the nail bed following injury, they may cause tenderness, elevation of the nail bed and nail dystrophy. The treatment is careful resection (Zook, 1986).

There are several alternatives for dealing with total absence of the nail, with its consequent aesthetic or functional defects.

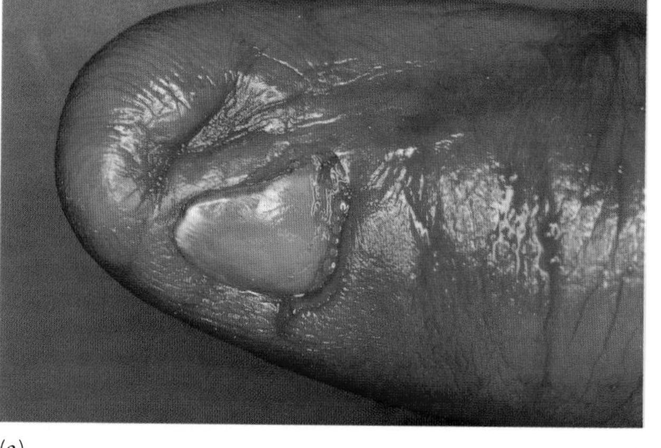

(a)

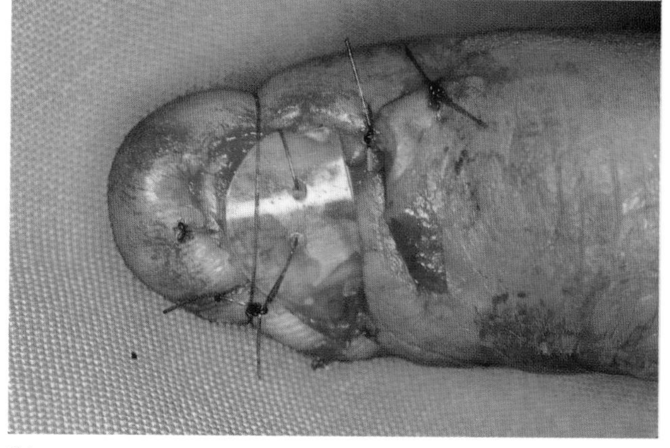

(b)

Fig. 10.70. (a & b) Removal of the nail plate and realignment of post-traumatic dystrophy (courtesy of P. Maksène, Toulon, France).

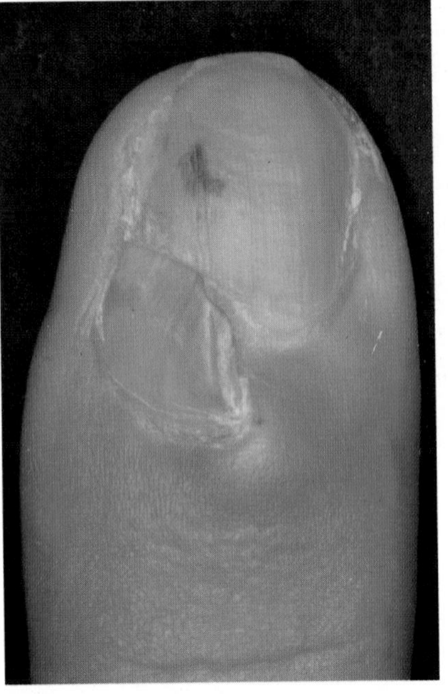

Fig. 10.71. Post-traumatic matrix deformity with 'overlying, second' nail.

In the absence of surgery, at least in women, the keratinized zone of the nail bed, or an epidermal graft which has ensured its healing, may be slightly improved by the application of nail polish. Alternatively, an artificial nail should be set in place. This latter is well 'set in' if a proximal nail fold and proximal groove are created by means of a thin graft. Unfortunately, the newly formed 'cul-de-sac' inevitably regresses. The artificial nail must be set with glue or surgical varnish. This frequently leads to complications. In Dufourmentel's hands (1974) this technique provided satisfactory results in 50% of those treated. This method requires a well-motivated patient who understands the pros and cons of the procedure. A fingertip prosthesis normally yields much better results.

Finally since the arrival of one-step microsurgical techniques, more ambitious results may be attempted by grafting the whole nail apparatus.

Hooked nail

Such nails may develop as one of the late effects of trauma to the nail apparatus (Figs 10.72(a) & (b); 10.73(a) & (b)). Crimped distal nail hood or parrot beak deformity reflects bowing of the nail bed from lack of support due to short bony phalanx or volar scar contracture (Rosenthal, 1983). The reforming nail obligingly follows the nail bed which had been used to achieve closure of an amputation. Treatment presents a most complex problem from the surgical point of view. When a hook nail is present, a decision must be made whether to add support to the nail bed.

There are several possible procedures.

1 Once the distal portion of the nail has been clipped, removal of the superfluous bed and its replacement by a split graft is usually definitive.

2 Retraction of the matrix and the nail bed (Dufourmentel, 1974) (Fig. 10.74): this is particularly suitable for hook-like nails and spatulate nails, when the length of the bone defect is less than 50%, because it uses two lateral flaps that correct the spatulate defect and cover the digital extremity.

3 Lengthening of the nail bed (Verdan, 1981). The procedure consists of lengthening the terminal phalanx with a shaped bone graft, covered on the palmar aspect with a cross-finger flap. Results are poor. One piece pedicled bone graft with palmar flap seems to be an improvement of Verdan's technique.

4 Reconstruction by removing the deformed nail plate, elevating the nail bed from the distal phalanx and supporting the straightened nail bed with longitudinal Kirschner wires has been reported as the 'antennae' procedure (Atasoy *et al.*, 1983).

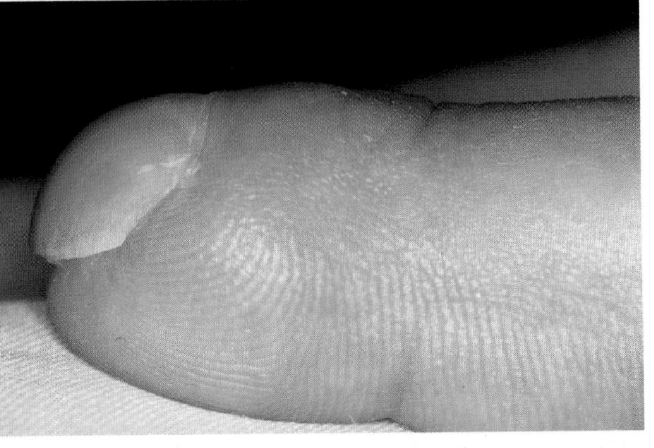

(a)

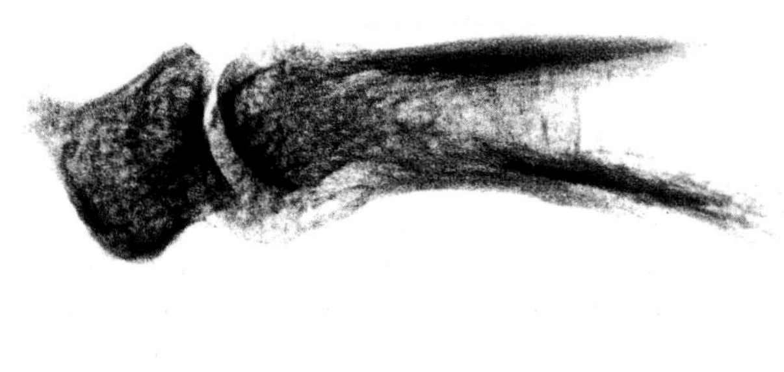

(b)

Fig. 10.72. (a & b) Clinical and radiological changes – shortening of the distal phalanx and hook nail deformity (traumatic).

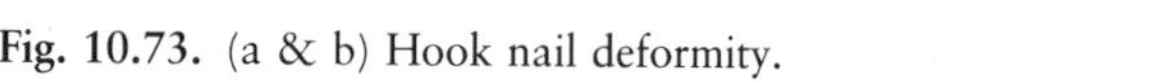

(a)

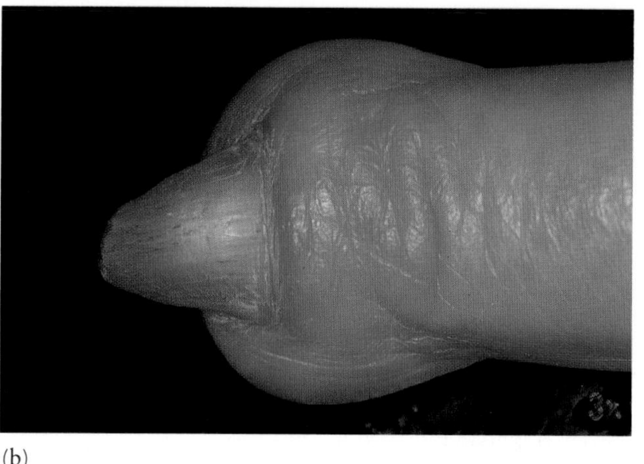

(b)

Fig. 10.73. (a & b) Hook nail deformity.

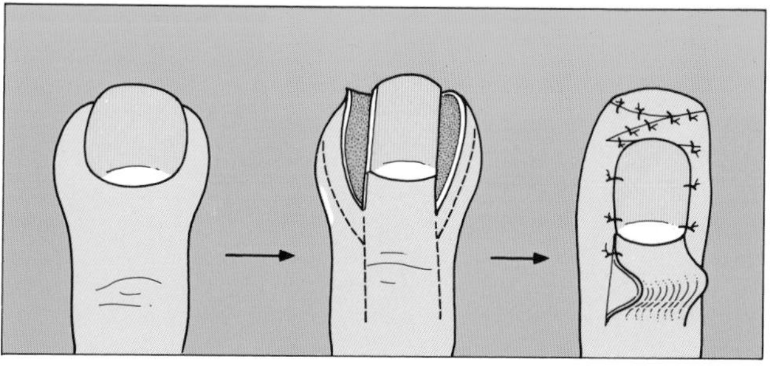

Fig. 10.74. Retraction of the nail matrix and nail bed for spatulate nail deformity (after C. Dufourmentel).

The cleft created by elevation of the bed is filled with a V-Y homodigital finger flap.

5 A composite graft from the second toe placed beneath the released nail bed may give good support and improve pulp substance (Buback, 1992).

6 Free transplants. Microsurgery may be carried out to reconstitute either the soft ungual apparatus alone (taken from the big toe) or the whole with a segment of the ungual phalanx. This complex procedure goes beyond the mere problem of reconstructing the nail apparatus.

Malaligned nail due to traumatic malposition (Fig. 10.75)

The treatment will vary according to the degree of deformity, ranging from plasty of the matrix to its total excision and replacement by a graft.

If tension has malaligned the direction of the proximal nail groove, the nail plate will grow in the same direction. It is important here to release the tension of the nail plate by replacement of the tip with a cross-finger flap, and/or a nail bed graft to allow the matrix to create a new nail plate that is not deformed by tension. Lateral deviation may be due to a full-thickness nail bed avulsion with displacement. After removal of the nail a full-thickness

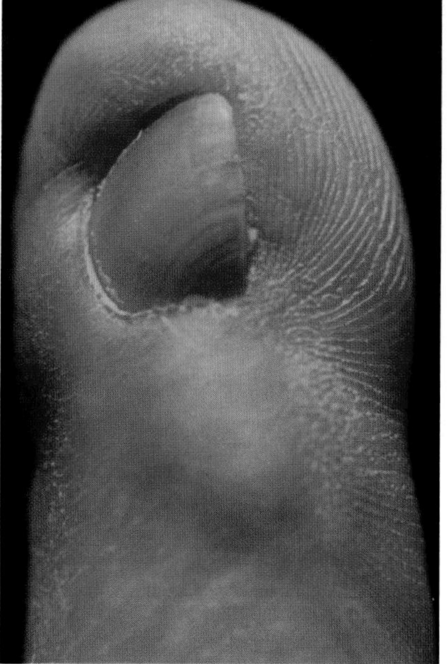

Fig. 10.75. Traumatic nail malalignment (courtesy of G. Cannata, Italy).

flap of nail bed and nail matrix is created down to the bone, the only attachment being the proximal portion of the matrix. The epidermis is excised in the direction of rotation of the flap. The flap is rotated into the correct longitudinal position. A wedge excision is taken from the area of transfer of the flap which is then sutured primarily creating a straight nail (Shepard, 1990). This technique is similar to the one used in the treatment of congenital malalignment of the big toenail.

Nail prosthesis (Fig. 10.76(a)–(c))

In a wide variety of cases, ranging from deformed nail to complete loss of the terminal phalanx, a silicone rubber, 'thimble-shaped' finger cover may be indicated. This prosthesis is easily fitted on the finger stump, encasing the

(a)

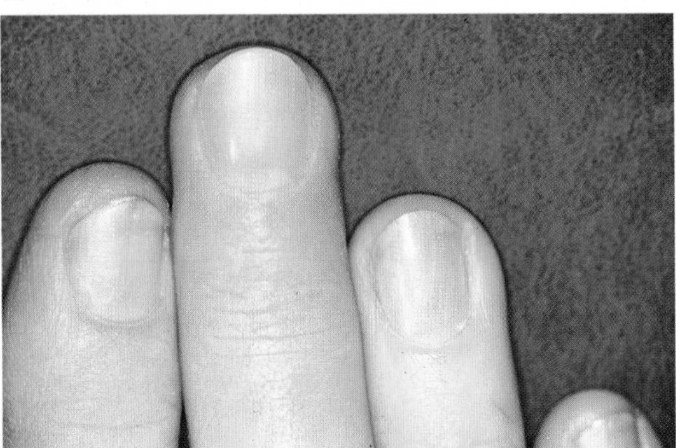

(c)

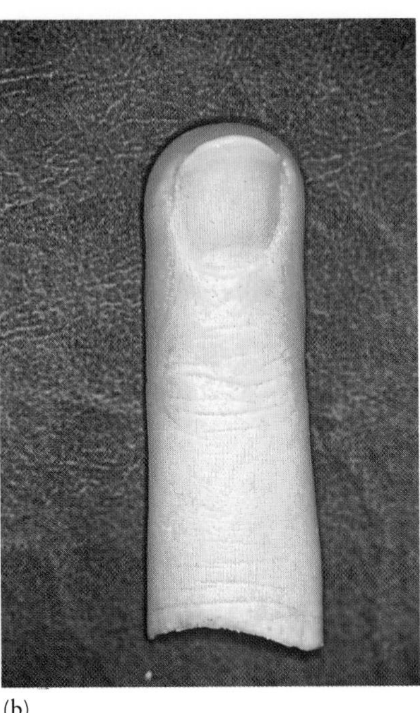

(b)

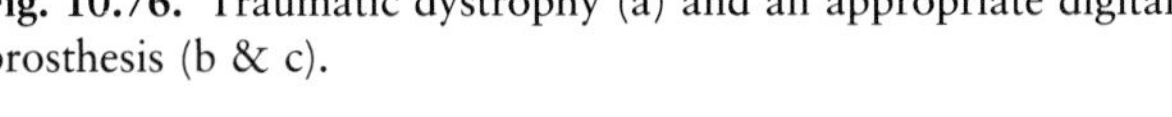

Fig. 10.76. Traumatic dystrophy (a) and an appropriate digital prosthesis (b & c).

entire distal phalanx; it must be fine and flexible to maintain pulp sensitivity and must have the same marking and colouring as the finger. The fixation is excellent and the nail form takes nail varnish well (Pillet, 1981). These devices, called PHP (Pillet hand prosthesis), are available in many countries (see Table 10.4). When there has been loss of tissues from the distal phalanx, 'submini' digital prosthesis can also help (Beasley & de Beze, 1990).

Repeated minor trauma

Self-inflicted injury (Figs 10.77–10.80)

The fingernails are subject to minor trauma which may result from occupational factors or the habit of nail picking or biting (Figs 10.77–10.79). In childhood, over 50% at some stage bite or pick some or all of the fingernails. This generally lasts for no more than 1–2 years. In many ways onychophagia is analogous to childhood trichotillomania, though the latter typically occurs in a younger age group. Those individuals who persist with the nail biting habit through adolescence into adult life (no more than 1–2%) may become almost obsessively destructive and on some fingers very little nail plate may remain (Fig. 10.79). The idea that nail biting is a 'nervous' trait is falaceous and quite misplaced; also the frequency of nail biting (and its severity) is not related to social class or occupation. In many successful adults, severe nail biting phases are related to periods of concentration and constructive activity. There is no objective evidence to link nail biting to mental subnormality or psychiatric disease (see Chapter 6).

If nail biting persists into late teens, the prognosis is poor and it may persist at least into middle life. The loss of permanent teeth is often the reason for nail biting to cease. Many nail biters can control the habit for short periods; others concentrate only on individual fingernails – either preserving one or two unbitten, or attacking one nail very destructively, often a thumb or one hand (Singer & Gibson, 1988). Nail biting and picking are a possible cause of longitudinal melanonychia (Fig. 10.81) (Baran, 1990). The cuticles are usually pushed back and biting causes pressure damage on the base of the nail. Minor traumas to the matrix may result in local areas of incomplete keratinization. Punctate leuconychia disappears as the nail grows out.

Picking and breaking tissue from the proximal and lateral nail folds is even more common than nail biting, though the two often coexist.

The commonest complication is nail plate deformity

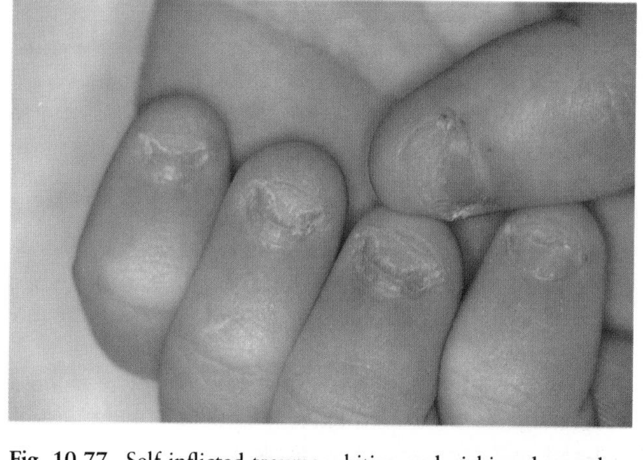

Fig. 10.77. Self-inflicted trauma – biting and picking dystrophy.

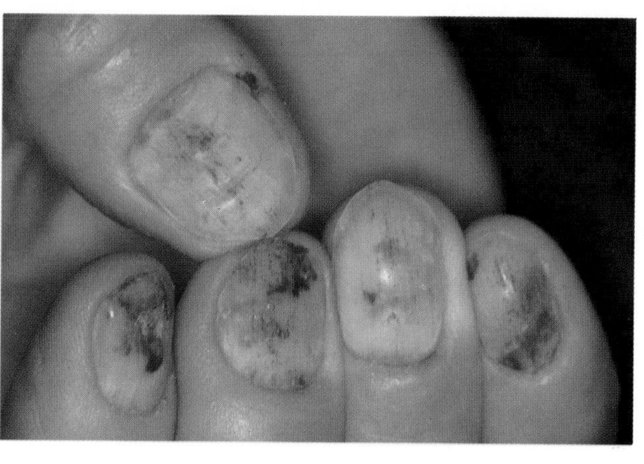
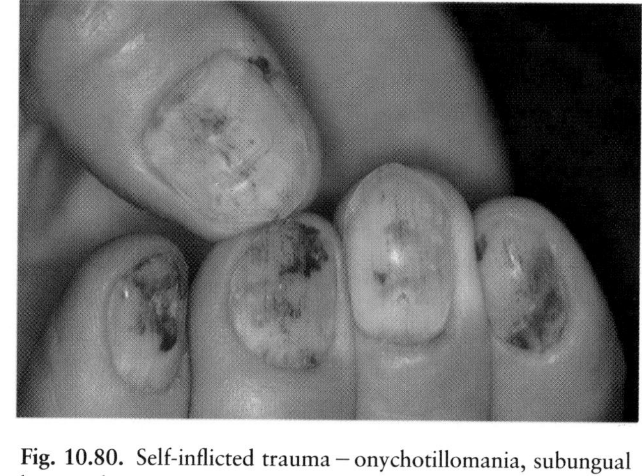

Fig. 10.80. Self-inflicted trauma – onychotillomania, subungual haemorrhages.

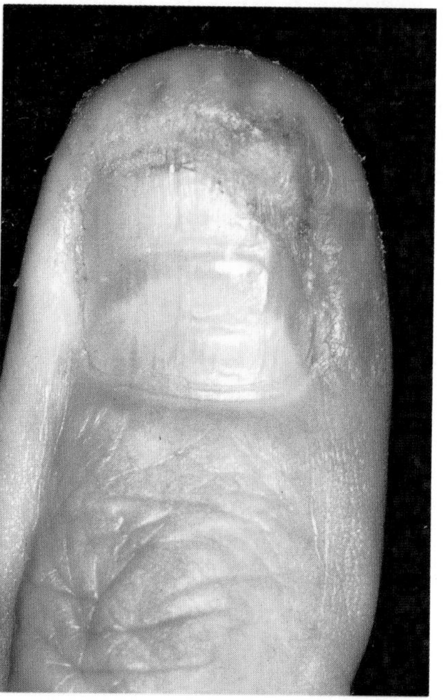

Fig. 10.78. Self-inflicted trauma of nail and periungual tissue.

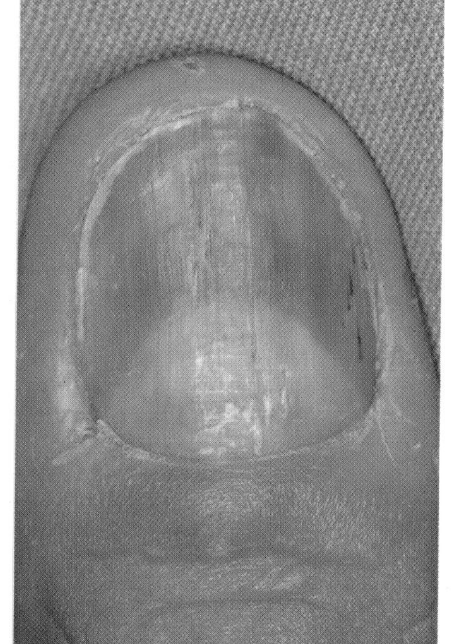

Fig. 10.81. Self-inflicted trauma – longitudinal melanonychia.

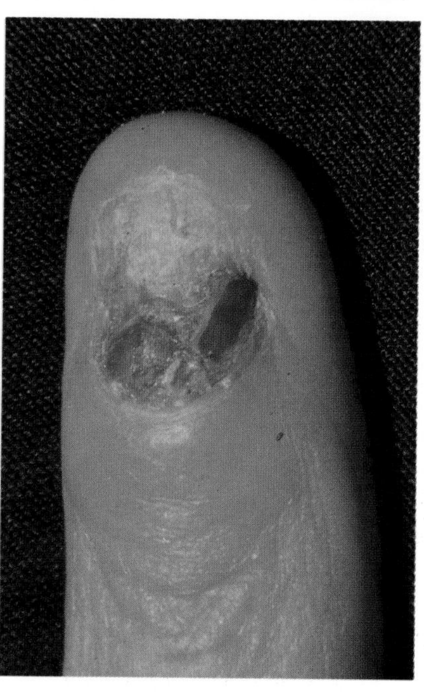

Fig. 10.79. Self-inflicted trauma – severe biting dystrophy.

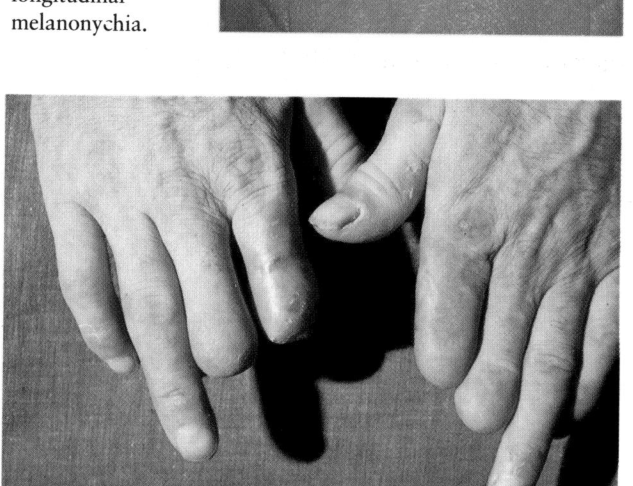

Fig. 10.82. Self-inflicted trauma – schizophrenic individual (courtesy of A. Bourloud, Belgium).

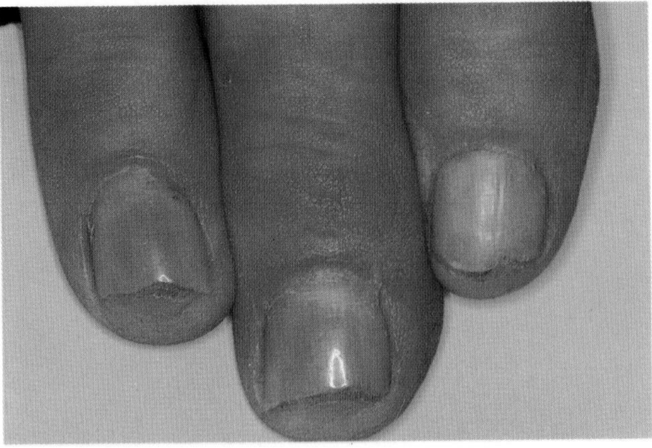

Fig. 10.83. Self-inflicted trauma – shiny 'buffed' nail due to itching in mycosis fungoides.

Table 10.4. Addresses from which PHP devices are available

United States	*Canada*
Asheville Hand Center 34 Granby Street Asheville, NC 28801 704/258-0847	The Workers' Compensation Board 115 Torbarrie Road Downsview, Ontario M3L 1G8 416/244-1761 – Ext. 257
Rocky Mountain Hand Rehabilitation Center Building 2 – Suite 600 2005 Franklin Street Denver, CO 80205 303/839-1694	Sunny Brook Aids-For-Living Centre University of Toronto 2075 Bayview Avenue Toronto, Ontario M4N 3M5 416/480-4259
Department of Orthpedics and Rehabilitation University of Miami P.O. Box 016960 Miami, FL 33104 305/549-6416	*France* Centre de Prothese Plastique P.O.M. 32 rue Godot de Mauroy 75009 Paris, France 1-742-5523
Pillet Hand Prostheses, Ltd. P.O. Box 63 Old Chelsea Station New York, NY 10113 212/206-7840	*Italy* Centro Protesi Estetiche Clinica Santa M.G. Rossello Vis Naselli Feo 4 17100 Savona, Italy 019/366-2123
Hand Rehabilitation Center 901 Walnut Street Philadelphia, PA 19107 215/629-0980	*Switzerland* Clinique Longeraie 9 Avenue de la Gare 1003 Lausanne, Switzerland 021-203 304

with centrally pronounced transverse ridges, called washboard nails (MacAulay, 1966), sometimes simulating Heller's median canaliform dystrophy. It is quite rare for nail biters and pickers to induce sufficient damage to cause scarring, but pterygium has been recorded, as well as secondary bacterial infection and episodes of acute paronychia – well over 80% of patients requiring surgical treatment for acute paronychia are 'biters or pickers'. Osteitis has been reported (Waldmann, 1991; Tosti *et al.*, 1993). Periungual warts are a common complication.

Onychotillomania is a more destructive type of self-mutilation of the nail apparatus; it is akin to dermatitis artefacta of the skin and, unlike nail biting, may well have associated psychological or psychiatric problems (see Chapter 6). Nevertheless, gouging nails with an instrument, biting the proximal part of the nail plate and indifference to the outcome may be indications of a pathological process (Colver, 1987).

However, other less clearly defined nail plate changes progressing to total destruction of the nails may be self-induced and are sometimes falsely claimed to be due to occupational exposure (Norton, 1987). Ronchese (1953) reviewed numerous examples that he encountered in compensation claims and he coined the term 'onychopathomimia'. Occlusive therapy may prevent irreversible changes, but once severe damage has been done to the subungual tissue there will always be abnormal keratinization and scarring (Colver, 1987).

Schizophrenics may rarely cause severe nail apparatus damage to themselves (Fig. 10.82). In the Lesh–Nyhan syndrome severe self-damage may be seen as well as in congenital insensitivity-to-pain syndrome (Thompson *et al.*, 1980) and in patients suffering C4 complete spinal cord injury (Dahlin *et al.*, 1985).

Finally, playing with the 'Frisbee' toy may produce repeated minor damage – the Frisbee nail (Jillson, 1979). Overzealous manicuring may lead to horizontal ridging identical to that caused by self-inflicted trauma and worn-down nail or 'usure des ongles' (Chapter 2) may be occupational or due to scratching (atopic dermatitis, mycosis fungoides, etc.) (Fig. 10.83).

Subungual haemorrhage

Repeated trauma between shoe and toe may occur in tennis (Gibbs, 1973), ball games, climbing, skiing, etc., and may cause black discoloration under the toenails due to subungual haemorrhage (Fig. 10.84(a) & (b)). Sudden starts, stops and abrupt changes in direction appear to be the cause. High-heeled shoes may produce the same disorder.

There may be associated lateral ridging, splitting and onycholysis. Oedema and throbbing pain may appear. When the cause is not obvious, clues to exclude the possible diagnosis of melanoma are: (i) the existence of similar discoloration on a contralateral or adjacent toe (Gibbs, 1980); (ii) the toenail affected is generally the most prominent one, i.e. the first or second toe, and blood seeps through the opening created by paring the affected nail in very recent cases. This condition is attributed to trauma between toenails and footwear.

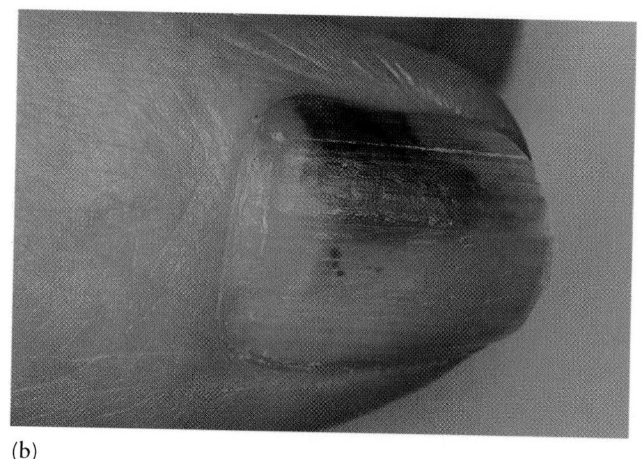

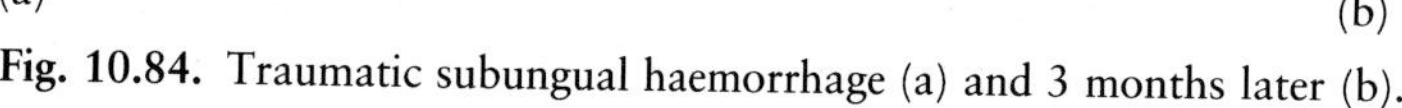

(a) (b)

Fig. 10.84. Traumatic subungual haemorrhage (a) and 3 months later (b).

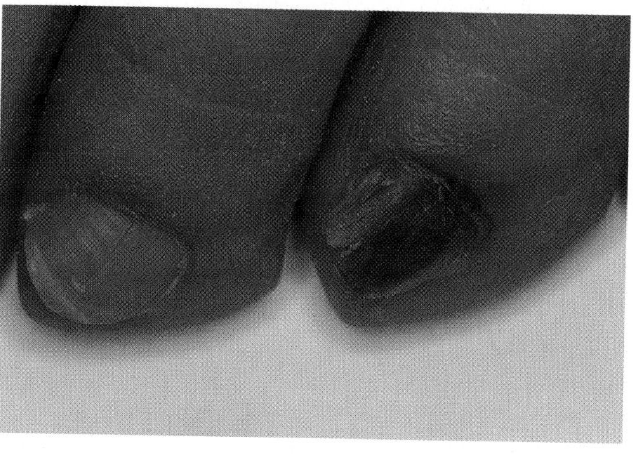

Fig. 10.85. Traumatic longitudinal melanonychia.

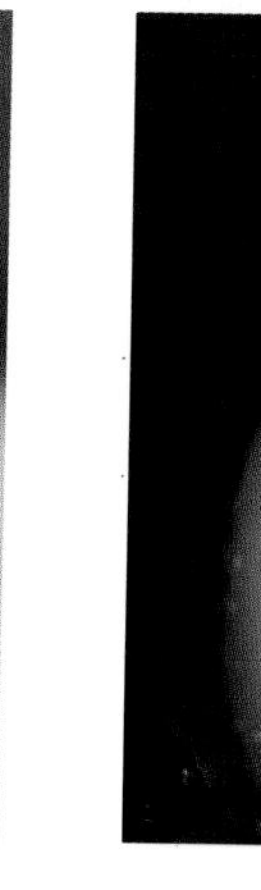

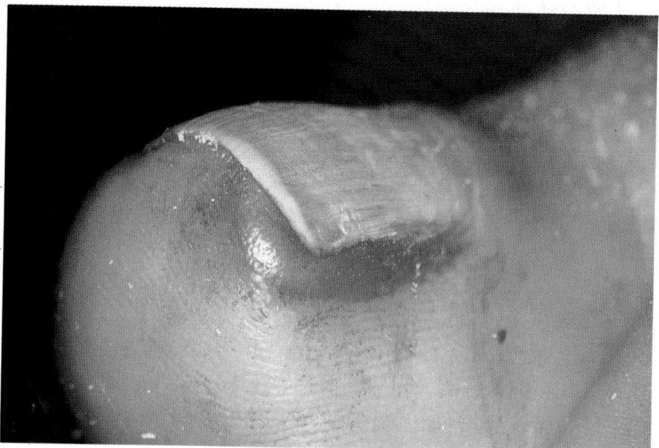

Fig. 10.86. Traumatic (exercise-induced) bulla.

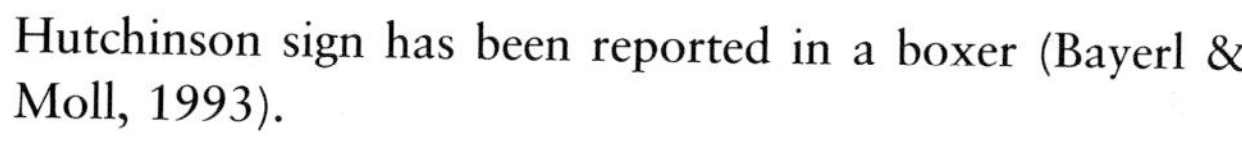

It may be advisable to check that the signs of trauma recede. Within a few months there is distal displacement of the pigmented area as the toenail grows out. Non-migrating subungual haematoma is rare. In joggers, the occurrence of haematoma on the more lateral toenails has been noted (Scher, 1978). Rather than sudden changes in motion, joggers' toe appears to be due to the constant pounding of the foot on the running surface. In fact, this condition may also result from the trauma of the footwear on the toes.

Self-inflicted anonychia of the toenails is associated with small or absent nails and crushing due to traumatic bleeding (Hurley & Balu, 1982).

Frictional melanonychia

Frictional melanonychia of the toes (Fig. 10.85) initiated by repeated trauma from footwear has been described as a new entity (Baran, 1987). Its proper recognition should help to rule out brown streaks due to malignant melanoma. Frictional longitudinal melanonychia with pseudo-Hutchinson sign has been reported in a boxer (Bayerl & Moll, 1993).

Traumatic onycholysis

Diagnosis of traumatic onycholysis due to minor repeated trauma is generally easy, even in the absence of a blackish hue. The case history usually indicates the aetiology of the onycholysis which may not be evident from clinical examination. Occasionally the nail plate may be lifted by a bulla after strenuous exercise in new footwear (Fig. 10.86); it often occurred with platform shoes (Almeyda, 1973). There is a distinct type of mild traumatic onycholysis generally affecting the big toe. In most cases one sees some orthopaedic anomaly of the foot, which may not be obvious to the patient (Baran & Badillet, 1982). When onycholysis presents laterally rather than on the distal or medial aspect, the second toe is often found to override the lateral part of the big toenail (Fig. 10.87). This condition is fully developed when shoes are worn. In some cases, in profile, dorsiflexion of the big toe is

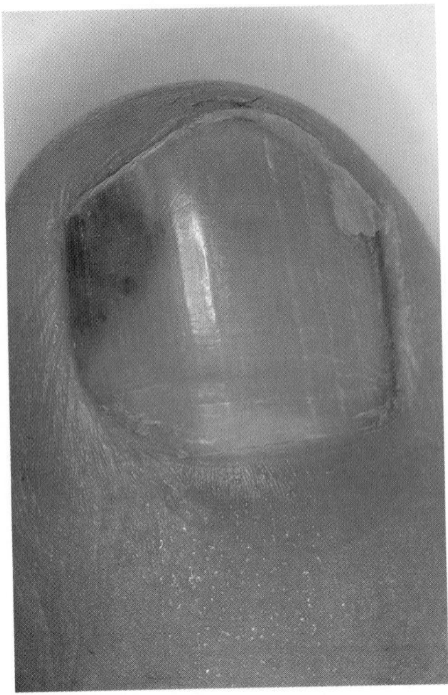

Fig. 10.87. Traumatic onycholysis of the left great toenail due to overriding second toe.

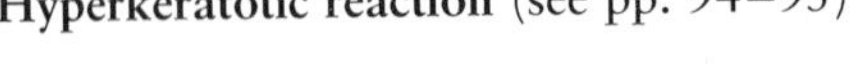

evident. Repeated mechanical trauma between the toe and the upper part of the shoe involves the distal and medial area of the nail plate. Additional common abnormalities may be the cause of mild traumatic onycholysis of the big toe, including a large central hyperkeratotic thickening of the 'ball' of the foot, or of its medial aspect, flat foot, 'sag' foot; sometimes high heels and narrow and slanting shoes may promote onycholysis.

When the second toe is longer than the first one (Morton's toe) this may produce nail dystrophy as a result of mechanical malfunction.

Therapy should be directed to the cause: alleviate the pressure and help to restore proper balance to the foot. Shoes should be properly fitted; padding or accommodative shields may be helpful (Montgomery & Lorascio, 1966). Examination of the feet on a plantarscope may demonstrate the distribution of the weight on the plantar surface. Overriding of the toes can be corrected by the use of silicone rubber orthodigital splints with an interdigital wedge moulded directly onto the toes (Fig. 10.88(a) & (b)). A silicone rubber toecap may efficiently protect the great and/or the second toenail. Sorbothane, a viscoelastic absorbing material, is widely used in running shoes to avoid damage from repeated minor trauma.

Hyperkeratotic reaction (see pp. 94–95)

Anatomical abnormalities and mechanical changes in foot function may well cause hyperkeratosis in the nail area. Subungual hyperkeratosis lifts up the nail plate (Fig. 10.89). Sometimes repeated minor trauma, for example from flat, narrow, pointed shoes, results in pressure on the distal toes: this may produce a subungual corn of the distal nail bed, a localized hyperkeratosis of the adjacent pulp, and nail thickening or thinning. Associated splitting or elevation of the nail may be present. Subungual corn (heloma or onychoclavus) is an entity first described by Thierry (1888) as 'durillon sous-unguéal' in relatively young people (Fig. 10.90(a),(b) & (c)). Typically, the corn affects the great toe and appears as a painful dark spot under the nail (Gilchrist, 1979), resembling a foreign body. Treatment of the subungual corn consists of removing a section of the nail and excising the hyperkeratotic tissue. In lesser toes, 'end' corn occurs under the pulp of a hammer toe below the nail tip (Jahss, 1979). The treatment is that of the hammer toe. Histological examination can rule out subungual melanoma. Pathological changes are identical to corns in other sites. A large parakeratotic plug extends towards the bone, the epidermis being acanthotic at the margins but rather thinned in the depth of the lesion.

Development of hyperkeratotic tissue in varying degrees, on the periungual folds or in the lateral nail grooves, in response to repeated minor trauma, is very common. This condition, which may be diffuse or localized as a corn, is called onychophosis (Fig. 10.91). It involves mainly

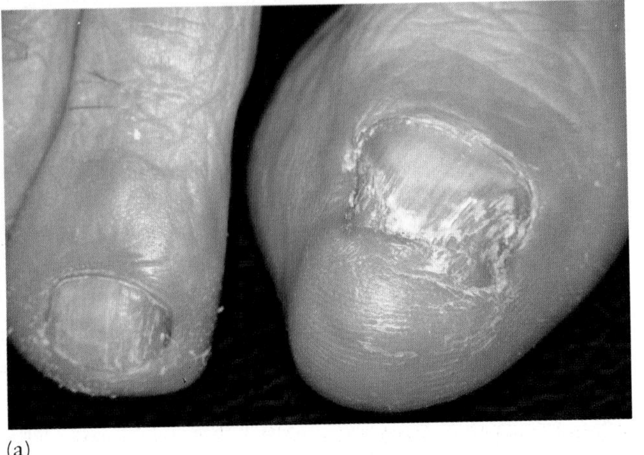

(a)

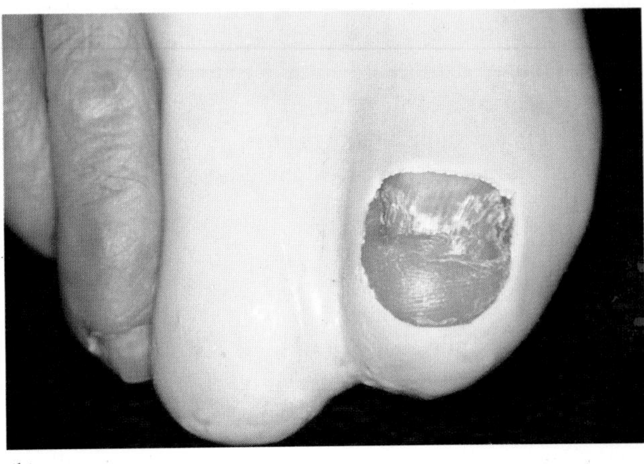

(b)

Fig. 10.88. Overriding of the toes (a) can be corrected by a silicone rubber orthodigital splint (b).

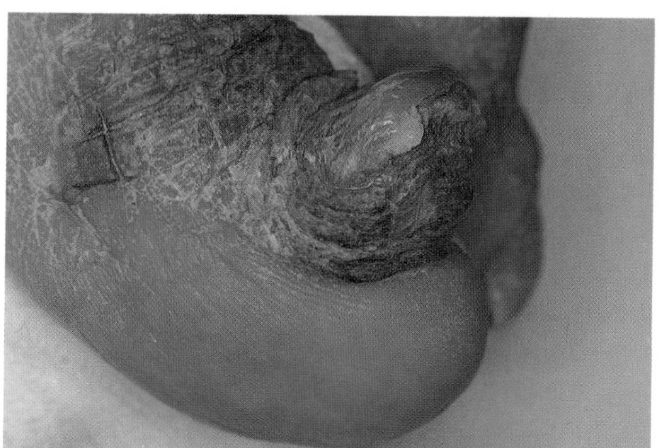

Fig. 10.89. Subungual hyperkeratosis due to repeated trauma.

the first and the fifth toes. Treatment consists of removal of the hard masses, the relief of any pressure exerted by the nail, and the provision of a comfortable shoe.

Lateral pressure can result in loss of normal nail grooves, hypertrophy of the matrix, thickening of the nail plate and onychogryphosis.

Chronic pressure on the growing nail can cause malalignment and is often seen in toenails from ill-fitting shoes (Guy, 1990). This condition is different from hallux valgus.

Subungual exostosis

Subungual exostosis is not uncommon in physically active individuals, particularly young adults, e.g. dancers and soccer players.

Onychogryphosis

The nail in onychogryphosis is severely distorted, thickened and interferes with the wearing of shoes (Fig. 10.92). The thick and spiralated nail can be managed either by conservative or surgical methods, depending on the medical status of the patient (Douglas & Krull, 1981).

Conservative management is especially useful in feet 'at high risk', i.e. patients with peripheral vascular disease and diabetes. Occasionally the pressure on the onychogryphotic nail will initiate subungual gangrene.

Treatment consists of trimming the thickened nail by means of an electric drill and burrs and the removal of subungual keratoses. A face mask and gloves should be worn in order to restrict exposure to the nail grindings. Periodical clipping and trimming of the dystrophic nail are usually sufficient to keep the condition under control.

Chemical nail destruction using 40% urea or 50% potassium iodine under occlusion usually renders the onychogryphosis soft enough to make it trimmable with ordinary scissors. Repeated applications are often necessary,

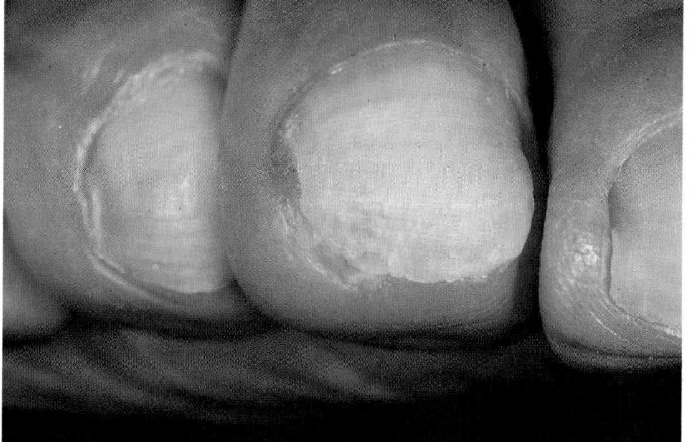

(a)

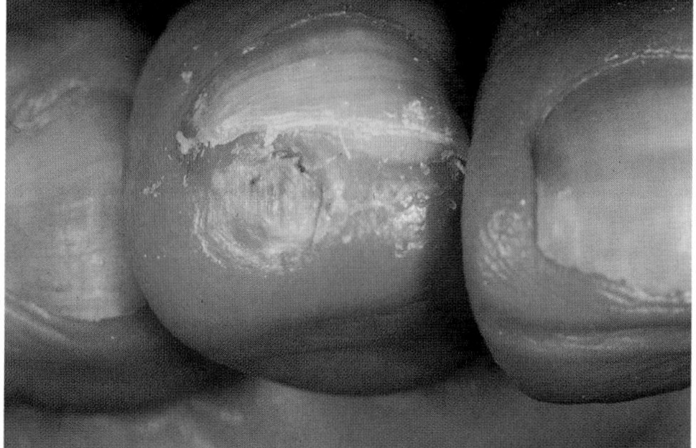

(b)

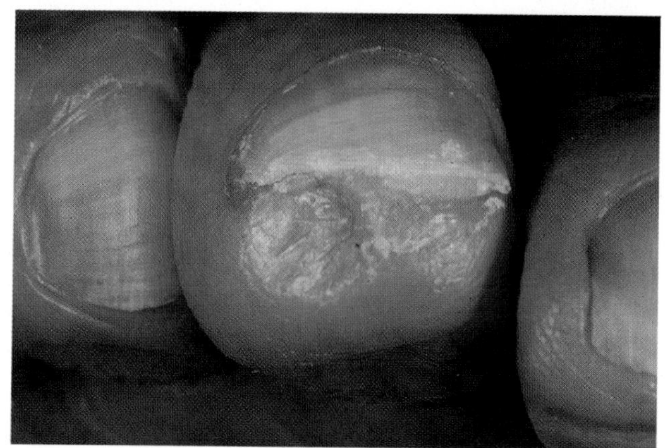

(c)

Fig. 10.90. Subungual corn (heloma) (a); after partial nail avulsion (b), and after removal of the corn (c) (courtesy S. Goettmann, Paris).

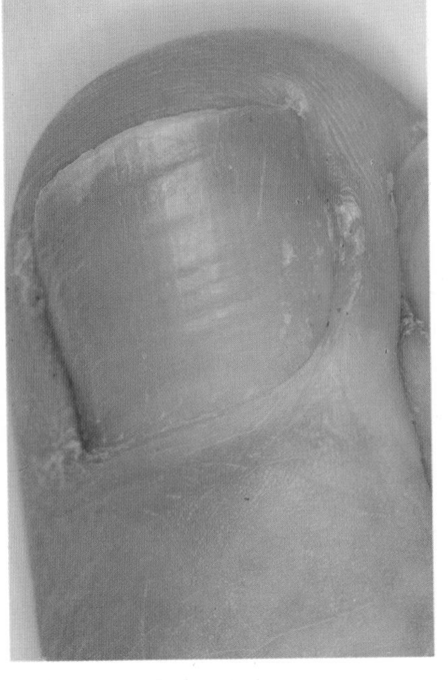

Fig. 10.91. Periungual (lateral) hyperkeratosis from repeated minor trauma – onychophosis.

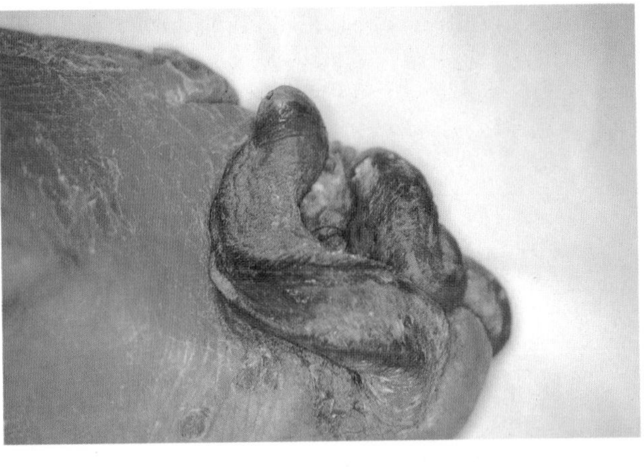

Fig. 10.92. Onychogryphosis.

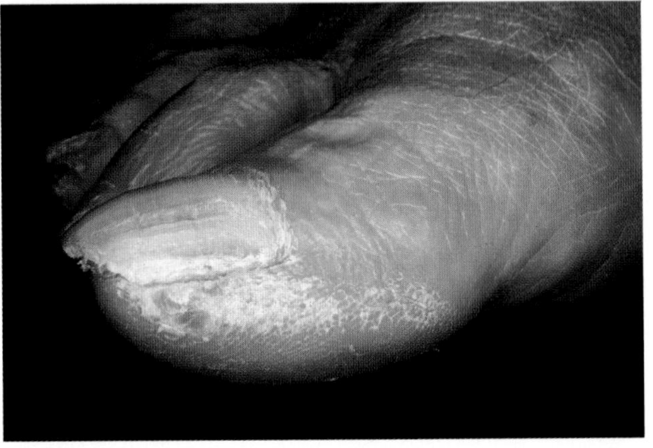

Fig. 10.93. Hallux valgus associated with hyperkeratosis of the lateral nail fold and adjacent nail bed.

which is time consuming. Simple nail avulsion of onychogryphotic toenails offers symptomatic relief in the majority of patients, particularly in the elderly population in whom the use of a tourniquet may be contraindicated (Greig *et al.*, 1989).

When palliative relief is short lasting, or when the patient is dissatisfied with the appearance of the nail plate, permanent eradication may be indicated in order to remove the nail permanently. The use of phenol is the safest and easiest method to destroy all the germinative cells which contribute to the nail plate. Up to 2 min application with firm pressure to the matrix area, 15 s to the under sides of the proximal nail fold, a further 30 s to the under sides of the proximal nail fold, and a further 30 s to the nail bed and sulci are average application times (Dagnall, 1981); post-operative pain is minimal. The patient may need dressings for up to 6 weeks before healing is complete. The use of daily povidone-iodine foot baths eliminates the post-matricectomy bacterial proliferation that tends to delay wound healing (Rinaldi *et al.*, 1982).

A 10% solution of sodium hydroxide is an alternative (Brown, 1981), with application for 20–25 s with a cotton-tipped applicator thinned out to no more than one-third the usual amount of cotton wool. Its action may be instantly stopped by flooding the area with a 3% solution of acetic acid.

Surgical resection of the matrix is usually done by avulsing the nail plate; two incisions starting from the nail grooves are then made on the proximal nail fold which is raised upwards; dissection of its undersurface is carried out, followed by resection of the entire matrix including proximally, the portion separated from the proximal nail fold, and distally, the portion that contains the lunula (Johnson & Ceilley, 1979). In some cases, the matrix is not the sole nail-forming tissue and ablation of the matrix is supplemented by excision of the nail bed which usually requires additional surgery to the distal phalanx (Douglas & Krull, 1981). Due to the matrix shape, recurrences or nail spicules often develop after surgical matricectomy.

CO_2 surgical laser has proved of value in treating the matrix and nail bed after the onychogryphotic nail has been avulsed (Kaplan *et al.*, 1976).

Old people are often unable to cut their own thick hard toenails and are hampered by failing eyesight. Prevention, by proper nail trimming in a home-care foot health programme, is clearly the best method of treatment (Gilchrist, 1979).

Hallux valgus

This deformity may cause pronounced changes in the nail apparatus, including hyperkeratosis of the tibial nail fold (Fig. 10.93) and the distal–medial subungual area; recalcitrant ingrowing toenail with granulation tissue in the lateral nail groove and adjacent nail bed of the great toe; lateral deviation of the big toenail resulting in lateral pincer nail; and laterally 'wound' screw-shaped onychogryphosis (Fabry, 1983).

References

Almeyda J. (1973) Platform nails. *Br. Med. J.* **1**, 176.

Andrus C.H. (1980) Instrument and technique for removal of subungual foreign bodies. *Am. J. Surg.* **140**, 588.

Atasoy E. (1982) Reversed cross-finger subcutaneous flap. *J. Hand Surg.* 7, 481–483.

Atasoy E., Ioakimidies E., Kasdon M.L. *et al.* (1970) Reconstruction of the amputated fingertip with a triangular volar flap. *J. Bone Joint Surg.* **52**, 921.

Atasoy E., Godfrey A. & Kalisman M. (1983) The 'antenna' procedure for the hook-nail deformity. *J. Hand Surg.* **8a**, 55–58.

Baran R. (1986) Removal of the proximal nail fold. Why, when, how? *J. Dermatol. Surg. Oncol.* **12**, 234–236.

Baran R. (1987) Frictional longitudinal melanonychia: A new entity. *Dermatologica* **174**, 280–284.

Baran R. (1990) Nail biting and picking as a possible cause of longitudinal melanonychia. *Dermatologica* **181**, 126–128.

Baran R. & Badillet G. (1982) Primary onycholysis of the big toenail: review of 113 cases. *Br. J. Dermatol.* **106**, 529–534.

Baran R. & Bureau H. (1981) Surgical treatment of recalcitrant chronic paronychias of the fingers. *J. Dermatol. Surg. Oncol.* 7, 106–107.

Barfod B. (1972) Reconstruction of the nail fold. *Hand* **4**, 85.

Bayerl C. & Moll I. (1993) Longitudinal melanonychia with Hutchinson sign in a boxer. *Hautarzt* **44**, 476–479.

Beasley R.W. & de Beze G (1990) Prosthetic substitution for finger nails. *Hand Clin.* **6**, 105–112.

Brown F.C. (1981) Chemocautery for ingrown toenails. *J. Dermatol. Surg. Oncol.* 7, 331.

Bubak P.J., Richey M.D. & Engraw L.H. (1992) Hook nail deformity repaired using a composite toe graft. *Plast. Reconstr. Surg.* **90**, 1079–1082.

Colver G.B. (1987) Onychotillomania. *Br. J. Dermatol.* **117**, 397–399.

Dagnall J.C. (1981) The history, development and current status of nail matrix phenolisation. *Chiropodist* **36**, 315–324.

Dahlin P.A., Van Buskirk N.E., Novotny R.W. *et al.* (1985) Self-biting leading to multiple finger amputations following spinal cord injury. *Paraplegia* **23**, 306–318.

Douglas M.C. & Krull E.A. (1981) Diseases of the nails. In: *Current Therapy*, ed. Conn, p. 712. W.B. Saunders, Philadelphia.

Dufourmentel C. (1974) Problème esthétiques dans la reconstruction des moignons douloureux. In: *Les Mutilations de la Main*, p. 109. Monographie du groupe de la main, Expansion Scientifique, Paris.

Fabry H. (1983) Haut-und Nagelveränderungen bei Hallux valgus. *Akt. Derm.* **9**, 77–79.

Foucher G., Marin Braun F. & Smith D.J. (1991) Custom made free vascularized compound toe transfer for traumatic dorsal loss of the thumb. *Plast. Reconst. Surg.* **87**, 310–313.

Gibbs R.C. (1973) Tennis toe. *Arch. Dermatol.* **107**, 918.

Gibbs R.C. (1980) *Skin Diseases of the Feet*, 2nd edn, p. 200. Warren H. Green Inc, St Louis, Missouri.

Gibbs R.C. (1985) Toenail disease secondary to poorly fitting shoes or abnormal biomechanics. *Cutis* 399–400.

Gilchrist A.K. (1979) Common foot problems in the elderly. *Geriatrics.* **34**, 67.

Greig J.D., Anderson J.H., Ireland A.J. *et al.* (1989) Simple avulsion of onychogryphotic toenails: a justifiable treatment? *Postgrad. Med. J.* **65**, 741–742.

Guy R.K. (1990) The etiologies and mechanisms of nail bed injuries. *Hand Clin.* **6**, 9–19.

Haneke E. (1991) Cirurgia de las uñas. *Monogr. Dermatol.* **4**, 408–423.

Haneke E. & Baran R. (1991) Nails: surgical aspects. In: *Aesthetic Dermatology*, eds Parrish L.C. & Lask G.P., pp. 236–247. McGraw Hill, New York.

Haneke E. & Tosti A. (1993) Sea-urchin granuloma of the nail organ (in press).

Hart R.G. & Kleinert H.E. (1993) Fingertip and nail bed injuries. *Emerg. Med. Clin. North Amer.* **11**, 755–765.

Hayes C.W. (1974) One-stage nail fold reconstruction. *Hand* **6**, 74–75.

Hoffman S. (1973) Correction of a split nail deformity. *Arch. Dermatol.* **108**, 568.

Hornstein O.P. & Haneke E. (1980) Granulomatöse Reactionen der Haut. In: *Verhandlungen der Deutschein Gesellschaft für Pathologie*, 64, Jagung, Fischer-Verlag, Stuttgart, pp. 180–193.

Hurley P.T. & Balu V. (1982) Self-inflicted anonychia. *Arch. Dermatol.* **118**, 956–957.

Jahss M.H. (1979) Geriatric aspects of the foot and ankle. In: *Clinical Geriatrics*, 2nd ed. Rossman I.J.B., p. 638. Lippincott, Philadelphia.

Jillson O. (1979) The Frisbee nail. *J. Am. Acad. Dermatol.* **1**, 163.

Johnson D.B. & Ceilley R.I. (1979) A revised technique for ablation of the matrix of a nail. *J. Dermatol. Surg. Oncol.* **5**, 642.

Johnson R.K. (1971) Nail plasty. *Plast. Recontr. Surg.* **42**, 275.

Kaplan I., Labandter C.B. & Labandter H. (1976) Onychogryphosis treated with the CO_2 surgical laser. *Br. J. Plast. Surg.* **29**, 102.

Kleinert H.E., Putcha S.M., Ashbell T.S. *et al.* (1967) The deformed fingernail, a frequent result of failure to repair nail bed injuries. *J. Trauma* 7, 117.

Kutler W. (1947) A new method for fingertip amputations. *J. Am. Med. Assoc.* **133**, 29.

MacAulay W.L. (1966) Transverse ridging of the thumbnails. *Arch. Dermatol.* **93**, 421–423.

Martin B.F. & Platts M.M. (1959) A histological study of the nail region in normal human subjects and in those showing splinter haemorrhages of the nail. *J. Anat.* **93**, 323.

Matsuba H.M. & Spear S.L. (1988) Delayed primary reconstruction of subtotal nail bed loss using a split-thickness nail bed graft on decorticated bone. *PRS*, **81**, 440–443.

McCash C.R. (1956) Free nail grafting. *Br. J. Plast. Surg.* **8**, 19.

Montgomery R.M. & Lorascio W.V. (1966) Padding and devices for foot comfort. *Arch. Dermatol.* **93**, 739.

Morrison W.A. (1990) Microvascular nail transfer. *Hand Clin.* **6**, 69–77.

Norton L. (1987) Self-induced trauma to the nails. *Cutis* **40**, 223–227.

Ogo K. (1987) Does the nail bed really regenerate? *Plast. Reconstr. Surg.* **80**, 445–447.

Pillet J. (1981) The aesthetic hand prosthesis. *Orthop. Clin. N. Am.* **12**, 961–969.

Recht P. (1976) Fingertip injuries and a plea for the nail. *J. Dermatol. Surg. Oncol.* **2**, 327.

Rinaldi R., Sabia M. & Gross J. (1982) The treatment and prevention of infection in phenol alcohol matricectomies. *J.*

Am. Podiatr. Assoc. **72**, 453.
Rodboard S. (1968) Treatment of injury of the root of the nail. *J. Am. Med. Assoc.* **205**, 940.
Ronchese F. (1953) Occupational nail marks, true and false. *Indust. Med.* **22**, 45–48.
Rose E.H. (1980) Nail plasty utilizing a free composite graft from the helixal rim of the scar. *PRS* **66**, 23–29.
Rosenthal E.A. (1983) Treatment of finger tip and nail bed injuries. *Orthop. Clin. N. Am.* **14**, 675–697.
Saito H., Suzuki Y., Fukino *et al.* (1983) Free nail bed graft for treatment of nail bed injuries of hand. *J. Hand Surg.* **8**, 171–178.
Scher R.K. (1978) Jogger's toe. *Int. J. Dermatol.* **17**, 719.
Schernberg F. & Amiel M. (1985) Etude anatomo-clinique d'un lambean unquéal complet. *Ann. Chir. Plast. Esth.* **30**, 217–231.
Seckel B.R. (1986) Self-advancing silicone rubber splint for repair of split nail deformity. *J. Hand Surg.* **11**, 143–144.
Shepard G.H. (1983) Treatment of nail bed avulsion with split-thickness nail bed grafts. *J. Hand Surg.* **8**, 48–54.
Shepard G.H. (1990) Nail grafts for reconstruction. *Hand Clin.* **6**, 79–103.
Singer P. & Gibson G. (1988) Unilateral dystrophy secondary to nail biting. *Cutis* **42**, 491–192.
Stone O.J. & Mullins J.F. (1963) The distal course of nail matrix hemorrhage. *Arch. Dermatol.* **88**, 186.
Thierry M. (1888) Durillon sous-unguéal. *Rev. Chir.* **8**, 423.
Thompson C.C., Park R.I. & Prescott G.H. (1980) Oral manifestations of the congenital insensitivity-to-pain syndrome. *Oral Surg. Oral Med. Oral Pathol.* **50**, 220–225.
Tosti A., Peluso A.M. Bardazzi *et al.* (1994) Phalangeal osteomyelitis due to nail biting. *Acta. Derm. Venereol.* (in press).
Van Beek A.L., Kassan M.A., Adson M.H. *et al.* (1990) Management of acute fingernail injuries. *Hand Clin.* **6**, 23–38.
Verdan C. (1981) Plastic surgery and claw-nail. In: *The Nail*, ed. Pierre M., p. 93. Churchill Livingstone, Edinburgh.
Waldmann B.A. (1991) Osteomyelitis caused by nail biting. *Pediatr. Dermatol.* **7**, 189–190.
Yong F.C. & Teoh L.C. (1992) Nail bed reconstruction with split-thickness nail bed grafts. *J. Hand Surg.* **17b**, 193–197.
Zook E.G. (1986) Complications of the perionychium. *Hand Clin.* **2**, 407–427.
Zook E.G. (1988) The perionychium. In: *Operative Hand Surgery*, ed. Green D.P., pp. 1331–1375. Churchill Livingstone, New York.
Zook E.G. (1990) Discussion of 'Management of acute nail bed avulsions'. *Hand Clin.* **6**, 57–58.

Miscellaneous nail dystrophies

Narrowing of the nail

This method has evolved from knowledge obtained over many years using lateral longitudinal biopsy techniques. We have found longitudinal matrix narrowing useful for the treatment of:

1 ingrowing toenail;
2 longitudinal melanonychia involving the lateral third of the nail plate;
3 longitudinal splitting of the nail at the lateral aspect;
4 tumours located at the lateral aspect;
5 racquet thumb.

The so-called wedge excision as depicted in most textbooks of minor surgery is obviously *not* suited for narrowing the nail: it involves removal of the lateral nail fold (Bennett, 1976) and has to include the lateral matrix horns; these however, are left in most instances.

Reference

Bennett R.G. (1976) Technique of biopsy of nails. *J. Dermatol. Surg. Oncol.* **2**, 325.

Congenital and/or hereditary nail disorders

Aplastic or dysplastic lesions, produced by restricting amniotic bands, are not amenable to surgery. Tight syndactyly of the Apert type, where the treatment is that of the syndactyly, is beyond the scope of this section.

Congenital absence of the nail

In congenital absence of the nail, Zook (1990) suggests an excision of the skin in the shape of a nail on the dorsal distal surface of the fingertip and application of split-thickness skin graft to simulate a nail. If desired, full-thickness grafts can be placed proximally to simulate the lunula and distally to mimic the white area, distal to the hyponychium. Koshima *et al.* (1988) performed free vascularized nail graft utilizing microneurovascular techniques in congenital absence of fingernail.

Pachyonychia congenita

This condition is rarely limited to the nails (Chang *et al.*, 1994). Whether the primary site of the pathological process is located in the nail bed (Forsling *et al.*, 1973; Shelley, 1974), the hyponychium (Kelly & Pinkus, 1958) or the matrix (Thomsen *et al.*, 1982) is still debatable. A few patients may require excision of the undersurface of the proximal nail fold and the entire subungual tissues in order to achieve permanent total removal of the nail. Full-thickness grafting (Cosman *et al.*, 1964) or split-skin grafting (White & Noon, 1977) achieve good results. According to Thomsen *et al.* (1982) the most effective and rapidly performed, and the most acceptable method, lies in vigorous curettage and electrofulguration of the matrix and nail bed. CO_2 has been suggested. Healing proceeds by secondary intention. Phenol cautery may be a useful alternative and can easily be repeated (Haneke, 1985).

Racquet thumbs

A short, broad terminal phalanx of the thumb results in a short and wide nail plate that usually lacks lateral nail folds. The aesthetic appearance may be improved by

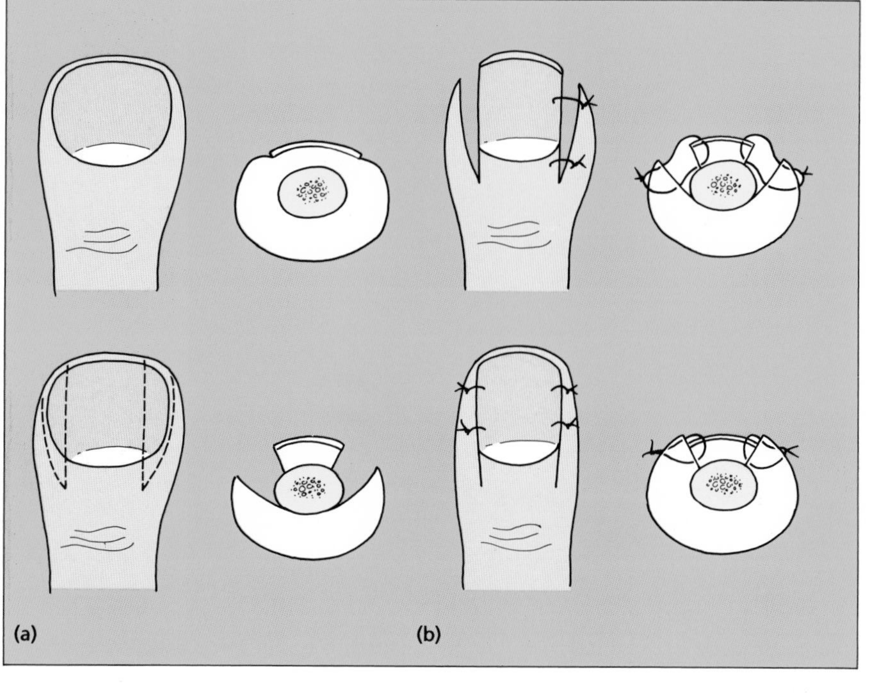

Fig. 10.94. Surgical treatment of racket thumb (from Haneke, 1985 with permission).

narrowing the nail plate and creating lateral nail folds (Fig. 10.94(a) & (b)).

Lateral-longitudinal nail biopsies are performed on both sides of the thumbnail. The lateral soft aspects of the distal phalanx are dissected from the bone, and back stitches are used to create lateral nail folds. The needle is run into the lateral aspect about 2–3 mm volar to the plane of the nail bed bone interface, through the nail bed and plate, and back again through the lateral thumb skin, which upon knotting will be elevated, thus forming a lateral nail fold. Nail groove epithelium develops by secondary intention (Haneke 1985, 1988).

Congenital malalignment of the big toenail

(see Chapter 2)

References

Chang A., Lucker G.P.H., van de Kerkhof P.C.M. *et al.* (1994) Pachyonychia congenita in the absence of other syndrome abnormalities. *J. Am. Acad. Dermatol.* (in press).

Cosman B., Sysmonds F.C. & Crikelair G.F. (1964) Plastic surgery in pachyonychia congenita and other dyskeratoses. *Plast. Reconstr. Surg.* **33**, 226.

Forsling B., Nylen B., Swanbeck G. *et al.* (1973) Pachyonychia congenita, a histologic and microradiographic study. *Acta Derm. Venereol.* **53**, 211.

Haneke E. (1985) Behandlung einiger Nagelfehlbildungen. In: *Fehlbildungen Nävi, Melanome*, eds Wolff H.H., Schmeller W. pp. 71–77, Springer Verlag, Berlin.

Haneke E. (1988) Reconstruction of the lateral nail fold after lateral longitudinal nail biopsy. In: *Surgical Gems in Dermatology*, Robins P., ed. Journal Publ. Group, New York, pp. 91–93.

Kelly E.W. & Pinkus H.N. (1958) Report of a case of pachyonychia congenita. *Arch. Dermatol.* **77**, 724.

Koshima I., Soeda S., Takase T. *et al.* (1988) Free vascularized nail grafts. *J. Hand Surg.* **13A**, 29–32.

Shelley W.B. (1974) Pachyonychia congenita. In: *Consultations in Dermatology*, Vol. II, p. 136. W.B. Saunders, Philadelphia.

Thomsen R.J., Zuehlke R.L. & Beckman B.L. (1982) Pachyonychia congenita. Surgical management of the nail changes. *J. Dermatol. Surg. Oncol.* **8**, 24.

White R.R. & Noon R.B. (1977) Pachyonychia congenita (Jadassohn–Lewandowki syndrome). Case report. *Plast. Reconstr. Surg.* **59**, 855.

Zook E.G. (1990) The perionychium. *Hand Clin.* **6**, 21.

Ingrowing toenails

Ingrowing toenail is a common, painful condition, multifactorial in its aetiology, and most frequently seen in adolescents and young adults. The main factors producing the condition are hereditary, or constitutional, imbalance between the width of the nail plate and that of the nail bed (Haneke, 1978, 1986), or overcurvature of the nail plate (Haneke, 1992). Additional factors may be medial rotation of the toe, thinner nails and thicker nail folds (Langford *et al.*, 1989). Sweating, convex cutting of the nail, and pointed-toe and high-heeled shoes are only participating factors. This is confirmed by the successful results of surgery, which corrects the discrepancy between the broad nail plate and narrow nail bed, and by the high recurrence rate found with conservative treatment. Certain constitutional features are more common in the group of patients with ingrowing toenails: these include tall stature, hyperhidrosis of hands and feet, and the 'unguis incarnatus syndrome' (Steigleder & Stober-

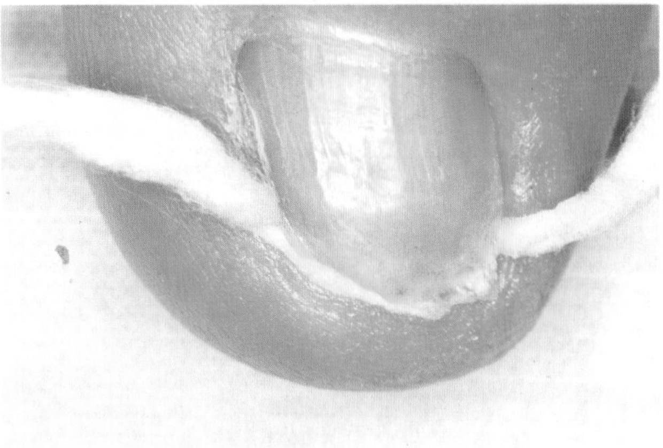

Fig. 10.95. Ingrowing toenail – separation of ingrowing nail edge from adjacent soft tissue (courtesy of G. Cannata, Italy).

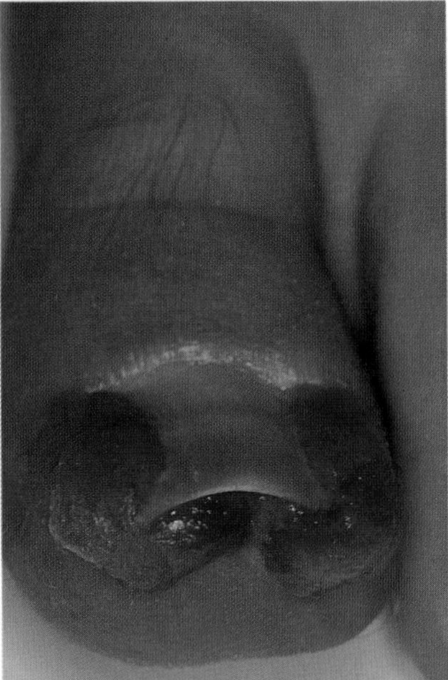

Fig. 10.96. Ingrowing toenail – excessive bilateral growth of granulation tissue.

Münster, 1977); they require special management (Reszler & Mari, 1981). There are five major types of ingrowing toenails:

1 subcutaneous ingrowing toenail;
2 hypertrophy of the lateral nail fold;
3 inward distortion of the nail;
4 distal nail embedding;
5 ingrowing toenail in infancy.

Subcutaneous ingrowing nail (juvenile ingrowing nail)

An ingrowning toenail is created by impingement of the nail plate into the dermal tissue of the lateral nail fold. It often appears as a result of improper trimming of the nail. A 'lacerating' spicule of the nail margin grows into the soft tissue surrounding the side of the nail, acts as a foreign body, and produces irritation and inflammation with pain from perforation of the nail groove epithelium.

Treatment for the early stage is conservative. The foot is soaked daily in lukewarm water with povidone-iodine antisepsis or with potassium permanganate (1 : 10 000 dilution). In mild cases, separating the offending nail edge from the adjacent soft tissue with a wisp of absorbent cotton coated with collodion, gives immediate relief of pain (Fig. 10.95). The collodion which fixes the cotton in place permits bathing (Ilfeld, 1991).

To increase pliability of the nail, its centre may be ground down until it is quite thin and the pink nail bed shines through (Maeda *et al*., 1990). Notching a 'V' in the end of the nail may also relieve the pressure at the corners. In fact it is essential to search for and to remove the lateral spike acting as a foreign body, under local anaesthesia. Subsequently, a small piece of povidone-iodine gauze is forced under the same edge, so that as the nail grows forwards, its lateral margin will not impinge on the soft tissue of the lateral nail fold.

The nail must be cut 'square' and the sharp 'corners' smoothed away with an emery board. Conservative management requires a high degree of compliance – recurrences are frequent.

Granulation stage (Fig. 10.96)

The nail groove may be involved along its entire length developing excess granulation tissue. It becomes filled with 'proud flesh' extending under the nail and involving a portion of the nail bed. This, together with the swollen lateral nail fold, overlaps the nail plate and since infection is almost always present, pus may exude from the nail groove.

Occasionally steroids covered by 'Blenderm' tape may control this condition if infection is not present, but when the large new mass is covered with surface epithelium, it will require curettage under local anaesthesia. This enables the 'fish hook' part of the nail to be removed and the acute inflammation of the lateral nail fold to be treated. This may be completed by antibiotic and sublesional injection of steroid suspension. Simple avulsion of the big toenail in the initial management (Murray & Bedi, 1975) has so high a recurrence rate that it should not be carried out (Haneke, 1978, 1986; Palmer & Jones, 1979). Moreover, the pulp of the hallux is pushed dorsally during weight bearing and the distal nail groove is obliterated by the developing of a distal nail fold (Fowler, 1958). When the newly formed nail advances it becomes embedded in the unsupported pulp which has pressed round the plate distally. Despite the treatments recurrences are still very frequent, which will therefore need a definitive procedure to be carried out.

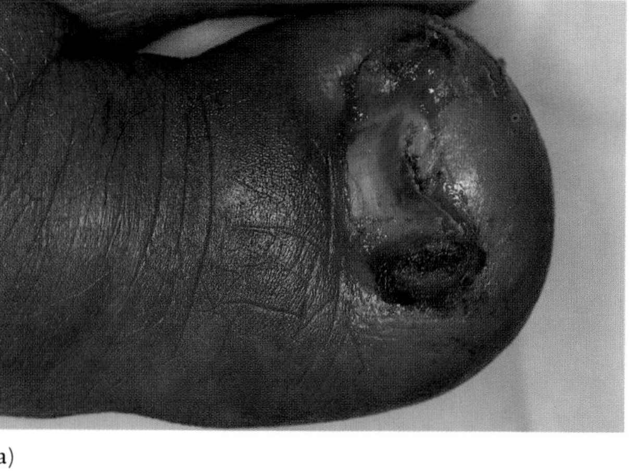

(a)

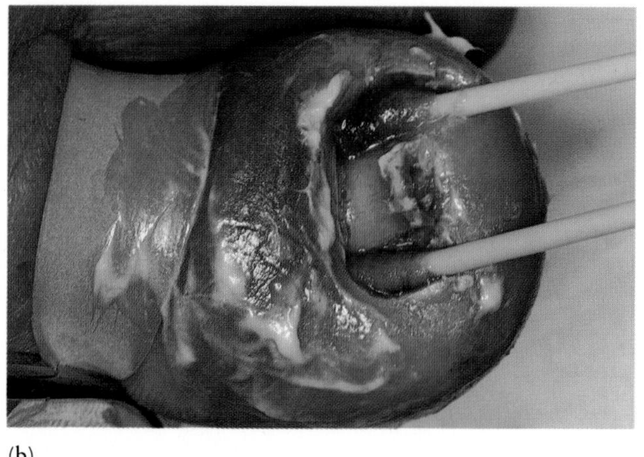

(b)

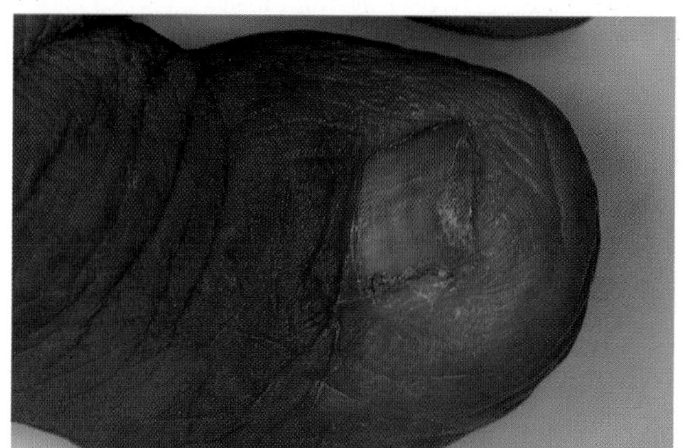

(c)

Fig. 10.97. Lateral nail plate excision for recalcitrant ingrowing nail: (a) before treatment; (b) during phenolic treatment; and (c) late stage many months after healing.

Definitive procedure

Since the nail plate seems too wide for its underlying bed, the logical treatment is aimed at correcting this disparity by the selective matrix excision which permanently narrows the nail. A lateral nail strip is freed from the proximal nail fold, nail bed and matrix with a Freer septum elevator, then cut longitudinally and extracted. This partial nail avulsion may be immediately followed by phenol cauterization, an easy and efficient technique which can be used even when the affected region is infected (Dagnall, 1976a) (Fig. 10.97(a), (b), (c)).

It is essential to work on a bloodless field since blood inactivates phenol. The haemostasis is accomplished with a tourniquet and the blood carefully cleaned from the space under the proximal nail fold using sterile gauze. The surrounding skin is protected with petroleum jelly and the freshly made solution of liquefied phenol (88%) has to be rubbed in vigorously for 3 min in order to achieve a complete eradication of the matrix horn epithelium. This is then neutralized with 70% alcohol. Since the nail plate is elevated slightly when the lateral nail strip is cut, the liquefied phenol usually seeps 1–2 mm under the adjacent nail plate, causing lateral onycholysis. This may be partly prevented by rubbing the phenol into the matrix in a rotating motion, moving outward at the nail margin and matrix.

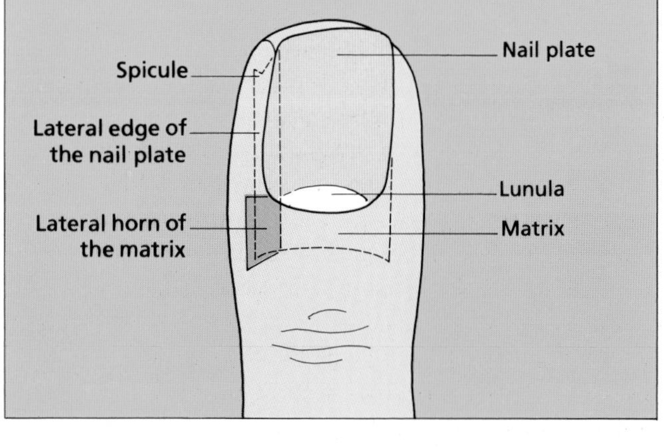

Fig. 10.98. Ingrowing nail – lateral nail excision and removal of matrix horn.

Post-operative pain is minimal since phenol has a considerable local anaesthetic action. It is also antiseptic. The matrix epithelium is sloughed off and there is usually slight oozing for 2–4 weeks. Daily foot baths with

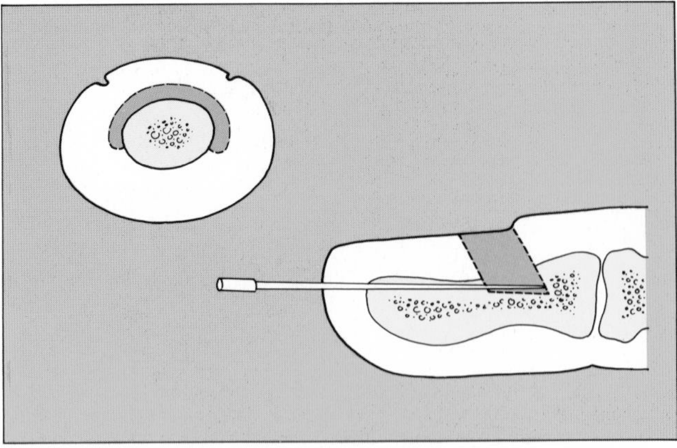

Fig. 10.99. See Fig. 10.100 – the No. 1 needle is inserted as shown to delineate the limits of the nail matrix (after R.T. Austin, UK).

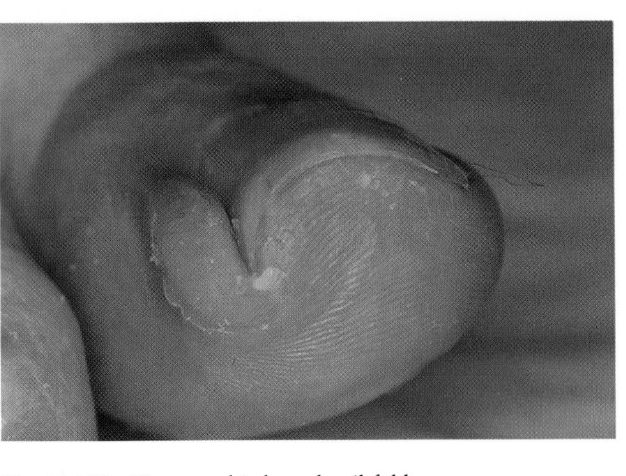

Fig. 10.100. Hypertrophic lateral nail fold.

povidone-iodine antisepsis will avoid infection and accelerate healing.

The major drawbacks of this procedure are twofold: (i) the length of time required for healing; (ii) the prolonged drainage caused by the chemical burn induced by the caustic properties of phenol. Rinaldi *et al.* (1982) have demonstrated that infection may also be a significant cause of the exudation. Poor home care may even be responsible for periostitis (Gilles *et al.*, 1986), which may therefore result indirectly from phenol use as well as directly if the procedure is preceded by matrix curettage for example. Using 10% sodium hydroxide (Brown, 1981) instead of phenol is an alternative.

For more experienced surgeons, definitive cure can be obtained by selective lateral matrix excision, which may be performed at the same time or preferably 1 month after the lateral strip of nail has been removed. The remaining granulation tissue is gently curetted, and if infection is severe, oral antibiotic is given and continued for a short time post-operatively. The proximal nail fold is incised obliquely in an angle of about 110°. The incision is opened with fine hooks exhibiting the lateral matrix horn which has to be carefully dissected and excised from the base of the distal phalanx (Haneke, 1978, 1984) (Fig. 10.98). A No. 1 needle is inserted along the floor of the lateral nail groove until it is arrested by the terminal phalanx. This will serve as a marker for the limits of the matrix (Austin, 1970; Haneke, 1988) (Fig. 10.99).

The authors do not recommend total ablation of the matrix and nail bed resulting in permanent eradication of the nail organ – which has been advocated in the past (Quenu, 1887; Zadik, 1950) despite the high rate of recurrence (Murray & Bedi, 1975). If decided this procedure is carried out 1 month after nail ablation; the proximal nail fold is reflected after lateral incision exposing the matrix epithelium. Using Austin's technique to determine the most proximo-lateral limits of the matrix, a rectangu-

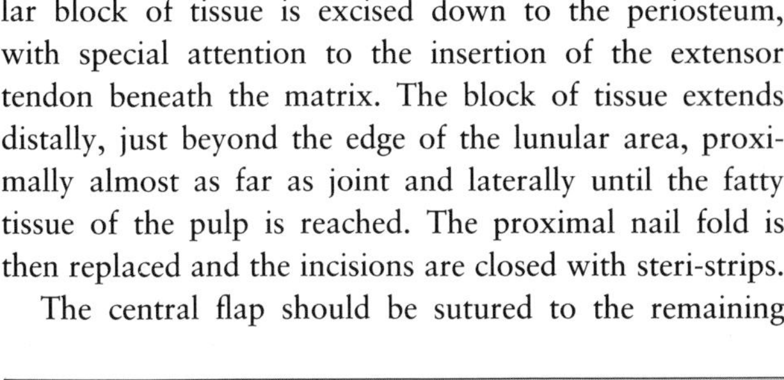

lar block of tissue is excised down to the periosteum, with special attention to the insertion of the extensor tendon beneath the matrix. The block of tissue extends distally, just beyond the edge of the lunular area, proximally almost as far as joint and laterally until the fatty tissue of the pulp is reached. The proximal nail fold is then replaced and the incisions are closed with steri-strips.

The central flap should be sutured to the remaining

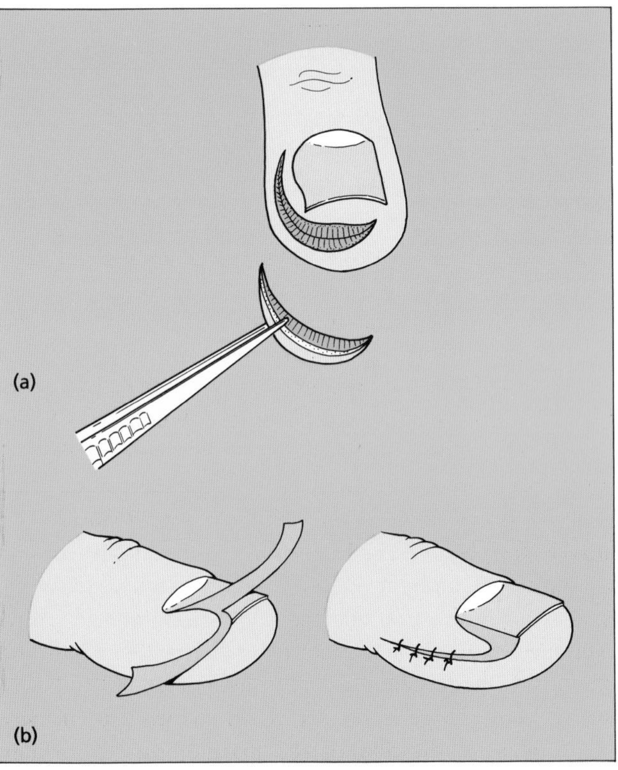

Fig. 10.101. (a) An elliptical wedge of tissue is removed to relieve pressure on the lateral nail fold. (b) A longitudinal wedge, the base of which is at the distal end of the lateral nail fold, is removed and the resultant flap is sutured to the side of the tip of the toe.

distal nail bed only if this can be achieved without tension of the flap. Murray (1979) prefers in many cases to leave the flap free and dress the area with paraffin gauze. If the lateral grooves are deep, the lateral nail folds are excised and the skin edges are sutured to the edges of the nail bed.

The terminal Syme operation

This procedure is still more radical (Thompson & Terwilliger, 1951). It entails the removal of matrix and nail bed with amputation of the distal half of the terminal bone. The ridged skin of the pulp is then pulled dorsally and sutured over the defect of the former matrix. This operation produces a shortened, bulbous big toe (Murray, 1979). This is now absolutely unacceptable, both functionally and cosmetically. These operations are unnecessary mutilating surgery if the more conservative methods have been learned and used correctly.

Hypertrophic lateral nail fold (Fig. 10.100)

Hypertrophic lateral nail fold usually accompanies long-standing ingrowing nails. The nail, generally, looks normal and the soft tissue appears to be at fault when the lip of the lateral nail fold overgrows the nail plate. Inflammation occurs deep beneath the hypertrophied tissue. Therefore, the treatment consists in narrowing the nail plate by phenol cauterization of the lateral nail horn of the matrix. If the hypertrophic tissue does not regress after 2 months, treatment of the soft tissue is then advised. The authors favour an elliptical wedge of tissue taken from the lateral wall of the toe and its disto-lateral portion. This pulls the lateral nail fold away from the offending lateral nail edge (Fig. 10.101(a)).

If lateral nail fold hypertrophy is pronounced its removal has been suggested. In Bose's technique (1971), the point of a No. 11 blade is inserted under the lateral nail fold half way along the nail. The nail fold is then transfixed, so that the point of the blade emerges at a distance of 5–7 mm from the nail fold. The blade is advanced distally in a straight line, cutting the fold, which exposes the distal half of the side of the nail. This cut fold is steadied with forceps: the direction of the blade is reversed, and the proximal part of the fold cut in such a way that the slices of tissue so removed thin out gradually. Any arterial haemorrhage is arrested with electrocautery. The wound is covered with petroleum gauze and the dressing is changed daily until the wound heals by granulation, in approximately 3–4 weeks.

The authors prefer Tweedie and Ranger's procedure (1985), which consists of making a transposition flap of the nail wall. The technique starts as in the previous one but the proximal part of the lateral nail fold is not cut. The flap which is created is then transposed inferiorly and

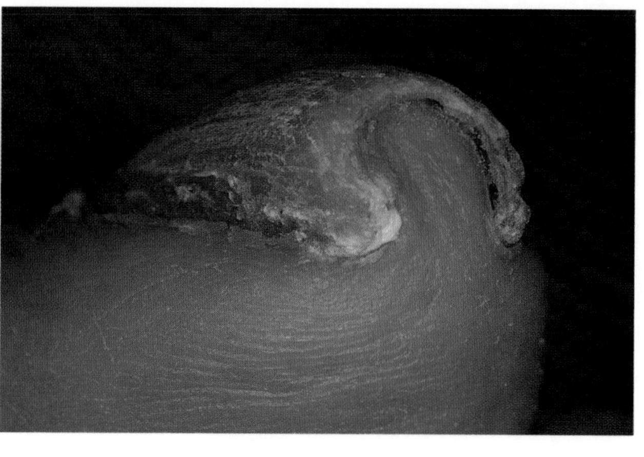

Fig. 10.102. Pincer nail deformity.

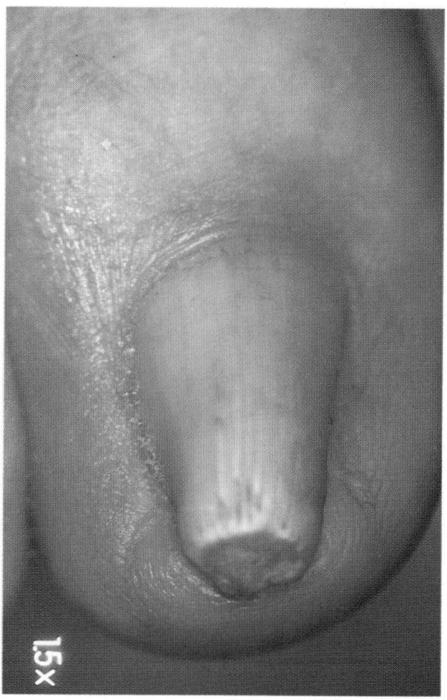

Fig. 10.103. Trumpet nail.

sutured in place with 4-0 nylon sutures. The excess of tissue is cut away (Fig. 10.101(b)).

Inward distortion of the nail plate (**transverse overcurvature, pincer nail, trumpet nail, unguis constringens, omega nail**)

Pincer nail is a dystrophy characterized by transverse overcurvature that increases along the longitudinal axis of the nail and reaches its greatest extent at the distal part, leading to trumpet nails (Baran, 1974) (Figs 10.102 & 10.103). The edges constrict the nail bed tissue and dig into the lateral grooves. Although pain is not severe in most cases, it may sometimes be excruciating. In patients whose nail plate is involved only at the lateral edge, pain will be felt in the lateral nail groove, simulating an ingrowing toenail. In overcurvature affecting the entire nail,

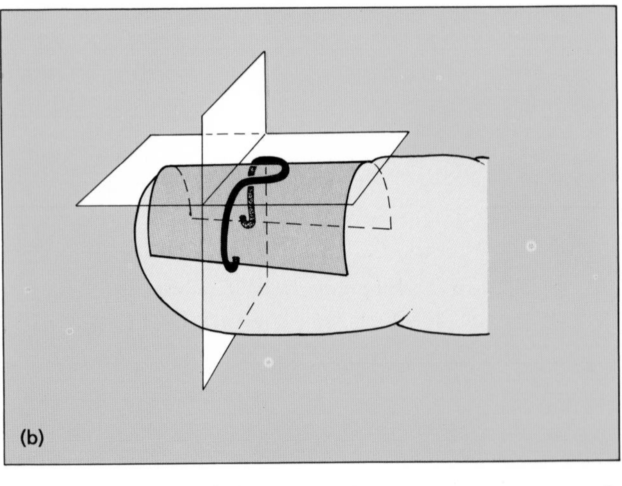

(a)

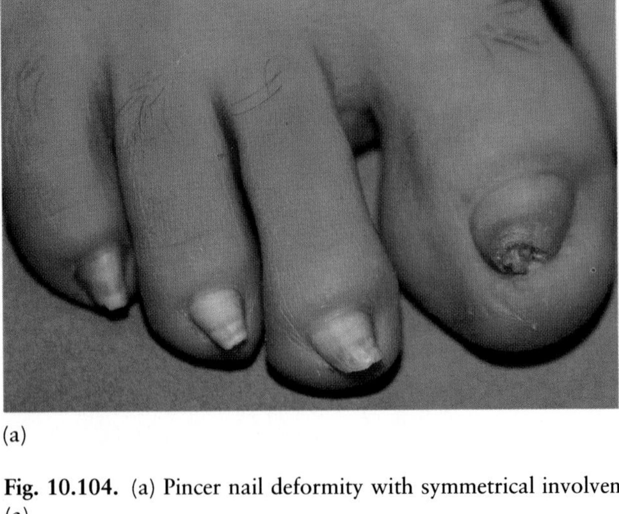

Fig. 10.104. (a) Pincer nail deformity with symmetrical involvement of several toes. (b) 'Brace' method to correct the overcurvature of (a).

the patients have pain along the lateral nail grooves as well, but on occasion they may develop pain specifically under the midpoint of the distal nail edge, dorsal to the distal phalangeal tuft (Douglas & Krull, 1981).

Two varieties of overcurvature can be distinguished (Haneke, 1992).

1 Asymmetrical involvement of usually only the halluces. The major causes are foot deformities and osteoarthritis.

2 Symmetrical involvement of several toes, usually with lateral deviation of the long axis of the hallux nails and medial deviation of the lesser toenails (Fig. 10.104(a) & (b)). This is probably genetically determined.

The pincer nail syndrome (Sorg *et al.*, 1989) includes gryphosis of finger and toenails in combination with acroosteolytic shortening of the end-phalanx and destructive arthrosis of the terminal joints of the digits. Since deformation of the nail is sometimes accompanied by marked pain, definitive cure may be necessary.

Particularly in the genetic form, X-ray films usually show a wider base of the terminal phalanx, often even exhibiting lateral osteophytes. Hyperostosis is also frequently seen on the dorsal tuft of the terminal phalanx, due to traction from heaped-up nail bed which is firmly attached to the bone by collagen fibres (Haneke, 1992).

The pathogenesis of pincer nail is described in Chapter 2.

Conservative management

Clipping. Clipping down the lateral edge of the inward distorted nail plate as proximally as is comfortable may be facilitated by emollients such as 3% salicylic acid in petrolatum. This is applied to the nail edge for 2–3 days before the procedure is undertaken.

Grooving. For the treatment of early cases, grooving of the nail plate with a burr extending forwards from the area of the lunula and terminating at the free edge may be of some help. A central single groove or a series of grooves running parallel to each other should be cut. The latter are cut covering the whole of the dorsal surface of the nail plate. If the nail is greatly thickened, grinding down the thickness may diminish the pressure. This procedure may alleviate the pain, however it increases the overcurvature.

Orthonyx (nail brace technique) (Dagnall, 1976b) (Fig. 10.104(b)). Orthonyx is the term coined by Fraser (1967) to describe the field of mechanical correction. This method is based on maintaining tension in the nail plate. The lateral nail grooves are cleaned in order to clear the space under the sides of the nail for the wire. A brace is constructed to fit the curved plate exactly; then, at one selected point, a minute 'adjustment' (a slight bend) is made to the brace and it is fitted to the plate. The nail plate is weaker than the stainless steel wire and the nail will conform to the shape of the brace. Gradually, a series of 'adjustments' are made and almost imperceptibly the curvature decreases. The nail plate will be flattened painlessly within a period of 6 months (Farnsworth, 1972). This technique has been successfully employed in overcurvature of fingernails associated with arthritis of the distal joint (R. Baran, unpublished data), but was followed by recurrence within a few weeks in other cases (E. Haneke, unpublished).

Unfortunately, pathogenesis of overcurvature explains why neither nail brace technique, nor repeated nail avulsion, will definitely cure the condition. Instead some patients report even that nail avulsion exacerbated their difficulties.

Surgical treatment (Fig. 10.105(a),(b) & (c))

Surgery cannot remove the lateral osteophytes to restore a normal matrix shape. After bilateral partial nail avulsion, the lateral matrix horns are treated as described above for

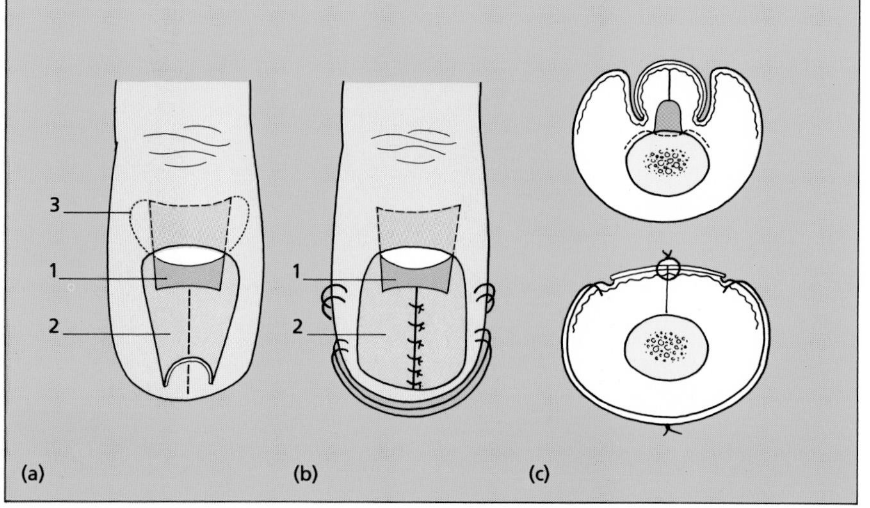

Fig. 10.105. (a) **1**: Nail plate after narrowing and removal of distal two-thirds; **2**: nail bed; **3**: matrix horn. Removal of lateral matrix horns, bilateral nail strip removal and flattening and spreading of remaining nail plate on previously separated nail bed (b & c) – the enclosed hyperostosis is removed with a bone rongeur (c).

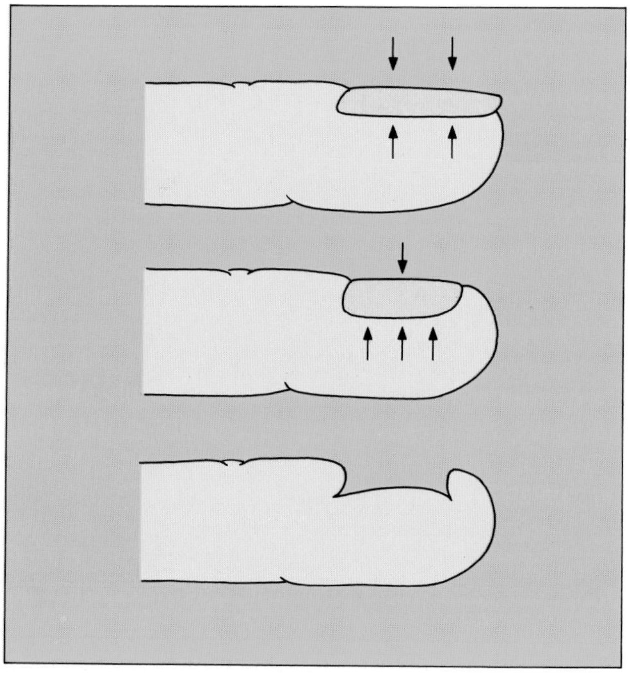

Fig. 10.106. Distal nail embedding – may occur after nail avulsion and regrowth (adapted from Fowler, 1958).

subcutaneous ingrowing toenails; the distal two-thirds of the nail are carefully removed. Then a longitudinal median incision of the nail bed is carried down to the bone. While doing this, one can usually feel the dorsal traction osteophyte. The entire nail bed is dissected from the phalanx and the dorsal tuft removed with a bone rongeur. The nail bed is spread and sutured with 6-0 PDS atraumatic stitches and kept in this position by using reversed tie-over sutures that pull the lateral nail folds apart. To prevent the sutures from cutting through the lateral nail folds, small rubber tubes are placed into the lateral grooves and the threads laid over them. These stitches are left for 18–21 days to allow the nail bed to adhere in the restored form (Baran & Haneke, 1987; Haneke & Baran, 1991).

Distal nail embedding (Fig. 10.106)

Particularly in the great toe, a distal wall may develop after nail avulsion or nail shedding following tennis toe for example. The nail in its normal position counteracts the forces that are exerted during walking. Due to lack of

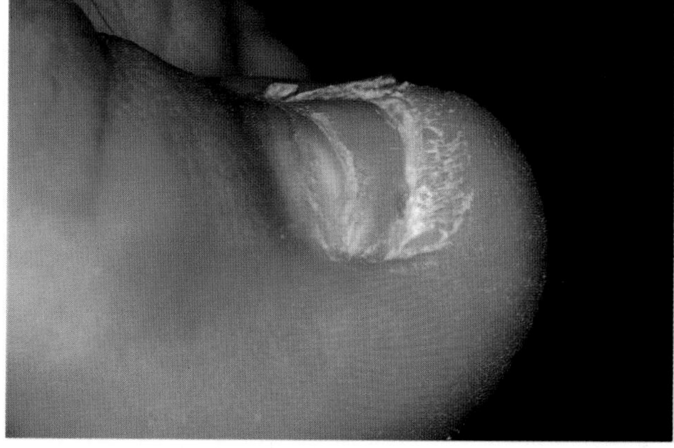

(a)

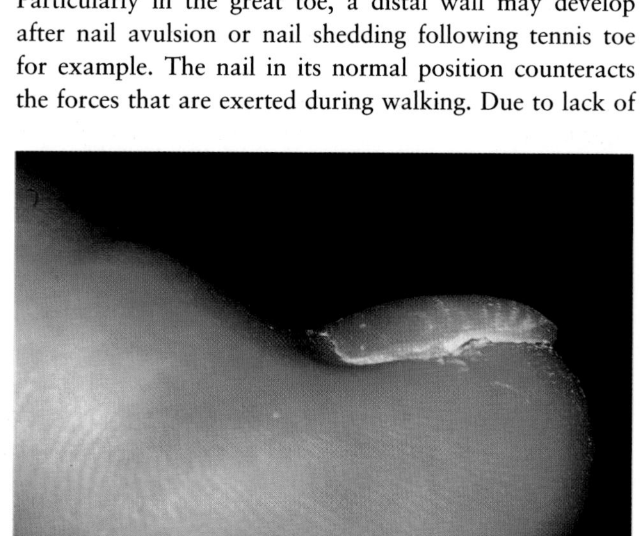

(b)

Fig. 10.107. Distal nail embedding (a) acrylic sculptered nail anchored into the embedded nail plate (b).

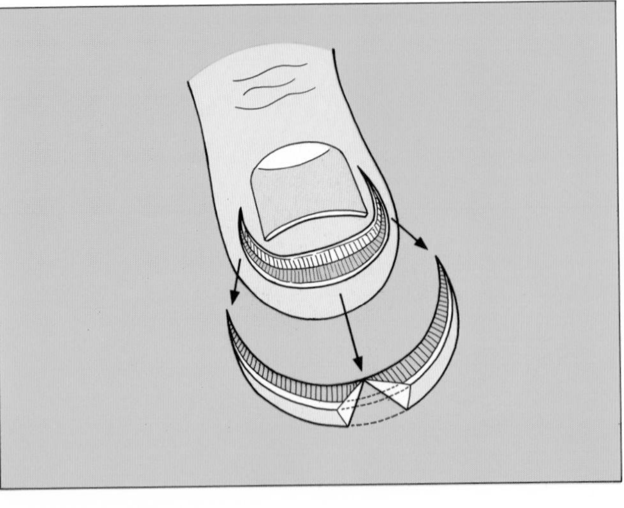

Fig. 10.108. Dubois' technique.

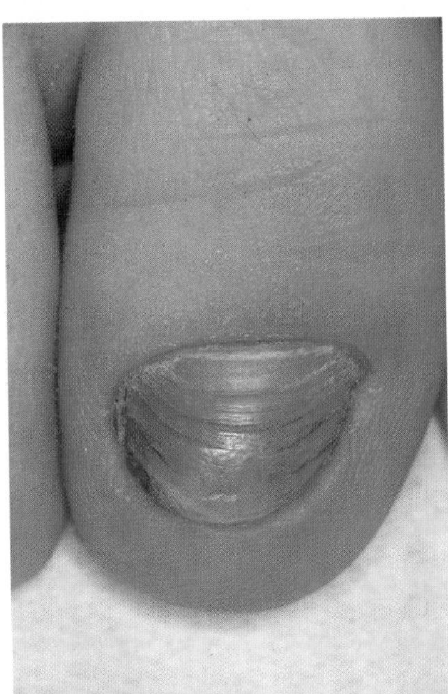

Fig. 10.110. Distal toenail embedding with normally directed nail.

counter pressure, the plantar portion of the hallux pulp becomes distorted dorsally when the foot rolls up and the body weight presses on the tip of the big toe during walking. The terminal phalanx looks shorter and the distal wall interferes with the growth of the newly formed nail plate (Fig. 10.107(a) & (b)). When the distal wall cannot be reversed by massaging back in a distal–plantar direction, the anchoring of an acrylic sculptured nail on the stump nail may enable it to overgrow the heaped up distal tissue. Should this procedure not be effective, a crescent-shaped wedge excision becomes necessary. A fish-mouth incision is carried out parallel to the distal groove around the tip of the toe, starting and ending 3–5 mm proximal to the end of the lateral nail fold. A second incision is then done to yield a wedge of 4–8 mm at its greatest width and

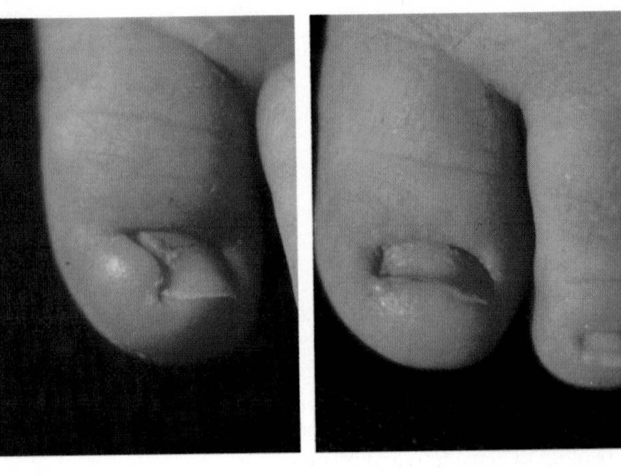

Fig. 10.109. Congenital hypertrophic lip of the great toe and its spontaneous correction (right) (courtesy of Ceccolini, Bulogna, Italy).

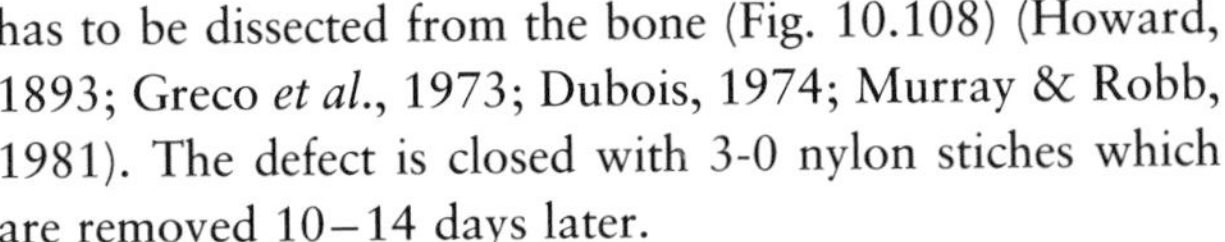

has to be dissected from the bone (Fig. 10.108) (Howard, 1893; Greco *et al.*, 1973; Dubois, 1974; Murray & Robb, 1981). The defect is closed with 3-0 nylon stiches which are removed 10–14 days later.

Ingrowing toenail in infancy

There are three kinds of ingrowing toenail in infancy before age 12 (Baran, 1989).

1 Congenital hypertrophic lip of the hallux (Fig. 10.109). In contrast to the hypertrophic lateral nail fold observed in adults, the congenital hypertrophic lip of the hallux disappears *spontaneously* after several months (Rufli *et al.*, 1992).

2 Distal toenail embedding with normally directed nail (Fig. 10.110). Conservative management is the rule. In those rare cases where permanent improvement has not been obtained by 1 year of age, a circular soft tissue resection should be performed in an identical manner as in adults.

3 Congenital malalignment of the big toenail (Baran *et al.*, 1979, 1983) (Fig. 10.111(a) & (b)) (see Chapter 3).

Should an operation be decided in this often misdiagnosed condition a crescent wedge-shaped resection must be carried back proximal to and below the nail bed and nail matrix (Fig. 10.110(c)). The crescent has to be much larger on the medial than on the lateral aspect. A small, triangular area is also excised at the start of the lateral incision line, thereby enabling the whole nail apparatus to be swung over the resected area so that it can be realigned and then sutured. When the nail deviation is medial instead of lateral, in contrast to the usual type, the crescent has to be larger on the lateral aspect than on the medial one, and a small triangular area is also excised at the start of the medial incision line thereby enabling the whole nail apparatus to be swung over the resected area, in order

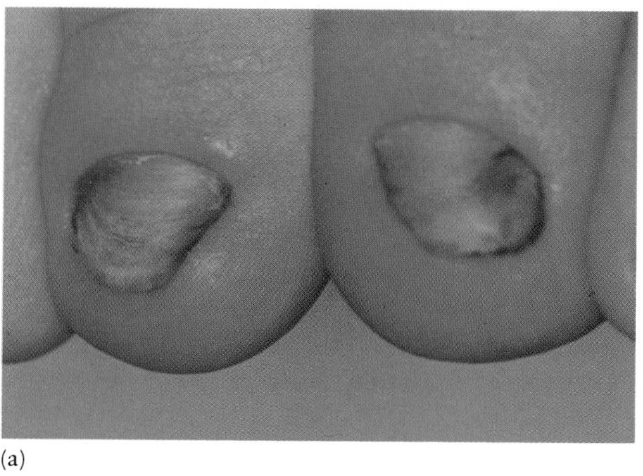
(a)

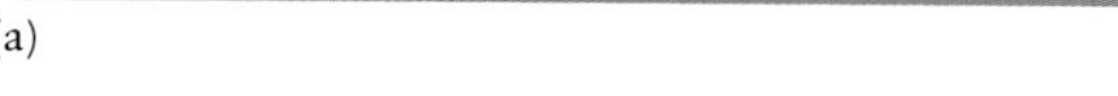

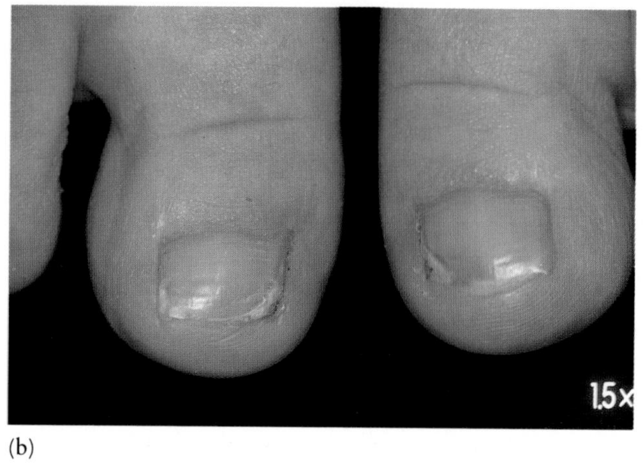

(b)

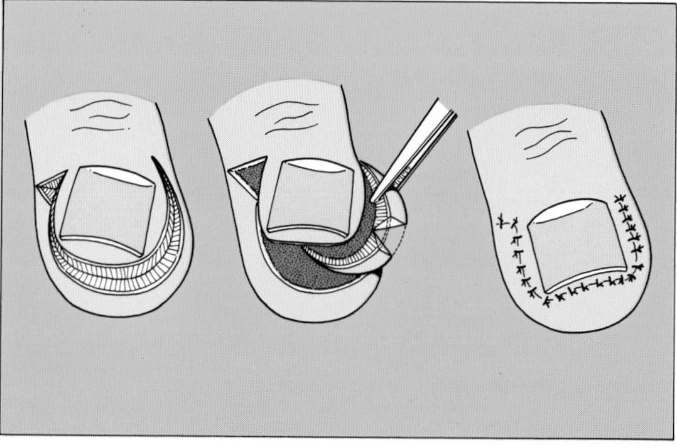
(c)

Fig. 10.111. Congenital malalignment of the great toenails before (a) and after correction (b) using procedure in (c).

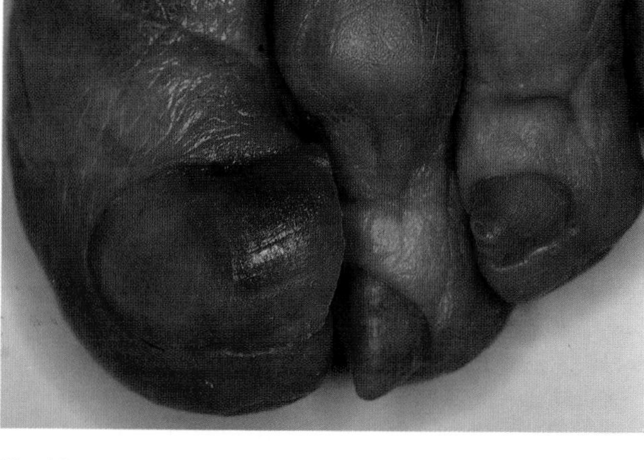

Fig. 10.112. Congenital malalignment – untreated, in an elderly subject.

that it can be realigned and then sutured (Baran & Bureau, 1983). If performed in motivated adults, this operation has given improvement and even complete recovery in some cases (Fig. 10.112).

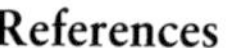

References

Austin R.T. (1970) A method of excision of the germinal matrix. *Proc. Roy. Soc. Med.* **63**, 757–758.

Baran R. (1974) Pincer and trumpet nails. *Arch. Dermatol.* **110**, 639.

Baran R. (1989) The treatment of ingrowing toenails in infancy. *J. Dermatol. Treat.* **1**, 55–57.

Baran R. & Bureau H. (1983) Congenital malalignment of the big toe-nail as a cause of ingrowing toe-nail in infancy. Pathology and treatment (a study of thirty cases). *Clin. Exp. Dermatol.* **8**, 619–623.

Baran R. & Haneke E. (1987) Surgery of the nail. In: *Skin Surgery*, eds Epstein E. & Epstien E. Jr. W.B. Saunders, Philadelphia.

Bose B. (1971) A technique for excision of nail fold for ingrowing toenail. *Surg. Gyn. Obstet.* **132**, 511.

Brown F.C. (1981) Chemocautery for ingrown toenails. *J. Dermatol. Surg. Oncol.* **7**, 331.

Dagnall J.C. (1976a) The history, development and current status of nail matrix phenolisation. *Chiropodist* **36**, 315–324.

Dagnall J.C. (1976b) The development of nail treatments. *Br. J. Chirop.* **41**, 165.

Douglas M.C. & Krull E.A. (1981) Diseases of the Nails. *Conn's Current Therapy*, ed., p. 712. W.B. Saunders, Philadelphia.

Dubois J.Ph. (1974) Un traitement de l'ongle incarné. *Nouv. Presse Med.* 3, 1938.

Farnsworth F.C. (1972) A treatment for convoluted nails. *J. Am. Podiat. Assoc.* **62**, 110.

Fowler A.W. (1958) Excision of the germinal matrix: A unified treatment for toenail and onychogryphosis. *Br. J. Surg.* **45**, 382.

Fraser A.R. (1967) Orthonyx: theory and practice. *Br. J. Chirop.* **32**, 229.

Gilles G.A., Dennis K.J. & Harkless L.B. (1986) Periostitis associated with phenol matricectomies. *JAPA* **76**, 469–472.

Greco J., Kiniffo H.V., Chanterelle A. *et al.* (1973) L'attaque des parties molles, secret de la cure chirurgicale de l'ongle incarné. Un point de technique. *Ann. Chir. Plast.* **18**, 363.

Haneke E. (1978) Chirurgische Behandlung des Unguis incarnatus. In: *Operative Dermatologie*, ed. Salfed K. Springer, Berlin.

Haneke E. (1986) Surgical treatment of ingrown toenails. *Cutis* **37**, 251–256.

Haneke E. (1992) Etiopathogénie et traitement de l'hypercourbure transversale de l'ongle du gros orteil. *J. Méd. Esth. Chir. Dermatol.* **19**, 123–127.

Haneke E. & Baran R. (1991) Nails: surgical aspects. In: *Aesthetic Dermatology*, eds Parish L.C. & Lask G.P. McGraw Hill, New York.

Howard W.R. (1893) Ingrown toenail; its surgical treatment. *N. Y. Med. J.* 579.

Ilfeld F.W. (1991) Ingrown toenail treated with cotton collodion insert. *Foot Ankle* **11**, 312–313.

Langford D.T., Burke C. & Robertson K. (1989) Risk factors in onychocryptosis. *Br. J. Surg.* **76**, 45–48.

Maeda N., Mizuno N.M. & Ichikawa K. (1990) Nail abrasion: A new treatment for ingrown toenails. *J. Dermatol.* **17**, 746–749.

Murray W.R. (1979) Onychocryptosis. Principles of non-operative and operative care. *Clin. Orthop. Rel. Res.* **142**, 96.

Murray W.R. & Bedi B.S. (1975) The surgical management of ingrowing toenail. *Br. J. Surg.* **62**, 409.

Murray W.R. & Robb J.E. (1981) Soft-tissue resection for ingrowing toenails. *J. Dermatol. Surg. Oncol.* **7**, 757.

Palmer B.V. & Jones A. (1979) Ingrowing toenails: the results of treatment. *Br. J. Surg.* **66**, 575.

Quenu M. (1887) Des limites de la matrice de l'ongle. Applications au traitement de l'ongle incarné. *Bull. Soc. Chir. Paris* **13**, 252.

Reszler M. & Mari B. (1981) Beitrag zum Unguis incarnatus-Syndrom. *Z. Hautkr.* **56**, 172.

Rinaldi R., Sabia M. & Gross J. (1982) The treatment and prevention of infection in phenol alcohol matricectomies. *JAPA* **72**, 453.

Rufli T., Von Schulthess A. & Itin P. (1992) Congenital hypertrophy of the lateral nail folds of the hallux. *Dermatology* **184**, 296–297.

Steigleder G.K. & Stober-Münster J. (1977) Das Syndrom des eingewachsenen Nagel. *Z. Hautkr.* **52**, 1225.

Thompson C. & Terwilliger C. (1951) The terminal Syme operation for ingrown toenail. *Surg. Clin. N. Am.* **31**, 575.

Tweedie J.H. & Ranger I. (1985) A simple procedure with nail preservation for ingrowing toenails. *Arch. Emerg. Med.* **2**, 149–154.

Zadik F.R. (1950) Obliteration of the nail bed of the great toe without shortening the terminal phalanx. *J. Bone Joint Surg.* **32B**, 66.

Complications of nail surgery

(Haneke & Baran, 1993)

Proper examination of the patient before performing nail surgery and correct technique may help avoid the commonest complications and rule out high-risk patients.

Bleeding

With simple procedures such as nail avulsion or punch biopsy, haemostasis is easily accomplished during operation simply by pressure on the lateral aspects of the digit. For more elaborate techniques an exsanguinating tourniquet can be made with a surgical glove. The rubber on the tip of the finger to be operated on is cut across and the glove is rolled down the finger.

If bleeding persists a Penrose drain is secured with a haemostat. The tourniquet should not be kept in place for more than 15 min, otherwise there is a risk of gangrene; therefore for longer procedures it has to be released for some minutes every 15 min. Hydropneumatic tourniquets are much less traumatizing than rubber tubes.

Post-operatively bleeding may be extensive, particularly after the release of the tourniquet. However, because the vessels involved are small, the bleeding can usually be controlled by direct pressure. Oxidized cellulose (oxycel, surgicel, gelfoam) and a dab of aluminium chloride (35%) solution may be applied if these methods prove to be unsatisfactory.

Pain

There is considerable individual variation in pain threshold. Pre-operative sedation is helpful in most patients undergoing nail surgery. Atarax (hydroxyzine) may be given – 25 mg the previous evening and repeated 2 h prior to the operation.

During operation, pain is due to poor anaesthesia.

Post-operatively, dressings must be padded to avoid injury and sealed with papertape, anchored in longitudinal pattern. The extremity should be elevated to reduce oedema, which is frequent, and pain which is decreased when the arm is put in a sling. The foot has to be elevated to 30° and the patient kept recumbent for 48 h. Pain may be significant, and therefore analgesia with acetaminophen with codeine should be available, mainly for special techniques such as cryosurgery. The addition of marcaine at the completion of the surgery is advisible, together with 0.4 ml dexamethasone in the original anaesthesia site, if there is no infection (Salasche & Peters, 1985).

Infection

Pre-operatively: strict aseptic procedures are similar to those used when performing any cutaneous surgery with local application of antiseptic solutions. The use of a sterile surgical glove, with the appropriate digit removed, will provide an aseptic covering for the rest of the patient's hand. Infection should be controlled since the consequences of extensive digital cellulitis may be severe. Tetanus toxoid for lesions of the toes should be discussed and advised especially in farmers, for example, as well as the use of prophylactic antibiotics for surgical patients with prosthetic cardiac valves or compromised circulation.

Post-operative infection can happen where infection was latent and not suspected prior to the operation. When infection is present, the organism should be cultured and treated immediately with antibiotics and antiseptic soaks. Post-operative infection has significant morbidity in the distal phalanx including felon, compartmental cellulitis and lymphangitis and osteomyelitis.

Necrosis

Necrosis, even without patent infection, may be seen when sutures are too tight and not removed in due time.

Recurrences

Recurrences will depend on the nature of the original lesions.

Permanent residual defects

These may lead to unsightly scarring.

1 Matrix involvement: crush injuries leave many small pieces of subungual tissue. If these fragments are not incorporated into the repair, some may grow independently and cause nail horns or spicules that must be removed.

2 In operations involving the lunula border it is cosmetically important to maintain the curvilinear configuration of the distal lunula which plays an important role in shaping the free edge of the nail plate.

3 Nail deformities have occurred from drilling the nail plate for the release of subungual haematoma and from rough or careless removal of the nail to expose the bed. Nail deformities may also occur from the use of vicryl sutures in nail bed repair. These sutures, if too large, dissolve too slowly and are still present during the new nail growth. This can produce an area of onycholysis and ridging in the nail.

Unpredictable complications

Two cases of reflex sympathetic dystrophy have been reported following a correct biopsy of the nail bed (Ingram *et al.*, 1987; Haneke, 1992). The appearance of an epidermoid implantation cyst in an operation scar is another unfortunate example of unpredictable complication (Baran & Bureau, 1988; Nakajima *et al.*, 1990). Self-resolving deformation of the nail following elastic band traction is unusual in the post-operative management of flexor tendon injuries (Hoddinot & Matthews, 1989). Ingrowing of a big toenail recurring several months after a successful toe-to-thumb transfer should suggest the possible complication and treatment of the nail before the transfer (Sadr & Schenck, 1982).

References

Baran R. & Bureau H. (1988) Two post-operative epidermoid cysts following realignment of the hallux nail. *Br. J. Dermatol.* **119**, 245–247.

Haneke E. (1992) Sympathische Reflexdystrophie (Sudeck-Dystrophie) nach Nagelbiopsie. *Zbl. Haut. Geschl. Kr.* **160**, 263.

Haneke E. & Baran R. (1993) Nail surgery. In: *Complications in Dermatologic Surgery*, ed. Harahap M. Springer, Berlin.

Hoddinot C. & Matthews J.P. (1989) Deformation of the nail following elastic band traction – A case report. *J. Hand Surg.* **14B**, 23–24.

Ingram G.J., Scher R.K. & Lally E.V. (1987) Reflex sympathetic dystrophy following nail biopsy. *J. Am. Acad. Dermatol.* **16**, 253–256.

Nakajima T., Yoshimura Y. & Yoneda K. (1990) Open treatment with drainage for ingrowing toenail. *Surg. Gynecol. Obstet.* **170**, 223–224.

Sadr B. & Schenck R.R. (1982) Ingrowing nail of a transplanted toe. *Hand* **14**, 337–338.

Salasche S.J. & Peters V.J. (1985) Tips on nail surgery. *Cutis* **35**, 428–438.

Infection

The hand's reaction to infection is dominated by anatomical considerations. The first stage in treatment of hand or foot infection is accurate and prompt diagnosis (Haussman & Lisser, 1992). Radiographs are required to identify foreign bodies, bone lesions, associated fractures and gas formation.

Infection of the nail folds

It is represented by inflammation, swelling and abscess formation. It can be either acute or chronic.

Acute paronychia

Minor trauma is a frequent cause of this infection and surgical treatment may be necessary. Acute paronychia may follow a break in the skin (e.g. if a hangnail is torn), a splinter under the distal edge of the nail, a prick from a thorn in a lateral groove, or sometimes from an infection secondary to a haematoma. When it spreads superficially around the proximal nail fold it has been nicknamed a 'runaround' (bulla repens or rodens). The infection starts

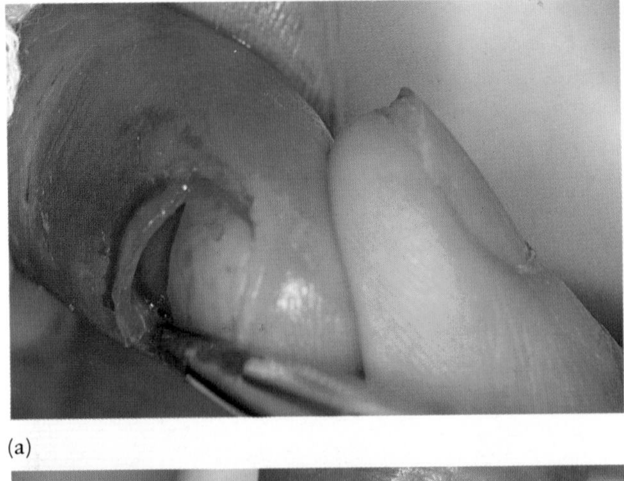

(a)

(b)

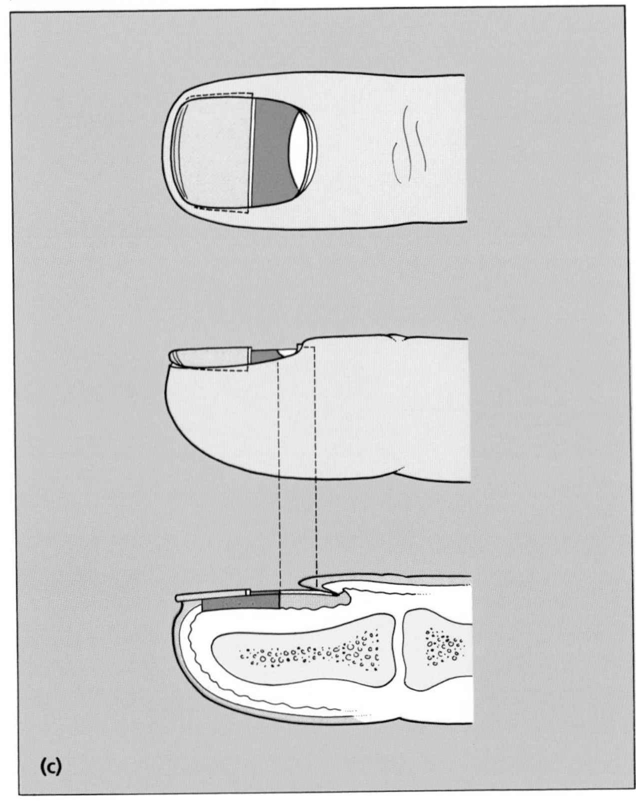

(c)

Fig. 10.113. Acute paronychia: removal of proximal nail (a & b); (c) shows the areas removed in red.

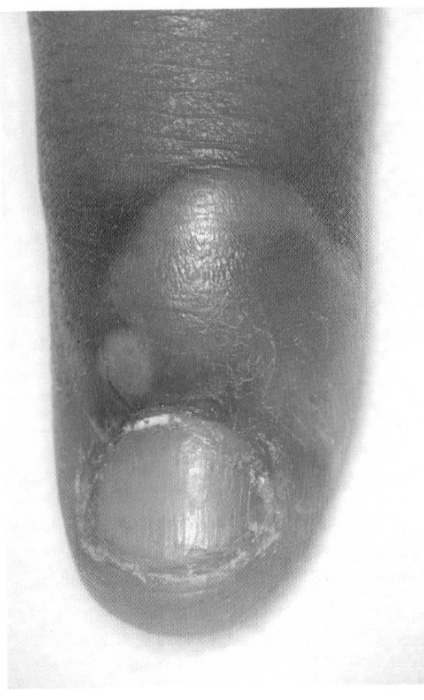

Fig. 10.114. Bullous pyoderma associated with acute paronychia.

in the paronychium at the side of the nail with local redness, swelling and pain. At this stage medical treatment is indicated: wet compresses (Burow's solution) or alcoholic baths and appropriate systemic antibiotic therapy are given. Because the continuation of antibiotics may mask developing pathology which can damage the nail apparatus, if acute paronychia does not show clear signs of response to penicillinase-resistant antibiotics within 2 days, then surgical treatment should be instituted (Vilain *et al.*, 1978), using proximal block anaesthesia. A penrose drain can be used as a tourniquet at the base of the digit but with suppuration infections, exsanguination of the finger should be accomplished by hand elevation only. Localization of the purulent reaction may take several days and during this time throbbing pain is always a major symptom. The collection of pus may easily be seen through the nail or at the paronychial fold. A bead of pus may present in the periungual groove. In the absence of visible pus, the 'gathering' gives rise to tension and classically the lesion should be incised at the site of maximum pain, not necessarily at the site of the maximum swelling. In practice, Bunell's technique is easy, successful and favoured by the authors: the base of the nail (the proximal third) is removed by cutting across with pointed scissors (Boyes, 1964) (Fig. 10.113(a),(b),(c)). A non-adherent gauze wick is laid under the proximal nail fold. If the infection in the paronychium remains restricted to one side, removal of the homologous lateral part of the nail is sufficient. Bacterial culture and sensitivity studies are of great importance. The bacteria most commonly found in acute paronychia are staphylococci (sensitive to second generation cephalosporins) and less commonly, β-haemolytic streptococci and Gram-negative enteric bac-

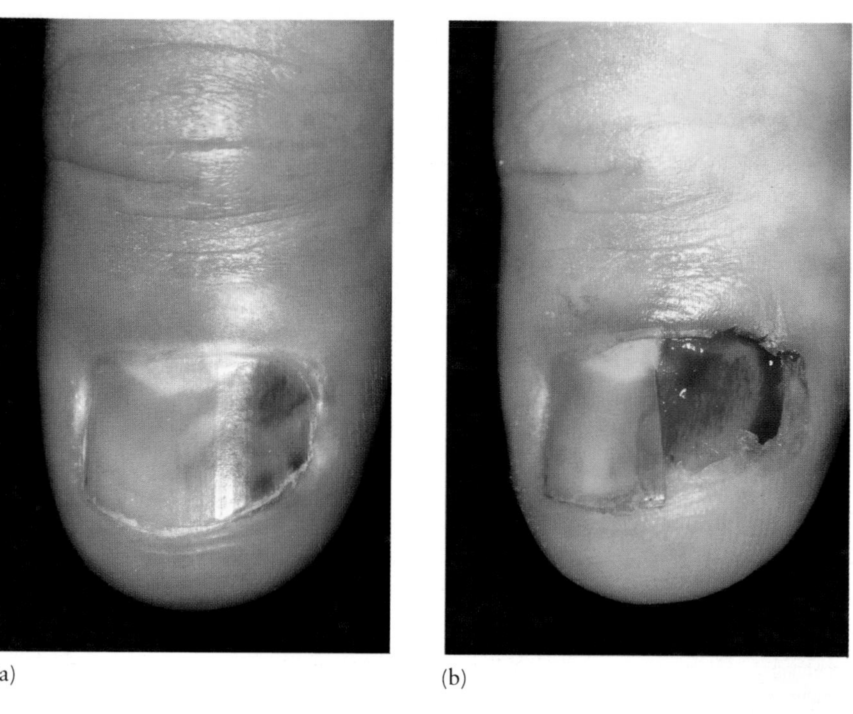

(a) (b)

Fig. 10.115. (a) Acute paronychia with subungual spread. (b) Removal of nail overlying purulent area.

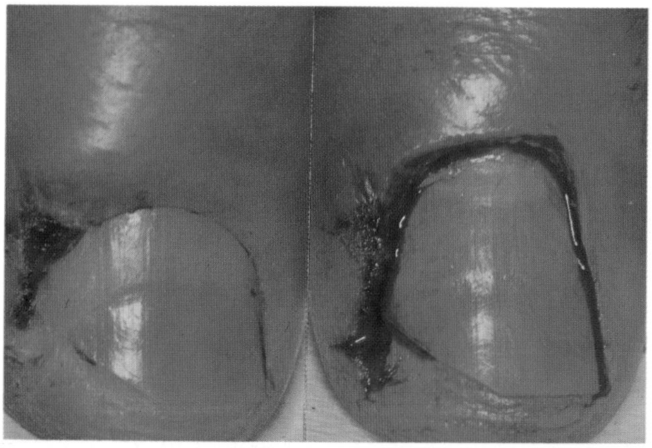

(a)

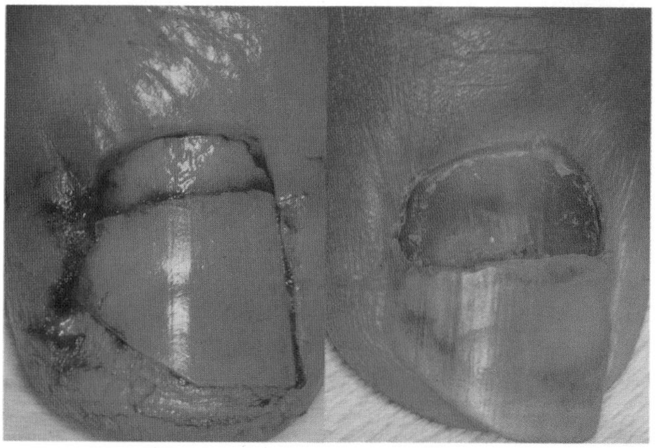

(b)

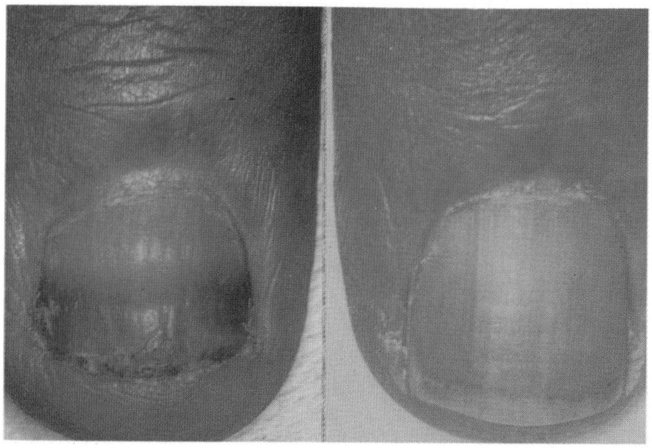

(c)

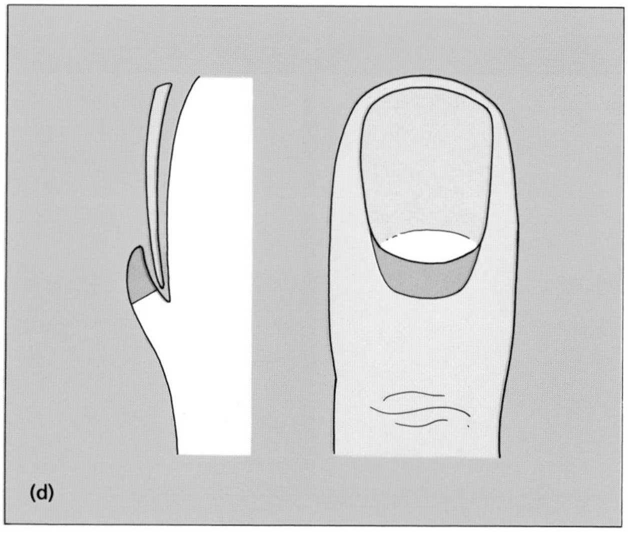

(d)

Fig. 10.116. (a) Chronic paronychia, (b) excision of the proximal nail fold, proximal nail excised and (c) subsequent good healing of the treated area, regrowth of the nail plate (e, f). (d) Diagram showing the proximal nail fold removed.

teria. Empirical antibiotic therapy should cover both aerobes and anaerobes (Brown & Young, 1993). Should surgical intervention be delayed the pus will track around the base of the nail under the proximal nail fold and inflame the matrix; it may then be responsible for transient or permanent dystrophy of the nail plate. It is essential to note that the nail matrix of a child is particularly fragile and can be destroyed within 48 h of acute bacterial infection. The pus may also separate the nail from its loose, underlying attachment proximally. The firmer attachment of the nail at the distal border of the lunula may offer some temporary resistance to the spread of the pus. In cases of extension under part of the distal nail bed, the whole nail base is removed and enough nail removed distally to fully expose the involved nail bed (Lowden, 1964).

Often the patient presents with a localized abscess adjacent to the cuticle. The superficiality of the abscess is readily apparent by the greenish discoloration; drainage may be carried out by lifting the cuticle and excising the epidermal layer over the infection without anaesthesia (Keyser *et al.*, 1990).

Sometimes, the evacuation of bullous pyoderma brings to light a narrow sinus (Fig. 10.114). This may be part of a 'collar stud' abscess which communicates with a deeper, necrotic inoculation zone. This must be exposed and excised. Bacterial cultures and systemic antibiotic therapy are always necessary.

If the infection in the paronychium remains restricted to one side, removal of the homologous lateral part of the nail is sufficient (Fig. 10.115) and a small wick of Betadine gauze is used to promote drainage.

If acute paronychia accompanies ingrowing nail, the treatment must be supplemented by removing all offending portions of the nail plate. After surgery, the dressing is kept moist with saline or antiseptic soaks. This should be changed daily after soaking in antiseptic until the purulent discharge stops. The finger, hand and forearm should ideally be raised and splinted for 2–3 days.

In acute paronychia it is common for only one nail to be involved. In chronic or subacute paronychia, whose flares may mimic acute paronychia, one or several fingernails may be infected. The differential diagnosis includes:

1 paronychial involvement of the fingernails accompanying chronic eczema and herpetic whitlow – the latter has been reported in association with bacterial abscess (Hurst *et al.*, 1991);

2 psoriasis and Reiter's disease, which may also involve the proximal nail fold.

Chronic paronychia

Chronic paronychia manifests as a red painless swelling with secondary retraction of the perionychial tissue. This results from loss of the cuticle and separation of the nail plate from the undersurface of the proximal nail fold. In recalcitrant cases, the thickened nail fold may be excised under regional block anaesthesia and anaemia (Baran & Bureau, 1981) (Fig. 10.116(a)–(f)). A Freer septum elevator is inserted into the proximal nail groove under the proximal nail fold to protect the matrix and extensor tendon. A No. 15 Bard-Parker blade or No. 67 Beaver blade is used to excise en-bloc a crescent-shaped full thickness skin, 4 mm at its greatest width, which extends from one lateral nail fold to the other. This includes the swollen portion of the proximal nail fold, with the septum elevator moved according to the tip of the scalpel to prevent the matrix from being inadvertently cut. A bevel incision prevents sustaining excision of the nail producing tissues of the proximal nail fold, responsible for the normal shine of the nail plate. Subsequently the area is dressed with an antibiotic preparation. Complete healing, by secondary intention, and restoration of the proximal nail fold, with its adherent cuticle, will take place in less

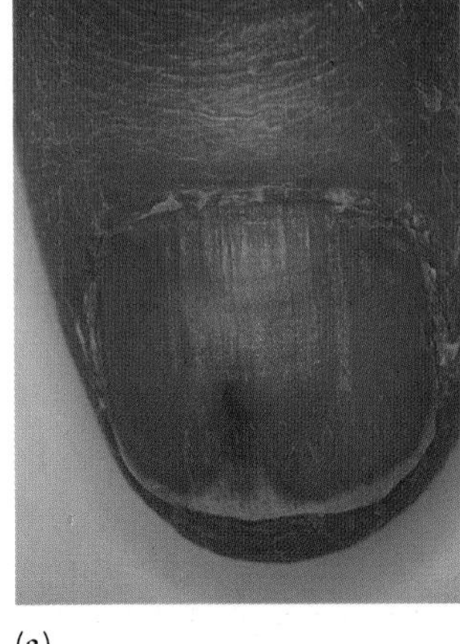
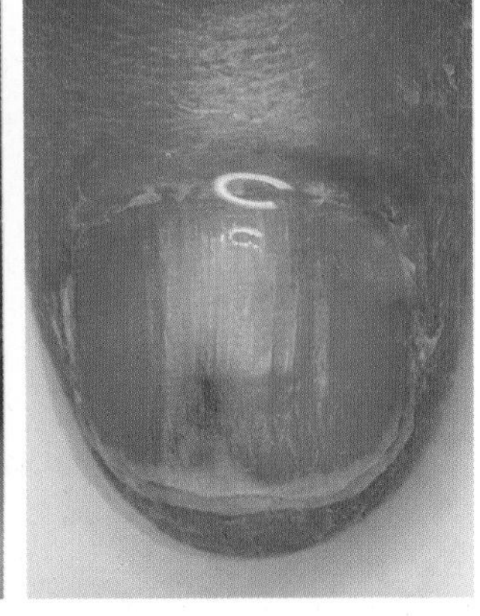

(a)

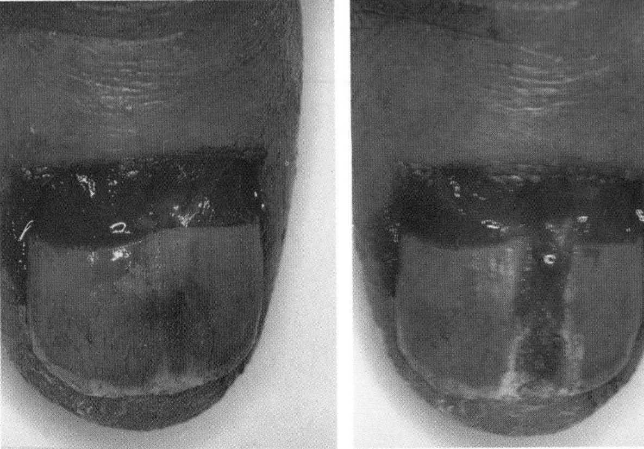
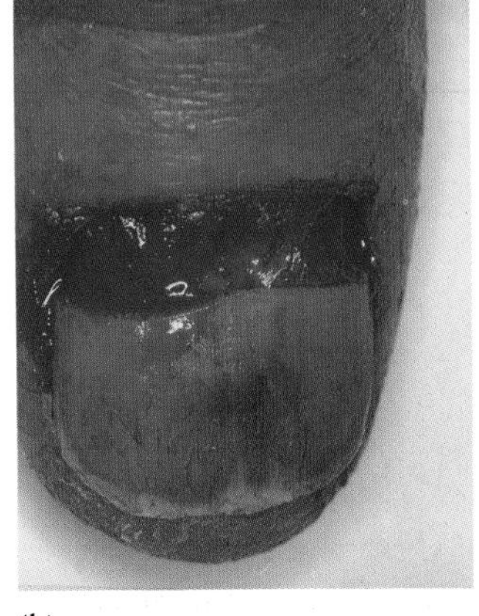

(b)

Fig. 10.117. Subungual infection (a) and parts of nail removed (b) for removal of the pus and drainage.

than 1 month. The nail fold is generally slightly retracted compared with the original one.

The author's technique is derived from Keyser and Eaton's crescentic marsupialization procedure (1976). It is simpler and more likely to be curative and functionally and cosmetically satisfactory. It is only used in severe cases when all else has failed. In patients who experience repeated acute painful flares associated with chronic paronychia, removal of the base of the nail plate is useful (Baran, 1981). Nail removal completing the marsupialization technique provides also better results in hands (Bednar & Lane, 1991).

Subungual infection

In subungual infection, palpation will generally define the most painful area and give a reasonable indication for the site of 'fenestration' of the nail plate. A U-shaped piece of the distal nail plate is excised in the region loosened by the pus and debridement of the affected nail bed area carried out (Fig. 10.117(a) & (b)). The yellow colour of the subungual pus will sometimes be an adequate guide for partial nail avulsion. Soaking the finger in antiseptic solutions, such as chlorhexidine, twice daily and dressing with wet compresses usually results in rapid healing.

Lacerations of the nail bed represent a violation of the cutaneous barrier to bacterial contamination of the underlying bone. If the latter is fractural, it will often extend through the adjacent skin, resulting in an open fracture (Fox, 1992).

Granulatomatous purulent nail bed inflammation

In lectitis purulenta et granulomatosa (Runne *et al.*, 1978) the nail bed of all the fingers may be affected by lenticular polycyclic macules surrounded by a yellowish area. These are visible through the normal nail plate. After nail avulsion, the nail bed reveals large masses of granulomatous tissue with marked acanthosis, parakeratosis and subcorneal haemorrhage. There is prominent polymorphonuclear leucocyte inflammation with proliferation of blood vessels. The condition results in permanent damage such as onycholysis and thickening of the nail.

Purulent inflammation of the nail bed of the great toe, probably secondary to repeated minor trauma from hiking shoes, was observed in a 68-year-old man. The nail covered a grossly enlarged terminal phalanx. It was discoloured and 'floated' on a 'serosanguinous' nail bed. It was easily removed, exposing large masses of granulation tissue on the nail bed, lateral sulci and nail walls. Biopsies taken from the nail bed and lateral nail wall showed a very dense, diffuse inflammatory cell infiltrate composed of granulocytes, lymphocytes and abundant eosinophils, in some areas giving the appearance of eosinophil abscess formation; eosinophil degranulation subsequently led to intensely eosinophilic, hyalin collagen fibres. The nail bed epithelium was either absent or spongiotic. Healing after nail avulsion was uneventful (Haneke, unpubl.).

References

Baran R. (1981) Nail growth direction revisited (Why do nail grow out instead of up?) *J. Am. Acad. Dermatol.* **4**, 78–82.

Baran R. & Bureau H. (1981) Surgical treatment of recalcitrant chronic paronychia of the fingers. *J. Dermatol. Surg. Oncol.* 7, 106–107.

Bednar M.S. & Lane L.B. (1991) Eponychial marsupialization and nail removal for surgical treatment of chronic paronychia. *J. Hand Surg.* **16A**, 314–317.

Brown D.M. & Young V.L. (1993) Hand infections. *South. Med. J.* **86**, 56–66.

Fox I.M. (1992) Osteomyelitis of the distal phalanx following trauma to the nail. A case report. *J. Am. Pod. Med. Assoc.* **82**, 542–544.

Haussman M.R. & Lisser S.P. (1992) Hand infections. *Orthop. Clin. N. Am.* **23**, 171–185.

Hurst L.C., Gluck R., Sampson S.P. *et al.* (1991) Herpetic whitlow with bacterial abscess. *J. Hand Surg.* **16A**, 311–314.

Keyser J.J. & Eaton R.G. (1976) Surgical cure of chronic paronychia by eponychial marsupialization. *Plast. Reconst. Surg.* **58**, 66.

Keyser J.J., Littler J.W. & Eaton R.G. (1990) Surgical treatment of infections and lesions of the perionychium. *Hand Clin.* **6**, 137–153.

Lowden T.G. (1964) Prevention and treatment of hand infections. *Postgrad. Med. J.* **40**, 247.

Runne U., Goertz E. & Weese A. (1978) Lectitis purulenta et granulomatosa. *Z. Hautkr.* **53**, 625.

Vilain R., Leviet D., Mitz V. *et al.* (1978) Le panaris, le praticien, les antibiotiques et le chirurgien. *Nouv. Presse Med.* **7**, 2161.

The management of diabetic and high-risk patients (Patterson & Hunter, 1989)

There are several conditions which place patients in the high-risk group. These and their associated problems, include:

- diabetes mellitus with neuropathy: increased incidence of infection and gangrene;
- peripheral vascular disease: gangrene;
- diseases of the nervous system – motor and sensory impairment: infection, gangrene;
- steroid therapy: infection;
- anticoagulant therapy: bleeding;
- prosthetic cardiac valve: infection of the prosthesis.

The toenails should be cut after the bath, when the nails are in a soft condition. They should be cut straight and not too short. It is unwise to use a sharp instrument to clean the subungual area of the free edge of the nail. If infection is not promptly controlled, it may, within a very short space of time, proceed to rapidly advancing cel-

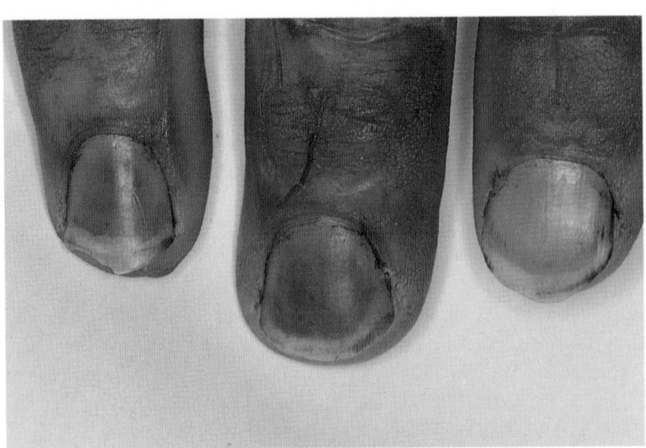

Fig. 10.118. Burns – brownish-yellow discoloration.

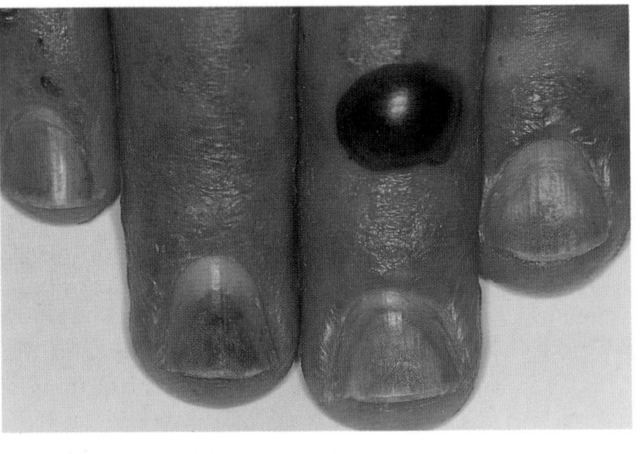

Fig. 10.119. Burns – nail bed involvement with onycholysis (may be permanent).

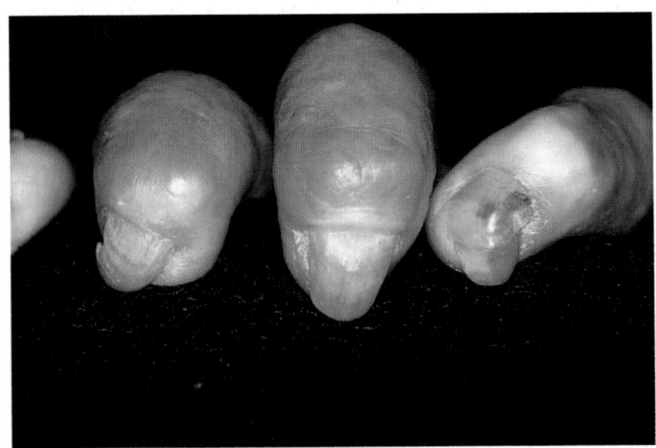

Fig. 10.120. Burns – scarring with nail dystrophy.

lulitis, invasion of bony tissue and gangrene and necessitate amputation. Infection must be treated aggressively and antibiotic therapy started empirically, without awaiting the bacteriology report. Penicillinase-resistant penicillin, erythromycin, or clindamycin should be prescribed. Prophylactic antibiotic cover for surgical patients with prosthetic cardiac valves or compromised circulation is the rule and may be considered appropriate if blood sugar control is not perfect (Middleton & Webb, 1992). Partial or total nail avulsion with chemical (liquefied phenol BP) ablation of the nail matrix is the most common and least traumatic procedure. Minimum use of adhesive padding and strapping as well as avoidance of constricting dressing and appliances are recommended.

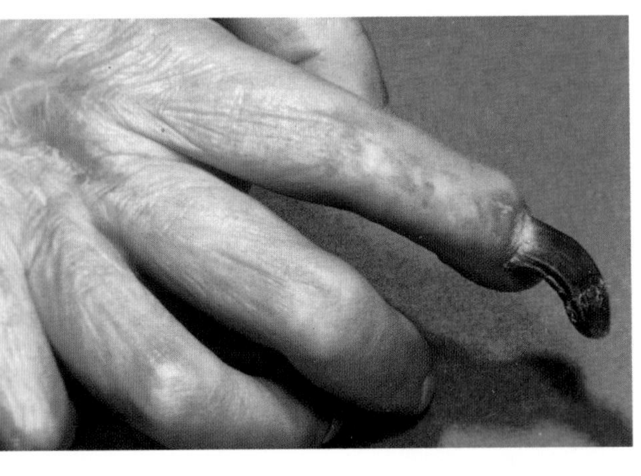

Fig. 10.121. Burns – black nail due to Hiroshima bomb blast (courtesy of Mr Takahashi, President Hiroshima Peace Memorial Museum).

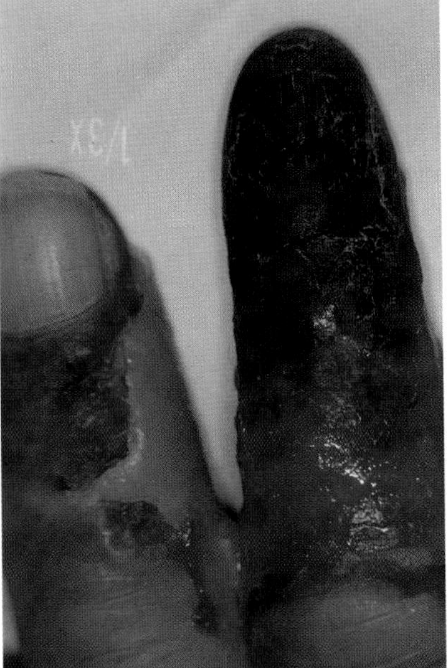

Fig. 10.122. Burns – acute inflammatory changes which lead to severe nail apparatus scarring (courtesy of A. Tosti, Bologna, Italy).

References

Middleton A. & Webb F. (1992) Toenail surgery for diabetic patients. *Diabetic Med.* 9, 680–684.

Patterson R.S. & Hunter A.M. (1989) The management of diabetic and other high risk patients. In: *Common Foot Disorders*, 3rd edn, eds Neale D. & Adams I.M., pp. 137–149. Churchill Livingstone, Edinburgh.

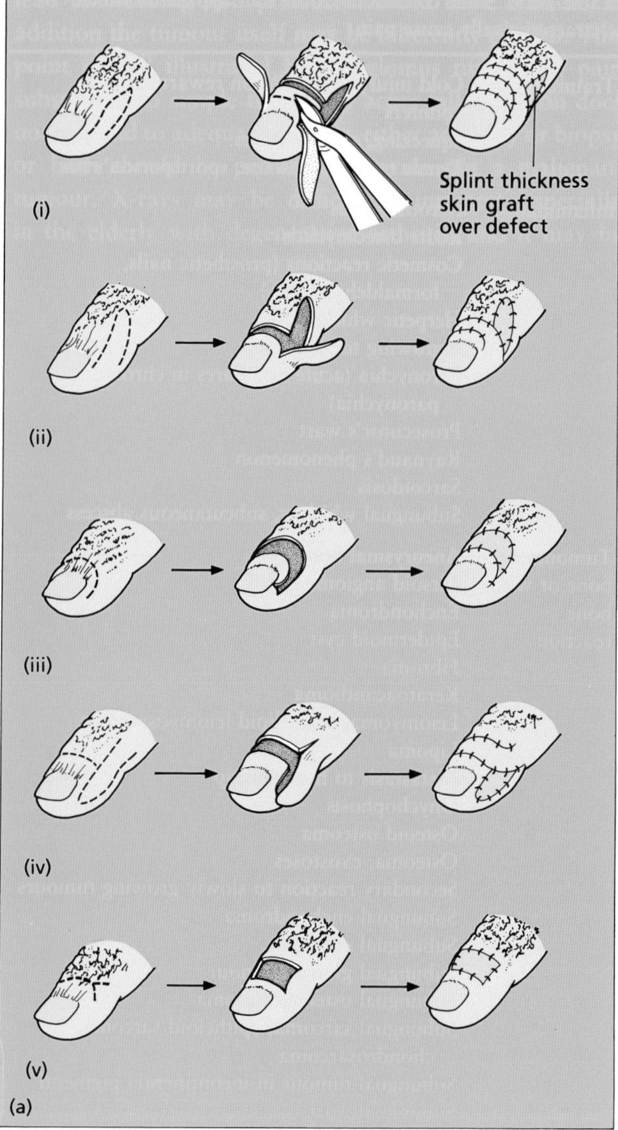

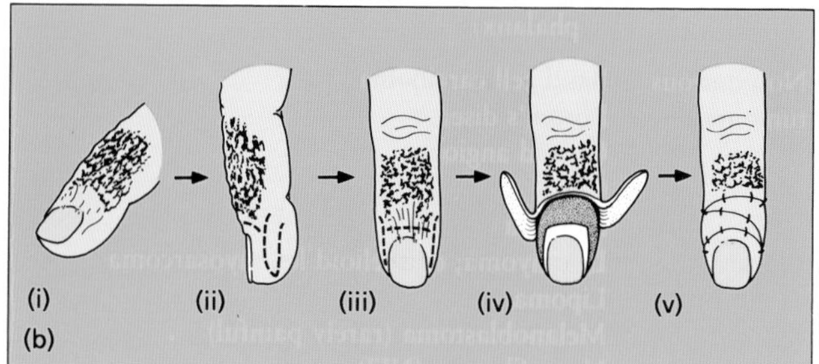

Fig. 10.123. (a) Summary of previous techniques (b) (i) Nail fold burn scar deformity. (ii) and (iii) Design of flaps. The curve of the nailfold is incorporated into the flap design. The base is designed to minimize dog-ears. (iv) Flaps elevated. A small amount of tissue is left at the distal nail base to suture flap. (v) Completed reconstruction. The donor sites are closed primarily (courtesy of B.H. Achauer, USA, with permission).

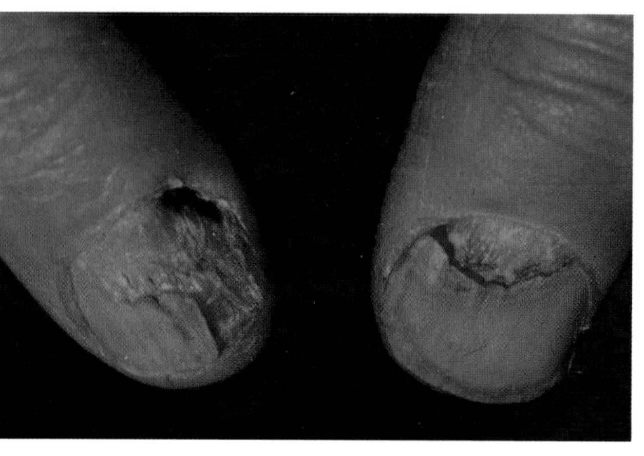

Fig. 10.124. Hydrofluoric acid burns involving the nail apparatus.

Burns

Nail involvement relates to the severity of the burn, the final result depending on this and other factors such as the site and the depth of the dermal structures involved, the presence of infection, the possibility of keloid formation and the promptness of treatment.

The signs produced will vary with the degree of the burn; with slight thermal injury, the nail plate turns a brownish-yellow colour (Jeune & Ortonne, 1979) (Fig. 10.118), nail bed involvement may result in transient or permanent onycholysis (Fig. 10.119) and burns of the matrix will lead to loss of the nail, which will be replaced by a dystrophic brownish nail (Figs 10.120 & 10.121). The extent of the dystrophy reflects the degree of matrix destruction. Involvement of the proximal nail fold (Fig. 10.122) and its following synechiae are among the most severe consequences and are very difficult to correct. However Barfod's technique (1972) or improved procedures derived from this techniques (Achauer, 1990) (Fig. 10.123) may give acceptable results. Otherwise, early excision and grafting in severe cases of burns will produce better results.

References

Achauer B.M. (1990) One-stage reconstruction of the postburn nailfold contracture. *Plast. Reconstr. Surg.* 85, 937–941.

Barfod B. (1972) Reconstruction of the nail fold. *Hand* 4, 85.

Jeune R. & Ortonne J.P. (1979) Chromonychia following thermal injury. *Acta Derm. Venereol.* 59, 91.

Chemical burns

The damage produced by chemical burns is dependent on the concentration of the irritant and its duration of action. Unlike thermal or electric burns, the destruction will con-

Guy (1990) has summarized well, pathophysiologically, the main signs induced by tumours in the nail area. They may cause bulbous enlargement of the fingertips with nail clubbing due to bone splaying and pressure under the main body of the nail bed. Most benign tumours cause nail deformation due to chronic pressure at some point on the matrix. Tumours involving the proximal nail fold may cause chronic matrix pressure from above and produce longitudinal grooving or fissuring of the nail. Some tumours (soft or hard) may also occur under the matrix, exerting pressure upward and causing ridging or even anonychia when they are under the matrix, and onycholysis when they are beneath the nail bed.

Neoplasia of the nail area may be benign, benign but aggressive, or malignant (Salasche & Garland, 1985). Nail deformation most often denotes benignity, while partial or total nail destruction denotes malignancy.

A history of trauma, associated infection, the screening effect of the nail, modification of tumour behaviour produced by the highly specialized nail anatomy and variations in pigmentation, are all factors which may mislead the diagnostician (Préaux, 1978).

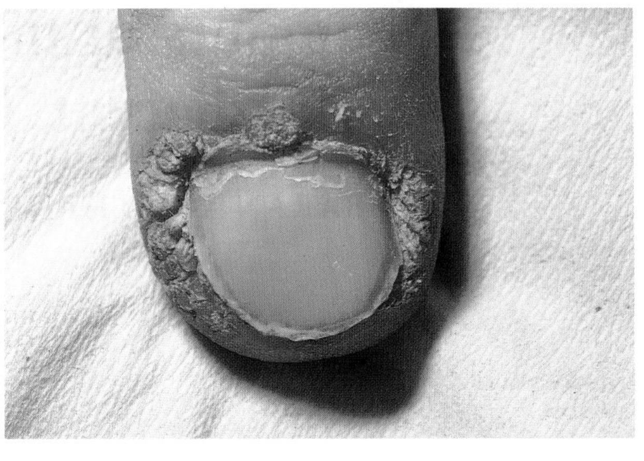

Fig. 11.1. Periungual warts – nail plate unaffected.

References

Guy R.J. (1990) The etiologies and mechanisms of nail bed injuries. *Hand Clin.* 6, 9–19.

Préaux J. (1978) Les tumeurs de la région unguéale des doigts. Problèmes diagnostiques. *Cutis* 2, 481–492.

Salasche S.J. Garland L.D. (1985) Tumors of the nail. *Dermatol. Clin.* 3, 501–519.

Epithelial tumours

Benign

Warts

Common warts are caused by human papilloma viruses of different DNA types. They are benign, weakly contagious, fibroepithelial tumours with a rough keratotic surface (Figs 11.1–11.6). Warts typically affect periungual tissues; when they involve the hyponychium, proximal subungual growth may raise the nail plate. The latter is not usually damaged though fissuring may be seen associated with tenderness. Longitudinal grooving is a rare sign. Tender nodular lesions are equally rare (Holland *et al.*, 1992). Subungual warts, if painful, may mimic glomus tumours. The nail plate is not often affected, but surface ridging may occur, dislocation of the nail being exceptional.

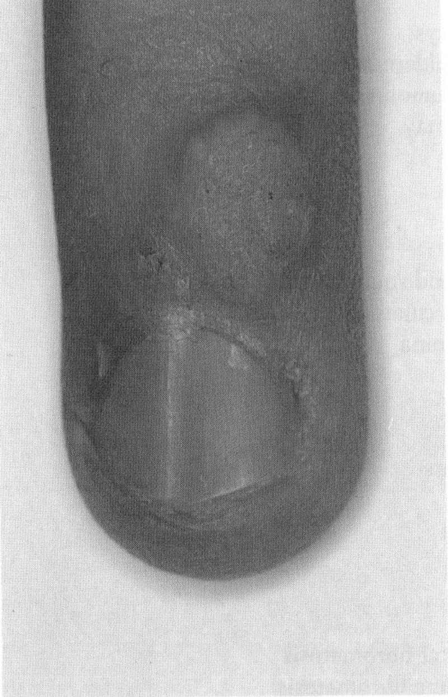

Fig. 11.2. Wart proximal to the nail apparatus – pressure on the matrix has caused a depression ('gutter') on the nail plate.

Biting, picking and tearing of the nail and nail walls are common habits in subjects with periungual warts. This type of trauma is responsible for the spread of the warts and contributes to their resistance to treatment (Figs 11.1 & 11.3).

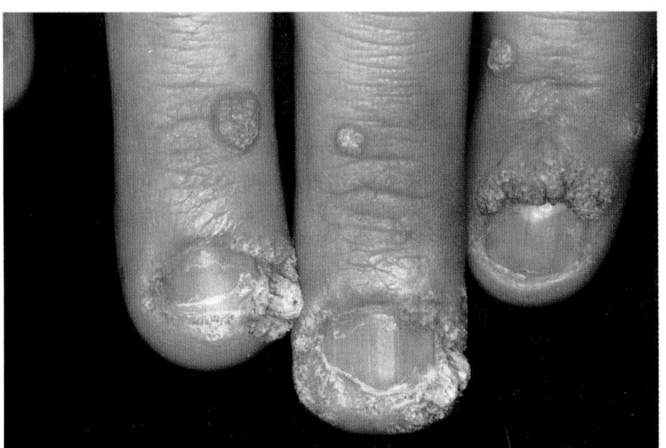

Fig. 11.3. Multiple periungual warts – more common in nail biters and cuticle/lateral nail wall 'pickers'.

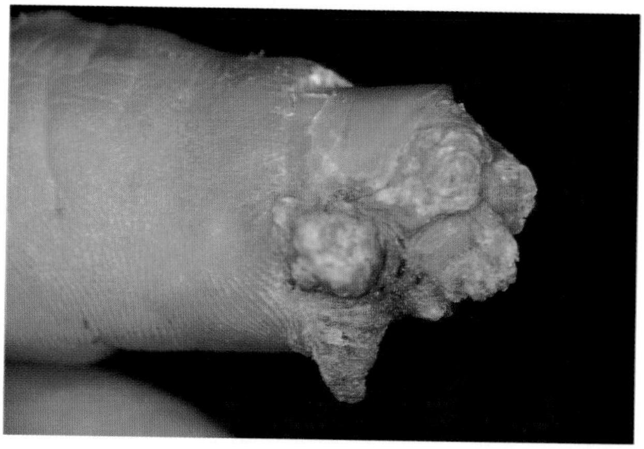

Fig. 11.4. Multiple warts distorting the nail apparatus – most frequently seen in immunosuppressed individuals.

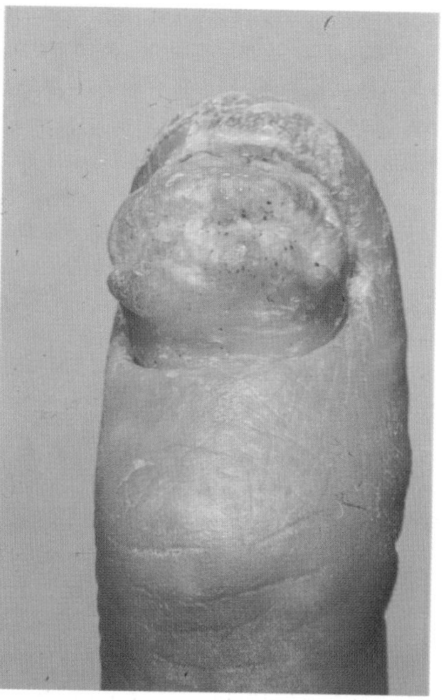

Fig. 11.6. Nail bed wart – massive distal subungual involvement.

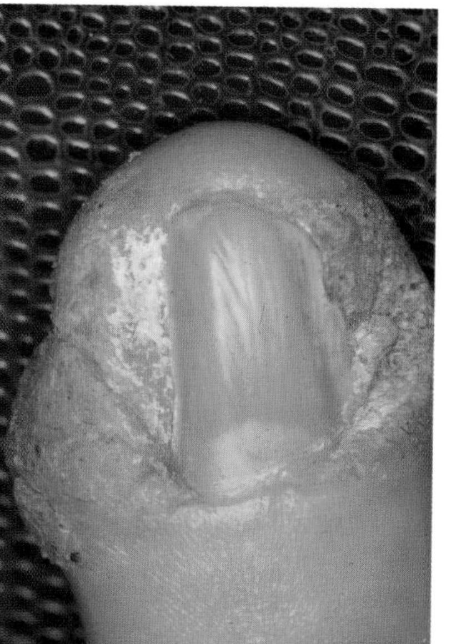

Fig. 11.5. Nail apparatus warts – lateral nail folds and adjacent nail bed involved.

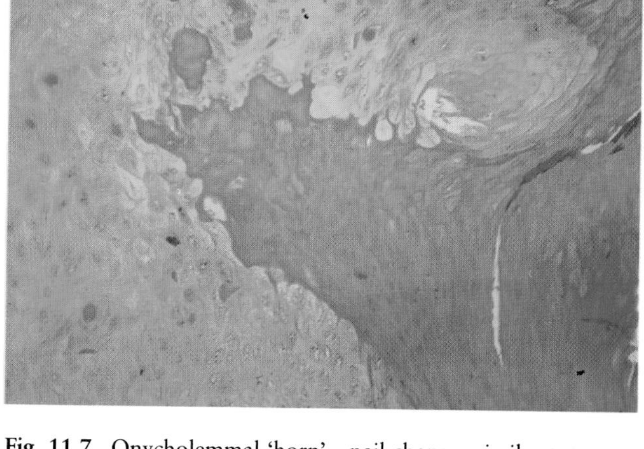

Fig. 11.7. Onycholemmal 'horn' – nail changes similar to proliferating trichilemmal cyst.

Bone erosion from verruca vulgaris has been observed (Shapiro *et al.*, 1961; Gardner & Acker, 1973; Plewig *et al.*, 1973; Shah *et al.*, 1976; Kumar *et al.*, 1980). However some of these cases may have been keratoacanthomas since the latter, as also epidermoid carcinoma, are sometimes clinically indistinguishable from verruca vulgaris.

The histopathology of subungual and periungual warts is similar to that of common warts. Cytopathogenic effects are not as marked as in plantar warts. An inflammatory infiltrate may be present when the wart has been traumatized repeatedly. Histologic examination may be necessary to differentiate extensive periungual warts from verrucous Bowen's disease, even early squamous cell carcinoma.

Periungual warts, particularly when located on the hyponychium, may be rather inconspicuous, presenting only a slightly thickened skin-coloured area which after immersion in water, swells and turns white more rapidly than the surrounding skin. Histological studies are then needed for accurate diagnosis, showing considerable thickening of the epidermis, vacuolization of the granular layer and a loose basket-weave-like horny layer (E. Haneke, unpubl.).

Tuberculosis cutis verrucosa (butcher's nodule, prosector's warts) may seldom pose differential diagnosis difficulties, but it is very rare in the periungual area. Haneke (1983) described a warty growth in the proximolateral nail groove which he termed 'onycholemmal horn' (Fig. 11.7); the histology was similar to proliferating trichilemmal cyst.

When mucinous syringometaplasia involves the distal nail bed, clinical resemblance to verrucae is stricking. Biopsy reveals a focal invagination of the epidermis lined by squamous epithelium, with one or several eccrine ducts leading into the invagination. The eccrine duct epithelium contains mucin-laden goblet cells, and there is mucinous syringometaplasia of the underlying eccrine coils (Scully & Assad, 1984).

Differential diagnosis includes also onychophosis affecting a lateral fold of the toenails, subungual filamentous tumour, amyloidosis subungual vegetation, subungual corn (heloma), verrucous epidermal naevus, inflammatory linear verrucous epidermal naevus (ILVEN), and multicentric reticulohistiocytosis. With longstanding warty lesions, Bowen's disease must always be considered and an appropriate biopsy taken.

Treatment of periungual warts is often frustrating. Warts have a finite natural life span but the duration may exceed the patience of the victim or physician (Shelley, 1972). X-ray and radium treatment have become obsolete. Samman (1979) recommends saturated monochloroacetic acid; this is applied sparingly, allowed to dry and then the wart covered with 40% salicylic acid plaster cut to the size of the wart and held in place with adhesive tape for 2–3 days. After 1–2 weeks most of the warts can be removed and this sometimes painful procedure repeated. Subungual warts are treated similarly, after cutting away the overlying part of the nail plate. Recalcitrant warts may respond to 2% dinitrochlorobenzene (DNCB) vaselinum; however, DNCB is mutagenic for *Salmonella* in the Ames test and therefore can no longer be recommended and should be replaced by diphenciprone (Orrecchia *et al.*, 1988) or squaric acid dibutylester (Iijima & Otsuka, 1993). Some authorities recommend the use of cantharidin (0.007%); Cantharone is applied to the lesions and covered by plastic tape for 24 h. The resultant blister should be re-treated at 2 week intervals, three to four times if necessary. Tkach (1989) suggests a trick to using cantharidin for warts: avoid blister formation which may spread the wart, a similar complication occurring with liquid nitrogen. After applying cantharidin, the wart is covered with paper tape. The patient is given an alcohol sponge and instructed to wipe off the cantharidin in 2 h. If there is not enough reaction, the cantharidin is left on progressively longer with subsequent visits. For children Cantharon is diluted 1:1000 with a 1:1 mixture of isopropyl alcohol and acetone and may be left on the skin longer.

Shumer and O'Keefe (1983) strongly recommend bleomycin for recalcitrant warts; it is given intralesionally 1 μ per 10 ml at 2 week intervals. Transitory (Baran, 1985) or permanent (Miller, 1984; Urbina Gonzalez *et al.*, 1986) nail dystrophy following intralesional injections of bleomycin for a periungual wart has been reported. Vasospastic effects such as permanent Raynaud's phenomenon from intralesional therapy may occur even when using reduced dose (Epstein, 1991). The authors favour the following technique.

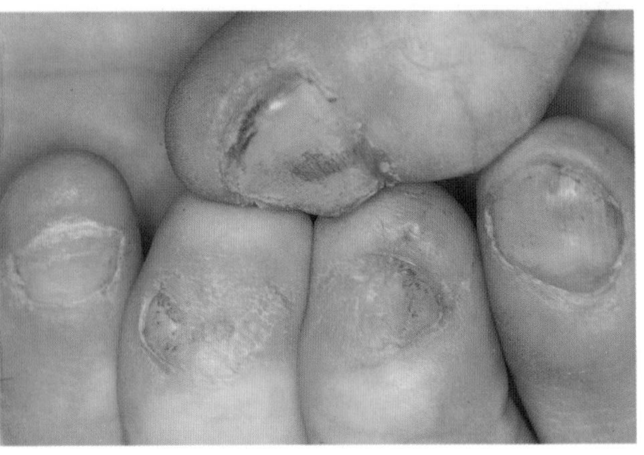

Fig. 11.8. Nail apparatus scarring following overzealous cryosurgery.

With a multiple puncture technique under local anaesthesia with a bifurcated vaccination needle to introduce bleomycin sulphate (1 μm/ml sterile saline solution) into warts, Shelley and Shelley (1991) obtained elimination of 92% of a random series of 258 warts after a single treatment.

Surgical treatment should be avoided if possible. Liquid nitrogen is often used Kuklik (1984). It may cause blistering with the blister roof containing the epidermal wart component if the treatment succeeds. However, when treating the proximal nail fold freezing must not be prolonged since one may easily damage the matrix; this may result in circumscribed leuconychia or even nail dystrophy (Fig. 11.8). Though scarring is rare, permanent onychatrophy with pterygium formation has been reported (Baran, 1985a). Particular side effects of cryosurgery include pain, secondary bacterial infection (rare), Beau's lines, onychomadesis, nail loss and subungual oedema, often worse in the very young and very old. Many side effects are avoidable if the freeze times used are carefully controlled, and prophylactic analgesic and subsequent anti-inflammatory treatment is carried out (Dawber *et al.*, 1992). Oral aspirin 600 mg three times daily, beginning 2 h before and for 3 days after treatment, is helpful. Pretreatment application of clobetasol propionate cream (Kersey, 1988), beneath 'Blenderm' tape reduces the inflammatory response to the freeze. Massages with this steroid may be continued twice daily for 3 days.

Destruction using curettage and electrodesiccation may produce considerable scarring. Recently infrared coagulation, argon and carbon dioxide laser treatments have been used with some success, but permanent nail dystrophy is possible after ablation of periungual warts (Olbright *et al.*, 1987; Street & Roenigh, 1990).

Many lay and medical people have 'tricks' for attempting to cure warts. Litt (1978) suggests 'wrapping' followed 2 weeks later by the careful application of liquified phenol, then a drop of nitric acid to the lesion. The fuming and spluttering that occurs looks efficaceous and the wart turns brown.

Since the incubation period of human warts may be up to several months, careful observation, even after seemingly successful therapy, is necessary to allow for early treatment of newly growing warts.

References

Baran R. (1985a) Brachytelephalangie révélée à l'occasion de dystrophies unguéales induites par cryothérapie. *Ann. Dermatol. Venereol.* **112**, 365–367.

Baran R. (1985b) Onychodystrophie induite par injection intralésionnelle de bléomycine pour verrue périunguéale. *Ann. Dermatol. Venereol.* **112**, 463–464.

Dawber R.P.R., Colver G.B. & Jackson A. (1992) *Cutaneous Cryosurgery*, pp. 30–38. Martin Dunitz, London.

Epstein E. (1991) Intralesional bleomycin and Raynaud's phenomenon. *J. Am. Acad. Dermatol.* **24**, 785–786.

Gardner L.W. & Acker D.W. (1973) Bone destruction of a distal phalanx caused by periungual warts. *Arch. Dermatol.* **107**, 275–276.

Haneke E. (1983) Onycholemmal horn. *Dermatologica* **167**, 155–158.

Hayes M.E. & O'Keefe E.J. (1986) Reduced dose of bleomycin in the treatment of recalcitrant warts. *J. Am. Acad. Dermatol.* **15**, 1002–1006.

Holland T.T., Weber C.B. & James W.D. (1992) Tender periungual nodules. *Arch. Dermatol.* **128**, 105–110.

Iijima S. & Otsuka F. (1993) Contact immunotherapy with squaric acid dibutylester for warts. *Dermatology* **187**, 115–118.

Kersey P.J.W. (1988) The cold injury response. Natural history and modification by clobetasol propionate in human subjects. Presented at the British Dermatological Surgery Group at the BAD Meeting, London.

Kuflik E. (1984) Cryosurgical treatment of periungual warts. *J. Dermatol. Surg. Oncol.* **10**, 673–676.

Kumar B., Shazma S.C. & Kaur S. (1980) Phalangeal erosions with subungual warts. *Ind. J. Dermatol. Venereol.* **46**, 166–168.

Miller R.A.W. (1984) Nail dystrophy following intralesional injections of bleomycin for a periungual wart. *Arch. Dermatol.* **120**, 963–964.

Litt J.Z. (1978) Don't excise – exorcise. Treatment for subungual and periungual warts. *Cutis* **22**, 327–333.

Olbright S.M., Stern R.S., Tang S.V. *et al.* (1987) Complications of cutaneous laser surgery, a survey. *Arch. Dermatol.* **123**, 345–349.

Orrechia G., Douville H., Santagostino L. *et al.* (1988) Treatment of multiple relapsing warts with diphenciprone. *Dermatologica* **177**, 225–231.

Plewig G., Christophers E. & Braun-Falco O. (1973) Mutilierende subunguale Warzen: Abheilung durch Methotrexat. *Hautarzt* **24**, 338–341.

Samman P.D. (1979) The nails. In: *Textbook of Dermatology*, 3rd edn, eds Rook A., Wilkinson D.S. & Ebling F.J.G., pp. 1838–1844. Blackwell Scientific Publications, Oxford.

Scully C. & Assad A. (1984) Mucinous syringometaplasia. *J. Am. Acad. Dermatol.* **11**, 503–508.

Shah S.S., Kothari U.R., Dhoshi H.V., Bhat A.C. & Bhalodia G.C. (1976) Erosion of phalanx by subungual wart. *Ind. J. Dermatol. Venereol. Leprol.* **42**, 185–186.

Shapiro L., Flushing N.Y. & Stoller N.M. (1961) Erosion of phalanges by subungual warts, report of a case. *J. Am. Med. Assoc.* **176**, 379.

Shelley W.B. (1972) *Consultations in Dermatology*, p. 13. W.B. Saunders, Philadelphia.

Shelley W.B. & Shelley E.D. (1991) Intralesional bleomycin sulfate therapy for warts: A novel bifurcated needle puncture technique. *Arch. Dermatol.* **127**, 234–236.

Shumer S.M. & O'Keefe E.J. (1983) Bleomycin in the treatment of recalcitrant warts. *j. Am. Acad. Dermatol.* **9**, 91–96.

Street M.L. & Roenigh R.K. (1990) Recalcitrant periungual verrucae: The role of carbon dioxide laser vaporisation. *J. Am. Acad. Dermatol.* **23**, 115–120.

Tanenbaum M.H. (1971) Onychodystrophy after topically applied fluorouracil for warts. *Arch. Dermatol.* **103**, 225–226.

Tkach J.R. (1989) Finding and inventing alternative therapies. How I do it. *Dermatol. Clin.* **7**, 1–18.

Urbina-Gonzales F., Cristobal-Gil M. & Aguilar Martinez A. (1986) Cutaneous toxicity of intralesional bleomycin administration in the treatment of periungal warts. *Arch. Dermatol.* **122**, 974–975.

Subungual papilloma

Subungual papillomata were briefly reviewed by Heller (1927) who stressed that papilloma is only a descriptive term and does not define a single entity. The history and morphology appear to vary in almost every case. Subungual papillomatosis may be seen in systemic amyloidosis (Chapter 6).

Reference

Heller J. (1927) Die Krankheiten der Nägel. In: *Handbuch der Haut-und Geschlechtskranheiten* (Hrsg. J. Jadassohn), Bd. VIII/pp. 2, 150–172. Spezielle Dermatologie, S.

Eccrine poroma

Eccrine poroma is a benign proliferation most common on the non-hairy parts of the foot. This tumour, approximately 0.5–3 cm in diameter, originating in hyponychial or volar–plantar skin, is always single, pink, soft and grows slowly. Typically it is superficial, often protruding or sessile, but occasionally it may project into the dermis. It may invade the nail bed and uplift the plate (Zaias, 1990). When surrounding the nail, the distal phalanx appears enlarged and the nail dislocated (Arenas, 1987) (Fig. 11.9). The differential diagnosis includes eccrine angiomatous hamartoma (Gabrielsen *et al.*, 1991) presenting as a painful tumour of the dorsal aspect of the distal phalanx leading to its amputation, pyogenic granuloma, amelanotic melanoma, viral wart, histiocytoma, and carcinoma. Treatment consists of excision – histological examination is essential.

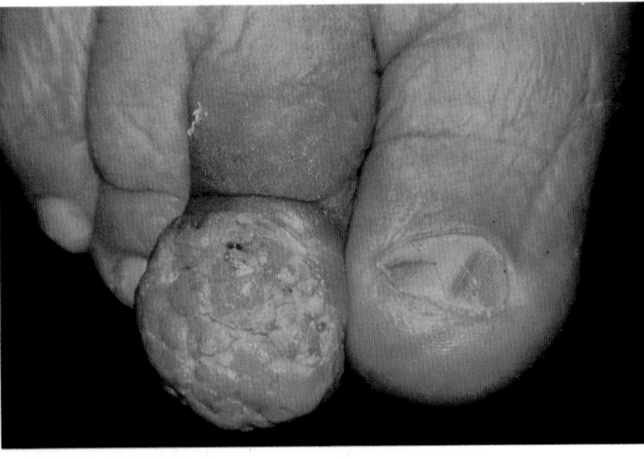

Fig. 11.9. Eccrine poroma of the nail apparatus (courtesy of R. Arenas, Mexico).

References

Arenas R. (1987) *Dermatologia, Atlas, Diagnostico y Tratamiento*, pp. 539–540. McGraw Hill, Mexico.

Gabrielsen T.O., Elgjo K. & Sommerschild H. (1991) Eccrine angiomatous hamartoma of the finger leading to amputation. *Clin. Exp. Dermatol.* **16**, 44–45.

Zaias N. (1990) *The Nail in Health and Disease*, p. 220. Appleton & Lange, Norwalk, Conn.

Keratoacanthoma

Subungual and periungual keratoacanthomata may occur as solitary or multiple tumours (Figs 11.10–11.13). This is a rare benign, but rapidly growing, seemingly aggressive tumour usually situated below the edge of the nail plate or in the most distal portion of the nail bed. More than 16 cases have been reported in the English literature (Ronchese, 1970; Stoll, 1980; Cramer, 1981; Keeney *et al.*, 1988); however, the diagnosis was not definitely confirmed in all cases (Stoll, 1980) since many lesions were inadequately biopsied and others persisted for more than 1 year. Keratoacanthoma is said to arise from hair follicle

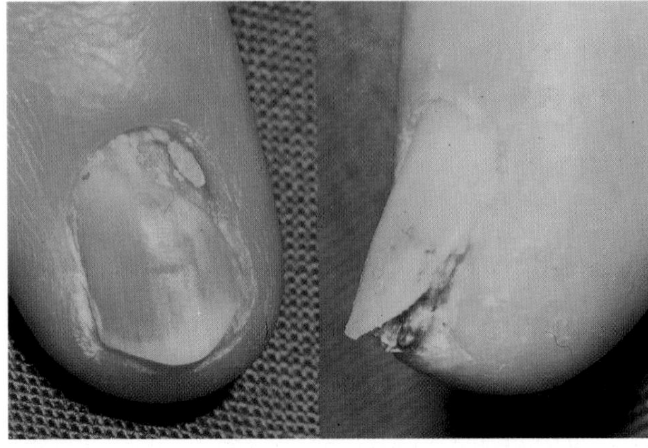

Fig. 11.10. Keratoacanthomas of the nail – subungual origin.

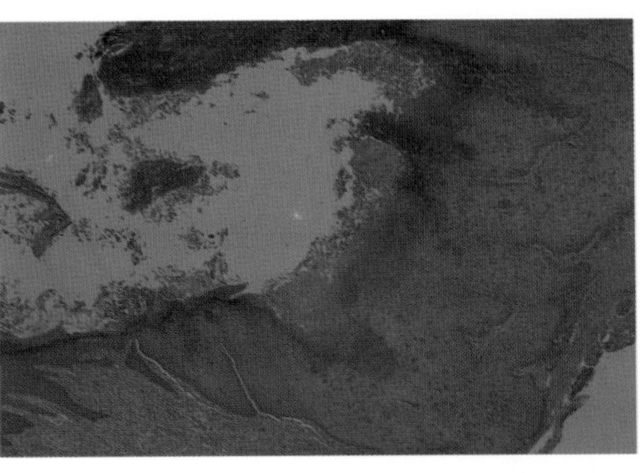

Fig. 11.11. Keratoacanthoma – low power microscopy to show 'architecture' of the lesion (see Fig. 11.10).

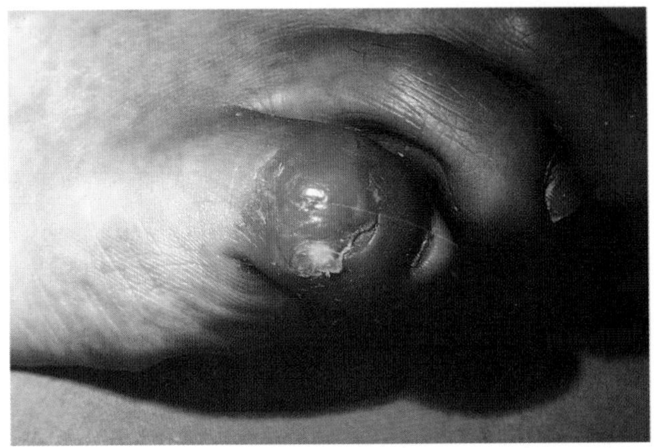

Fig. 11.12. Distal digital keratoacanthoma distorting the proximal nail structures and thus the nail plate (courtesy of O. Hilker & M. Winterscheidt, Germany).

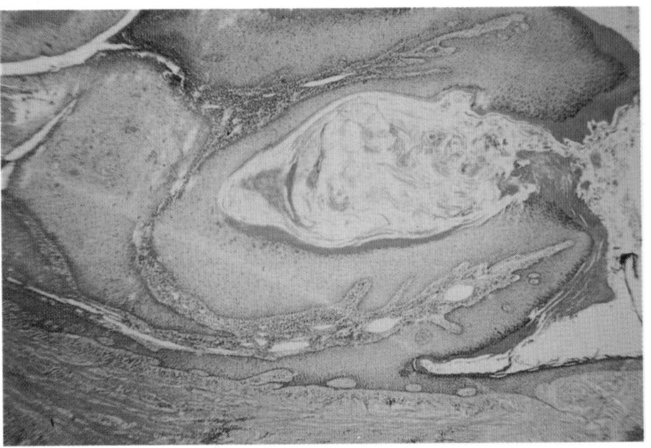

Fig. 11.13. Low-power histological 'architecture' of lesion – type as in Fig. 11.12.

epithelium, but there are no hair follicles in the subungual regions.

The lesion may start as a small and painful keratotic nodule visible beneath the free edge, growing rapidly to

Table 11.1. Differences between keratoacanthoma (KA) on the skin and under the nails (adapted from Stoll, 1980)

	KA on skin	Subungual KA
Growth direction	More horizontal	More vertical
Infiltrate	Many neutrophils and eosinophils	Less neutrophils and eosinophils, no fibrosis at base
Bone erosion	Usually none	Rapid
Duration	9–12 m	Longer if not treated
Spontaneous regression	Frequent	Infrequent
Symptoms	No pain	Pain

Table 11.2. Differentiation between subungual keratoacanthoma and squamous cell carcinoma (adapted from Norton, 1980)

	Subungual KA	Subungual carcinoma
Sex	M > F	M > F
Age	35–65	60–80
Incidence	Very rare	Relatively common
Growth rate	Rapid	Slow
Duration of symptoms	Short	Long
History of trauma	Rarely	Sometimes
Tumour mass	Always present	Often not present
Bone invasion	Early	Late
Radiography	Bone erosion	Late bone destruction
Multiple tumours	Common	Rare

1–2 cm diameter within 4–8 weeks (Fig. 11.10). The typical gross appearance, as a dome-shaped nodule with a central plug of horny material filling the crater, is not often seen subungually although histology of an adequate biopsy specimen will clearly show the characteristic pattern (Table 11.1). Less frequently the tumour grows out from under the proximal nail fold (Fig. 11.10), which becomes inflamed, and may cover or surround it with a cushion of swollen tissue (Gonzales-Ensenat *et al.*, 1988). Spontaneous regression is exceptionally observed in this area. The tumour soon erodes the bone and this may be demonstrated radiologically as a fairly well-defined, crescent-shaped lytic defect of 'tuft' adjacent to the overlying nail bed. Reconstitution of the bony defect can be expected (Levy *et al.*, 1985; Pellegrini & Tompkins, 1986). A case of multiple familial keratoacanthoma (Hilker & Winterscheidt, 1987) (Fig. 11.12) showed no tendency towards spontaneous involution, in contrast to Mittal *et al.*'s (1984) case associated with polyarthritis. Familial subungual keratoanthoma has been reported in association with ectodermal dysplasia (Shatkin *et al.*, 1993).

Whether trauma plays a role in subungual keratoacanthoma (Ronchese, 1970) or there is a relationship to exposure to steel wool has not been shown conclusively (Fisher, 1990).

Diagnosis of subungual keratoacanthoma depends on the rapid growth, its erosion of bone and characteristic histology. Clinical differentiation from squamous cell carcinoma remains nonetheless difficult (Shapiro & Baraf, 1970; Bräuninger & Hoede, 1986).

Staining with involucrin has been advocated for distinguishing between keratoacanthoma and squamous cell carcinoma (Smoller *et al.*, 1986). In addition, the surface receptors for lectins are not present in the latter and keratoacanthoma demonstrates a lectin-binding profile similar to that found in the normal epidermis (Ramirez-Bosca *et al.*, 1988) (Table 11.2). Transforming growth factor α expression may be a more valuable marker of epithelial differentiation and may help distinguish between these two tumours (Ho *et al.*, 1991).

Histopathology of subungual keratoacanthoma differs slightly from that of the skin (Figs 11.11 & 11.13). In this particular location, the tumour is more narrow but deeply infiltrating. It shows a marked shoulder with an epidermal lip, a central crater filled with keratin, and the tumour cells are large, pale and often develop keratohyalin granules. This feature corresponds with filaggrin expression as revealed by immunohistochemistry. However, neither involucrin, cytokeratin and filaggrin expression nor staining for the lectin peanut agglutinin allow keratoacanthoma to be distinguished from subungual squamous cell carcinoma. Their staining is too variable to enable differentiation between keratoacanthoma and squamous cell carcinoma on immuno- and lectin-histochemical stainings alone (Vigneswaran *et al.*, 1989). Recently, an antibody directed against transforming growth factor α was shown to give different staining patterns in keratoacanthoma and squamous cell carcinoma (Ho *et al.*, 1991), but further studies are needed to establish its discriminating value. Histologically perineural invasion by keratoacanthoma may be a risk factor for recurrence (Wagner *et al.*, 1987).

Treatment of keratoacanthoma

Management of subungual keratoacanthoma ranges from conservative local excision to amputation, but aggressive ablative surgery as the initial intervention for this benign condition should be discouraged. Pellegrini and Tompkins (1986) reviewed 18 cases reported in the literature revealing that 86% of the lesions treated by curettage eventually required conservative amputation.

The patient should be followed for an adequate period of time to rule out recurrence since regrowth has been reported as late as 22 months after treatment. If the tumour recurs, further curettage or amputations of the distal phalax may be done judged by the amount of bone destruction and function (Patel & Desai, 1989). Chemosurgery has been advocated (Moreno-Gimenez *et al.*, 1987). Retinoids may be beneficial in keratoacanthoma (Yoshikawa *et al.*, 1985). Eruptive keratoacanthomas have responded to oral etretinate 1 mg/kg/day with complete resolution. Recurrence can occur after cessation of treatment, requiring maintenance therapy (10 mg on alternative days), however this mode of treatment is more effective as prophylaxis in multiple keratoacanthoma. 5-Fluorouracil has also been used, either injected into the lesion or applied as a 20% ointment three times daily for 3–4 weeks (Bennet *et al.*, 1985). Intralesional bleomycin may be tried in the distal nail area (Sayama & Tagami, 1983) as well as methotrexate.

References

Bräuninger W. & Hoede N. (1986) Subunguales Keratoakantom. *Hautarzt* **37**, 270–273.

Bennet R., Epstein E. & Goette D. (1985) Current management using 5FU. *Cutis* **36**, 218–236.

Cramer S.F. (1981) Subungual keratoacanthoma. A benign bone-eroding neoplasm of the distal phalanx. *Am. J. Clin. Pathol.* **75**, 425–429.

Fisher A.A. (1990) Subungual keratoacanthoma: Possible relationship of exposure to steel wool. *Cutis* **46**, 26–28.

Gonzales-Ensenat A., Vilalta A. & Torras H. (1988) Kerato-acanthome péri et sous-unguéal. *Ann. Dermatol. Venereol.* **115**, 329–331.

Hilker O. & Winterscheidt M. (1987) Familiäre multiple Keratoakanthome. *Z. Hautkr.* **62**, 284–289.

Ho T., Horn T. & Finzi E. (1991) Transforming growth factor α expression helps to distinguish keratoacanthomas from squamous cell carcinomas. *Arch. Dermatol.* **127**, 1167–1171.

Keeney G.L., Banks P.M. & Linscheid R.L. (1988) Subungual keratoacanthoma. Report of a case and review of the literature. *Arch. Dermatol.* **124**, 1074–1076.

Levy D.W., Bonakdarpour A., Putong P.B. *et al.* (1985) Subungual keratoacanthoma. *Skeletal Radiol.* **13**, 287–290.

Mittal R., Mittal R.L., Chopra A. *et al.* (1984) Polyarthritis with atypical keratotic nodular dermatosis or polyarthritis with multiple keratoacanthoma. *Dermatologica* **169**, 199–202.

Moreno-Gimenez J.C., Lerma Puerta E., Sanchez Conejo-Mir J. *et al.* (1987) Queratoacantoma subungual. *Actas Derm. Sif.* **78**, 561–564.

Parker C.M. & Hanke W.C. (1986) Large kerato-acanthoma in difficult locations treated with intralesional 5FU. *J. Am. Acad. Dermatol.* **14**, 770–777.

Patel M.R. & Desai S.S. (1989) Subungual keratoacanthoma in the hand. *J. Hand Surg.* **14A**, 139–142.

Pellegrini V.D. & Tompkins A. (1986) Management of subungual keratoacanthoma. *J. Hand Surg.* **11A**, 718–724.

Ramirez-Bosca A., Reano A. & Valcuende-Cavero F. (1988) Lectin-binding sites in squamous cell carcinomas and keratoacanthomas. *Acta Derm. Venereol.* **68**, 480–485.

Ronchese F. (1970) Subungual keratoacanthoma. *Chron. Dermatol.* **1**, 3–4.

Sayama S. & Tagami H. (1983) Treatment of kerato-acanthoma with intralesional bleomycin. *Br. J. Dermatol.* **109**, 449–452.

Shapiro L. & Baraf C.S. (1970) Subungual epidermoid carcinoma and keratoacanthoma. *Cancer* **25**, 141–152.

Shatkin B.T., Hunter J.G. & Song I.C. (1993) Familial subungual keratoacanthoma in association with ectodermal dysplasia. *Plast. Reconstr. Surg.* **92**, 528–531.

Smoller B.R., Kwan T.H., Said J.W. *et al.* (1986) Keratoacanthoma and squamous cell carcinoma of the skin: Immunohistochemical localization of involucrin and keratin proteins. *J. Am. Acad. Dermatol.* **14**, 226–234.

Stoll D.M. (1980) Subungual keratoacanthoma. *Am. J. Dermatopathol.* **2**, 265–271.

Vigneswaran N., Haneke E. & Hornstein O.P. (1989) Are differences in filaggrin expression suitable for discriminating benign, premalignant and malignant skin lesions? *Path. Res. Pract.* **184**, 402–409.

Wagner R.F., Cottel W.I. & Smoller B.K. (1987) Perineural invasion associated with recurrent sporadic multiple self-healing squamous carcinomas. *Arch. Dermatol.* **123**, 1275–1276.

Yoshikawa K., Hirano S. & Kato T. (1985) A case of eruptive kerato-acanthoma treated by oral etretinate. *Br. J. Dermatol.* **112**, 579–583.

Dysgenetic tumours

Subungual keratotic incontinentia pigmenti tumours

Incontinentia pigmenti (IP) or Bloch–Sulzberger syndrome is a multi-organ disease with an X-linked dominant inheritance which affects females and usually is lethal in males. Independent sporadic cases resembling X-autosomal translocations involving the same X-chromosome breakpoint have been reported but recent DNA probes have failed to confirm this localization (Harris *et al.*, 1988). There are three clinical stages of skin changes: a linear erythematovesiculous and bullous reaction, which is present at birth, is then followed by a second stage of verrucous lesions which gradually disappear. The third stage is characterized by a 'splashed or whorled' pigmentation in a pattern which follows Blaschko's lines.

From 15 to 26 years of age painful subungual keratotic tumours (Mascaro *et al.*, 1985; Simmons *et al.*, 1986) (Fig. 11.14) or warty periungual tumours (Moss & Ince, 1987) can appear as a manifestation of IP. It is usually the fingers which are involved. The keratotic subungual mass produces dystrophy or simple onycholysis of the nail

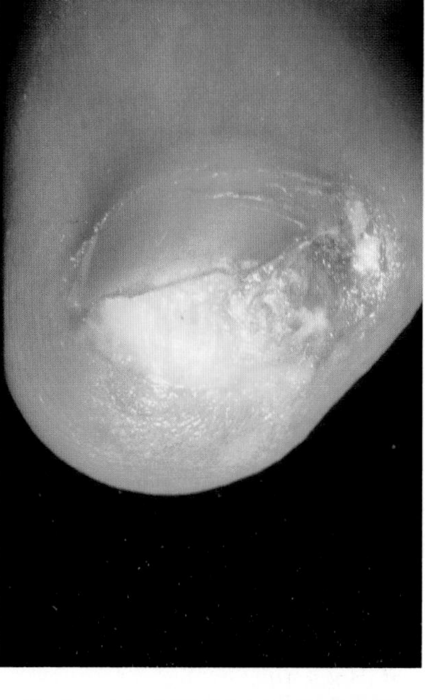

Fig. 11.14. Incontinentia pigmentii – painful, warty subungual tumour (courtesy of J.M. Mascaro, Barcelona, Spain).

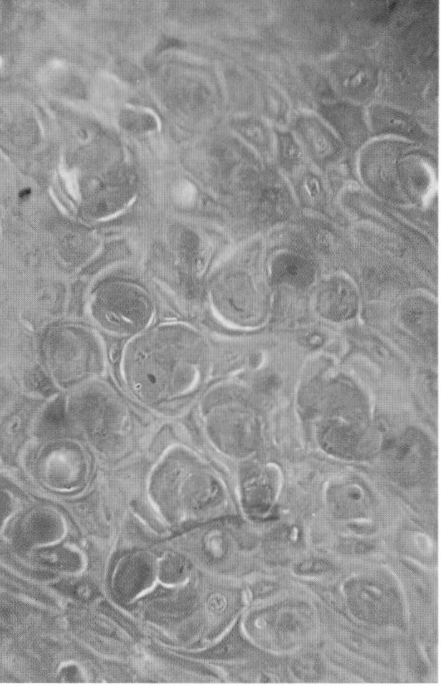

Fig. 11.15. Incontinentia pigmentii – dyskeratotic cells.

which is displaced from its bed. Erythema and swelling of the fingertip are found at the border of the lesion. The tumour may be sited only on the subungual proximal nail area leading to the destruction of a portion of the nail plate, or on the proximal nail fold with tender swellings which are smooth proximally and warty distally (Moss & Ince, 1987; Adenvian *et al.*, 1993). The tumours destroy the distal bony phalanx. They may disappear spontaneously after several months leaving small scars on the pulp just under the free edge of the nail at the site of a warty lesion (Moss & Ince, 1987). Hartmann and Danville (1976) reported the case of a 30-year-old woman with painful subungual tumours from the age of 20 years. The keratotic lesions resulted in nail dystrophy and scalloped bone deformities of the terminal phalanges of the fingers. On two occasions regression followed pregnancy. Eight fingernails and one toenail were affected over a 20-year period in a female who developed her first lesion at 16 (Hermanns & Pierard, 1986).

Histological examination of the tumours shows a verrucous or pseudoepitheliomatous hyperplasia of the epidermis where dyskeratotic cells are found at all levels (Fig. 11.15). Differential diagnoses include warts, epidermoid cysts, subungual fibromas, squamous cell carcinoma and, most important, keratoacanthoma which is clinically and histologically undistinguishable.

Despite spontaneous resolution being likely, the patient may require treatment because of pain (Nurse, 1979) and disability. Management by electrodesiccation and curettage, or surgical excision, is usually successful but permanent nail atrophy occurs. A course of retinoids should therefore be strongly considered despite possible recurrence (Bessems *et al.*, 1988).

References

Adenvian A., Townsend P. & Peachy R. (1993) Incontinentia pigments manifesting as painful periungual and subungual tumours. *J. Hand Surg. (UK)* **18B**, 6679.

Bessems P.J.M., Jagtman B.A. & Van de Staak W. (1988) Progressive, persistent, hyperkeratotic lesions in incontinentia pigmenti. *Arch. Dermatol.* **124**, 29–30.

Harris A., Shelley L., Haan E. *et al.* (1988) The gene for incontinentia pigmenti: failure of linkage studies using DNA probes to confirm cytogenetic localization. *Clin. Genet.* **34**, 1–6.

Hartmann D.L. & Danville P.A. (1976) Incontinenta pigmenti associated with subungual tumours. *Arch. Dermatol.* **112**, 535–542.

Hermanns J.F. & Pierard G.E. (1986) Onychodystrophie hypertrophique de l'incontinentia pigmenti. *Nouv. Dermatol.* **5**, 421.

Mascaró J.M., Palou J. & Vives P. (1985) Painful subungual keratotic tumours in incontinentia pigmenti. *J. Am. Acad. Dematol.* **13**, 913–918.

Moss C. & Ince P. (1987) Anhidrotic and achromians lesions in incontinenta pigmenti. *Br. J. Dermatol.* **116**, 839–849.

Nurse D.S. (1979) Help-wanted: Incontinentia pigmenti. *Schoch Lett.* **29**, 3.

Simmons D.A., Kegel M.F., Scher R.K. *et al.* (1986) Subungual tumours in incontinentia pigmenti. *Arch. Dermatol.* **122**, 1431–1434.

Verrucous epidermal naevus

Involvement of the distal phalanx and nails by verrucous epidermal naevi is rare. Onset may be from birth, or later. This history, together with the linear arrangement, usually make differentiation from extensive warts relatively easy.

Verrucous epidermal naevi are as a rule asymptomatic, except when they impinge upon the proximal nail fold, where they may cause recurrent paronychia and distort

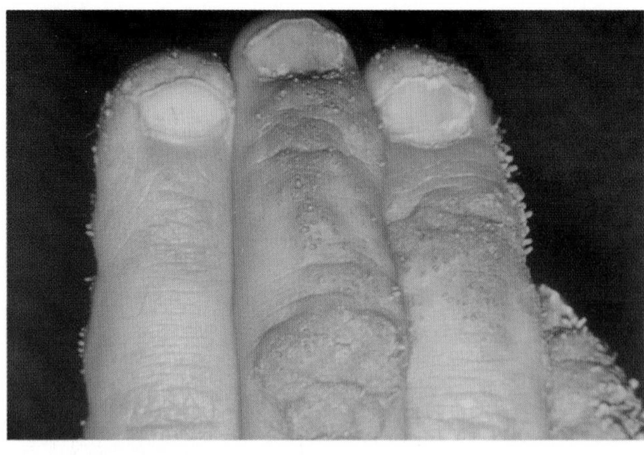

Fig. 11.16. Verrucous epidermal naevus – some splitting and ridging of the nails.

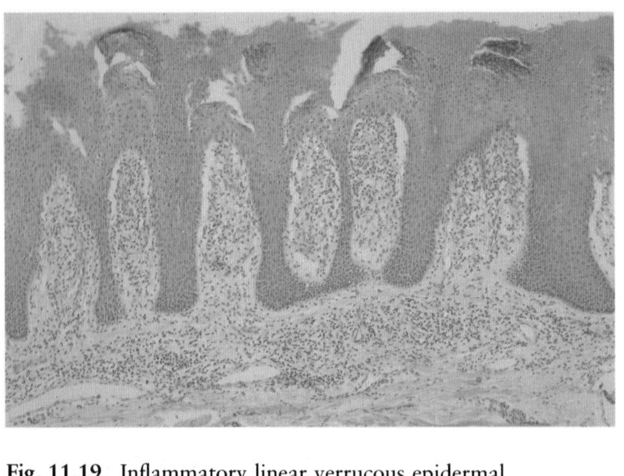

Fig. 11.19. Inflammatory linear verrucous epidermal naevus – histological slide; marked dermal chronic inflammatory changes.

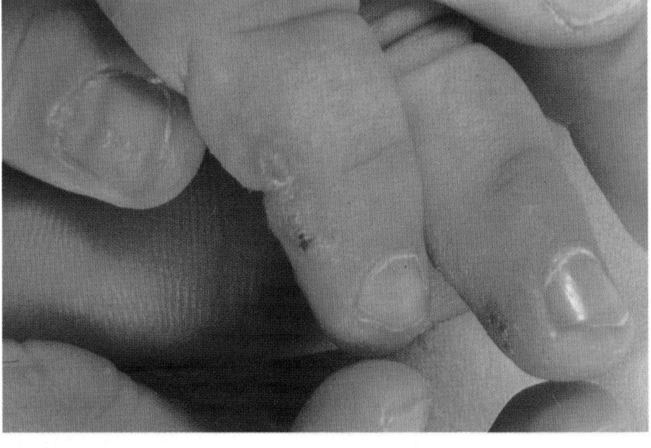

Fig. 11.17. Inflammatory linear verrucous epidermal naevus – only slight nail involvement (courtesy of A.J. Landwehr).

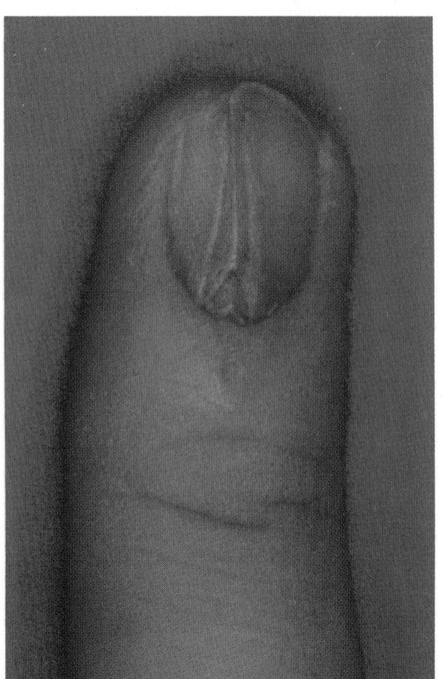

Fig. 11.18. Inflammatory linear verrucous epidermal naevus – severe central nail dystrophy.

the nail (Rook *et al.*, 1986). Involvement of the nail bed causes ridging (Fig. 11.16) splitting, discoloration or dystrophy.

Linear verrucous epidermal naevus may belong to the epidermal naevus syndrome (Solomon *et al.*, 1968). Differential diagnosis includes lichen striatus and ILVEN (Figs 11.17–11.19) (see Chapter 5).

Histopathology shows papillomatosis with hyperkeratosis giving a wart-like appearance. However, HPV-type cytopathic effects are lacking. In the matrix and nail bed the typical epithelium is no longer discernible and the verrucous naevus does not produce a normal nail plate.

References

Rook A., Wilkinson D.S., Ebling F.J.G., Champion R.H. & Burton J.L. (1986) *Textbook of Dermatology*, 4th edn., p. 170. Blackwell Scientific Publications, Oxford.

Solomon L.M., Fretzin D.F. & Dewald R.L. (1968) The epidermal nevus syndrome. *Arch. Dermatol.* 97, 273–285.

Keratin cysts

Implantation epidermoid cyst (synonyms: keratin, squamous epithelial or traumatic cysts)

Epidermoid cysts in the terminal phalanx of the digits are usually secondary to heavy trauma, with implantation of epidermis into subcutaneous tissue or even into the bone. The trauma may have been many years before and is not always remembered. Post-operative epidermoid cysts may occur in the proximity of scars (Baran & Bureau, 1989) (Fig. 11.20).

The distal phalanx gradually enlarges and clubbing becomes evident. Pain is of late onset and it results from compression of the bone and may eventually lead to a fracture; shooting pain without bone involvement was

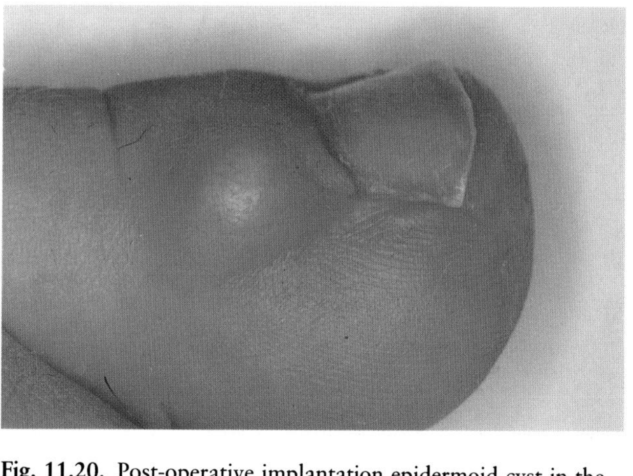

Fig. 11.20. Post-operative implantation epidermoid cyst in the postero-lateral nail fold.

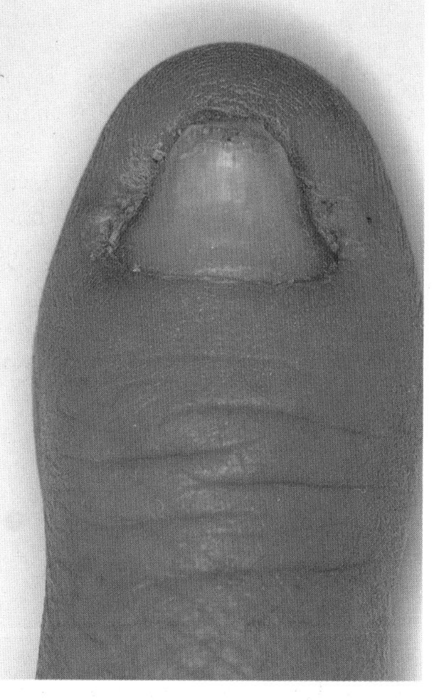

Fig. 11.21. Pincer nail deformity due to epidermoid cyst.

described in one case (Yung & Estes, 1980). Acquired pincer nail is an unusual presentation (Baran & Broutard, 1989) (Fig. 11.21).

Intraosseous epidermoid cysts (Fig. 11.22) are solitary lesions twice as frequently in men as in women. Pain and swelling of the terminal phalanx are the most frequent clinical signs. The lesions appear as round, osteolytic zones embedded in the bone (Figs 11.22 & 11.23) without trabecules or sclerosis (cf. enchondroma), or as a marginal defect of cortical substance of bone (Drewes *et al.*, 1985). The clinical and radiological differential diagnosis may be very difficult (Schajowicz *et al.*, 1970). Nuclear magnetic resonance imaging shows a cystic lesion with a smooth wall (Wu, 1992). Treatment is by enucleation of the lesion including its entire membrane. This can usually be achieved with a lateral L-shaped incision. Bone transplants are not necessary.

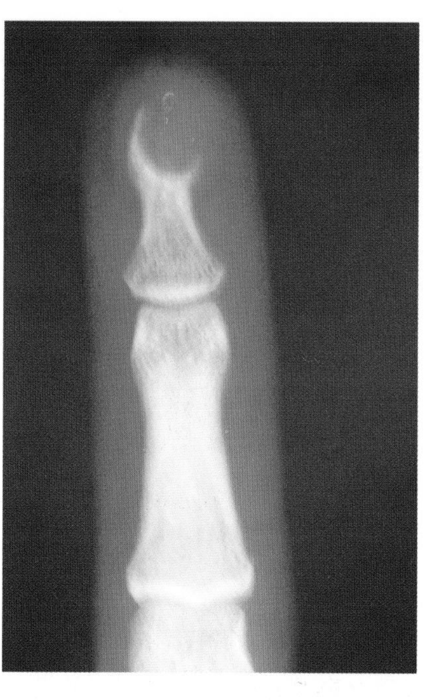

Fig. 11.22. Intraosseous epidermoid cyst – X-ray changes in terminal phalanx.

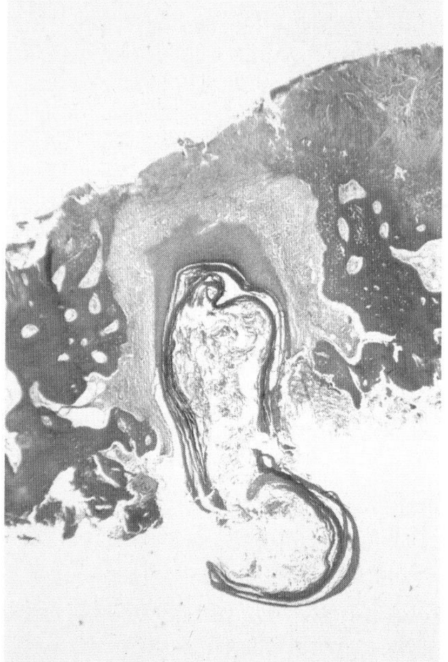

Fig. 11.23. Intraosseous epidermoid cyst – histological changes (see Fig. 11.22).

Histopathology shows a simple epidermoid cyst filled with orthokeratin and lined with a thin epidermis (Fig. 11.24). However, if remnants of matrix epithelium are displaced into the subcutaneous tissue, the cyst may also contain areas resembling trichilemmal cyst epithelium (Haneke, 1983).

References

Baran R. & Broutard J.C. (1989) Epidermoid cyst of the thumb presenting as a pincer nail. *J. Am. Acad. Dermatol.* **19**, 143–144.

Baran R. & Bureau H. (1989) Two post-operative epidermoid cysts following realignment of the hallux nail. *Br. J. Der-*

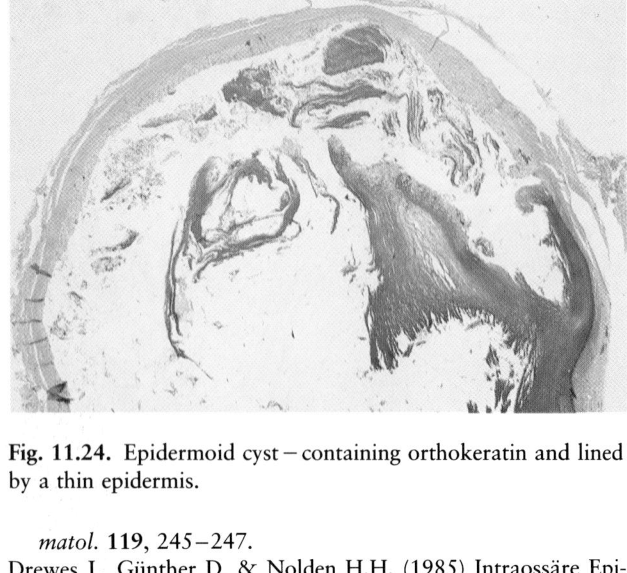

Fig. 11.24. Epidermoid cyst – containing orthokeratin and lined by a thin epidermis.

matol. **119**, 245–247.

Drewes J., Günther D. & Nolden H.H. (1985) Intraossäre Epidermiszysten der Finger und Zehen. *Akt. Chir.* **20**, 171.

Haneke E. (1983) Onycholemmal horn. *Dermatologica* **167**, 155–158.

Samman P.D. (1959) The human toenail, its genesis and blood supply. *Br. J. Dermatol.* **71**, 296–302.

Schajowicz F., Aiello C.A. & Slullitel I. (1970) Cystic and pseudo cystic lesions of the terminal phalanx with special reference to epidermoid cyst. *Clin. Orthop. Rel. Res.* **68**, 84–92.

Wu K.K. (1992) Epidermoid cysts of the foot: with or without bone involvement. *J. Foot Surg.* **31**, 203–206.

Yung W. & Estes S.A. (1980) Subungual epidermal cyst. *J. Am. Acad. Dermatol.* **3**, 599–601.

Subungual epidermoid inclusions

Subungual epidermoid inclusions (epidermal buds; Zaias, 1990) develop from the ridges of the nail bed epithelium. Although histologically indistinguishable from subungual epidermoid cysts, they usually remain microscopic. Exceptionally, they become large enough to produce symptoms, such as swelling of the nail bed. Trauma is a possible cause (Samman, 1959). They occur especially with finger clubbing but without the associated dystrophy (Lewin, 1969).

In contrast to the two main varieties which spare the nail bed, a new form of subungual epidermoid inclusion has been reported in eight cases (Fanti & Tosti, 1989). The most striking clinical features of this is subungual hyperkeratosis associated with shortened and dystrophic nail plate (Fig. 11.25). Onycholysis was observed in one case. A history of trauma is frequent, but the condition is symptomless. In all cases, the biopsy reveals marked hyperplasia of the nail bed, and epidermoid cysts in the dermis (Fig. 11.26). Onychomycosis and psoriasis are the main differential diagnosis.

References

Fanti P.A. & Tosti A. (1989) Subungual epidermoid inclusions: report of 8 cases. *Dermatologica* **178**, 209–212.

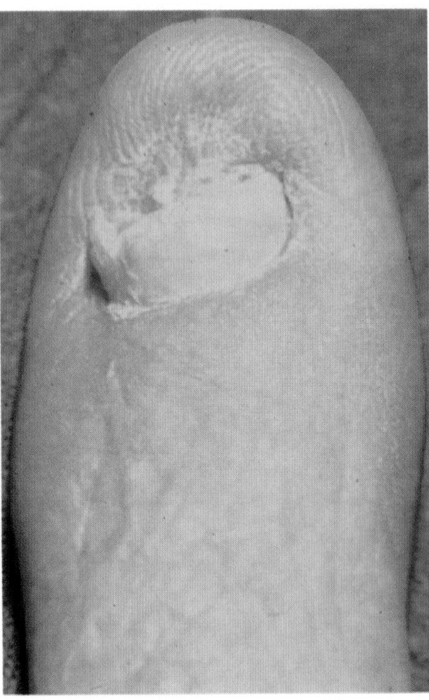

Fig. 11.25. Subungual epidermoid inclusions – dystrophic nail.

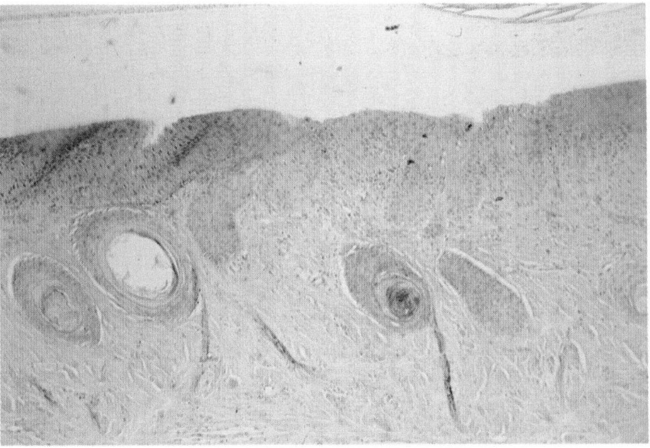

Fig. 11.26. Subungual epidermoid inclusions – nail bed epithelial hyperplasia and dermal epidermoid cysts. Histology of Fig. 11.25 (courtesy of P.A. Fanti & A. Tosti, Bologna, Italy).

Lewin K. (1969) Subungual epidermoid inclusion. *Br. J. Dermatol.* **81**, 671–675.

Samman P.D. (1959) The human toenail, its genesis and blood supply. *Br. J. Dermatol.* **71**, 296–302.

Zaias N. (1990) *The Nail in Health and Disease*, p. 218. Appleton & Lange, Norwalk, CT.

Fibroepithelial tumours (see Fibrous tumours)

Onychomatricoma (filamentous tufted tumour in the matrix of a funnel-shaped nail) (Baran & Kint, 1992)

Four main clinical signs are striking enough to arouse suspicion of this condition.

1 A yellow coloration of variable width along the entire

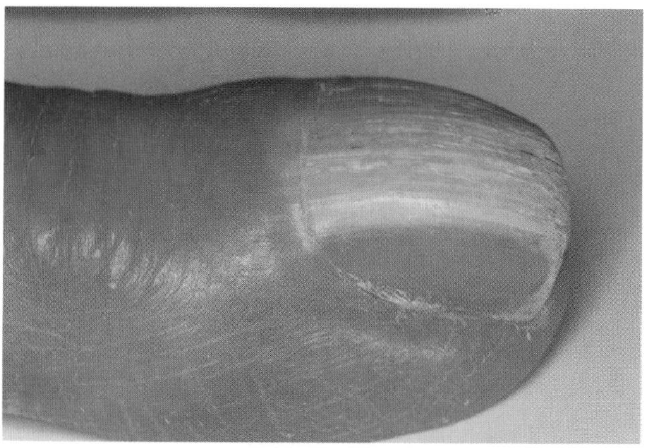

Fig. 11.27. Onychomatricoma.

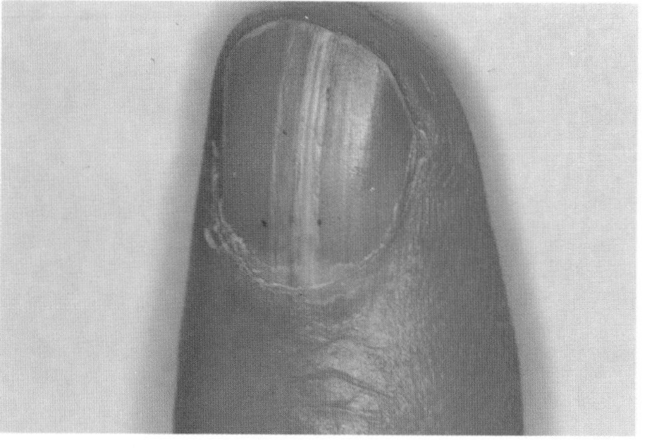

Fig. 11.28. Onychomatricoma.

length of the nail plate, leaving a single or double portion of normal pink nail; with splinter haemorrhages in the yellow area involving the proximal nail region (Figs 11.27 & 11.28).

2 More prominent ridging of the affected nail, than of a normal one from the same patient.

3 A tendency toward transverse overcurvature of the affected nails which becomes increasingly pronounced when the yellow colour is more extensive.

4 Nail avulsion exposes a tumour emerging from the matrix region while the nail appears as a flat funnel, storing filamentous digitations in holes in its proximal section (Figs 11.29 & 11.30).

The tumours all have the same histological features and consist of epithelial proliferations related to the nail matrix or to the surrounding epidermis. The lobules are delineated by normal basal cells and composed of keratinocytes (Fig. 11.31). A narrow column of dense elongated cells with dark nuclei can be seen centrally. These are similar in structure to keratinizing matrix cells. After elimination of these parakeratotic cells, an invagi-

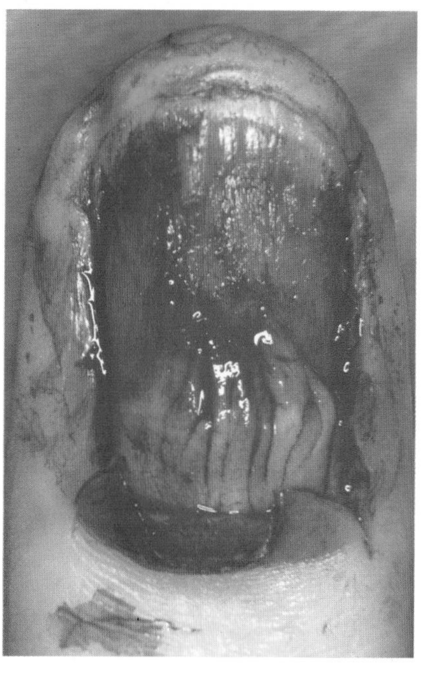

Fig. 11.29. Onychomatricoma – emerging nail tumour visible after nail avulsion.

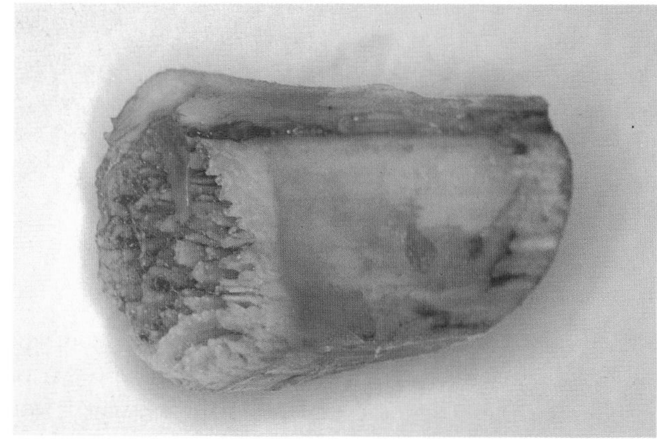

Fig. 11.30. Onychomatricoma – nail plate undersurface showing in its proximal region the holes storing the filamentous digitations.

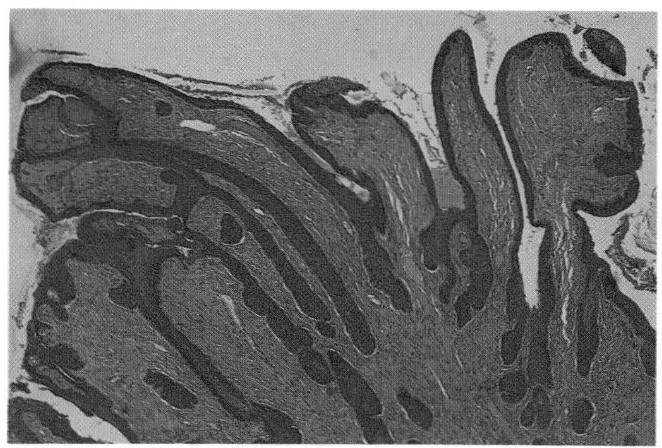

Fig. 11.31. Onychomatricoma – biopsy, showing epithelial proliferations with the lobules surrounded by normal basal cells.

nation resembling the infundibulum of a hair follicle remains in the cell strands. These invaginations probably correspond to the small hollows found clinically in all of the lesions. The collagen is loose around the epithelial lobules and contains no mucin.

Reference

Baran R. & Kint A. (1992) Onychomatrixoma. *Br. J. Dermatol.* **126**, 510–515.

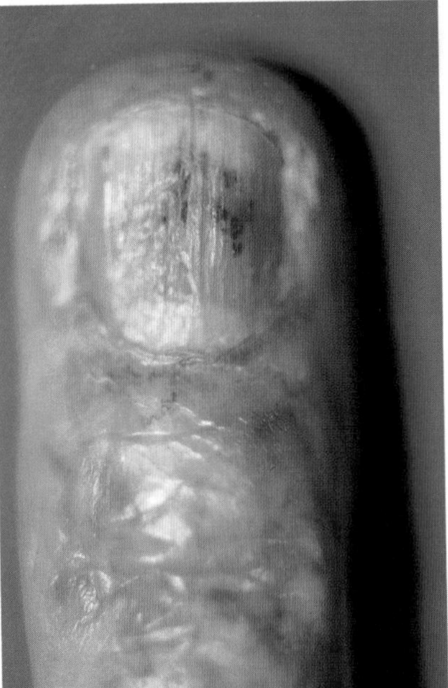

Fig. 11.32. Radiodermatitis – chronic changes many years after X-irradiation for psoriasis.

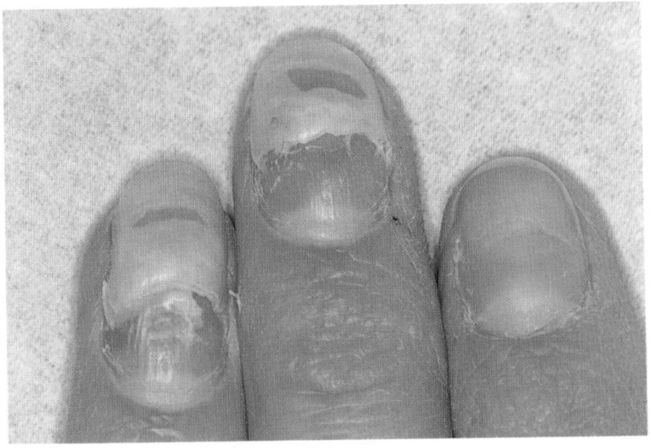

Premalignant tumours

Actinic keratosis

Actinic keratosis is the commonest precancerous lesion of the skin. Although the nail provides only partial protection of the nail bed from solar damage, as judged by the occurrence of subungual keratoacanthoma and squamous cell carcinoma (Norton, 1980), actinic keratoses are very rare in the subungual area. They usually present as cutaneous 'horns' on the proximal nail fold. Since, however, only about one-third of cutaneous horns overlie actinic keratoses, each lesion must be biopsied or completely excised. Common warts, Bowen's disease, squamous cell carcinoma, chronic radiodermatitis, arsenical keratoses and keratoacanthoma may also give rise to such cutaneous horns.

Fig. 11.33. Acute radiodermatitis – progressive nail shedding.

Arsenical keratoses

Arsenical keratoses are due to a high content of arsenic in water or wine, or to iatrogenic arsenic ingestion. Microscopically, they cannot definitely be differentiated from other types of keratoses such as actinic keratoses. Keratotic papules and plaques develop on the periungual skin or nail bed. The latter may also become diffusely hyperkeratotic. Nail dystrophy subsequently develops. All patients with signs of chronic arsenical poisoning must be carefully examined and followed-up, since arsenic has a high carcinogenic potential in various organs.

Reference

Norton L.A. (1980) Nail disorders. *J. Am. Acad. Dermatol.* **2**, 451–467.

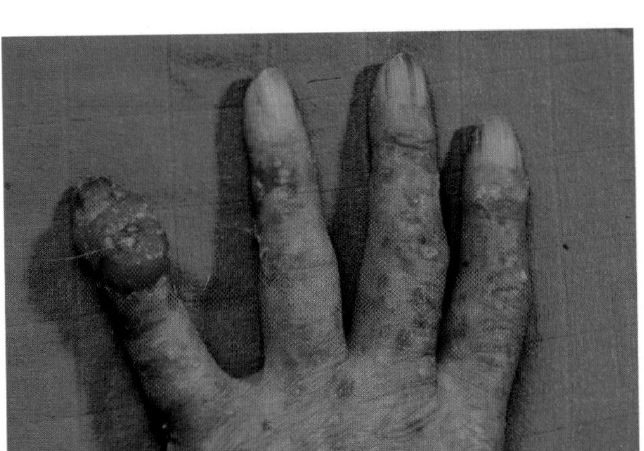

Fig. 11.34. Radiodermatitis – late changes including squamous carcinoma of the nail apparatus.

Radiodermatitis (Figs 11.32–11.36)

Acute necrosis of the fingertip, nail apparatus and the distal phalanx can occur from massive radiation overdose. Chronic effects have been seen after the treatment of eczema, psoriasis (Fig. 11.32), onychomycosis, and in health care workers before the institution of proper precautions (Guy, 1990).

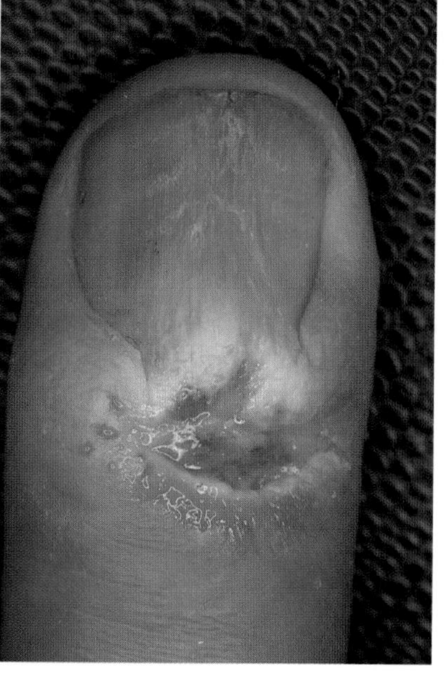

Fig. 11.35. Ulceration (benign), pterygium formation and nail plate dystrophy – late changes of X-irradiation.

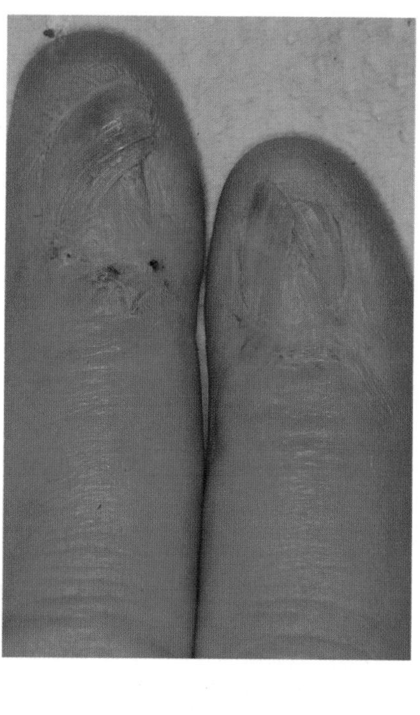

Fig. 11.36. X-irradiation-induced scarring and nail plate distortion (courtesy of B. Richert, Belgium).

Ionozing radiation may cause loss of nails (Gallaghar *et al.*, 1955) (Fig. 11.33) as well as late changes associated with chronic radiodermatitis (Messite *et al.*, 1957); this may lead to skin cancer up to 30 years after exposure (Fig. 12.34). The earliest signs are longitudinal ridging and brittleness. Later, the surrouding skin appears sclerotic and atrophic with telangiectasia and hyperkeratosis. Ulceration may occur, slow in evolution and failing to heal (Fig. 11.35). The nail plates become dull, slightly opaque with a brownish hue, and may become variably thickened and distorted (Fig. 11.36) with splitting of the distal edges. The nail bed develops fine, red, longitudinal striations which proceed into punctate 'charcoal' patches. A verrucous lesion appearing on the hyponychium or adjacent nail bed may herald the development of malignant change. Hyperkeratosis of the nail bed elevates the nail and causes pain. Paronychia-like flares are quite common. Pseudoclubbing is unusual (Richert & de la Brassine, 1993). Occupational radiodermatitis from ^{192}Ir exposure was reported from Spain (Condé-Salazar *et al.*, 1986). After an acute episode, an asymptomatic period of several months may follow; the typical picture of chronic radiodermatitis then appears.

Treatment depends on the size and location of the keratotic lesions. For small nail bed lesions, curettage may be efficient after a U-shaped piece of the distal nail has been excised. En-bloc excision of the nail apparatus with healing by secondary intention (de Dulanto & Camacho, 1979), or Mohs' fresh tissue technique which spares the normal surrounding tissue, are treatments of choice. The defect can be covered with a free graft or a flap (Lagrot & Greco, 1978).

References

Condé-Salazar L., Guimaraens D. & Romero L.V (1986) Occupational radiodermatitis from Ir-192 exposure. *Contact Derm.* **15**, 202–204.

De Dulanto F. & Camacho F. (1979) Radiodermatitis. *Acta Derm. Sif.* 70, 67–94.

Gallaghar R.G., Zavon M. & Doyle H.N. (1955) Radioactive contamination in a radium therapy clinic. *Publ. Health Rap.* 70, 617–624.

Guy R.J. (1990) The etiologies and mechanisms of nail bed injuries. *Hand Clin.* **6**, 9–20.

Lagrot F. & Greco J. (1978) Les lésions des ongles dans les radiodermites chroniques des mains. *Cutis (France)* **2**, 507–528.

Messite J., Troisi F.M. & Kleinfeld M. (1957) Radiological hazards due to X-radiation in vetenarians. *Arch. Ind. Health* **16**, 48–51.

Richert B. & de la Brassine M. (1993) Subungual chronic radiodermatitis. *Dermatology* **186**, 290–293.

Malignant epithelial tumours

When dealing with malignant nail tumours four features should always be taken into account: variation in nail colour, nail plate deformity, partial or total disappearance of the nail plate, and periungual soft tissue dystrophy.

Epidermoid carcinoma of the nail apparatus

Bowen's disease and squamous cell carcinoma

These are considered together as epidermoid carcinoma for reasons described below (Figs 11.37–11.48).

Bowen's disease is a non-aggressive malignant

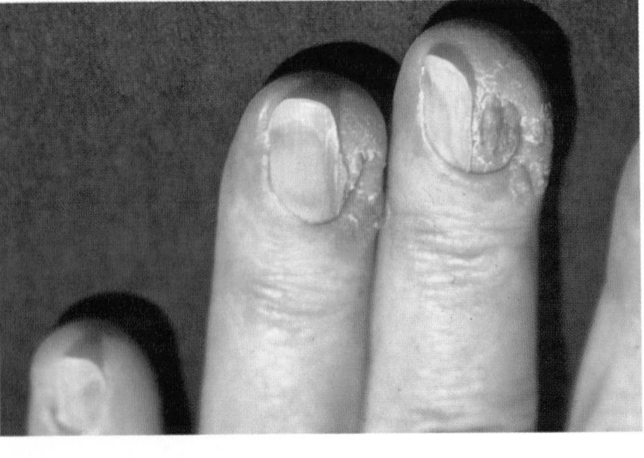

Fig. 11.37. Epidermoid carcinoma. Bowen's disease, *in situ*, variety (two digits affected) (courtesy of D. Gormley, Los Angeles, USA).

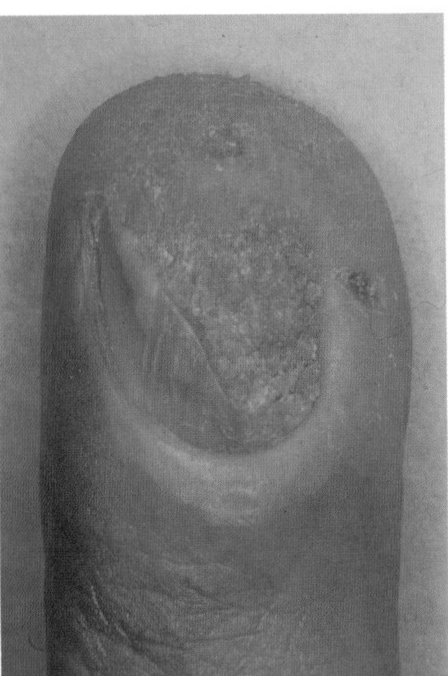

Fig. 11.39. Epidermoid carcinoma *in situ* – white cuticle area and nail dystrophy (courtesy of N. Zaias, Miami, USA).

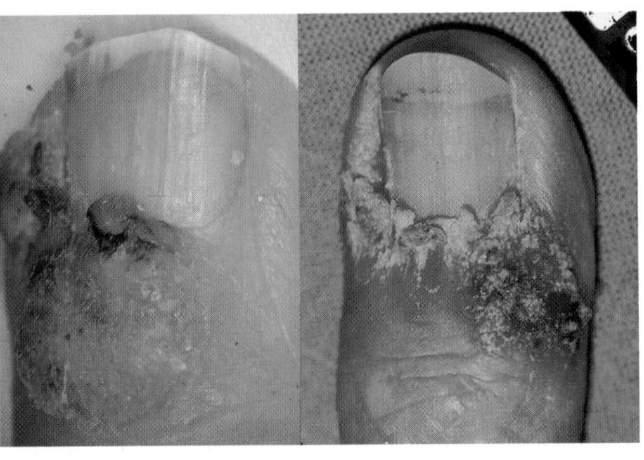

Fig. 11.38. Epidermoid carcinoma *in situ* – periungual warty proliferation.

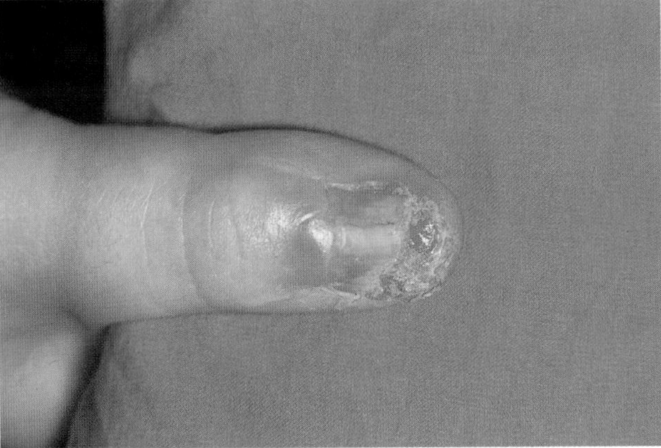

Fig. 11.40. Epidermoid carcinoma *in situ* – marked inflammatory changes.

condition (the first recognized example of carcinoma *in situ*) which has been of interest for several reasons.

1 The increasing awareness of its frequency from many recent publications.

2 The identification of new clinical patterns such as longitudinal melanonychia (Baran & Simon, 1988).

3 Our experience indicating that Bowen's disease of the fingernail structures should always be regarded as a potentially 'polydactylous' process with the passage of time (Baran & Gormley, 1988; McGrae *et al.*, 1993) (Fig. 11.37).

4 Finally the possibility of a link with HPV types 16, 34 and 35 which has shed new light on the aetiology of this type of cancer (Fig. 11.44).

Bowen's disease of the nail apparatus is a distinctive type of squamous cell carcinoma that differs from other variants. However, some authors prefer to avoid the use of the term Bowen's disease for *in situ* epidermoid carcinoma occurring beneath the nail plate, because: (i) it is not always easy to separate invasive from *in situ* carcinoma; (ii) it cannot be overemphasized that a biopsy specimen showing Bowen's disease does not exclude the possibility of invasive carcinoma in other areas of the lesions.

The malignant process may develop in the epithelium of the periungual area as well as in the subungual tissues.

Periungual involvement includes: hyperkeratotic or papillomatous growth (Fig. 11.38); erosions, scaling and fissuring of the nail folds and nail bed (Figs 11.40–11.42); whitish cuticle area (Zaias, 1990) (Fig. 11.39); periungual swelling from deep tumour proliferation, with erythema caused by inflammation due to infection; fissuring or ulceration of the lateral nail groove, sometimes crusted with granulation-like tissue beneath the scab (Fig. 11.42).

Subungual involvement was constant in the 12 cases

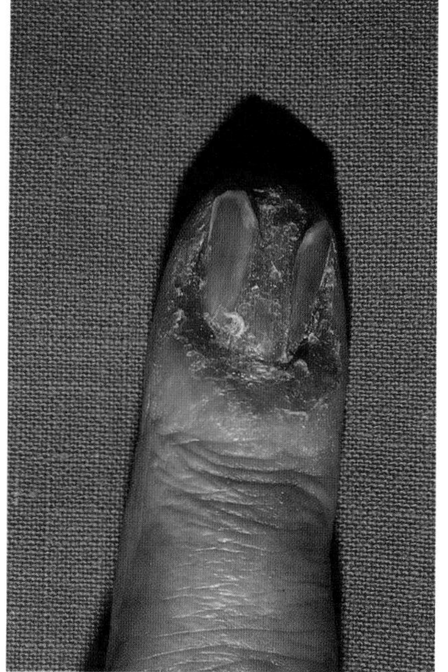

Fig. 11.41. Epidermoid carcinoma *in situ* – marked inflammatory changes.

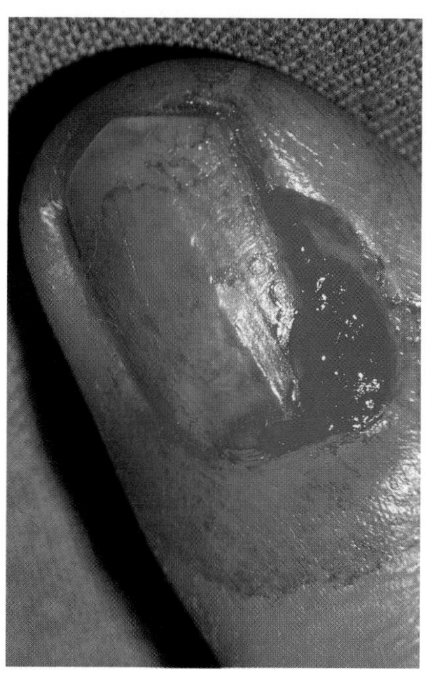

Fig. 11.42. Epidermoid carcinoma *in situ* – lateral ulcerated variety (courtesy of G. Moulin, Lyon, France).

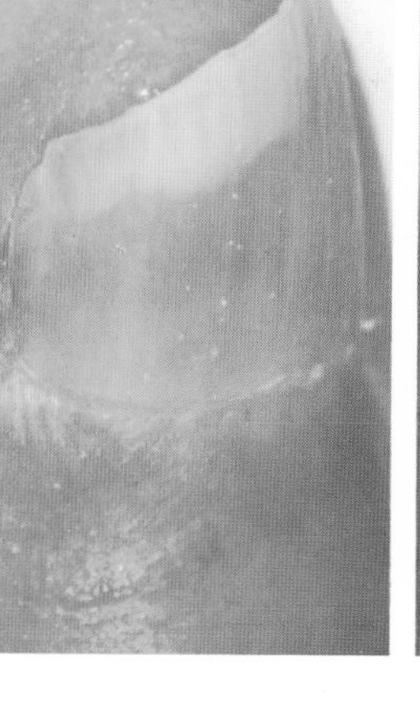

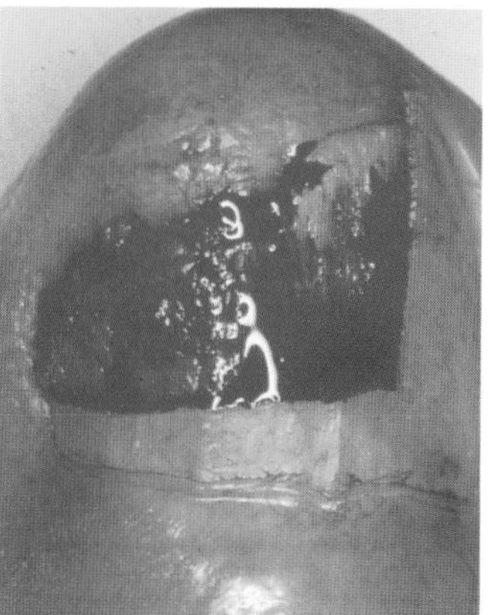

Fig. 11.43. Epidermoid carcinoma *in situ* – surface onycholysis with subungual 'granulation' and oozing.

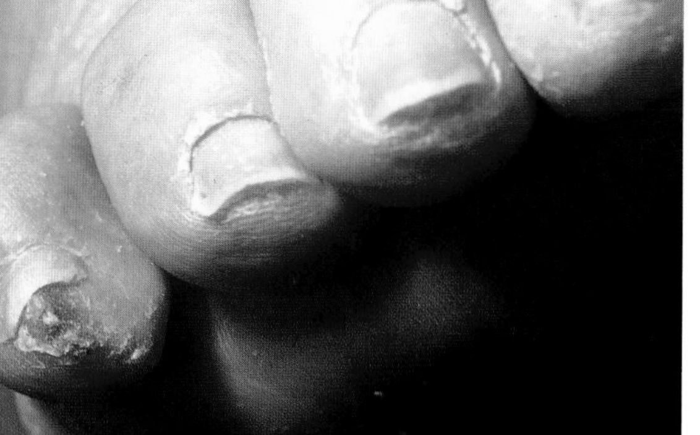

Fig. 11.44. Epidermoid carcinoma – invasive 'warty' growth (possibly due to HPV virus).

described by Guitart *et al.* (1990). It may present with onycholysis and nail clipping of the non-adherent portion of the nail plate shows hyperkeratosis or oozing ulceration of the nail bed (Fig. 11.43). The appearance of longitudinal melanonychia, with normal pattern (Saijo *et al.*, 1990) or abnormal pattern (Baran & Simon 1988; Baran & Eichmann, 1993), is a recent finding. The nail plate may become dystrophic, even ingrowing; or there may be partial or total nail loss which implies that the malignant process has developed in the nail matrix. Localized pain may be noted, for example when the patient dials a phone number.

The presence of nodularity, ulceration or bleeding indicates that the carcinoma has become invasive (Mikhail, 1984) (Figs 11.45 & 11.46). Bone involvement is seen in less than 20% (Salasche & Garland, 1985; Long & Espinella, 1978). Metastases have been reported mainly in patients with hereditary ectodermal dysplasia (Campbel & Keokarn, 1966; Mauro *et al.*, 1972).

The key to diagnosis is the histological examination (Fig. 11.48). The picture is identical with that of Bowen's disease of other skin areas. The most important feature is the intact basement membrane.

Bowen's disease has been reported in individuals between the ages of 20 and 90, the incidence being highest in the 50–69 year range. The tumour grows slowly and the duration of signs and symptoms from onset to the time of diagnosis has varied from several months to 18 years. The diagnostic biopsy is often delayed because of the patient's reluctance, technical difficulties, or because the physician has failed to suspect the disease. The digits of the hand are significantly more frequently affected than the toes, the thumbs being the commonest site.

Fig. 11.45. Epidermoid carcinoma with longitudinal melanonychia along the lateral edge of the nail.

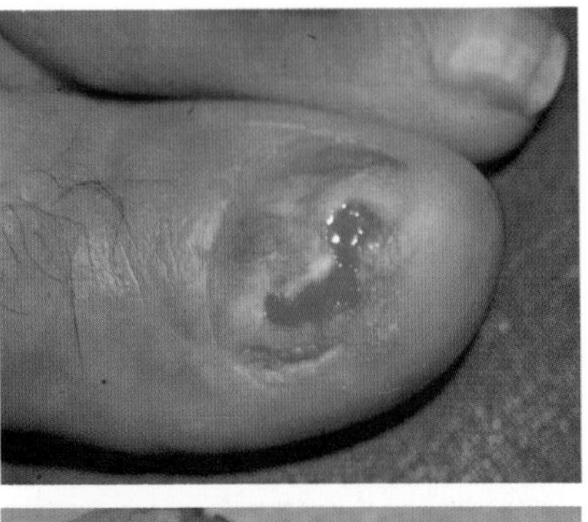

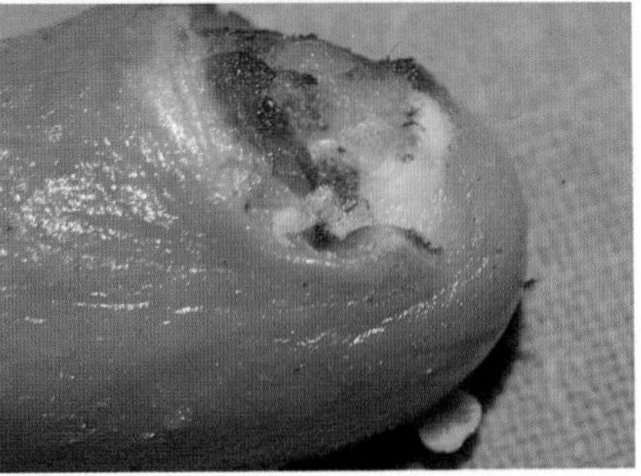

Fig. 11.46. Epidermoid carcinoma – ulceration and bleeding.

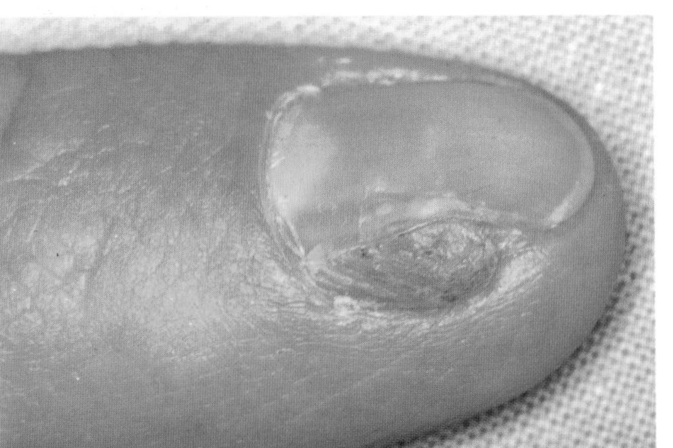

Fig. 11.47. Epidermoid carcinoma – mimicking acquired periungual fibrokeratoma.

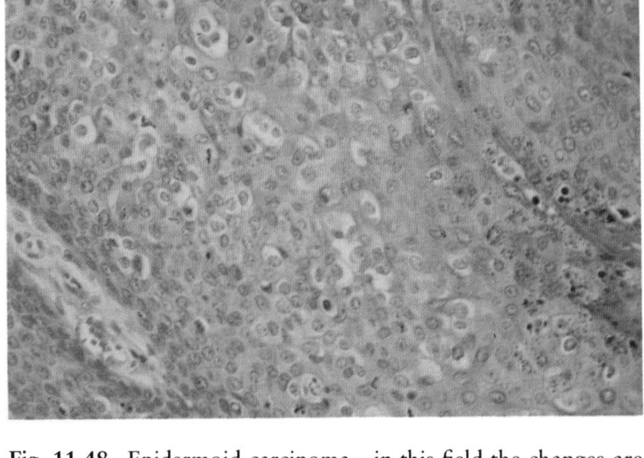

Fig. 11.48. Epidermoid carcinoma – in this field the changes are *in situ* (Bowen's disease).

The neoplastic process most commonly originates in the nail folds or nail grooves and may thus clinically mimic infections and other chronic inflammatory conditions.

Differential diagnosis. The signs are often mistaken for chronic inflammatory conditions, including bacterial infections (Bizzle, 1992) as well as pyogenic granuloma nail dystrophy, verruca vulgaris, subungual exostosis, malignant melanoma, glomus tumour and subungual keratoacanthoma, and even acquired ungual fibrokeratoma (Haneke, 1991; Baran & Perrin, 1994 and Figs 11.47 & 11.48).

The aetiology of subungual epidermoid carcinoma remains unclear. Arsenic cannot be excluded, e.g. in older psoriatic patients. Trauma and chronic paronychia have been cited as aetiological factors, but the most important factor is exposure to X-ray (physicians, dentists, patients). This may be followed by radiodermatitis (de Dulanto & Camacho, 1979) which is, with discovery of HPV infection, the most common factor for the development of squamous cell carcinoma (Guitart *et al.*, 1990). HPV-16, -34 (Kawashima *et al.*, 1986) and -35 (Rüdlinger *et al.*, 1989) have been detected in epidermoid carcinoma *in situ* and invasive types. The HPV genome was found in eight out of 10 periungual lesions by dot-blot analysis of frozen tissue; six of these were related to HPV-16 (Moy *et al.*, 1989). Using the polymerase chain reaction to detect human papillomavirus in formalin-fixed, paraffin-embedded specimens of periungual squamous cell carcinoma, Ashinoff *et al.* (1991) found that five of the seven periungual lesions contained HPV-16. *In situ* hybridization failed to identify HPV in any of these patients' tumours.

This finding prompts one to speculate whether genital–digital transmission of the virus occurs or whether the carcinomas may be the product of malignant transformation of warts. In Rüdlinger *et al.*'s case (1989), Bowen's disease of the nail apparatus and bowenoid papulosis of the anogenital area revealed an identical HPV-35 infection. Since the patient suffered from long-lasting pruritus of the anogenital area, scratching may have resulted in autoinoculation. However, in the case of Bowen's disease reported by Ostrow *et al.* (1989), the HPV-16 DNA was discovered in a solitary subungual warty lesion and the integration of the HPV-16 DNA appears, so far, to be closely associated with the progression of a premalignant lesion to a malignant one.

Treatment. The need for complete removal of the lesion cannot be overemphasized.

1 The best treatment is Mohs' micrographic surgery technique allowing adequate excision with maximal preservation of normal tissue and function. This can be performed with routine instrumentation as well as with the CO_2 laser in a focused beam incisional mode – this avoids bleeding and ensures minimal post-operative discomfort for the patient.

2 Excisional surgery may be used in some cases or for complete removal of the nail apparatus, healing being by secondary intention, grafting or flap (Haneke, 1991).

3 Electrosurgery is a therapeutic alternative in a minority of selected cases.

4 Liquid nitrogen cryosurgery may give good results in experienced hands (Dawber *et al.*, 1992).

References

Ashinoff R., Junli J., Jacobson M. *et al.* (1991) Detection of HPV DNA in squamous cell carcinoma of the nail bed and finger determined by polymerase chain reaction. *Arch. Dermatol.* **127**, 1813–1818.

Baran R. & Eichmann A. (1993) Longitudinal melanonychia associated to Bowen disease. *Dermtology* **186**, 159–160.

Baran R. & Gormley D. (1988) Polydactylous Bowen's disease of the nail. *J. Am. Acad. Dermatol.* **17**, 201–204.

Baran R. & Perrin C. (1994) Pseudo-acquired fibrokeratoma of the nail apparatus: A new clue for diagnosing Bowen disease. *Acta Dermato. Venereol.* (in press).

Baran R. & Simon C. (1988) Longitudinal melanonychia: A symptom of Bowen's disease. *J. Am. Acad. Dermatol.* **18**, 1359–1360.

Bizzle P.G. (1992) Subungual squamous cell carcinoma of the thumb marked by infection. *Orthopedics* **15**, 1350–1352.

Campbel J. & Keokarn T. (1966) Squamous-cell carcinoma of the nail bed in epidermal dysplasia. *J. Bone Joint Dis.* **48**, 92–99.

Dawber R.P.R., Colver G.B. & Jackson A. (1992) *Cutaneous Cryosurgery*, 1st edn, pp. 78–82. Martin Dunitz, London.

De Dulanto F. & Camacho F. (1979) Radiodermatitis. *Acta Derm. Sif.* **70**, 67–94.

Guitart J., Bergfeld W.F., Tuthull R.J. *et al.* (1990) Squamous cell carcinoma of the nail bed: a clinicopathological study of 12 cases. *Br. J. Dermatol.* **123**, 215–222.

Haneke E. (1991) Epidermoid carcinoma (Bowen's disease) of the nail simulating acquired ungual fibrokeratoma. *Skin Cancer* **6**, 217–221.

Kawashima M., Jablonska S., Favre M. *et al.* (1986) Characterization of a new type of human papillomavirus found in a lesion of Bowen's disease of the skin. *J. Virol.* **57**, 688–692.

Long P.I. & Espinella J.L. (1978) Squamous cell carcinoma of the nail bed. *J. Am. Med. Assoc.* **239**, 2154–2155.

McGrae J.D., Greer C. & Manos M. (1993) Multiple Bowen's disease of the fingers associated with HPV type 16. *Int. J. Dermatol.* **32**, 104–107.

Mauro J.A., Maslyn R. & Stein A.A. (1972) Squamous-cell carcinoma of nail bed in hereditary ectodermal dysplasia. *NY State J. Med.* **72**, 1065–1066.

Mikhail G. (1984) Subungual epidermoid carcinoma. *J. Am. Acad. Dermatol.* **11**, 291–298.

Moy R.L., Eliezri Y., Nuovo G.J., Zitelli J.A., Bennett R.G. & Silverstein S. (1989) Human papillomavirus Type 16 DNA in periungual squamous cell carcinomas. *J. Am. Med. Assoc.* **261**, 2669–2673.

Ostrow R.S., Shaver M.A., Turnquist S. *et al.* (1989) Human papillomavirus-16 DNA in a cutaneous invasive cancer. *Arch. Dermatol.* **125**, 666–669.

Rüdlinger R., Grob R., Yu Y. & Schnyder U.W. (1989) Human papillomavirus-35 positive bowenoid papulosis of the anogenital area and concurrent with bowenoid dysplasia of the periungual area. *Arch. Dermatol.* **125**, 655–659.

Saijo S., Kato T. & Tagami H. (1990) Pigmented nail streak associated with Bowen's disease of the nail matrix. *Dermatologica* **181**, 156–158.

Salasche S.S. & Garland L.D. (1985) Tumour of the nail. *Dermatol. Clin.* **3**, 501–519.

Zaias N. (1990) *The Nail in Health and Disease.* Appleton & Lange, Norwalk, CN.

Epithelioma cuniculatum

Epithelioma cuniculatum is a rare, slow-growing, but locally destructive, low-grade epithelioma of squamous cell origin (Figs 11.49–11.51). It has been reported in three patients with thumb involvement and in one patient with raquet thumb (Haneke & Baran, 1990). Distolateral onycholysis and paronychia of the corresponding side (Fig. 11.49) was observed by McKee *et al.* (1986) in a 38-year-old woman; it had been present for at least 18 months. The second case started in a similar fashion. Progressively the inflammatory features were accompanied by subungual purulent material leading to disappearance of the nail plate. The nail bed was covered with multiple 'holes' extruding toothpaste-like, 'foul-smelling', yellow-white material (Magnin *et al.*, 1986). The patient of Coldiron *et al.* (1986) presented with a verrucous growth of the distal portion of the thumb. It was a friable mass erupting from the pulp. A biopsy revealed that the entire pulp was involved down to the bone. The great toe (Hitti *et al.*, 1987) and fifth toe (Tosti *et al.*, 1992) may be involved with loss of the nail.

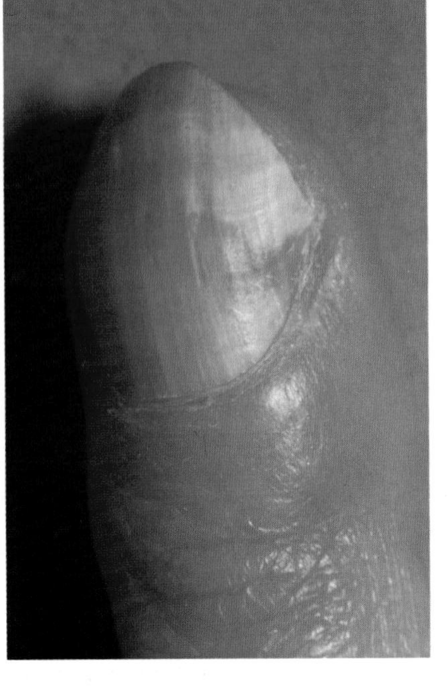

Fig. 11.49. Epithelioma cuniculatum—onycholysis (courtesy of R. Staughton, London, UK).

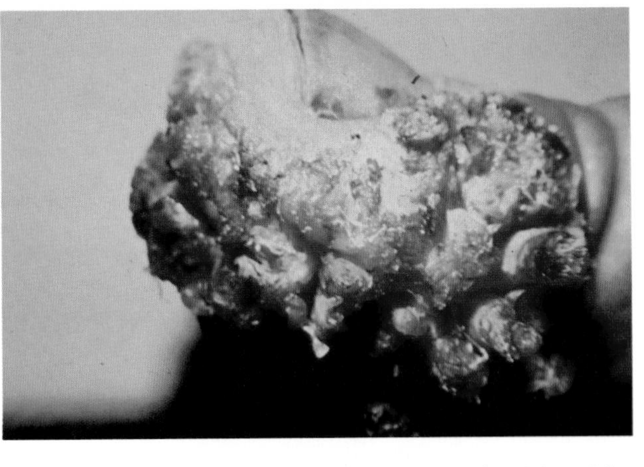

Fig. 11.50. Epithelioma cuniculatum (courtesy of L. Jaimovich, Buenos-Ayres, Argentina).

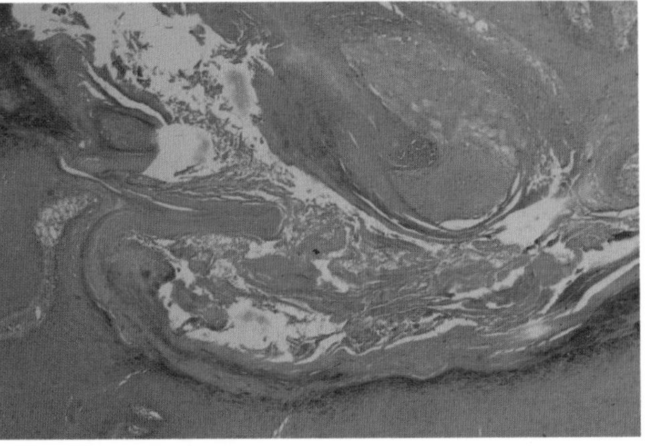

Fig. 11.51. Epithelioma cuniculatum – histological changes.

The radiography of most patients shows erosion or disappearance of the distal third of the phalanx.

Carcinoma cuniculatum is a rare variant of verrucous carcinoma (Fig. 11.50) characterized by a system of epithelium-lined tunnels in the tumour. Histology (Fig. 11.51) shows a proliferation of epithelial cell complexes with squamous differentiation, formation of fistulae filled with keratinous debris, and a pushing border rather than frank invasion. Mitoses are rare, as are dyskeratoses. Usually, there is marked focal hypergranulosis. Cellular atypia is usually not pronounced and the lesion may be misdiagnosed as pseudoepitheliomatous hyperplasia.

Immunohistochemistry using antibodies to different cytokeratins, involucrin and filaggrin as well as lectin histochemistry with peanut agglutinin only reflect the high degree of differentiation (Haneke & Baran, 1990). Filaggrin is present where keratohyalin can be seen in haematoxylin and eosin (H&E) stained section, and involucrin is also expressed by the major part of the tumour cells. PNA binding is variable with both completely positive and negative areas. Neuraminidase digestion unmasks the Friedreich–Thomsen antigen thus rendering all tumour cells positive (E. Haneke, unpublished data).

Differential diagnosis includes verrucae (even histologically) and keratoacanthoma, which exhibits rapid growth and clinically aggressive behaviour.

Epithelioma cuniculatum should not be confused with squamous cell carcinoma as it is verrucous and histologically shows little anaplasia. Pseudoepitheliomatous hyperplasia shows very irregular, jagged, papillomatous down growths when compared with epithelioma cuniculatum (Coldiron *et al.*, 1986).

Successful treatment may require Mohs' histographic surgery because of its 'tissue-sparing' capacity. Amputation is usually not necessary.

References

Coldiron B.M., Brown F.C. & Freeman R.G. (1986) Epithelioma cuniculatum of the thumb: a case report and literature review. *J. Dermatol. Surg. Oncol.* **12**, 1150–1154.

Cowen P. (1983) Epithelioma cuniculatum. *Aust. J. Dermatol.* **24**, 83–85.

Haneke E. & Baran R. (1990) Epithelioma cuniculatum. ISDS meeting, Florence, Italy (Abstr. p. 55).

Hitti I.F., Sadowski G., Statsinger A.L. *et al.* (1987) *Cutis* **39**, 250–252.

Magnin Ph., Label M.G., Schroh R. *et al.* (1986) Carcinoma cuniculatum localizado en el ledra subungual. *Rev. Arg. Dermatol.* **67**, 68–72.

McKee R., Wilkinson J.D., Black M.M. *et al.* (1986) Carcinoma (epithelioma) cuniculatum: a clinico-pathological study of nineteen cases and review of the literature. *Histopathology* **5**, 425–436.

Tosti A., Morelli R., Fanti P.A. *et al.* (1993) Carcinoma cuniculatum of the nail apparatus, report of 3 cases. *Dermatology* **186**, 217–221.

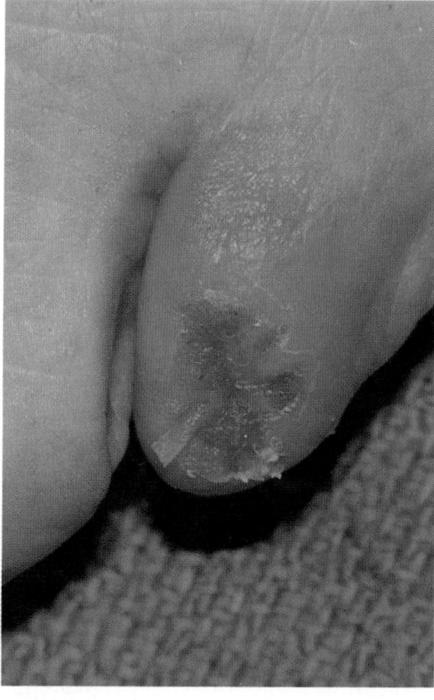

Fig. 11.52. Basal cell carcinoma of the fifth toe (courtesy of G.R. Mikhail, Detroit, USA).

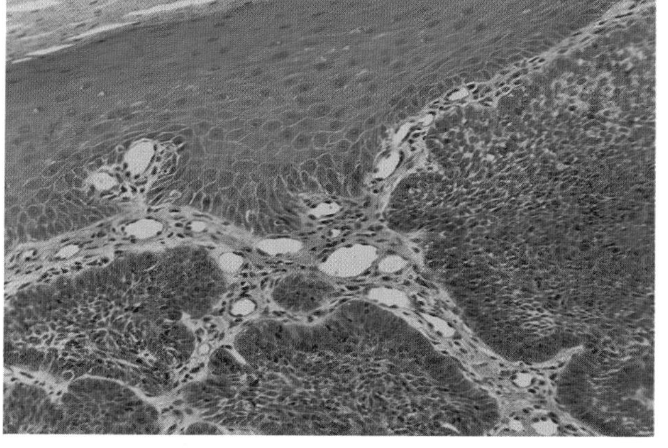

Fig. 11.53. Basal cell carcinoma – case seen in Fig. 11.52, histological changes.

Basal cell carcinoma (basalioma)

Although basal cell carcinoma is the most common malignant skin tumour, it is exceptionally rare in the subungual region (Figs 11.52 & 11.53). Only 13 cases have been reported since the first description by Eisenklam (1931).

The usual presentation is a chronic paronychia or a periungual eczematous process, often associated with ulceration, granulation tissue, and pain. Acquired longitudinal melanonychia in a white patient as the only manifestation of subungual basal cell carcinoma is unique (Rudolph, 1987).

Basal cell carcinoma may be present for many years before diagnosis.

In most cases the lesions have occurred on the fingers, except for one lesion on a fifth toe (Mikhail, 1985) (Fig. 11.52), and involvement of the great toe (Zaias, 1990) developing into a large ulcerating mass (Waldman & Jacobs, 1986).

The diagnosis can only be made by histological examination (Fig. 11.53).

References

Eisenklam D. (1931) Über subunguale Tumouren. *Wien Klin. Wschr.* **44**, 1192–1193.

Mikhail G.R. (1985) Subungual basal cell carcinoma. *J. Dermatol. Surg. Oncol.* **11**, 1222–1223.

Rudolph R.I. (1987) Subungual basal cell carcinoma presenting as longitudinal melanonychia. *J. Am. Acad. Dermatol.* **16**, 229–233.

Waldman M.H. & Jacobs L.A. (1986) Malignant tumours of the foot. A report of 2 cases. *J. Am. Podiatr. Assoc.* **76**, 345.

Zaias N. (1990) *The Nail in Health and Disease*, p. 225. Appleton & Lange, Norwalk, CN.

Porocarcinoma

Periungual porocarcinoma is exceptional. Requena *et al.* (1990) reported on a patient exposed to X-rays for many years which resulted in chronic radiodermatitis of several digits on both hands. He displayed an ulcer in the lateral nail fold of the right third digit which extended into the nail bed (Fig. 11.54). The histology was consistent with malignant eccrine poroma (Fig. 11.55).

Another case originating in the lateral nail fold of the third finger of the right hand of a 77-year old man was described by Van Gorp and Van der Putt (1993). The patient presented with a very painful induration on the radial side of the distal portion of the finger. During excision, the tumour showed infiltrative growth into the long phalanx.

References

Requena L., Sanchez M., Aguilar P. *et al.* (1990) Periungual porocarcinoma. *Dermatologica* **180**, 177–180.

Van Gorp J. & Van der Putt S.C.J. (1993) Periungual eccrine porocarcinoma. *Dermatology* **187**, 67–70.

Soft tissue tumour

Fibrous tumour

There are many different types of fibromas which may develop in the subungual and periungual area. These may represent true entities in themselves, or merely be variants of the same process. These fibrous tumours comprise a large variety of clinical types ranging from fibrous dermatofibroma to digital fibrokeratoma. This contrasts markedly with the uniformity of the histology of the fibrous tumours. This is an argument in favour of Koenen's tumour, acquired fibrokeratoma and dermatofibroma

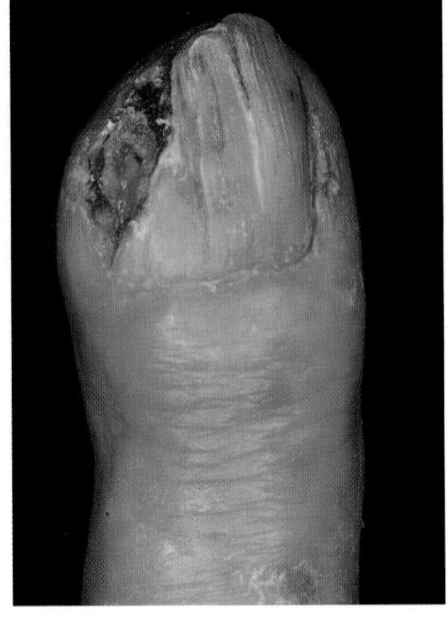

Fig. 11.54. Malignant eccrine poroma.

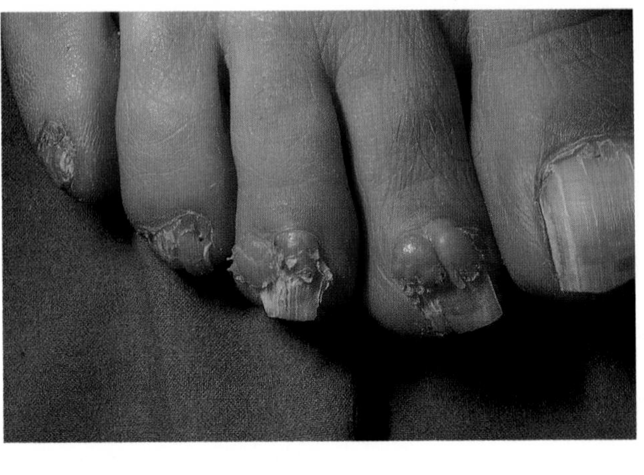

Fig. 11.56. Koenen's tumours of tuberous sclerosis.

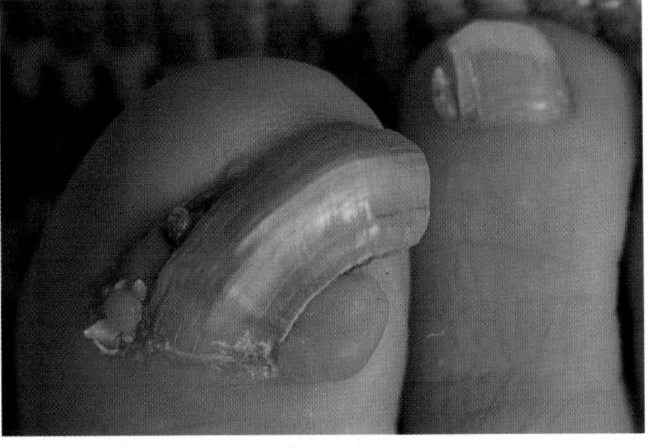

Fig. 11.57. Koenen's tumours of tuberous sclerosis.

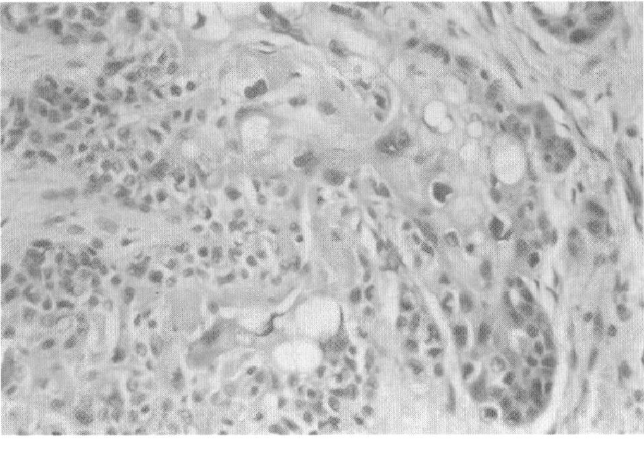

Fig. 11.55. Malignant eccrine poroma – histological changes (courtesy of L. Requena, Madrid, Spain).

being part of a 'clinical continuum' (overlapping), though the location of the origin of fibroplastic proliferation could offer a clue to the diagnosis (Baran *et al.*, 1994). For all these reasons, fibrokeratoma, a fibroepithelial tumour, is studied with the various fibrous tumours (Figs 11.56–11.76).

What follows hopes to document and make some sense of the literature in the field – it looks complex, but if one ignores clinical variability and sticks to pathology, it is probably quite simple!

Koenen's tumours

Koenen's periungual fibromata develop in 50% of the cases of tuberous sclerosis (epiloia or Bourneville–Pringle disease) and are, consequently, as frequent as renal ham-

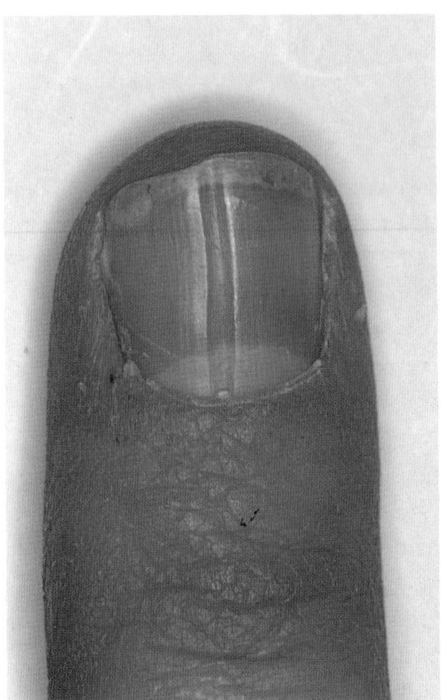

Fig. 11.58. Koenen's tumour – small lesion under the proximal nail fold causing a groove in the nail plate.

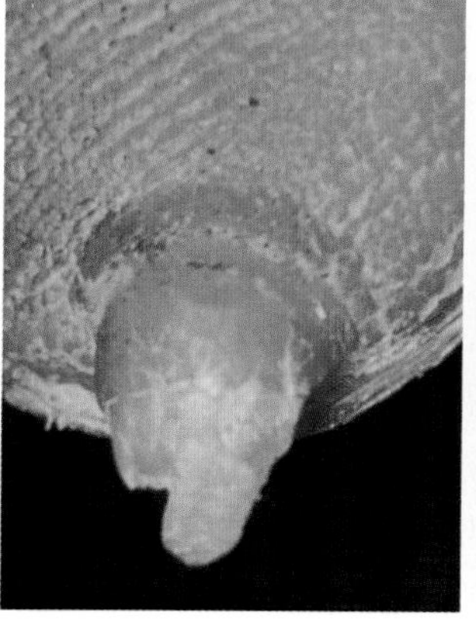
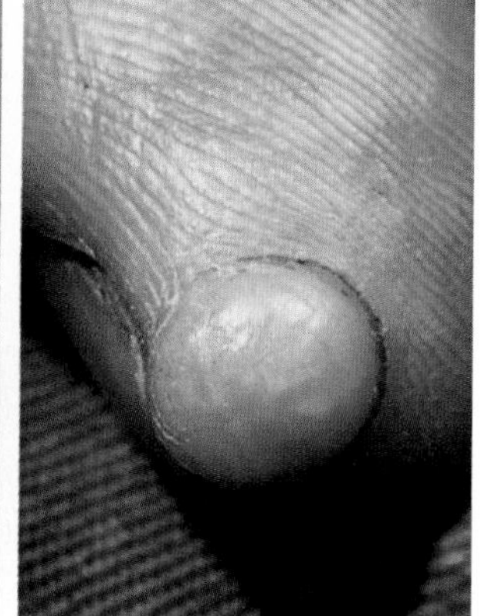

Fig. 11.59. Acquired digital fibrokeratoma.

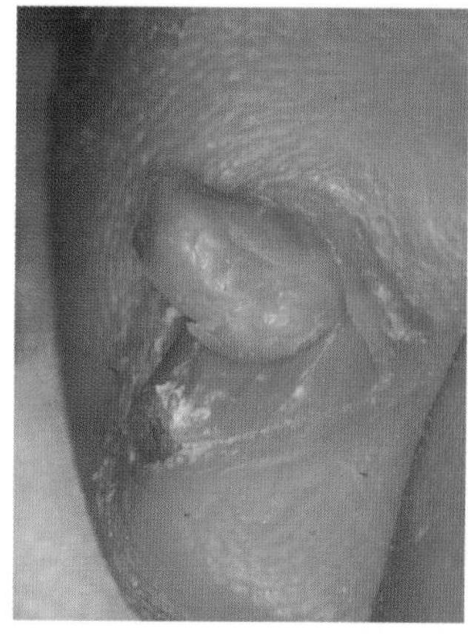
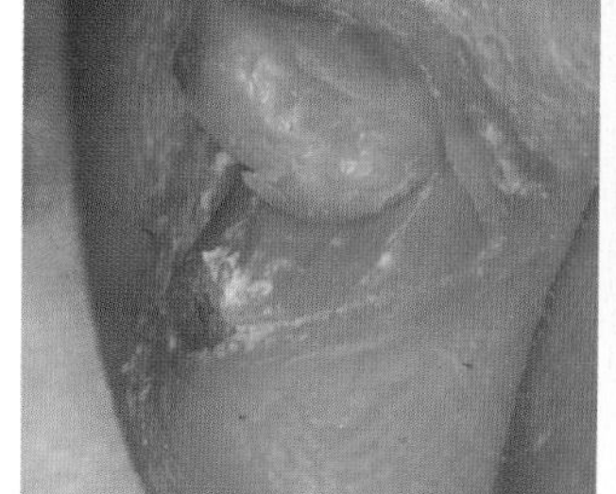
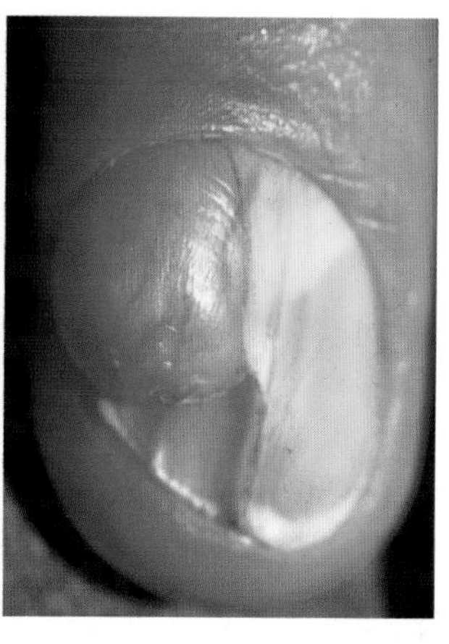

Fig. 11.60. Garlic-clove fibroma.

artomata. They usually appear between the ages of 12 and 14 years and increase progressively in size and number with age. Individual tumours are small, round, flesh-coloured, and asymptomatic, with a smooth surface (Figs 11.56 & 11.57).

The tip of the tumour may be slightly hyperkeratotic, and resemble fibrokeratoma. They grow out of the nail fold, eventually overgrowing the nail bed and destroying the nail plate. Depending on their location, they may cause longitudinal depression of the nail plate. Even tiny hyperkeratotic lesions in the cuticle area may produce identical longitudinal nail grooves and have the same significance as Koenen's tumours (Colomb *et al.*, 1976) (Fig. 11.58). Excessively large tumours are often painful and should be excised at their base.

In the Koenen's tumours we have examined (Kint & Baran, 1988) two portions were distinguishable: a small distal segment with loose collagen and many blood vessels and a larger proximal part composed of dense collagen bundles and fewer capillaries. No neural or glial appearance (Nickel & Reed, 1962) or arteriovenous anastomoses (Knoth & Meyhöfer, 1957) could be found. It thus appears that Koenen's tumour can be considered as a particular type of fibrokeratoma which can be subdivided according to its clinical appearance, location, and origin, into the following subtypes.

1 Fibrokeratomas originating from the dermal connective tissue. These are post-traumatic or appear spontaneously and are usually located on the fingers (acquired digital fibrokeratoma).

2 Fibrokeratomas originating from the proximal nail fold or the surrounding connective tissue. They are located in the nail fold and can be hereditary (tuberous sclerosis) or acquired (for example, garlic-clove fibroma).

Circumscribed storiform collagenoma (Metcalf *et al.*, 1991), recently described in Cowden's disease, is a fibrotic nodule. Its histological features include a whorled appear-

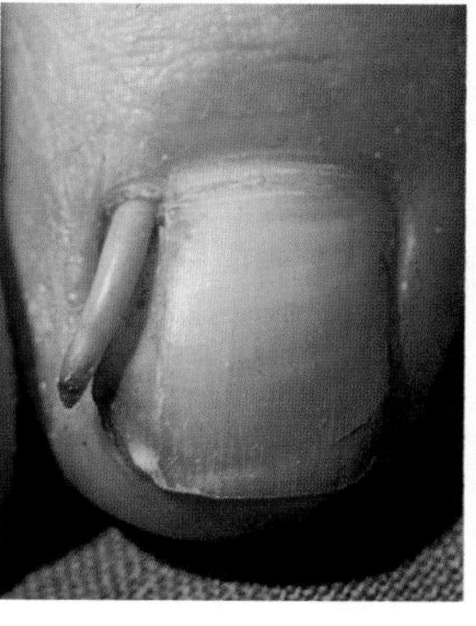
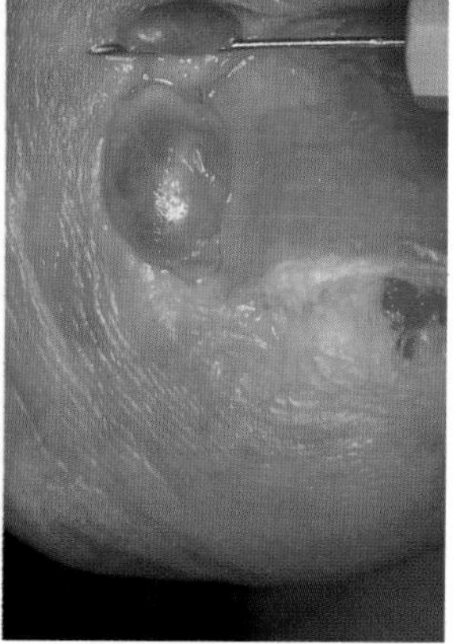

Fig. 11.61. Acquired periungual fibrokeratoma.

ance of sclerotic hyalinized collagen bundles separated by mucin-containing clefts, similar to fibroma. However, the bands of collagen are sharply demarcated from the surrounding normal skin in sclerotic hypocellular fibroma and the lesions are almost acellular.

Koenen's tumours are cured by simple excision. Usually, no suture is necessary. Tumours growing out from under the proximal nail fold are removed after reflecting the proximal nail fold back by making lateral incisions down each margin in the axis of the lateral nail grooves. Subungual fibromas are removed after avulsion of the corresponding part of the nail plate.

References

Baran R., Perrin C., Baudet J. & Requena L. (1994) Clinical and histological patterns of dermatofibromas (true fibromas) of the nail apparatus. *Clin. Exp. Dermatol.* in press.

Colomb D., Racouchot J. & Jeune R. (1976) Les lésions des ongles dans la sclérose tubéreuse de Bourneville isolées ou associées aux tumeurs de Koenen. *Ann. Dermatol. Syphil.* **103**, 431–437.

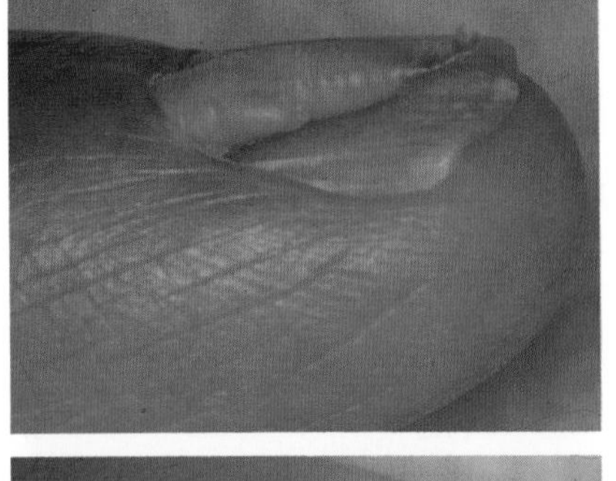

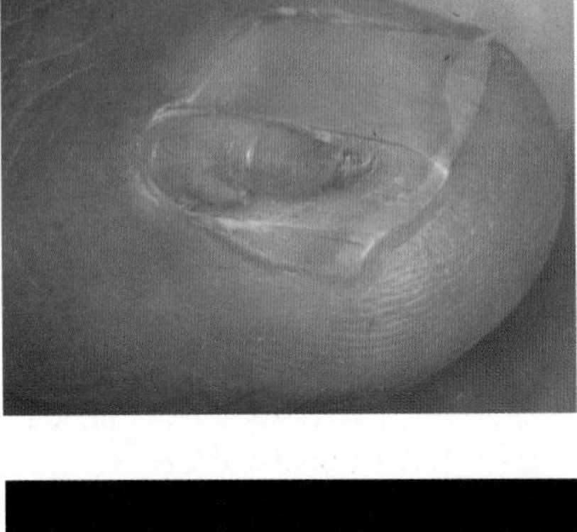

Fig. 11.62. Acquired fibrokeratoma – causing a longitudinal nail plate depression (courtesy of I. Kikuchi, Japan).

Fig. 11.63. Acquired periungual fibrokeratoma – after operative removal (top); low-power histological (Masson stain) changes (bottom).

Kint A. & Baran R. (1988) Histopathologic study of Koenen tumours. *J. Am. Acad. Dermatol.* **18**, 369–372.

Knoth W. & Meyhöfer W. (1957) Zur Nosologie des Adenoma sebaceum Typ Balzer, der Koenenschen Tumoren und des Morbus Bourneville-Pringle. *Hautarzt* **8**, 359–366.

Metcalf J.S., Maize J.S. & LeBoit P.E. (1991) Circumbscribed storiform collagenoma. *Am. J. Dermatopathol.* **13**, 122–129.

Nickel W.R. & Reed R.J. (1962) Tuberous sclerosis. Special reference to the microscopic alterations in the cutaneous hamartomas. *Arch. Dermatol.* **85**, 209–224.

Acquired periungual fibrokeratoma

Acquired periungual fibrokeratoma is probably identical to acquired digital fibrokeratoma (Bart *et al.*, 1968) (Fig. 11.59) and garlic-clove fibroma (Steel, 1965; LoBuono *et al.*, 1979) (Fig. 11.60). They are acquired, benign, spontaneously developing, asymptomatic nodules with a hyperkeratotic tip and a narrow base which occur mostly in the periungual area (Fig. 11.61) or elsewhere on the fingers. They may be double and even triple. Takino and Mitoh (1983) reported a case in which the lesion was located beneath the nail and visible under the free margin of the great toenail. Most periungual fibrokeratomas emerge from the most proximal part of the nail sulcus, growing on the nail and causing a sharp longitudinal depression (Kikuchi *et al.*, 1978) (Figs 11.62 & 11.63).

Trauma is thought to be a major factor initiating acquired periungual fibrokeratoma. Biopsy is mandatory for the diagnosis of nail tumours: Haneke (1991) then Baran and Perrin (1994) described a case of Bowen's disease simulating acquired ungual fibrokeratoma (Fig. 11.47).

Histological examination of 50 cases of acquired digital fibrokeratoma (Kint *et al.*, 1985) disclosed three histological variants: (i) a tumour composed of thick dense and closely packed collagen bundles (Fig. 11.64); (ii) a variant

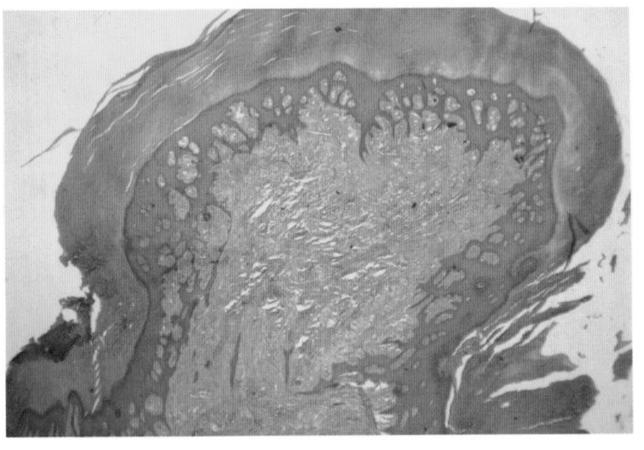

Fig. 11.64. Acquired periungual fibrokeratoma type 1.

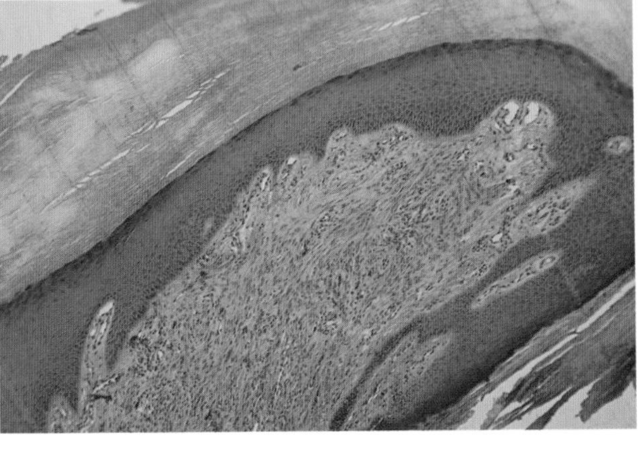

Fig. 11.65. Acquired periungual fibrokeratoma type 2.

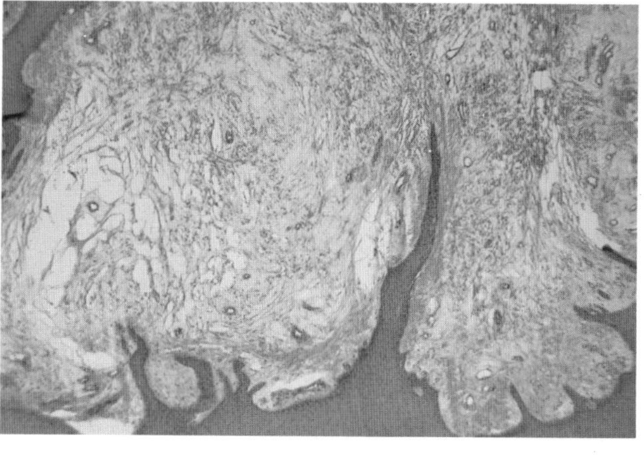

Fig. 11.66. Acquired periungual fibrokeratoma, type 3.

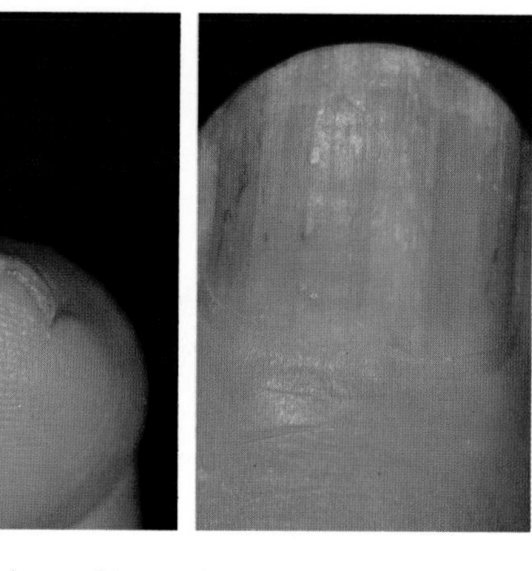
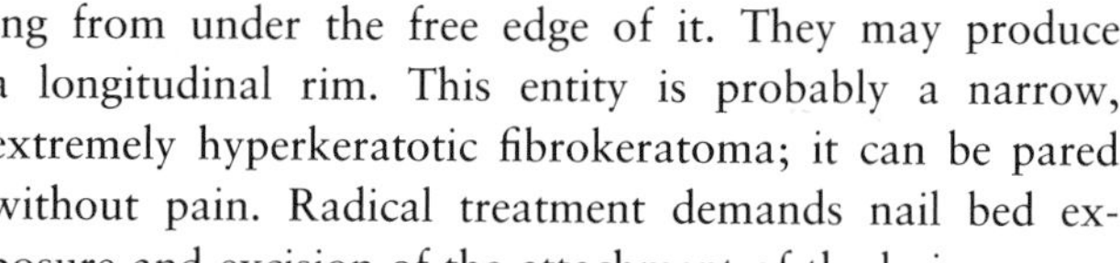

Fig. 11.67. Distal subungual keratosis.

with an increased number of fibroblasts in the cutis (Fig. 11.65); and (iii) a type with an oedematous and poorly cellular structure (Fig. 11.66). The acquired digital fibrokeratoma is thought to be made up of newly formed collagen. The acanthosis of the epidermis is probably secondary to the dermal changes.

Immunohistochemistry shows that the fibroblasts are vimentin positive and many of them stain with HHF-35, a monoclonal antibody said to be specific for muscle actin.

Surgical treatment is the same as for Koenen's tumours and will depend on the size and location of the fibroma.

The differential diagnosis of acquired periungual fibroma includes fibroma, keloid, Koenen's tumour, recurring digital fibrous tumour of childhood, dermatofibrosarcoma, fibrosarcoma, acrochordon, cutaneous horn, Bowen's disease, eccrine poroma, pyogenic granuloma, verruca vulgaris and exostosis (Cahn, 1977).

Invaginated fibrokeratoma with matrix differentiation
(Perrin & Baran, 1994)

Two cases of a variant of a fibrokeratoma involving the ventral aspect of the proximal nail fold have been seen. They have three characteristic features.

1 Proximal to the normal matrix, and in the same axis, there is epithelial invagination.

2 The floor of this infolding acts as an accessory matrix without a granular layer, and gives rise to a pseudonail made of keratin, similar to the normal nail plate.

3 This accessory nail apparatus, lying on a dermal fibrous nodule, is sharply demarcated from the surrounding dermis, having a large base which narrows to its tip, giving the typical appearance of an incipient fibrokeratoma – type I in Kint *et al.*'s (1985) classification.

Subungual filamentous tumour

Subungual filamentous tumours are thread-like horny subungual lesions growing with the nail plate and emerging from under the free edge of it. They may produce a longitudinal rim. This entity is probably a narrow, extremely hyperkeratotic fibrokeratoma; it can be pared without pain. Radical treatment demands nail bed exposure and excision of the attachment of the lesion.

Histology shows a subungual rim of keratinous substance in an irregular whorled arrangement. The nail bed may show a single slight papillomatous projection with marked hypergranulosis.

References

Baran R. & Perrin C. (1994) Invaginated fibrokeratoma with matrix differentiation. *Br. J. Dermatol.* (in press).

Baran R. & Perrin C. (1994) Pseudo-acquired fibrokeratoma of the nail apparatus: A new clue for Bowen disease. *Acta Derm. Venereol.* (in press).

Bart R.S., Andrade R., Kopf A.W. & Leider M. (1968) Acquired digital fibrokeratomas. *Arch. Dermatol.* **97**, 120–129.

Cahn R.L. (1977) Acquired periungual fibrokeratoma. *Arch. Dermatol.* **113**, 1564–1568.

Haneke E. (1991) Epidermoid carcinoma (Bowen's disease) of the nail simulating acquired ungual fibrokeratoma. *Skin Cancer* **6**, 217–221.

Kikuchi I., Ishii Y. & Inoue S. (1978) Acquired periungual fibroma. *J. Dermatol.* **5**, 235–237.

Kint A., Baran R. & De Keyser H. (1985) Acquired (digital) fibrokeratoma. *J. Am. Acad. Dermatol.* **12**, 816–821.

LoBuono P., Jothikumar T. & Kornblee L. (1979) Acquired digital fibrokeratoma. *Cutis* **24**, 50–51.

Steel H.H. (1965) Garlic-clove fibroma. *J. Am. Med. Assoc.* **191**, 1082–1083.

Perrin C. & Baran R. (1993) Invaginated fibrokeratoma of the nail apparatus (in press).

Takino C. & Mitoh Y. (1983) A case of acquired ungual fibroma located beneath the nail. *Jap. J. Clin. Dermatol.* **37**, 57–62.

Distal subungual keratosis (Baran *et al.*, 1993)

Distal subungual keratosis is a small horny lesion originating from the hyponychium, resembling a form fruste of the subungual filamentous tumour (Fig. 11.67). It may be traced clinically and histologically as far as the lunula

Table 11.3. Differential diagnosis of ungual true fibroma with other fibrous tumours of the nail apparatus

Sclerotic fibroma (Rapini *et al.*, 1989)	*Leiomyoma* (Requena & Baran, 1994; Fitzpatrick *et al.*, 1990)
Well circumscribed Overlying epidermis thin	Muscle stains red with Masson Trichom (in contrast, fibroma stains blue)
Collagen bundle in a 'whorl-like' pattern	Leiomyoma is labelled by smooth muscle actin and desmin (Lever, 1983)
Fibroma of tendon sheath Well circumscribed	*Recurrent infantile digital fibromas* First year of life
Attachment to tendon or tendon sheath	Characteristic inclusion bodies visualized with phosphotungstic acid haematoxylin stain (Lever, 1983)
Gradual transition between cellular and more hyalinized areas	
Pleomorphic fibroma Multinucleated cells with large hyperchromatic nuclei	*Rudimentary supernumerary digits* Present at birth Involvement of the fifth digit Multiple nerve bundles within the dermal core
Keloid (Ackerman, 1978; Lever, 1983; Mehregan, 1986) Well circumscribed Papillary dermis normal Hypocellular areas admixed with more cellular areas	

and is clearly demonstrated by magnetic resonance imaging (MRI) (Goettmann, personal communication).

Fibrous dermatofibromas or 'true' fibromas (Table 11.3) (Baran *et al.*, 1994)

Fibromas usually develop as painless slow-growing nodular tumours (Figs 11.68–11.76). They may be spherical or oval in shape, and either firm or rubbery in consistency. They can develop in any epidermal structure of the nail apparatus and may move freely or remain fixed (Butler *et al.*, 1960). Fibromas may become cherry shaped and lift the nail in the distal subungual area (Fig. 11.68). In addition to deformity of the nail, displacement of the finger pulp and erosion of the distal phalanx may lead to the necessity for amputation. The tumour is smooth on the dorsal aspect of the proximal fold, or on the nail bed, and more often spherical (resembling a small pea) than ovoid. The fibroma may also be spherical on the lateral nail fold but without the collar of slightly elevated skin seen in acquired periungual fibrokeratoma.

Fibroma of the matrix results in nail dystrophy. Therefore clinical features are variable according to the anatomical site on the matrix, ranging from simple thinning of the nail plate to a longitudinal canal: the latter is sometimes partially covered by nail keratin to form a tunnel-like structure (Figs 11.71 & 11.74).

Lebouc (1889) described a plexiform fibroma of the nail bed which had developed after severe trauma. Heller (1902) described a sub- and periungual fibroma, the size of a pigeon egg. Histologically, fibromata are composed of hypocellular reticular nodules composed of very dense connective tissue bundles with elastic fibres present which are ill-defined and are similar in all patients. Factor XIIIa was negative in the core of the tumours but in one case the papillary dermis above the tumour showed a slight increase in factor XIIIa cells surrounding the vessels.

Two types of dermatofibroma are classically described (Lever & Schaumber-Lever, 1983): fibroma (or fibrous dermatofibroma) and histiocytoma. In the latter, uncommon in the nail apparatus, histiocytic proliferation is sometimes associated with an angiomatous component, most often referred to as sclerosing haemangiomas. Rupp *et al.* (1957) reported a unique case with darkening of the right great toenail, slight oedema, moderate erythema, and thickening of the nail, which proved to be a tumour

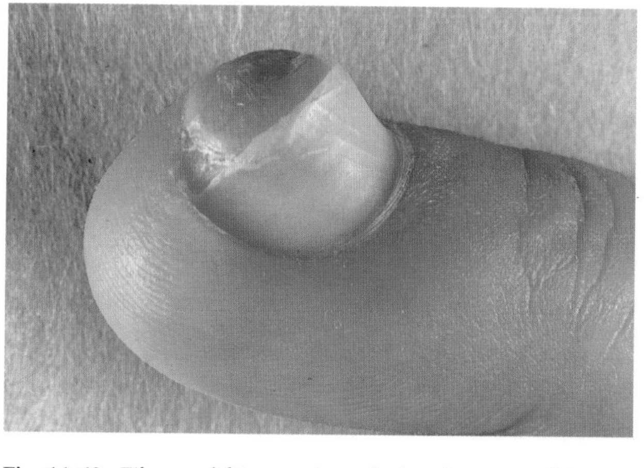

Fig. 11.68. Fibroma lifting up the nail plate (courtesy of S. Goettmann, Paris, France).

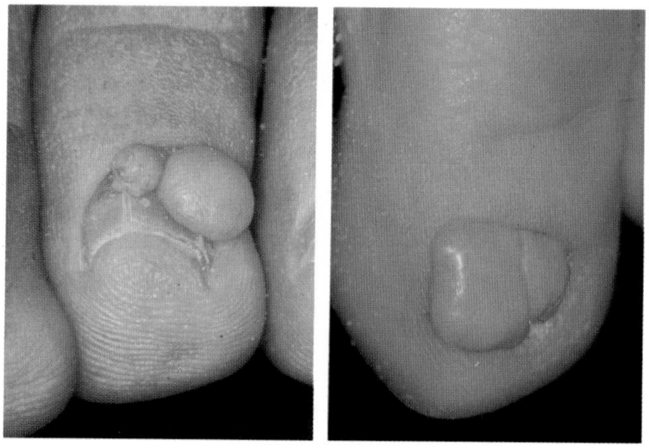

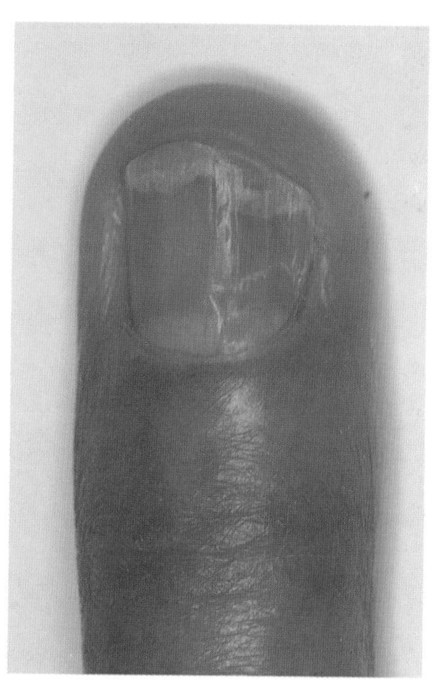

Fig. 11.71. Fibroma – nail dystrophy.

Fig. 11.69. Fibromata.

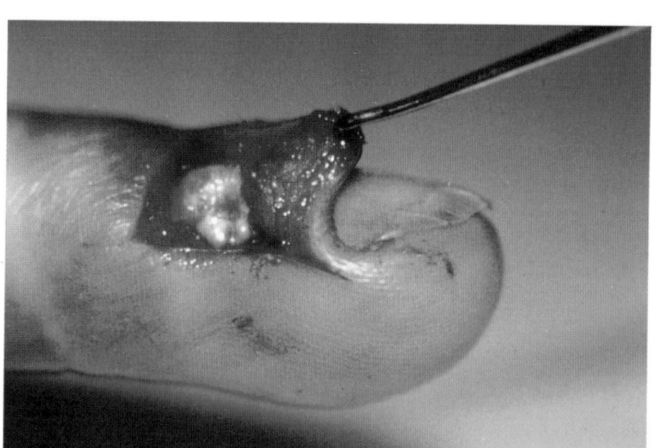

Fig. 11.72. Fibroma (Fig. 11.71), at operation.

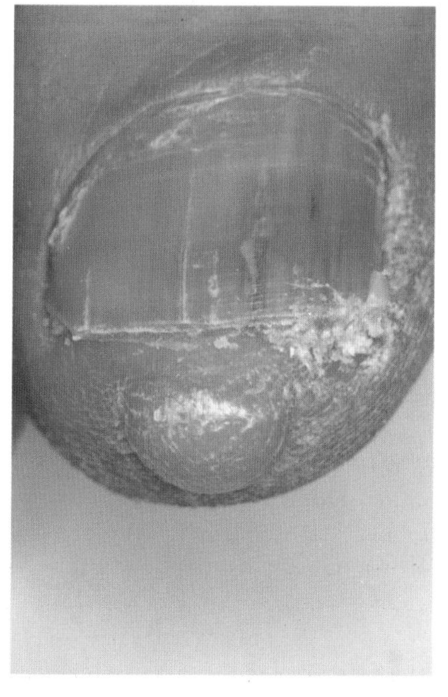

Fig. 11.70. Fibroma with distal nail plate fissuring.

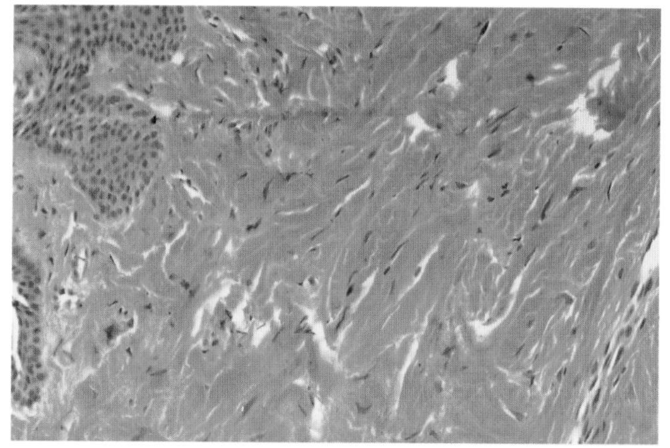

Fig. 11.73. Fibroma (Fig. 11.70).

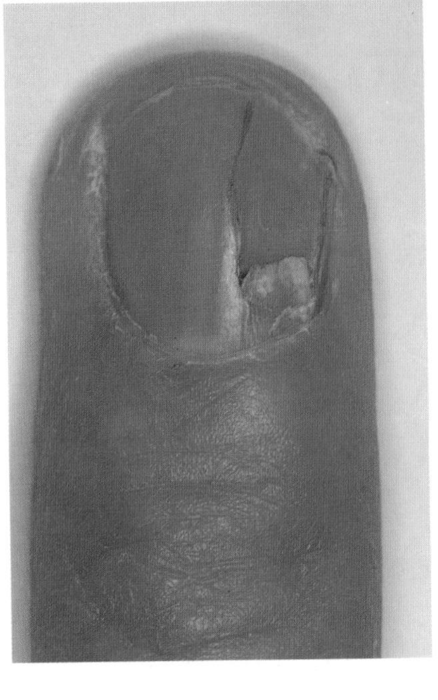

Fig. 11.74. Fibroma – nail dystrophy.

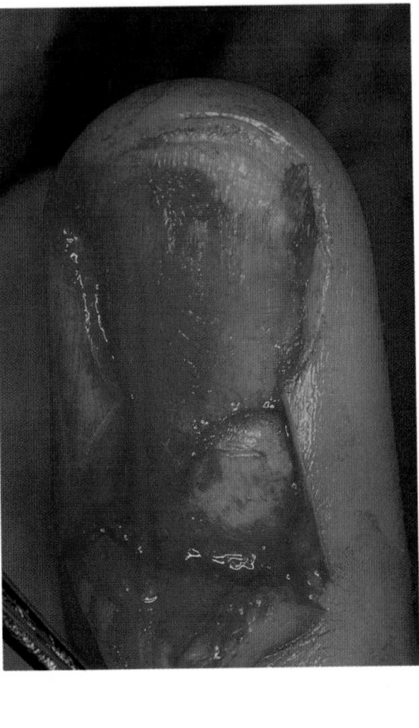

Fig. 11.75. Fibroma (11.74), at operation.

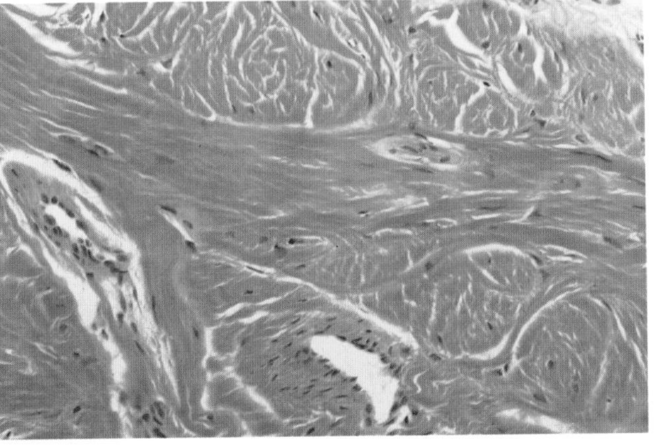

Fig. 11.76. Fibroma (11.74) – dermal microscopy.

mass within the distal phalanx. Focal erosion of the dorsal cortex with extension of the mass into the lower dermis was present. This was, histologically, a benign fibrous histiocytoma clinically mimicking a melanoma. Reed and Elmer (1971), in a review of 28 cases of solitary acral fibrous tumours, distinguished three histological varieties: (i) acquired fibrokeratoma; (ii) irritation fibroma; and (iii) fibroma molle.

This classification is difficult to apply in our experience and should probably be discarded; in support of this, several authors have used periungual fibroma and periungual fibrokeratoma as interchangeable or synonymous (Yasuki, 1985; Kojima *et al.*, 1987).

Three main histological clues distinguish isolated 'true' fibroma from AFK and from other tumours of the nail apparatus: (i) the lesions are composed of areas of very thick, hypocellular, hyalinized collagen bundles, in a haphazard array; (ii) there is an ill-defined nodule situated mostly in the reticular dermis; (iii) the elastic fibres are most often absent or scarce.

Several connective tissue lesions are easily ruled out (Table 11.3): hypertrophic scar and keloid, and the sclerosing type of giant cell tumour of tendon sheath. Leiomyoma is extremely rare. Recurrent infantile digital fibroma shows characteristic eosinophilic cytoplasmic inclusion bodies. Rudimentary supernumerary digits, at birth, have multiple nerve bundles within the dermal core. Some other connective tissue tumours should be mentioned: (i) circumscribed storiform collagenoma, often described in Cowden's disease, but the subungual fibrotic nodule reported by Sigel (1974) in a case of Cowden's disease was not explored histologically; (ii) dermatomyofibroma; (iii) desmoid tumours have not been described in the nail apparatus; and (iv) acquired digital fibrokeratoma is typically characterized by external finger-like projections with hyperkeratosis at the distal portion, while hereditary digital fibrokeratoma (Koenen's tumors) can appear as similar, but less hyperkeratotic, dome-shaped tumours, clinically very similar to fibroma. However, in contrast to fibroma, coarse hyalinized fibres are not present and there is no typical deep dermal nodule (Lever & Schaumber-Lever, 1983; Mehregan, 1986).

A case of 'osteoid fibroma' of the tip of the right little finger in a 10-year-old girl was described by Stein (1959).

References

Baran R., Perrin C.H., Baudet J. & Requena L. (1994) Clinical and histological patterns of desmatofibromas of the nail apparatus. *Clin. Exp. Dermatol.* (in press).

Butler E.D., Hamill J.P., Seipel R.S. & de Lorimier A.A. (1960) Tumours of the hand. *Am. J. Surg.* 100, 293–302.

Fitzpatrick J.E., Mellette J.R., Hwang R.J. *et al.* (1990) Cutaneous angiolipoleiomyoma. *J. Am. Acad. Dermatol.* **23**, 1093–1098.
Heller E. (1902) Zur Kenntnis der Fibrome und Sarkome an Hand und Fingern. Inaugural-Dissertation, Leipzig.
Kojima T., Nagano T. & Uchida M. (1987) Periungual fibroma. *J. Hand. Surg.* **12A**, 465–470.
Lebouc L. (1889) Etude clinique et anatomique sur quelques cas de tumeurs sous-unguéales. Thèse pour le doctorat en médecine, pp. 1–34, G. Steinheil, Paris.
Lever W.F. & Schaumburg-Lever G. (1983) *Histopatology of the Skin*, 7th edn. JB Lippincott, Philadelphia.
Mehregan A.M. (1986) *Pinkus' Guide to Dermatohistopathology*, 4th edn. Appleton Century-Crofts, Norwalk, CT.
Rapini R.P. & Golitz L.E. (1989) Sclerotic fibromas of the skin. *J. Am. Acad. Dermatol.* **20**, 266–271.
Reed R.J. & Elmer L.C. (1971) Multiple acral fibrokeratomas. Discussion of classification of anal fibrous nodules. *Arch. Dermatol.* **103**, 286–297.
Requena L. & Baran R. (1994) Angioleiomyoma of the finger. *J. Am. Acad. Dermatol.* **29**, 1043–1044.
Rupp M., Khalluf E. & Toker C. (1987) Subungual fibrous histiocytoma mimicking melanoma. *J. Am. Pod. Med. Assoc.* 3, 141–142.
Sigel J.M. (1974) Tuberous sclerosis (forme fruste) vs. Cowden syndrome. *Arch. Dermatol.* **110**, 476–477.
Stein A.H. (1959) Benign neoplastic and nonneoplastic destructive lesions in the long bones of the hand. *Surg. Gynec. Obstet.* **109**, 189–197.
Yasuki Y. (1985) Acquired periungual fibroid keratoma. *J. Dermatol.* **12**, 349–356.

Keloid

Hypertrophic scars and keloids result from injuries to the nail fold or nail bed and may produce disturbances in the nail unit (Heller, 1927) (Figs 11.77 & 11.78). Keloid exhibits hyalinized collagen bundles (Ackerman, 1978); the fibroblasts are contiguous with and parallel to the thick collagen bundles which are separated from the epidermis by nearly normal papillary dermis (Lever, 1983; Mehregan, 1986). Additionally, keloids are well circumscribed and elastic fibres are not present. In fresh hypertrophic scars, collagen fibres and fibroblasts are aligned parallel to the surface of the skin, and the epidermis is not hyperplastic (Ackerman, 1978). Leiomyomas are rare in the nail apparatus. In this disease, the muscle fibres are often difficult to distinguish from collagen. Aniline blue stain and more recently the indirect immunoperoxidase method with anti-desmin, distinguish muscle (red, desmin positive) from collagen (blue, desmin negative) (Lever, 1983).

References

Ackerman A.B. (1978) *Histologic Diagnosis of Inflammatory Skin Diseases*. Lea & Febiger, Philadelphia.
Heller J. (1927) Die Krankheiten der Nägel. In: *Handbuch der Haut-und Geschlechtskrankheitsen* (Hrsg. J. Jadassohn), Bd VIII/2: Spezielle Dermatologie, S.150–172.
Mehregan A.M. (1986) *Pinkus' Guide to Dermatohistopathology*, 4th edn. Appleton-Century-Crofts, Norwalk, CT.

Knuckle pads

Knuckle pads (Fig. 11.79) are asymptomatic, persistent, flesh-coloured, keratotic, nodular plaques occurring on the dorsal surface of the interphalangeal joints. Histology shows hyperkeratosis and an increase in the thickness of the collagen bundles (Mulvaney *et al.*, 1985).

Reference

Mulvaney M.S., Salasche S.J. & Hayes T.J. (1985) Differential diagnosis of multiple acral nodules. *J. Assoc. Milit. Derm.* **11**, 24–27.

Fibromatosis

Infantile digital fibromatosis (recurring digital fibrous tumours of childhood, benign juvenile digital fibromatosis) (Reye, 1965)

Recurring digital fibrous tumours (RDFT) (Fig. 11.80) are round, smooth, dome-shaped, shiny (Oñate-Cuchet *et al.*,

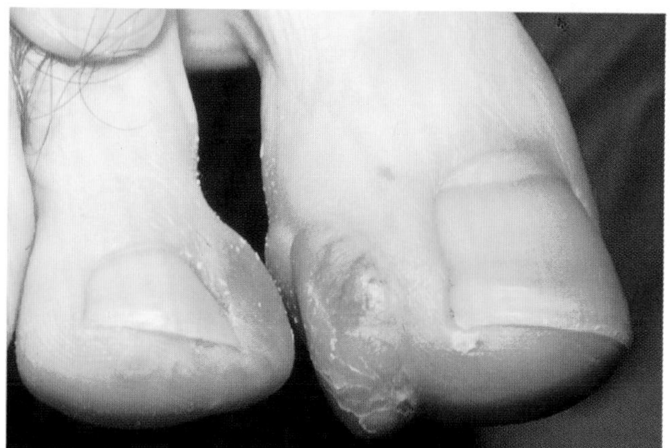

Fig. 11.77. Keloid from electrosurgery of a periungual wart.

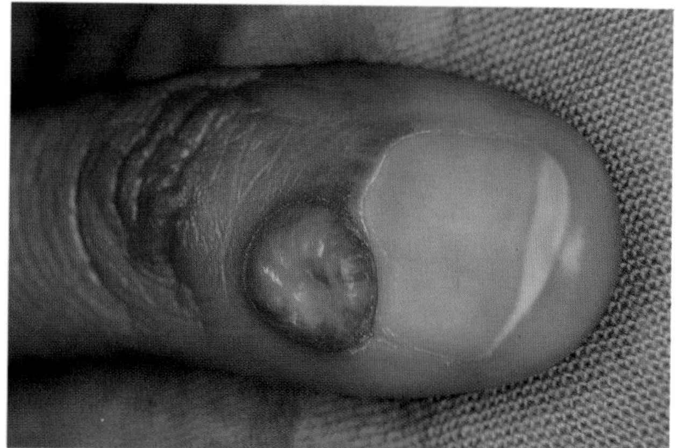

Fig. 11.78. Keloid (courtesy of S. Salasche, USA).

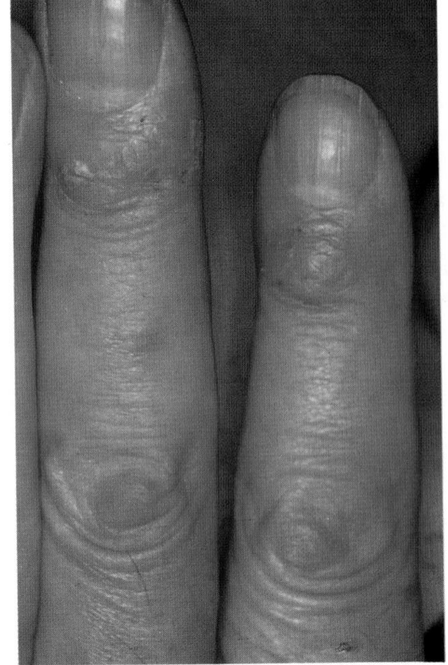

Fig. 11.79. Knuckle pads.

1989), firm, tense dermal nodules, with reddish or livid-red colour; they are usually located on the dorsal and axial surfaces of the fingers and toes, characteristically sparing the thumbs and great toes. They may be present at birth or develop during infancy. A single case was described in an adult (Sarma & Hoffman, 1980). Fingers are more often affected than toes. On reaching the nail unit, they may elevate the nail plate leading to dystrophy but not destruction. The tumour may cause considerable distortion of the digits. Often the tumour is multicentric occurring on several digits (Fig. 11.80).

Ryman and Bale (1985) reported 30 cases, seen over a 36-year period. There were 20 females and 10 males. The fingers and toes were equally affected. Multiple lesions occurred in 50% of patients, more often in the fingers, especially on adjacent fingers; two patients had bilateral lesions. Dabney *et al.* (1986) and Piñol-Aguadé *et al.* (1971) observed firm plantar nodules in one of their three cases with infantile digital fibromatosis.

Recurrence occurs in 60% after excision surgery; it should therefore be attempted only if functional impairment is present. Excessive growth was treated by amputation of the involved digit in some cases (Poppen & Niebauer, 1977). Surgery necessitates deep dissection to the fascial and tendinous areas in an effort to avoid recurrences. It can be mutilating. As metastasis has never been recorded, the amputations sometimes performed in the past (38 of 115 cases to 1985) can no longer be justified (Ryman & Bale, 1985).

Conservative treatment is most logical since the lesions have a natural course—a tumoural stage, followed by spontaneous resolution, showing why it is not found in

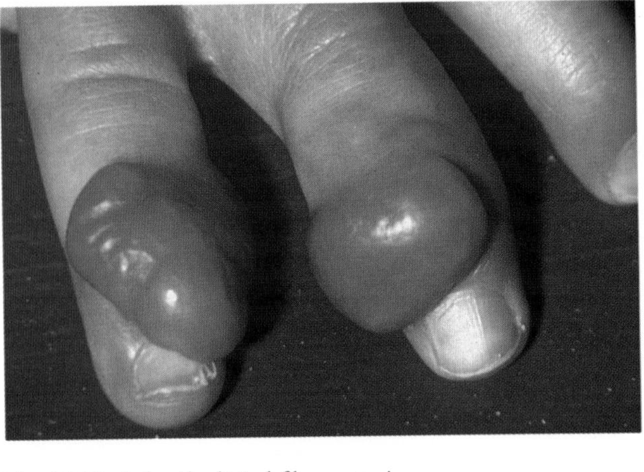

Fig. 11.80. Infantile digital fibromatosis.

adults (Sangueza & Jove, 1983). Cryosurgery may accelerate this natural course.

Histologically (Fig. 11.81), in about 2% of the fibroblasts, paranuclear inclusion bodies can be seen in properly fixed specimens using stains such as iron haematoxylin, methyl green-pyronin, and phosphotungstic acid-haematoxylin (Mehregan, 1981). Zina *et al.* (1986) studied two cases of Reye's tumour by electron microscopy and immunohistochemistry (IHC), using rabbit anti-actin sera. The tumour cells were typical myofibroblasts, containing inclusion bodies and bundles of microfilaments. IHC has shown that the paranuclear inclusions consist of actin fibres.

Differential diagnosis includes, on clinical grounds, pseudo-infantile digital fibromatosis with hypertrophic lateral lips of the great toe in early infancy, fibrosarcoma and neurofibrosarcoma. Cerebriform connective tissue naevus (Bauer & Eisen, 1985) (Fig. 11.82) should also be ruled out. Progressive thickening of the soles of the feet was accompanied in a 10-year-old girl by fleshy, cerebriform elevations over the plantar surfaces with extension onto the sides and dorsal aspect of several toes. The most striking biochemical abnormality is the marked reduction in the production of collagenase. Similar patients have been reported (Cohen & Hayden, 1979) associated with multiple hamartomas including linear epidermal naevi.

Histopathologically Reye's fibrous tumour may be confused with dermatofibroma, fibroma and scar tissue.

References

Bauer E.A. & Eisen A.Z. (1985) Biochemical changes in certain genodermatoses. *Clin. Dermatol.* 3, 135–142.

Cohen M.M. & Hayden P.W. (1979) A newly recognized hamartomatous syndrome. *Birth Defects* **5B**, 291–296.

Dabney K.W., MacEwen G.D. & Davis N.E. (1986) Recurring digital fibrous tumour of childhood. Case report with long-term follow-up and review of the literature. *J. Ped. Orthop.* **6**, 612–617.

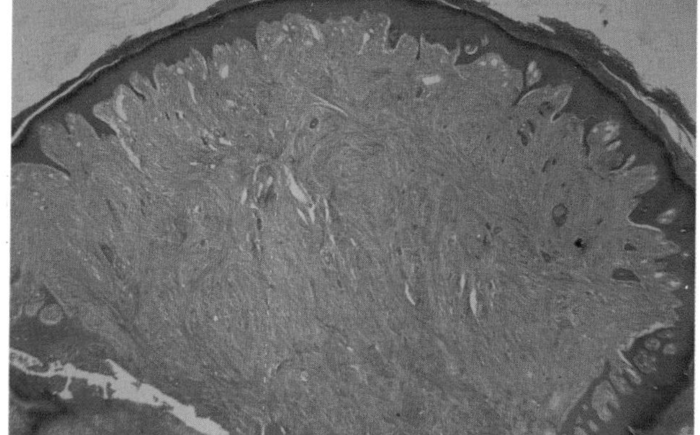

Fig. 11.81. Infantile digital fibromatosis – low magnification histological appearance.

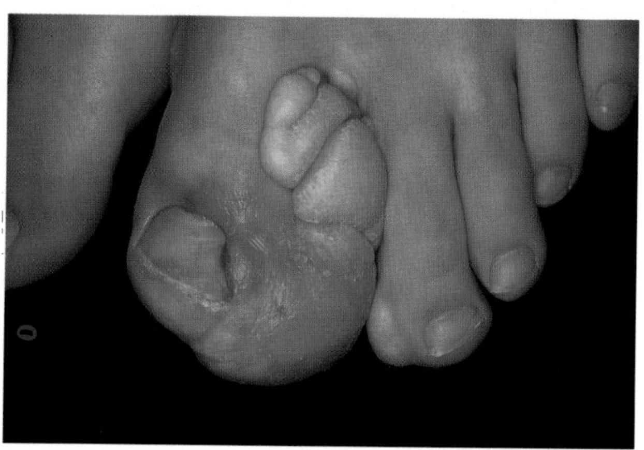

Fig. 11.82. Cerebriform connective tissue naevus (courtesy of E.A. Bauer, Stanford, USA).

Kowalczuk A.M., Villalba L.I., Galarza M. *et al.* (1983) Fibromatosis digital infantil. *Arch. Argent Dermatol.* **33**, 343–347.

Mehregan A. (1981) Superficial fibrous tumors in childhood. *J. Cut. Pathol.* **8**, 321–334.

Mulvaney M.S., Salasche S.J. & Hayes T.J. (1985) Differential diagnosis of multiple dermal acral nodules. *J. Assoc. Milit. Dermatol.* **11**, 24–27.

Oñate-Cuchet M.J., Vargas Castrillon J., Sanchez Gomez-Coronada P. *et al.* (1989) Fibromatosis digital recurrente infantil. *Actas Derm.-Sif.* **80**, 15–18.

Poppen N.K. & Niebauer J.J. (1977) Recurring digital fibrous tumour of childhood. *J. Hand Surg.* **2**, 253–255.

Reye R.D.K. (1965) Recurring digital fibrous tumours of childhood. *Arch. Pathol.* **80**, 228–231.

Ryman W. & Bale P. (1985) Recurring digital fibromas of infancy. *Aust. J. Dermatol.* **26**, 113–117.

Sangueza P. & Jove N. (1983) Fibromatosis digital infantil recidivante. *Med. Cut. ILA* **XI**, 307–310.

Sarma D.P. & Hoffman E.D. (1980) Infantile digital fibroma-like tumour in an adult. *Arch. Dermatol.* **116**, 578.

Zina A.M., Rampini E., Fulcheri E. *et al.* (1986) Recurrent digital fibromatosis of childhood. An ultrastructural and immunohistochemical study of 2 cases. *Am. J. Dermatopathol.* **8**, 22–26.

Juvenile hyaline fibromatosis II

Juvenile hyaline fibromatosis II is the name introduced by Kitano *et al.* (1972) to describe the condition previously reported as molluscum fibrosum, mesenchymal dysplasia (Puretić syndrome), systemic hyalinosis and fibromatosis (Figs 11.83 & 11.84). It is characterized by skin lesions, muscle weakness, and flexion contractures of large joints. Both multiple large tumours and small pink or pearly papules or nodules with a translucent appearance and a gelatinous consistency are found in the head and neck region, on the trunk and at the tip of the digits, where acroosteolysis may be seen. Clubbing has been observed (Camarosa & Moreno, 1987).

The tumours are characterized by 'chondroid' cells

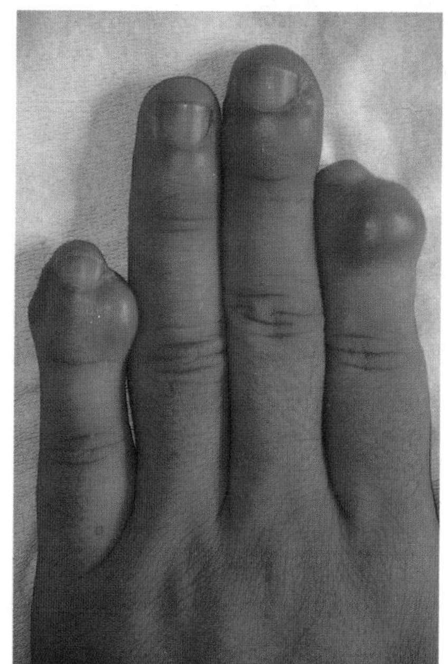

Fig. 11.83. Juvenile hyaline fibromatosis II.

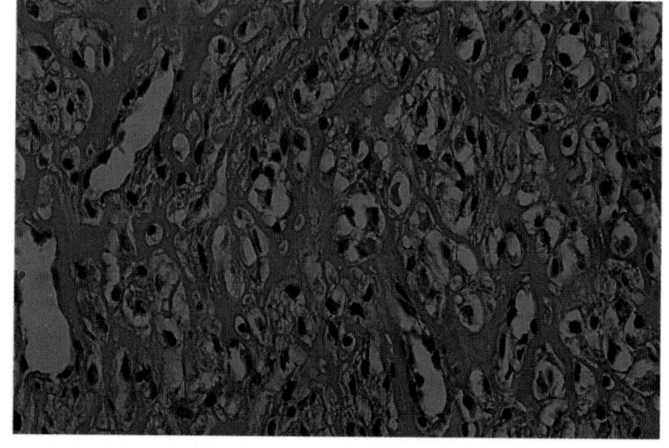

Fig. 11.84. Juvenile hyaline fibromatosis – 'chondroid' cells within eosinophilic substance.

within an eosinophilic substance (Finlay *et al.*, 1983) (Fig. 11.84). Excision of cutaneous lesions is almost always followed by local recurrences (Kan & Rogers, 1989).

Juvenile hyaline fibromatosis is inherited as an autosomal recessive trait.

References

Camarosa J.G. & Moreno K. (1987) Juvenile hyaline fibromatosis. *J. Am. Acad. Dermatol.* **16**, 881–883.

Finlay A.Y., Ferguson S.D. & Holt P.J.A. (1983) Juvenile hyaline fibromatosis. *Br. J. Dermatol.* **108**, 609–616.

Kan A.E. & Rogers M. (1989) Juvenile hyaline fibromatosis: an expanded clinicopathologic spectrum. *Pediatr. Dermatol.* **6**, 68–75.

Kitano Y., Horiki M. & Aoki T. (1972) Two cases of juvenile hyalin fibromatosis. Some histological, electron microscopy and tissue culture observations. *Arch. Dermatol.* **106**, 877–883.

Dermatofibrosarcoma protuberans

A 31-year-old black women gave a history of the presence of 13-month-old mass on her left non-dominant thumb. The nail was asymmetrical (2 × 1 × 1 cm). A pink, firm, multilobulated, and painful mass involved the palmar aspect of the digit. The fibrous growth of rubbery consistence was surrounded by a well-circumscribed skin (Coles *et al.*, 1989). X-ray showed mild irregularity of the anterior cortex of the terminal phalanx. Histology showed intertwining fibrocellular bands forming a storiform pattern.

Reference

Coles M., Smith M. & Rankin E.A. (1989) An unusual case of dermatofibrosarcoma protuberans. *J. Hand. Surg.* **14A**, 135–138.

Vascular tumours

Benign

Haemangiomas (Figs 11.85 & 11.86)

Haemangiomas of the nail bed and tip of the digit are extremely rare. They exhibit the classic course with fast growth and slow spontaneous involution.

Capillary malformation (port-wine stains and telangiectases) (Fig. 11.87)

Capillary malformations are developmental defects present from birth, and usually permanent. They may look violet through the nail. Paradoxically, when the colouration of the angioma is pronounced, true leuconychia can be observed (Fig. 11.88) (Enjolras & Riché, 1990).

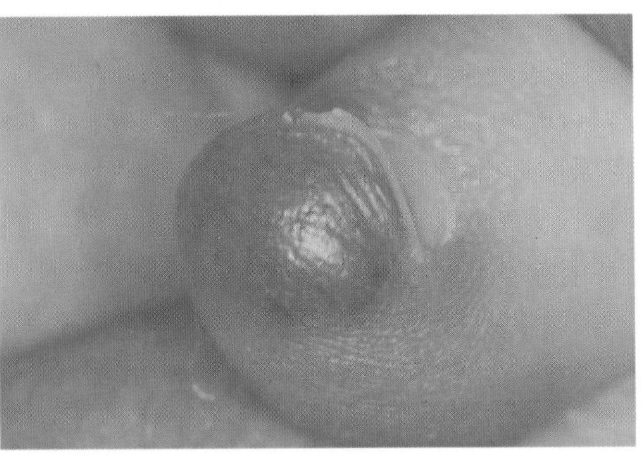

Fig. 11.85. Subungual haemangioma.

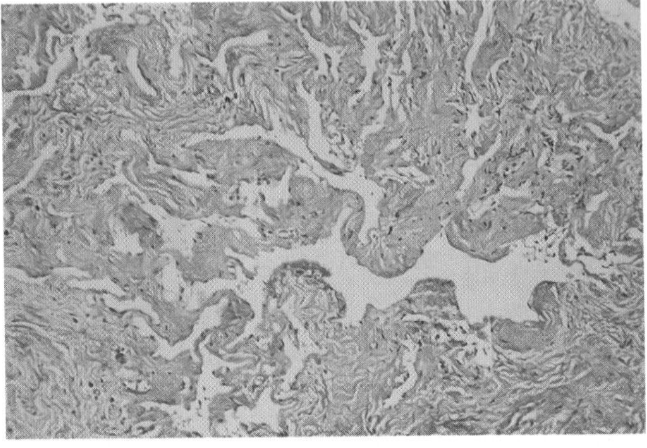

Fig. 11.86. Subungual haemangioma; histological changes.

Venous malformations

Venous malformations of the nail apparatus are rare and should be left untreated. The shape of the nail may remain normal but the nail bed is blue (Enjolras, 1990) (Fig. 11.89). It may blacken in becoming thrombotic (Fig. 11.90). Venous malformations may arise in the bone or soft tissue. When primary in the bone they have a characteristic radiological appearance of linear striations parallel to the shaft of the bone. Soft tissue venous malformations are more common lesions and may be radiographically manifested by local soft tissue masses, phleboliths in the soft tissue, and pressure erosion of the underlying bone (Monses & Murphy, 1984). Histopathology shows ectatic capillary or venous channels with normal-looking endothelial cells. Heller's case with 'angioelephantiasis' probably represented Klippel–Trenaunay's syndrome, i.e. a capillary and venous complex combined malformation (Figs 11.91 & 11.92), or a Parkes–Weber syndrome, i.e. a limb overgrowth syndrome due to arteriovenous fistula. The bed of the thumb was dark blue and four toenails were reduced to keratotic plugs (Heller, 1927).

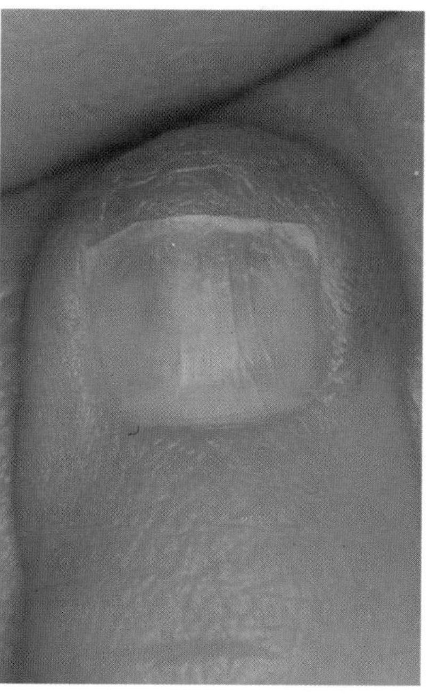

Fig. 11.87. Port-wine stain.

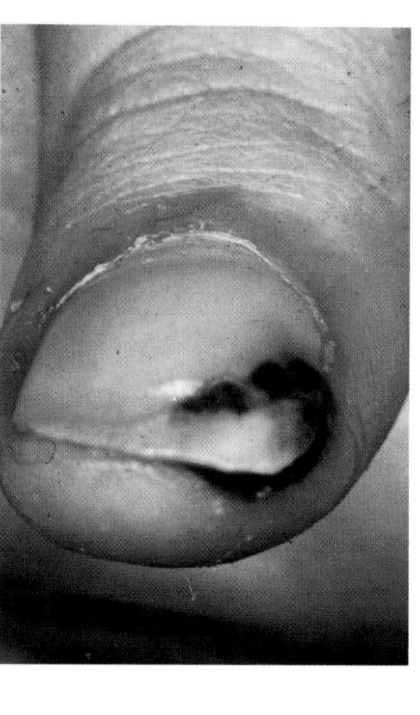

Fig. 11.90. Blackening due to spontaneous thrombosis in a 10-year-old child.

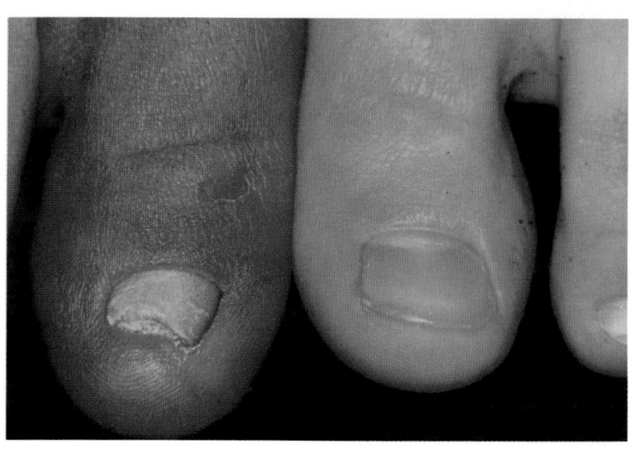

Fig. 11.88. Paradoxical leuconychia in the midst of an angioma.

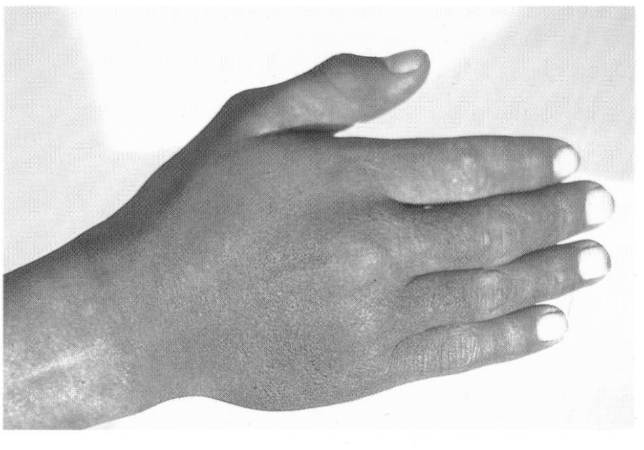

Fig. 11.91. Klippel–Trenauney syndrome – very prominent leuconychia.

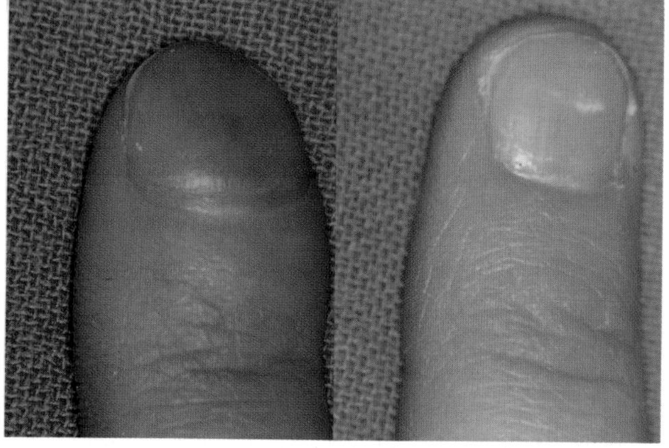

Fig. 11.89. Venous malformation showing blue nail bed (left).

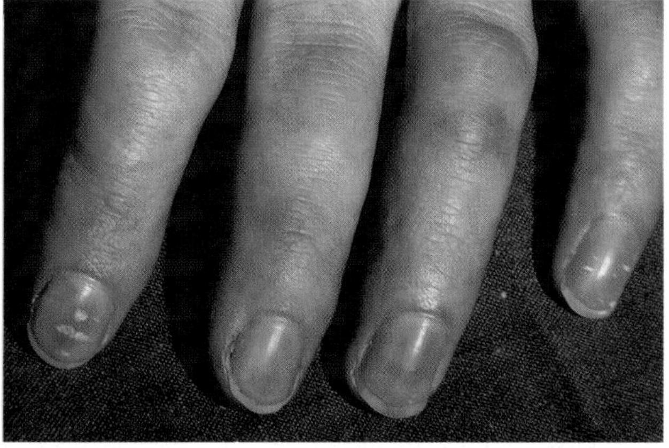

Fig. 11.92. Klippel–Trenauney syndrome – 'venous' colour of the subungual area.

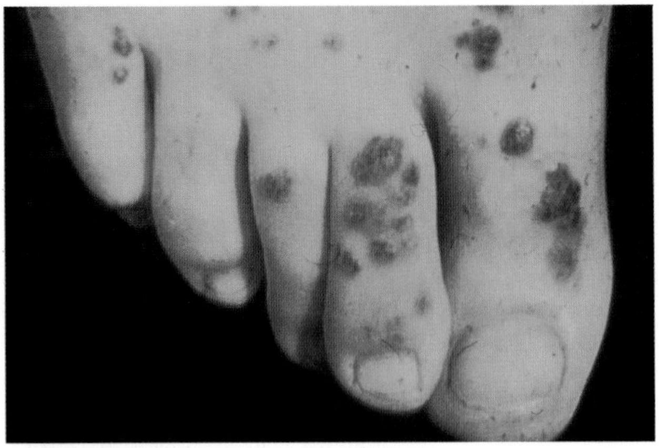

Fig. 11.93. Angiokeratoma (Mibelli) (courtesy of S. Weinberg, New York, USA).

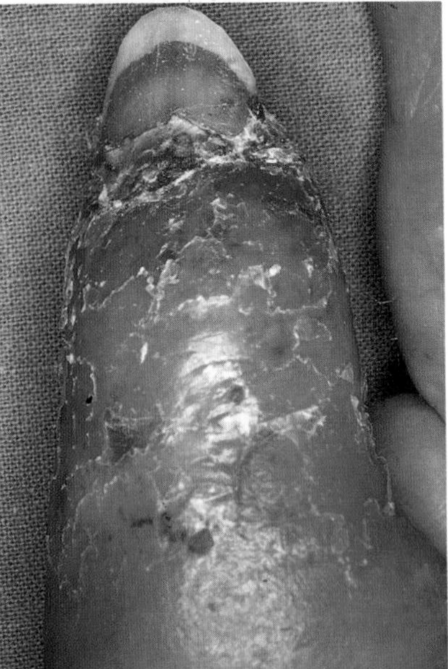

Fig. 11.94. Arteriovenous fistula (courtesy of O. Enjolras, Paris, France).

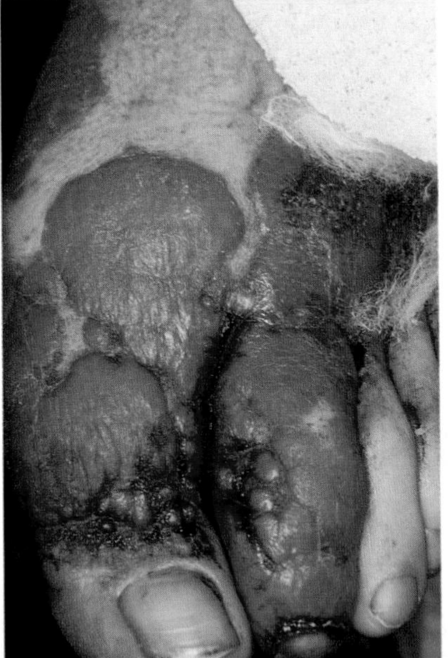

Fig. 11.95. Pseudo-kaposi syndrome.

References

Enjolras O. & Riché M.C. (1990) *Hémangiomas et Malformations Vasculaires Superficielles*. Medsi/McGraw-Hill, New York, Paris.

Monses B. & Murphy W.A. (1984) Distal phalangeal erosive lesions. *Arth. Rhum.* 27, 449–455.

Angiokeratoma circumscriptum (Fig. 11.93)

Dolph *et al.* (1981) described a 12-year-old girl with a raised, firm, bluish-purple nodule over the dorsal aspect of the distal index joint. It enlarged with the concomitant appearance of several black dots at the periphery. Histology showed a typical angiokeratoma. The authors listed several tumours in the differential diagnosis, malignant melanoma being the most important.

Reference

Dolph J.L., Demuth R.J. & Miller S.H. (1981) Angiokeratoma circumscriptum of the index finger in a child. *Plast. Reconst. Surg.* 67, 221–223.

Acquired subungual superficial capillary angioma (Baran & Perrin, 1994)

Sometimes mimicking longitudinal melanonychia, the clinical lesions appear in adult life, usually as a longitudinal narrow band of subungual haematoma, brown or black, often interrupted. The origin of the band is located in the proximal nail bed, less commonly in the lunula. In a single case, we observed double banding. After nail avulsion a very tiny elevation marks the origin of the band.

Histology shows only capillary haemangioma. A 3 mm punch excisional biopsy is the treatment of choice. We did not observe any recurrence in our six patients.

Periungual and subungual arteriovenous tumours (cirsoid aneurysms)

A firm, bluish, vascular nodule has been reported in the lateral nail fold of the left little finger with histological findings consistent with cirsoid aneurysm (Fig. 11.97) (Burge *et al.*, 1986). In four cases an apparent vascular tumour involved the subungual tissue (Fig. 11.98). This painless lesion is distinguished from pyogenic granuloma by the prolonged history without enlargement or bleeding, while the absence of exquisite tenderness differentiates it clinically from glomus tumour. Cirsoid aneurysm should be considered in the differential diagnosis of causes of

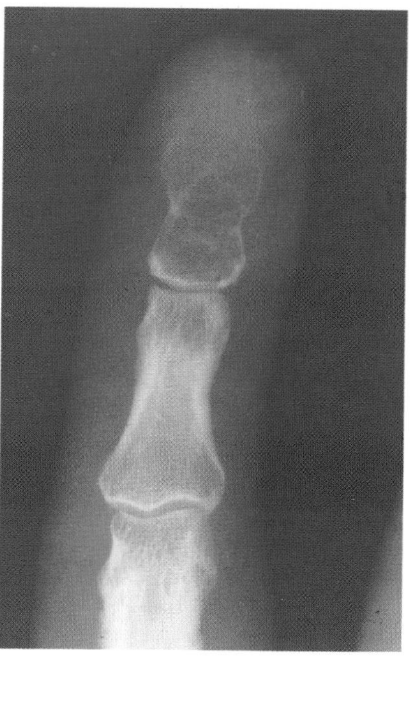

Fig. 11.96. Arteriovenous fistula – aneurysmal bone cyst, X-ray changes.

a longitudinal red line with distal fissuring in the nail (Fig. 11.99).

Reference

Burge S.M., Baran R., Dawber R.P.R. & Verret J.L. (1986) Periungual and subungual arteriovenous tumours. *Br. J. Dermatol.* **115**, 361–366.

Digital arteriovenous malformation

In digital arteriovenous malformation the digit and the nail bed have a purple hue with progressive resorption of the distal phalanx and shrinking of the nail plate presenting a slight transverse overcurvature (Fig. 11.95), worsening from childhood to adolescence may be associated with bone overgrowth and macrodactyly. Pseudo-Kaposi's syndrome can be seen (Enjolras & Riché, 1990) (Fig. 11.95).

Arteriovenous fistulae may occur in the distal phalanx of young people (Figs 11.94 & 11.95). They are rapidly growing, painful lesions with marked, bulbous enlargement of the fingertip. Aneurysmal bone cyst is a distinct clinical entity separated from haemangiomas of bone and from other tumours in which giant cells are also a prominent feature. It has been named aneurysmal bone cyst because the contour of the affected bone suggests a 'blow-out' type of distention which resembles the saccular protrusion of the walls of an aneurysm, and also because cystic blood-filled spaces are encountered at surgery. On X-ray, the phalanx may be excessively enlarged and almost completely occupied by osteolytic tissue simulating a malignant tumour (Schajowicz *et al.*, 1970) (Fig. 11.96). MRI allows the specific diagnosis of aneurysmal bone cysts to be made (Schmutz *et al.*, 1988).

References

Enjolras O. & Riché M.C. (1990) *Hémangiomes et Malformations Vasculaires Superficielles*. Medsi/McGraw-Hill, New York.

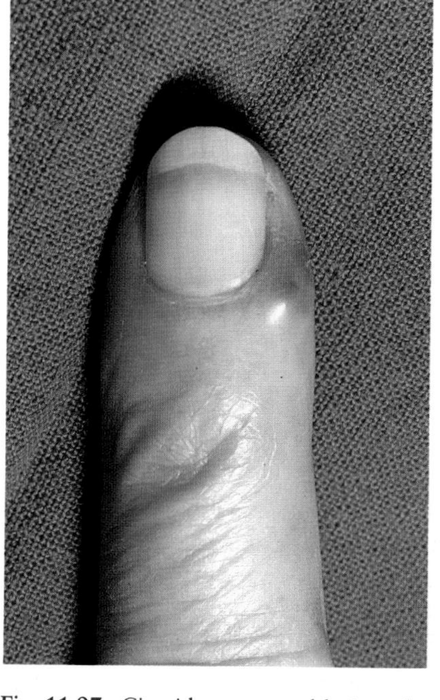

Fig. 11.97. Cirsoid aneurysmal lesion of the lateral nail fold.

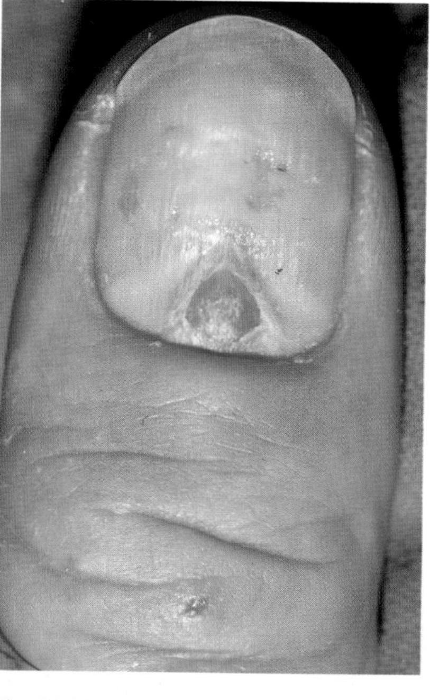

Fig. 11.98. Pyogenic granuloma after a penetrating wound.

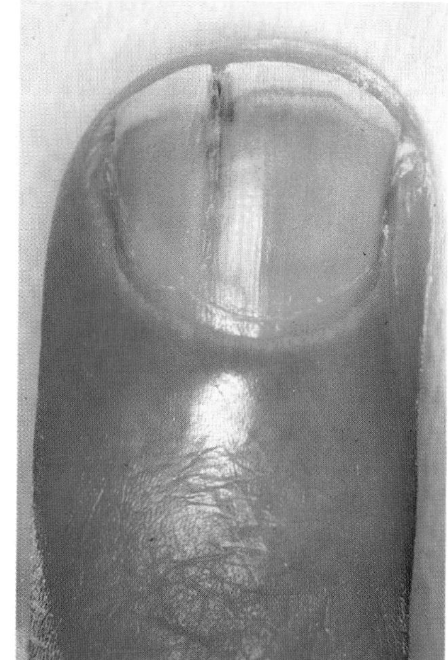

Fig. 11.99. Cirsoid aneurysm – nail dystrophy at the end of a longitudinal red 'streak'.

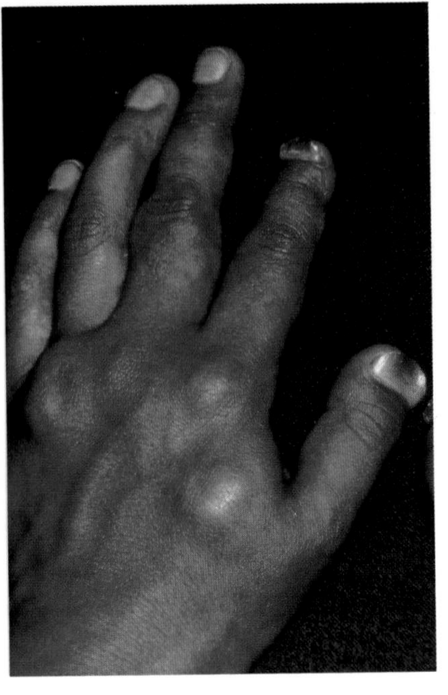

Fig. 11.100. Blue rubber bleb naevi (courtesy of L. Tamayo, Mexico).

Heller J. (1927) Die Krankheiten der Nägel. In: *Handbuch der Haut-und Geschlechts-krankheitsen* (Hrsg J. Jadassohn), Bd VIII/2: Spezielle Dermatologie, S. 150–172.

Schajowicz F., Aiello C. & Slullitel I. (1970) Cystic and pseudocystic lesions of the terminal phalanx with special reference to epidermoid cysts. *Clin. Orthop. Rel. Res.* **68**, 84–92.

Schmutz J.L., Cuny J.F., Duprez A. *et al.* (1988) Kyste osseux anévrismal d'un orteil. *Rech. Dermatol.* **1**, 679–681.

Epithelioid haemangioma

Weiss and Enzinger (1982) proposed the term 'epithelioid haemangioendothelioma' to describe an unusual tumour of soft tissue having an epithelioid appearance. These tumours pursue a clinical course between that of a haemangioma and that of a conventional angiosarcoma. Similar neoplasms occur in other sites such as the lung, liver and bone.

Epithelioid haemangioma, masquerading as a paronychia, was described in a 42-year-old female who had a 6-month history of progressive swelling and some tenderness of the left great toe. The toe was diffusely swollen, the pulp was bluish-red and there was increased curvature of the nail of the left big toe. On X-ray a large lytic lesion of the distal phalanx was shown without any reactive new bone formation and with expansion of the proximal end of the phalanx and an associated large soft tissue mass. The tumour was multicentric, as seen on a bone isotope scan (Kennedy *et al.*, 1990).

Histopathology of curetted tissue showed numerous vessels of varying size and development, many with large epithelioid endothelial cells. The associated inflammatory infiltrate contained foci of eosinophils (Kennedy *et al.*, 1990). Because of its rare occurrence, the tumour may be misdiagnosed as a metastatic carcinoma or other neoplasm (Tsuneyoshi *et al.*, 1986).

References

Kennedy C.T.C., Burton P.A. & Cook P. (1990) Swollen toe due to epithelioid haemangioma of bone. *Br. J. Dermatol.* **123** (Suppl. 37), 85–89.

Tsuneyoshi M., Dorfman H.D. & Bauer T.W. (1986) Epithelioid hemangioendothelioma of bone. A clinicopathologic, ultrastructural, and immunohistochemical study. *Am. J. Surg. Pathol.* **10**, 754–756.

Weiss S.W. & Enzinger F.M. (1982) Epithelioid haemangioendothelioma. A vascular tumor often mistaken for a carcinoma. *Cancer* **50**, 970–981.

Pseudopyogenic granuloma (histiocytoid haemangioma)

Avenel *et al.* (1982) described a 40-year-old woman with angiomatous nodules affecting the fingertip, lateral nail folds and nail bed. The histological and ultrastructural changes were consistent with a diagnosis of pseudopyogenic granuloma (Wilson-Jones & Bleehen, 1969; Rosai *et al.*, 1979; Verret *et al.*, 1983); Dannaker *et al.* (1989) reported a case with simultaneous cutaneous and bone involvement of histiocytoid hemangiomas. The patient, a 31-year-old Mexicano-American man, presented with nail changes including onycholysis of the distal area, longitudinal splitting, subungual and periungual erythema, and paronychial swelling with purulent drainage. Biopsy specimens showed a proliferation of histiocytoid endothelial cells with intracytoplasmic vacuoles and associated vascular lumen formation. Radiation therapy resulted in significant clinical improvement.

The collective term histiocytoid haemangioma (Rosai *et al.*, 1979) encompasses a spectrum of diseases that share histologic features characterized by distinctive histiocytoid endothelial cells. Several incompletely defined cutaneous and extracutaneous vascular tumours, including atypical pyogenic granuloma, pseudopyogenic granuloma, papular angioplasia, angiolymphoid hyperplasia with eosinophilia, Kimura's disease, and inflammatory arteriovenous haemangioma, have been included in this group. Radiation therapy results in significant clinical improvement.

References

Avenel M., Verret J.L. & Fortier P. (1982) Finger localisation of Wilson–Jones pseudo-pyogenic granuloma. Case Presentations in XVI Congressus Int. Derm. Tokyo 1982, p. 38. University of Tokyo Press, Japan.

Dannaker C., Piacquadio D., Willoughby C.B. & Goltz R.W. (1989) Histiocytoid hemangioma: A disease spectrum. *J. Am. Acad. Dermatol.* **21**, 404–409.

Rosai J., Gold J. & Landy R. (1979) Histiocytoid haemangiomas. *Human Pathol.* **10**, 707–729.

Verret J.L., Avenel M., François H., Baudoin M. & Alain P. (1983) Hémangiomes histiotycoides des pulpes digitales. *Ann. Dermatol. Venereol.* **110**, 251–257.

Wilson-Jones E. & Bleehen S.S. (1969) Pseudo pyogenic granuloma. *Br. J. Dermatol.* **81**, 804–816.

Acral pseudolymphomatous angiokeratoma of children (APACHE)

Ramsay *et al.* (1983) described five children (four females, one male) between the ages of 2 and 13 years who developed a unilateral eruption of multiple angiomatous papules on the extremities (in four patients on the feet and in one patient on the hand). The lesions were red-violaceous, discrete, irregularly shaped papules, 1–4 mm in size with a hyperkeratotic collar occurring over acral sites (Fig. 11.101). The provisional diagnosis in three of the patients was angiokeratoma of Mibelli, but the lesions were more numerous and chilblains were not a feature. The lesions have persisted, with some decrease in size, during follow-up periods of up to 16 years.

Histological findings consist of epidermal hyperkeratosis and a dense lymphoid infiltrate present throughout the dermis, extending from the subcutis to the dermo-epidermal junction, but without involving the epidermis. There are equal numbers of B- and T-cells and the T-suppressor phenotype cell (CD8) outnumbered helper phenotype T-cell (CD4) (Ramsay *et al.*, 1990). In one patient the lesions were destroyed by curettage and did not recur.

Hara *et al.* (1991) reported a 14-year-old Japanese girl presenting multiple lesions in a linear fashion on one finger, with involvement of the medial aspect of the nail as partial onycholysis. The histology corresponded to that of a pseudolymphoma but there was a lack of prominent thickened capillaries. There were epidermal changes consisting of liquefaction degeneration of the basal cells with predominance of T-lymphocytes CD4 at the upper portion of the infiltrate and CD8 the lower.

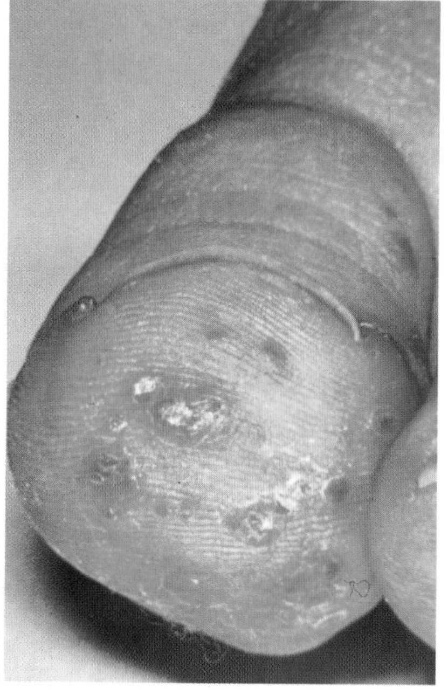

Fig. 11.101. Acral pseudolymphomatous angiokeratoma of children (APACHE) (courtesy of M. Dahl, Newcastle, UK).

References

Hara M., Matsunaga J. & Tagami H. (1991) Acral pseudolymphomatous angiokeratoma of children (APACHE): a case report and immunohistological study. *Br. J. Dermatol.* **124**, 387–388.

Ramsay B., Dahl M.G.C., Malcolm A.J., Soyer H.P. & Wilson-Jones E. (1983) Acral pseudolymphomatous angiokeratoma of children (APACHE). *Br. J. Dermatol.* **119** (Suppl. 33), 13.

Ramsay B., Dahl M.G.C., Malcom A.J. & Wilson-Jones E. (1990) Acral pseudolymphomatous angiokeratoma of children. *Arch. Dermatol.* **126**, 1524–1525.

Pyogenic granuloma (granuloma telangiectaticum, botryomycoma)

Pyogenic granuloma is a benign eruptive haemangioma typically following a minor penetrating skin injury. It starts around the nail with a minute red papule which rapidly grows to the size of a pea or even a cherry. Its surface may become eroded by necrosis of the overlying epidermis. Crusting may mimic malignant melanoma although the typical 'collarette' can usually be seen. Pyogenic granuloma is commonly located at the proximal nail fold (Fig. 11.102) but may develop distally (Fig. 11.103) in the hyponychium region with onycholysis or in the nail bed after a penetrating wound of the nail plate (Figs 11.98 & 11.104). Tenderness and a ready tendency to bleed are characteristic features. Extensive granulation tissue due to an ingrowing toenail is a variant of pyogenic periungual granuloma, and it also has been observed in patients treated with aromatic retinoids (Baran, 1990). Differential diagnosis also includes cavernous angioma, pseudopyogenic granuloma, haemangiosarcoma and amelanotic melanoma. Histological investigation of the specimen is therefore essential. Therapy should be as simple as possible to avoid disfiguring scars or nail deformity. Pyogenic granuloma may be removed by excision at its base followed by application of Monsel's or aluminium chloride solution. The use of lasers is also curative.

Reference

Baran R. (1990) Retinoids and the nails. *J. Dermatol. Treat.* **1**, 151–154.

Glomus tumour

The glomus tumour was first described by Wood (1812) as a painful subcutaneous 'tubercle'. Several cases were

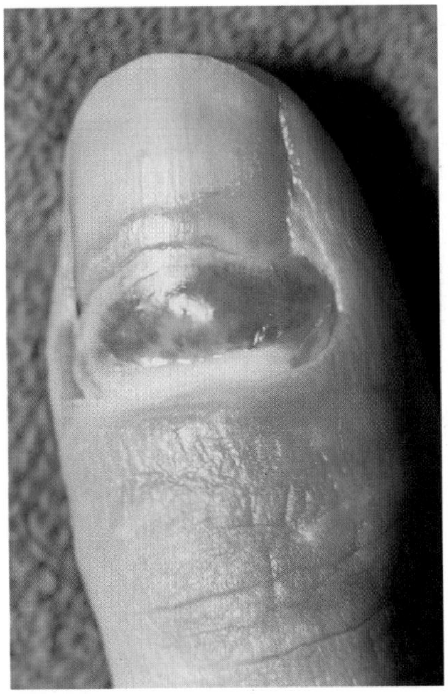

Fig. 11.102.

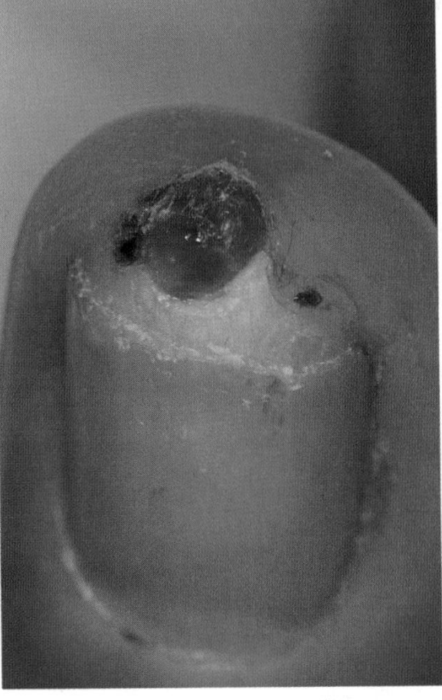
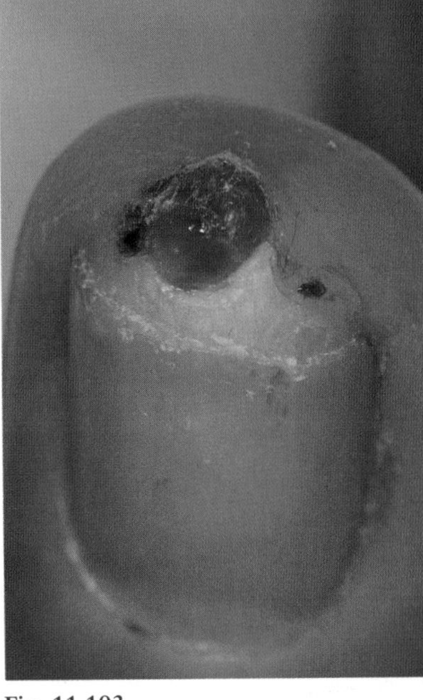

Fig. 11.103.

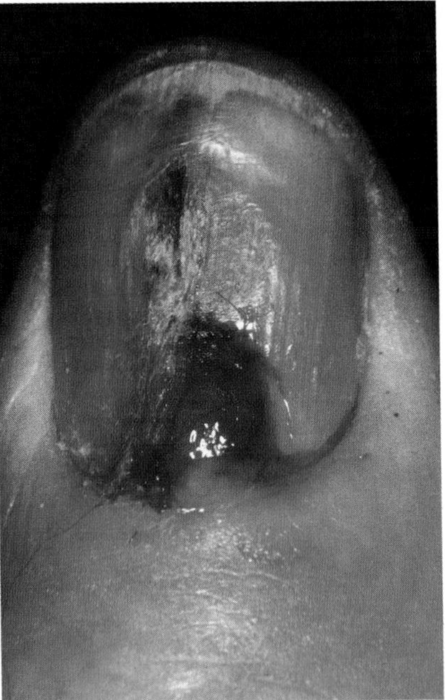

Fig. 11.104.

Fig. 11.102–11.104. Pyogenic granuloma.

described as malignant angiosarcomas or colloid sarcoma until Barré and Masson (1924) published their investigation on two glomus tumours.

Seventy-five per cent of glomus tumours occur in the hand, especially in the fingertips, and particularly in the subungual area (Figs 11.105–11.107). One to two per cent of all hand tumours are glomus tumours (Rettig & Strickland, 1977). The average age of patients at diagnosis ranges from 30 to 50 years (Carroll & Berman, 1972). Men are less frequently affected than women.

The glomus tumour is characterized by intense, often pulsating pain that may be spontaneous or provoked by the slightest trauma. Even changes in temperature, especially from warm to cold, may trigger pain radiating up to the shoulder. Sometimes the pain is worse at night. A tourniquet placed at the base of the digit stops the pain.

The tumour is seen through the nail plate as a small bluish to reddish-blue spot several millimetres in diameter, rarely exceeding 1 cm in diameter (Fig. 11.105). A nail with an erythematous focus that does not blanch totally with pressure and is associated with pain probably represents a glomus tumour. Sometimes it causes a slight rise in surface temperature; this can be detected by thermography. One-half of the tumours cause minor nail deformities, ridging and fissuring being the commonest (Figs 11.105 & 11.106). About 50% cause a depression on the dorsal aspect of the distal phalangeal bone or even a cyst visible on X-ray (Fig. 11.107). Enlargement of the thickened nail and of the purple soft tissues with moderate pain of the fourth right finger was present for 20 years in a 95-year-old woman (Watelet *et al.*, 1986). Probing and transillumination may help to localize the tumour if it is not clearly visible through the nail. If the tumour cannot be localized clinically or on X-ray, arteriography should be performed; this will reveal a star-shaped telangiectatic zone useful for diagnosis and localization of the tumour (Natali *et al.*, 1966; Camirand & Giroux, 1970; Priollet, 1985) (Fig. 11.108). MRI has been shown to help in the diagnosis of a glomus tumour of the fingertip (Figs 11.109–11.111) (Jablon *et al.*, 1990; Holzberg, 1992).

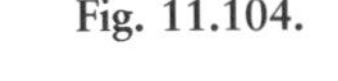

Many patients give a history of trauma. The most common misdiagnoses are neuroma, causalgia, gout and arthritis. These have resulted in disastrous therapeutic attempts such as posterior rhizotomy and amputation (Rettig & Strickland, 1977).

Histology (Figs 11.112 & 11.113) shows a highly differentiated, organoid tumour. It consists of an afferent arteriole, vascular channels lined with endothelium and surrounded by irregularly arranged cuboidal cells with round dark nuclei and pale cytoplasm. Primary collecting veins drain into the cutaneous veins. Myelinated and non-myelinated nerves are found and may account for the pain. The tumour is surrounded by a fibrous capsule. Since all the elements of the normal glomus are present, the glomus tumour may be considered a hamartoma rather than a true tumour.

Immunohistochemistry of glomus tumours showed that the glomus cells were positive for vimentin, a 42 kD muscle actin (with HHF 35) and smooth muscle actin (CGA 7), but negative for desmin, factor VIII-related

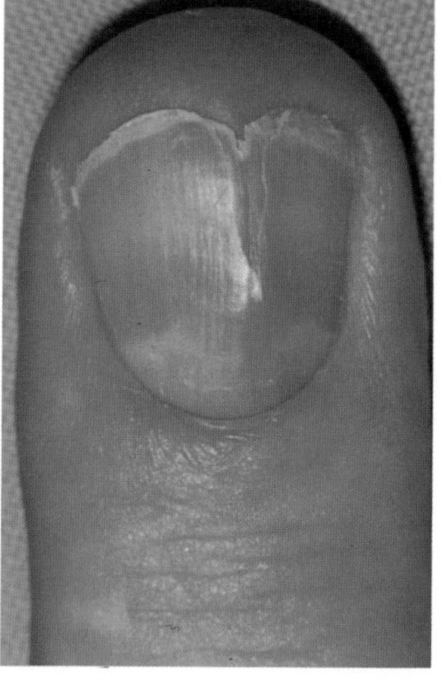

Fig. 11.105. Glomus tumour.

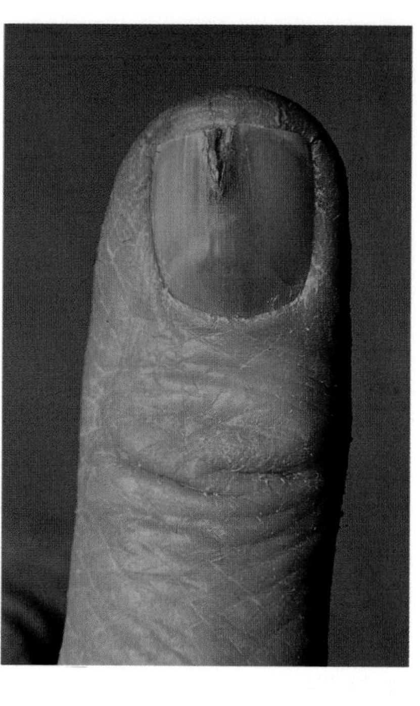

Fig. 11.106. Glomus tumour.

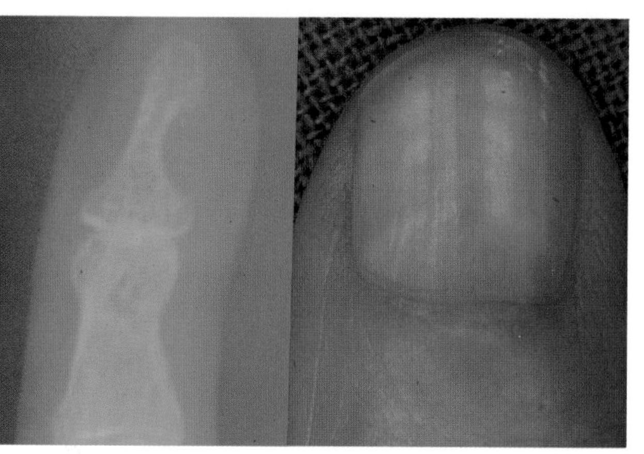

Fig. 11.107. Glomus tumour – depression on the dorsal surface distal phalanx shown radiologically (bottom).

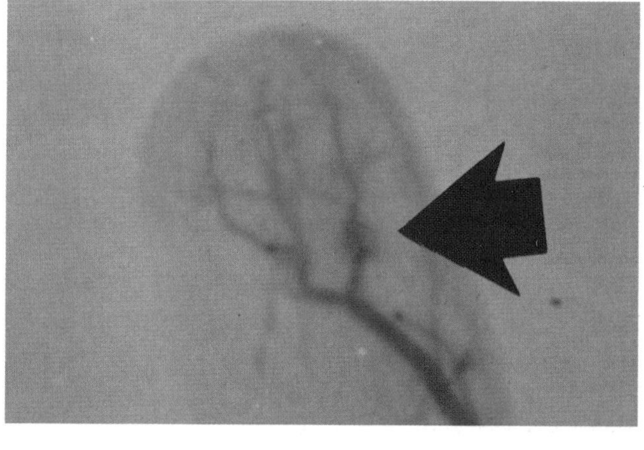

Fig. 11.108. Glomus tumour – arteriogram (courtesy of P. Priollet, Paris, France).

antigen and several neural markers; however, nerve fibres contained protein S-100, Leu-7 antigen (HNK-I, 110 kD), neuron-specific enolase and neurofilaments (Herbst *et al.*, 1991). The endothelium clearly stains with factor VIII-related antigen, β_2-microglobulin and the lectin *Ulex europaeus* agglutinin (UEA) I, whereas only a few endothelial cells of the glomus tumour bind PNA, in contrast to normal nail bed vessels the endothelial cells of which do not stain for PNA at all (E. Haneke, unpublished data).

The only treatment is surgical removal. Small tumours may be removed by punching a 6 mm hole into the nail plate (Fig. 11.114(a),(b),(c)) incising the nail bed, and enucleating the lesion. The small nail disc is put back in its original position as a physiological dressing. Larger tumours may be treated after removal of the proximal half of the nail plate; those in lateral positions are removed by an L-shaped incision parallel to and 4–6 mm on the volar side of the lateral nail fold (Fig. 11.115). The nail bed is carefully dissected from the bone until the tumour is reached and extirpated. Extirpation is usually curative although the pain may take several weeks to disappear (Jepson & Harris, 1970). Recurrences occur in 10–20% of cases (Carroll & Berman, 1972) and may represent either incomplete excision or tumour overlooked at the initial operation, or newly developed tumours (Cornell, 1981). More extensive surgery than is often carried out might achieve more first-time cures (Varian & Cleak, 1980). Amputation of the distal phalanx is exceptionally needed (Watelet *et al.*, 1986).

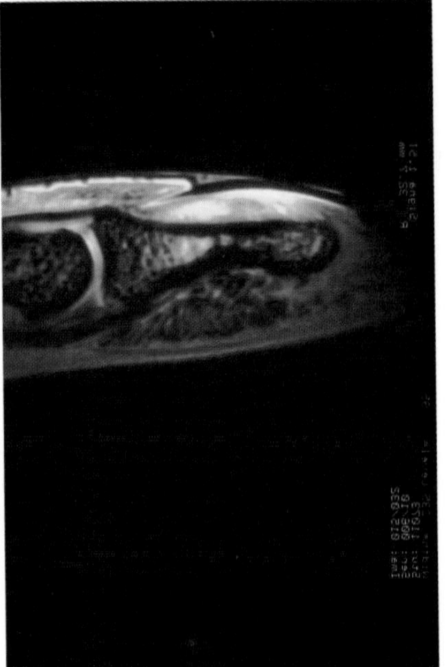

Fig. 11.109. Magnetic resonance image – normal.

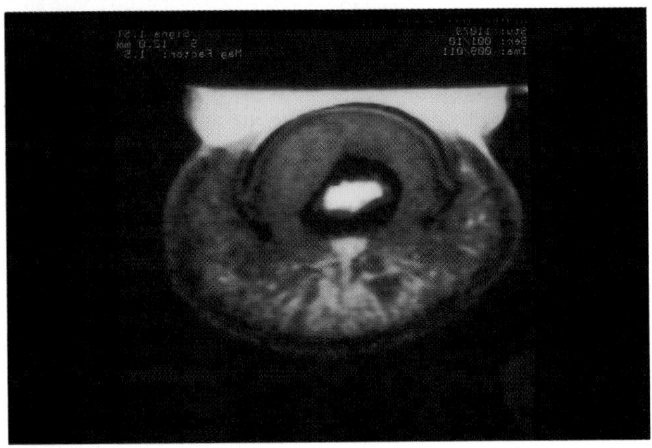

Fig. 11.110. MRI – L. lateral glomus.

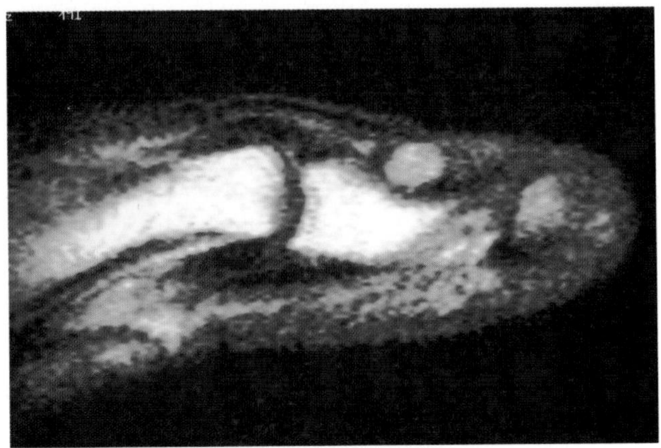

Fig. 11.111. MRI showing a nodular (white) glomus body atop the terminal phalanx (courtesy of S. Goettmann, Paris, France).

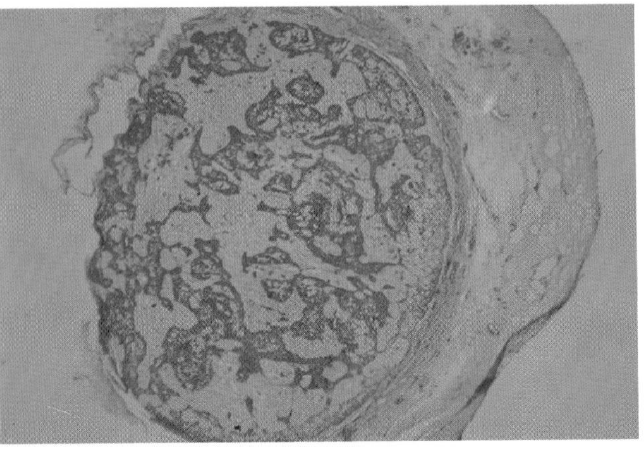

Fig. 11.112. Glomus tumour – low-power microscopy.

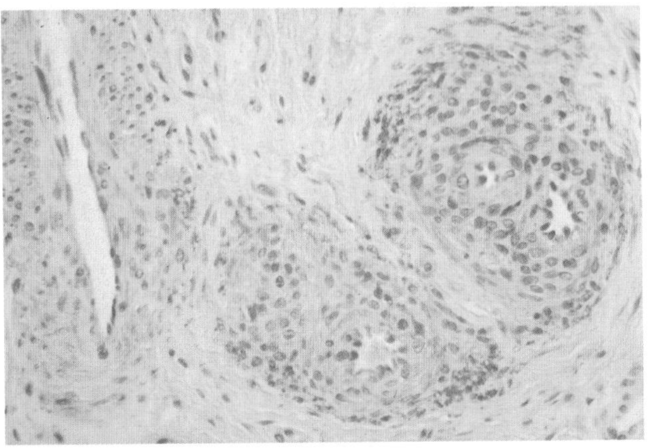

Fig. 11.113. Glomus body – normal, cf. Fig. 11.112 (S-100 stain).

References

Barré J.A. & Masson P. (1924) Etude anatomo-clinique de certaines tumeurs sous-unguéales douloureuses (tumeurs du glomus neuro-myo-artériel des extrémités). *Bull. Soc. Fr. Dermatol. Syphil.* **31**, 149–159.

Camirand P. & Giroux J.M. (1970) Subungual glomus tumour. *Arch. Dermatol.* **102**, 677–679.

Carroll R.E. & Berman A.T. (1972) Glomus tumours of the hand. *J. Bone Joint Surg.* **54A**, 691–703.

Cornell S.J. (1981) Multiple glomus tumours in one digit. *Hand* **13**, 301–302.

Herbst W.M., Nakayama K. & Hornstein O.P. (1991) Glomus tumours of the skin: an immunohistochemical investigation of the expression of marker proteins. *Br. J. Dermatol.* **124**, 172–176.

Holzberg M. (1992) Glomus tumor of the nail. A 'red herring' clarified by magnetic resonance imaging. *Arch. Dermatol.* **128**, 160–162.

Jablon M., Horowith A. & Bernstein D.A. (1990) Magnetic resonance imaging of a glomus tumour of the fingertip. *J. Hand Surg.* **15A**, 507–509.

Jepson R.P. & Harris J.D. (1970) Glomus tumours. *Med. J. Aust.* **2**, 452–454.

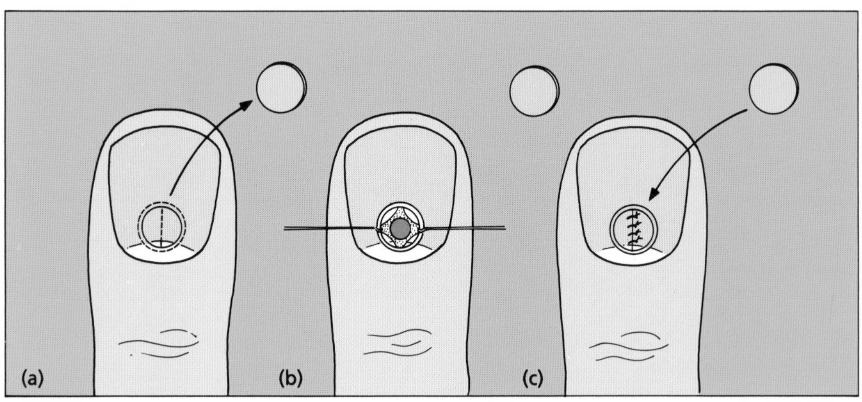

Fig. 11.114. Diagram to show sequence of events in the removal of a glomus tumour through the nail.

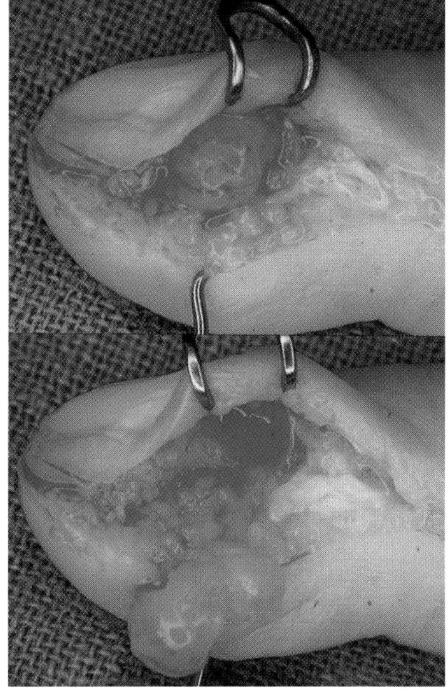

Fig. 11.115. Glomus tumour – removal through a lateral incision.

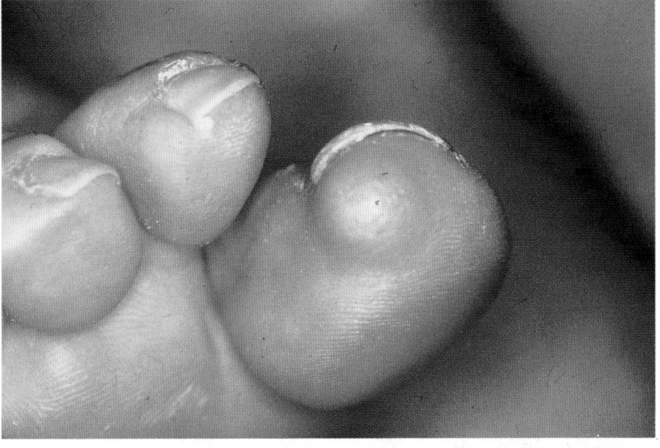

Fig. 11.116. Angioleiomyoma.

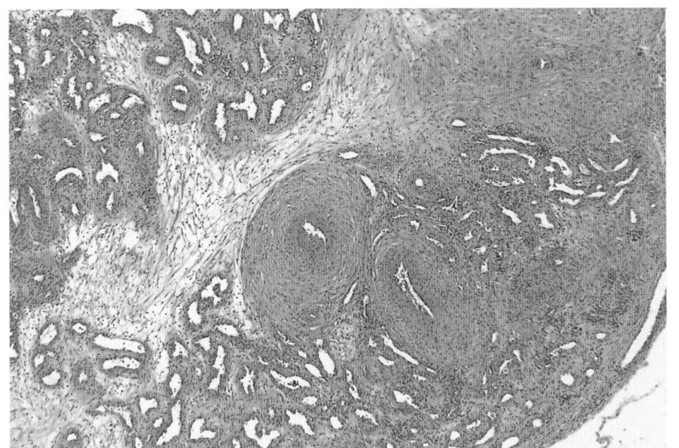

Fig. 11.117. Angioleiomyoma – histological changes; bundles of fibres interspersed with arterial and venous vessels.

Natali J., Ecarlat B., Vinardi G. & Batissen F. (1966) Artériographie d'une tumeur glomique. *J. Chir. (Paris)* **92**, 481–484.

Priollet P., Pernes J.M., Laurian C. *et al.* (1985) Intérêt de l'artériographie dans l'exploration des tumeurs glomiques sous-unguéales. *J. Mal. Vascul.* **10**, 363–365.

Rettig A.C. & Strickland J.W. (1977) Glomus tumour of the digits. *J. Hand Surg.* **2**, 261–265.

Varian J.P.W. & Cleak D.K. (1980) Glomus tumours in the hands. *Hand* **12**, 293–299.

Watelet F., Menez D., Pageaut G. *et al.* (1986) Tumeur glomique sous-unguéale. Un cas de forme inhabituelle. *Rev. Chir. Orthop.* **72**, 509–510.

Wood W. (1812) On painful subcutaneous tubercle. *Edin. Med. J.* **8**, 283.

Blue rubber bleb naevus (Fig. 11.100)

Blue rubber bleb naevus of the hand and fingers may be accompanied by leuconychia.

Angioleiomyoma (Figs 11.116 & 11.117)

Lebouc (1889) described a case of subungual leiomyoma of the great toe. The pea-sized tumour consisted mainly of bundles of fibres intermingled with arterial and venous vessels. The muscular layer of the vessels was heavily hypertrophic, sometimes actually obliterating the lumen.

Smooth muscle bundles were also found without vascular structures.

Conolly (1980) showed a clinical and radiological picture of a leiomyoma presenting as a slow-growing tumour of the fingertip of a male aged 54 years. We have observed an apparently similar case in a young lady. The distal third of the nail plate was elevated and dystrophic. After avulsion of the nail plate, a small tumour was then seen directly distal to the lunula. Histology showed numerous blood vessels with a unique cushion-like hypertrophy of the smooth muscle which did not form a circular muscularis media layer. The patient had never experienced pain (E. Haneke, unpublished data). We have also reported on a case, clinically identical to a fibroma of the tip of the great toenail (Requena & Baran, 1993).

Clinically it is not possible to rule out cutaneous angiolipoleiomyoma (Fitzpatrick *et al.*, 1990), a tumour histologically well circumscribed with a well-defined fibrous pseudo-capsule and composed of smooth muscle, vascular spaces, connective tissue and mature fat.

References

Conolly W.B. (1980) *A Colour Atlas of Hand Conditions*, p. 167. Wolfe Medical Publications, London.

Fitzpatrick J.E., Mellette J.R., Hwang R.J. *et al.* (1990) Cutaneous angiolipoleiomyoma. *J. Am. Acad. Dermatol.* **23**, 1093–1098.

Lebouc L. (1989) Etude clinique et anatomique sur quelques cas de tumeurs sous-unguéales. Thèse pour le doctorat en médecine, pp. 1–34. G. Steinheil, Paris.

Requena L. & Baran R. (1994) Angioleiomyoma of the finger. *J. Am. Acad. Dermatol.* **29**, 1043–1044.

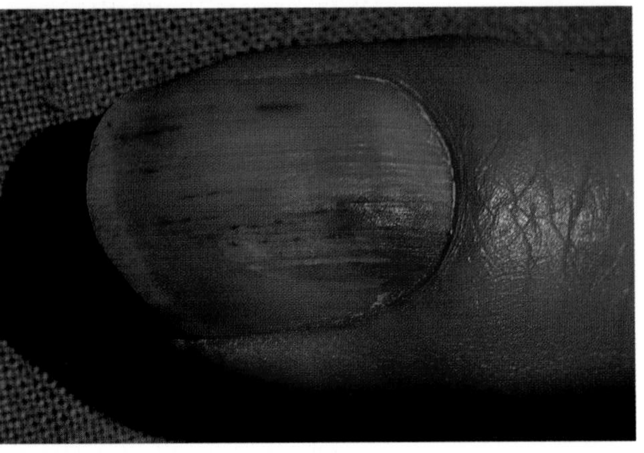

Fig. 11.118. Kaposi's sarcoma.

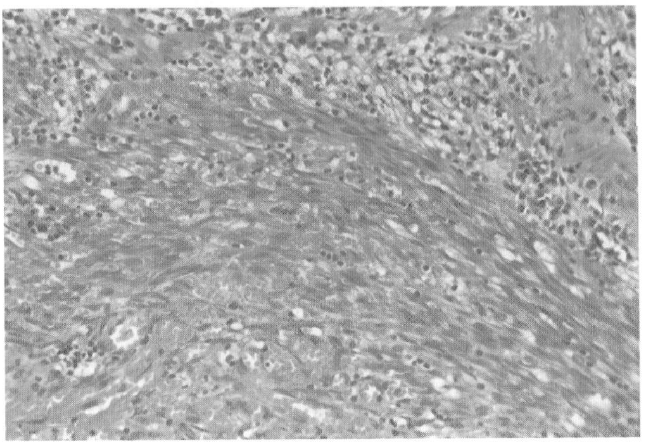

Fig. 11.119. Kaposi's sarcoma; histological changes.

Malignant

Kaposi's sarcoma

Kaposi's haemorrhagic sarcoma may involve the nail unit (Figs 11.118 & 11.119) causing elevation or deformation of the nail plate (Zaias, 1990). König (1899) described the case of a 61-year-old man with 'angiosarcoma multiplex' in the distal phalanges of three toes who later developed metastases in the gastrocnemius regions. Most cases described before 1920 as subungual angiosarcoma (Kolaczeck, 1878; Kraske, 1887) were probably glomus tumours.

Kaposi's sarcoma can involve the nail region in patients with aquired immune deficiency syndrome (AIDS).

References

Kolaczeck J. (1878) Über das Angio-Sarkom. *Dtsch. Z. Chir.* **9**, 1–48.

König F. (1899) Über multiple Angiosarkome. *Langenbecks Arch. Klin. Chir.* **59**, 600–614.

Kraske P. (1887) Über subunguale Geschwülste. *Münch. Med. Wschr.* **34**, 889–891.

Zaias N. (1990) *The Nail in Health and Disease*. Appleton & Lange, Norwalk, CT.

Malignant haemangioendothelioma

A 55-year-old-man who worked with polyvinyl chloride presented with a 3-month history of an ulcerating lesion affecting the nail bed of his third left toe. Histological examination showed malignant haemangioendothelioma (Davies *et al.*, 1990). This rare tumour is more commonly found in the liver where it has been reported to arise in association with exposure to the vinyl chloride monomer.

Reference

Davies M.F.P., Curtis M. & Howat J.M.T. (1990) Cutaneous haemangioendothelioma: possible link with chronic exposure to vinyl chloride. *Br. J. Indust. Med.* **47**, 65–67.

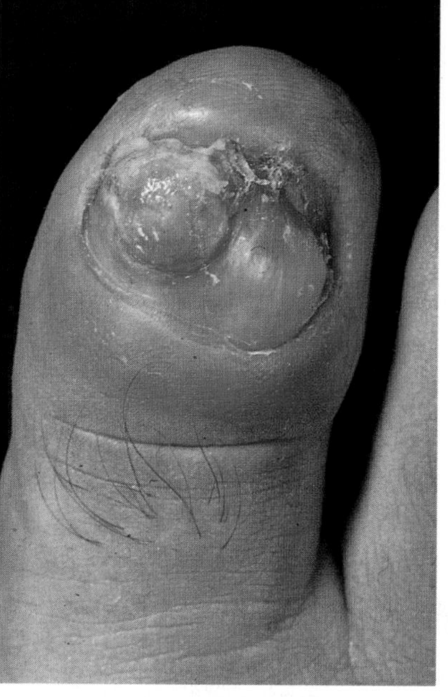

Fig. 11.120. Neurofibroma Recklinghausen (courtesy of U. Runne, Germany).

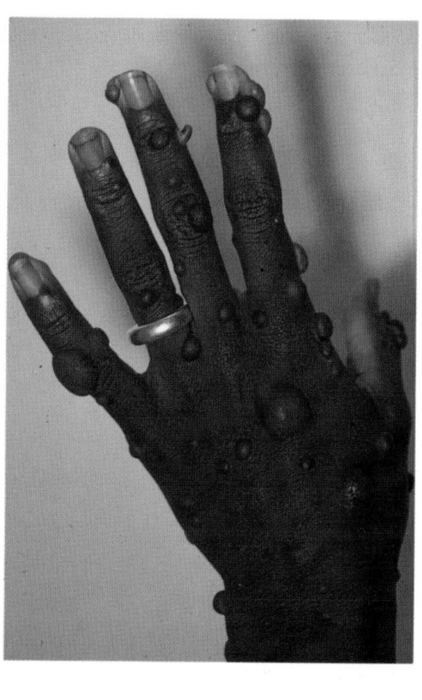

Fig. 11.123. Intradermal blue naevi presenting as pseudoneurofibromata (courtesy of B. Cavelier–Baloy, Paris, France) (see p. 492).

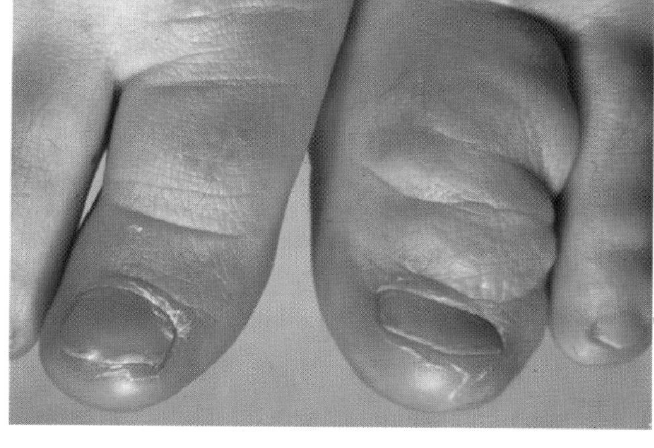

Fig. 11.121. Neurofibroma – diffuse lesion distorting the nail apparatus distal to it.

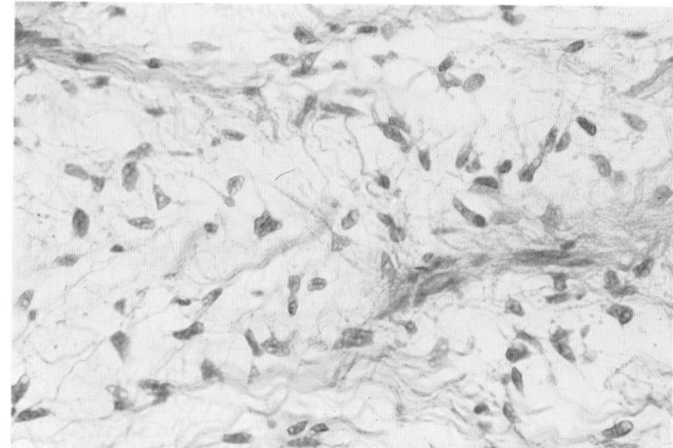

Fig. 11.122. Neurofibroma of the nail apparatus showing histological changes.

Neuroendocrine tumour

Merkel cell tumour

Merkel cell tumours on a toe is reported in a teenage girl (Goldenhersh *et al.*, 1992). The tumour clinically masqueraded as granulation tissue associated with an ingrown nail. On the medial aspect of the left great toe, at the junction of the lateral nail fold and the nail bed, there was a deep red, focally ulcerated granular nodule. On cut section of the specimen, a poorly delineated tumour consisting of brown haemorrhagic tissue and measuring 0.7 cm in diameter was identified.

The tumour cells were present in dense sheets, and focally were arranged in a trabecular pattern at all levels of the dermis and in the superficial subcutaneous fat.

Reference

Goldenhersh M.A., Prus D., Ron N. *et al.* (1992) Merkel cell tumor masquerading as granulation tissue on a teenager's toe. *Am. J. Dermatopathol.* **14**, 560–563.

Tumours of peripheral nerves

Neurogenic tumours of the terminal phalanx are very rare (Figs 11.120–11.132).

Neuroma

Post-injury neuromas are produced by the numerous nerve fibres in the nail bed (Fig. 11.132). They may cause tenderness, elevation of the nail bed and nail dystrophy. The treatment is careful resection with preservation or reconstruction of the nail bed (Zook, 1988).

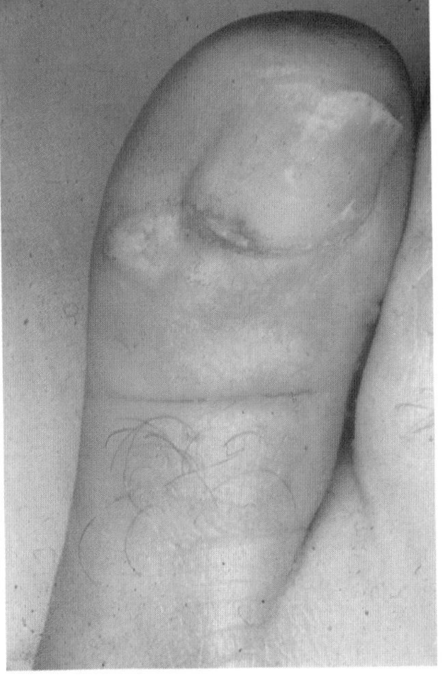

Fig. 11.124. Granular cell tumour (courtesy of L. Requena, Madrid, Spain).

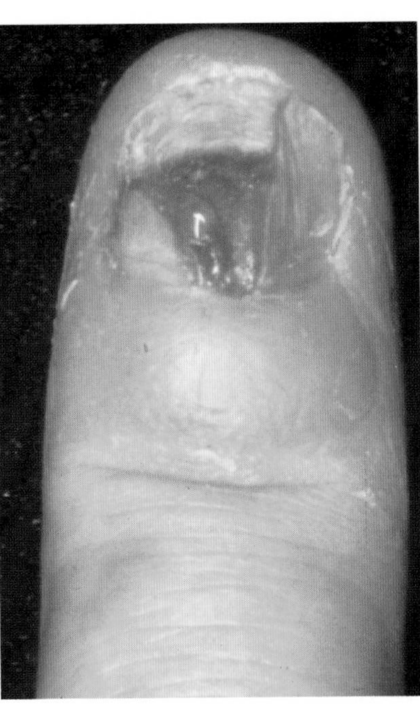

Fig. 11.126. Malignant granular cell tumour (courtesy of A. Urabe, Japan).

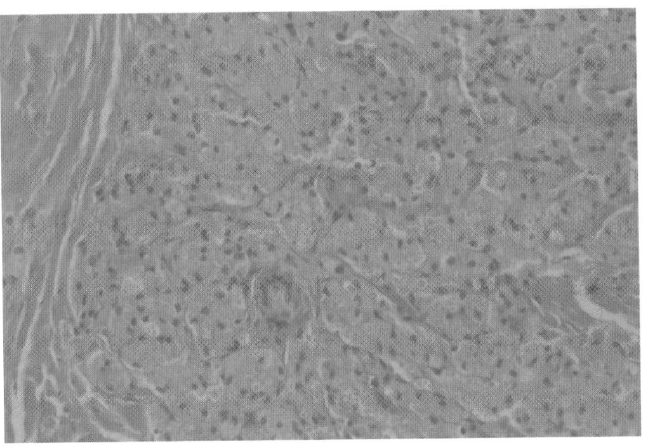

Fig. 11.125. Granular cell tumour; histology – clusters of tumour cells surrounded by strands of collagen fibres.

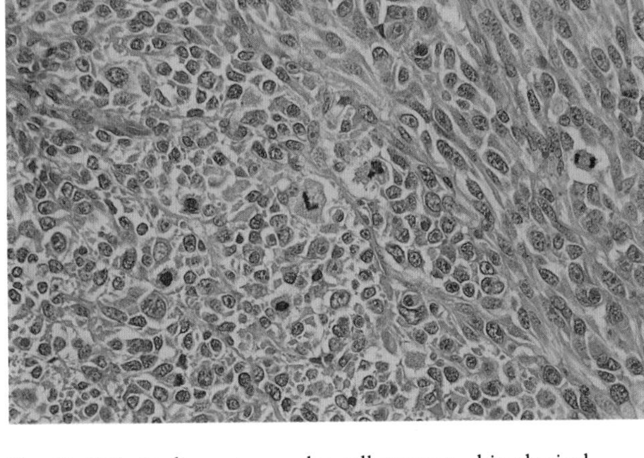

Fig. 11.127. Malignant granular cell tumour – histological changes.

Neurofibromas

Neurofibromas in Recklinghausen's neurofibromatosis (NF type I) seldom occur in the nail region (Figs 11.120 & 11.121). When located in the proximal nail fold they may produce a longitudinal depression (Zaias, 1990), or even mimick Koenen's tumours (Fig. 11.120) (Fröhlich, 1939); a subungual location may cause onychodystrophy (Runne & Orfanos, 1981). Exploratory nail plate removal may be a diagnostic aid for treating this painful tumour (Shelley & Shelley, 1986). Diffuse neurofibroma of the distal phalanx of a thumb was shown to enlarge both the fingertip and the nail without causing gross nail deformity (Zaias, 1980). We observed similar signs on the distal phalanx of the great toe. Papules associated with intradermal naevi may resemble Recklinghausen's disease which can be ruled out by immunohistochemistry (Fig. 11.123; see p. 492).

Systematized multiple fibrillar neuromas

These were observed by Altmeyer and Merkel (1981). Involvement of the tips of several fingers resulted in thickening of the periungual tissue without nail plate abnormalities.

'Pacinian' neuroma

A plexiform 'Pacinian' neuroma was observed in the distal phalanx of an 11-year-old boy. The tumour was asymptomatic but inhibited complete flexion of the distal interphalangeal joint. The nail plate was normal. Histology

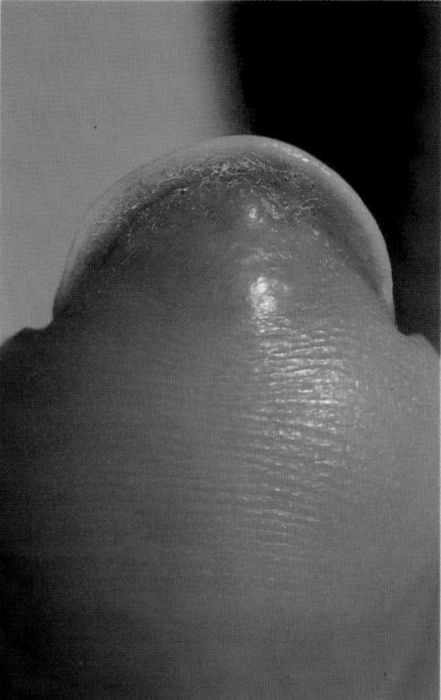

Fig. 11.128. Glioma (courtesy of J. Preaux, Paris, France).

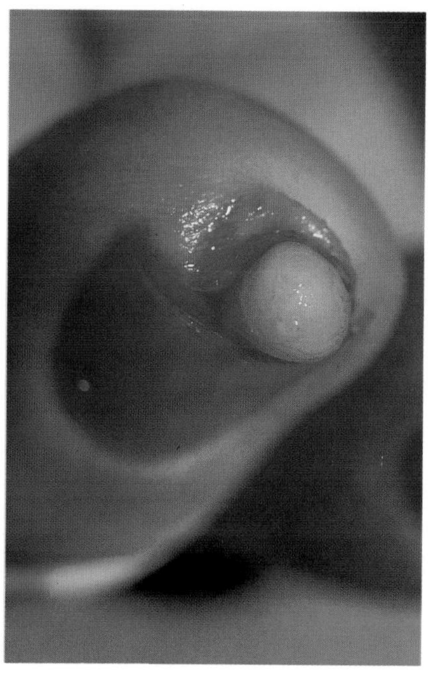

Fig. 11.129. Glioma (same patient as in Fig. 11.128).

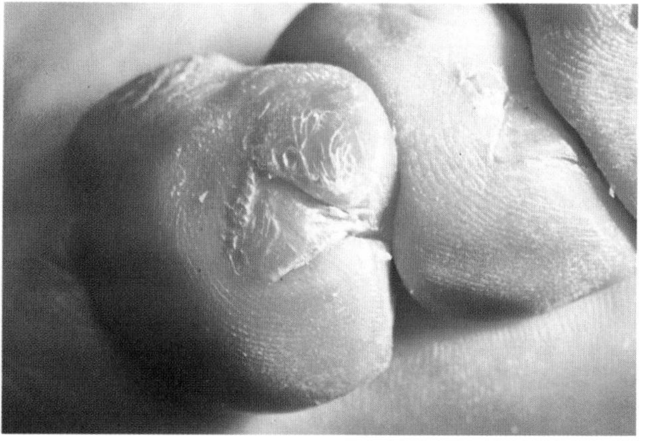

Fig. 11.130. Schwannoma (courtesy of A. Tosti, Bologna, Italy).

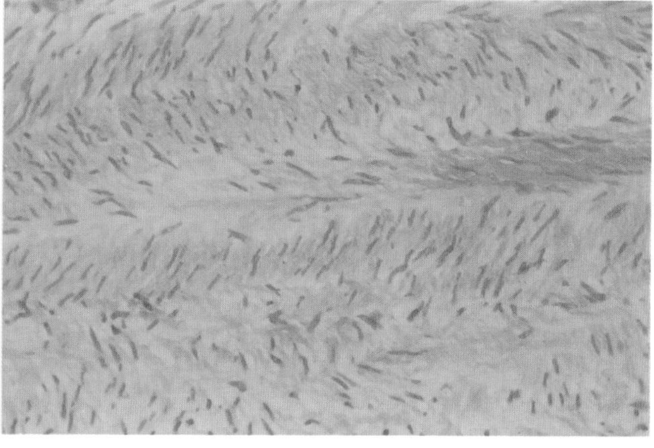

Fig. 11.131. Schwannoma – histological changes from Fig. 11.130 lesion.

showed unusual connective tissue structures resembling Pacini's corpuscles (Altmeyer, 1979).

Runne (1977) described a case of multiple mucosal neuroma syndrome with marked thickening of the proximal nail folds which were shown to contain neuromas.

Granular cell tumour

Hasson *et al.* (1991) reported on tender verrucous periungual growth located deeply medially in the proximal nail fold of the great toe in a 35-year-old female and producing a longitudinal groove of the nail plate (Fig. 11.124). Histology showed well-circumscribed clusters of tumour cells surrounded by strands of collagen fibres. The tumour cells were large with round or oval and centrally located nuclei and pale cytoplasm filled with faintly eosinophilic fine granules (Fig. 11.125). The lesion was surgically excised.

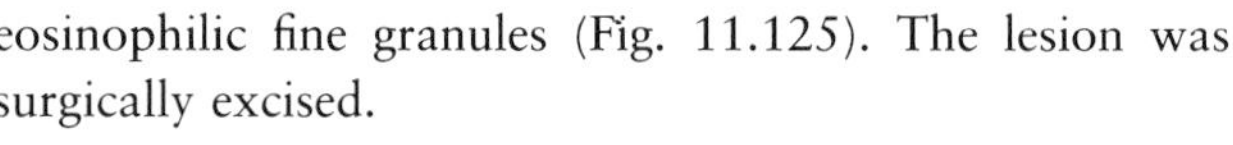

Malignant granular cell tumour (Urabe *et al.*, 1991)

A reddish nodule that reached a size of 5 mm in diameter and destroyed the nail developed under the nail of the right index finger of a 51-year-old Japanese woman (Fig. 11.126). It recurred 2 years after resection and was firm, partly eroded and 25 mm in diameter when the finger was amputated. Multiple metastases appeared 6 months later and the patient eventually died. Histopathology of the primary and recurrent tumour as well as a metastasis (Fig. 11.127) revealed polygonal cells with eosinophilic granular cells, mitoses, some multinucleated giant cells and in the metastasis, anaplastic cells. Immunohisto-

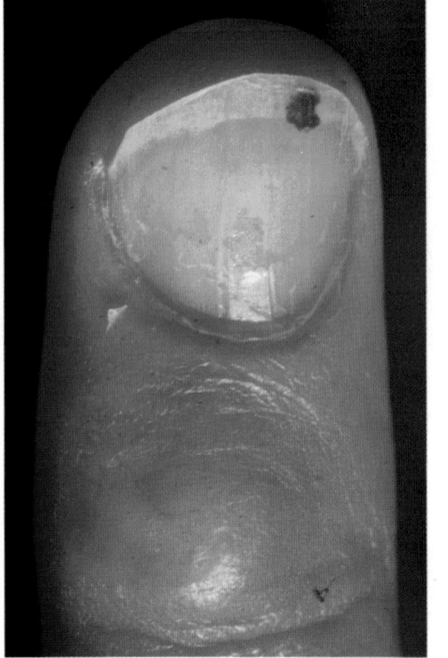

Fig. 11.132. Neuroma (proximal to proximal nail fold).

chemistry (protein S-100, Leu 7, vimentin) and electron microscopy confirmed the diagnosis of malignant granular cell tumour.

Glioma, neurilemmoma, schwannoma
(Figs 11.128–11.131)

These only rarely occur in a subungual position (Figs 11.128 & 11.129). A pigmented cutaneous lesion extending into the nail bed of the right index finger of a 71-year-old woman was the unique presentation of malignant melanocytic schwannoma (Elder *et al.*, 1981). The superficial pigmented portion of the primary tumour consisted of epitheloid and somewhat spindled cells above the white spindle cell portion demonstrating the biphasic nature of the lesion.

Post-section neuroma (Fig. 11.132) may occur due to focal nerve trunk damage.

So-called rudimentary supernumerary digits

The so-called rudimentary supernumerary digit is usually present at birth, often bilaterally symmetrical and almost always located at the base of the metacarpophalangeal joint. The lesion is distinguished by the finding of multiple nerve bundles within the dermal core and especially at the proximal base of the nodule.

References

Altmeyer H. (1979) Histologie eines Rankenneuroms mit Vater-Pacini-Lamellenkörper ähnlichen Strukturen. *Hautarzt* **30**, 248–252.

Altmeyer H. & Merkel K.H. (1981) Multiple systematisierte Neurome der Haut und der Schleimhaut. *Hautarzt* **32**, 240–244.

Elder D.E., Ainsworth M.A., Goldman L.I. *et al.* (1981) Malignant melanocytic schwannoma. In: *Pathology of Malignant Melanoma*, ed. Ackerman A.B., pp. 251–261. Masson Publishing USA, New York.

Fröhlich W. (1939) Fibromatosis subungualis. *Derm. Wschr.* **109**, 1211–1212.

Hasson A., Arias M.C., Guttierez A. *et al.* (1991) Periungual granular cell tumour. A light-microscopic, immunohistochemical and ultrastructural study. *Skin Cancer* **6**, 41–46.

Runne U. (1977) Syndrom der multiplen Neurome mit metastasierendem medullärem Schilddrüsenkarzinom ('Multiple mucosal neuroma-syndrome'). *Z. Hautkr.* **52**, 299–301.

Runne U. & Orfanos C.E. (1981) The human nail. *Curr. Prob. Dermatol.* **9**, 102–149.

Shelley E.D. & Shelley W.B. (1986) Exploratory nail plate removal as a diagnostic aid in painful subungual tumours:

Table 11.4. Differential features of exostosis, osteochondroma, enchondroma and epidermoid cyst (Norton, 1980)

Tumour	Age	Sex ratio	History of trauma	Rate of growth	X-ray
Exostosis	20–40	F:M 2:1	Occasionally	Moderate	Trabeculated osseous growth with expanded distal portion covered with radiolucent fibrocartilage
Osteochondroma	10–25	M:F 2:1	Often	Slow	Well-defined sessile bone growth with hyaline cartilage cap
Enchondroma	20–40	M = F	Often	Rapid	Lobulated bone cyst showing radiolucent defect, bone expansion, and flecks of calcification
Epidermoid cyst	8–83	M:F 2:1	Almost always	Rapid	Radiolucent cyst: no calcification

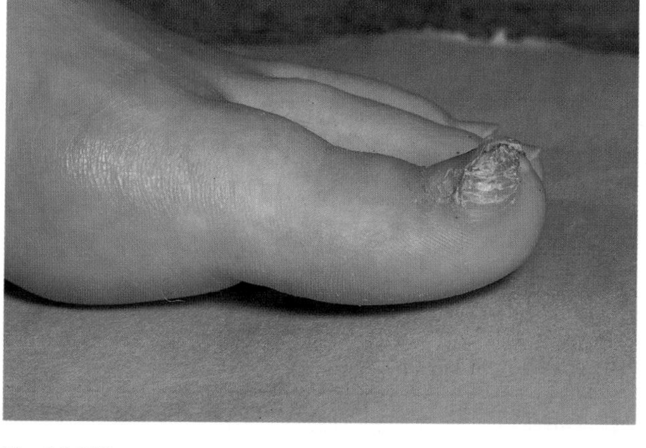

Fig. 11.133.

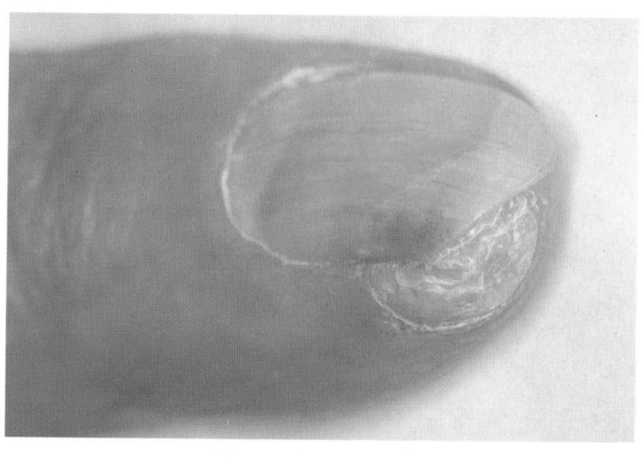

Fig. 11.135.

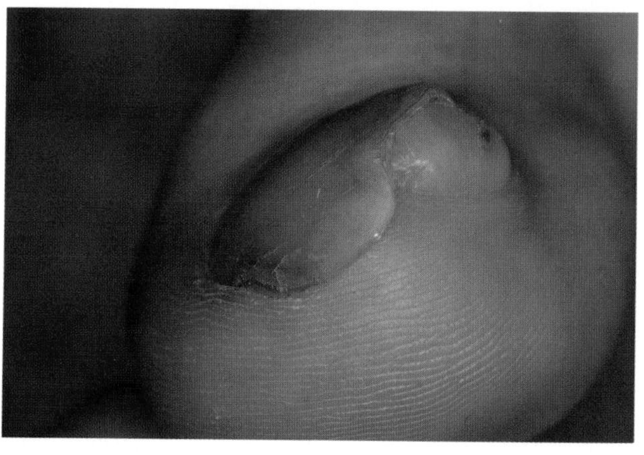

Fig. 11.134.

Fig. 11.133–135. Subungual exostosis.

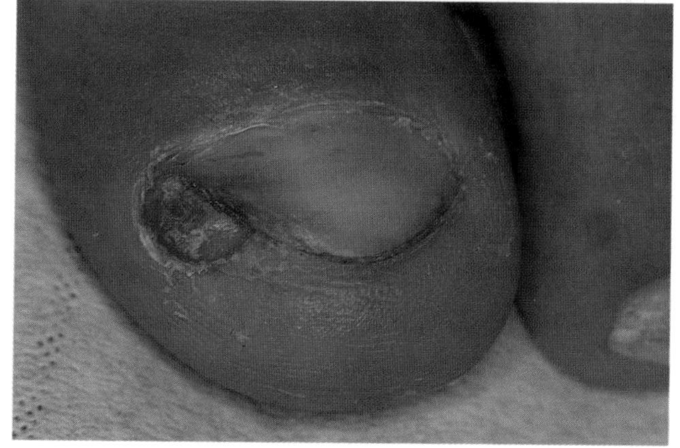

Fig. 11.136. Exostosis – lateral nail bed lesion.

glomus tumour, neurofibroma, and squamous cell carcinomas. *Cutis* **38**, 310–312.

Urabe A., Imayama S., Yasumoto S. *et al.* (1991) Malignant granular cell tumor. *J. Dermatol.* **18**, 161–166.

Zaias N. (1990) *The Nail in Health and Disease*, 2nd edn. Appleton & Lange, Norwalk, CT.

Zook E.G. (1988) Complications of the perionychium. *Hand Clin.* **2**, 407–427.

Osteocartilaginous tumours

Benign tumours

Exostosis

Subungual exostoses are not true tumours but outgrowths of normal bone or calcified cartilaginous remains (Figs 11.133–11.139). Whether or not subungual osteochondroma (Apfelberg *et al.*, 1979) is a different entity is not clear. Norton (1980) listed differential features (see Table 11.4).

Subungual exostoses are painful osseous growths which elevate the nail (Figs 11.133–11.135). They are particularly frequent in young people and mostly located in the great toe (Kato, 1990; Haneke, 1991, 1992) (Fig. 11.136), though subungual exostoses may also occur in lesser toes and less commonly in the thumb or index fingers (Baran & Sayag, 1978; Carroll *et al.*, 1992). They start as small elevations of the dorsal aspect of the distal phalanx and may eventually emerge from under the nail edge or destroy the nail plate. If the nail is lost, the surface becomes eroded and secondarily infected, sometimes mimicking an ingrowing toenail. Walking may be painful (Pambor & Neubert, 1971).

James (1988) reported a case arising from the ventral aspect of the distal phalanx of the left index finger and causing enlargement of the fingertip. Proximal nail groove pain associated with bilateral exostoses on the proximal medial aspect of the base of the distal hallux phalanges is unusual (Chinn & Jenkin, 1986).

Lemont and Christman (1990) presented a new classification for subungual exostoses, genetic and acquired types. This was based on the pathology, radiographic appearance, location, and age. They stated that the genetic subungual exostosis (type I) appears in the second and third

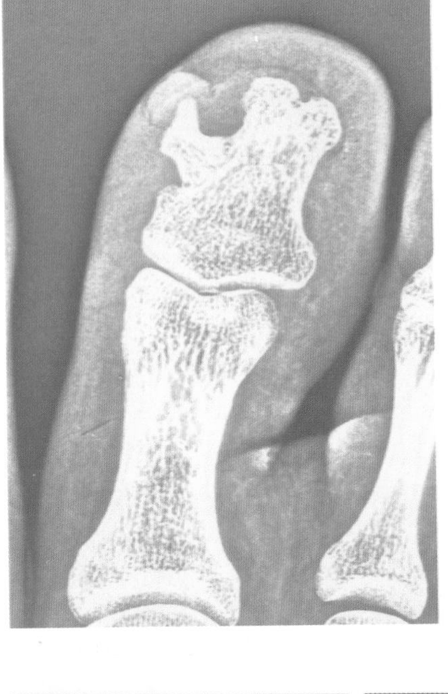

Fig. 11.137. Exostosis – clearly visible on X-ray.

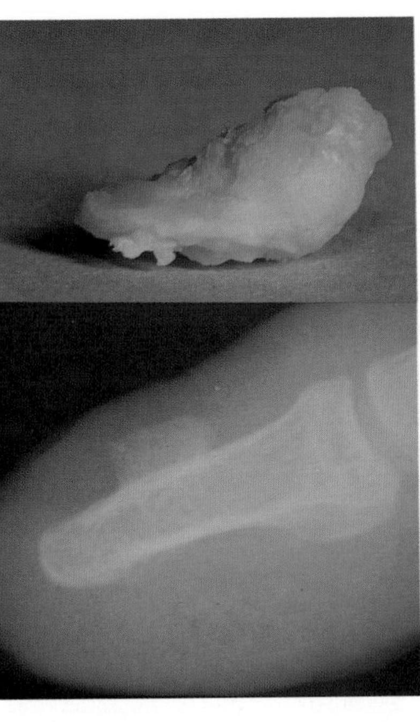
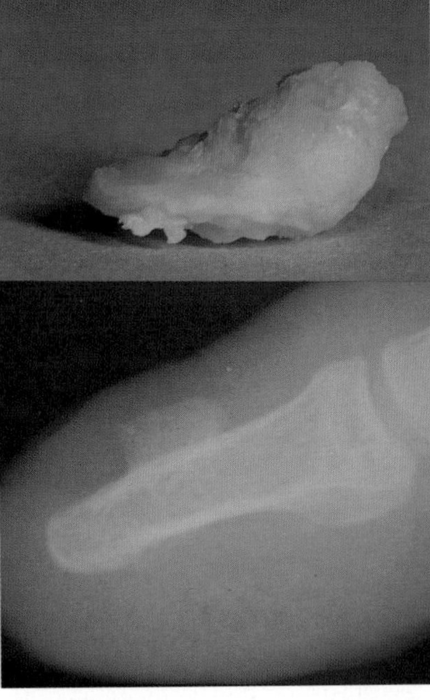

Fig. 11.139. Exostosis – the removed lesion (top); X-ray of lesion *in situ* (bottom).

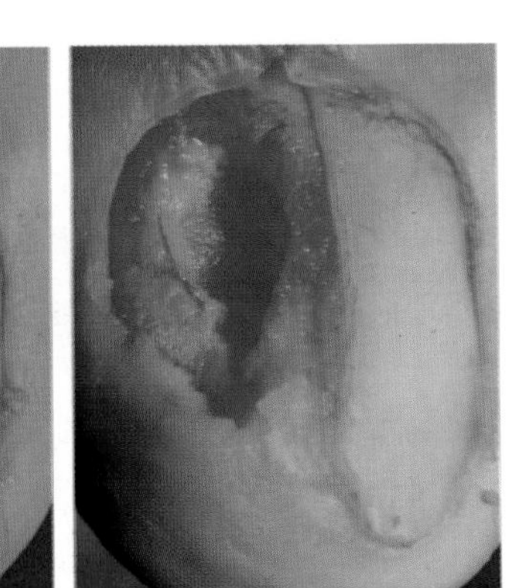

(a) (b)

Fig. 11.138. Exostosis – exposed after removal of the overlying nail (a); (b) shows the removal complete.

Fig. 11.140. Multiple exostes syndrome – radiological appearance.

decades of life, paronychia is frequent and only the medial aspect of the nail bed is hypertrophic. The acquired subungual exostosis (type II), in their study, is observed from the fourth through the sixth decade of life with a distal dorsal and central ungual tuberosity location and without cartilage covering. The nail plate appears as an inverted U, with nail bed hypertrophy being apparent. This type II is in fact equivalent to the so-called subungual hyperostosis, a condition often observed in pincer nail that is accompanied by a blunt or sharp protuberance at the distal and dorsal aspect of the terminal phalanx. This hyperostosis may be due to an abnormal positional relationship between the first metatarsal and hallux, with secondary osteoarthritis. Trauma appears to be a major causative factor (Sebastian, 1977) though some authors claim that a history of trauma is only occasionally found in subungual exostosis (Norton, 1980) (see Table 11.4).

The triad of pain (the leading symptom), nail deformation and radiographic features is usually diagnostic (Fig. 11.137). The exostosis is an ill-defined, trabeculated, osseous growth with an expanded distal portion covered with radiolucent fibrocartilage (Figs 11.138–11.140).

Histology shows a proliferative fibrocartilaginous cap that merges into mature trabecular bone at its base. Electron microscopy reveals that the tumour is composed of two types of cells: one rich in cell organelles including rough endoplasmic reticulum, well-developed Golgi apparatus, and glycogen granules; the other cell with few such cell organelles. The former cells seem to be osteoblasts actively engaged in bone formation, and the latter

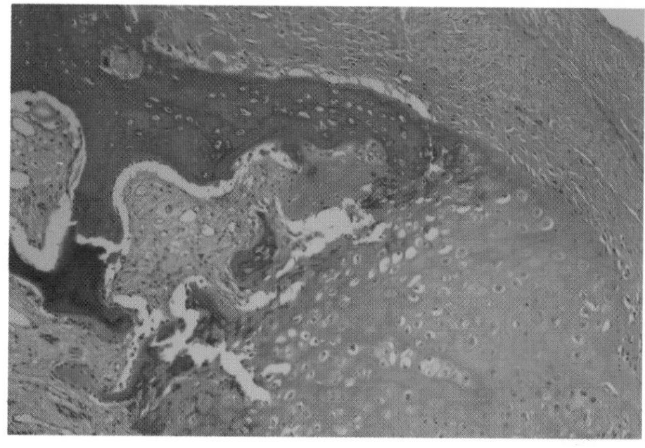

Fig. 11.141. Subungual osteochondroma; histological changes clearly different from subungual calcification.

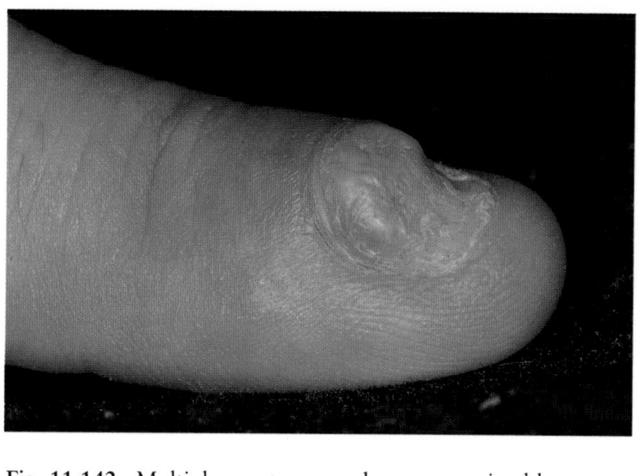

Fig. 11.142. Multiple exostoses syndrome – proximal bony swelling with anonychia (see Fig. 11.140).

to be osteocytes related to those situated deeper in bone matrix in normal bone. However, ossification or calcification in subungual exostosis is rather minimal, and osteocytes in this disorder may lack the capacity to elaborate compact bone.

Osteochondroma

Osteochondroma, commonly evoking the same symptoms, is said to be commoner in men. There is also often a history of trauma (Apfelberg *et al.*, 1979). Its growth rate is slow. X-ray shows a well-defined circumscribed pedunculated or sessile bone growth projecting from the dorsum of the distal phalanx with a hyaline cartilage cap. It must be differentiated from primary subungual calcification, particularly seen in older women, and secondary subungual calcification (Fig. 11.141) due to trauma and psoriasis (Fischer, 1982).

A unique case of osteochondroma on the ulnar side of the distal phalanx of the small finger and penetrating the skin and the nail was described by Ganzhorn *et al.* (1981).

Therapy consists of curettage (Senff *et al.*, 1987) or excision of the excess bone under full aseptic conditions. The nail plate is partially removed and a longitudinal incision is made in the nail bed. When possible, we prefer to remove the tumour by an L-shaped or a fish-mouth incision, in order to avoid avulsion of the nail plate. The osseous growth with its cartilaginous cap is carefully dissected using fine skin hooks to avoid damage to the fragile nail bed and the tumour is removed with a fine chisel.

References

Apfelberg D.B., Druker D., Maser M. & Lash H. (1979) Subungual osteochondroma. *Arch. Dermatol.* **115**, 472–473.

Baran R. & Sayag A. (1978) Exostose sous-unguéale de l'index. *Ann. Dermatol. Venereol.* **105**, 1075–1076.

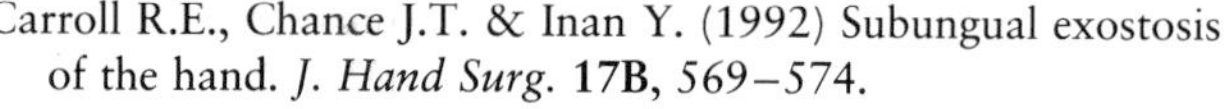

Carroll R.E., Chance J.T. & Inan Y. (1992) Subungual exostosis of the hand. *J. Hand Surg.* **17B**, 569–574.

Chinn S. & Jenkin W. (1986) Proximal nail groove pain associated with an exostosis. *J. Am. Pod. Med. Assoc.* **76**, 506–508.

Fischer E. (1982) Subunguale Verkalkungen. *Fortschr. Röntgenst.* **137**, 580–584.

Ganzhorn R.W., Bahri G. & Horowitz M. (1981) Osteochondroma of the distal phalanx. *J. Hand Surg.* **6**, 625–626.

Haneke E. (1991) Cirugía dermatológica de la región ungueal. *Mon. Dermotol.* **4**, 408–423.

Haneke E. (1992) Etiopathogénie de l'hypercourbure transversale de l'ongle du gros orteil. *J. Med. Esth. Chir. Dermatol.* **29**, 123–127.

James M.P. (1988) Digital exostosis causing enlargement of the fingertips. *J. Am. Acad. Dermatol.* **19**, 132.

Kato H., Nakagawa T., Suji T. *et al.* (1990) Subungual exostosis clinicopathological and ultrastrutural studies of 3 cases. *Clin. Exp. Dermatol.* **15**, 429–432.

Lemont H. & Christman R.A. (1990) Subungual exostosis and nail disease and radiologic aspects. In: *Nails: Therapy, Diagnosis, Surgery*, eds Scher R. & Daniel C.R., pp. 250–257. Saunders, W.B. Philadelphia.

Norton L.A. (1980) Nail disorders. *J. Am. Acad. Dermatol.* **2**, 451–467.

Pambor M. & Neubert H. (1971) Tumorartige Begleitreaktionen der Haut bei Exostosen der Zehenendphalangen (Zur Differentialdiagnose par – und subungualer Tumoren). *Derm. Mschr.* **157**, 532–537.

Sebastian G. (1977) Subunguale Exostosen der Grosszehe, Berufsstigma bei Tänzern. *Dermatol. Mschr.* **163**, 998–1000.

Senff H., Kuhlwein A. & Janner M. (1987) Subungual exostosis. *Z. Hautkr.* **62**, 1401–1404.

Stieler W., Reinel D., Jänner M. & Haneke E. (1989) Ungevöhuliche Lokalisation einer subungualen exostose. *Akt. Dermatol.* **15**, 32–34.

Multiple exostoses syndrome (MES) (diaphysial aclasis)

MES is a hereditary disorder affecting the enchondral skeleton during the period of growth in a variety of ways – generally 'close to the knee and far from the elbow'.

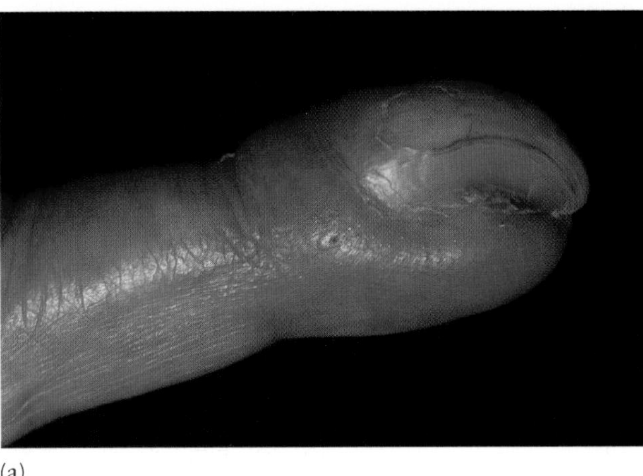

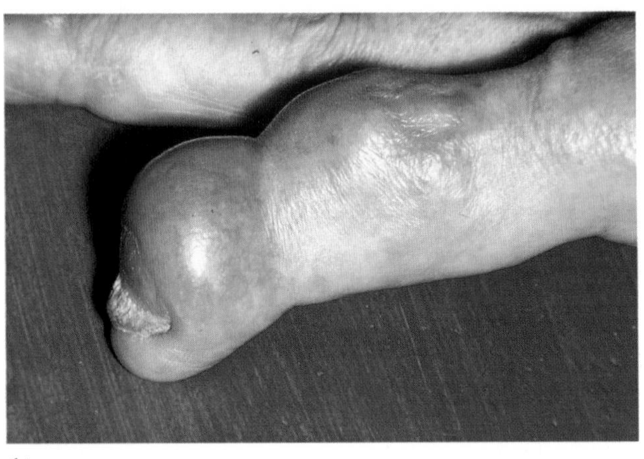

(a) (b)

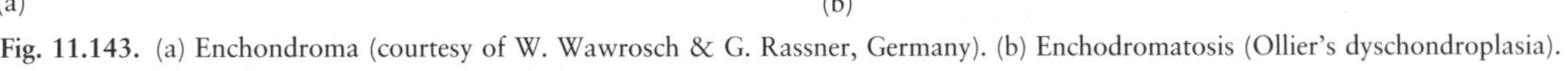

Fig. 11.143. (a) Enchondroma (courtesy of W. Wawrosch & G. Rassner, Germany). (b) Enchodromatosis (Ollier's dyschondroplasia).

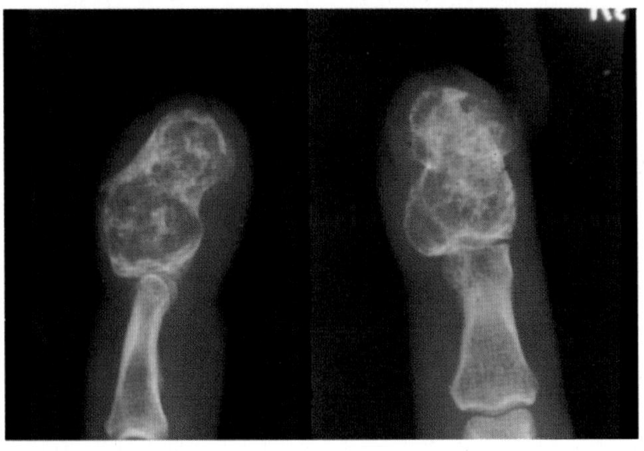

Fig. 11.144. Enchondroma.

Fig. 11.145. Enchondroma – X-ray showing expansion of the distal phalanx and irregular, spotty calcification – see Fig. 11.143.

It is characterized by thickening and deformity of the growing bone with the formation of numerous cartilage-capped exostoses clustered around the areas of most active growth (Figs 11.140 & 11.142).

A 16-year-old boy presented with anonychia of his left index finger caused by a firm non-tender nodule affecting the proximal two-thirds of the nail bed and the lunula with resultant slight elevation of the proximal nail fold (Fig. 11.142). The outgrowth had started 2 years earlier. A lateral X-ray revealed an exostosis (Fig. 11.140). His sister, aged 12, presented with multiple exostoses of the hands, clearly visible radiologically. They were located on the ventral aspect of the middle phalanx of the right index finger and the dorsal aspect of the distal phalanx of the right fifth digit and the first, second and third left digits, where they slightly lifted up the nail plate (Baran & Bureau, 1991).

Laugier *et al.* (1964) reported two cases in the French literature. In the first, exostosis of the base of the distal phalanx of the fourth finger of a 10-year-old boy resulted in a lateral deviation of the nail plate. Several fingers were affected in an 11-year-old girl presenting with various physical signs including a bump at the base of the right index nail, an overcurvature of the lateral aspect of the nail of the right middle finger, a red linear longitudinal line with a distal fissure on the right fifth fingernail, and distal fissures arranged in a fanwise manner on two other nails.

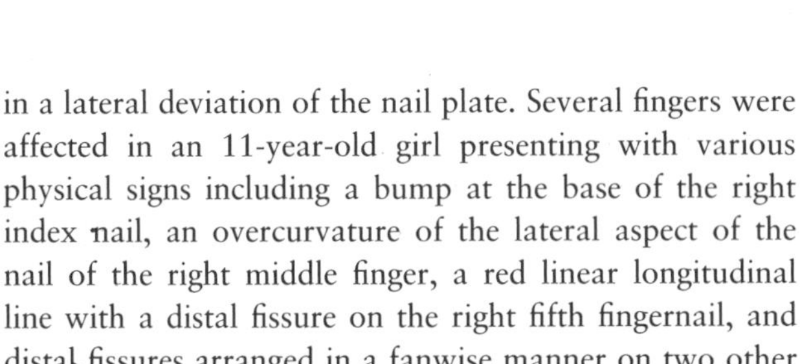

Recently Hazen and Smith (1990) reported a type with prominent elevation of the proximal portion of the nail and corresponding nail fold of several fingers by firm and non-tender nodules. In Del Rio *et al.*'s report (1992) nail plate deformity consisted of malalignment, longitudinal dystrophy and swelling of the proximal nail fold on several fingers that had developed slowly since birth.

When the disease involves the distal phalanx it seems to affect most often several digits simultaneously. Such a distribution should therefore suggest MES with the possible risk of malignant changes to chondrosarcoma in from 1 to 25% (Solomon, 1974), this is despite the absence of malignancy reported in this location and in childhood (Smith, 1988).

References

Baran R. & Bureau H. (1991) Multiple exostoses syndrome presenting with anonychia on a single finger. *J. Am. Acad. Dermatol.* **25**, 333–335.

Del Rio R., Naveorra E., Ferrando J. & Mascarŏ J.M. (1992) Multiple exostoses syndrome presenting as nail malalignment and longitudinal dystrophy of fingers. *Arch. Dermatol.* **128**, 1655–1656.

Hazen P.G. & Smith D.E. (1990) Hereditary multiple exostoses: Report of a case presenting with proximal nail fold and nail swelling. *J. Am. Acad. Dermatol.* **22**, 132–134.

Laugier P., Gille P., Gondy B. *et al.* (1964) Maladie exostosante avec lésions unguéales (2 cas). *Bull. Soc. Fr. Dermatol. Syphil.* **71**, 338.

Smith D.W. (1988) *Recognizable Patterns of Human Malformation. Genetic, Embryologic and Clinical Aspects.*, 4th edn. W.B. Saunders, Philadelphia.

Solomon L. (1974) Chondrosarcoma in hereditary multiple exostosis. *S. Afr. Med. J.* **48**, 671–676.

Enchondroma

Solitary enchondroma of the distal phalanx is rare. It is a painful tumour which expands the finger (Figs 11.143 & 11.144). It may present clinically as paronychia (Shelley & Ralston, 1964; Pastinszky & Dévai, 1968; Wawrosch & Rassner, 1985) or as clubbing with thickening, discoloration and longitudinal ridging of the nail (Yaffee, 1965). A 'fungus-shaped', white tumour may lift the overlying nail plate (Carjaval *et al.*, 1987). X-ray reveals a well-defined radiolucent defect with expansion of the distal phalanx or spotty calcification (Schajowicz *et al.*, 1970) (Fig. 11.145). The enchondroma is typically located at the base of the distal phalanx abutting onto the articular surface (Monsees & Murphy, 1984). Pathological fractures may occur as a result of continuous thinning of the bony cortex.

Chondroma involving the distal phalanx of the hand was monostotic in three cases and polyostotic in 30 cases in Takigawa's review (1971). Chondrosarcoma may arise in a preexisting enchondroma (Bellinghausen *et al.*, 1983).

Histology shows hyaline cartilage proliferation with irregularly arranged cells (Fig. 11.146).

Treatment is required to prevent further enlargement of the enchondroma and because of its symptoms. The tumour is enucleated under full aseptic precautions. Curettage followed by autologous cancellous bone grafting usually yields the best results – the ilium can be recommended as a good donor site for such grafting. However, all lesions do not necessarily need such an operation as some cases undergo spontaneous resolution.

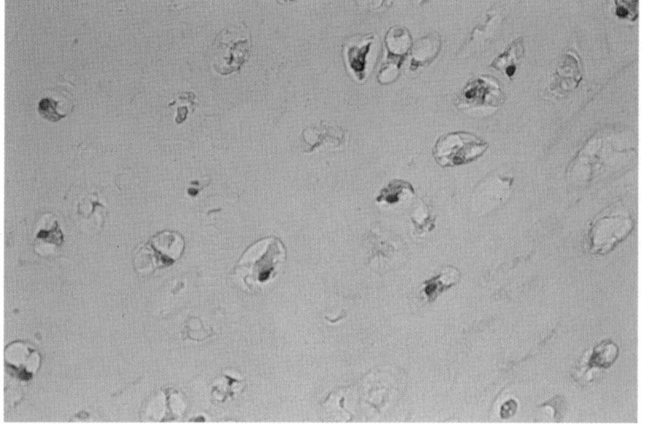

Fig. 11.146. Enchondroma – hyaline cartilage proliferation with irregularly arranged cells (see Figs 11.143 & 11.145).

Enchondromatosis (Ollier's dyscondroplasia)

Enchondromatosis results from cartilage failing to undergo normal ossification in asymmetrical fashion (Fig. 11.143).

Maffucci's syndrome (enchondromatosis, or dyschondroplasia with multiple soft tissue haemangiomas)

In Maffucci's syndrome multiple subcutaneous angiomas and hard cartilaginous nodules of epiphyseal lines develop in childhood, due to masses and columns of uncalcified cartilage causing unequal growth of bones and delayed healing of the easily sustained bone fractures (Figs 11.147

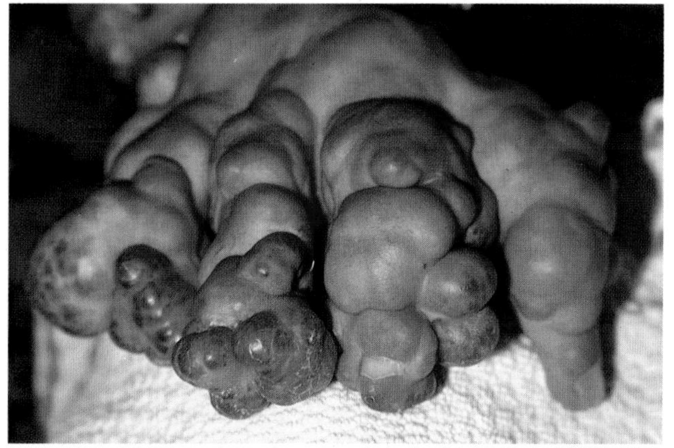

Fig. 11.147. Maffucci's syndrome (courtesy of D. Tilsley).

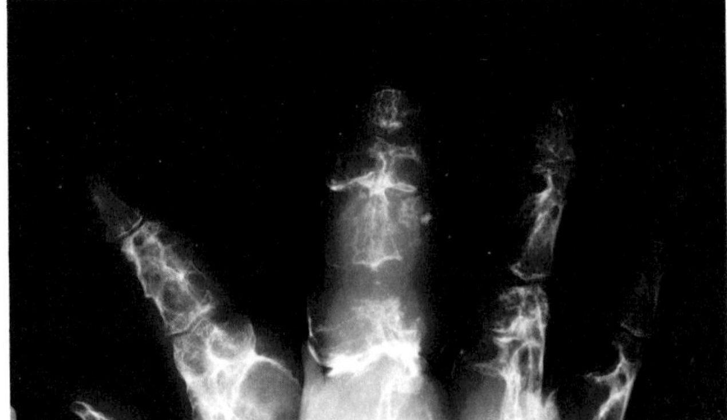

Fig. 11.148. Maffucci's syndrome – X-ray changes (courtesy D. Tilsley).

& 11.148). The hands and feet may be transformed into useless masses (Steudel, 1892; Hackenbroch, 1922).

The differential diagnosis of subungual chondroma (Ayala *et al.*, 1983) includes most tumours occurring in a subungual location, such as subungual exostosis, pyogenic granuloma, common wart, glomus tumour, epidermoid cyst, keratoacanthoma, melanoma, neurofibroma and sarcoma; the distinction between chondroma and low-grade chondrosarcoma is one of the most difficult to be made histopathologically (Gottschalk & Smith, 1963).

Involvement of the terminal phalanx may result in gross deformity, dystrophy or loss of the nail (Tilsley & Burden, 1981). The most important complication is the high frequency of chondrosarcoma (Lewis & Ketcham, 1973), or angiosarcoma.

References

Ayala F., Lembo G. & Montesano M. (1983) A rare tumour. Subungual chondroma. *Dermatologica* **167**, 339–340.

Bellinghausen H.W., Weeks P.M., Young L.V. & Gilula L.A. (1983) Chondrosarcoma of distal phalanx. *Orthop. Rev.* **12**, 97–100.

Carvajal L., Uraga E., Garcia I. *et al.* (1987) Tumours of the hallux: myxoma, osteochondroma and enchondroma. *Skin Cancer* **2**, 197–201.

Gottschalk R.G. & Smith R.T. (1963) Chondrosarcoma of the hand. *J. Bone Joint Surg.* **45A**, 141–150.

Hackenbroch M. (1922) Über Olliersche Waschstumsstörung und Chondromatose des Skeletts. *Fortschr Röntgen.* **30**, 432–440.

Lewis R.J. & Ketcham A.S. (1973) Maffucci's syndrome; functional and neoplastic significance. *J. Bone Joint Surg.* **55A**, 1465.

Monses B. & Murphy W.A. (1984) Distal phalangeal erosive lesions. *Arth. Rhem.* **27**, 449–455.

Pastinszky I. & Dévai J. (1968) Paronychia et onychodystrophia enchondromatosa. *Börgyögy. Vener. Szle.* **44**, 176–178.

Schajowicz F., Aiello C. & Slullitel I. (1970) Cystic and pseudocystic lesions of the terminal phalanx with special reference to epidermoid cysts. *Clin. Orthop. Rel. Res.* **68**, 84–92.

Shelley W.B. & Ralston E.L. (1964) Paronychia due to enchondroma. *Arch. Dermatol.* **90**, 412–413.

Steudel (1892) Multiple Enchondrome der Knochen in Verbindung mit venösen Angiomen der Weichteile. *Beitr. Klin. Chir.* **8**, 503–521.

Takigawa K. (1971) Chondroma of the bones of the hand. *J. Bone Joint Surg.* **53A**, 1591–1600.

Tilsley D.A. & Burden P.W. (1981) A case of Maffucci's syndrome. *Br. J. Dermatol.* **105**, 331–336.

Wawrosch W. & Rassner G. (1985) Monströses Enchondrom des Zeigefingerendgliedes mit Nageldeformierung. *Hautarzt* **36**, 168–169.

Yaffee H.W. (1965) Peculiar nail dystrophy caused by an enchondroma. *Arch. Dermatol.* **91**, 361.

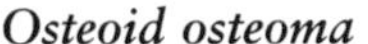

Osteoid osteoma

Osteoid osteoma (Jaffé, 1935) is a distinct clinical and pathological entity, rare in the distal phalanx (Rosborough, 1966). About 8% of all osteoid osteomata occur in the phalanges, and 1–2% of hand tumours are osteoid osteomata (Fig. 11.149); however, its location in the distal phalanx is quite rare (Aulicino *et al.*, 1981) with index predominance. Osteoid osteoma causes swelling of the distal phalanx or even enlargement of the entire tip, and clubbing, thickening or enlargement of the nail may be associated. The skin is either normal in colour or faintly violaceous. Increased sweating of the area has been described. Palpation with a blunt probe may help to localize the tender tumour on pressure. A nidus, characterized by a small area of rarefaction with surrounding sclerosis, is demonstrable radiologically in most cases and has been likened to a 'sleigh-bell' (Foucher *et al.*, 1987) (Fig. 11.150); it is located in the medulla, in the cortex, or subperiosteally with a very thin covering of bone over the nidus (Sullivan, 1971). However, symptoms generally precede radiographic changes by several months. A radionuclide bone scan of the affected region is useful. The hypervascularization, explaining the nail thickening, can

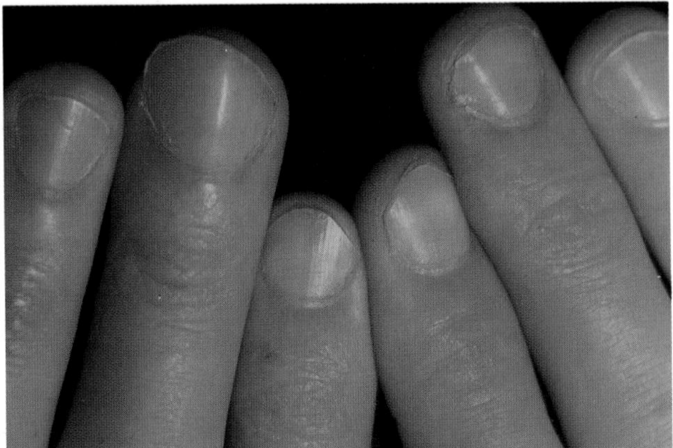

Fig. 11.149. Osteoid osteoma – third left digit in figure (courtesy of G. Foucher, Strasbourg, France).

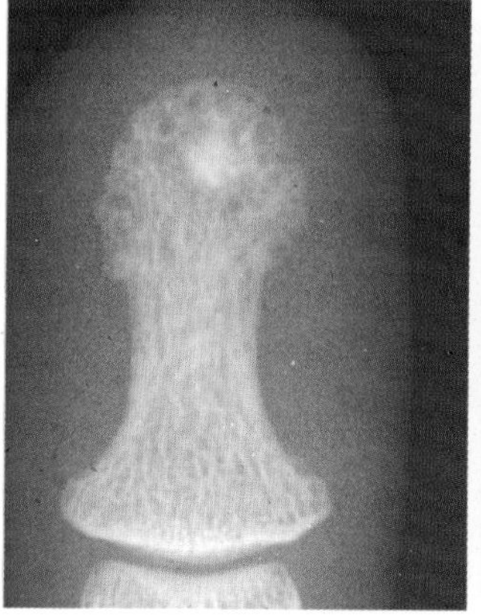
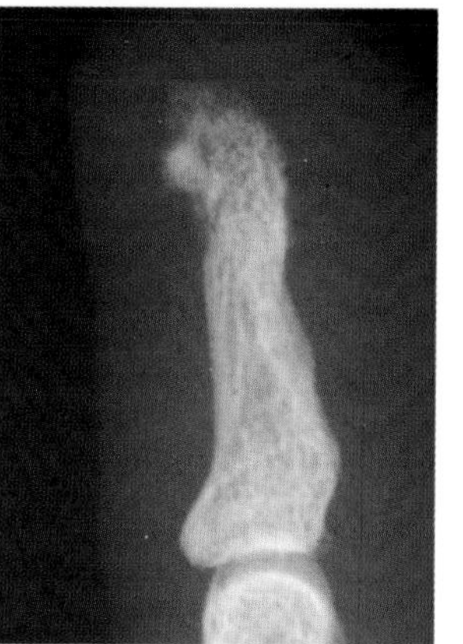

Fig. 11.150. Osteoid osteoma – X-ray changes.

be demonstrated by arteriography (Lindbom *et al.*, 1960; Sullivan, 1971), by thermography (O'Hara *et al.*, 1975), or by scintigraphy (Braun *et al.*, 1980). Young patients may have premature fusion of the adjacent epiphysis. Histologically, the nidus is a meshwork of osteoid trabeculae with varying degrees of mineralization in a background of vacular fibrous connective tissue. When they appear in the distal phalanx they present unusual diagnostic difficulties due to (i) atypical radiological appearance; (ii) presence of soft tissue enlargement and nail deformity; (iii) small size of the distal phalanx and consequent close approximation of lesions to the nail and distal interphalangeal joint (Bowen *et al.*, 1987). The sex incidence is 2:1 male: female. They appear in young adults but Szabó and Smith (1985) reported one case which had probably existed since birth.

Osteoid osteoma usually evokes a 'nagging' pain, accentuated at night, which is poorly localized. Local tenderness is present in about half of the cases. There is no evidence of inflammation or systemic toxicity.

Treatment is by en-bloc resection through a fish-mouth incision. Curettage may fail to eradicate the lesion. Radiography does not seem to be helpful in deciding whether the whole lesion has been removed. After therapy the swelling regresses, normal nail regrows and the pain gradually disappears. There are cases, however, in which digital enlargement persists after removal of the lesion, therefore reducing the soft tissue and narrowing the nail when the lesion is removed has been advocated.

Relief of pain by salicylates is characteristic. However, symptoms may vary considerably. Naproxen or aspirin (Saville, 1980; Brown *et al.*, 1991) given in low doses may prevent the pain of osteoid osteoma, offering useful non-surgical treatment since spontaneous regression leading even to complete cure is possible (Foucher *et al.*, 1987).

The differential diagnosis includes glomus tumour, implantation epidermoid cyst, sclerosing osteitis of Garré, localized cortical bone abscess, syphilitic dactylitis, tuberculosis, chondroma and arteriovenous fistula. It is not possible to differentiate between osteoid osteoma and benign osteoblastoma (less painful, less sclerosis) on histological grounds alone (Table 11.5).

Table 11.5. Differentiation between osteoid osteoma and benign osteoblastoma

	Osteoid osteoma	Osteoblastoma
Size	<1 cm in diameter	Slow progressive enlargement
Symptoms	Painful	Less painful
X-ray	Considerable reactive bone and sclerosis	Less sclerosis
Location	Long bones	Flat bones
Hostology	Indistinguishable	

References

Aulicino P.L., DuPuy T.E. & Moriarity R.P. (1981) Osteoid osteoma of the terminal phalanx of finger. *Orthop. Rev.* **10**, 59–63.

Bowen C.V.A., Dzus A.K. & Hardy D.A. (1987) Osteoid osteomata of the distal phalanx. *J. Hand Surg.* **12B**, 387–390.

Braun S., Chevro A., Tomeno B. & Durand-Kulas R. (1980) Les ostéomes ostéoides phalangiens. *Méd. Hyg. (Genève)* **38**, 1222–1229.

Brown R.E., Russel J.B. & Zook E.G. (1991) Osteoid osteoma of the distal phalanx of the finger: A diagnostic challenge. *Plast. Reconsti. Surg.* **90**, 1016–1021.

Foucher G., Lemarechal P., Citron N. *et al.* (1987) Osteoid osteoma of the distal phalanx. A report of four cases and review of the literature. *J. Hand Surg.* **12B**, 382–386.

Jaffé H.L. (1935) Osteoid osteoma. A benign osteoblastic tumor composed of osteoid and atypical bone. *Arch. Surg.* **31**, 709–728.

Lindbom A., Lindvall N., Sodenberg G. & Spujt H. (1960) Angiography in osteoid osteoma. *Acta Radiol. Stockholm* **54**, 327–333.

O'Hara J.P., Tegmeyer C., Sweet D.E. & MacCue F.C. (1975) Angiography in the diagnosis of oesteoid osteoma of the hand. *J. Bone Joint Surg.* **57A**, 163–166.

Rosborough D. (1966) Osteoid osteoma: report of a lesion in the teminal phalanx of a finger. *J. Bone Joint Surg.* **48B**, 485–487.

Saville P.D. (1980) A medical option for the treatment of osteoid osteoma. *Arth. Rheum.* **23**, 1409–1411.

Stein A.H. (1959) Benign neoplastic and nonneoplastic destructive lesions in the long bones of the hand. *Surg. Gynec. Obstet.* **109**, 189–197.

Sullivan M. (1971) Osteoid osteoma of the fingers. *Hand* **3**, 175–178.

Szabó R.M. & Smith B. (1985) Possible congenital osteoid osteoma of a phalanx; case report. *Am. J. Bone Joint Surg.* **67**, 815–816.

Solitary bone cyst

Solitary bone cyst of the distal phalanx is exceptional. Goldsmith (1966) reported on a clubbing nail deformity overlying a bulbous distal end of the left second toe which was tender. X-ray examination revealed an expanded distal phalanx with an ultra-thinned cortex and cystic-like loss of substance in the main body of bone.

Reference

Goldsmith E. (1966) Solitary bone cyst of the distal phalanx. A case report. *J. Am. Pod. Assoc.* 56, 69–70.

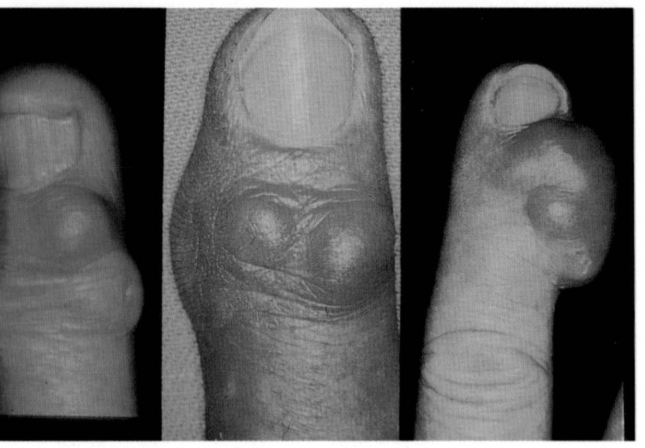

Fig. 11.151. Giant cell tumour (benign synovioma).

Malignant tumours

Chondrosarcoma

See p. 473.

Synovial tumours

Giant cell tumour (benign synovioma, benign xanthomatous giant cell tumours, villo-nodular pigmented synovitis)

Giant cell tumour is a neoplasm derived from the tendon sheath or the joint synovia. It is the second most common subcutaneous tumour of the hand. It is more frequent in females than in males. On the digits (Fig. 11.151), it usually occurs on the dorsum of the distal interphalangeal joint and commonly appears as a solitary, often lobulated slow-growing, skin-coloured and smooth-surfaced nodule which tends to feel firm and rubbery. The tumour may enlarge to the size of a cherry and may cause pain on flexion by virtue of its dimensions. Only rarely does the tumour interfere with the nail unit. In the region of the lateral nail fold, periodic inflammation and drainage may occur (Norton, 1990). In contrast to malignant synovioma, no calcification is demonstrable on X-ray (Wright, 1951).

Histopathology (Fig. 11.152) shows a cellular tumour composed of histiocytic and fibroblastic cells with a variable number of giant cells and some foam cells in a hyalin stroma. Siderophages may give the tumour a brown appearance.

Differential diagnosis includes ganglion, which tends to feel more cystic (aspiration or transillumination), fibroma of the tendon sheath (Chung & Enzinger, 1979), implantation epidermal cyst, fibrokeratoma, rheumatoid nodule, multicentric reticulohistiocytosis, metastatic tumour, tendinous xanthoma, chondro- or osteosarcoma, and reticulohistiocytoma, whose histology may be indentical to giant cell tumour. Granuloma annulare (Fig. 11.153) and erythema elevatum diutinum (Fig. 11.154) should also be ruled out.

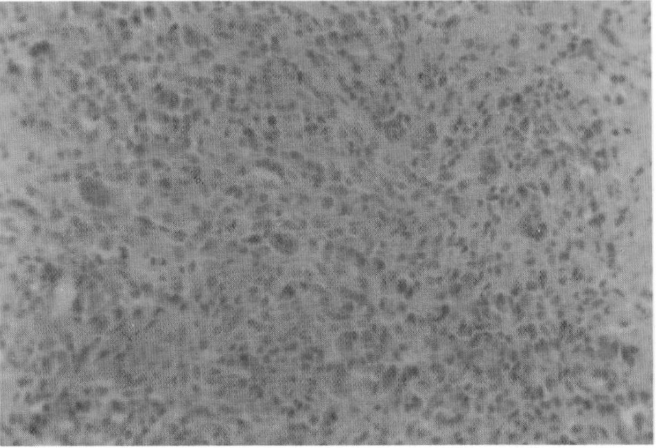

Fig. 11.152. Giant cell tumour – mainly histiocytic and fibroblastic cells and some giant cells and foam cells in a hyaline stroma.

Treatment is by careful surgical removal. An oblique incision along the greatest axis of the tumour enables the multi-lobulated lesion to be exposed. It may penetrate the extensor tendon. Complete removal is necessary to prevent recurrences.

Giant cell tumour may involve the distal bony phalanx of young adults. The most common complaint is pain that may be noted suddenly in the hand, following relatively mild trauma (Averill *et al.*, 1980). A painful lesion is always tender to palpation, sometimes with a palpable bony mass at the site of the lesion. Radiologically the lesions often show extensive destruction of the cortical and cancellous bone with one-third of the tumours expanding the cortex so that the bone widens to two to three times its normal diameter. Fracture of the cortex or complete destruction of the bone may be seen. In no case has stippling or calcification been present within

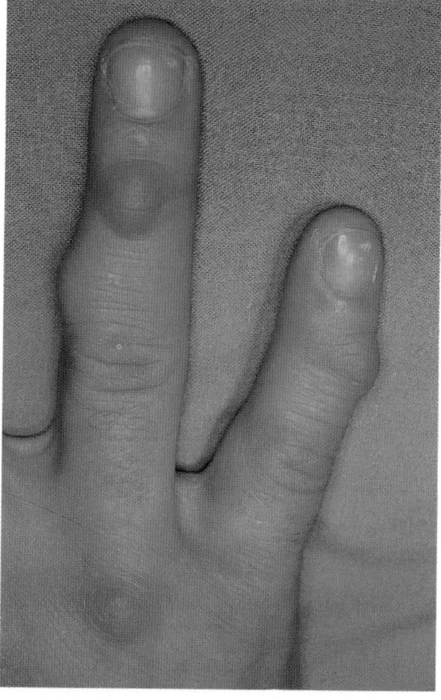

Fig. 11.153. Granuloma annulare (courtesy of S. Salaschie, USA).

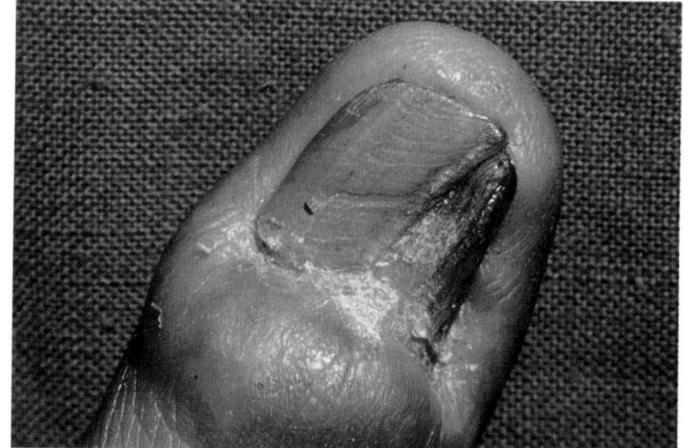

Fig. 11.154. Erythema elevatum diutinum (courtesy of G. Moulin, Lyon, France).

the tumour. The tumour tissue is vascular, friable and reddish-brown. Since there is an 18% incidence of multicentric foci of giant cell tumours of the hand, bone scan is advised when these tumours occur (Averill *et al.*, 1980).

Histological examination is necessary to confirm the diagnosis.

Curettage was found ineffective as a method of treatment. Local resection is recommended. Amputation is not necessary except for extreme cases.

References

Averill R.M., Smith R.J. & Campbell C.J. (1980) Giant-cell tumors of the bones of the hand. *J. Hand Surg.* 5, 39–50.

Chung E.B. & Enzinger F.M. (1979) Fibroma of tendon sheath. *Cancer* **44**, 1945–1954.

Norton L.A. (1990) Tumors. In: *Nails: Therapy, Diagnosis, Surgery*, eds Scher & Daniel, pp. 202–213. W.B. Saunders, Philadelphia.

Schwartz R.A. & Southwick G.J. (1979) Solitary multinodular giant cell tumor of tendon sheath. *J. Surg. Oncol.* **12**, 191–197.

Wright C.J.E. (1951) Benign giant-cell synovioma. An investigation of 85 cases. *Br. J. Surg.* 38, 257–271.

Lipoma

Stein (1959) described a lipoma of the distal phalanx of the thumb causing a tender and painful swelling, and destruction of the distal bony phalanx. We have seen a lipoma (Baran, 1984) located in the lateral nail fold of a finger. The tumour underwent slow growth; histologically it resembled naevus lipomatodes superficialis. A subungual lipoma of the ring finger (Higashi, 1988) deformed the nail which became hemispherical with ridging and loss of lustre. The tumour mimicked fibroma (Fig. 11.155).

References

Baran R. (1984) Periungual lipoma: an unusual site. *J. Dermatol. Surg. Oncol.* **10**, 32–33.

Higashi N. (1988) Subungual lipoma. *Hifu* **30**, 447–448.

Stein A.H. (1959) Benign neoplastic and nonneoplastic destructive lesions in the long bones of the hand. *Surg. Gynec. Obstet.* **109**, 189–197.

Sarcoma

Sarcomas arising in the fingertip are very rare. The disease has usually been present long before the diagnosis is made and the lesion treated; a very painful oozing growth sheds the nail plate or grows out from under the nail.

Phalangeal sarcoma with osteolytic lesions may enlarge the distal phalanx to three times its normal size and present with a warm and extremely painful clinical appearance, similar to paronychia (Marcove & Charosky, 1972). Osteogenic sarcoma arising in the distal phalanx of the thumb of a dentist after chronic intermittent exposure to X-ray irradiation is unique (Carrol & Godwin, 1956). Recurrent keratotic material progressed and replaced two-thirds of the nail bed. Metastases into regional lymph nodes occurred very early. Therefore, excisional biopsy of all ulcerating lesion is the only effective treatment.

Due to its rarity, osteogenic sarcoma is not often considered in the differential diagnosis of phalangeal tumours. 'Florid reactive periostitis of the tubular bones of the hands and feet' (Spjut & Dorfman, 1981), a benign lesion which may simulate osteosarcoma, should be ruled out. This benign 'fibro-osseous pseudotumour' of the digits occurs in the soft tissue of young adults. It may, microscopically, resemble myositis ossificans (Dupree & Enziger, 1986).

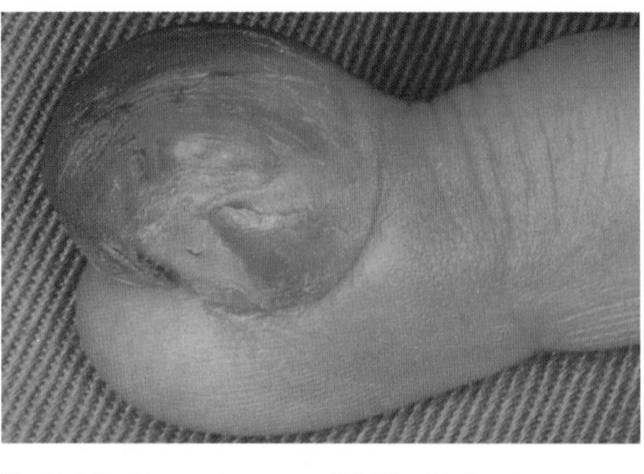

Fig. 11.155. Lipoma (courtesy of N. Higashi, Japan).

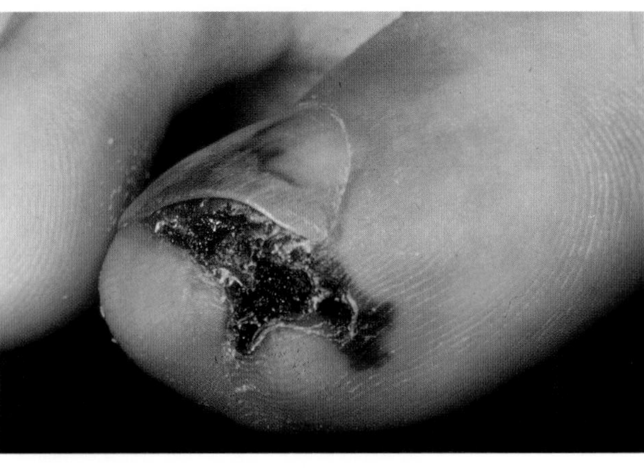

Fig. 11.156. Epitheloid sarcoma (courtesy of J. Revuz, Paris).

(a)

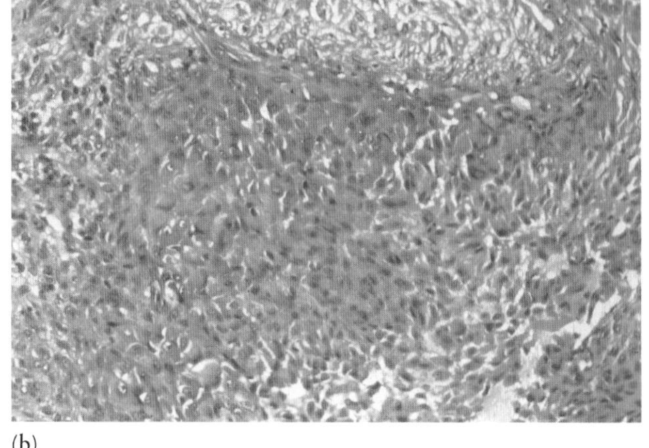

(b)

Fig. 11.157. Epitheloid sarcoma – histological changes showing many eosinophilic cells and proliferation of plump epithelial cells blending with fusiform cells.

Epithelioid sarcoma usually occurs in the soft tissues of adults. It may arise from the synovia of the distal interphalangeal joint and cause 'diffuse swelling' (Zanolli *et al.*, 1992), or mimic hard ganglion cysts. This spreads to affect the dorsal aspect of the tip of the digit (Fig. 11.156). Diagnosis is difficult and often delayed. Although the majority of the patients were otherwise asymptomatic, pain and tenderness was a complaint of some. An ulcerated tumour of the dorsum of the digit may recur in the stump and eventually metastasize to lymph nodes and lungs.

Histologically the individual cells usually display a striking eosinophilia and grow as nodular proliferations of plump, epithelial appearing cells blending with fusiform cells (Chase & Enzinger, 1985) (Fig. 11.157(a) & (b)).

Differential diagnosis includes necrobiotic granuloma, giant cell tumour, malignant fibrous histiocytoma, squamous cell carcinoma, malignant melanoma, synovial sarcoma and epithelioid haemangioendothelioma.

Hartert (1913) described a case of xanthomatous giant cell sarcoma of the foot secondarily involving the terminal phalanx of the fifth toe.

Epithelioid leiomyosarcoma

A 63-year-old man had a non-traumatic avulsion of this right great toenail after a 3-week history of pain. Histopathological examination showed a neoplasm composed mainly of interlacing bundles of spindle cells with indistinct cell borders, eosinophilic cytoplasm and pleomorphic nuclei. Immunohistological stains were positive for desmin and muscle-specific actin, but negative for S-100, HMB 45, cytokeratin, carcinoembryonic and factor VIII-related antigens. The diagnosis was epitheloid leiomyosarcoma (Bryant, 1992).

Differential diagnosis includes necrobiotic granuloma, giant cell tumour, malignant fibrous histiocytoma, squamous cell carcinoma, malignant melanoma, synovial sarcoma and epithelioid haemangioendothelioma.

Hartert (1913) described a case of xanthomatous giant cell sarcoma of the foot secondarily involving the fifth toe and its terminal phalanx.

Fibrosarcoma usually arises superficially as a hard, fixed, painful tumour, but may present as a deep swelling, often reaching a large size, with a tendency to invade the skin and neighbouring tissues. The tumour may grow slowly over a period of many years and then show rapid growth; or it may be rapidly invasive from the start. Metastases to the lung and, less commonly, to regional nodes occur early. Amputation offers the best chance for cure (Butler *et al.*, 1960).

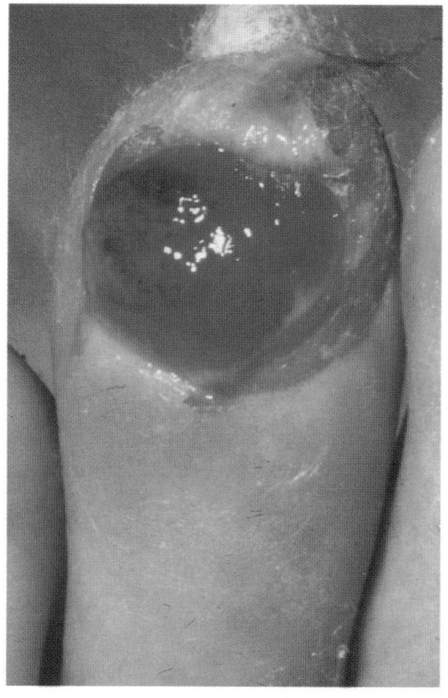

Fig. 11.158. Haemangioendothelioma.

Chondrosarcoma

In chondrosarcoma, pain and swelling are common symptoms (Gargan *et al.*, 1984). In contrast patients with benign cartilaginous tumours of bone rarely have pain, unless pathologic fracture has occurred (Dahlin & Salvador, 1974).

Radiologically a chondrosarcoma is a large and well-defined lesion with expanded bone contours and endosteal 'scalloping'. Cortical destruction and extra-osseous extension with tiny calcifications in clusters are indicative of active and more aggressive lesions (Bellinghausen *et al.*, 1983).

Although the incidence of malignant transformation of a solitary enchondroma is less than 1%, it may be as high as 50% in Ollier's disease and 18% in Maffucci's syndrome. The risk of malignant changes in the multiple exostoses syndrome varies from of 1 to 25%, but there is no report of malignancy in the distal phalanx.

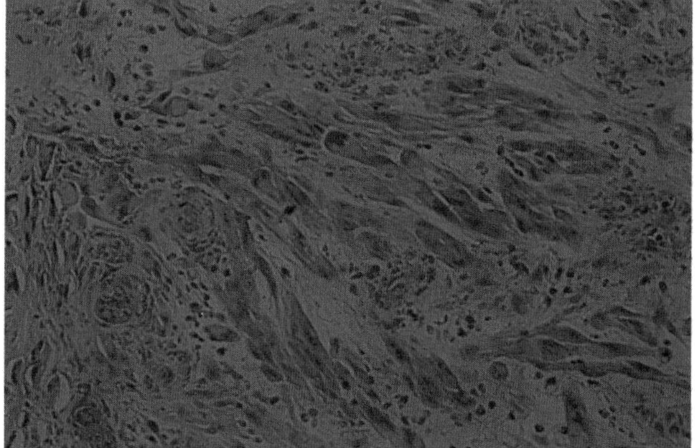

Fig. 11.159. Haemangioendothelioma – histological changes (courtesy of M.F.P. Davies, UK).

Haemangiosarcoma (haemangioendothelioma)

This malignant tumour of blood vessels is quite rare. The size of the tumour ranges from that of a pea to that of a plum. It is dark or bluish-red, moderately soft and non-tender. Davies *et al.* (1990) reported on a cutaneous haemangioendothelioma developed on a toenail bed of a patient who had worked with polyvinyl chloride (Fig. 11.158). Histology showed plump cells in a loose connective tissue stroma (Figs 11.159 & 11.160). Some were clumped; others formed capillary-sized channels with open lumina. Cellular pleomorphism and bizarre mitotic figures were marked and reticulin fibers were frequent.

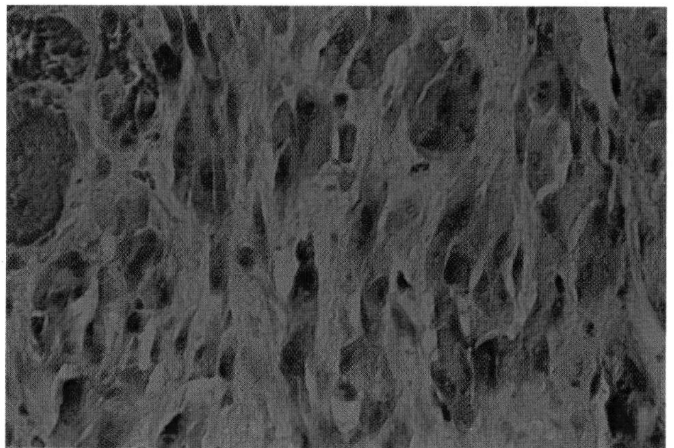

Fig. 11.160. Haemangioendothelioma – histological changes (see also Fig. 11.159).

Ewing's sarcoma

When the bone is primarily involved, it is designated as Ewing's sarcoma (Dick *et al.*, 1971). This presents with a painless swelling with appearance of ulceration of the tip of the digit. Park *et al.* (1992) saw a 15-year-old girl for a lobulated, dome-shaped (2.5 cm in diameter) denuded mass on the distal phalanx of the right middle finger which had increased in size for a 14-month period. X-rays reveal a lytic lesion of the distal phalanx. Biopsy is the key to the diagnosis. Radical resection is the treatment of choice.

References

Bellinghausen H.W., Weeks P.M., Young L.V. *et al.* (1983) Roentgen Rounds 64. Chondrosarcoma. *Orthop Rev.* **XII**, 97–100.

Butler E.D., Hamil J.P., Seipel R.S. *et al.* (1960) Tumors of the hand. A ten-year survey and report of 437 cases. *Am. J. Surg.* **100**, 293–302.

Bryant J. (1992) Subungual epithelioid leiomyosarcoma. *South Med. J.* **85**, 560–561.

Carroll R.E. & Godwin J.T. (1956) Osteogenic sarcoma of phalanx after chronic Roentgen-ray irradiation. *Cancer* **9**, 753–755.

Chase D.R. & Enzinger F.M. (1985) Epithelioid sarcoma. *Am. J. Surg. Pathol.* **9**, 241–263.

Dahlin D.C. & Salvador A.H. (1974) Chondrosarcomas of the bones of the hands and feet. A study of 30 cases. *Cancer* **34**, 755–760.

Davies M.F.P., Curtis M. & Howat J.M.T. (1990) Cutaneous hemangioendothelioma: possible link with chronic exposure to vinyl chloride. *Br. J. Industr. Med.* **47**, 65–67.

Dick H.M., Francis K.C. & Johnston A.D. (1971) Ewing's sarcoma of the hand. *J. Bone Joint Surg.* **53A**, 345–348.

Dupree W.B. & Enziger F.M. (1986) Fibro-osseous pseudotumour of the digits. *Cancer* **58**, 2103–2109.

Gargan T.J., Kanter W. & Wolfort F.G. (1984) Multiple chondrosarcomas of the hand. *Ann. Plast. Surg.* **12**, 542–546.

Hartert W. (1913) Zur Kenntnis der pigmentierten riezenzellenhaltigen Xanthosarcome an Hand und Fuss. *Beitr. Klin. Chir.* **84**, 546–562.

Heller J. (1927) Die Krankheiten der Nägel. In: *Handbuch der Haut-und Geschlechtskrankheiten* (Hrsg J Jadassohn), Bd VIII/2: Spezielle Dermatologie, 150–172.

Kennedy C.T.C., Burtun P.A. & Cook P. (1990) Swollen toe due to epithelioid haemangioma of bone. *Br. J. Dermatol.* **123** (Suppl. 37), 85–89.

Marcove R.C. & Charosky C.B. (1972) Phalangeal sarcomas simulating infections of the digits. *Clin. Orthop. Rel. Res.* **83**, 224–231.

Park S.D., Koh M.O., Jeon B.K. *et al.* (1992) *Euring Sarcoma of the Finger.* Book of Abstracts, 18th World Congress of Dermatology. New York June, 12–18.

Spjut J.H. & Dorfman H.D. (1981) Florid reactive periostitis of the tubular bones of the hands and feet. *Am. J. Surg. Pathol.* **5**, 423–433.

Tsuneyoshi M., Dorman H.D. & Bauer T.W. (1986) Epithelioid hemangioendothelioma of bone. A clinicopathologic, ultrastructural and immunohistochemical study. *Am. J. Surg.* **10**, 754–764.

Zanolli M.D., Wilmoth G., Show J.A. *et al.* (1992) Epithelioid sarcoma: Clinical and histologic characteristics. *J. Am. Acad. Dermatol.* **26**, 302–305.

Degenerative tumours

Myxoid pseudocysts of the digits

(Figs 11.161–11.170)

The many synonyms for this lesion reflect its controversial nature: dorsal finger cyst, synovial cyst, recurring myxomatous cyst; cutaneous myxoid cyst (Johnson *et al.*, 1965; Sonnex *et al.*, 1982); dorsal distal interphalangeal joint ganglion (Newmeyer *et al.*, 1974); digital mucinous pseudocyst (Goldman *et al.*, 1977), focal myxomatous degeneration (Zaias, 1990); mucoid cyst (Armijo, 1981). Whereas some authors regard it as a synovial cyst most now believe it to be a degenerative lesion.

Myxoid pseudocysts occur more often in women. They are typically found in the proximal nail fold of the fingers and rarely on toes. The lesions are usually asymptomatic varying from soft to firm, cystic to fluctuant, and may be dimpled, dome-shaped or smooth-surfaced (Figs 11.161–11.168). Transillumination confirms their cystic nature. They are always located to one side of the midline and rarely exceed 10–15 mm in diameter. The skin over the lesion is thinned and may be verrucous or even ulcerated. Rarely paronychial fistula may develop beneath the proximal nail fold (Fig. 11.168) and exceptionnally under the nail plate. Longitudinal grooving results from pressure on the matrix. Subungual digital mucinous pseudocyst may produce a nail dystrophy and discoloration without abnormalities of the periungual skin (Westrom & Findlay, 1986). Identical dystrophy may be observed when it is located beneath the matrix. Degenerative, 'wear and tear' osteoarthritis, frequently with Herberden's nodes, is present in most cases.

Spontaneous rupture or manipulation with a needle will release a thick, clear, gelatinous fluid (Fig. 11.164). This decompresses the matrix and nail growth is normal until the cyst refills. Purulent drainage due to infection and development of septic arthritis of the distal interphalangeal joint has been reported (Rangarathnam & Linscheid, 1984).

Histopathology reveals the pseudocystic character (Fig. 11.169). Cavities without synovial lining are located in an ill-defined fibrous capsule. The structure is essentially myxomatous with interspersed fibroblasts. Areas of myxomatous degeneration may merge to form a multilobular pseudocyst. In the cavities, a jelly-like substance is found which stains positively for hyaluronic acid. Goldman *et al.* (1977) found a mesothelial-like lining in the stalk connecting the pseudocyst with the distal interphalangeal joint. Kleinert *et al.* (1972) suggested that the lesion arises from the joint capsule as do ganglia in other areas (Fig. 11.167). Electron microscopy and immunohistochemistry did not reveal a synovial lining of the pseudocyst (Haneke, 1986).

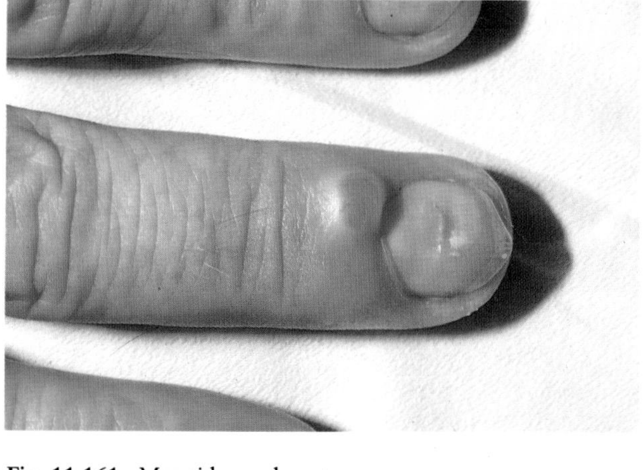

Fig. 11.161. Myxoid pseudocyst.

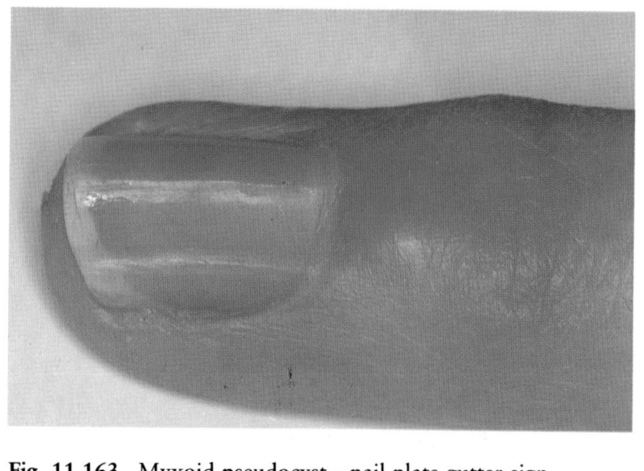

Fig. 11.163. Myxoid pseudocyst – nail plate gutter sign.

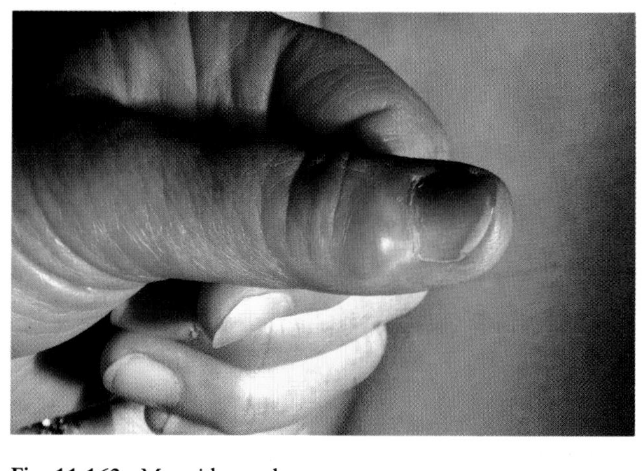

Fig. 11.162. Myxoid pseudocyst.

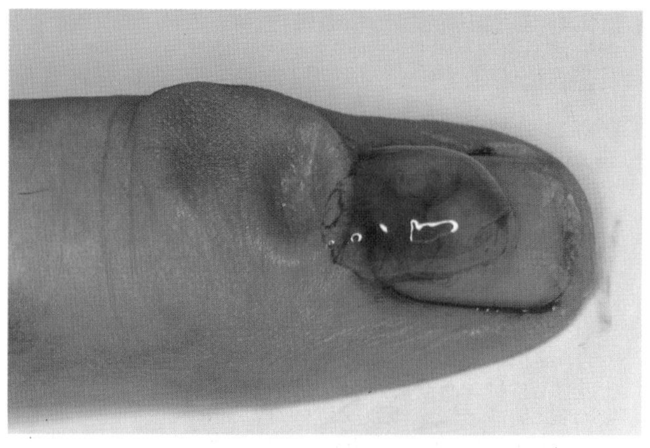

Fig. 11.164. Myxoid pseudocyst – gelatinous contents exuded after pricking the lesion.

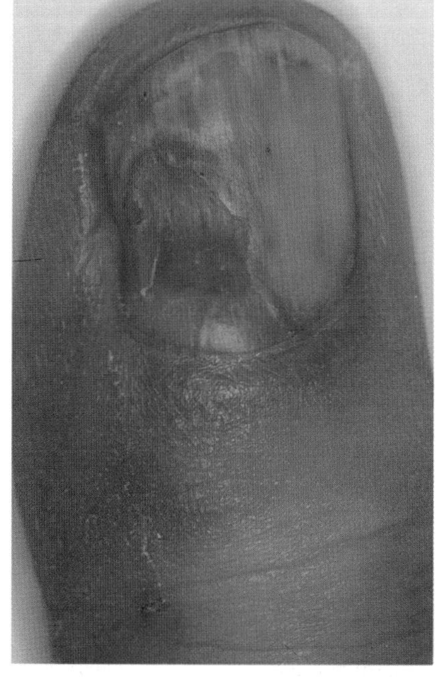

Fig. 11.165. Myxoid pseudocyst located beneath the matrix nail dystrophy.

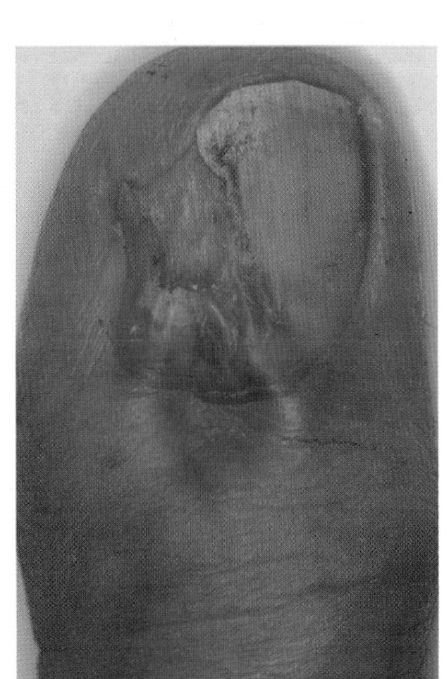

Fig. 11.166. Myxoid pseudocyst – same patient after evacuation of the gelatinous fluid.

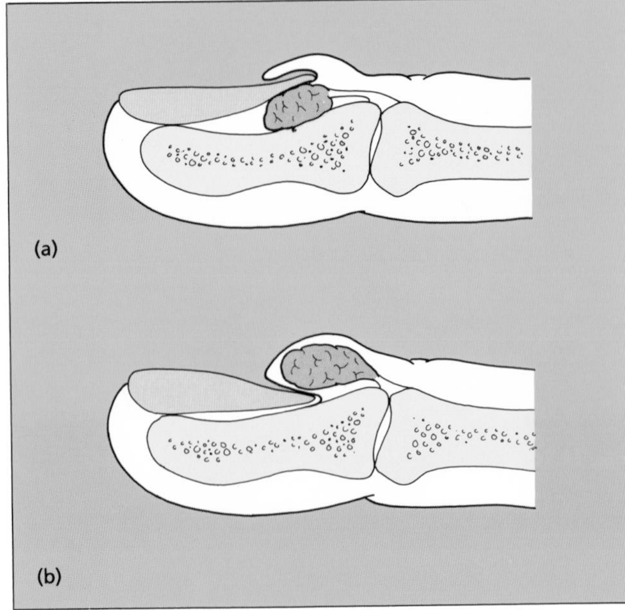

Fig. 11.167. Myxoid pseudocyst – showing types of attachment to the distal interphalangeal joint (after E. Zook).

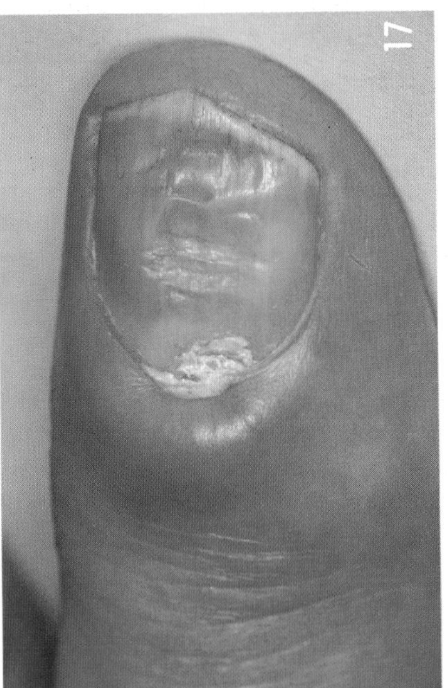

Fig. 11.168. Myxoid pseudocyst – mimicking chronic paronychia.

A multitude of treatments have been recommended, including repeated incision and drainage, simple excision, multiple needlings and expression of contents (Epstein, 1979), X-rays (5 Gy, 50 k, Al 1 mm, three times at weekly intervals), electrocautery, chemical cautery with nitric acid, trichloracetic acid or phenol, massages or injection of proteolytic substances, hyaluronidase, steroids (flurandrenolone tape (Ronchese, 1970) or injections), freezing with liquid nitrogen, dioxide laser vaporization

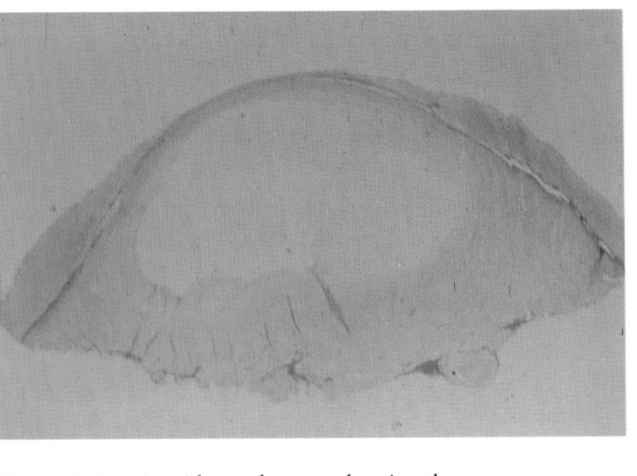

Fig. 11.169. Myxoid pseudocyst – showing the gross microscopic appearance.

(Huerter *et al.*, 1987), radical excision and even amputation (Kleinert *et al.*, 1972). Tomoda *et al.* (1982) reported a case that had had more than 20 recurrences each treated by incision, the cyst eventually moving from the characteristic dorsal, to a subungual position, producing an ulcer in the nail plate.

Kleinert *et al.* (1972) recommend the careful extirpation of the lesion. A tiny drop of methylene blue solution mixed with fresh hydrogen peroxide is injected into the distal interphalangeal joint at the volar joint crease. The joint will accept only 0.1–0.2 ml of dye (Newmeyer *et al.*, 1974). This clearly identifies the pedicle connecting the joint to the cyst and also the cyst itself which may look like a subcutaneous teno-arthro-synovial 'hernia' (Armijo, 1981). This procedure sometimes reveals occult satellite cysts. The incision line is drawn on the finger including a portion of the skin directly over the cyst and continuing proximally in a gentle curve to end dorsally over the joint (Fig. 11.170(a)). The lesion is meticulously dissected from the surrounding soft tissue and the pedicle traced to the joint capsule and resected. Dumb-bell extension of cysts to each side of the extensor tendon is easily dissected by hyperextending the joint. *Osteophytic spurs adjacent to the joint* must be removed with a fine chisel or bone rongeur. Sonnex *et al.* (1982) used liquid nitrogen cryosurgery with an 86% cure rate: the field treated included the cyst and the adjacent proximal area to the most distal transverse skin creases overlying the terminal joint. Two freeze/thaw cycles were carried out, each freeze time being 30 s after the ice field had formed, the intervening thaw times being at least 4 min; if this method is adopted then longer freeze times must be avoided or permanent matrix damage may occur. Salasche (1984) suggested nail fold excision for posterior nail fold distal lesions. The injection of a sclerosing agent, such as 1%

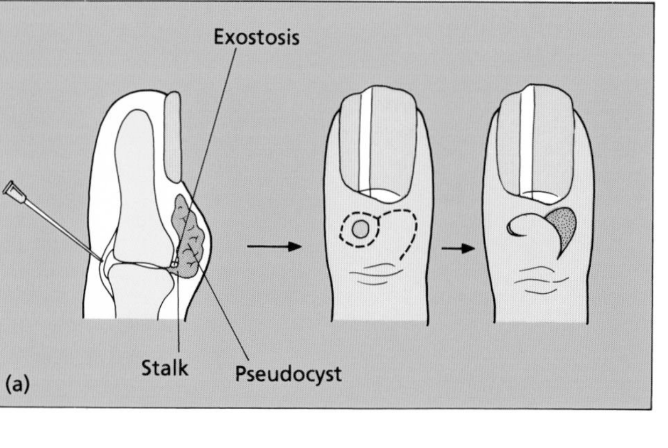

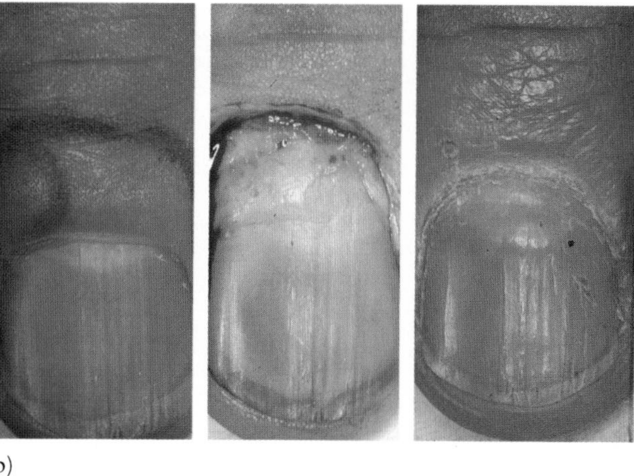

Fig. 11.170. (a) Myxoid pseudocyst – diagram showing one method of removal. (b) Removal of pseudocyst located in the distal part of the proximal nail fold.

sodium tetradecyl sulphate into mucoid pseudocysts may well have superseded the previous treatments (Audebert, 1989). After the cyst has been pierced and its jelly-like material expressed 0.10–0.20 ml is injected, painlessly. One single procedure may be enough. A second or a third one can be performed at monthly intervals.

References

Armijo M. (1981) Mucoid cysts of the fingers. *J. Dermatol. Surg. Oncol.* 7, 31–22.

Audebert C. (1989) Treatment of mucoid cysts of fingers and toes by injection of sclerosant. *Dermatol. Clin.* 7, 179–182.

Epstein E. (1979) A simple technique for managing digital mucous systs. *Arch. Dermatol.* **115**, 1315–1316.

Goldman J.A., Goldman L., Jaffe M.S. & Richfield D.F. (1977) Digital mucinous pseudocysts. *Arth. Rheum.* **20**, 997–1002.

Haneke E. (1986) Dorsal finger cyst. Soc. Cut. Ultrastruct. Res.-Eur. Soc. Skin Biol. Meeting, Paris, Abstract 43.

Huerter C.J., Wheeland R.G., Bailin P. *et al.* (1987) Treatment of digital myxoid cysts with carbon dioxide laser vaporisation. *J. Dermatol. Surg. Oncol.* **13**, 723–727.

Johnson W.C., Graham J.H. & Helwig E.B. (1965) Cutaneous myxoid cyst: a clinico-pathological and histochemical study. *J. Am. Med. Assoc.* **191**, 15–20.

Kleinert H.E., Kutz J.E., Fishman J.H. & McCraw L.H. (1972) Etiology and treatment of the so-called mucous cyst of the finger. *J. Bone Joint Surg.* **54A**, 1455–1458.

Newmeyer W.L., Kilgore E.S. & Graham W.P. (1974) Mucous cyst: the dorsal distal interphalangeal joint ganglion. *Plast. Reconstr. Surg.* **53**, 313–315.

Rangarathnam C. & Linscheid R. (1984) Infected mucous cyst of the finger. *J. Hand Surg.* **9a**, 245–246.

Ronchese F. (1970) Treatment of myxoid cyst with fluorandrenolone tape. *Rhode Island Med. J.* 57, 154–155.

Salasche S.J. (1984) Myxoid cyst of the proximal nail fold, a surgical approach. *J. Dermatol. Surg. Oncol.* **10**, 35–39.

Sonnex T.S., Leonard J., Ralfs I. & Dawber R.P.R. (1982) Myxoid cysts of the finger: treatment by liquid nitrogen spray cryosurgery. *Br. J. Dermatol. Suppl.* **107**, 21.

Tomoda T., Ono T., Ohyama K. & Kojo Y. (1982) Subungual myxoid cysts producing an ulcer in the nail plate. *Jap. (Rinsho) Dermatol.* **9**, 451.

Westrom D.R. & Findlay R.F. (1986) Subungual mucinous pseudo-cyst. *J. Dermatol. Surg. Oncol.* **12**, 558–559.

Zaias N. (1990) *The Nail in Health and Disease.* Appleton & Lange, Norwalk, CT.

Myxoma

Eisenklam (1931) described a pea-sized subungual myxoma elevating the nail of the great toe of a 65-year-old woman. Subsequently Sanusi (1982) reported a case presenting with a growth at the tip of the right thumb; this has gradually increased in size, raising and distorting the nail. X-ray examination showed an osteolytic lesion surrounded by sclerotic edges. Myxoma in a subungual position differs from the exceptional myxoma affecting the distal bony phalanx, which has only been described in the toe. A firm pea-sized tumour involving the distal portion of the lateral nail wall of the right thumb was observed by Donzel and Martel (1991) in a 58-year-old male with normal bony phalanx (Figs 11.171 & 11.172).

Armijo (1981) reported a case of a large myxoma of the dorsal aspect of the terminal segment of the middle finger allegedly developing 2 years after injury. The patient presented with a pinkish-violet, somewhat translucent, firm tumour. It was widely excised and the defect covered with a full-thickness skin graft. Injection of methylene blue solution did not demonstrate a cystic space or communication with the joint.

Armijo (1981) listed the salient differences between cutaneous myxoma and myxoid pseudocyst (Table 11.6). The differential diagnosis includes a group of neoplasms in which myxomatous change is a prominent secondary feature and a variety of conditions characterized by

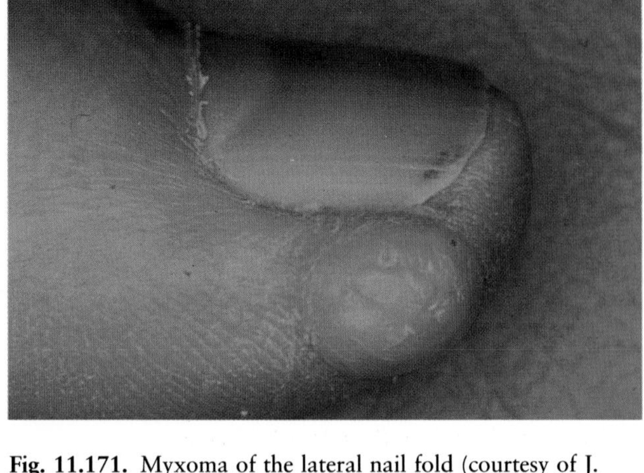

Fig. 11.171. Myxoma of the lateral nail fold (courtesy of J. Martel, France).

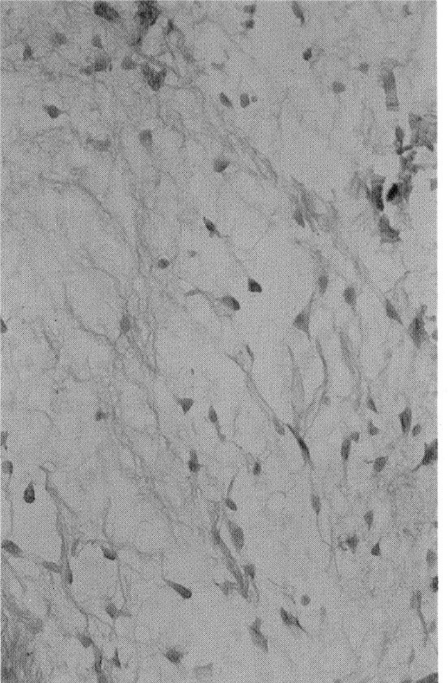

Fig. 11.172. Myxoma – histological appearance.

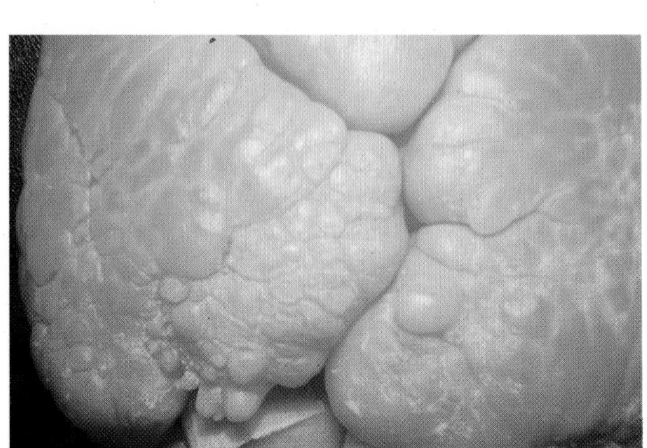

Fig. 11.173. Severe 'pretibial' myxoedema hiding the nails (courtesy of P. Lazar, Chicago).

Table 11.6 Differential diagnosis of myxoid cyst and cutaneous myxoma (Armijo, 1981)

	Cutaneous myxoma	Myxoid cyst
Radiography	Negative	Exostosis (at times)
Newmeyer test	Negative	Positive
Histology	Focal mucinosis	Cysts in contiguity covered by synovial, fibrotic, areolar, or adipose membranes
Anatomical position	Intradermal	Subcutaneous
Histogenesis	Hyperproduction of hyaluronic acid by fibroblasts and decreased or failure of production of collagen	Herniation of tendon sheaths or joint linings
Cause	Trauma (?)	Inflammatory osteoarticular processes
Treatment	Excision and repair by graft	Excision including exostosis if present and repair by flap

mucinous degeneration of the skin or soft tissues (Sanusi, 1982).

Carjaval *et al.* (1987) reported the case of a 43-year-old woman presenting a slow-growing subungual tumour of the left hallux lifting the nail and occupying all the subungual surface with mild pain on pressure. Biopsy of this greyish white myxoid tumour showed small amount of spindle-shaped cells and stellate cells in the dermis.

Pretibial myxoedema

The pink or flesh-coloured mucinous plaques may involve the dorsal aspect of the foot and exceptionally the toes partially hiding the nails (Fig. 11.173).

References

Armijo M. (1981) Mucoid cysts of the fingers. *J. Dermatol. Surg. Oncol.* 7, 317–322.

Carvajal L., Uraga E., Garcia I. *et al.* (1987) Tumours of the hallux: myxoma, osteochondroma and enchondroma. *Skin Cancer* **2**, 197–201.

Donzel J.P. & Martel J. (1991) Myxome digital du pouce droit. *Nouv. Dermatol.* **10**, 706–707.

Eisenklam D. (1931) Über subunguale Tumoren. *Wien. Klin. Wschr.* **44**, 1192–1193.

Sanusi D. (1982) Subungual myxoma. *Arch. Dermatol.* **118**, 612–614.

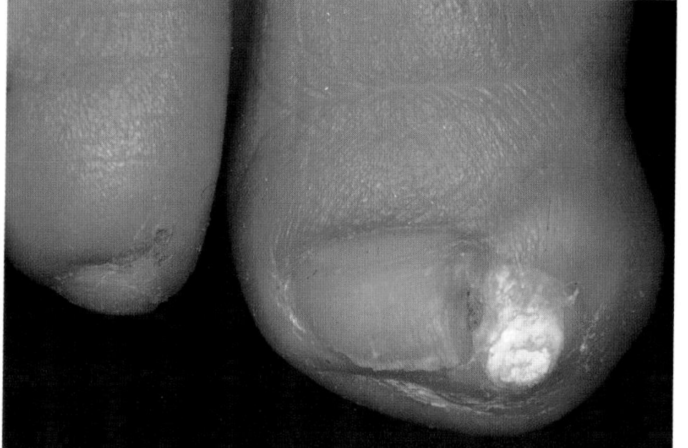

Fig. 11.174. Cutaneous calculi (courtesy of P. Souteyrand, Clermont-Ferrand, France).

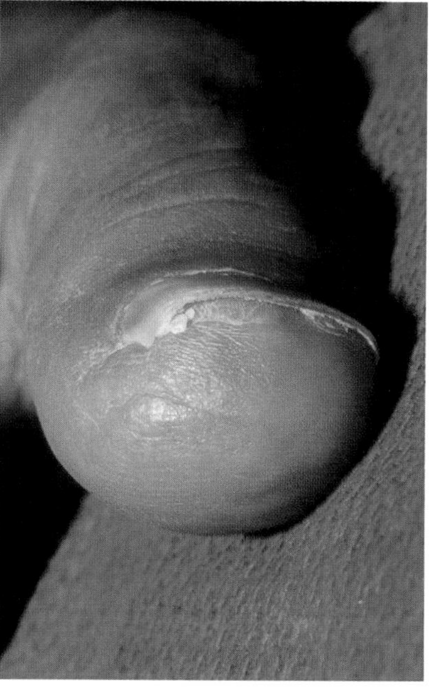

Fig. 11.175. Oxalate granuloma (courtesy of B. Sina, Baltimore, USA).

Subungual calcifications

Primary subungual calcification in the normal nail bed of the digits is occasionally seen in the elderly, especially women (Fischer, 1982). The frequency decreases from the second to the fifth digit. In about 10% the subungual calcifications are combined with similar subungual calcifications of the toes (Fischer, 1983a). Soft tissue calcification at the margin of the distal phalanges of the fingers occurs in 7% of normal adults and results from mechanical injury of the collagen fibres close to their insertion into the margin of the tuberosity (Fischer, 1983b). In the normal toenail bed they begin in women during their thirties and reach an incidence of 47% in their eighties. These calcifications appear in men up to 20 years later, with an incidence of only 4% in old age. The first toe is involved three times more often than the fifth toe (Fischer, 1984). Secondary subungual calcification occurs occasionally after trauma and in psoriasis (Fischer, 1982).

References

Fischer E. (1982) Subungulale Verkalkungen. *Fortschr. Röntgenstr.* **137**, 580–584.

Fischer E. (1983a) Subunguale Verkalkungen im normalen Nagelbett der Finger. *Hautarzt* **34**, 625–627.

Fischer E. (1983b) Weichteilverkalkungen am Rand der Tuberositas phalangis distalis der Finger. *Fortschr. Röntgenstr.* **139**, 150–157.

Fischer E. (1984) Subunguale Verkalkungen im normalen Nagelbett der Zehen. *Radiologe* **24**, 31–34.

Cutaneous calculi (calcinosis cutis circumscripta)

Winer (1952) first recognized 'solitary congenital nodular calcification of the skin' as a distinct entity. These quite rare lesions presented from birth, as slowly enlarging hard yellowish-white warty nodules at the side of a finger or toenail (Fig. 11.174). In fact they are not always solitary and frequently not congenital (Woods & Kellaway, 1963). The distal aspect of the involved digit may appear erythematous, with a solid chalky-white, well-circumscribed lesion, not tender to palpation. Radiographs demonstrate a radiopaque mass, consisting of multiple calcified fragments located adjacent to the distal phalanx (Mendoza *et al.*, 1990) in a subepidermal location histologically.

References

Mendoza L.E., Lavery L.A. & Adam R.C. (1990) Calcinosis cutis circumscripta. A literature review and case report. *J. Am. Pod. Med. Assoc.* **80**, 97–99.

Winer L.H. (1952) Solitary congenital nodular calcification of the skin. *Arch. Dermatol. Syphil.* **66**, 204–211.

Woods B. & Kellaway T.B. (1963) Cutaneous calculi. *Br. J. Dermatol.* 75, 1–11.

Oxalate granuloma

Several pink, lightly keratotic, tender subungual nodules affecting two digits associated to multiple tiny tender, yellow-tan papules on several fingertips were reported in a 46-year-old white man with chronic renal failure treated by haemodialysis for 20 years (Fig. 11.175). Biopsy specimen of a subungual nodule showed in the dermis a corymbiform arrangement of calcium oxalate cystals surrounded by foreign body granulomas (Figs 11.176 & 11.177) (Sina & Lutz, 1990).

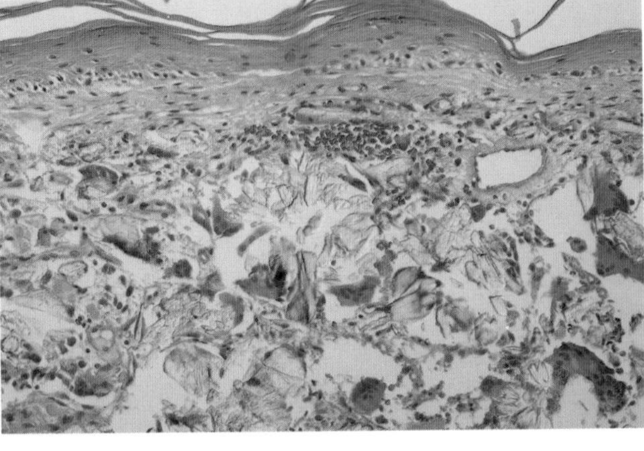

Fig. 11.176. Oxalate granuloma – many crystals surrounded by granuloma cells (courtesy of B. Sina, USA).

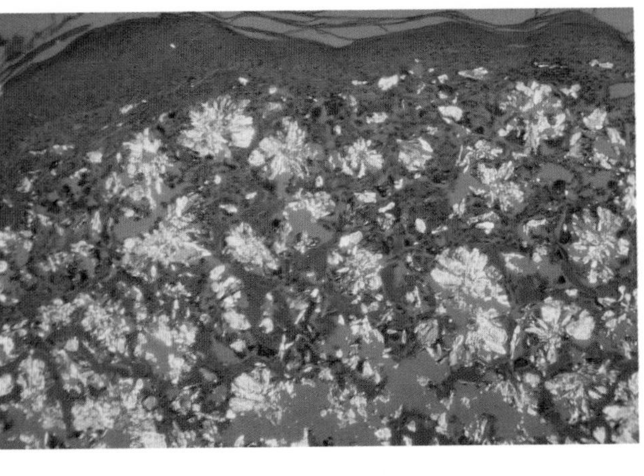

Fig. 11.177. Oxalate granuloma – micrograph showing the crystals within the dermis (courtesy of B. Sina, USA).

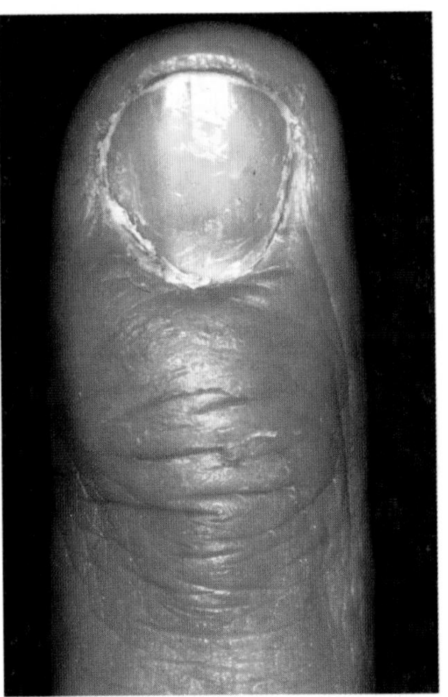

Fig. 11.178. Xanthoma of nail folds and dorsum of digit (courtesy of A. Tosti, Bologna, Italy).

Reference

Sina B. & Lutz L.L. (1990) Cutaneous oxalate granuloma. *J. Am. Acad. Dermatol.* **22**, 316–317.

Histiocytic and metastatic processes

Histiocytic processes

Xanthoma (Figs 11.178 & 11.179)

Keller (1960) reported a case of hypercholesterolaemic xanthomatosis in a 61-year-old woman exhibiting pseudo-Koenen's tumours periungually in the second and third toes.

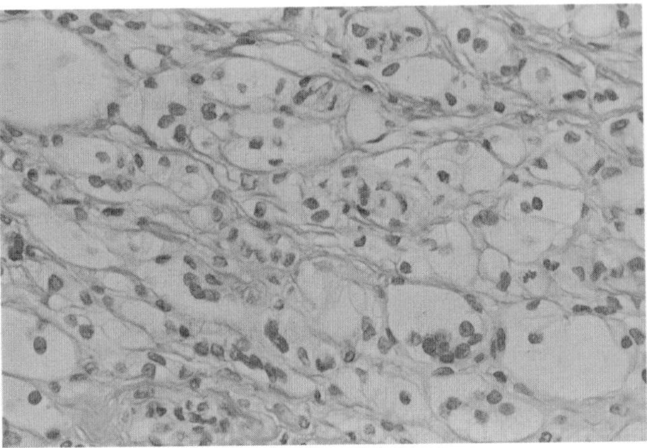

Fig. 11.179. Xanthoma (courtesy of A. Tosti, Bologna, Italy).

Reference

Keller P. (1960) Hypercholesterinämische Xanthomatose. *Derm. Wschr.* **141**, 336–337.

Verruciform xanthoma

Verruciform xanthoma is a rare skin condition characterized histologically by uniform epithelial acanthosis without atypia and foam cells within elongated dermal papillae. Verruciform xanthoma also occurs, rarely, as a secondary reaction in lesions with marked epidermal hyperplasia, such as epidermal naevus and ILVEN. Chyu *et al.* (1987) reported a 36-year-old Black woman with verruciform xanthoma on the toes of a lymphoedematous leg. This was a recurrent yellow-brown tumour on the right first toe present for 18 months, slowly increasing in size, as a 2 cm yellowish, fungating, verrucous nodule involving the proximal nail fold. It was asymptomatic until its size interfered with the fit of her shoe.

Multiple verruciform xanthomas (Mountcastle & Lupton, 1989) presented with a fingernail which was severely dystrophic and for the most part absent. The remaining part of the lesion measured 1 × 1.5 cm and appeared verrucous, with some crusted exudate that encompassed the nail bed.

References

Chyu J., Medenica M. & Whitney D.H. (1987) Verruciform xanthoma of the lower extremity-report of a case and review of literature. *J. Am. Acad. Dermatol.* **17**, 695–697.

Mountcastle E.A. & Lupton G.P. (1989) Verruciform xanthomas of the digits. *J. Am. Acad. Dermatol.* **20**, 313–317.

Juvenile xanthogranuloma

Juvenile xanthogranuloma is a benign, self-limited, histiocytic, proliferative disorder most frequently seen in children. In Frumkim *et al.*'s case (1987) a progressive deformity of the second toenail developed after trauma leading to a brown, opaque nail lifted from the nail bed and resembling onychogryphosis. After nail avulsion, the whole nail bed and the matrix were seen to be occupied by a round, yellow, soft tumour 6 mm in diameter. Histology revealed lipidized macrophages intermingled with lymphocytes, eosinophils, foam cells and giant cells of the foreign body and touton types. The latter exhibited the characteristic 'wreath' of nuclei.

Reference

Frumkin A., Roytan M. & Johnson S. (1987) Juvenile xanthogranuloma underneath a toenail. *Cutis* **40**, 244–245.

Metastases

Metastases to the fingertip or nail region (Figs 11.180–11.186) are quite rare (about 116 cases reported; Baran & Tosti, 1993) and are often initially misdiagnosed as acute infection in and around the nail apparatus and treated as such by incisions. These lesions may be the first manifestation of an internal neoplasm (Camiel *et al.*, 1969).

Most metastatic tumours affect the bone first with subsequent spread to soft tissues. Primary soft tissue metastases of the distal digit may secondarily involve the underlying bone.

The symptoms and signs of metastases are very variable and include dusky red painful or painless swelling (Figs 11.181 & 11.182), expansile pulsation, pseudoclubbing (Hödl, 1980) (Fig. 11.183), nail dystrophy, and changes simulating acute (Cohen & Buzden, 1993) or chronic paronychia, a finger infection such as felon or osteomyelitis, and even benign lesions such as glomus tumour (Wu & Guise, 1978) and early rheumatoid arthritis. A clinical picture of necrotizing vasculitis involving the nail

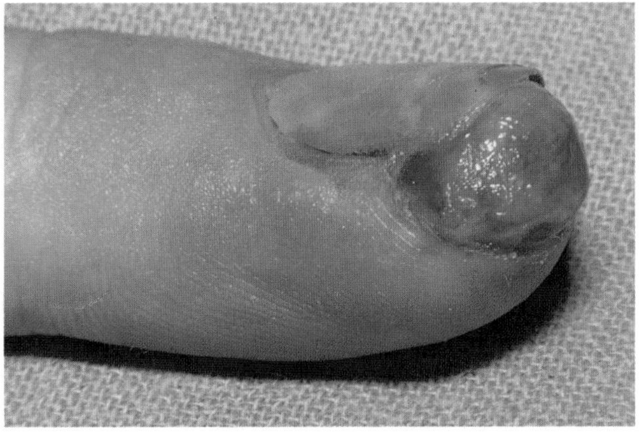

Fig. 11.180. Metastasis – from a chondrosarcoma (courtesy of D. Lambert, Dijon, France).

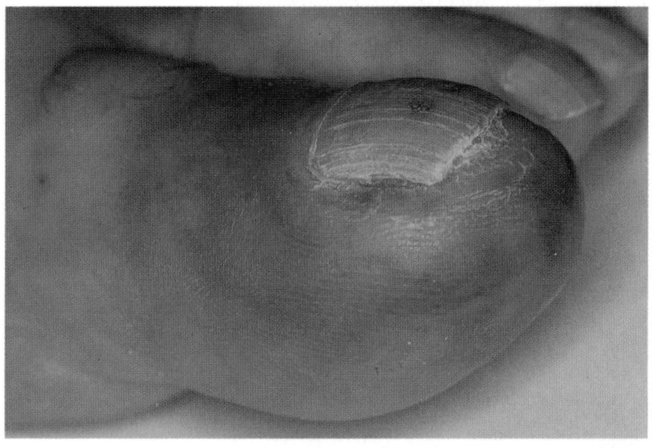

Fig. 11.181. Metastasis – lung carcinoma.

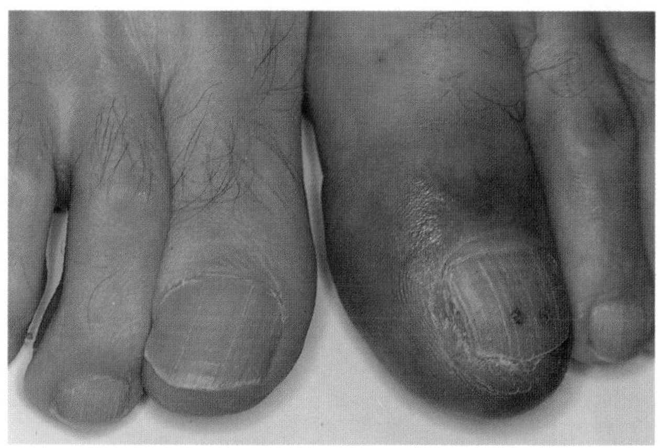

Fig. 11.182. Metastasis – lung carcinoma.

area was mimicked by metastatic hypopharyngeal carcinoma (Nigro *et al.*, 1992). Whatever symptoms occur, the signs increase out of proportion to the pain, and in the absence of injury or infection this should suggest the

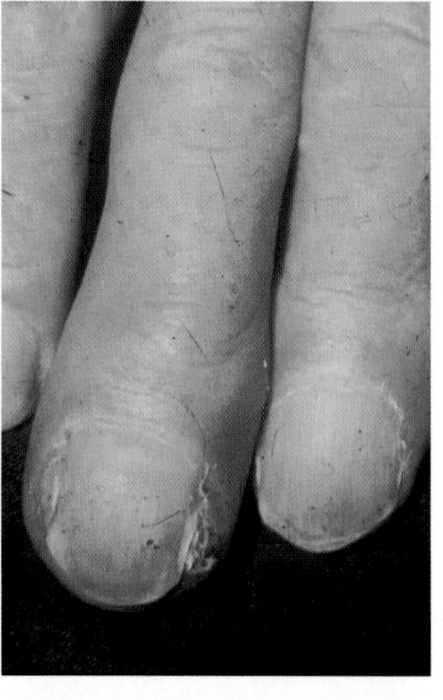

Fig. 11.183. Metastasis – bronchial carcinoma (courtesy of S. Hödl, Graz, Austria).

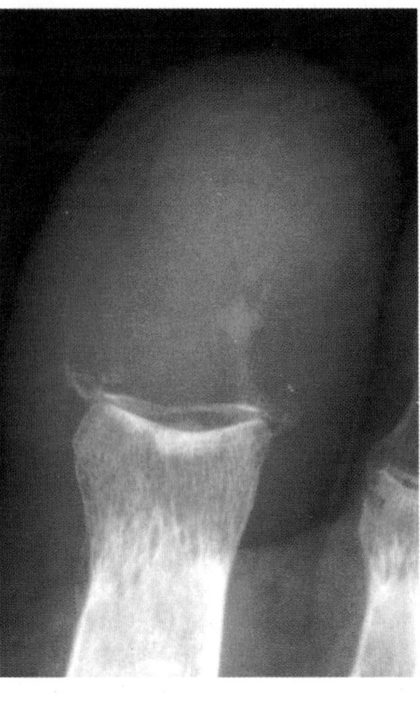

Fig. 11.184. Metastasis – distal phalanx bronchial carcinoma.

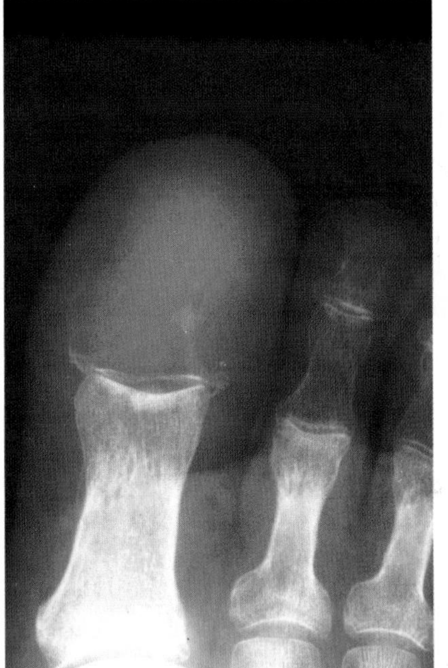

Fig. 11.185. Metastasis – distal phalanx bronchial carcinoma.

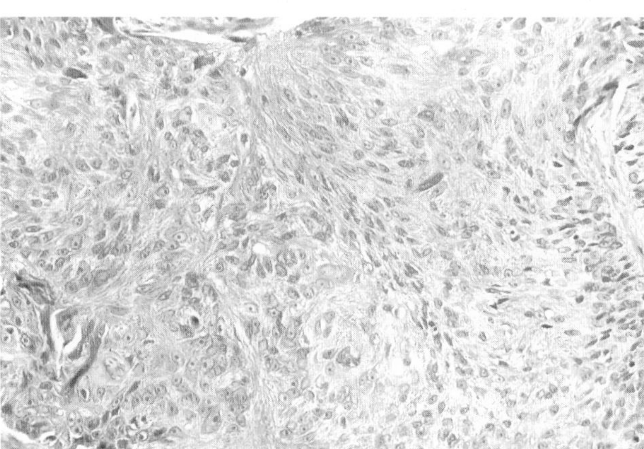

Fig. 11.186. Metastasis from bronchial carcinoma.

possibility of metastases (Baran & Tosti, 1993). With the passage of time, a reddish-purple nodule in the distal nail bed, hyponychial region may become ulcerated (Fig. 11.180)

X-rays usually show an osteolytic focus (Figs 11.184 & 11.185) which may resemble spina ventosa or osteomyelitis. Distal phalangeal metastases usually do not cross the articular surface; in fact they characteristically preserve a thin margin of subchondral cortical bone and sometimes a 'blown-out' cortical shell (Monsees & Murphy, 1984). Aspiration or incision biopsy is necessary to classify the tumour and exclude a primary bone growth (Dick *et al.*, 1971) but even this may fail to reveal the true nature of the primary lesion.

Bronchial carcinoma most frequently (50% of cases) produces phalangeal metastases (Figs 11.183 & 11.186). The other primary sites include breast (15% in female), kidney, colon, rectal and parotid gland carcinoma (Falkinburg & Fagan, 1956), seminoma (Gartmann, 1958), melanoma producing mainly polydactylic longitudinal melanonychia (Kolmsee & Schultka, 1972; Zaun, 1980; Retsas & Samman, 1983), neuroblastoma, plasmocytoma, chondrosarcoma; also skin and adrenal glands.

References

Baran R. & Tosti A. (1994) Metastatic bronchogenic carcinoma to the terminal phalanx of the big toe. Report of two cases with review of 116 non-melanoma metastatic tumors to the distal digit. *J. Am. Acad. Dermatol.* (in press).

Barnett L.S. & Morris J.M. (1969) Metastases of renal-cell carcinoma simultaneously to a finger and a toe. *J. Bone Joint Surg.* **51A**, 773–774.

Camiel M.R., Aron B.S., Alexander L.L., Benninghoff D.L. & Minkowitz S. (1969) Metastases to palm, sole, nailbed, nose, face, and scalp from unsuspected carcinoma of the lung. *Cancer* **23**, 214–220.

Cohen P.R. & Buzdar A.U. (1993) Metastatic breast carcinoma mimicking an acute paroxychia of the great toe: case report and review of subungual metastases. *Am. J. Clin. Oncol.* **16**, 86–91.

Dick H.M., Francis K.C. & Johnston A.D. (1971) Euring's sarcoma of the hand. *J. Bone Foot Surg.* **161**, 545–552.

Falkinburg L.W. & Fagan J.H. (1956) Malignant mixed tumor of the parotid gland with a rare metastasis. *Am. J. Surg.* **91**, 279–282.

Gartmann H. (1958) Seminommetastasen der Haut. *Derm. Wschr.* **138**, 828–829.

Hödl St. (1980) Fingermetastasen bei Bronchuscarcinom. *Akt. Derm.* **6**, 249–254.

Kolmsee I. & Schultka O. (1972) Keratoma palmare et plantare dissipatum hereditarium, Pachyonychia congenita und Hypotrichosis lanuginosa, malignes Melanom, Möller-Huntersche Glossitis, Vasculitis allergica superficialis (Bildberichte). *Hautarzt* **23**, 459–460.

Monsees B. & Murphy W.A. (1984) Distal phalangeal erosive lesions. *Arth. Rheum.* **27**, 449–455.

Nigro M.A., Chieregato G. & Castellani L. (1992) Metastatic hypopharyngeal carcinoma mimicking necrotizing vasculitis of the skin. *Cutis* **49**, 187–188.

Retsas S. & Samman P.D. (1983) Pigment streaks in the nail plate due to secondary malignant melanoma. *Br. J. Dermatol.* **108**, 367–370.

Wu K.K. & Guise E.R. (1978) Metastatic tumours of the hand: a report of six cases. *J. Hand Surg.* **3** 271.

Zaun H. (1980) Krankhafte Veränderungen des Nagels. *Beitr. Derm.* **7**, 9–10, 50–60.

Melanocytic lesions

Benign

Subungual melanocytic lesions (Figs 11.187–11.200)

Melanocytes (Fig. 11.187) are present in the nail matrix and nail bed although they usually remain functionally (relatively) inactive in Caucasians particularly in the nail bed. When they become active and produce melanin in amounts that can no longer be degraded by the keratinocytes of the matrix, melanin will continuously be enclosed in the growing nail plate to give rise to a longitudinal light brown to black band (Figs 11.188–11.190). A rapid enlargement of a subungual pigmented lesion may be seen as a stripe that is wider in its proximal part; estimation of the nail growth rate and measurement of the difference in width proximally and distally allows an exact calculation of the growth of the pigment-producing lesion to be made. Pigmented lesions in the nail bed usually do not cause longitudinal melanonychia but shine through the nail as a greyish–brown–black spot.

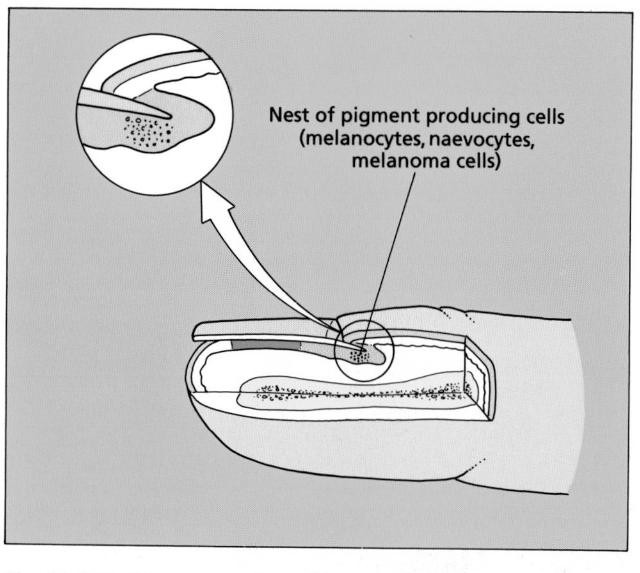

Fig. 11.187. Diagram to show the main site of functionally active melanocytes in health and disease.

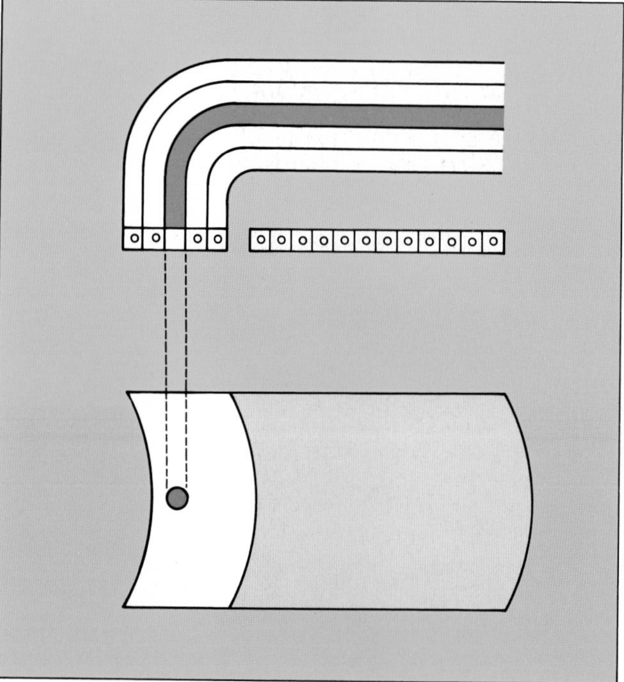

Fig. 11.188. Diagram relating matrix sites of melanocytes and the levels in the nail plate that their pigment will reside in.

Longitudinal melanonychia may be due to benign melanocytic hyperplasia, lentigo simplex, melanocytic naevus, atypical melanocytic hyperplasia and acral lentiginous melanoma. There are many conditions causing non-melanin nail pigmentation (see Chapter 2); in contrast, approximately 25% of subungual melanomas are amelanotic.

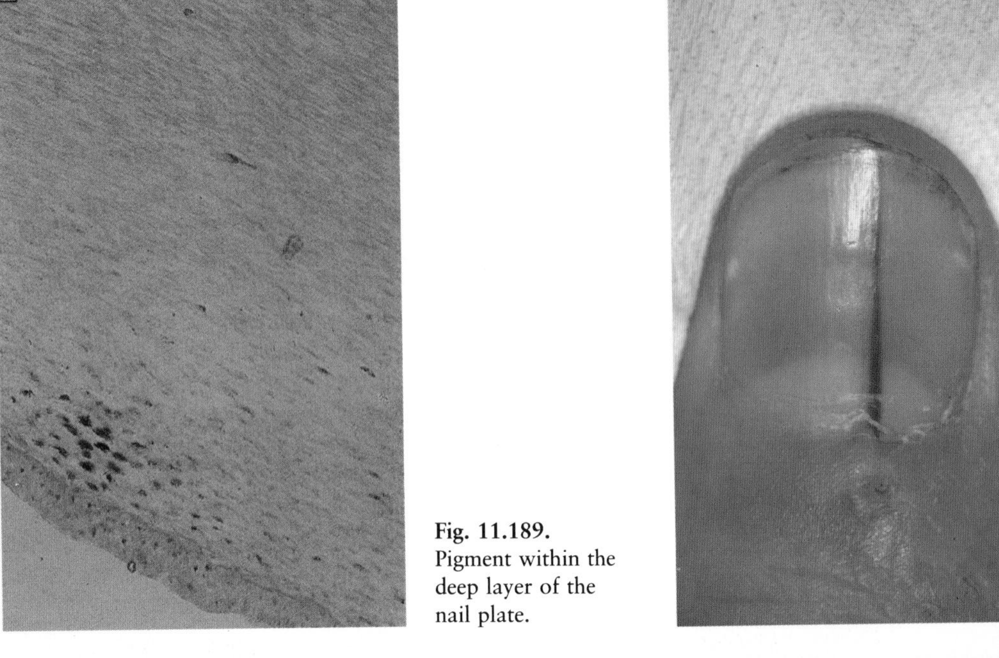

Fig. 11.189. Pigment within the deep layer of the nail plate.

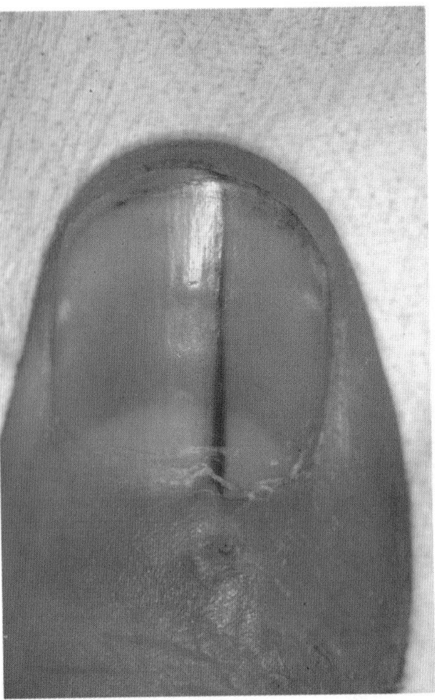

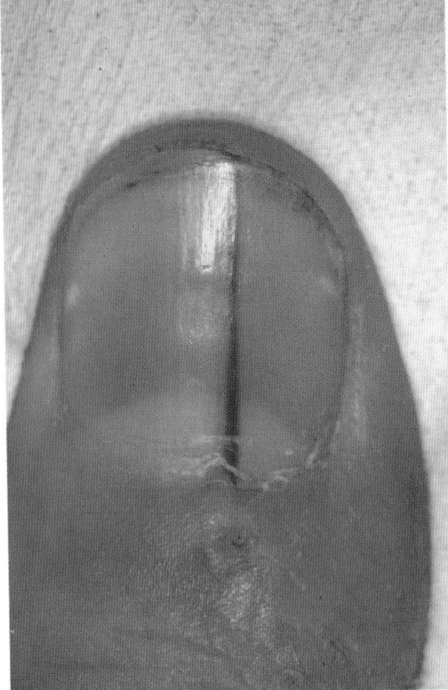

Fig. 11.190. Longitudinal melanonychia. Proximal widening of the band should make the clinician suspicious.

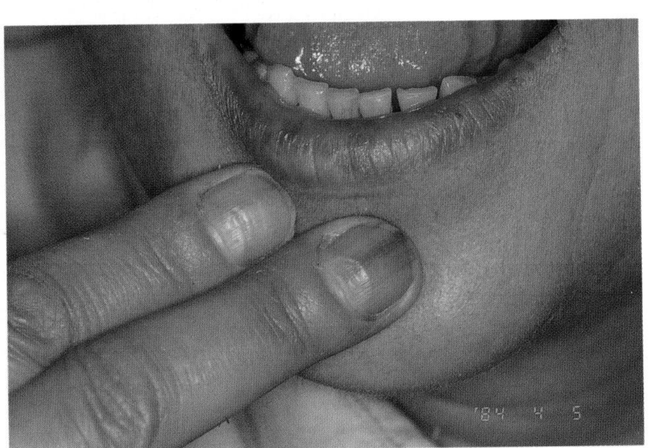

Fig. 11.191. Laugier–Hunziker syndrome – nail and lip pigmentation.

Fig. 11.192. Laugier–Hunziker syndrome – nail and lip pigmentation.

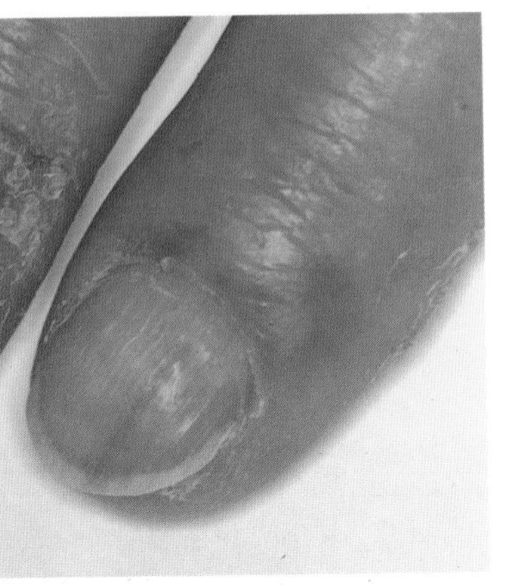

Fig. 11.193. Laugier–Hunziker syndrome – longitudinal melanocytic and periungual changes showing pseudo-Hutchinson's sign, i.e. not malignant melanoma.

Fig. 11.194. Laugier–Hunziker syndrome – showing normal-looking melanocytes.

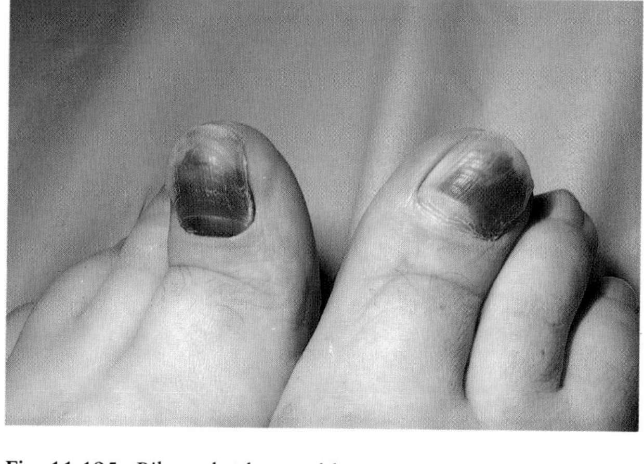

Fig. 11.195. Bilateral subungual haematoma – obvious haemorrhage and clearly not melanoma.

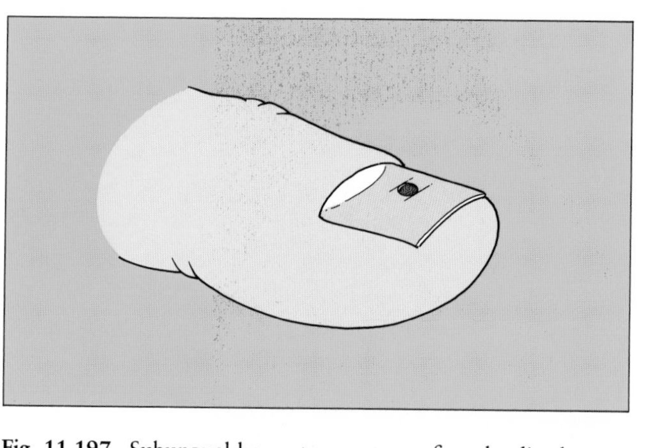
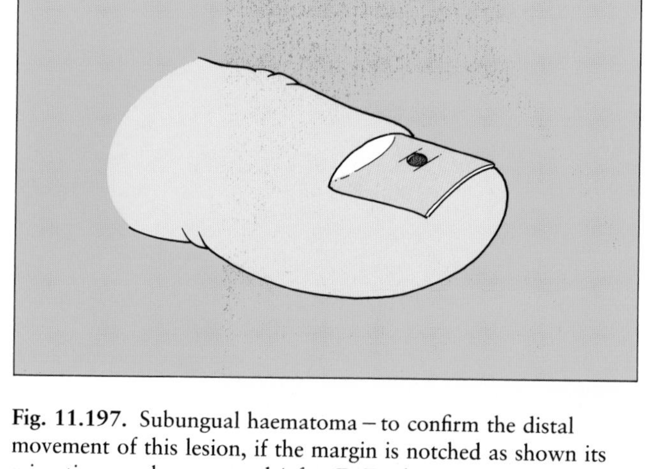

Fig. 11.197. Subungual haematoma – to confirm the distal movement of this lesion, if the margin is notched as shown its migration can be measured (after E. Zook).

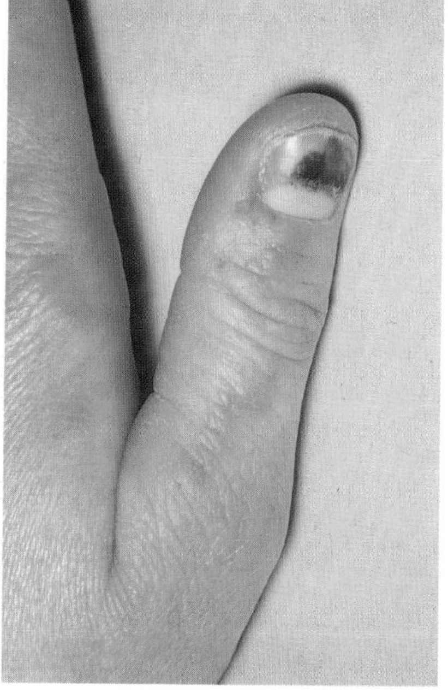

Fig. 11.196. Subungual haematoma.

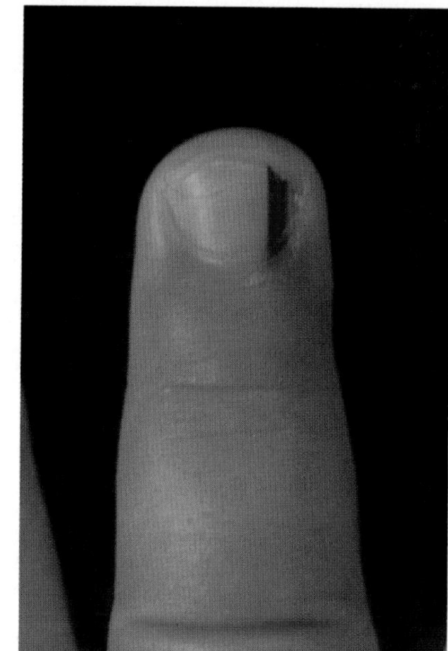

Fig. 11.198. Congenital naevus – pseudo-Hutchinson's sign without malignant melanoma.

Benign melanocytic hyperplasia

Benign melanocytic hyperplasia is due to an increase in melanocyte activity and/or number causing a circumscribed pigmented macule in the matrix. Melanocytic hyperplasia in the matrix may also be induced by repeated trauma such as friction and X-irradiation. A circumscribed increased number of normal looking melanocytes is found in the matrix in the Laugier–Hunziker–Baran syndrome (Figs 11.191–11.194) (Haneke, 1991).

Longitudinal melanonychia (LM) (see also Chapter 2)

LM is characterized by a brown or black longitudinal streak within the nail plate (Figs 11.190–11.193). LM results from increased melanin deposition in the nail plate. This deposition may result from greater melanin synthesis by normally non-functional matrix melanocytes or from an increase in the total number of matrix melanocytes that synthesize melanin (Fig. 11.187); in either instance, melanocytes may be normal or abnormal. Melanocytes in the distal portion of the nail matrix are more numerous and more strongly dopa-positive than melanocytes in the proximal matrix. Probably as a result of greater melanocyte density and activity, LM usually originates in the distal matrix, a fortunate circumstance because permanent nail plate deformity is less common when surgery is performed in the distal rather than in the proximal matrix. The more proximal the origin, the more superficial is the melanin within the nail plate. Histology enables one to identify the site of origin of pigmentation in LM within the matrix by staining nail plate clipping with Fontana–

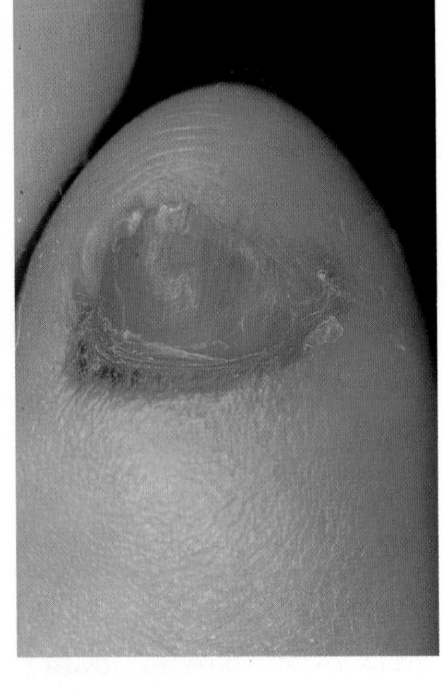

Fig. 11.199. Congenital naevus – pseudo-Hutchinson's sign without malignant melanoma.

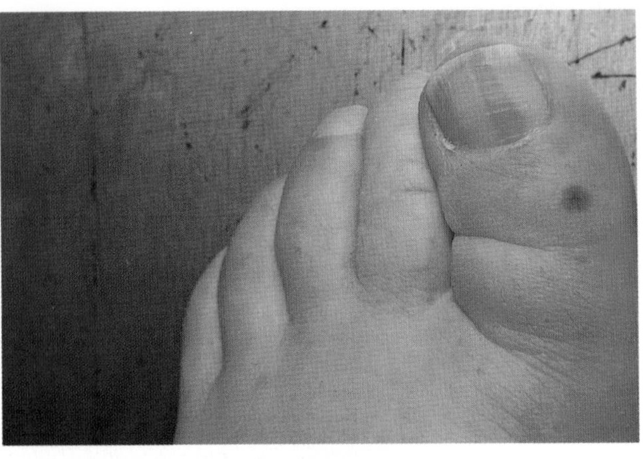
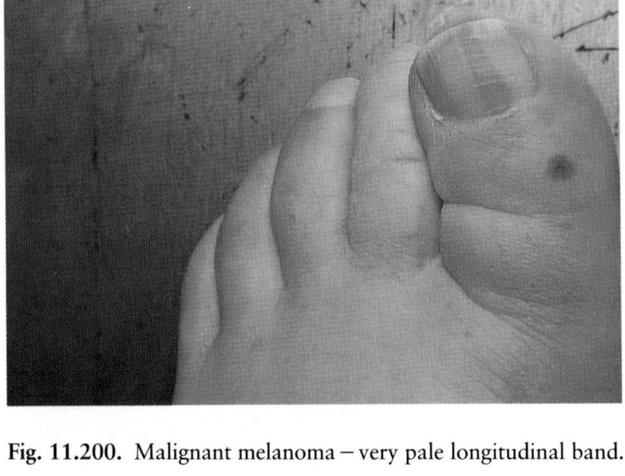

Fig. 11.200. Malignant melanoma – very pale longitudinal band.

Fig. 11.201. Malignant melanoma – broad, widening band in a black person.

Masson's argentaffin reaction. When distal matrix origin seems likely, the cuticle can sometimes be retracted proximally to confirm the distal origin of LM without incision of the proximal nail fold.

LM is common in darkly pigmented persons. LM occurs in 77% of African-Americans over 20 years of age and in almost 100% older than 50 years; the thumbs and index fingers are most frequently involved. LM occurs in 10–20% of Japanese; the thumbs, index and middle fingers are most frequently involved in this group. LM is also common in Hispanic and other dark-skinned groups. Among Whites, LM is unusual.

The distribution of LM between digits coincides with relative digital use; LM is more common in frequently used fingers. The thumb, always used in grasping, is the digit that most often demonstrates LM. The index, middle, fourth, and fifth fingers are employed with diminishing frequency for grasping objects and demonstrate a correspondingly lower incidence of LM. More frequently used digits are also subject to greater trauma. Several authors (Roberts, 1984) have implicated trauma in the pathogenesis of subungual melanoma (SM).

To distinguish the small number of patients with SM (Figs 11.200–11.221) from the very much larger group of patients with 'non-specific' LM is difficult. Both are similar in several ways. In the hand, each arises most often in the thumb, index fingers or both. LM has been reported to precede the onset of SM and may be an early sign of SM. Both are more common in dark-skinned individuals.

The distribution of LM and SM is remarkably similar. In the hand, both usually occur in the thumb or thumb and index finger, as noted earlier. SM develops slightly more often on the hand than on the foot. Forty-five per cent to 60% of SM arise on the hand; 40–55% arise on the foot. On the foot, SM usually occurs in the great toe. Is the incidence of SM higher in the thumb and great toe because each digit is subject to greater trauma; because LM, which commonly occurs on the thumb (and presumably the great toe), is a precursor of SM; or because the thumb and great toe occupy relatively large surface areas and afford greater opportunity for SM to develop?

LM may represent an early sign of SM: in a Japanese study, 31% of SM started as LM and became ulcerated or painful several years later (Takematsu *et al.*, 1985). A report from Belgium showed six of 10 White patients with SM who described as their first sign a longitudinal pigmented band of nail (Nogaret *et al.*, 1986). Other authors have reported similar findings.

Approximately 3% of malignant melanomas in White persons are SM. In the Japanese, the proportion of SM

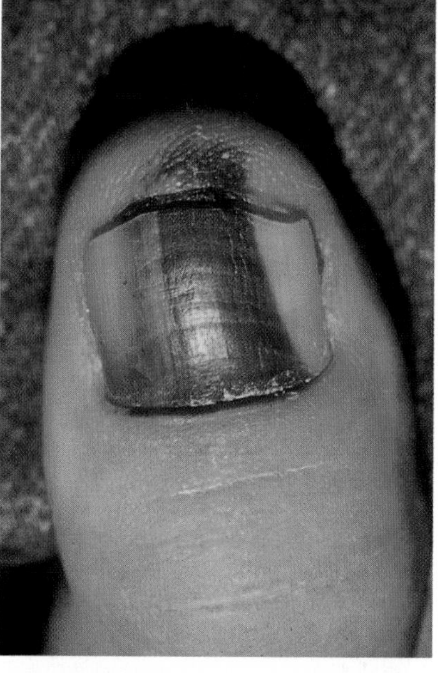

Fig. 11.202. Malignant melanoma with Hutchinson's sign.

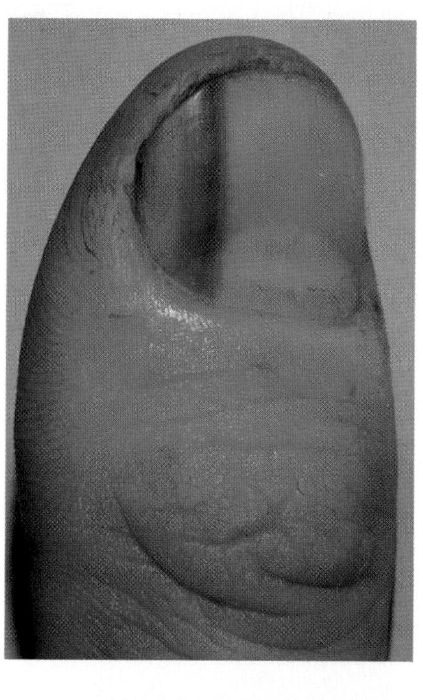

Fig. 11.203. Melanoma *in situ* (courtesy of P. Kechijian, New York, USA).

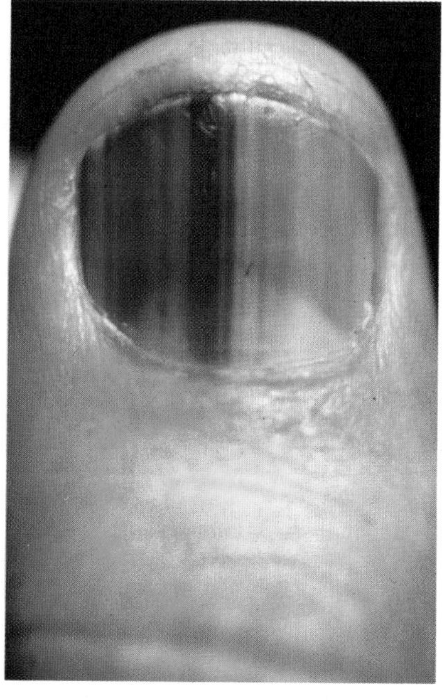

Fig. 11.204. Melanoma *in situ*.

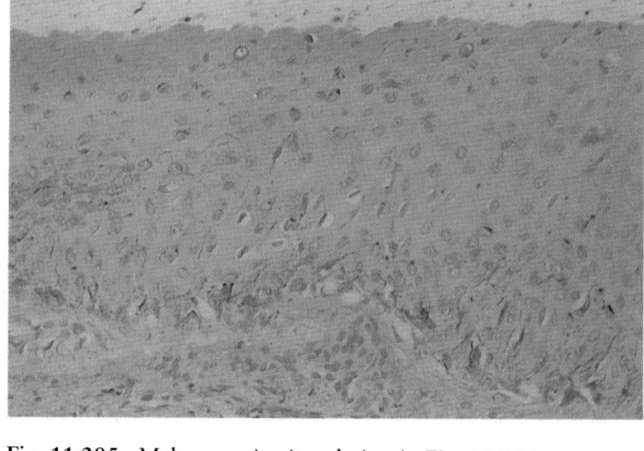

Fig. 11.205. Melanoma *in situ* – lesion in Fig. 11.204.

was similar to that in Whites in two studies (Obata *et al.*, 1979; Takahashi & Seiji, 1983) and higher, 10%, in a third (Miura & Jimbow, 1985). In African-Americans the proportion of SM was higher and varied from 15% to 20% (Collins, 1984). The proportion among Chinese (17%) was similar to that in African-Americans. The 33% proportion in a small study of American Indians was also high. In general, when melanoma occurs in dark-skinned persons, the melanoma is more likely to arise in the nail apparatus, whereas melanoma in light-skinned individuals is less likely to arise in the nail apparatus.

A thorough history and physical examination should enable the various exogenous causes of a single band of LM to be distinguished. The most common pigmented lesion is subungual haematoma and is easily distinguished from LM. It usually migrates distally and its proximal margin is gently curved in a transverse direction. If the nail plate is notched with a scalpel at the proximal margin of the band, distal migration of the haematoma can be accurately measured as the nail plate grows (Fig. 11.197). Non-migratory haematomas and foreign bodies, however, do not follow this rule and require more extensive evaluation (see Chapter 10).

Periungual spread of pigmentation to the proximal and lateral nail folds is called Hutchinson's sign (Figs 11.207 & 11.214). It is the most important indicator of SM. When this sign is present, SM is the presumptive diagnosis. This sign, however, particularly when subtle, is not absolutely pathognomonic for SM. Occasionally, LM that

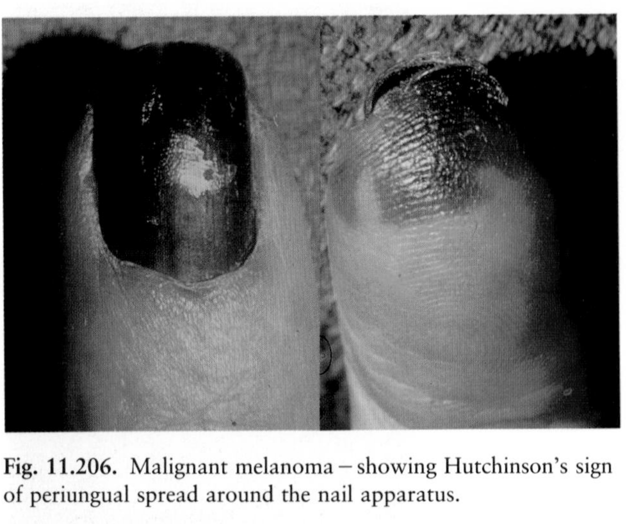

Fig. 11.206. Malignant melanoma – showing Hutchinson's sign of periungual spread around the nail apparatus.

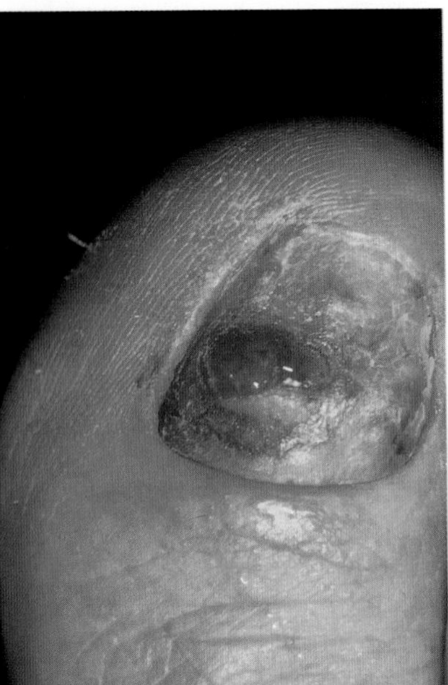

Fig. 11.208. Melanoma – severe dystrophy with very little pigmentation.

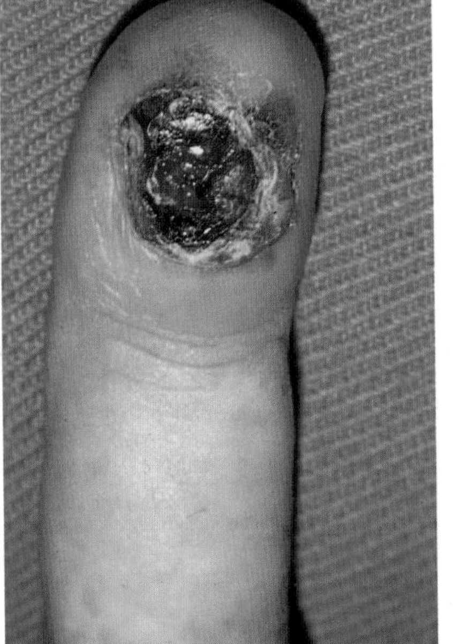

Fig. 11.207. Nodular melanoma with destruction of the nail plate.

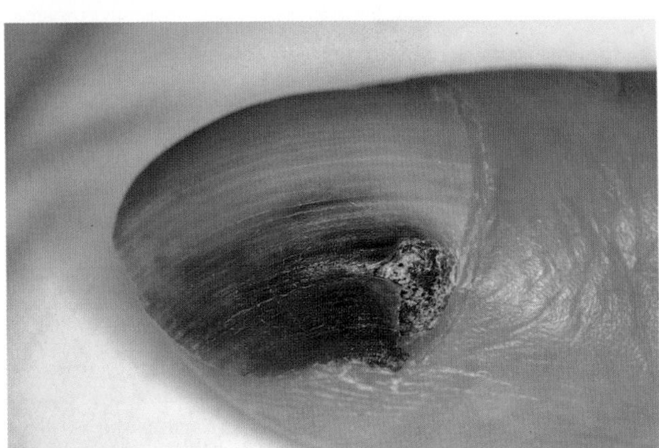

Fig. 11.209. Benign due to pseudomonas, mimicking melanoma – lateral subungual lesion.

is dark brown simulates pigmentation of the overlying cuticle and proximal nail fold. The pigmentation is visible because of the cuticle and proximal nail fold's relative transparency and not because of melanin deposition within these tissues. This sign, the pseudo-Hutinchson's sign, can be identified by careful inspection. In good lighting, it is usually possible to establish whether pigment is present within the periungual tissues or beneath them in the underlying nail plate.

1 Periungual spread of pigmentation without subungual melanoma may occur in the Laugier–Hunziker syndrome (Fig. 11.192) (Baran & Barrière, 1986), a disorder recognizable by the association of LM with macular pigmentation of the lips and mouth (Figs 11.191 & 11.192) (Dupré & Viraben, 1990; Haneke, 1991).

2 Periungual pigmentation of a congenital naevus of the nail region (Figs 11.198 & 11.199) and periungual recurrence of pigmentation after nail surgery for a naevus (Kopf, 1981).

3 LM and periungual hyperpigmentation after X-ray therapy for finger dermatitis (Shelley *et al.*, 1964).

4 Pigmented bands and periungual hyperpigmentation resulting from malnutrition (Bisht & Singh, 1962) and some drugs.

5 LM and periungual hyperpigmentation have been described in association with minocycline therapy (Mooney & Bennet, 1988).

6 The theoretic association of LM with acral pigmentation in Peutz–Jeghers syndrome.

7 LM and pigmentation of the distal pulp have been reported in patients with AIDS even before the institution of systemic treatment (Gallais *et al.*, 1992).

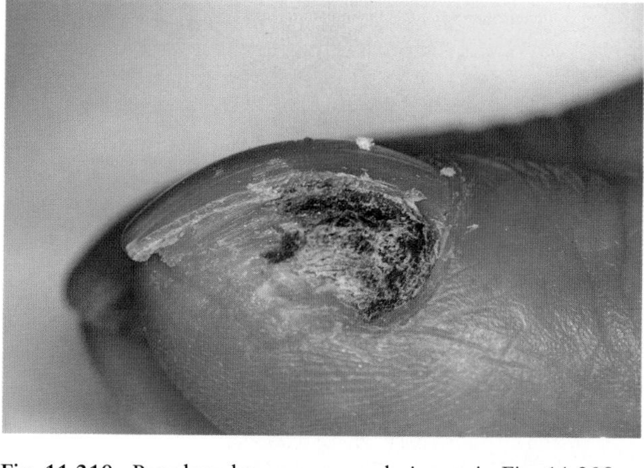

Fig. 11.210. Pseudomelanoma – same lesion as in Fig. 11.209, overlying nail plate removed.

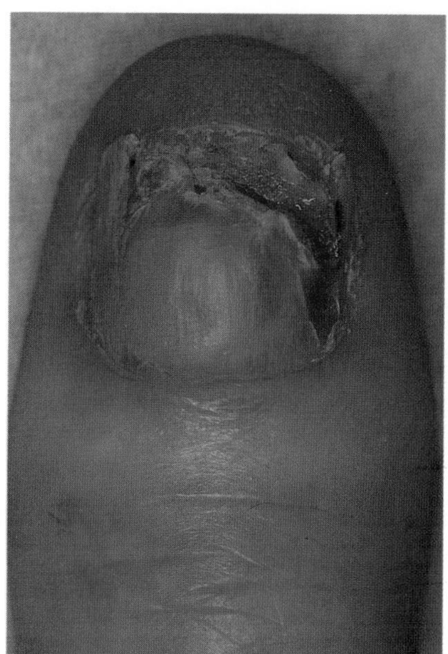

Fig. 11.212. Melanoma – periungual and subungual inflammatory signs but 'amelanotic'.

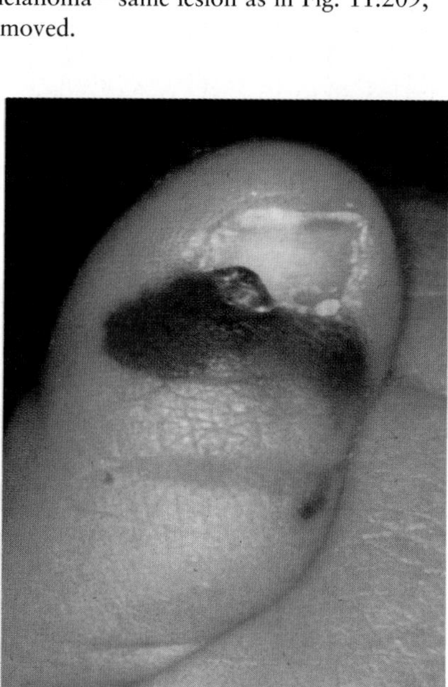

Fig. 11.211. Blue naevus, pseudomalignancy (courtesy of Kerl, Graz, Austria).

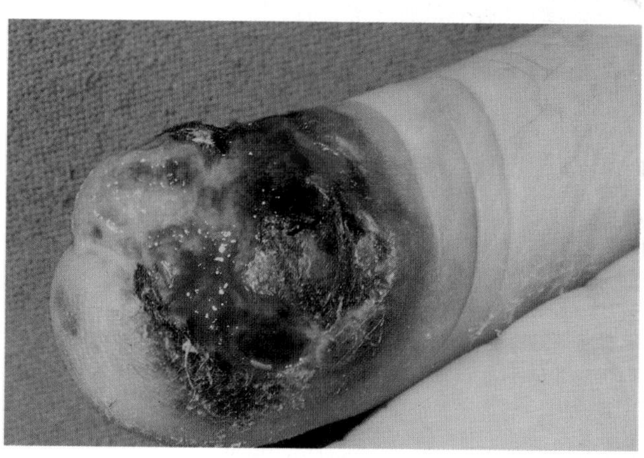

Fig. 11.213. Melanoma – late stage.

8 'Naevoid nail area melanosis' observed in Japanese children may undergo spontaneous regression and even complete disappearance (Kikuchi *et al.*, 1992).
9 LM and periungual pigmentation in a boxer (Bayerl & Moll, 1993). Friction and pressure had been acting on this patients' nails during boxing for the past 40 years.

Periungual extension of pigmentation therefore is a very important, but not always specific sign of SM. However, the absence of Hutchinson's sign does not imply benignity.

Other clues to the diagnosis of SM can be important. The clinician should be suspicious when LM:

1 begins in a single digit of a person during adult life; however, melanonychia due to SM has even been observed in children;
2 develops abruptly in a previously normal nail plate;
3 becomes suddenly darker or wider (Fig. 11.201);
4 occurs in either the thumb, index finger, or great toe;
5 occurs in a person who gives a history of digital trauma (Fig. 11.216);
6 occurs singly in the digit of a dark-skinned patient, particularly if the thumb or great toe is affected;
7 demonstrates blurred, rather than sharp, lateral borders;
8 occurs in a person who gives a history of malignant melanoma;
9 occurs in a person in whom the risk for melanoma is increased (e.g. dysplastic naevus syndrome) (Kechijian, 1991);
10 is accompanied by nail dystrophy, such as partial nail destruction or complete disappearance (Fig. 11.219).

Other signs are noteworthy, but not necessarily helpful, in establishing the likelihood of malignancy.

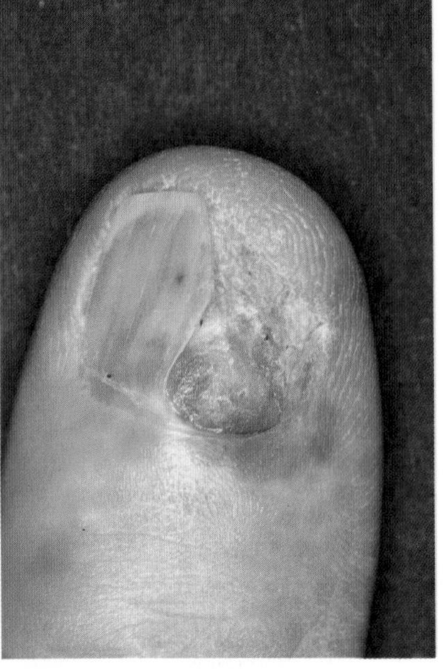

Fig. 11.214. Melanoma – 'amelanotic' but Hutchinson's sign present.

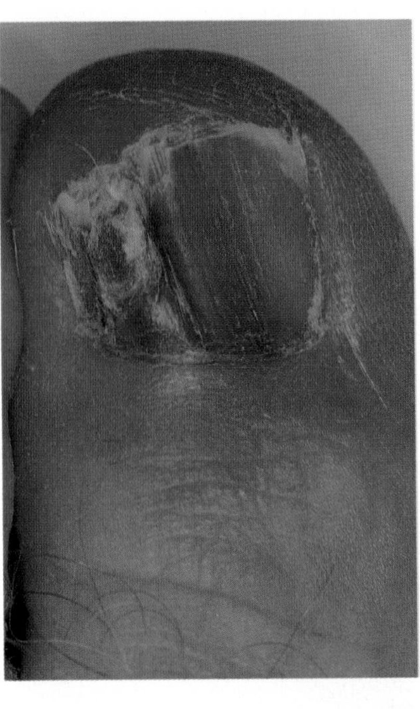

Fig. 11.215. Melanoma – nail dystrophy occurring.

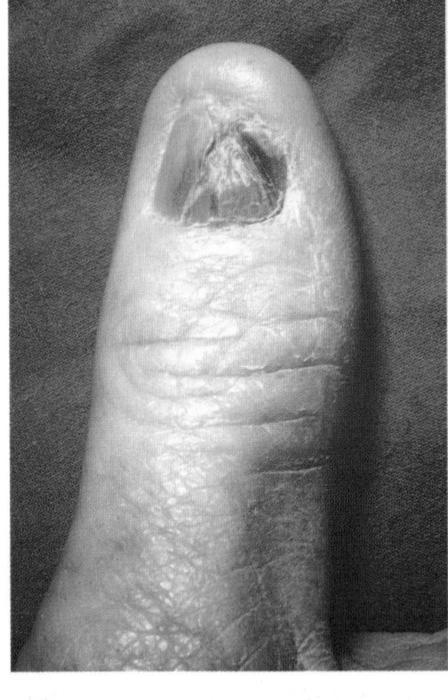

Fig. 11.216. Melanoma – longstanding nail dystrophy preceded this, following trauma.

Fig. 11.217. Melanoma – late stage.

1 Although amelanotic SM is not rare lightly pigmented bands of LM (Fig. 11.200) rarely represent SM; the pathologist may have difficulty even visualizing the melanin and melanocytes that constitute light-banded LM.
2 Darker shades of brown do not necessarily represent SM because naevi and melanoma may manifest identical shades of brown. In white persons, black bands may be an important clue to SM; in African-Americans, however, 'jet-black' bands are not unusual. Theoretically, colour variegation suggests SM; however, variegation is common in persons with multiple 'benign' LM.
3 Wide bands suggest SM (Figs 11.201 & 11.204); however, the critical width that signifies SM has yet to be established.
4 Bands that do not extend distally to the free edge of the nail are unlikely to represent SM because they do not take their origin from the nail matrix. However, they may represent metastatic melanoma or LM arising from the nail bed.

The management of Black patients with pigmented bands can be difficult. Although multiple nails demonstrate LM, there may be substantial variability in the colour and width of bands within a single nail plate and among different nails in the same patient. Whether LM in a thumb or great toe represents SM or racial variation is not necessarily easily determined by history and inspection alone. Change in the morphology of LM, in particular

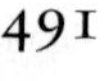

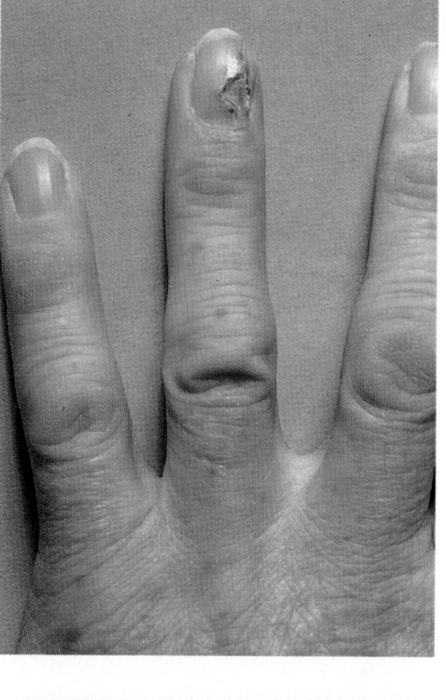

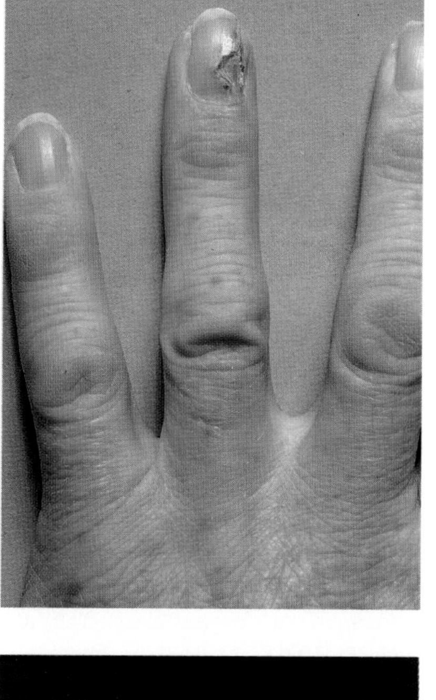

Fig. 11.218. Melanoma – relatively amelanotic with nail dystrophy.

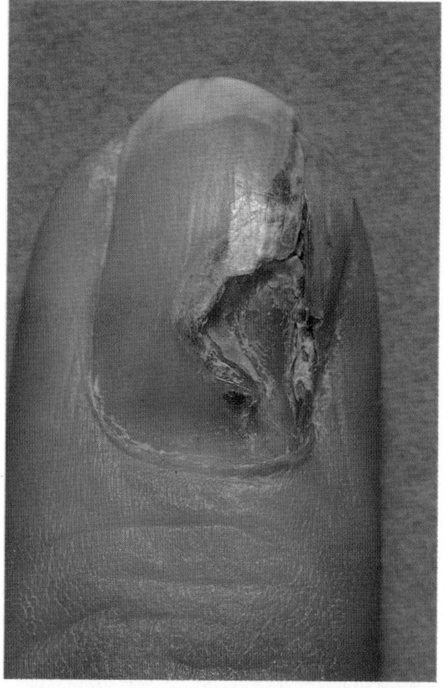

Fig. 11.219. Melanoma – this dystrophic variety was preceded by LM of 2 years duration.

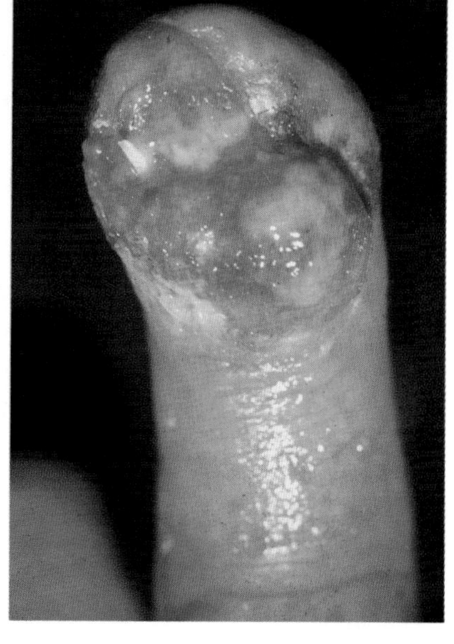

Fig. 11.220. Melanoma – amelanotic.

Fig. 11.221. Melanoma – amelanotic.

widening and darkening, is the most important clue to the possibility of SM in these patients (Fig. 11.201).

Polydactylic bands of LM are usually not neoplastic in origin although multiple SM has been observed (Leppard *et al.*, 1974). A drug history and complete general review to exclude possible systemic disorders and a thorough examination of the skin and nails to rule out nail infection and associated cutaneous disorders will usually reveal an underlying cause of multiple LM.

Frequently, despite meticulous evaluation, the aetiology of LM remains obscure, and biopsy becomes necessary. There is no consensus among dermatopathologists regarding the melanocytic causes of LM. The following represents an attempt to organize the causes into a practical list: (i) proliferation of normal melanocytes; (ii) acquired melanocytic naevus; (iii) congenital melanocytic naevus; (iv) proliferation of atypical melanocytes; (v) recurrent or persistent melanocytosis with histologic features that may simulate SM; (vi) melanoma *in situ* (Figs 11.203–11.205); (vii) SM; (viii) metastatic melanoma.

Lentigo simplex and melanocytic naevus

Lentigo simplex is characterized by a considerable increase in highly active melanocytes accompanied by epidermal hyperplasia. The nature of the underlying melanotic lesion responsible for the pigmented band cannot be determined by clinical examination alone. The same holds true for subungual melanocytic naevi (Figs 11.198 & 11.199). On histological examination they show nests of naevus cells in the rete ridges with melanin pigmentation of varying intensity. Ohtsuka *et al.* (1978) reported a case of congenital naevocytic naevus of the tip of the little finger in a Japanese female infant. This caused discoloration, hypercurvature and subungual hyperkeratosis giving rise to an appearance similar to the nail of a monkey. Congenital subungual naevi are usually excised to prevent the rare occurrence of secondary malignant melanoma (Coskey *et al.*, 1983); the management of 'naevoid nail area melanosis' in Japanese children (Kikuchi *et al.*, 1993) is currently under debate. There is still therefore a great deal of controversy regarding: (i) the malignant potential of small congenital naevi; (ii) the malignant potential of subungual naevi; and (iii) the relationship of childhood lentigines to the evolution of naevi and to the development of melanomas (Wong *et al.*, 1991).

Pseudo-Recklinghausen intradermal naevi

Abnormal naevoblast migration may mimic neurofibromatosis (Lycka *et al.*, 1991). Hundreds of papules and nodules on both feet and toes were intradermal naevi. A close clinical presentation was shown in a Black male (Cavelier-Balloy *et al.*, 1992) (Fig. 11.123). The main difference was in the presence of only blue naevi. Leu 7 and myelin basic protein were negative which also ruled out neurofibromatosis (Gray *et al.*, 1990).

Malignant melanoma

Atypical melanocytic hyperplasia and SM

Atypical melanocytic hyperplasia shows an increased number of melanocytes with larger, hyperchromatic, pleomorphic nuclei, more prominent nucleoli, increased mitoses, and long branching dendrites. Thus, atypical melanocytic hyperplasia may be considered to be incipient malignant melanoma *in situ* (Figs 11.203–11.205) (Kopf & Waldo, 1980; Kamino & Ackerman, 1981).

Melanomas of the nail region are now better understood (Dawber & Colver, 1991) since the identification and analysis of acrolentiginous melanoma (ALM), the most frequent type (Clark *et al.*, 1979; Feibleman *et al.*, 1980). Superficial spreading melanoma (SSM) is rare. Existence of nodular melanomas is debatable in the subungual area despite Milton's *et al.* (1985) findings in Australia (seven cases out of a total of 30), and Miura and Jimbow's (1985) questionnaire survey of 108 cases of SM in Japan, indicating that ALM was present in 80% of cases, nodular melanoma in 15% and SSM in 5%. Some cases are not classifiable for two main reasons: (i) there may be a histological transition between SSM and ALM (Sondergaard & Tejan, 1980) indicating a close biological relationship between the two types; (ii) poor quality of the biopsy specimen.

Approximately 2–3% of melanomas in Caucasians, and 15–20% in black people are located in the nail apparatus (Oropeza, 1976). However since malignant melanoma is rare in black people, the number of nail melanomas in Caucasians and black people does not significantly differ. In Caucasians, most patients have a fair complexion, light hair, and blue or hazel eyes. There is no sex predominance. The mean age is 60 years. Most tumours are located on the thumbs and great toes, but develop more commonly on the foot than on the hand. Melanomas are often asymptomatic, pain and bleeding being rare. The clinical appearence of the tumour varies (Figs 11.200–11.221) (Patterson & Helwig, 1980; Dawber & Colver, 1991), but half of the patients note a mass below the nail, usually associated with partial destruction of the nail, or total loss (Figs 11.207 & 11.208).

Periungual infection, ulceration of the nail bed, and granulation tissue occur in about one-third of the patients. In another third, discoloration of the nail area is the presenting sign.

1 Some lesions begin as longitudinal melanonychia. This pigmented (brown to black) linear streak of variable width runs through the whole length of the visible nail (Figs 11.200–11.202). After some months or years, the borders of the band widen, become blurred and ulceration appears.

2 A spot can appear in the matrix, nail bed or nail plate. This may vary in colour from brown to black and may be homogeneous or irregular. It is seldom painful.

3 Less frequently seen is the Hutchinson's sign (1886) (Figs 11.207 & 11.214), an irregular brown-black pigmentation of the matrix, nail bed, nail plate, and surrounding tissues. It represents the radial growth phase of subungual melanoma and has proved to be a valuable clue to the clinical diagnosis of malignancy (Kopf, 1981) after the pseudo-Hutchinson's sign has been ruled out (Figs 11.192, 11.198 & 11.199). Its presence means that the entire nail apparatus must be removed (without prior incisional biopsy). This technique enables serial sections to be examined which is particularly important in acral lentiginous melanoma in which histology may be difficult to interpret. The radial growth phase of malignant melanoma in the subungual region is easily confused histologically with junctional naevus and the clinician must be wary of a benign histological report in any subungual lesion showing Hutchinson's sign. The vertical phase with its abrupt onset when compared temporally with the slowly evolving radial growth phase is manifested by the focal appearance of a discrete blue, black or pink nodule in subungual tumours causing partial or total permanent

destruction of the nail plate (Clark *et al.*, 1979) (Fig. 11.213).

Approximately 25% of melanomas are amelanotic (Figs 11.220 & 11.221) and may wrongly suggest the diagnosis of pyogenic granuloma, inflammatory granulation tissue, ingrowing nail or mycobacterial infection with nail dystrophy. The risk of misdiagnosis is therefore particularly high in these cases. The rare cases of spontaneous regression of the pigment and even total disappearance of malignant melanoma are debatable.

Malignant melanoma must be considered in the differential diagnosis in all patients affected by unexplained chronic paronychia, whether painful or not, torpid granulomatous ulceration of the proximal nail fold, pseudoverrucous keratotic alterations of the nail bed and lateral nail groove and persistence of a lesion following trauma of the nail (Shukla & Hughes, 1989).

SM may also be simulated by subungual haematoma which is not rare and may even be present without a history of severe trauma (Figs 11.195 & 11.196). It may follow repeated minor trauma which escapes the patient's attention such as in tennis toe or following trauma from hard ski boots. Haematoma following a single episode of trauma usually grows out in one piece rather than as longitudinal streak due to the latter continuously producing pigment; but SM following a single injury to the digit was observed in eight cases after an interval of between 9 months and 7 years (Roberts, 1984). Repeated trauma may cause difficulties in differential diagnosis (Dawber & Colver, 1991) and non-migrating haematoma should be ruled out. Alkiewicz and Pfister (1976) suggest that the lesion should be examined with a loup, after it has been covered by a drop of oil. The pigmented nail should be clipped and tested with the argentaffin reaction in order to rule out melanin pigmentation. Subungual haemoglobin is not degraded to haemosiderin and is therefore Prussian blue negative. Scrapings or small pieces of the nail boiled with water in a test tube gives a positive benzidine reaction with conventional haemostix. The difference between blood and melanotic pigment, sometimes rather difficult to discern by routine histological methods, is easily seen by ultrastructural techniques – iron pigment is mainly intercellular while melanin is intracellular (Achten, 1982).

Histopathology of SM

SM is a particular form of acrolentiginous melanoma. This type of melanoma is defined by its location on palms, soles and under the nails rather than by specific microscopic morphology; however, some authors distinguish subungual nodular melanoma and subungual SSM from acrolentiginous melanoma (Miura & Jimbow, 1985; Takematsu *et al.*, 1984; Diepgen *et al.*, 1991).

It is also very important to stress that the majority of patients suffering from SM have undergone some minor surgery before the diagnosis of SM was made. This may have been a consequence of patient neglect or medical misdiagnosis, false biopsy techniques or inadequate histopathological technique and knowledge. Thus the importance of proper biopsy (Fig. 11.225 & Chapter 10) and histopathology for prognosis assessment cannot be exaggerated.

There is usually no difficulty in the histopathological diagnosis of advanced invasive SM. Most subungual acrolentiginous melanomas exhibit a lentiginous pattern with pleomorphic, often dendritic, atypical melanocytes being arranged singly or in irregular clusters in the basal and suprabasal epithelial layers (Figs 11.222–11.224). Sheets of melanoma cells, either spindle, epithelioid, polygonal, small, dendritic, or bizarre and pleomorphic, extend from the epithelium into the dermis. Large round melanoma cells are dispersed throughout the entire epidermis in the pagetoid (SSM-like) pattern. The nodular pattern is rare and shows subepidermal tumour cells usually with little junctional cell complexes, and at least part of the overlying epithelium is necrotic. Mixed features of lentiginous and pagetoid patterns are not rare. The lentiginous type of SM may exhibit a dense population of atypical melanocytes in the basal epithelial layers which may give rise to artificial bulla formation due to lack of cohesion between melanoma cells and nail bed and matrix epithelium upon sectioning; it is also one cause of nail atrophy in SM (Haneke, 1986). Melanoma cells migrating up to the superficial matrix layers may be included in the nail plate and can be seen microscopically, sometimes even in nail clippings. Subungual nodular melanoma with no junctional component may be difficult to distinguish from lymphoma, anaplastic and small cell carcinoma as well as other malignant tumours including metastases all of which are rare in this location; also a lichenoid infiltrate in SM may mimic lichen planus. Immunohistochemical demonstration of protein S-100 or another melanoma marker such as HMB 45 aids in making the correct diagnosis.

The most difficult problem in subungual pigmented lesions is to differentiate benign melanocytic hyperplasia that may eventually develop into benign junctional or compound naevus, from the earliest changes of SM. One has always to keep in mind that there are many well-documented cases of SM with histories longer than 20 or 30 years. These cases often started with a light-brown longitudinal stripe in the nail. We have seen two cases of SM *in situ* with only very pale longitudinal melanonychia; however, both pigmented bands were wider than 5 mm.

In case of a pigmented spot in the matrix or nail bed, the lesion should be completely excised and serial and step sections are mandatory. It is common to see only a few

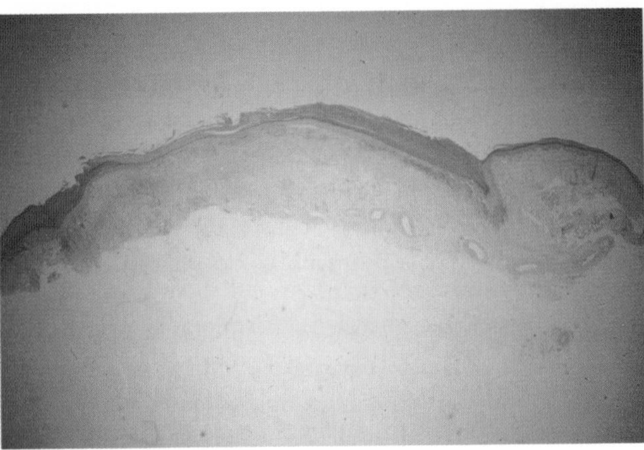

Fig. 11.222. Melanoma – low-power view; section from a longitudinal nail biopsy.

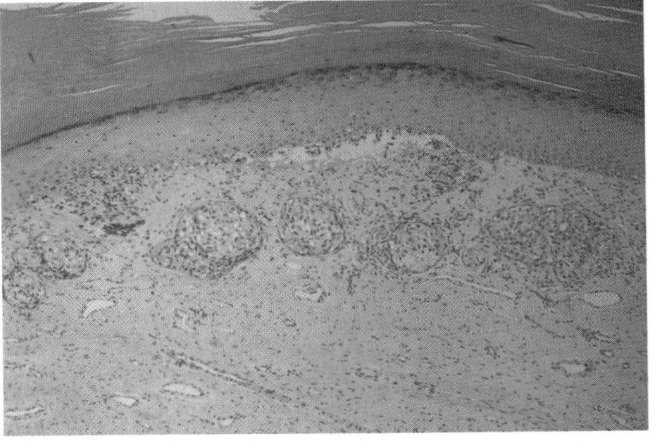

Fig. 11.223. Melanoma – junctional involvement and nests of melanoma cells in the dermis; see Fig. 11.222, proximal nail bad and adjacent matrix area.

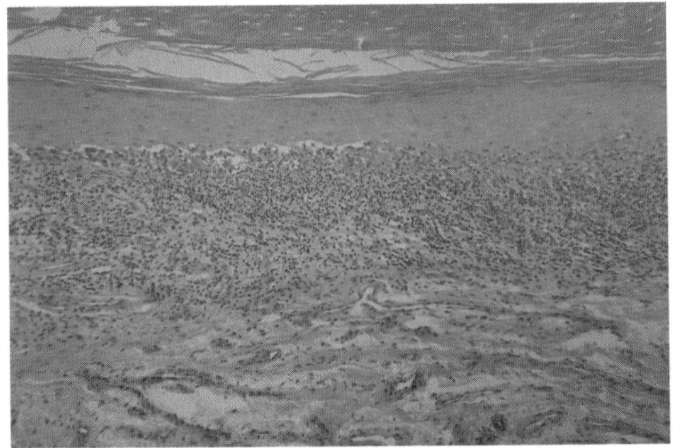

Fig. 11.224. Melanoma (see Figs 11.222 & 11.223) – infiltrate in the upper dermis from the middle and distal nail bed. The lichenoid appearance is not diagnostic of melanoma, which was present more proximally.

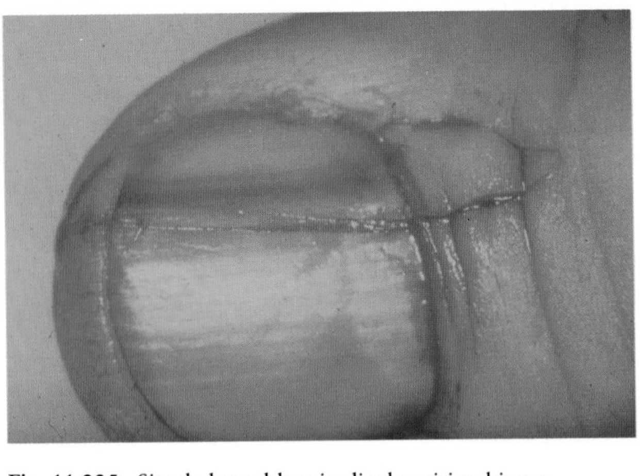

Fig. 11.225. Simple lateral longitudinal excision biopsy technique for longitudinal melanonychia if melanoma is suspected.

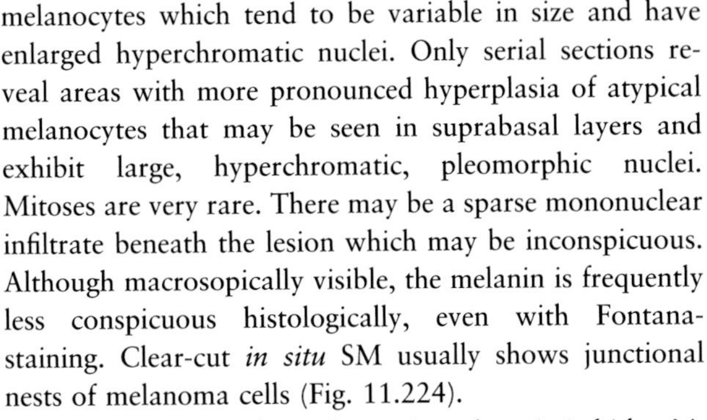

melanocytes which tend to be variable in size and have enlarged hyperchromatic nuclei. Only serial sections reveal areas with more pronounced hyperplasia of atypical melanocytes that may be seen in suprabasal layers and exhibit large, hyperchromatic, pleomorphic nuclei. Mitoses are very rare. There may be a sparse mononuclear infiltrate beneath the lesion which may be inconspicuous. Although macrosopically visible, the melanin is frequently less conspicuous histologically, even with Fontana-staining. Clear-cut *in situ* SM usually shows junctional nests of melanoma cells (Fig. 11.224).

Histopathology of Hutchinson's melanotic 'whitlow' is virtually identical with the lentiginous pattern of acrolentiginous melanoma *in situ* of palms and soles (Kerl *et al.*, 1981). Atypical melanocytes, often polygonal or even dendritic, are dispersed mainly in the basal layer of the periungual epidermis with relatively few cells being localized suprabasally (Fig. 11.205).

Histopathology is crucial for the diagnosis of any melanin-induced pigmentation in, under, or around the nail. Both the biopsy techniques and histological techniques, the number of serial and step sections as well as the expertise of the investigating dermatopathologist are crucial for the correct diagnosis. However, the clinician is central to accurate management, because he or she must decide whether to biopsy or not, how to do it, to whom to send the specimen and to mark the tissue correctly so that orientation will be possible in the laboratory. Neither gender, localization, nor age must influence the decision for biopsy since SM does occur on fingers of great 'aesthetic' importance; and even in children (Kato *et al.*, 1989).

Prognosis of SM (see Table 11.7)

The diagnosis of nail melanoma is commonly delayed by several years: fingernail and pigmented tumours are

Table 11.7. Survival rates of ungual melanomas

Authors	Period	%
Das Gupta & Brasfield (1965)	5 years	38
Graham (1979)	5 years	50
Panizzon & Krebs (1980)	5 years	25
Patterson & Helwig (1980)	5 years	16
Krementz *et al.* (1982)	5 years	63
Takematzu *et al.* (1985)	5 years	40
Blessing *et al.* (1991)	5 years	41
Rigby *et al.* (1992)	10 months	29
Paul *et al.* (1992)	5 years	51 (fingers 57) (toes 48)
	10 years	28 (fingers 41) (toes 22)

usually diagnosed and treated the earliest. Hence it follows that the prognosis of toenail melanoma is worse than that of fingernails.

Recently reported series of ungual melanomas (Blessing *et al.*, 1991) have shown that many patients with advanced invasive tumours had been inadequately biopsied prior to definitive therapy. Two independent series reporting 124 British nail melanoma patients had a mean Breslow depth of 4.7 mm giving evidence of unfortunate neglect by patients and physicians of nail lesions. These studies also demonstrated that tumour thickness is the single most important prognostic factor on which further significant factors such as mitotic activity and vascular invasion depend. At the time of treatment, the melanoma subtype itself, whether acral lentiginous, superficial spreading, or nodular melanoma, is not significantly associated with prognosis although acral lentiginous melanomas often have a history of many years or even decades and the development of nodular ungual melanomas is frequently very rapid.

The experience from recently published series of (sub)ungual melanomas with very thick tumours is in contrast to our experience of more than 20 *in situ* and early SM; however, any acquired longitudinal melanonychia or any periungual pigmentation, no matter how light it appeared to us, was totally removed and examined histopathologically using a large number of serial sections. There was no difference in the survival of Park *et al's* (1992) patients (100) treated with local/proximal interphalangeal joint amputation compared with those having more proximal amputations. Because nearly 70% of these tumours arose on the thumb or hallux, it is concluded that, provided adequate clearance could be obtained, less radical excision should be performed for these lesions to maintain maximum function. Early treatment of any 'melanoma-suspicious' lesion is mandatory to improve the cure rate and to enable a more conservative surgical approach to be carried out.

Malignant melanoma in childhood

Malignant melanoma is exceptional in childhood. Lyall (1967) reported on a pigmented spot of the tip of the right middle fingernail of a 12-month-old male. Soyer and Kerl (1984) found on the dorsum of the left big toe of a 4-year-old girl a slightly infiltrated black area well demarcated with a small periungual nodule. In the neighbouring skin several pinhead-sized satellite nodules were found with lymph nodes of the left groin. Histology showed lymph node metastases of the blue naevus combined with a junctional naevus, but this was not malignant melanoma (Fig. 11.211). There are a few reports of malignant melanoma in Oriental children. Ohno *et al.* (1988) presented the case of a 7-year-old girl with LM and seen at 27 with a deformed nail and Hutchinson's sign. Histology revealed malignant melanoma and lymph node metastases. Mori and Futui (1993) reported the case of LM starting at age 9 (following an injury at age 4) and developing SM at age 32. Kato *et al.* (1989) published three cases of LM revealing melanoma *in situ*.

Malignant melanoma in deeply pigmented races

Because of its frequency in deeply pipmented races, LM is not the usual presenting sign as observed in Caucasians. However, the pigmented band shows an indistinct border, sometimes widens rapidly (Fig. 11.201), and the longitudinal streak becomes jet black rather than the normal brown. The diagnosis may be aided by comparison with the brown streaks in other nails or by the occurrence of Hutchinson's sign.

Malignant melanoma in transplant recipients

Of clinical importance is the development of malignant melanomas in transplant recipients. Merkle *et al.* (1991) reported a slowly enlarging tumour on the tip of the middle finger in a 59-year-old man. This verrucous and erosive non-pigmented tumour involving the distal nail bed was a nodular malignant melanoma in a patient treated with corticosteroids and azathioprine and who had undergone kidney transplantation 7 years earlier.

The diagnosis of malignant melanoma may be made only by maintaining a high index of suspicion with any persistent nail bed lesion, irrespective of the presence of pigmentation. Incisional biopsy should be performed in all suspected cases, followed by urgent definitive treatment (Winslet & Tejan, 1990).

Recent advances in the management of malignant melanoma have been made through knowledge of determinants such as primary depth of invasion, thickness, presence of ulceration, status of regional lymph nodes (Daly *et al.*, 1987).

Spontaneous regression of melanocytic lesions
(Ceballos & Barnhill, 1993)

LM

LM, as a symptom of the 'naevoid nail area melanosis' observed in Japanese children, may present spontaneous regression and even may disappeare (Kikuchi *et al.*, 1993). The histological features of these pigmented lesions are lacking. We have reported a case with progressive fading of LM due to a nail matrix naeves in a child (Tosti *et al.*, 1994).

Melanoma of the nail apparatus

Pathologists now more readily recognize the subtle features of histological regression since step sections through the entire block are more often being done. Regression was found in 27.1% of SSM and 17.4% of lentigo maligna melanomas and was not identified in nodular melanomas (Trau *et al.*, 1983). Histological regression, however, played only a marginal role as a prognostic factor in SSM, deriving its significance mainly from its close relationship to the thickness of the melanoma.

References

Achten G. (1982) What's new about normal and pathologic nail. *Abstracts in XVI Int. Congress Dermatol. Tokyo*, pp. 17–18.

Alkiewicz J. & Pfister R. (1976) *Atlas der Nagelkrankheiten* Schattauer Verlag, Stuttgart.

Baran R. & Barrière H. (1986) Longitudinal melanonychia with spreading pigmentation in Laugier–Hunziker syndrome: a report of two cases. *Br. J. Dermatol.* **115**, 707–710.

Bayer C. & Moll I. (1993) Longitudinal melanonychia with Hutchinson sign in a boxer. *Hautarzt* **44**, 476–479.

Bisht D.B. & Singh S.S. (1962) Pigmented bands on nails: a new sign in malnutrition. *Lancet* **1**, 1175–1181.

Blessing K., Kernohan N.M. & Park K.G.M. (1991) Subungual malignant melanoma – Clinicopathological features of 100 cases. *Histopathology* **19**, 425–429.

Cavelier-Balloy B., Aractingi S., Verola O. *et al.* (1992) Naevus géant congénital avec naevi bleus multiples disséminés. Presented at 'Journées Dermatologiques de Paris', Poster **115**, 18–21 Mars.

Ceballos P.I. & Barnhill R.L. (1993) Spontaneous resolution of cutaneous tumours. In: *Advances in Dermatology*, Eds Callen R., Dahl M. *et al.*, Ch. 8. Mosby, St Louis.

Clark W.H., Bernardino E.A., Reed R.J. & Kopf A.W. (1979) Acral lentiginous melanomas. In: *Human Malignant Melanoma*, eds Clark W.H., Goldman L.I. & Mastrangero, pp. 109–124. Grune & Stratton, New York.

Collins R.J. (1984) Melanomas in the Chinese among southwestern Indians. *Cancer* **55**, 2899–2902.

Coskey R.J., Magnel T.D. & Bernarcki E.G. (1983) Congenital subungual naevus. *J. Am. Acad. Dermatol.* **9**, 747–751.

Daly J.M., Berlin R. & Urmacher C. (1987) Subungual melanoma: a 25-year review of cases. *J. Surg. Oncol.* **35**, 107–112.

Das Gupta T. & Brasfield R. (1965) Subungual melanoma. *Ann. Surg.* **161**, 545–552.

Dawber R.P.R. & Colver G.B. (1991) The spectrum of malignant melanoma in the nail apparatus. *Semin. Dermatol.* **10**, 82–88.

Diepgen T.L., Schell H., Müller A. *et al.* (1991) Maligne Melanome an den Akren-Häufigkeit, Klinik und Prognose. *Z. Hautkr.* **66**, 631–636.

Dupré A. & Viraben R. (1990) Laugier's disease. *Dermatologica* **181**, 183–186.

Feibleman C.E., Stoll H. & Maize J.C. (1980) Melanomas of the palm, sole, and nailbed: A clinicopathologic study. *Cancer* **46**, 2492–2504.

Gallais V., Lacour J.P.H. Perrin C. *et al.* (1992) Acral hyperpigmentated macules and longitudinal melanonychia in AIDS patients. *Br. J. Dermatol.* **126**, 387–391.

Graham W.P. (1973) Subungual melanoma. *Penn. Med.* **76**, 56.

Gray M.H., Smoller B.R., McNult N.S. *et al.* (1990) Neurofibromas and neurotized melanocytic nevi are immunohistochemically distinct neoplasm. *Am. J. Dermatopathol.* **12**, 234–241.

Haneke E. (1986) Pathogenese der Nagel dystrophie beim subungualen Melanom. *Verh. Dtsch. Ges. Path.* **70**, 484.

Haneke E. (1991) Laugier-Hunziker-Baran-Syndrom. *Hautarzt* **42**, 512–515.

Hutchinson J. (1986) Melanosis often not black: Melanotic whitlow. *Br. Med. J.* **1**, 491.

Kerl H., Hödl S. & Stettner H. (1981) Acral lentiginous melanoma. In: *Pathology of Malignant Melanoma*, pp. 217–242, ed. Ackerman A.B. Mason, New York.

Kato I., Usuba Y., Takematsu H. *et al.* (1989) A rapidly growing pigmented nail streak resulting in diffuse melanosis of the nail. *Cancer* **64**, 2191–2197.

Kechijian P. (1991) Subungual melanoma *in situ* presenting as longitudinal melanonychia in a patient with familial dysplastic nevi. *J. Am. Acad. Dermatol.* **24**, 283.

Kikuchi I., Inoue S., Sakaguchi E. *et al.* (1993) Nevoid nail area melanosis in childhood (cases which showed spontaneous regression). *Dermatology* **186**, 88–93.

Krementz E.T., Reed R.J. & Coleman W.P. *et al.* (1982) Acral lentiginous melanoma; a clinico-pathlogical entity. *Ann. Surg.* **195**, 632.

Kopf A.W. (1981) Hutchinson's sign of subungual malignant melanoma. *Am. J. Dermatopathol.* **3**, 201–202.

Lycka B., Krywonis N. & Hordinsky M. (1991) Abnormal nevoblast migration mimicking neurofibromatosis. *Arch. Dermatol.* **127**, 1702–1704.

Lyall D. (1967) Malignant melanoma in infancy. *J. Am. Acad Dermatol.* **202**, 1153.

Leppard B., Sanderson K.V. & Behan F. (1974) Subungual malignant melanoma. Difficulty in diagnosis. *Br. Med. J.* **1**, 310–312.

Merkle T., Landthaler M., Eckert F. *et al.* (1991) Acral verrucous malignant melanoma in an immunosuppressed patient after kidney transplantation. *J. Am. Acad. Dermatol.* **24**, 505–506.

Milton G.W., Shaw H.M. & McCarthy W.H. (1985) Subungual malignant melanoma. A disease entity separate from other forms of cutaneous melanoma. *Aust. J. Dermatol.* **26**, 61–64.

Miura S. & Jimbow K. (1985) Clinical characteristics of subungual melanoma in Japan: case report and questionnaire survey of 108 cases. *J. Dermatol. (Tokyo)* **12**, 393–402.

Mooney E & Bennet R.G. (1988) Periungual hyperpigmentation mimicking Hutchinson's sign associated with minocycline administration. *J. Dermatol. Surg. Oncol.* **14**, 1011–1013.

Mori T. & Fukui V. (1993) A case of malignant melanoma originating from subungual pigmented lines which had existed since childhood. *Rinsho. Dermatol.* **35**, 808–809.

Nogaret J.M., André J., Parent D. *et al.* (1986). Le mélanome des extrémités: diagnostic méconnu et traitement délicat. Revue des 20 observations. *Acta Chir. Belg.* **86**, 238–244.

Obata M., Kato T. & Seiji M. (1979) Eight cases of subungual melanoma. *Jpn. J. Clin. Dermatol.* **33**, 515–521.

Ohno M., Veda M. & Mishima Y. (1988) Subungual malignant melanoma. Especially on precursor lesions of ALM and nodular melanoma. *Hifu Rinsho* **30**, 1041–1048.

Ohtsuka H., Hori Y. & Ando M. (1978) Naevus of the little finger with a remarkable nail deformity. *Plast. Reconstr. Surg.* **61**, 108–111.

Oropeza R. (1976) Melanomas of special sites. In: *Cancer of the Skin*, eds Andrade R., Gumpert S.L., Popkin G.L. & Rees T.D., Vol. 2, pp. 974–987. W.B. Saunders, Philadelphia.

Panizzon R. & Krebs A. (1980) Das subunguale maligne melanom. *Hautarzt* **31**, 132–140.

Park K.G.M., Blessing K. & Kernohan N.M. (1992) Surgical aspects of subungual malignant melanoma. *Ann. Surg.* **216**, 692–695.

Patterson R. & Helwig E.B. (1980) Subungual melanoma: a clinical pathological study. *Cancer* **46**, 2074–2087.

Rigby H.S. & Briggs J.C. (1992) Subungual melanoma: a clinico-pathological study of 24 cases. *Br. J. Plast. Surg.* **45**, 275–278.

Roberts A.H.N. (1984) Subungual melanoma following a single injury. *J. Hand Surg.* **9B**, 328–330.

Shah M.P. & Goldsmith H.S. (1971) Malignant melanoma in the North American Negro. *Surg. Gynecol. Obstet.* **133**, 437–439.

Shelley W.B., Rawnsley H.M. & Pillsbury D.M. (1964) Post-irradiation melanonychia. *Arch. Dermatol.* **90**, 174–176.

Shukla V.K. & Hughes L.E. (1989) Differential diagnosis of subungual melanoma from a surgical point of view. *Br. J. Surg.* **76**, 1156–1160.

Sondergaard K. & Tejan J. (1990) Subungual amelanotic melanoma: diagnostic pitfall. *Postgrad. Med. J.* **66**, 200–202.

Soyer H.P. & Kerl H. (1984) Congenital blue naevus with lymph node metastases and Klippel–Trenaunay syndrome. European Society of Pediatric Dermatology. Clinical case reports. *Dia-Klinik*, pp. 28–29.

Takahashi M. & Seiji M. (1983) Acral melanoma in Japan. *Pigment Cell* **6**, 150–166.

Takematsu H., Obata M., Tomita Y. *et al.* (1984) Subungual melanoma. A clinicopathological study of 16 Japanese cases. *Cancer* **55**, 2725.

Tosti A., Baran R., Marelli R. *et al.* (1994) Progressive fading of longitudinal melanonychia due to a nail matrix naevus in a child. *Arch. Dermatol.* (in press).

Trau H., Kopf A.W., Rigel D.S. *et al.* (1983) Regression in malignant melanoma. *J. Am. Acad. Dermatol.* **8**, 363–368.

Winslet M. & Tejan J. (1990) Subungual amelanotic melanoma: diagnostic pitfall. *Postgrad. Med. J.* **66**, 200–202.

Wong D.E., Brodkin R., Rickert R. & McFalls S.G. (1991) Congenital melanonychia. *Int. J. Dermatol.* **30**, 278–280.

Index

Page numbers in *italic* refer to figures and tables

absence of middle phalanges with hypoplastic nails *320*
acanthosis nigricans 200, 232, *332*, *339*
acetanilid 246
acetonitrile 291
acid burns 414
acquired immune deficiency syndrome *see* AIDS
acral arteriolar ectasia 94
acral dermatitis, psoriasis mimicry 143–4
acral pansclerotic morphoea 214
acral pseudolymphomatous angiokeratoma of children (APACHE) 453
acral pustular psoriasis 144–5
acral pustulosis
  acute 145–6
  differential diagnosis 145–6
acral skin necrosis 247
Acremonium spp 101, 102
acrocephalosyndactyly *326*
acrocyanosis 181, *182*
  cold haemagglutinin disease 179
  erythromelalgia 183
acrodermatitis enteropathica 195, *332*, *339*
acrodysostosis *326*
acrogeria *320*
acrokeratoelastoidosis 172
acrokeratosis paraneoplastica 143, 229–30
acrokeratosis verruciformis 167–9, *331*
acrolentiginous melanoma 492, 493, 494
acromegaly 197
acroosteolysis 37, 38, *129*, 170–1, *172*
  familial 171
  hyperparathyroidism 198
  idiopathic 171
  longitudinal 171
  neurosensory loss 171
  occupational *276*
  with osteoporosis *325*
  pseudoxanthoma elasticum 179
  radionecrosis 171
  transverse 171
acropachy 35
acropachydermodactyly, psoriatic 146–7
acroparaesthesia 171
acropustulosis
  oil patches 139
  psoriasis 143, 144–5
acrorenal-ocular syndrome 191
acrosclerosis *180*, *181*, 264
acrylic materials 267
  nail preparation 279
  nail sculpturing 291
  photopolymerizable resin 267
  premixed gels 291
  UV curable monomers 275
actinic keratosis 430
acyclovir 125
adipose genital syndrome 196
adrenal disease 197
adrenocorticotrophic hormone (ACTH) 253
adriamycin *255*, 257
ADULT syndrome *307*
adult T-cell leukaemia *235*
advancement flaps 378, *379*, 381, *382*
AEC syndrome 302, *307*
AIDS 223–4
  congenital malformations 330
  disseminated lichenoid papular dermatosis 156
  fluconazole use 116
  Kaposi's sarcoma 458
  longitudinal melanonychia 488
  psoriasis 142
  scabies 132
  total nail dystrophy 106
ainhum *185*
albendazole 134
alcoholism 330
algodystrophy *see* reflex sympathetic dystrophy
alkalis 270
  burns 414
alkaptonuria 201
allergic contact dermatitis *see* dermatitis
alopecia areata 52, *164*, 165–7
  hair regrowth 167
  leuconychia 78
  nail biopsy 166
  nail fragility 62
  pits 135
  surface alterations 165
  twenty-nail dystrophy 53, 166
  twenty-nail dystrophy of childhood 91, 92
alopecia mucinosa *see* follicular mucinosis
alopecia universalis, onychodystrophy and total vitiligo 166
alstroemeria 266
aluminium 4
  nail composition 81
  preterm infant nail content 30
aluminium chloride 63
aminoethylethanolamine-containing soldering flux 272
aminogenic alopecia deficiency *339*
ammoniated mercury ointment 281
amodiaquine 251
amorolfine 114
amphotericin B 119
amputation 372
  traumatic fingertip 380–1, *382*
amrinone 247
amyloidosis 203–4, *332*
  macular *341*
anaemia 78, 226
  iron-deficiency 196
  pernicious *333*
  sickle cell 226
anaesthesia 346–52
  agents 347
  bloodless field technique 351
  central local distal digital 347–8
  digital nerve block 348
  digital sites *349*
  general 352
  intravenous regional anaesthesia 351–2
  median nerve block 349
  metacarpal block 348
  peripheral nerve block 347–9
  radial nerve block 350
  regional 349–52
  toe nerve blocks 350, *351*
  transthecal digital block 348–9
  ulnar nerve block 349–50
  wing block 347, *348*
  wrist block 349–50
androgens 252
aneurysm, clubbing 177
aneurysmal bone cyst 451
angiokeratoma circumscriptum 450
angioleiomyoma 457–8
angioma *333*
angiosarcoma, subungual 458
anhidrotic and hypohidrotic ectodermal dysplasias 302, *307*
aniline 251
anonychia 45–6, 297–9
  atrophica 46
  isolated 298
  nail sculpturing *290*, 291
  with other symptoms 297–9
  pseudo-amputee appearance *299*
  self-inflicted 391
ANOTHER syndrome *307*
annular constriction *see* pseudo-ainhum
anti-inflammatory agents 246
antibiotics, high-risk patients 411–12
antibody 34βE12 8
antibody HHF35 9
anticoagulants 251
anticonvulsant drugs 239
antifungal agents
  oral 115–16
  topical 117
antifungal therapy 31
antihistamines 259
antimalarial agents *68*, 251–2
antimicrobial agents 243–5
antimycotics 32
antirheumatic drugs *69*
aortic regurgitation 177
aphalangia, congenital 44
apical dysplasia of fingers *309*
apical epidermal ridge (AER) 4
aplasia cutis *332*
  congenita *309*
  with dystrophic nails *309*
AREDYLD syndrome *307*
argon laser 420
argyria 249, *250*
arsenic 248–9, 272
  occupational poisoning 279
  poisoning 76
arsenical keratoses 430
arterial catheters, splinter haemorrhages 184
arterial obliteration, periungual tissues 178
arteriovenous fistula 448, *450*, 451
  distal phalanx 451

arteriovenous tumours 450–1
arthritis
  degenerative 95
  psoriatic 146
arthrospores, onychomycosis 106
artificial nails 267, 268
  preformed 291
  traumatic nail dystrophy 386
Aspergillus spp 101, 102, 106
  itraconazole 116
aspirin 246
asthma 188
atrichia with nail dystrophy *309*
atrophic nails, occupational *276*, *278*
avulsion, traumatic *375–7*
azathioprine *255*
azidothymidine 224, 245
azotaemia 190
AZT *see* azidothymidine

B27 antigens 147
β-blockers 246–7
  gangrene 179
  psoriasis exacerbation 142
Bacillus fragilis 84
bacterial endocarditis
  petechiae 177
  splinter haemorrhages 184
bacterial infections
  infants 84
  occupational 272–4
Bacteroides 84
Bamberger–Pierre–Marie syndrome *see* hypertrophic osteoarthropathy, pulmonary
Bantu porphyria 202
Barfod's technique 413
basal cell carcinoma 437
Bazex syndrome 229
Beau's lines 50–1
  acrokeratosis paraneoplastica 230
  AIDS 224
  alopecia areata 165, 166
  bullous pemphigoid 162
  cancer chemotherapy 83, 254
  cardiac disorders 178
  drug-induced erythroderma 239
  exposure to abnormal cold 182
  febrile illness 225
  gastrointestinal disorders 193
  hypoparathyroidism 197
  infants 83
  latent onychomadesis *57*
  leprosy 128
  malaria 225
  menstrual cycle relationship 199
  nail growth interference *27*
  nail volume measurement 26, *27*
  pemphigus 163
  syphilis 127
beautification of nails 285
Behçet's disease 223
belt buckle patina 272
benoxaprofen 246
benzodiazepines 239
benzophenone-2 281, 293
Berk–Tabatznik syndrome *326*
bifonazole 117, 118, 119
big toenail
  avulsion 398
  fungal infection 96
  mould infection 96
biliary cirrhosis 192
biopsy of nail area 5, 352–63
  bands 3–6 mm wide 361–2
  double punch technique *353*
  en bloc excision 362
  examination 363
  lateral longitudinal *355*, *358*, 358
  lateral third of nail plate 358
  limitations *354*
  longitudinal 6, 17, *353*, 355
  longitudinal melanonychia 357
  metastases 482
  methods *357–62*
  midportion 358, *359*
  nail matrix–nail bed *355*, *358*
  neonatal anabolic disorders 81
  periungual pigmentation *357*, 358
  proximal nail fold *355–6*
  punch 354, 360, 362
  releasing flap method 361
  specimens 363
  stage method 360–1
  techniques *353–6*
  thin band *359–61*
  transverse elliptical excision 361, 362
  transverse matrix *353*, *355*
  treatment after 362–3
  tumours 415
biotin 260
black disease 131
black foot disease 249
blancophore fluorochromatin 5–6
Blaschko's lines, pigmentation 424
blastomycosis, primary cutaneous 275
bleeding
  post-operative 406
  surgical complication 406
bleomycin 253, 254, *255*, 257, 420
blistering diseases, neonates 83
blistering distal dactylitis (BDD) 90–1
Bloch–Sulzberger syndrome 424
blood dyscrasias, nail colour modification 72
blood groups 226
  essential thrombocythaemia 226
  haemoglobinopathies 226
  polycythaemia 226
blue digit syndrome 178
blue naevus *489*
blue rubber bleb naevi *452*, 457
bone
  abnormalities 4
  relationship with nail 4
  solitary cyst 470
Bose's technique 401
Bourneville–Pringle disease 438
Bowen's disease 32, 96, 431–5, 440
  human papilloma virus 435
  periungual involvement 432
  subungual involvement 432–3
brachydactylia 43
brachydactyly
  anonychia 298
  with nail dysplasia *320*
  pseudohypoparathyroidism 198
brachymorphism-onychodysplasia-dysphalingism syndrome *320*
brachyonychia 42
bradydactyly 298
Brazilian pemphigus foliaceus 163
breast cancer, androgen therapy 252
breast carcinoma 233
brittle nails 61–2
  gastrointestinal disorders 193
  haemodialysis 189
  hypoparathyroidism 197
  occupational *276*
  swelling factor 63
broad nails
  hereditary *326–7*
  pseudoclubbing 327
5-bromodeoxyuridine *255*
bronchial carcinoma 188
  metastases 482
bronchial tumours 229
bronchiectasis 38, 187
bryozoans 269
Buerger's disease 178
bulla
  repens 407
  rodens 407
  traumatic 391
bullous dermatosis of haemodialysis 189
bullous lesions
  self-inflicted 83
  zinc deficiency 195
bullous pemphigoid *161*, 162–3
Bunell's technique 408
Bureau–Barriere's non-familial mutilant ulcer acropathy 206
burns 264, *412*, 413
  chemical 413–14
buspirone 240

C3 163
cachexia 196
cadavers, nail growth 27–8
cadmium 30
calcification, subungual 479
calcinosis cutis circumscripta 479
calcium
  channel blockers 247
  hyperparathyroidism 197, 198
  nail content 62
  oxalate 479
calculi, cutaneous 479
cancer chemotherapeutic agents 253–5, *256*, 257
cancer chemotherapy, Beau's lines 83
Candida infection 64, 65, 98
  bacterial involvement 113
  chronic fungal paronychia 112, 113
  congenital malformations 330
  Darier's disease 168
  diabetes 199
  DLSO 101
  histopathology *110*
  immunodeficiency 221
  infant 84–5
  itraconazole 116
  ketoconazole 115
  kidney transplant recipients 190
  laboratory culture 107
  occupational 275
  onycholysis 58
  onychomycosis 100–1, 119–20
  parathyroid disease 197
  paronychia 85, 104
  SWO 102
  TDO 104, *105*, *106*
  thumb sucking 85
  see also chronic mucocutaneous candidiasis (CMC)
cantharidin 420
cantharone 420
capillaroscopes 210
capillary
  acquired subungual angioma 450
  malformations 448
  microscopy 210–12
captopril 247
carbamazepine 330
carbocaine 347
carbon monoxide 248
carcinoid tumours 229
carcinoma
  cuniculatum 436
  in situ 32
  of nail apparatus 96
cardiac disorders 176–7
  bacterial endocarditis 177, *178*
cardiac failure, lunula effects 177
cardiovascular drugs 246–7
carotene 259
carpal tunnel syndrome 51, 207
  vibrating power tools 266
cartilage–hair hypoplasia *325*

Castelman tumour 233
causalgia 208
CD1-antigen 229
CD4/CD8 in APACHE syndrome 453
cement dermatitis 269, *270*
central nervous system acting drugs 239–40
cephalexin 89, 114, 244
cephaloridine 244
cephalosporin 244
cerebral gigantism 197
cervical rib syndrome 207
chancre 127
CHANDS syndrome *309*
CHARGE association *320*
chemicals
  discolouration of nails 65
  irritants 270–2, 280
  nail damage 62
  sensitizers 279–80
chemotherapy, uraemic half-and-half nail 77
chilblains *see* perniosis
CHILD syndrome 142
children
  blistering distal dactylitis (BDD) 90–1
  impetigo 89–90
  nail composition 81–2
  toxic shock syndrome 91
  twenty-nail dystrophy 91–2
chlorambucil 235
chloramphenicol 244
chloride 30
chlorine 81
chloroform 134
chloroquine 31, 251, 252
cholesterol 29
  microemboli 178
  sulphate 30
chondrodysplasia
  punctata *309*
  X-linked dominant 54
chondroectodermal dysplasia *307*
chondroitin sulphate 9
chondroma 467
  subungual 468
chondrosarcoma 467, 473
  metastases *481*
Christ–Siemens–Touraine syndrome 302, *307*
chromium salts 251
chromoblastomycosis 123
chromonychia 63–4
  alopecia areata 166
  psoriasis 139
chromosome
  anomalies *319*
  localization 317, *318*
chronic lymphocytic leukaemia 234–5, 235
chronic mucocutaneous candidiasis (CMC) *110*, 119, 120, 221
  HIV infection 223
  hypoparathyroidism 198
  total dystrophic onychomycosis (TDO) 104, *105*, *106*
cicatricial pemphigoid 162
ciclopirox 114
cicloproxolamine 117
cigarette smokers 280
circulation disorders 178–85
  acrocyanosis 181
  cutaneous reactions to cold 182
  erythromelalgia 183
  perniosis 182
  Raynaud's disease/phenomenon 180–1
  splinter haemorrhages 183–4
  venous ischaemia 183
circumferential nail 43, 328
cirrhosis 191–2
  nail mineral content 30
  Terry's nail 77
cirsoid aneurysm 450, *451*
citrullinemia *339*
claw-like nail 43
claws 20, 21
cleido-cranial dysostosis *325*
clindamycin 86
clobetasol propionate cream 420
clofazimine 244
clonidine 247
Clostridium tetani 272, 414
clotrimazole 86, 117
cloxacillin 244
clubbing 35–8, 198
  acropachy, hippocratic nails 324
  AIDS 223
  aneurysm 177
  asthma 188
  asymmetric 36
  chronic mucocutaneous candidiasis (CMC) 104
  cirrhosis 191
  classification *38*
  congenital 36
  congenital cardiovascular diseases 176–7
  congenital heart disease *180*
  and cyanosis 176, 177
  diabetes 200
  diffuse chronic sarcoidosis 188
  familial 36
  gastrointestinal disorders 193
  hereditary *325*
  hypertrophic osteoarthropathy 37–8
  hypertrophic pulmonary osteoarthropathy 185
  laxative abuse 210
  lung neoplasm 231
  lupus erythematosus 164
  nail curvature 35
  neonates 82
  nerve damage 207
  neurovascular pathology 17
  pachydermoperiostosis 37–8
  pneumoconiotic lung disease 275
  purgative abuse 248
  radiological changes 36
  Raynaud's phenomenon *176*
  shell nail syndrome 38
  simple type 35–7
  stages 35
  ulcerative colitis 193–4
  vasodilatation 37
  venous stasis 183
CO_2 laser
  haemostasis 366
  onychogryphosis 394
  scarring 369
  uses 366
  warts 420
coal spots 264
Coat's syndrome *333*
cocaine 240
coccidomycosis 123
Cockayne–Touraine syndrome *335*
codeine 266–7
coffee plantation workers 275
Coffin–Siris syndrome 299, *307*
cold
  cutaneous reactions 182
  epiphyseal destruction in children 182
  haemagglutinin disease 179
  occupational injury 264
  perniosis 182
collagen disease 180, 210
collagen VII 9
collagenoma, circumscribed storiform 439
colour modification 63–4
  causes 64, *66–71*, *72*, *73*
  chemicals *69–70*
  cosmetics 67
  fungal *68*
  physical agents *67*
  systemic conditions 65–6, *72*, *73*
  tobacco *67*
  topical therapeutic agents 66
  traumatic causes *67*
  variations in elderly 94
  see also dyschromia; hyperpigmentation; pigmentation
concanavalin A 110
confidence 285
congenital anonychia 396
  phenytoin-induced 4
congenital disorders 4, 396–7
congenital erythropoietic porphyria 202
congenital hemidysplasia with ichthyosiform erythroderma and limb defects (CHILD syndrome) *320*
congenital hypertrophic lip of hallux 404
congenital hypoparathyroidism *308*
congenital insensitivity to pain 171, 206, *339*
  self-inflicted trauma 390
congenital malalignment of big toenail 88–9
congenital malformations
  drug-induced 330
  infection-induced 330
congenital naevus *485*, 488, 492
  pigmented *332*
congenital onychodysplasia
  digital ischaemia 17
  of the index fingers (COIF) 4, 299, 317, *320*, *321*, *322*, *323*
conidia, onychomycosis 106
connective tissue diseases 17, 210
  dermatomyositis 216, *217*
  fibroblastic rheumatism 220–1
  follicular mucinosis 220
  microscopic polyarteritis 219
  multicentric reticulohistocytosis 219–20
  osteoarthritis 221
  periarteritis nodosa 219
  rheumatoid arthritis 217–18
  systemic lupus erythematosus 215
  systemic sclerosis 213–14
  Wegener's granulomatosis 219
connective tissue naevus, cerebriform 446, *447*
contact dermatitis *see* dermatitis
copper 30
  acetate 272
  children's nail composition 81
  Wilson's disease 192
corn *see* heloma, subungual
corneocytes 14, 15, 62
cortical diaphysis, irregular thickening 36
corticosteroids
  eczema treatment 152
  topical psoriasis therapy 141
cortisone 253
cosmetic industry 285
  product experience reports 294
cosmetics
  adverse reactions 295
  hypoallergenic 294
Cowden's disease 234, 439, 444
craniofrontal dysplasia *320*
  nasal 299
CREST syndrome 192
  capillary changes 211
Crohn's disease 194–5, 222
Cronkhite–Canada syndrome 194
Crow–Fukase syndrome *see* POEMS syndrome
crush injury 372
  fractures 377–8
cryoglobulinaemia 228
cryosurgery 364–5
  warts 420
cryotherapy 264
Curth's modified profile sign 35–6

curved nail of the fourth toe 328
Cushing's syndrome 101, 197
cutaneous horns, actinic keratosis 430
cuticle 1, 2, 15
  remover 286, 293
  thickened 60
cyanoacrylate glue 279
  nail mending 289
  nail wrapping 290
cyanosis
  acral 177, *178*
  cholesterol microemboli 178
  congenital cardiovascular diseases 176
  digital 179
  lunula 226
  Raynaud's disease 180
cyclophosphamide 253, *255*
cyclosporin 259
  systemic psoriasis therapy 142
  topical psoriasis therapy 142
cystic fibrosis 30, 200
  nail composition 81, 185
cystine 62, 260
  nail content in koilonychia 40
cytochrome P450 115
cytosine arabinoside *255*, *257*

dacarbazine 253, *255*
dancers 266
dapsone 87, 245
Darier's disease 167–9
  acrokeratitis verruciformis 168
  congenital nail discolouration *332*
  dermatophyte infections 111
  leuconychia 78
  lines 167, *168*
  longitudinal leuconychia 76
  nail plate thickening 167
  recurrent pyoderma 169
  secondary infection 167–8
  subungual hyperkeratosis 60
daunorubicin 253, *255*
DDT 134
deafness, onychoosteodystrophy and mental retardation (DOOR) syndrome 298–9
dental personnel 267
dentooculocutaneous syndrome *308*
depilatories 280
dermatitis 52
  allergic contact 269, 279
  atopic 221
  contact 267, 293–4
  finger pulp 269
  hyponychial 143
  lichenoid 224
  rhus 266
  spongiotic 152, 166
  X-ray 264
dermatofibroma 437
  fibrous 442, 444
dermatofibrosarcoma protruberans 448
dermatological conditions
  nail colour effects *71*
  psoriasis 135–47
dermatomyositis 210, 212, *213*, 216, *217*, 229
dermatopathia pigmentosa reticularis *303*
dermatophyte infections
  DLSO 100
  nail colour 64–5
  occupational of toenails 275
  onycholysis 58
dermatophytosis, dry type 116
dermis layer 8
dermojet steroid injection 253
desmin 9
desmosomes 8
detergents 270
diabetes 199–200, *339*
  onychogryphosis risk 393
  patient management 411–12
diabetes mellitus 30, 199
  paronychia of toenails 113
diabetic neuropathy 30
  acroosteolysis 171
diabetic retinopathy 30
Diamond syndrome 198
diaphysial aclasis *see* multiple exostoses syndrome (MES)
dicyanide derivatives 269
digital arteriovenous malformation 451
digital ischaemia 178, 232
  acute 178
  chronic of lower limbs 178
  congenital onychodysplasias 17
digital necrosis 210
  occult neoplasm 232
  Raynaud's phenomenon 180
dimercaptosuccinic acid 259
dimethacrylates 267
dinitroorthocresol 272
dinobuton 272
diphenciprone 420
diphtheria, cutaneous 226
diquat 272
discoid lupus erythematosus 163–5, 211–12, *213*
disease
  loci 317
  prognostication by nail analysis 30
dishwashers 266
dishydrosis, leuconychia 78
disseminated intravascular coagulation 178–9
disseminated lichenoid papular dermatosis 156
distal finger lesions, dorsal exposure 364
distal groove 2, 3
distal and lateral subungual onychomycosis (DLSO) 98–102
  causes *110*
  dermatophyte infections 100
  discolouration 101
  epidermization of nail bed 110–11
  histopathology *108*, *109*
  non-dermatophyte moulds 119
  opaque streaks 98
  oral therapy 119
  primary 98–101
  secondary to onycholysis 101–2
  Trichophyton rubrum 99
  urea treatment 118
distal nail embedding 403–4, *405*
distal phalangeal bone, destructive changes 170
distal phalanx duplication 44
diuretics 259
dolichonychia 42
DOOR syndrome *309*
dorsal digital arteries 16
dorsal matrix 6, 23
dorsal nail apparatus 2
dorsal nail fold arch 16
double-edged nail 210
dressings, surgical 352, 362–3, 406
drug penetration 32
Dufourmentel's hands 386
dwarfism
  nanocephalic *326*
  short-limbed 221
dwarfism–brachydactyly syndrome *326*
dyscephalic-mandibulo-oculofacial syndrome of Hallerman–Streiff–Francois 299
dyschondroplasia with multiple soft tissue haemangiomas 467–8
dyschromia 63–4
  congenital/hereditary 330, *331–3*
  nail care products 293
  occupational 275, 277, 278, 279
  porphyria 202
  white nails 71
  see also colour modification; hyperpigmentation; pigmentation
dyskeratosis congenita 62, *303*, 312
dyslipoproteinaemia 200
dystelephalangy *325*

E-keratins 3
  nail plate 19, 29
eccrine poroma 421, *422*
  malignant 438
ectodermal dysplasia
  with abnormal papillar ridging *310*, *310*
  with hair and/or skin changes *309–11*
  with nail and teeth changes *307–9*
  with onychogryphosis *310*
  see also hereditary ectodermal dysplasia
ectopic nails 328–9
ectrodactyly–clefting (EEC) syndrome 302, *303*
eczema 151–2
  buckled nail 111
  hypertrophy of nail 46
  latent onychomadesis 51
  nail formation effects 62
  staphylococcal growth 113
  subungual hyperkeratosis 60
ED-AOHD syndrome *303*
eggshell nail, vitamin A deficiency 195
Ehlers-Danlos syndrome 42
Eikenella corrodens 86
electroradiosurgery 365
elkonyxis 54
embryology 297
embryopathies 297
emetine 245
enchondroma *462*, *466*, 467
  malignant transformation 473
enchondromatosis 467
endocrine disorders
  adrenal disease 197
  hypogonadism 196
  menstrual factors 199
  parathyroid disease 197–8
  pituitary disease 197
  pregnancy 199
  thyroid disease 198
enzyme detergent 280
epidemic encephalitis 209
epidermal naevus *332*
  syndrome 425
  verruciform xanthoma 480
epidermis 2
  nail bed 11
epidermis bullosa, disease types *337–8*
epidermoid carcinoma, subungual 96
epidermoid carcinoma of nail apparatus 431–5
  aetiology 434
  diagnosis 434
  treatment 435
epidermoid cysts *462*, *466*
  implantation 407, 426–7
  intraosseous 426–7
  orthokeratin containing 427, *428*
  post-operative 426, *427*
epidermoid inclusions, subungual 428
epidermolysis bullosa
  acquisita (EBA) 87
  atrophicans *336*
  dystrophica *335*, *336*
  infants/neonates 86–7
Epidermophyton floccosum 101, 103, *107*
epilepsy 209
epiloia 43, 438
epithelial keratins *see* E-keratins
epithelioma cuniculatum 435–6

epithelium, thickness 7
epitheloid haemangioma 452
epitheloid leiomyosarcoma 472–3
eponychium 15
  hyperkeratotic 111
epoxy resin 267–8, *278*
ergotamine 259–60
  gangrene 179
erysipeloid 272
erythema
  elevatum diutinum 173, 470, *471*
  multiforme *see* Stevens–Johnson syndrome
  periungual 199
erythroderma, drug-induced *52*, 239
erythromelalgia 183
erythromycin 89
erythropoietic protoporphyria *332*
escavenitis 269
ethyl methacrylate 291
ethyl-cyanoacrylate-containing glue 267
etoposide 253, *255*
etretinate
  acrokeratosis paraneoplastica treatment 230
  keratosis lichenoides chronica 162
  nail changes *241*
  palmoplantar keratoderma treatment 173
eunuchoidism 42, 46
  onychauxis 196
Ewing's sarcoma 473
exostosis *462*, 463–5, *466*
  classification 463–4
  multiple 465–7
  radiology *464*
  subungual 393
eyedrops 269

Fabry's disease 201
false nails 279
familial hypercholesterolaemia 200
farmyard pox 275
FDA, complaints handling 294–5
fetal alcohol syndrome 196
fibre glass, nail wrapping 290
fibroblastic rheumatism 220–1
fibroblasts, infantile digital fibromatosis 446
fibrokeratoma 356, 437, 438
  acquired 439, 440–1
  hereditary 439, 444
  invaginated 441
  subungual *440*
fibroma
  osteoid 444
  plexiform 442
  subungual 439
  ungual 205
  ungual true 442, *443*, 444
fibromatosis 445–8
fibronectin 9
fibrosarcoma 473
fibrous dermatofibroma 442, 444
fibrous histiocytoma 444
filaggrin 436
filamentous tumour, subungual 441
finger
  arterial supply 16
  arteritis 178
  vascular supply alteration 17
  venous drainage 17
  see also clubbing
fishermen 269
flexibility measurement 32
flexometer 32
fluconazole 116
fluorescent substances 249
fluorine 260
fluorouracil 145
  topical psoriasis therapy 141
5-fluoruracil 255, *256*, 257

focal dermal hypoplasia *303*, *310*
follicular mucinosis 220
food allergy 269
foreign bodies 378–9, *380*
formaldehyde 134, 268, 271–2
  nail hardeners 280, 289–90
Freer septum elevator 369, *370*
friable nails 61–2
friction 265
Fried's tooth and nail syndrome *308*
Frisbee nail 390
frontometaphyseal dysplasia *320*
frostbite 182, 264
fructose–lysine 30, 199
Fryns syndrome *320*
fucosidosis 202
fungal hyphae, onychomycosis 106
fungal infection 275
  discolouration of nails 64–5
  elderly 94, 96
  friable nails 62
  infants 84–5
  nail plate 13
  nail removal 116, 117
  oral agents 115–16
  sporotrichosis 122–3
  urea chemical treatment 116–18, 119
  see also onychomycosis
furosine 30, 199
Fusarium, chronic paronychia 113, 114
F. oxysporum 102
Fusibacterium 84

gamma heavy chain disease 228
gangrene 178, 184
  cholesterol microemboli 178
  diabetic foot 199
  digital 179
  erythromelalgia 183
  frostbite 182
  mercury toxicity 250
  peripheral 179
  phlyctenular 17
  systemic lupus erythematosus 215
  systemic scleroderma 213
  venous thrombosis 179
garlic-clove fibroma 439, 440
gastrointestinal disorders 193
  clubbing 193
  Crohn's disease 194–5
  Cronkhite-Canada syndrome 194
  Peutz–Jeghers–Touraine syndrome 194
  Plummer–Vinson syndrome 194
  ulcerative colitis 193–4
gelatin 260
gestational age assessment 82
giant cell
  tumour 470–1
  xanthomatous sarcoma 472, 473
gingival fibromatosis *339*
glass fibre 265
glioma *461*, 462
glomus bodies 9, 18
glomus tumour 415, 453–5, *456*, *457*
  immunohistochemistry 454–5
  radiology 33
  surgery 455, *457*
  ultrasound 33
glossopalatine ankylosis syndrome 299
gloves 281
  materials *280*
glucagonoma syndrome 229, 231
glutathione 195
glycoprotein 58
gold 250
  potassium cyanide 270
Goltz and Gorlin syndrome *303*
gonorrhoea 126–7
  primary cutaneous 125

  primary extragenital cutaneous 127
gorillas, oblique nail lines 21
Gottron's papules 216, *217*
gout 201
graft-versus-host disease 156, 214, 222
  yellow nail syndrome 186
grafting 375–6
  burns 413
  composite *378*
  congenital absence of nail 396
  free nail 377
  microsurgery for whole nail 386
  pachyonychia congenita 396
  scars 378
  split-thickness nail bed 383
granular cell tumour *460*, 461
  malignant *460*, 461–2
granulation of nail keratin 293
granuloma annulare 173, 470, *471*
Graves' disease 198
green nail syndrome 272
Greig cephalopolysyndactyly syndrome *326*
griseofulvin 110, 114, 115
grooming 285
gummata 128
Gunther's disease *see* congenital erythropoietic porphyria
Günther's syndrome *332*

Ha-1 8
habit-tic deformity 51
haemangioendothelioma 473–4
  malignant 458
haemangioma 448
  epitheloid 452
  histiocytoid 452
  multiple soft tissue with dyschondroplasia 467–8
  sclerosing 442
haemangiosarcoma 473–4
haematological disorders
  anaemias 226
  blood groups 226
  cryoglobulinaemia 228
  gamma heavy chain disease 228
  hereditary haemorrhagic telangiectasia 227
haematoma 372–3
  non-migrating subungual 391
  subungual 63, *485*, 493
haemochromatosis 40, 192, *331*
haemodialysis 189
  nail–patella syndrome 191
haemoglobinopathies 226
haemorrhage, nail bed 372
haemorrhage, subungual 390–1
  cystic fibrosis 200
  gastrointestinal disorders 193
  occupational 266
haemosiderin 63, 238
haemostasis, surgery 366, 406
Hailey–Hailey disease 169
  leuconychia 78
hair
  follicle 19–20
  splinters 265
  subungual *278*
hair follicle/nail unit homology *20*
hair–nail dysplasia *310*
hairdresser 265, 269, *278*
hairspray 280
hairy elbows syndrome *320*
half-and-half nails 190–1
Hallopeau–Siemens syndrome *335*
hallux, congenital hypertrophic lip 87
hallux valgus 394–5
  elderly 93, 94–5
haloprogin 117
Hand–Schuller–Christian disease 228
hangnail 60, 407

hapalonychia 61
hard nails 61
Hartnup disease 200
Hay–Wells syndrome *309*
hazards, non-occupational 279
  chemical irritants 280
  chemical sensitizers 279–80
  physical 279
  see also occupational hazards
heart disease, congenital *333*
heavy bag lifting *265*
heavy metal intoxication 248–51
Heberden's nodes 95, 221, 474
heloma 392, *393*
  subungual *95*
hemidesmosomes 8
hemionychogryphosis 23, 47–8
hemiplegia 206
Hendersonula toruloidea 98, 101
  chronic paronychia 113, *114*
  occupational infection 275
  onychomycosis 119
henna hair dye 280
Henoch–Schönlein purpura 191
heparin 251
hepatic disorders 191
  cirrhosis 191–2
  haemochromatosis 192
  Wilson's disease 192
hepatitis 115
hepatoerythropoietic porphyria 203
hepatolenticular degeneration 81, 192, *333*
hereditary disorders 297, 396–7
  anonychia 297
  clubbing of digits *325*
  haemorrhagic telangiectasia 227
  with nail involvement *340–1*
  nail–patella syndrome 299–300
  osteoonychodysplasia (HOOD) *see* nail–patella syndrome
  secondary nail changes 338, *339–40*
hereditary ectodermal dysplasias (HED) 301–2
  anhidrotic and hypohidrotic 302
  clubbing, acropachy, hippocratic nails 324
  hyperonychia, hyperplastic thick nails 323–4
  hypohidrotic 312
  with keratoderma palmoplantare and nail changes *303–7*
  metastases in Bowen's disease 433
  pachyonychia congenita 302, 311
  syndromes *332*
  trichothiodystrophy 312–13
  see also ectodermal dysplasia
heredofamilial amyloid polyneuropathy 204
herpes simplex infection 123, *124*, 125
  AIDS 223
  autoinoculation 123
  diagnosis 123, 125
  distal digital 123
  occupational hazards 275
  thumb sucking association 85–6
herpes zoster infection 125, 126
herpetic whitlow 86
  AIDS 223
  recurrent 123
hexadecanoic acid octadecyl ester 146
hidrotic ectodermal dysplasia 301, *302*, *303*
high-risk patients 411–12
hippocratic digits *see* clubbing
histidinaemia 200
histiocytic processes 480–1
histiocytoid haemangioma 452
histiocytosis X 228
HLA-A2 147
HLA-A3 154
HLA-A5 154
HLA-B7 154
Hodgkin's disease 237
homocystinuria 202
homografts 375
hooked nail 386–7
hooves 20, 21
hormones, therapeutic 252–3
HTLV-1 positive cutaneous T-cell lymphoma 237
human immunodeficiency virus (HIV) 85, 223–4
  SWO 102
  yellow nail syndrome 186
human papilloma virus 418
  Bowen's disease 435
  epidermoid carcinoma 434
  squamous cell carcinoma 434
Hutchinson's melanotic whitlow 494
Hutchinson's sign 357, 487, 492, 495
hyacinth bulbs *265*
hyalin bodies 164
hydantoin 330
hydrangea 266
hydrofluoric acid 270–1
  burns *413*, 414
hydroquinone 260
hydroxylamine 268
5-hydroxytryptamine antagonist 181
hydroxyurea 253, *256*
hyper- and hypopigmentation with dystrophic nails *304*
hyper–IgE syndrome 221, *339*
hyperbilirubinaemia 191
hypercholesterolaemic xanthomatosis 480
hyperglycaemia, diabetic 199
hyperhidrosis of hands and feet 397
hyperkeratosis 15
  eccentrica atrophicans *see* porokeratosis, of Mibelli
  fungal infection 96
  parakeratosis pustulosa 153
  periungual 393, *394*
  traumatic 392–3
hyperkeratosis, subungual 22, 59–60, 392–3
  acrocyanosis 181
  Darier's disease 167, *168*
  isolated *131*
  lichen planus 155
  lupus erythematosus 164
  pemphigus 163
  pityriasis rubra pilaris 150
  psoriasis *136*, 139
  psoriasis mimicry 143
  punctate keratoderma 173
hyperkeratotic hypertrophy of periungual tissues *160*, 161–2
hyperkeratotic lesions, toes of elderly 94, 95
hyperlipoproteinaemia 200
hyperonychia, hyperplastic thick nails 323–4
hyperostosis 95
hyperoxaluria 200
  primary 179
hyperparathyroidism, bone resorption 42
hyperpigmentation
  AIDS 224
  antimalarial agents 251–2
  cancer chemotherapeutic agents 253–4
  hypotrichosis and dystrophy of nails *304*
  palmoplantar keratosis and childhood blistering *304*
  pituitary disease 197
  pregnancy 199
  subungual lichen planus 155
  vitamin B_{12} deficiency 195
  see also colour modification; dyschromia; pigmentation
hyperthyroidism 198
hypertrophic osteoarthropathy
  confined to lower extremities 37
  pulmonary 37, 185
hypertrophy of the nail 46–8
hyperuricaemia 48, 201, *339*
hypoalbuminaemia 77, 188–9
hypocalcaemia 197
hypogammaglobulinaemia, congenital 221
hypogonadism 196
hypohidrotic ectodermal dysplasia 302, *308*, *311*
  with hypothyroidism *310*
hyponychium, 1, 2, 3, 10–11, 46
  cells 15
  crevice 11
  pityriasis rubra pilaris 150
  psoriasis mimicry by dermatitis 143
hypoparathyroidism 197
hypopituitarism 42, 197
hypoplastic nails 4
hypoplastic–enamel-onycholysis–hypohidrosis syndrome *304*
hypothyroidism 198
hypoxanthine-guanine phosphoribosyl-transferase deficiency 201

ibuprofen 246
ichthyosiform dermatosis with linear keratotic flexural papules *325*
ichthyosis
  dermatophyte infections 111
  follicularis with alopecia *310*
  onychogryphosis 47
  X-linked 30
ichthyosis follicularis-alopecia-photophobia syndrome *310*
idiopathic atrophy of the nails 157
ifosfamide *256*
IgA, bullous pemphigoid 161–2
IgG
  bullous pemphigoid 161–2
  pemphigus 163
IgM 163
ILVEN, verruciform xanthoma 480
imidazoles 114, 115
immunological disorders
  AIDS 223–4
  Behçet's disease 223
  graft-versus-host disease 222
  human immunodeficiency virus (HIV) 223–4
  primary deficiency syndromes 221
  therapeutic immunosuppression 222
  vitiligo 223
immunosuppression, therapeutic 222
impetigo 89–90
  bullous 89
  vesiculopustular 89
implantation epidermoid cyst 407, 426–7
incontinentia pigmenti *320*, *332*
  subungual keratotic tumours 424–5
infantile digital fibromatosis 445–6, *447*
infants
  bacterial infections 84
  Beau's line 83
  epidermolysis bullosa 86–7
  fungal infection 84–5
  impetigo 89–90
  ingrowing toenail 87–9
  koilonychia 82
infection
  subungual 411
  surgery 406–7
  see also Candida infection
infectious diseases 225
  cutaneous diphtheria 226
  malaria 225
inflammation, painful nail 414
inflammatory linear verrucous epidermal naevus (ILVEN) 159–60
infrared coagulation 420

ingrowing nail 41
  paronychia 410
ingrowing toenail
  blistering distal dactylitis 90–1
  clipping 402
  congenital hypertrophic lip of hallux 404
  congenital malalignment of big toenail 88–9, 404, *405*
  conservative treatment 398, 402
  distal embedding 87–8, 403–4, *405*
  elderly 94, *95*
  granulation stage 398
  grooving 402
  hypertrophic lateral nail fold 401
  infancy 87–9, 404–5
  inward distortion of nail plate 401–3
  phenolic treatment 399–400
  selective lateral matrix excision 400–1
  spinal cord injuries 2–6
  subcutaneous 398–401
  surgery 397–405
  surgical treatment 402–3
  susceptible groups 397
  terminal Syme operation 401
  toe-to-thumb transfer 407
  treatment in infancy 88
  types 398
injury classification 372
inoculation synovitis 379
intermediate matrix 7
  epithelium 7
  melanocyte activity 13
  rete ridges 7
intestinal leiomyosarcoma 233
intoxicants 248
  heavy metal 248–51
intrathoracic suppurative diseases 185
involucrin 9, 436
^{192}Ir exposure 431
iron 30
  fragile nails 63
  nail composition 62, 81
iron deficiency 40, 196
  koilonychia in infancy 82
ischaemic lesions, periungual 210
ischaemic necrosis 178–9
Iso–Kikuchi syndrome 23, 299
  hemionychogryphosis 48
  micronychia 44
  see also congenital onychodysplasia of the index fingers (COIF)
itraconazole 115–16, 119, 122

Jadassohn–Lewandowsky syndrome *see* pachyonychia congenita
Janeway lesions 177
jaundice 191
Job's syndrome 221
jogging 391
joint arthropathy *146*, 147
juvenile hyaline fibromatosis II 447–8
juvenile psoriatic arthritis 146
juvenile xanthogranuloma 229, 481

Kaposi's sarcoma 224, 458
Kashin–Beck disease 192
Kawasaki disease 225
keloid 445
keratin
  antibodies 8
  cysts 426–8
  fibre alteration in leuconychia 72
  granulation 293
  low sulphur 29
  nail content 62
  proximal nail fold 15
  structure change 62
  synthesis 3
keratin 1 8
keratin 7 8, 23
keratin 10 8
keratin 19 8–9
keratinocytes, Darier's disease 169
keratitis, ichthyosis and deafness *331*
keratoacanthoma 419, 422–4
  diagnosis 423
  trauma 423
  treatment 424
keratoderma
  with leuconychia totalis *305*
  palmoplantar 172, 301, *305–6*, *325*, *331*
  punctate 172–3
keratohyalin 150, 156, 157
keratosis
  actinic 430
  arsenical 430
  cristarum 60, 143
  distal subungual 441–2
  ichthyosis and deafness (KID) syndrome *304*
  lichenoides chronica *160*, 161–2
  punctata *57*
  subungual 93
ketanserin 18, 181
ketoconazole 114, 115, 119, 260
kindler's syndrome *306*
Kirschner wires 386
Klein's syndrome 299
Klippel–Trenaunay syndrome *333*, 448, *449*
Klippel–Trenaunay–Weber syndrome 43
knuckle pads 445, *446*
Koebner phenomenon 139, 140
  deep 144, 146
  rheumatoid arthritis 218
Koenen's tumour 205, 437, 438–9, 444, 480
koilonychia 39–40
  acroosteolysis 170
  at birth 3
  cardiac disorders 178
  classification *40*
  elderly 94
  haemochromatosis 192
  haemodialysis 189
  hereditary 328
  infants 40, 82
  neonates 82
  occupational *277*
  racial 40
  thyroid disease 198
Kutler V-Y advancement flap 378, *379*, 381
kwashiorkor 196

L-dopa 240
lacrimo-auriculo-dento-digital syndrome *304*
lamellar ichthyosis *306*
Langerhan's cells 8, 144
  histiocytosis 228–9
  papuloerythroderma 233
Larsen's syndrome *326*
larva migrans *133*, 134
laser
  doppler 34
  surgery 365–9, 420
lateral nail fold 1, 2, 15
  hypertrophic 401
lateral nail groove 2, 3
  loss in elderly 93
Laugier–Hunziker syndrome *484*, 488
  see also Laugier–Hunziker–Baran syndrome
Laugier–Hunziker–Baran syndrome 357, 485
lead 30, 250
  scalp lotion 281
lectitis purulenta et granulomatosa 58, 411
  oil patches 139
Leiner's disease 84
leiomyoma 445
  subungual 457, 458
leiomyosarcoma
  epitheloid 472–3
  intestinal 233
leishmaniasis *130*, 131, *273*
lentigo
  malignant melanoma 496
  simplex 491–2
leopard syndrome *331*
lepromatous leprosy 128, *129*, 130
  acroosteolysis 171
  clofazimine 244
  dapsone 245
leprosy 128, *129*, 130
  leuconychia 78
  neurological involvement 206
Lesch–Nyhan syndrome 201, 204, 207, *339*
  self-inflicted trauma 390
lethal syndrome with cloudy cornea, diaphragmatic and distal defects *321*
Letterer–Siwe disease 228
Leu-7 antigen 455
leuconychia 40, 71–2, 74–8
  acanthosis nigricans 232
  acquired forms 76
  acquired lichen planus 155
  acquired transverse 76
  angioma 448, *449*
  apparent 72, 76–7, 78
  blue rubber bleb naevi *452*, 457
  butchers' *278*
  cancer chemotherapy 83, 254
  cardiac disorders 178
  classification *78*
  complete *75*
  congenital 76, *331*
  dermatological forms 78
  distal 72, *75*
  endogenous 76
  febrile illness 225
  gastrointestinal disorders 193
  Hailey–Hailey disease 169
  longitudinal 75–6
  menstruation 199
  minor trauma 388
  nail growth 74
  occupational *277*
  pellagra 195
  psoriasis 137, *138*
  punctate 72, *75*, 76
  renal failure 189–90
  renal transplant rejection 190
  subtotal 72, 74–5
  sympathetic 208
  total 72, 74
  transverse 72, *75*, 210, 279
  transverse striate *75*
  trichophytica 102
  true 72, 74–6
  variegata *75*
leucovorin calcium 254, 255
leukaemias 234–5
leukopathia *see* leuconychia, apparent
levamisole 131
lichen nitidus 160
lichen planus 153–8
  with alopecia areata 166
  bullous 157
  dermatophyte infections 111
  diagnosis 157–8
  drug reactions 156
  dystrophica erosive 156
  hereditaria *339*
  idiopathic atrophy of the nails 157
  isolated nail dystrophy 157
  keratohyalin 156
  longitudinal grooves 154
  nail depression 154
  nail formation effects 62
  onychoschizia 54

lichen planus (*cont'd*)
pterygium *55*
scalp 156
subungual hyperkeratosis 60
treatment 158
twenty-nail dystrophy *53*, 157
twenty-nail dystrophy of childhood 91, 92
ulcerative 156, 157
lichen planus/lupus erythematosus overlap syndrome 159
lichen spinulosus 224
lichen striatus 39, 159–60
longitudinal splits 49
lichenoid trikeratosis *see* keratosis lichenoides chronica
lidocaine 347
light imaging 34
lipoblastomatosis 44
lipochrome 191
lipoid proteinosis 200
lipoma 471, *472*
liquid nitrogen 420
lithium
carbonate 240
psoriasis effects 142, *143*
local anaesthetics 268
longitudinal grooves 48–50
differential diagnosis 49–50
lichen planus 154
longitudinal ridges 50
Lovibond's profile sign 35, *36*
lung
cancer 185
carcinoma metastases *481*
neoplasm 231
neural reflex 185
pneumoconiotic disease 275
lunula 1, 2, 3, 7
alopecia areata 166
blue in Wilson's disease 192
cardiac failure effects 177
cyanosis 226
erythema 80
Iso–Kikuchi syndrome 23
nail shape relationship 23, *24*, *25*
nail–patella syndrome 299, *300*
red 166, 177
lupus erythematosus 55
chilblain 164
clubbing 164
hypertrophic 164
lichen planus/lupus erythematosus overlap syndrome 159
nail bed 164
unguium mutilans 163–4, 215
see also discoid *and* systemic lupus erythematosus
Lyell's syndrome *57*
lymphangitis 123
lymphatics 17
impaired drainage in yellow nail syndrome 186
lymphoedema 187
yellow nail syndrome 185, 186
with yellow nails *339*
lymphoma 235, *236*

macrodactylia fibrolipomatosis 44
macrodactyly *326*
macronychia 43–4
Maffucci's syndrome 43, 467–8, 473
magnetic resonance imaging 33
malaria 225
malignant acanthosis nigricans 229
malignant melanoma 357, 486–7, *488*, 492–6
amelanotic 493
childhood 495
in situ 492, 494
transplant recipients 495
malnutrition 196
mandibuloacral dysplasia *326*
manicure
apparatus *287*
professional 285
routine 286, 288
manicuring, overzealous *292*, 390
manicurists 267
marasmus 196
Marfan's syndrome 42
marsupialization procedure 411
matricectomy 365
electrode 365
nail plate dystrophy 367
matrix doubling syndrome 323
measles 51
mechloretamine 145
median nail dystrophy 48, 49
Mees' lines 76
arsenic poisoning 249
occupational 279
megadactyly 43, *44*
Meissner's corpuscles 9
melanin
deposition in nail plate 485
half-and-half nails 190
photoonycholysis prevention 238
melanocyte-stimulating hormone (MSH) 253
melanocytes 7
distribution 485
lichen planus 157
matrix sites *483*
melanocytic hyperplasia
atypical 492
benign 485
melanocytic lesions 483, *484*, 485–96
melanocytic naevus 491–2
melanogenesis 195
melanoma *488*, *489*
in situ *487*
markers 493
of nail apparatus 496
nodular *488*
melanoma, subungual 96, 486–8, 490, 491, 492
amelanotic 489, *490*, *491*
childhood 495
diagnosis 487–9
histopathology 493–4
incidence 486–7
prognosis 494–5
melanonychia 7–8
frictional 391
fungal 65, *68*
striata 259
melanonychia, longitudinal 13, 483, *484*, 485–91
aetiology 491
bands 3–6 mm wide 361–2
biopsy 357
black patients 490
Bowen's disease 433
causes *74*
childhood 495
distribution 486
en bloc excision 362
epidermoid carcinoma 433, *434*
frictional 391
incidence 486
lateral third of nail plate 358
lichen planus 154, 155, 157
midportion of nail plate 358
naevoid nail area melanosis 496
nail-biting/–picking 388, *389*
origin 361
periungual pigmentation *357*, 358
phototherapy-induced 32
pigmented races 495
polydactylic bands 491
progression to malignancy 488–90
progression to malignant melanoma 492
punch biopsy 360, 362
thin band 359–61
melanotic lesions, subungual 483
melanotrophic hormone 190
melphalan 253, *256*
membrane coating granules 8
menstrual factors 199
mepacrine 251
mercaptopurine *256*
mercury 249–50
Merkel cell 4
tumour 459
mesoderm, chick limb bud 4
metabolic disorders
alkaptonuria 201
amyloidosis 203–4
cystic fibrosis 200
diabetes 199–200
dyslipoproteinaemia 200
Fabry's disease 201
fucosidosis 202
gout 201
Hartnup disease 200
histidinaemia 200
homocystinuria 202
hyperoxaluria 200
Lesch–Nyhan syndrome 201
lipoid proteinosis 200
porphyria 202–3
metamphetamine 31
metastases 234, 481–2
methionine 260
methotrexate 114, 253, 254, 255, *256*
Reiter's syndrome 147
systemic psoriasis therapy 142
1-methylquinoxalinium-*p*-toluene sulphonate 267
miconazole 117
micronychia 43–4, 317, *322*
microscopic polyarteritis 219
microsurgery 381, *382*
free transplants 387
whole nail grafting 386
Milian's lilac arch 127
milker's nodules 274–5
mineral oil 270, *271*
minocycline 243
mitotane *256*
mitoxantrone *256*
mixed connective tissue disease 212
Moh's chemosurgery 364
Moh's surgery 435, 436
monilethrix 40
monoclonal IgG light chain gammopathy 235
monomyelocytic leukaemia 235
Morey and Burke's nail 77
Morton's toe 392
Morvan syndrome 205
motor oil 270
mountain sickness, chronic 183, 184
mucinous pseudocyst, subungual digital 474
mucinous syringometaplasia 419–20
mucocutaneous lymph node syndrome *see* Kawasaki disease
mucoviscidosis 81
Muehrcke's lines 189, 196
paired narrow white bands 77–8
multicentric reticulohistiocytosis 219–20, 233
multiple cartilaginous exostosis *339*
multiple exostoses syndrome (MES) 465–7
malignant change risk 467, 473
multiple myeloma 235
multiple sclerosis 209
mumps, nail growth 27, 28
Munro–Sabouraud microabscesses 144, 145
Musca domestica larvae 134

mutilant ulcer acropathy, acroosteolysis 171
Mycobacterium leprae 128
M. marinum 125, *273*, 274
M. tuberculosis 272
mycosis fungoides 235, *236*
  self-inflicted trauma *390*
mydriatic agent 269
myiasis, subungual 134
myxoedema, pretibial 478
myxoid cyst 34
  crysourgery 365
myxoid pseudocyst 95, 356, 478
  of the digits 474, *475*, 476–7
myxoma 477–8

naevoid nail area melanosis 489, 492, 496
naevus striatus symmetricus of the thumb 49
nail
  acquired atrophy 46
  anlage 3
  bank transplant 375, 381
  base coat 279, 288
  brace technique 402
  composition in cirrhosis 191
  consistency modification 61–3
  contour variations in elderly 94
  curvature in clubbing 35
  embedding 88
  examination 63–4
  extenders 294
  formation 7
  fragility 62–3
  free edge 23
  functions 19
  laquers for drug delivery 114
  measurement in neonates 81–2
  mending kit 289
  mineral constituents 29–30
  normal morphology 23
  permeability 32
  physical properties 31–2
  press-on colour 291, *292*
  prosthesis 387–8
  regeneration 22
  regrowth shape *25*
  sculpturing 290–1
  shedding *56*, *57*
  softening techniques 5–6
  strength 31–2
  synthetic covers 279
  thickness measurement with pulse echo ultrasound 33
  tooth and ear syndrome *304*
  traumatic malalignment 387
  varnish 279–80, 281, *286*
  wrapping 290
nail analysis
  disease prognostication 30
  exogenous materials 30–1
  forensic 30–1
nail apparatus
  anatomy 1–3
  development 297
  elderly 93
  electron microscopy 8
  embryology 3–4
  imaging 33–4
  immunohistochemistry 8–9
  melanoma 496
  morphogenesis 3
  nerve supply 18
  pertinax bodies 93
  physiology 21–8
  psoriasis mimicry 142–4
  regional anatomy 5–9
  tissue differentiation 3–4
  wart *419*
nail avulsion
  biopsy *353*
  Cordero's method 369–70
  distal 369, *370*
  donor nail bank transplant 370
  partial 370–1
  proximal 369–70
  proximal subungual onychomycosis 371
  total 369–70
nail bed 1, 2, 10–11
  ablation 367
  arteriovenous anastomoses 18
  avulsion 375–6, 387
  biopsy *353*
  bonding to nail plate 12
  capillaries in elderly 94
  drug penetration 32
  epidermis 11
  epithelium 7
  granulomatous purulent inflammation 411
  growth effects 23
  haemorrhage 372
  infolding 15
  interdigitation 15
  jaundice sign 191
  keratinization after avulsion 370
  longitudinal biopsy *353*, *355*
  lupus erythematosus 164
  proliferation 297
  red 226
  retraction 386, *387*
  separation from 58
  split thickness grafting 17
  sweat ducts 11
  vaporization 368
  wart *419*
nail bed-matrix flap 383
nail care
  adverse effects 292–5
  art 285–6
  benefits 292
  contact dermatitis 293–4
  discolouration 293
  granulation of nail keratin 293
  hardeners 289–90
  items for *287–8*, 289
  manicure routine 286, 288
  mending kits 289
  onycholysis 293
  preformed artificial nails 291
  premixed acrylic gels 291
  press-on colour 291, *292*
  ridging 293
  sculpturing 290–1
  wrapping 290
nail dystrophy
  acrocyanosis 181
  alopecia areata *165*
  anyloidosis 203
  bleomycin-induced 420
  bullous pemphigoid 162
  cardiac disorders 178
  cicatrizing 163
  drug-induced 4
  hereditary 297
  incontinentia pigmenti tumours 425
  nail sculpturing 291
  narrowing of nail 396
  peripheral vascular disease 17
  prosthesis 292
  pseudo-mycotic in vitiligo 166
  psoriatic 146
  sarcoidosis 188
  self-inflicted injury *389*
  traumatic 385–6
  X-ray 33
nail enamel 288
  allergens 294
  remover 288
nail fold 15
  biopsy 18
  dystrophy and CO_2 laser surgery 368
  erythema 210
  hypertrophic 87
  infection 407
  morphogenesis 3
  picking/breaking tissue 388
  telangiectasia 210
  tumours 48
  vessels 17–18
nail fold capillaries 17–18
  Crohn's disease 194–*5*
  early infancy 82
  microscopy 210–12
nail growth 21–3, *24*
  conditions of rapid 14
  direction 23, *24*
  in disease 27–8
  influences *28*
  linear in elderly 93–4
  local disease effects 28
  measurement 25–7
  nerve damage 207
  physiological factors 26–7
  pregnancy 199
  sex difference 27
  temperature effects 27
  total leuconychia 74
  volumetric 26
  yellow nail syndrome 186
nail hardeners 280, 289–90
  reactions to *289*
nail matrix 1, 2
  anatomy 6–9
  biopsy *353*
  cultured cell explants 21
  definition 21–3
  distortion in elderly 93
  excision for ingrowing toenails 400–1
  fibroma 442
  flow cytometry 21
  horn removal 399, 402–3
  injury 372
  kinetics 21
  leuconychia 71
  narrowing 396
  psoriasis 140
  psoriatic arthropathy 146
  retraction 386, *387*
  spongiotic dermatitis 92
  transverse biopsy *353*, *355*
  vaporization 367
nail plate 1, 2, 3, 11–15
  ablation 114
  ampullar dilatation *13*
  avulsion *347*
  bi-lamellar structure 13
  biochemical analysis 29–31
  chemical constitution 4
  colour modification 63–4
  composition 11–12, 62
  consistency variation in elderly 93, 94–*5*
  deformity from self-inflicted trauma 388, 390
  discolouration 280–1
  dystrophies 23
  electron microscopy *13*, 14–15
  epidermal ridges 10–11, *12*
  fungal infections 13
  growth 4
  hydration 62, 63
  hypoplasia 45
  inorganic analysis 29–31
  intercellular junctions 14
  inward distortion 401–3
  keratin fibrils 29
  keratin studies 22–3
  light microscopy 12–14
  longitudinal ridges *10*, 12
  mass analysis 21

- nail plate (*cont'd*)
  - modifications 54–60
  - nail matrix contributions 21–2
  - occupational destruction *276*
  - opaque streaks 98
  - primordium 4
  - psoriasis 139–40
  - retarded growth in elderly 93
  - soft tissue association *11*
  - soft tissue attachments 54–60
  - sunscreen effect 93
  - theories of origin *22*
  - thickness 12
  - thinning 62
  - transient thickening *385*
  - ultrasound 22
  - upper surface 12
- nail plate–nail bed adhesion absence 381
- nail surface modification 48–54
  - longitudinal grooves 48–50
  - longitudinal ridges 50
- nail surgery
  - anaesthesia 346–52
  - contraindications 345
  - imaging 346
  - instruments 346, *347*
  - patient examination 345–6
  - preoperative measures 346
- nail unit
  - basement membrane analysis *9*
  - comparative anatomy 19–21
  - hair comparison 19
  - phylogenetic comparisons 20–1
- nail-biting 42, 209, 388
  - herpes simplex infection 123
  - prognosis 388
- nail–patella syndrome 45–6, 49, 191, 299–300
  - bone 299, *300*
  - genetics 300
  - lunula 299, *300*
- nail-picking 388
- narcissus bulbs 265
- nasodigitoacoustic syndrome *326*
- nasopharyngeal carcinoma 233
- National Electronics Injury Surveillance System (NEISS) 295
- Neapolitan nail *77*
  - elderly 94
  - hemiplegia 206
- *Neisseria gonorrhoeae* 125
- Nelson's syndrome 197
- neonates
  - blistering diseases 83
  - epidermolysis bullosa 86–7
  - koilonychia 82
  - nail composition 81
  - nail dimensions 82
  - self-inflicted bullous lesions 83
  - *Veillonella* infection 83–4
- neoplastic disorders
  - breast carcinoma 233
  - Castelman tumour 233
  - Cowden's disease 234
  - digital ischaemia 232
  - glucagonoma syndrome 231
  - Hodgkin's disease 237
  - HTLV-1 positive cutaneous T-cell lymphoma 237
  - intestinal leiomyosarcoma 233
  - Langerhan's cell histiocytosis 228–9
  - leukaemias 234–5
  - lung neoplasm 231
  - lymphoma 235, *236*
  - metastases 234
  - multicentric reticulohistiocytosis 233
  - nasopharyngeal carcinoma 233
  - papuloerythroderma 232–3
  - plasmacytoma 235
- nephrosis 27
- nephrotic syndrome 189, 191
- *Nereis diversicolor* 269
- nerve damage 207
- nervous disorders 204
  - causalgia 208
  - congenital insensitivity to pain syndrome 206
  - hereditary 204
  - peripheral neuropathies 206–8
  - phacomatoses 205
  - reflex sympathetic dystrophy 208
  - spinal cord injuries 206
  - syringomyelia 205
- neurilemmoma 462
- neurofibroma *459*, 460
  - plexiform 43
- neurofibromatosis 205, *340*
- neuroma 385, 459–61
  - Pacinian 460–1
  - systematized multiple fibrillar 460
- Nezelof syndrome 221
- nickel 30
- nifedipine 18
- nigraemia *333*
- niridazole 134
- nitrogen
  - children's nail composition 81
  - mustard *256*
- nitrosurea 253, *256*
- nodular erythema with digital changes *325*
- nonoxyno-6 268
- North American Contact Dermatitis Group 295
- Norwegian scabies 131–2
  - adult T-cell leukaemia 235
  - AIDS 223
  - psoriasis mimicry 143
- nutritional disorders
  - fetal alcohol syndrome 196
  - iron deficiency 196
  - malnutrition 196
  - pellagra 195
  - selenium deficiency 196
  - vitamin A deficiency 195
  - vitamin B_{12} deficiency 195
  - vitamin C deficiency 195
  - zinc deficiency 195–6

- occupational disorders
  - perionychial tissue modifications 61
  - principal signs 275, *276–8*, 279
- occupational hazards 263, 264
  - bacterial infections 272–4
  - chemical irritants 270–2
  - chemical sensitizers 266–9, *270*
  - clinical reactions 264
  - disorder diagnosis 263–4
  - fungal infections 275
  - physical 264–6
  - radiodermatitis 431
  - systemic conditions 275
  - viral infections 274–5
- occupational stigmata 265
- ochronosis *332*
- octadecanoic acid octadecyl ester 146
- oculo-dentodigital AD or AR syndrome *304*
- oculo-tricho-dysplasia syndrome *304*
- Odland bodies *see* membrane coating granules
- odonto-thichomelic hypohidrotic ED *304*
- odontoonychodysplasia with alopecia *308*
- oil spot, psoriasis 138, 139
- old age 93–6
  - colour variations 94
  - fungal infection 96
  - hyperkeratotic lesions of toe nail 94, 95
  - ingrowing toenail 95
  - linear nail growth 93–4
  - nail apparatus 93
  - nail bed capillaries 94
  - nail contour variations 94
  - nail plate thickness 94–5
  - onychomycosis treatment in toenail 114
  - *Sarcoptes hominis* infection 132
  - splinter haemorrhages 94
  - toenail care 394
  - tumours in nail area 95–6
- Ollier's disease 473
- Ollier's dyschondroplasia *see* enchondromatosis
- Olmsted's syndrome *306*
- omega nail, ingrowing 401–3
- onions 269
- onychatrophy 45
- onychauxis 46
- onychia
  - punctata 52
  - syphilis 127
- onychoclavus 392
- onychocorneal band 12
- onychodermal band 1, *2*
- onychodystrophy, alopecia areata 165
- onychogryphosis 40, 46–7, 324, 393–4, 395
  - cardiac disorders 178
  - causes *48*
  - CO_2 laser surgery 366
  - elderly 94
  - fungal infection 47
  - gout 201
  - hereditary 47
  - hereditary nervous disorders 204
  - keratosis punctata 57
  - pemphigus 163
  - pityriasis rubra pilaris 150
  - rheumatoid arthritis 217, *218*
  - self-neglect 47
  - syphilis 127
  - traumatic 47
  - venous ischaemia 183
  - onychoheteropia 328–9
  - onycholemmal horn 419
  - onycholysis 12, *57*, 58
    - cancer chemotherapy 254, 255
    - candida 58
    - *Candida* infection 98, 119
    - cardiac disorders 178
    - chemical sensitizers 152
    - classification *59*
    - congenital *324*
    - diabetes 199
    - DLSO secondary to 101–2
    - elderly 94
    - hypothyroidism 198
    - lichen planus 155
    - nail growth 28
    - occupational *277*, 279
    - pemphigus 163
    - porphyria 202
    - post-traumatic 381, *383*
    - psoriasis *136*, 139
    - sculptured 58, *293*
    - self-inflicted 209
    - spongiotic dermatitis 152
    - squamous cell carcinoma of the lung 188
    - syphilis 127
    - toe nail loss 57
    - toes 58
    - traumatic 101, 391–2
    - yellow nail syndrome 186
  - onychomadesis *56*, *57*
    - cardiac disorders 178
    - hereditary nervous disorders 204
    - latent 51, *56*, *57*
    - lichen planus 154
    - recurrent 57
  - onychomatricoma 428–30
  - onychomycosis 97
    - arthrospores 106
    - *Candida* 100–1

conidia 106
culture 106–7
DLSO 98–102, *108*, *109*, *110*, 110–11, 118, 119
elderly 96
fungal hyphae 106
histopathology 107, *108*, 109–11
hypertrophy of nail 46
incidence 97
kidney transplant recipients 190
koilonychia 40
laboratory investigation 106–7, *108*, 109–11
nigricans 111
non-dermatophyte moulds 119
onycholysis 58
primary 118–19
proximal subungual 371
proximal subungual onychomycosis (PSO) 102–4, *109*, 111
proximal subungual white onychomycosis (PWSO) *98*, *109*, 110
pseudo-leuconychia 72
superficial black onychomycosis (SBO) 102
subungual keratosis 111
superficial white onychomycosis (SWO) *98*, 102, 111, 119
total dystrophic onychomycosis (TDO) 104, *105*, 106, *109*, *110*, 111, *112*
treatment 114–15
Zaias' classification 98
onychopachydermoperiostitis, psoriatic 146–7
onychopathomimia 390
onychophosis 93, 392–3, *394*
elderly 94
onychorrhexis 48
brittle nails 61
pemphigus 163
onychoschizia 14
lamellina *53–4*, 190
lichen planus 154
treatment 32
onychotillomania 209, *389*, 390
onychotrichodysplasia with neutropenia *310*
oral contraceptive pill 252
orange stick 266
orf 274, *275*
organic solvents 270
orthonyx 402
Osler–Rendu–Weber sydrome *see* hereditary haemorrhagic telangiectasia
Osler's nodes 177
osseous growth 463
osteo-onycho dysplasia *321*
osteoarthritis 95, 221
mucinous pseudocysts 474
osteoarthropathy, hypertrophic 177
osteoblastoma 469
osteochondroma *462*, *465*, *466*
osteoid osteoma 468–9
osteolysis, leprosy 128, *129*
osteomyelitis 209
atopic dermatitis 221
phalangeal 226
osteopenia 4
otoonychoperoneal syndrome 299, *325*
otopalatodigital syndrome *326*
oven cleaners 270
overcurvature of nails 328
transverse 401–3
overlapping toes 93
oxalate granuloma 479, *480*
oxalic acid 271

pachydermoperiostosis 37–8, 229, *325*
pachyonychia 46, 323–4
phacomatoses 205
pachyonychia congenita 302, *306–7*, 311, *312*, *332*, 396
hard nails 61
hypertrophy 46, *47*, 297
nail bed ablation 367, *368*
subungual hyperkeratosis 11
Pacinian neuroma 460–1
pain sensation loss 205
painful digital necrosis 228
painful nail 414–15
palmar arch 16
palmar Atasoy flaps 378
palmar digital arteries 16
palmoplantar keratoderma pemphigus 229
papilloma, subungual 421
papuloerythroderma 232–3
parakeratosis pustulosa 152–3
psoriasis mimicry 143
parakeratotic cells 4, 74, *75*
paramethadione 330
paraneoplastic disorders 229
acanthosis nigricans 232
acrokeratosis paraneoplastica 229
paranuclear inclusion bodies 446
paraquat 272
parathyroid
disease 197–8
extracts 253
paravaccinia virus 274
parenteral nutrition 195, 196
Parkes–Weber syndrome 448
Parkinson's disease 209
paronychia
acrocyanosis 181
acromegaly 197
acute 407–8, *409*, 410
antibiotic treatment 408, 410
bacterial 84, 113, 408
cancer chemotherapy 254
Candida infection 98
chronic 112–13, *114*, *119*, 410–11
diabetes 199
drug-induced 114
elderly 96
fungal 112–13
infant bacterial infections 84
manicuring faults 292
multiple inflammatory 127
nail sculpturing *290*
neonatal candidiasis 85
occupational *276*
PSO secondary to 104
psoriatic 135
subungual spread *409*, *410*
syphilitic 127
therapy in childhood 86
with thumb sucking 85–6
treatment in infancy 88
yellow nail syndrome 186
zinc deficiency 195
paronychial infection 272
occluded arteriographic findings 17
paronychial ulceration, occluded arteriographic findings 17
parrot's beak nail 43
systemic scleroderma 214
Pasteurella tularensis 274
patent ductus arteriosus 177
Patterson–Kelly–Brown syndrome *see* Plummer–Vinson syndrome
pedicle reconstruction 371
pediculosis 132
pellagra 195
peloprenoic acid 260
pemphigus 163
palmoplantar keratoderma 229
vegetans of Hallopeau 163
penicillamine 260
penicillin 89
Penicillium spp 101
periarteritis nodosa *213*, 219
perionychial tissue
distal fissures 61
inflammation with ingrowing toenail 88
modifications 60–1
perionychium, lupus erythematosus 164
peripheral heart of Masson 18
peripheral neuropathies 206–8
peripheral vascular disease
nail dystrophies 17
onychogryphosis risk 393
paronychia of toenails 113
surgical risk 411
periungual tissues
arterial obliteration 178
erythema 199
perniosis 182
acute 264
pertinax bodies 7, 93
petaloid nail 39
petechiae, bacterial endocarditis 177
Peutz–Jeghers syndrome 488
Peutz–Jeghers–Touraine syndrome 194, *325*, *333*
phacomatoses 205
phaeochromocytoma, acral skin necrosis 247
phalangeal atrophy, cortisone 253
phalangeal demineralization 36
phalanx, traumatic denudation 378
phenindione 251
phenobarbitone 330
phenol 399–400
formaldehyde resin 279
phenothiazines 240
phenylephrine 260
phenytoin 4, *332*
photochemotherapy, psoriasis treatment 141
photography 33–4
photoonycholysis 32, 58
drug-induced *237–8*
porphyria 202
quinine sulphate 252
quinolone therapy 244
photosensitizing drugs 32
Pierre Robin syndrome 329
pigment accumulation 63
pigmentation
alkaptonuria 201
azidothymidine 245
melanin-induced 494
minocycline 243
occupational 279
periungual *357*, 358, 488–9
syphilis 127
see also colour modification; dyschromia; hyperpigmentation
pili torti and onychodysplasia *310*
Pillet hand prosthesis (PHP) 388, *390*
pincer nail 41
acquired 426, *427*
deformity 170
ingrowing 401–3
pinta 65
pitting 52
alopecia areata 135, 165–6
lichen nitidus 160
pityriasis rosea 152
psoriatic 135, 136, 137, 139, 140
Reiter's syndrome 147
pituitary
disease 197
tumour 197
pityriasis
lichenoides acuta 172
rosea 52, 152
pityriasis rubra pilaris 150, *340*
hypertrophy of nail 46
psoriasis mimicry 143

pityriasis rubra pilaris (*cont'd*)
  subungual hyperkeratosis 11, 60
Pityrosporum ovale 223
plant exposure 265, 266
plasmacytoma 235
Plasmodium vivax 225
platonychia
  cardiac disorders 178
  elderly 94
  haemodialysis 189
  partial 367–8
pleonosteosis *326*
pleural cancer 185
pleural effusion, yellow nail syndrome 185
plexiform neurofibroma 205
plicated nail 41
Plummer–Vinson syndrome 194
Plummer's nails 198
POEMS syndrome 207–8, 233, 235
Pohl–Pincus line 51
poikiloderma congenita *321*
polarized light 34
poliomyelitis 209
polychlorinated biphenyls 330
  intoxication 248
polycythaemia 226
  vera 54
polydactyly 204
  anonychia 297
polyeponychia bolboides 60
polymyositis 212
polyonychia 204
polyvinyl chloride 275
popliteal pterygium syndrome *308*
porocarcinoma 437
porokeratosis *340*
  linear 169
  of Mibelli 169
porphyria 202–3
  congenital *332*
  cutanea tarda 43, 189, 202, *332*
  variegate 202
port-wine stain 448, *449*
potassium
  children's nail composition 81
  iodide 122
  permanganate 281
pottery workers 265
povidone-iodine 398
power tools 266
practolol 246
pre- and post-natal growth retardation, mental retardation and acral limb deficiencies *321*
prednisolone 235
  Reiter's syndrome 147
prednisone 87
pregnancy 199
  salbutamol 260–1
  systemic drugs 239
  warfarin effects 251, 330
pressure 265
preterm infants
  nail composition 81
  nail size 82
pretibial myxoedema 478
primary nail field 3
printing workers 267
progeria *321*, *332*
propanidid 268–9
propranolol 246
prosector's paronychia 272, *273*
prosector's wart 273
prosthesis, silicone rubber 387
protection, gloves 281
proteins
  high glycine/tyrosine 29
  high sulphur 29
  starvation 76
Proteus spp
  nail infection 65
  paronychia 113
Proteus syndrome 43
proximal groove 3
proximal nail fold 1, 2, 15, 23
  biopsy *355–6*
  capillary loops *17*
  diabetes mellitus 199
  dorsal flap 356
  junction with intermediate matrix 6
  psoriasis 139
  small lesion removal 356
  traumatic avulsion 376–7
  tumours 356
proximal subungual onychomycosis (PSO) 102–4, *109*, 111
  secondary to paronychia 104
proximal white subungual onychomycosis (PWSO) *98*, 102–4, *109*
  diagnosis 110
pseudoainhum 206, 305, 325
pseudo-Hutchinson's sign 391, *485*, *486*, 488
pseudo-Kaposi syndrome *450*
pseudo-Koenen's tumour 200
pseudo-leuconychia 72, *76*
pseudo-Recklinghausen intradermal naevi 492
pseudoclubbing *326–7*
  broad nails 327
  occupational acroosteolysis *276*
pseudohypoparathyroidism *326*
  brachydactly 198
pseudomacropychia 44
pseudomegadactyly 44
Pseudomonas
  with *Candida* infection 119
  Darier's disease 168
  green nail syndrome 272, *277*
  nail infections 65
  paronychia 112, 113
pseudoporphyria, haemodialysis 189
pseudopyogenic granuloma 452
pseudoxanthoma elasticum 179
psoralens *68*, 237, 238, 242–3
psoriasis 14, 135–47, *340*
  acral pustular *144–5*
  acropustulosis 143
  acute acral pustulosis 145–6
  acute nail abnormalities 139
  with alopecia areata 166
  associated with other disorders 142
  β-blockers 246
  Beau's lines 28
  chromonychia 139
  commensal fungi 111
  dermatophyte infection 138
  dermojet steroid injection 253
  diagnosis 139, 140
  discolouration *136*
  elkonyxis 54
  exacerbation by drugs 142
  family history 135
  fetal 135
  friable nails 62
  HIV infection 223
  hypertrophy of nail 46
  koilonychia 40
  leuconychia 78, 137, *138*
  longitudinal ridges 137
  mimicry in nail apparatus 142–4
  nail analysis 146
  nail bed involvement 138
  nail formation effects 62
  nail lesions 135
  occupational trauma 264
  oil spot 138, 139
  onychogryphosis 47
  onycholysis 58, *136*, 139
  onychoschizia 54
  osteolysis 144
  photo-therapy 32
  pits 135, 136, 137, 139, 140
  proximal nail fold involvement *137*
  Reiter's syndrome 147
  splinter haemorrhages 138
  staphylococcal growth 113
  subungual hyperkeratosis 60, *136*, 139
  therapy effects on nail growth *27*, *28*
  transverse depressions *137*
  treatment 140–2
  twenty-nail dystrophy 53
  twenty-nail dystrophy of childhood 91
psoriatic acropachydermodactyly 146–7
psoriatic arthritis 146
psoriatic arthropathy 42
  acroosteolysis 171
psoriatic onychopachydermoperiostitis 146–7
psychiatric disorders 209–10
psychological disorders 209–10
pterygium 49, 384
  dorsal *55*, *56*, *130*
  lichen planus 155, 156
  pemphigus 163
  self-inflicted 209
  toxic epidermal necrolysis 170
  vasospastic conditions 178
  ventral *55–6*
pterygium inversum unguis 11, *55–6*, 206, 246
  systemic scleroderma 214
pulse oximetry 259
punch biopsy 354
pup tent sign 155
puretic syndrome fibromatosis systemic hyalinosis *327*
PUVA therapy
  acute acral pustulosis 145
  keratosis lichenoides chronica 162
  photoonycholysis 238, 242
  psoriasis 141
  Reiter's syndrome 147
pycnodysostosis *325*
pyoderma 221
pyogenic granuloma 127, *241*, 242, 453, *454*
  excision 365
Pyrenochaeta unguium hominis 101

Quincke pulsation 177
quinidine 247
quinine sulphate 252
quinolones 244

rabies encephalomyelitis 209
racquet nails 42–3, 327
  acquired 170, 198
racquet thumb 42, 396–7
  epithelioma cuniculatum 435
radiation 259
  ionizing 264
  microwave 265
radiation penetration 32
radiocoagulation 365
radiodermatitis 264, 265, 430–1
  occupational 431
radiology 33
radiosurgery 365
radiotherapy, psoriasis 142
rapeseed oil, denatured 248
Rapp–Hodgkin syndrome 302
Raynaud's disease 180–1
  longitudinal splits 49
  transverse depressions 51
  treatment 181
Raynaud's phenomenon 18, 180–1
  acroosteolysis 171
  β-blockers 246
  clubbing *176*

cold injury 264
cryoglobulinaemia 228
digital necrosis 210
DLSO 101
occult neoplasm 232
preceding scleroderma 213
ventral pterygium *55*
vibrating power tools 266
razoxane *256*
Recklinghausen's disease *see* von Recklinghausen's disease
recurring digital fibrous tumours (RDFT) of childhood 445–6
red lunulae 80
disorders in patients *79*
reflex sympathetic dystrophy 208
Reiter's syndrome
elkonyxis *54*
HIV infection 223
pitting 147
psoriasis 142, 147
psoriasis mimicry 143
subungual hyperkeratosis 60
releasing flap method of biopsy 361
renal disorders
acrorenal-ocular syndrome 191
haemodialysis 189
half-and-half nails 190–1
Henoch–Schönlein purpura 191
leuconychia 189–90
Muehrcke's lines 188–9
nail–patella syndrome 191
transplantation 190
yellow nail syndrome and nephrotic syndrome 191
renal transplantation 190
half-and-half nails 190
resorcinol 281
respiratory disorders 185
asthma 188
bronchial carcinoma 188
hypertrophic pulmonary osteoarthropathy 185
respiratory manifestations 186
sarcoidosis 187–8
shell nail syndrome 187
yellow nail syndrome 185–7
reticulohistiocytosis 219–20, 233
retinal angioma with hair and nail defects *310*
retinoid therapy 28, 54, 240, *241*, 242
acute acral pustulosis 145
Hailey–Hailey disease 169
incontinentia pigmenti tumours *425*
keratoacanthoma 424
psoriasis 141
Reiter's syndrome 147
Reye's tumour 446
rheumatoid arthritis 212, *213*, 217–18
acroosteolysis 171
rheumatoid nodules 218
rheumatoid psoriasis 146
rheumatoid vasculitis 218
rhus dermatitis 266
ridged brittle fingernails 17
Rosenau's depressions 52
Rubinstein–Taybi syndrome *327*
Rüdiger syndrome *321*
runaround 407

S-100 protein 455, 493
Salamon syndrome *308*
salbutamol 261
sand paper nails *see* twenty-nail dystrophy
sarcoid bone disease 36
sarcoid dactylitis 187
sarcoid granuloma 188
sarcoidosis 187–8
sarcoma 471–2
epitheloid 472
osteogenic 471–2
phalangeal 471–2
Sarcoptes hominis infection 132
S. scabiei 131
scabies 131–2
associations of crusted *132*
Norwagian 131
subungual hyperkeratosis 60
scarring, surgery 407
Schamroth's sign 36
schizophrenia, self-inflicted trauma *389*, 390
schwannoma *461*, 462
sclerodactyly, occupational *275*
scleroderma *55*
acroosteolysis 171
with alopecia areata 166
proximal nail fold 211
Raynaud's phenomenon preceding 213
scleronychia, yellow nail syndrome 186
Scoggins' type ED *303*
Scopulariopsis brevicaulis 101, 107, 223
Scopulariopsis infections 106, *107*
scratching, self-inflicted trauma 390
screening service, postal 81
sculptured nails 294
scurvy 195
Scytalidium hyalinum 98, 101, 113
occupational infection 275
S. dimidiatum 102
see also Hendersonula toruloidea 98, 101
sea urchin granuloma *379*, *381*
sealants 267
Seckel's technique 383
selenium 30, 248
deficiency 82, 196
self-biting 206, 207
self-image 285
self-inflicted injury 209, 388, *389*, 390
self-mutilation 206
senile changes in nail 93
serrated koilonychia syndrome 39, *51*
serum triglycerides 30
severe combined immunodeficiency 221
Sézary syndrome 150, 235
subungual hyperkeratosis 60
shaft fracture 377–8
Sheehan's syndrome 197
shell nail syndrome 187
bronchial tumours 229
shiny nail, self-inflicted trauma *390*
shoes
fitting 94, 95, 390, 391, 392
running 392
shoreline nails *52*, 239
short nails 42–3
shoulder–hand syndrome 178
sickle cell anaemia 226
siderophages 470
silver 249, *250*
skeletal anomaly syndromes 317, 318
hypoplastic/atrophic nails with 317, *320–2*, *323*
sodium, children's nail composition 81
soft nails 61
soldering flux 272
solehorn (Solenhorn) 11, 22
solenonychia 49
solitary bone cyst 470
sorbothane 392
Sotos syndrome 197
spatulate nail deformity 386, *387*
Spiegler tumours
multiple malignant 43
and racquet nails *327*
spinal cord injuries 2–6
splint
orthodigital 392
silicone rubber 383
splinter 407
splinter haemorrhages *10*, 11, 183–4, 372
bacterial endocarditis 177
Buerger's disease 178
elderly 94
psoriasis 138
Raynaud's phenomenon 180
trichinosis 131
split dermal graft *375*
split nail deformity 381–3, *384*
non-traumatic 383
split-thickness graft
nail 376
nail bed 383
skin 384
skin in pachyonychia congenita 396
splitting 32
spongiotic dermatitis of nail matrix 92
spongiotic trachyonychia 53
spoon nail *see* koilonychia
sporotrichosis 114, 122–3
sportsman's toe 57
sportsmen 266
squamous cell carcinoma 423
elderly 96
invasive 32, 33
of nail apparatus 431–2
subungual in AIDS 224
X-irradiation 264, *265*
squaric acid dibutyl ester 167, 420
Staphylococcus aureus 90, 222
paronychia 112, 113
Staph. epidermis 11, 90
steatorrhoea 193
stereomicroscopes 210
steroid sulphatase 30
steroids
acrokeratosis paraneoplastica treatment 230
dermojet injection 253
ingrowing toenail granulation stage 398
lichen planus therapy 158
systemic 253
Stevens–Johnson syndrome 170
stub thumb with racquet nail *327*
subpapillary plexus visibility 210
Sucquet–Hoyer canal 18
sulphonamides 245
superficial black onychomycosis (SBO) 102
superficial spreading melanoma 492, 493, 496
superficial white onychomycosis (SWO) 64, *98*, 102, *109*, 111
non-dermatophyte moulds 119
treatment 119
supernumerary digits, rudimentary 462
surgery
acute paronychia 408, *409*, 410
bleeding control 352
burns 413–14
chronic paronychia 410
CO_2 laser 365–9
complications 406–7
congenital disorders 396–7
crush fractures 377–8
distal interphalangeal joint 364
dressings 352
epidermoid carcinoma of nail apparatus 435
fingertip amputation 380–1
foreign bodies 378–9, *380*
glomus tumours 455
granulomatous purulent nail bed inflammation 411
haematoma 372–3
haemostasis 366
hereditary disorders 396–7
hooked nail 386–7
incontinentia pigmenti tumours 425
infection 406–7

surgery (*cont'd*)
  ingrowing toenails 397–405, 399–401, 402–3
  lacerating wounds 374–7
  lesion mapping 364
  microscopically controlled 364
  nail avulsion 369–71
  nail dystrophies 385–6
  necrosis 407
  non-scalpel techniques 364–71
  pachyonychia congenita 396
  pain 406
  pedicle reconstruction 371
  post-operative care 352
  pterygium 384
  racquet thumbs 396–7
  recurrence 407
  residual defects 407
  split nail deformity 381–3
  subungual infection 411
  trauma 371–95
  traumatic avulsion 375–7
  traumatic denudation of terminal phalanx 378
sutures 407
swimming pool granuloma *273*, *274*
syndactyly 317
  anonychia 297, *298*
  Apert type 396
synovioma, benign 470
syphilis 127–8
  congenital 127
  occupational acquisition 274
  primary *126*, 127
  tertiary *126*, 128
syphilis, secondary 52, *126*, 127
  chromonychia *65*
  elkonyxis 54
syphilitic chancre 113
syphilitic whitlow of Hutchinson 127
syringomyelia 205
  acroosteolysis 171
systemic conditions
  discolouration of nails 65–6, *71*
  occupational 275
systemic drugs 259–61
  anti-inflammatory agents 246
  anticoagulants 251
  antihistamines 259
  antimalarial agents 251–2
  antimicrobial agents 243–5
  azidothymidine 245
  cancer chemotherapeutic agents 253–5, *256*, 257
  cardiovascular drugs 246–7
  central nervous system action 239–40
  discolouration of nails *65*, *69–70*
  early pregnancy 239
  erythroderma 239
  hormones 252–3
  intoxicants 248
  photoonycholysis 237–8
  psoralens 242–3
  purgatives 248
  retinoids 240, *241*, 242
systemic lupus erythematosus 210, *213*, 215
  capillary loops 211–12
  oil patches 58, 139
  splinter haemorrhages *183*
systemic scleroderma 180
systemic sclerosis 210, 213–14
  capillary changes 211
  occupational 275

T-cell lymphoma 235, *236*
T-keratins 3, 4
  antibody *8*
  hair content 19
  hair/nail differentiation function 20
  nail plate 19, 29
  ventral matrix 22
tabes dorsalis 209
  acroosteolysis 171
tall stature 397
talons 21
tarsiers 21
tegafur 253, *256*
telangiectasia 199, 448
  acrolabial *333*
  hereditary haemorrhagic 227
  homocystinuria 202
  nail fold 210
  periungual in cystic fibrosis 200
  rheumatoid arthritis 217
temperature sensation loss 205
tenascin 9
teratogens 239
terbinafine 31, 116
terminal Syme operation 401
Terry's nails 76–7
  cirrhosis 191–2
  and half-and-half nails 190
  pancreas carcinoma 229
  ulcerative colitis 194
p-tertiary butylphenol (PTBP) formaldehyde resin 268
tetanus
  prophylaxis 134
  risk 414
tetracycline 237, 243
tetradecanoic acid octadecyl ester 146
thallium 251
  occupational poisoning 279
  thiabendazole 134
thiazide diuretics 259
Thierry's tissue technique 14
thioglycollate 5, 280
thiourea 266
thoracic outlet syndrome 178
thorns 279, *380*, 407
thrombocythaemia, essential 226
thrombosis, spontaneous *449*
thumb deformity and alopecia *310*
thumb sucking 153
  Candida paronychia 113
  chronic paronychia 85–6
  herpes simplex infection 123
thyroid disease 198
tile-shaped nail 41
timolol maleate 247
tinea
  CO_2 laser surgery 368
  unguium 41
tioconazole 114
toenails
  intermediate matrix grafts 17
  onychomycosis treatment 114
  shoe contact trauma 390
  subungual haemorrhage 390–1
toes
  joggers 391
  nail fold capillary network 18
  overriding 392
  self-inflicted anonychia 391
tolnaftate 114
toluenesulphonamide formaldehyde resin 280
tooth
  development 298
  and nail syndrome *308*
total dystrophic onychomycosis (TDO) 104, *105*, 106, *109*, *110*, 111–12
Touraine–Solente–Golé syndrome *see* pachydermoperiostosis
tourniquet 406
toxic epidermal necrolysis 170, *225*, *227*
toxic oil syndrome 248
toxic shock syndrome 91
trachyonychia *see* twenty-nail dystrophy
transillumination 34
Transparent Yellow Lake 16901 281
transplant recipients, malignant melanoma 495
transverse depressions 51
transverse elliptical excision biopsy 361, 362
transverse grooves 50–1
  menstrual cycle 51
transverse overcurvature of nail 41–2
  types 42
trauma
  acute paronychia 407–8, *409*, 410
  avulsion 375–7
  bulla 391
  crush fractures 377–8
  delayed deformities 381–7
  denudation of terminal phalanx 378
  elkonyxis 54
  fingertip amputation 380
  foreign bodies 378–9, *380*
  functional anatomy 371
  glomus tumour 454
  haematomas 372–3
  hallux valgus 394–5
  hooked nail 386–7
  hyperkeratosis of nail folds 15
  hyperkeratotic reaction 392–3
  keratoacanthoma 423
  lacerating wounds 374–7
  longitudinal splits 49
  nail bed haemorrhage 372
  nail damage 62, 63
  nail injury classification 372
  nail malalignment 387
  nail prosthesis 387–8
  nails of elderly 94
  occupational 52
  onycholysis 381, *383*, 391–2
  onychomadesis in toes 57
  painful nail 414
  pedicle reconstruction 371
  perionychial tissue 60
  plant/wood 265
  pterygium 384
  repeated minor 388, *389*, 390–5
  self-induced 209
  self-inflicted injury 49, 388, *389*, 390
  shoe and toe 390, 392
  splinter haemorrhage 372
  split nail deformity 381–3, *384*
  subungual haemorrhage 390–1
  surgery 371–95
trench foot 264
triamcinolone
  acetonide 141–145
  yellow nail syndrome 186
trichinosis 131
  splinter haemorrhages 184
tricho-donto-dermal syndrome *308*
tricho-donto-osseous syndrome *308*
tricho-oculo-dermal vertebral syndrome *311*
tricho-rhino-pharyngeal syndrome *309*
trichocyte keratins *see* T-keratins
trichoonychotic hidrotic ectodermal dysplasia 39
  Trichophyton, spp 84, 103
  T. interdigitale 101, 102, 106, 107
  T. mentagrophytes 98
  T. rubrum 98, 99, 101, 102, 107
    graft-versus-host disease 222
    HIV infection 223
    occupational infection 275
    TDO *105*, 106
trichothiodystrophy *307*, *311*, 312–13
tricyclic antidepressants 240
trimethadone 330
triphalangy of thumbs and toes *309*
trumpet nail 41

  ingrowing 401–3
L-tryptophan 261
tuberculoid leprosy 128, 130
tuberculosis
  acute febrile 27
  verrucosa cutis 114, 273, 419
tuberous sclerosis *205*, *340*
  fibrokeratoma 439
  Koenen's tumours 438
tuft
  erythema 177
  fracture 377
tularaemia 274
tulip bulbs 266
tumours 418
  arteriovenous 450–1
  benign epithelial 418–30
  benign vascular 448, *449*, 450–5, *456*, 457–8
  cryosurgery 365
  degenerative 474, *475*, 476–9, *480*
  dysgenetic 424–6
  fibrous soft tissue 437–42, *443*, 444–8
  keratin cysts 426–8
  malignant epithelial 431–7
  malignant vascular 458–9
  Merkel cell 459
  nail area in elderly 95–6
  neuroendocrine 459
  osteocartilaginous 463–70
  painful nail 414–15
  peripheral nerves 459–62
  premalignant epithelial 430–1
  subungual epidermoid inclusions 428
  synovial 470–1
  verrucous epidermal naevus 425
tungiasis 133–4
Turner's syndrome 44, *335*
turpentine 134, 266
turtle-back fingernails 201
Tweedie and Ranger's procedure 401
twenty-nail dystrophy 52–3
  alopecia areata 166
  of childhood, 91–2
  familial *341*
  lichen planus 157
  longitudinal splits 49
  spongiotic inflammation 53
  vertical striated sandpaper 91

ulceration, nail region of elderly 93
ulcerative colitis
  clubbing 193–4
  gastrointestinal disorders 193–4
  Terry's nails 194
ulcers, systemic lupus erythematosus 215
ultrasound 33
ungual tufts 36
unguis constringens, ingrowing 401–3
unguis incarnatus syndrome 397
uraemic half-and-half nail 77
Urbach–Wiethe disease *see* lipoid proteinosis
urea chemical treatment 116–18

V-Y homodigital finger flap 387
valproic acid 330
vasodilatation, clubbing 37
Veillonella infection in newborn 83–4
venous ischaemia 183
venous malformation 448, *449*
venous thrombosis 179
ventral matrix 6
  primordium 3
Verdan's technique 386
verruca vulgaris 419
verruciform xanthoma 480–1
verrucosa necrogenica 273
verrucous epidermal naevus 425–6
  linear 425, *426*
vesiculobullous lesions 83
vibrating power tools 266
Vieira sign 163
vimentin 9, 454
vinyl chloride 248
  disease 171
vinyl chloride monomer 275
  malignant haemangioendothelioma 458
viral infections 274–5
vitamin A 261
  deficiency 195
vitamin B_{12} deficiency 195
vitamin C deficiency 195
vitamin E 186
vitiligo 166, 223
von Recklinghausen's disease 43, 205, *340*, *459*, 460

waffling technique 368
Waldenström's macroglobulinaemia 235
warfarin 251, 330
warts 418
  cryosurgery 420
  malignant transformation 432
  treatment 420
  verruca vulgaris 419
  viral 275
warts, periungual 209, 418, 419
  AIDS 223
  bleomycin treatment 254, 257
  CO_2 laser 366, *367*
  cryosurgery 365
  electroradiosurgery 365
  5-fluoruracil treatment 255
warts, subungual 418, 419
  CO_2 laser 366, *367*
  hyperkeratosis 60
washboard nail plates 49, 51
Weaver syndrome *321*
wedge excision 396, 404
weedkillers 272
Wegener's granulomatosis *213*, 219
Werner syndrome *322*
white finger syndrome 180
Williams elfin facies syndrome *322*
Wilson's disease *see* hepatolenticular degeneration
Wiskott–Aldrich syndrome 221
Wood's lamp examination 34, 64
worn-down nails 45
wounds, lacerating 374–7
  avulsive 375–7

X-ray
  dermatitis 264
  therapy 259
  tumours 415
xanthoma 480
xeroderma, talipes and enamel defect syndrome *309*
xeroradiography 33
xylocaine 351

yellow nail syndrome 111, 185–7
  bronchial tumours 229
  congenital *332*
  and nephrotic syndrome 191
  rheumatoid arthritis 217
yellow nails
  HIV infection 223
  occupational *277*, *278*
  tetracyclines 243

zidovudine *see* azidothymidine
Zimmerman–Laband syndrome 44, 298, *339*, *340*
zinc 30
  supplementation 187
zinc deficiency 51, 195–6
  Muehrcke's bands 77
Zinsser–Engman–Cole syndrome 221, *303*